INTEGRATED PRINCIPLES OF ZOOLOGY

John Shaw/Tom Stack & Associates.

INTEGRATED PRINCIPLES OF

ZOOLOGY

SEVENTH EDITION

CLEVELAND P. HICKMAN, Jr.

Professor of Biology
Washington and Lee University,
Lexington, Virginia

LARRY S. ROBERTS

Professor and Chairman, Department of Biological Sciences,
Texas Tech University,
Lubbock, Texas

FRANCES M. HICKMAN

Emeritus, Department of Zoology,
DePauw University,
Greencastle, Indiana

Original artwork by **WILLIAM C. OBER, M.D.** *Crozet, Virginia*

TIMES MIRROR/MOSBY COLLEGE PUBLISHING

ST. LOUIS · TORONTO · SANTA CLARA 1984

Editor: **Diane L. Bowen**
Assistant Editor: **Susan Dust Schapper**
Editorial Assistant: **Jackie Yaiser**
Manuscript Editor: **Patricia Tannian**
Designer: **William A. Seabright**
Production: **Susan Trail**

Front matter art *Early Autumn* by Ch'ien Hsuan, thirteenth century, ink and watercolor, courtesy Detroit Institute of Arts, Founders Society Purchase, General Membership and Donations Fund.

Front cover art *Monkey and Grasshopper* by Mori Sosen, late eighteenth century– early nineteenth century, ink and color on silk, Shinenkan Collection courtesy Joe D. Price.

Back cover art *Swallows and Waves* by Okamoto Shūki, nineteenth century, ink and color on paper, Shinenkan Collection courtesy Joe D. Price.

SEVENTH EDITION

Copyright © 1984 by Times Mirror/Mosby College Publishing
A division of The C.V. Mosby Company
11830 Westline Industrial Drive, St. Louis, MO 63146

Previous editions copyrighted 1955, 1961, 1966, 1970, 1974, 1979

Printed in the United States of America

Library of Congress Cataloging in Publication Data
Hickman, Cleveland P.
    Integrated principles of zoology.

    Bibliography: p.
    Includes index.
    1. Zoology. I. Roberts, Larry S., 1935-
II. Hickman, Frances Miller. III. Title.
QL47.2.H529 1984   591   83-11471
ISBN 0-8016-2173-9

TS/VH/VH 9 8 7 6 5 4 3 2 1   02/C/221

PREFACE

When we began work on this seventh edition of *Integrated Principles of Zoology,* we no longer hoped, as we had with previous editions, that this revision would come more easily than before. If anything, the ceaseless growth of biological information renders each new revision a greater challenge than its predecessor. To see how much zoology has changed, one merely needs to read an earlier edition of this book or of any other textbook in the biological sciences. In some instances (fortunately not many), yesterday's zoological truths have become today's myths. In other instances, the facts have not changed but their importance in the context of later advances has waned or waxed. In preparing a new edition, old material must be taken out and new material added, chapters must be reorganized, emphases must be changed, and errors must be corrected—all without allowing the resulting textbook to become larger than previous editions.

Because advances in biology are so rapid, authors may despair that even the most thoughtfully and carefully researched revision is mere writing in the sand. This edition is a statement of the status of zoological science at this particular time, which is soon to become the target of dissenting opinion. Author and instructor alike, however, can take comfort in at least the *relative* permanence of the general principles of biology summarize in Chapter 1. These cardinal principles are the cornerstones of biology, the fundamental concepts that have grown out of the work of many minds and have stood the test of time. Well-formulated principles are indispensable in helping us interrelate facts and apply biological knowledge. We encourage the reader to refer to these principles from time to time while progressing through the book.

We approached this revision with the same objectives established by the late Cleveland P. Hickman, Sr., in the first edition published 28 years ago: to present the concepts and principles of zoology simply and logically and to instill in the student an enduring enthusiasm for the wonderful world of animals. We have extensively revised the text for this edition, but to users of previous editions, the most visible changes will be the new format, the inclusion of many new full-color photographs and drawings, and the addition of chapter summaries and marginal notes.

Major changes in this edition

This edition, like past editions, is divided into five parts. Many of the changes in this revision reflect the suggestions and criticisms offered in response to a detailed questionnaire by more than 400 people, including both those who have used the text in their classes and those who have not. The following paragraphs describe only major changes in the text, but the entire book was carefully scrutinized and changes were introduced where they seemed required.

Part One consists of seven chapters that serve as an introduction to the living animal. Chapter 1 has been extensively rewritten, with new sections on the nature of science and the scientific method. Chapter 2, on the structure of living matter, has been revised to update the sections on electron pathways of atoms, dissociation theory and buffer action, the structure of water, and protein structure. An updated section on enzymes has been moved to this chapter from its previous position in Chapter 5. Chapter 4, which describes eukaryotic cell structure, membrane function, and mitosis, has been thoroughly revised and is illustrated with many new electron micrographs. Following the suggestions of several people who have used the text, Chapter 5, on cell physiology, has been completely rewritten. The chapter opens with a section on the application of the laws of thermodynamics to living systems and then explains how cells use adenosine triphosphate (ATP) to perform biochemical work. The discussion of cellular metabolism, which forms the main body of the chapter, has been recast to describe the stages of respiration in the same sequence as the oxidation of food molecules. This chapter includes a simplified explanation of the chemiosmotic mechanism, the currently favored hypothesis for coupling in ATP synthesis. Chapter 6, on the architectural patterns of animals, remains largely unchanged from the sixth edition except for a revised section on radial and spiral cleavage. Animal classification and phylogeny are treated in Chapter 7. Students who have been taught the principles of animal classification in a previous biology course should be required to read at least the closing sections of this chapter (pp. 154-161) before proceeding to Part Two.

Part Two, consisting of 20 chapters that form the core of many zoology courses, is a survey of the animal phyla from the single-celled protozoa to the most advanced mammal. This part has been given careful attention in the revision. Several of the chapters are illustrated with full-color photographs carefully selected for high information content.

Chapter 8 has been extensively rewritten. It incorporates the 1980 revision of protozoan classification published by the Society of Protozoologists, which recognizes seven protozoan phyla. A new section on form and function of protozoa has been included. In chapter 9 the treatment of the phylum Mesozoa has been modified and the phylum Placozoa and the class Sclerospongiae of the phylum Porifera have been added. Discussions of the class Cubozoa and the subclass Ceriantipatharia have been included in Chapter 10, and the description of coral reefs has been modified to include the parts of a typical reef. Chapter 11, on the acoelomates, has been updated and now includes the phylum Gnathostomulida. Chapter 12 has undergone a number of modifications, especially an updating of information on gastrotrichs and kinorhynchs. Chapter 13, concerning the molluscs, has been extensively reworked. This chapter particularly benefited from the suggestions of Dr. Kenneth Boss of Harvard University. It incorporates the classes Caudofoveata and Solenogastres in place of the Aplacophora and places these classes in perspective relative to the origin and early evolution of the molluscs. In Chapter 15 the section on pycnogonids has been rewritten, the section on spiders has been shortened, and the discussion of the Acari has been expanded to reflect the importance of their numbers of individuals and species. In Chapter 16 the newly described subclass (or class) Remipedia has been added to the discussion of the crustaceans. Chapter 17 (terrestrial mandibulates) has been reworked and shortened. The section on Pogonophora in Chapter 18 has been rewritten, and a marginal note on the remarkable giant pogonophoran *Riftia pachyptila* has been added. In all the chapters dealing with the invertebrates, we have tried to emphasize the form and function and the diversity of entire groups, while deemphasizing the form and function of particular representative types. Thus, we hope the student will have a more accurate impression of the phylum or class as a whole.

Chapter 22, the first of the six chapters dealing with the chordates, describes the general characteristics of chordates, their ancestry and evolution, and the protochordates. The descriptions of the morphology of amphioxus and the ammocoete larva have been greatly shortened because this material appears in the accompanying laboratory manual, *Laboratory Studies in Integrated Zoology*. Chapter 23, on the fishes, has been completely reillustrated with color photographs and new artwork. The sections on fish locomotion and reproduction have been rewritten, and we have once again reluctantly deferred to the restless fish taxonomists by updating fish classification. This has meant dropping Petromyzontes in favor of Cephalaspidomorphi for the lamprey class. Chapter 24, dealing with the amphibians, contains revised sections on the integument, coloration, and vision. Chapter 25, on the reptiles, has been extensively revised and shortened. The opening sections have been condensed, and the descriptions of the reptile orders have been rewritten to stress the many interesting adaptations that distinguish this important and fascinating group. Chapter 26 contains revised or new material on flightless birds, bird color, origin of bird flight, and mating systems. In Chapter 27, the final chapter of Part Two, the section on reproduction in the mammals has also been completely rewritten.

Part Three, on the activities of animal life, consists of six chapters dealing with the functional systems of animals and a closing chapter on animal behavior. Chapter 28, concerning support, protection, and movement, includes a new section on hydrostatic skeletons and revised descriptions of the sliding filament theory and excitation-contraction coupling. Several new illustrations have been added to help the student understand how skeletal muscle functions. Chapter 29 provides a comparison of the specialized circulatory, immune, and respiratory systems of animals. The section on the immune system has been totally rewritten and expanded to summarize in a few pages the current understanding of this exciting and fast-moving field. The explanations of heart excitation and the control of breathing have also been reworked. Chapters 32 and 33 consider the animal's internal coordinating systems: nervous and endocrine. Sections that have been revised and reillustrated include those on neuron and synapse function, chemoreception, pressure reception, hearing, equilibrium, mechanisms of hormone action, and calcium regulation. New material on fluid circulation in the brain and on brain neuropeptides has been added to those chapters. Chapter 34, on animal behavior, focuses on the basic concepts of instinctive and social behavior as they have been developed by ethologists and are currently understood.

The five chapters of Part Four deal with reproduction, development, genetics, and the evolutionary process. In discussing these traditional and fundamental subjects, we have included topics of special interest to students. For example, Chapter 35, on the reproductive process, explores the question "What good is sex?" to emphasize to the student that not all "easy" questions in biology have simple answers. Reproduction leads naturally into development, the subject of Chapter 36. The first half of the chapter focuses on the mechanisms of development (early embryology is discussed in Chapter 6), and the closing pages deal with the amniotic egg, human development, birth, and, in a thought-provoking discussion, human longevity and the aging process. Chapters 37 and 38, on genetics and evolution, have been completely revised to introduce new material on split genes, gene regulation in eukaryotes, recombinant DNA techniques, neutral mutations, and punctuated equilibrium and to update sections on the physical structure of the genetic material, Lamarckism, fossil dating, and the emergence of modern Darwinism. Both chapters have been reorganized to improve clarity and flow. Chapter 39, on human evolution, has been completely rewritten and reillustrated to incorporate the rich harvest of recent hominid fossil finds and to provide a view of the lively debate fueled by these discoveries.

The environment of animals is the theme of Part Five. Responding to criticisms that Chapter 40, on the biosphere, needed radical surgery, we have deleted much of the introductory material on the lithosphere, hydrosphere, and atmosphere, reworked the discussion of biomes, and rewritten the zoogeography section to include the current debate over dispersal versus vicariance as explanations for animal distribution. Chapter 41, on ecology, has been revised to include an explanation of K-selection and r-selection and a new section on the recent fascinating discoveries of animal communities living adjacent to deep-sea thermal vents, a world independent of solar energy. The final chapter, Chapter 42, explores the causes of animal extinction, an issue that affects our values and culture, as well as our natural environment.

Distinctive features

Some of the special features of this edition are the following:

- Numerous photographs of animals, many in full color, have been selected from the files of many professional photographers and biologists; these were chosen mainly to illustrate adaptations rather than merely for visual appeal.
- This edition contains hundreds of original drawings by artist-biologist-physician William C. Ober, all carefully researched and designed for accuracy and maximum value as learning aids.
- Reference lists at the ends of the chapters have been thoroughly edited, updated, and annotated to help students and instructors supplement their reading. A separate annotated list of *Scientific American* articles is given for many chapters.
- Throughout Part Two, derivations of the generic names of animals are given where they first appear in the text. In seeing how scientific names are devised, students quickly grasp the use of classical roots in nomenclature and find scientific names easier to remember.
- The text has been augmented with marginal notes that provide interesting sidelights without interrupting the narrative.
- Chapter summaries have been added to help students draw out underlying themes.
- An extensive glossary provides the pronunciation, derivation, and definition for each term.
- An annotated historical appendix, unique to this textbook among zoology and biology texts, lists key discoveries in zoology. Books and publications that have greatly influenced the development of zoology are listed separately. Many readers have found this appendix an invaluable reference to be consulted long after completing their formal training in zoology.
- The companion laboratory manual, *Laboratory Studies in Integrated Zoology*, is closely correlated with this text.
- The instructor's manual, prepared by Steele Lunt of the University of Nebraska especially for this edition, summarizes the key points of each chapter and provides test questions and a list of appropriate visual aids.

Acknowledgments

We have depended on many people for advice and criticism in the preparation of this edition. Especially helpful were the hundreds of individuals who responded to a detailed questionnaire and whose advice guided our approach to this revision. In addition to these unnamed but deeply appreciated contributors, experts in various fields read part of the manuscript. Reviewers who read large portions of the book and to whom we extend special thanks are Martyn L. Apley, Western State College of Colorado; John Dixon, University of Wisconsin at Eau Claire; Robert P. Higgins, Smithsonian Institution; William R. Teska, Furman University; and James A. MacMahon, Utah State University. Two of Dr. Hickman's colleagues at Washington and Lee University graciously responded to his request for help: Brown Goehring patiently and meticulously clarified the discussion of inorganic chemistry in Chapter 2, and Peter Bergstrom offered valuable suggestions for the revision of the chapters on animal behavior and birds. Rebecca Emmons of the University of Virginia, Pete Diffley of Texas Tech University, and Royal Ruth of the University of Alberta contributed enormously to the extensive revision of the immune system section of Chapter 29. Others to whom we extend our appreciation for reading and commenting on specific chapters are Stanley L. Miller, University of California at San Diego (Chapter 3); Joseph Nelson, University of Alberta (Chapter 23); James Ashe, Watamu, Kenya (Chapter 25); Kenneth Boss, Harvard University (Chapter 13); and Bryan Fuller, Texas Tech University (Chapter 37). Edward I. Coher, Southampton College, provided help with Chapter 20.

Locating the hundreds of photographs used in this edition would have been impossible without the cooperation of many professional photographers and biologists. We especially thank Leonard L. Rue, III, who, beginning with the fifth edition, opened his files of thousands of superb wildlife photographs for our examination. Other professional photographers who provided us with large selections of their best work are Jim and Kathy Church, Gilroy, Calif.; John H. Gerard, Alton, Ill.; Daniel Gotshall, Los Osos, Calif.; Cy Hampson, Sidney, B.C.; Rick Harbo, Nanaimo, B.C.; Jeffrey L. Rotman, Somerville, Mass.; Kjell Sandved, Smithsonian Institution; Bo Tallmark, Uppsala, Sweden; and D.P. Wilson, Plymouth, England. Biologist-photographers who responded to our specific requests for photographs are Stuart and Jeanne Altmann, University of Chicago; Javier Andrada, Seville, Spain; Nell Bolen, Lexington, Va.; William P. Braker, John G. Shedd Aquarium; Timothy G. Branning, San Pedro, Calif.; Margaret Butschler, Vancouver, B.C.; Fred Grassel, Woods Hole, Mass.; Lynne Houck, University of Chicago; J.E. Lloyd, University of Florida; Kenneth Lorenzen, University of California at Davis; Leif Marking, National Fisheries Research Laboratory; Frank Moore, Oregon State University; Murray Newman, Vancouver Public Aquarium; David Pilbeam, Harvard University; and Peter C.H. Pritchard, Florida Audubon Society. Many fine electron micrographs were graciously supplied by J.D. Berlin, Texas Tech University; P.P. Graziadei and Edward Morrison, Florida State University; Richard G. Kessel, University of Iowa; Diane R. Nelson, East Tennessee State University; J.P. Revel, California Institute of Technology; Arthur W. Spira, University of Calgary; Mary E. Todd and A. Wayne Vogl, University of British Columbia; and C.L.F. Woodcock, University of Massachusetts.

Finally, the book would not have progressed to its present form without the help of the conscientious staff of Times Mirror/Mosby College Publishing. We especially thank our editors Diane Bowen and Susan Schapper, who shepherded the manuscript through its early stages; Kay Kramer, who oversaw the book's design; and manuscript editor Patricia Tannian.

Cleveland P. Hickman, Jr.
Larry S. Roberts
Frances M. Hickman

Rod Planck/Tom Stack & Associates.

CONTENTS

DETAILED CONTENTS

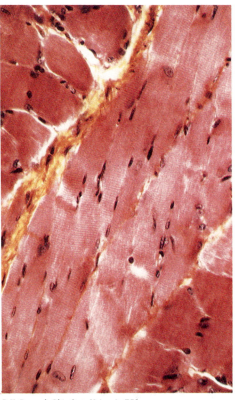

R.K. Burnard, Ohio State University/BPS.

M. Timothy O'Keefe/Tom Stack & Associates.

Tom Stack.

Rod Planck/Tom Stack & Associates.

Tom Stack.

Alan G. Nelson/Tom Stack & Associates.

Gary Milburn/Tom Stack & Associates.

Gary Milburn/Tom Stack & Associates.

PART FOUR   CONTINUITY AND EVOLUTION OF ANIMAL LIFE

John Gerlach/Tom Stack & Associates.

Tom Stack.

PART ONE

Green darner *Anax junius.*

INTRODUCTION TO
THE LIVING ANIMAL

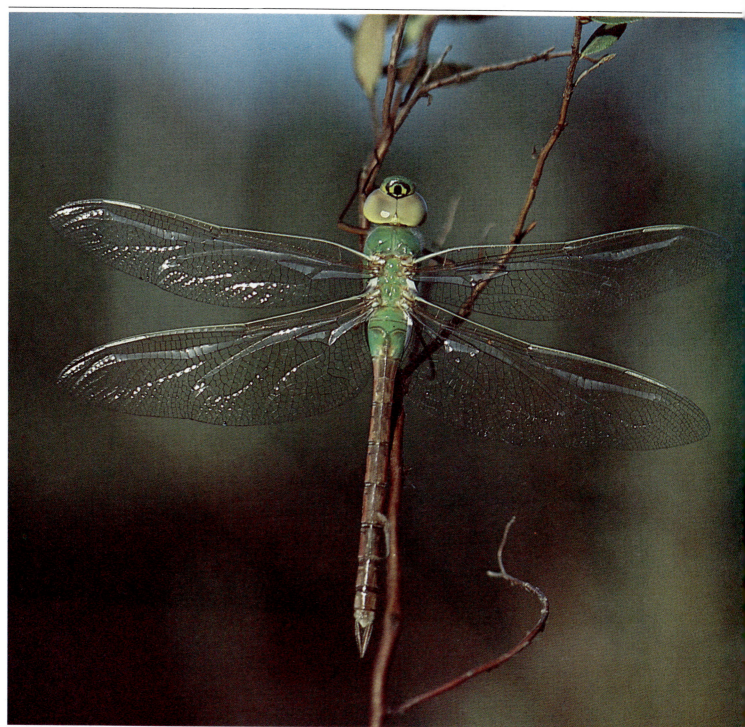

Photograph by C.P. Hickman, Jr.

In these seven chapters we discuss the basic nature of life as we understand it today. So far as can be determined, the same physical and chemical laws of the nonliving world also apply to the living. The essential difference appears to lie in the organization of the elementary materials of the nonliving into the highly specific architecture of the living. In its simplest form, life is associated with a heterogeneous substance constructed of organic macromolecules. From this substance has evolved an organizational hierarchy of cells, tissues, organs, organisms, and, finally, the vastly complex community of life, the ecosystem. The living animal's activity, growth, reproduction, and use of its environment require a still further organization of energy processes beyond that encountered in the strictly nonliving world.

CHAPTER 1

LIFE General Considerations and Biological Principles

Early morning sun strikes a green frog in a Michigan pond.

Photograph by C.P. Hickman, Jr.

Figure 1-1

Although both the living and the nonliving are subject to the same physical and chemical laws, living things are distinguished by a complex of unique structural and functional patterns that are unknown in the nonliving world. **A,** Bobwhite quail *Colinus virginianus.* **B,** Hermit crab *Coenbita compressus.*

Photographs by C.P. Hickman, Jr.

Zoology (Gr., *zōon,* animal, + *logos,* discourse on, study of) is the study of animals and, more than that, it is the scientific study of animals. It is commonly considered a subdivision of an even broader science, biology (Gr., *bios,* life, + *logos,* discourse on, study of), the study of all life. The panorama of animal life, how animals function, live, reproduce, and interact with their environment, is exciting, fascinating, and awe inspiring. A complete understanding of all phenomena included in zoology is beyond the ability of any single person, perhaps of all humanity, but the satisfaction of knowing as much as possible is worth the effort. In the chapters to follow, we hope to give the student an introduction to this science and to share our excitement in the pursuit of it.

In this chapter we briefly discuss zoology as a science, the concept of organic evolution, and a number of principles that will be developed in the rest of the book. These principles will provide conceptual unity to the knowledge that has accumulated about animals.

ZOOLOGY: THE SCIENTIFIC STUDY OF ANIMALS
Biology as the Study of Life

We begin our discussion with two very difficult questions: what is life, and what is an animal? At first these questions seem easy. Anyone, after all, can tell the difference between a rock and a robin, or between a toad and a tree. However, absolute definitions are not nearly as easy.

The question "What is life?" is one that many biologists have considered almost unanswerable. We must define life in terms of attributes that we associate with it. Several biological manifestations clearly distinguish the living from the nonliving. The essential differences between the two appear to be organization, metabolism, growth, adaptability, irritability, reproduction, and interaction with the environment. As we have learned more about the structural and organizational properties of living matter, it has become increasingly apparent that the living and the nonliving share the same kind of chemical elements and that both are subject to the law of conservation of energy. Few biologists today hold to the vitalistic view, prevalent not so many years ago, that living things are endowed with an inexplicable vital force. The accumulating weight of scientific evidence indicates that life is governed by physical and chemical laws, even though we still may be far from understanding the complex fabric of life as a whole.

Organization

Nonliving matter is organized at least into atoms and molecules and often has a higher degree of organization as well. However, atoms and molecules are combined into patterns in living organisms that have no counterparts in the nonliving. Combinations of certain large molecules (macromolecules) are unique to life: the proteins, fats, carbohydrates, and nucleic acids. Such combinations of common elements, which are highly improbable on thermodynamic grounds, and which are themselves nonliving, provide dynamic systems of coordinated chemical and physical activities when they are organized as they are in cells. Many of the macromolecules are organized into the various structures of the cell, where the thousands of chemical reactions take place. Others, although produced in the cell, may exit from it and become nonliving structural components of the organism (for example, hair, nails, and supporting structures) or function in communication with other cells (for example, hormones).

Metabolism

Metabolism is the collective name given the essential chemical processes that go on in living cells and organisms, including digestion, production of energy (respiration), and synthesis of molecules and structures. It is the sum of the constructive (anabolic) and destructive (catabolic) reactions.

Growth

All living organisms grow in size during the course of their lives, although single-celled organisms may simply divide into one or more new cells, so that their absolute increase in size is very limited. Many organisms undergo considerable growth and development, then eventually become senescent and die.

Adaptability

An individual organism has the ability to adjust to changes in its environment, although the range of the adjustment in particular cases may be quite narrow. The *ability* to make specific adjustments may be considered an adaptation and is heritable. Every organism is the product of thousands of adaptations evolved by its ancestors.

Irritability

Irritability is the ability to respond to stimuli in the environment. The stimulus and response may be simple, such as a bacterium moving away from or toward a light source or away from a noxious substance, or quite complex, such as a bird responding to a complicated series of signals in a courtship ritual.

Reproduction

Some individual organisms may be unable to reproduce or replicate themselves, although they are undeniably alive. Nevertheless, the ability to reproduce is present in the population of those organisms and of course is necessary for the continued existence of the population.

Interaction with the environment

A further important characteristic of living organisms is the intimate, reciprocal relationship between them and their environment. Life and the environment are inseparable. The evolutionary history of the organism has placed it in a specific environment that has determined the structural, functional, and behavioral properties of the organism. The environment is fit for the organism, and the organism is fitted to the environment and responds to its changes. The interaction between the living and the nonliving has determined the character of life on earth and the character of the earth itself. Each has deeply marked the other.

Almost every criterion of life has its counterpart in the nonliving world.

Figure 1-2

Mating green treefrogs *Hyla cinerea*. Reproduction, perhaps the ultimate objective of the life process, is indispensable for the survival of a species.
Photograph by C.P. Hickman, Jr.

Figure 1-3

Some animals, such as this flagellate protozoan *Euglena,* occupy the dividing line between animals and other living organisms.

Courtesy Claude Taylor III.

Some nonliving systems are even capable of a limited amount of metabolism or reproduction. However, only living things have combined these properties into unique structural and functional patterns.

Zoology as Biology

The question "What is an animal?" may be answered somewhat more definitely than "What is life?", but difficulty arises at the dividing line between animals and other living things. Animals are organisms comprised of one or more cells in which most of the material for inheritance is collected in membrane-enclosed structures (nuclei); which cannot use light energy to produce organic compounds; and in which the cells are not enclosed by cell walls. This definition separates animals from bacteria, which do not have their genetic material enclosed in nuclei and have cell walls, and from fungi, which have cell walls. It also separates animals from plants, which use the energy of light (usually from the sun) to incorporate carbon dioxide from the atmosphere into organic compounds; these become building blocks for the cell and provide energy for other reactions. Animals are unable to do this and must depend on plants to capture the energy of the sun and make it available as organic compounds to the animals. The attributes on which these distinctions are based seem clear enough—certainly as applied to toads and trees—but cases exist in which the difference between plants and animals is not at all clear. For example, *Euglena* (p. 180) exists in a transition zone, functioning as an animal in the dark and a plant in the light; some varieties have completely lost the ability to use light energy. Are *Euglena* plants or animals? Some authors prefer the five-kingdom arrangement (p. 157), with organisms such as *Euglena* placed with many other single-celled organisms in a separate kingdom, the Protista. Even so, we often find ourselves referring to the "plantlike" protistans and the "animal-like" protistans.

Principles of Science

We emphasized in the first sentence of this chapter that zoology is the scientific study of animals. Certain historical aspects of the development of modern science, particularly as it relates to zoology, will be discussed in other parts of this book, but a basic understanding of zoology requires an understanding of what science is, what it is not, and how knowledge is gained by the scientific method.

Nature of science

What we call science, in the modern sense, has arisen recently in human history, really within the last 200 years or so. Even in that span of time, the pace of discovery and accumulation of knowledge concerning our world and universe have been expanding as the number of scientists has grown and as the sophistication of our instruments and the power of our analyses have increased. Thus, scientific discoveries have changed human lives enormously from what they were 100, or even 20, years ago. Even the most primitive societies in the most remote locations have hardly remained untouched. Nevertheless, many, perhaps most, people in such highly developed countries as the United States and Canada have little or no notion of the real nature of science. Eloquent testimony to the truth of this is that on March 19, 1981, the governor of Arkansas signed into law the

Balanced Treatment for Creation-Science and Evolution-Science Act (Act 590 of 1981). The enactment of this law led to a historic lawsuit tried in December 1981 in the court of Judge William R. Overton, U.S. District Court, Eastern District of Arkansas. The suit was brought by the American Civil Liberties Union on behalf of 23 plaintiffs, including a number of religious leaders and groups representing several denominations, individual parents, and educational associations. The plaintiffs contended that the law was a violation of the First Amendment to the U.S. Constitution, which prohibits "establishment of religion" by the government. This prohibition includes passing a law that would aid one religion or prefer one religion over another. On January 5, 1982, Judge Overton permanently enjoined the State of Arkansas from enforcing Act 590.

Considerable testimony during the trial dealt with the nature of science. Some witnesses defined science simply, if not very informatively, as "what is accepted by the scientific community" and "what scientists do." However, on the basis of other testimony by scientists, Judge Overton was able to state explicitly these essential characteristics of science:

1. It is guided by natural law.
2. It has to be explanatory by reference to natural law.
3. It is testable against the empirical world.
4. Its conclusions are tentative, that is, are not necessarily the final word.
5. It is falsifiable.

The pursuit of scientific knowledge must be guided by the physical and chemical laws that govern the state of existence and interactions of atoms, sub-atomic particles, molecules, and so on. Scientific knowledge must explain what is observed by reference to natural law without requiring the intervention of any supernatural being or force. One may believe, as many scientists do, that the universe was brought into existence by the action of a supernatural being, but such a belief is neither within the realm of science nor contradictory to the tenets of science. We must be able to observe events in the real world, directly or indi-rectly, for them to have scientific value, and testing of hypotheses and theories must be accessible to our senses or to instruments that can measure the events. If we draw a conclusion relative to some event, we must always be ready to discard or modify our conclusion if it is inconsistent with further observations. As Judge Overton stated, "While anybody is free to approach a scientific inquiry in any fashion they choose, they cannot properly describe the methodology used as sci-entific, if they start with a conclusion and refuse to change it regardless of the evidence developed during the course of the investigation."

Scientific method

The manner in which a scientist seeks to gain new knowledge or explain natural phenomena is known as the scientific method. It has sometimes been described as ordinary common sense raised to a higher level and applied systematically. The first step is **observation.** The scientist observes a series of events, often indirectly by means of instruments. Frequently, the events are "observed" by reading descriptions of the observations made by other scientists as recorded in the scien-tific literature. By use of instruments or literature, the scientist may observe oth-erwise inaccessible events, such as those too small to be seen or those that may have taken place many years previously. After considering the observations, the scientist seeks to generalize about them, that is, to make a statement of explana-tion about the observations, such as their cause, mechanism, and relationship to

Figure 1-4

Scientific instruments are extensions of the scientist's senses. The electron micro-scope allows us to visually explore the structure of cells, such as the fine struc-ture of this arterial cell seen magnified 19,000 times.

Electron micrograph courtesy M.E. Todd.

each other. This statement becomes the **hypothesis.** To have any scientific value, the hypothesis must then be tested. On the basis of the hypothesis, the scientist must make a **prediction** about future observations. The scientist must say, "If my hypothesis is a valid explanation of past observations, then future observations ought to have certain characteristics." If the observations do have such characteristics, they constitute evidence in favor of the hypothesis and the hypothesis gains strength as an explanation of the events. In experimental science the "future observations" are in the form of experiments. An **experiment** is a manipulative process by which a prediction made on the basis of the hypothesis can be tested. A certain condition or manipulation is applied to an entity (such as a plant, an animal, a container of a substance, or a body of water), and the results are observed. If the results are as predicted, the hypothesis is supported (not proved), but if the results are otherwise, the hypothesis is invalidated. The results, usually called **data** (sing., **datum**), are evidence for or against the hypothesis. The condition or manipulation that has been applied and is being tested is referred to as the **experimental variable.** To have confidence that the experimental variable is responsible for the effect observed, another entity just like the first one must be subjected to all the conditions that prevailed during the experiment *except* the experimental variable. This part of the experiment is called the **control.** The difference observed between the experimental subject and the control is thus the effect of the experimental variable. In practice an experiment is almost never performed on a single entity, such as an individual plant or animal, but on a group of individuals; therefore there are an experimental group and a control group. Furthermore, the experiment is usually repeated a number of times. The more data obtained, the more confidence can be placed in the conclusion about the hypothesis.

Not all scientific knowledge is gained by means of experiments. Much science is descriptive, but the scientific method is applied nevertheless and the steps are similar. Observations are made, a hypothesis is formed, predictions are made on the basis of the hypothesis as to what the results of further observations should be, and data are collected that may support or disprove the hypothesis. For example, suppose we examine several individual organisms and compare them with published descriptions of such organisms (initial observations). Based on these observations, we form a hypothesis that the organisms represent a new species, that is, a species that has never before been described in the literature. We collect and examine more of the same kinds of individuals from other locations, and we find that they are distinct from other known species. These data support our hypothesis. Alternatively, we may find that there are many intergrading individuals and that our specimens cannot be reliably distinguished from a species already known. In the latter case, our test requires us to discard the hypothesis.

If a hypothesis is supported by a great deal of data, and particularly if it is very powerful—explains a wide variety of related phenomena—the hypothesis may attain the status of a **theory.** We emphasize that the meaning of the word "theory," when used by scientists, is not "speculation" as it is in ordinary English usage. The failure to make this distinction has been prominent in the creationism versus evolution controversy. The creationists have spoken of evolution as "only a theory," as if it were little better than a guess. In fact, the theory of evolution is supported by such massive evidence that most biologists view repudiation of evolution as tantamount to repudiation of reality. Nonetheless, evolution, along with other theories in science, has not been *proved* in a mathematical sense but is testable, tentative, and falsifiable. It has been tested for more than 120 years, and to date there is no scientific evidence that it is false; indeed, organic evolution is accepted as the cornerstone of biology. On the other hand, although much has been learned about the *mechanisms* of evolution, they continue to be explored and clarified.

Concept of Organic Evolution

Organic evolution explains the diversity of modern organisms, their characteristics, and their distribution as the historical outcomes of change from previously existing forms. The doctrine of organic evolution holds that all existing forms of life have descended over an enormous span of time from a single, simple, cellular, protoplasmic mass that arose spontaneously, probably in the sea. The possibility that life has arisen more than once is not excluded, however. Organic evolution refers to the change of life forms over many generations through time and is an aspect of the larger view of **inorganic evolution,** which is concerned with the development of the physical universe from unorganized matter. The principal alternative interpretation for the diversity of life is that of special creation, which holds that all life forms were divinely created much as we find them today. However, the study of biology must account for the physical evidence that life has evolved and changed over time. This evidence, which included the thousands of fossils found in all parts of the world, is not consistent with special creation. Since the late nineteenth century, the principal concern of scientists has not been whether evolution occurs but how it occurs.

Evolutionary theory is strongly identified with Charles Robert Darwin, one of the most important figures in the history of human culture. Darwin and Alfred Russel Wallace simultaneously presented the first credible explanation of the occurrence of evolution, the **principle of natural selection.** The supporting evidence for the principle, so lucidly and forcibly presented by Darwin in his book *On the Origin of Species* (1859), established his undisputed preeminence in evolutionary theory. Darwin's theory generated a storm of controversy between those who supported his ideas and those who opposed them. The major weakness in the theory—ignorance of the mechanisms that underlie hereditary change—was removed at the beginning of the twentieth century, when knowledge of genetics expanded and scientists began to learn about the mechanisms of inheritance and mutations.

Natural selection is the guiding force of evolution. The principle is founded on the observed facts that no two organisms are exactly alike; that some variations, at least, are inheritable; that all groups tend to overproduce their kind; and that because more individuals are reproduced than can survive, there is a struggle for existence among them. In this struggle, according to Darwin, organisms possessing variations that make them better adapted to the environment will survive. If, because of their survival, they have more offspring than do those with less favorable variations, their inheritable characteristics will appear in greater proportion in the next generation. Continuation of this natural selection will produce continuous evolutionary change. Natural selection therefore is based on **adaptations**—those characteristics possessed by an organism that enable it to survive and reproduce in its environment. The idea of *fitness* is embodied in the well-known nineteenth-century phrase, "survival of the fittest."

Figure 1-5

Modern evolutionary theory is strongly identified with Charles Robert Darwin who, with Alfred Russel Wallace, provided the first credible explanation of evolution—natural selection. This photograph of Darwin was taken in 1854 when he was 45 years old.

Courtesy American Museum of Natural History.

With the discovery of genes and chromosome systems at the turn of the century and the recognition that genes were self-reproducing, operative units of heredity, the mechanism of inheritable variation became understandable. Genes can undergo sudden, spontaneous, and random changes called **mutations.** Mutations are the ultimate source of new variation. Natural selection acts to encourage the spread of some mutations while repressing the spread of others. *Mutations are the raw material of evolution; natural selection provides direction.*

The essence of natural selection is reproductive success. Because of genetic differences between individuals within a population, some have more progeny that live to reproduce than do others. This means that the "winning" genes become common in the population, while others are selected against and become rare or absent. Evolution is a continuing process in which chance variations are constantly interacting with the environment to determine individual success. This leads to the evolution of individual adaptations and to the gradual modification of a group of organisms as a whole. The evolutionary process is all-pervasive. Every feature of life as we know it today—the vast diversity of life on earth; every adaptation; every aspect of structure, function, and behavior of every organism— has been shaped by the unrelenting pressure of natural selection. Many biologists now believe that several other processes also play significant roles in evolution: recombination, the founder effect, genetic drift, and punctuated equilibria. These are discussed in Chapter 38.

——SOME IMPORTANT BIOLOGICAL PRINCIPLES AND CONCEPTS

A principle or generalization is a statement of fact that has a wide application and can be used to formulate other principles and concepts. Like the other sciences, biology has a number of fundamental principles and assumptions, although they may not lend themselves to the mathematical exactness of the physical sciences. Well-formulated principles are indispensable to help us organize our thinking, see important relationships, and form basic conclusions from the awesome mass of factual material with which we are confronted. These principles are products of the scientific method and have been tested by many workers over long periods of time. Inevitably, some will be subject to revision and new interpretation in the light of new knowledge.

Inevitably also, any such list compiled by other zoologists might have a different organization or emphasis, or even the addition or deletion of certain points, depending on the background and training of those individuals. Nonetheless, there would be significant agreement on the principles that demonstrate the essential unity of the organism and the integration of all biological systems.

Statements of principles are necessarily condensed, and many terms used here, although defined in the glossary, will be fully explained in later chapters. *The student is not expected to memorize the principles at this point, but rather should assimilate them gradually while progressing through the book and beginning to interrelate information.* References to the principles will be made in later chapters, where they will have significant application and will be better understood. Some are so well accepted that they form a part of the conceptual scheme of virtually all biologists. Others are of more recent development and have yet to be thoroughly integrated into the science.

Application of Physical and Chemical Principles

1. Living systems and their constituents obey physical and chemical laws. All living systems are subject to the same physical and chemical laws as are nonliving systems. Within the cells of any organism, the living substance is comprised of a multitude of nonliving constituents: proteins, nucleic acids, fats, carbohydrates, waste metabolites, crystalline aggregates, pigments, and many others, all of which are composed of molecules and their constituent atoms. Living substance (protoplasm) is alive because of the highly complex organization of these nonliving substances and the way they interact with one another, just as a watch is a timepiece only when all of its gears, springs, and bearings are organized in a particular way and interact with one another. Neither the gears of a watch nor the molecules in protoplasm can interact in any way that is contrary to universal physical laws. Consequently, the more completely we can understand the functioning of protoplasm and its constituents on the basis of chemical principles, the more completely we can understand the phenomena of life (Chapter 2).

2. All organisms capture, store, and transmit energy. Of the many physicochemical principles pertinent to the maintenance of life, the laws governing energy and its transformations (thermodynamics) are central. The first law of thermodynamics is the **law of conservation of energy.** This says that *energy can be neither created nor destroyed, although it may be transformed from one form to another.* All aspects of life require energy in some form, and the energy to support life on earth flows from the fusion reactions in our sun and reaches the earth in the form of light and heat. Sunlight is captured by green plants and transformed by the process of photosynthesis into chemical bond energy. Chemical bond energy is a form of potential energy that can be released when the bond is broken; the energy is then used to perform electrical, mechanical, and osmotic tasks in the cell. Energy made and stored in plants is used by animals that eat the plants, and these animals may in turn provide energy for other animals that eat them.

Ultimately, all the energy transformed and stored by the plants will again be transformed, little by little, and dissipated as heat. This is in accord with the second law of thermodynamics, which otherwise might seem to be violated by living systems. This law states that *there is a tendency in nature to proceed toward a state of greater molecular disorder* or **entropy.** Thus, the high degree of molecular organization in living cells is attained and maintained *only* as long as energy fuels the organization. The ultimate fate of materials in the cells is degradation and dissipation of the chemical bond energy as heat, thereby approaching greater molecular disorder, or randomness (Chapters 5 and 41).

3. There is a biochemical and molecular unity of living systems. Given that living systems are subject to universal physicochemical laws and that a particular molecule or element has the same characteristics, whether it is in a bacterial cell or an elephant cell, it should not be surprising that living systems possess a high degree of molecular and biochemical unity. All cells require chemical constituents to serve the biochemical functions of food utilization and energy transformation and the hereditary functions of genetic replication. Despite the occurrence of more than 170 amino acids in nature, only 20 are used almost ubiquitously as building blocks of active proteins in living organisms. Deoxyribonucleic acid, the hereditary material of life, is constructed from only four particular nitrogenous bases, in addition to certain sugar phosphate units. The macromolecules used in energy

Figure 1-6

Fusion reactions in the sun support all life on earth.
Photograph by C.P. Hickman, Jr.

transformations often show remarkable consistency in structure. The same sequences of metabolic reactions to release the stored energy in chemical bonds occur over an enormous variety of unrelated organisms, and the reactions often differ only in detail (Chapters 2 and 5).

___ Concept of Evolution

4. Animals evolve by the mechanism of natural selection. That existing organisms have evolved by organic evolution from preexisting organisms through the mechanism of natural selection constitutes one of the great unifying principles of all biology. This concept has already been introduced and will be discussed further in Chapter 38. Evolution by means of natural selection allows us to ask two fundamental questions about any biological phenomenon or characteristic: "What is its function?" and "How did it evolve?"

The idea of function is unique to biology among the sciences. By function we do not mean "purpose" in the sense of consciously directed objective, but the way in which a particular characteristic helps an organism or a population to survive and reproduce. For example, the function of legs or limbs in particular animals may be locomotion, food gathering, food handling, copulation, respiration, or even a combination of these. The legs help the animal to survive and reproduce; hence they have **adaptive value,** that is, they are an **adaptation.** By the same token, the function of a particular enzyme may be to help derive the energy from a food molecule, or an entire metabolic sequence of reactions may have such a function, and they can thus be viewed as adaptations. A living organism is a bundle of adaptations, some of which may be widely possessed by a great variety of organisms, and some of which are narrow, or specialized, adaptations, helping the organism to survive in its particular habitat (Chapter 38).

5. All organisms are adapted to their habitat. Environmental conditions vary from one habitat to another, and these conditions constitute **selective factors** or **pressures,** which favor the survival of organisms with certain characteristics over others; that is, they favor the survival of those organisms that are better adapted to a specific environment. Thus, over the generations, organisms with adaptations suitable for a particular habitat (special adaptations) evolve because of persistent selection by environmental pressures (Chapters 7 to 27 and 38).

6. Animals that have many morphological characters in common share a common descent. Since existing animals have evolved from preexisting ones, it is highly probable that those having many morphological characteristics in common share a common ancestor. The more characters organisms have in common, the more closely they are related, and the closer they are to their common ancestor. The phylogenetic scheme forms the basis for modern classification of animals. A few common characters shared by two groups may have limited significance because of the possibility of **convergent evolution;** similar selective pressures may have selected for the evolution of similar adaptations in unrelated groups. However, when common characters are homologous—similar in origin—the evidence for relationship is strong (Chapters 7 to 27).

7. The embryos of animals tend to resemble the embryos of their ancestors. Studies of the embryogenesis of animals in the context of evolution resulted in the observation that embryos often go through stages resembling their ancestors, which led to

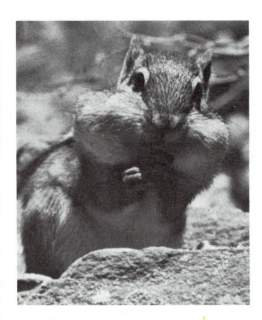

Figure 1-7

A living organism is a bundle of adaptations. An eastern chipmunk fills its pouches with food to be stored for winter use.

Photograph by L.L. Rue, III.

the formulation of the **biogenetic law.** As originally conceived, it was believed that the embryonic stages of an animal were similar to the adult stages of its phylogenetic ancestors: the **principle of recapitulation,** or the idea that ontogeny (the life history) repeats phylogeny (the ancestral history). This viewpoint assumed that all evolutionary advancements were added to the terminal stages of the life histories of organisms. Although subsequent observation has shown that this interpretation is incorrect, there is nevertheless a tendency for early developmental patterns to become more or less stabilized in successive ontogenies of later descendants (**paleogenesis**). Thus, a modern restatement of the biogenetic law would be that *embryos of animals tend to go through stages resembling the embryos of their ancestors.* This tendency is demonstrated mostly in the least specialized members of animal groups. It is not well demonstrated and may not be evident at all in specialized members for two reasons: embryos are just as subject to natural selection as are adults and so may show embryonic adaptations, and adult adaptations often begin their development in the embryonic stages. Therefore any similarity to ancestral embryos may be completely obscured. Paleogenesis is important, nevertheless, because study of the less highly specialized or modified members of a group may provide evidence of phylogenetic relationships with other groups (Chapters 7 and 36).

8. Evolution is irreversible. An evolutionary generalization of wide applicability is sometimes known as **Dollo's law:** that with the possible exception of short intervals and in a very restricted sense, evolution is a one-way process, or is irreversible. An evolutionary path once taken cannot be retraced. A consequence of this fact is that the possible range of adaptations possessed by descendant groups is predetermined and limited by the array of adaptations possessed by their ancestors. Accordingly, each major group of animals usually has a basic adaptive pattern that may have determined its evolutionary divergence. For example, in the phylum Mollusca—a very large group of animals with over 100,000 living species—there is a certain array of characteristics that, if figuratively extrapolated backward, suggests a hypothetical ancestral mollusc. Most investigators of molluscs agree that the hypothetical ancestral mollusc must be very much like the actual ancestral mollusc and that all living molluscs, from the tiny snail to the giant squid, are but elaborations on the ancestral pattern. Thus, the adaptive radiation of present-day molluscs, although enormous, is strictly limited by the characteristics of their ancient ancestor (Chapters 8 to 27, 38).

Biogenesis

9. Life comes from life. Certainly a basic principle of the widest possible applicability is the concept that all organisms come from preexisting organisms, or the **principle of biogenesis.** This is in contrast to the notion that life can spring from inanimate matter, that is, abiogenesis or spontaneous generation—a concept that is now discredited. That living organisms could be spontaneously generated was widely accepted until the experiments of several workers, including Pasteur, were carried out. Pasteur showed that when nutrient broth was boiled in flasks with S-shaped necks, thus sterilizing the medium, no bacterial growth subsequently occurred in the broth because the S-shaped neck prevented entry of bacteria on dust particles from the air. If the S-shaped neck was broken off, bacterial colonies rapidly developed.

Modern biologists have recognized, however, that while the principle of

Figure 1-8

Whelk *Busycon.* A living mollusc is an elaboration of an ancestral pattern. Photograph by C.P. Hickman, Jr.

Figure 1-9

All animals and plants are composed of cells that, even in their simplest form, are enormously complex structures. This section of amphibian intestine reveals that it is composed of a variety of cell types.
Photomicrograph by F.M. Hickman.

biogenesis applies now, it was not always so. Life must have originated on earth from nonliving matter at least once, perhaps several times. But of course, conditions were far different in the primeval seas than they are now (Chapter 3).

10. Reproduction is a property of living systems. A corollary of the principle of biogenesis is the ability of living organisms to reproduce. Reproduction is a unique and ubiquitous property of living systems. This principle becomes self-evident when one considers the alternatives (Chapter 35).

Cell Theory

11. Cells are the fundamental and functional units of life. The cell theory, or **cell doctrine** as it is often called, is another of the great unifying concepts of biology. All animals and plants are comprised of cells and cell products. New cells come from division of preexisting cells, and the activity of a multicellular organism as a whole is the sum of the activities of its constituent cells and their interactions.

Despite great variation in size (although most cells are between 0.5 and 40 μm in diameter), shape, and function, all cells are basically similar in structure. It is a remarkable fact that living forms, from amebas and unicellular algae to whales and giant redwood trees, are formed from this single type of building unit (Chapter 4).

12. Cells contain differentiated and functionally interdependent structures. The cell is surrounded by a membrane, and in plants also by a cell wall secreted by the cell. Within the cell are various structures referred to as **organelles.** In plant and animal cells there are a number of organelles bounded by membranes, including a **nucleus,** a relatively large structure containing the hereditary material. The material and structures outside the nucleus are collectively called the **cytoplasm.** In addition to the membranous organelles in the cytoplasm, there are particulate structures, proteins in colloidal suspension, and smaller molecules in solution; there also may be other substances, such as lipid (fat). The cells of bacteria and blue-green algae lack membrane-bound organelles, and their nuclear area is not surrounded by a membrane (Chapter 4).

Gene Theory

13. All organisms inherit a structural and functional organization from their progenitors: the principle of hereditary transmission. This generalization involves the laws of heredity and applies to all living things. The highest and lowest types of animals have the capacity for reproducing their own kind and transmitting their characteristics to their offspring. What is inherited by an offspring is not necessarily an exact copy of the parent; heredity is not as simple as that. What is inherited is a certain type of organization that, under the influence of developmental and environmental forces, gives rise to a certain expressed result. Many potentialities may be inherited, but those that are actually expressed are much more limited (Chapters 35 and 37).

14. The gene is the fundamental unit of inheritance, and inheritance obeys Mendel's laws. The gene is a bit of coded information that confers the potential for expression of a certain characteristic on the cell or organism. The genes are borne on structures called **chromosomes;** each chromosome bears many genes. With certain notable exceptions, the nucleus of each animal cell has two sets of chromosomes (**diploid condition**), with pairs of chromosomes bearing the genes for the same set of characteristics. The two genes for a particular characteristic, one on each member of a pair of homologous chromosomes, are described as allelic genes, or **alleles.** Only one of the alleles may result in the production of an expressed characteristic in the organism (the dominant allele), although both are present in each cell and either may be passed on to the progeny.

During the production of the sex cells (**gametes: sperm** and **ova**), the number of chromosomes is halved (**haploid condition**), with each gamete receiving one of each of the homologous pairs of chromosomes. Thus, each gamete has only one of each kind of gene. This is the **law of segregation,** first formulated by Gregor Mendel in 1866.

Mendel's second law, the **law of independent assortment,** implies that the likelihood of an individual progeny inheriting a particular allele is the result of chance alone. Although each gamete has a full haploid set of chromosomes, which chromosome of each of the homologous pairs is actually passed to a particular gamete is completely random; that is, it is independent of the other homologues passed to that gamete. Of course, all of the genes on the same chromosome tend to be inherited together and do not assort independently (Chapter 37).

15. Gene frequencies in a population can remain stable under certain conditions. When the female gamete (ovum) is fertilized by the male (sperm), a fusion of their nuclei restores the number of chromosomes to the diploid condition. Thus, the progeny receive one set of chromosomes from each parent and, consequently, have two genes for each trait. However, in the population as a whole, there may be several other alleles for the same trait, and the frequency of occurrence of a given gene can be expressed as a fraction of one (one equals the whole population, or the frequencies of all the alleles added together). It might be expected that if the frequency of a gene in a population were very low, the allele would eventually disappear. However, it can be shown that, provided certain conditions are met, the gene frequencies of all alleles in a population remain constant. This is the **Hardy-Weinberg law,** which operates under certain specific conditions (Chapter 38).

16. Gene frequencies in a population can change. The presence of numerous alleles, or combinations of alleles, in a population provides variability in the characteristics possessed by the individuals in that population. Clearly, if some of these characteristics are helpful to survival and reproduction of those individuals, they will provide a disproportionate share of their genes to the next generation. If selective pressures are strong, gene frequencies in a population may change markedly over time. Thus, *natural selection influences gene frequencies.*

Furthermore, the genes themselves may change; that is, the coded information in a gene may undergo a molecular alteration so that the trait produced by that gene is different. This is a **mutation.** Mutations are the ultimate source of biological variation. Mutations may produce genetic effects that are helpful in terms of natural selection, or they may be detrimental. They may be induced by artificial means, such as x-rays or radioactivity, or by a variety of chemical agents, but their natural causes are largely obscure. Mutations may occur in somatic (body) cells, but only mutations in germ cells, which give rise to gametes, will be inherited by the next generation. The frequencies of genes with detrimental effects may be reduced over time, or they may be constant if the rate of mutation offsets the negative selective value of its effect.

Figure 1-10

Walrus bulls. Gene frequencies within a population remain stable unless disturbed by natural selection, mutation, genetic drift, or migration.
Photograph by L.L. Rue, III.

Figure 1-11

James Watson and Francis Crick with one of their models of DNA.

From James D. Watson, *The Double Helix*, Atheneum, New York, 1968; copyright 1968 by James D. Watson; reprinted by permission of the publisher.

Genetic drift is a change in gene frequency by chance alone. This can occur when the population is small, and "sampling errors" can accumulate, thus changing gene frequencies in the population over time (Chapters 37 and 38).

17. DNA is the substance that contains the inherited information. We have referred to the gene as a "bit of coded information." The discovery of the nature of the code and how the code is translated into the expression of a characteristic is among the great triumphs of modern biology. The genetic material on the chromosomes is **deoxyribonucleic acid (DNA)**. This is a high–molecular weight substance composed of many units of a sugar phosphate (deoxyribose phosphate) and many units of four nitrogenous bases (adenine, guanine, thymine, and cytosine, abbreviated A, G, T, and C, respectively). In 1953 James Watson and Francis Crick suggested a **double helix model** for DNA, for which abundant evidence has subsequently accumulated. According to the Watson-Crick model, two very long strands of sugar phosphate units are connected together, and the strands twist around each other in a double helix form. Projecting toward each other between the two strands are the nitrogenous bases. When a precisely scaled molecular model was constructed, it was found that adenine would fit opposite thymine and cytosine would fit opposite guanine, but other combinations would not fit in the available space. This suggested a hypothesis for DNA replication: the strands could unwind, and each could serve as a template for the synthesis of the complementary strand, resulting in two double helices exactly the same as the preexisting one (Chapters 2 and 37).

18. The genetic code is in the linear order or sequence of bases on the DNA strand. The Watson-Crick model implied that the genetic code would lie in the linear order of the nitrogenous bases: A, G, T, and C. As mentioned previously, proteins are constructed of 20 different amino acid building blocks. Assuming that the order of bases in DNA represented a code for the order of amino acids in a protein, it was clear that some combination of bases must code for one protein, since there are only four bases but 20 amino acids. The minimum number of bases to provide a sufficient number of different combinations to specify each of the amino acids is three, as suggested by Francis Crick in 1961. Subsequent research has substantiated Crick's hypothesis. The genetic code is based on triplets of nitrogenous bases along the DNA molecule. Each triplet, called a **codon,** codes for a single amino acid, and the codons do not overlap. The genetic code is apparently universal; that is, the same codon or sequence of three nitrogenous bases codes for the same amino acid in all organisms (Chapter 37).

19. Transcription and translation of genetic information are mediated by RNA. Although the transmission of genetic information and the nature of the genetic code now seem to us at once ingenious and astonishingly simple, they fall far short of explaining how the cell reads the code and translates it into cell products and structures. Nevertheless, much progress has been made in elucidating these critical processes. They depend on molecules of **ribonucleic acid (RNA),** a substance somewhat similar to DNA except that ribose is present in its strand instead of deoxyribose, and uracil is present instead of thymine. There are three principal types of RNA: **messenger RNA (mRNA), transfer RNA (tRNA),** and **ribosomal RNA (rRNA).** Molecules of mRNA are synthesized alongside strands of DNA in the chromosome, using the DNA as a template and thus transcribing the code from the DNA to the mRNA. The mRNA moves out of the nucleus into the cytoplasm where it interacts with submicroscopic particles called **ribosomes.** Ribosomes are constructed of about 50% protein and 50% rRNA. The molecules of tRNA provide the translation function. The various types bind with specific amino acids. At a particular position in a specific tRNA molecule there is a triplet sequence of nitrogenous bases, the **anticodon,** which is complementary to the codon sequence in the mRNA. Ribosomes move along the strand of mRNA, positioning the molecules of tRNA according to the codon-anticodon specificity, and the amino acid attached to the tRNA is reattached to the chain of amino acids being assembled into a protein. The specificity or kind of protein is determined by the sequence of amino acids in it, and this depends on the sequence of codons in DNA as transcribed and translated by the RNA system (Chapter 37).

20. A gene constitutes the information needed to synthesize an enzyme: the "one gene–one enzyme" principle. A gene, then, may be redefined as a series of codons of DNA that result in the production of a particular protein. The physical and chemical properties of the protein depend on the ordinal sequence of its amino acids. The properties of many proteins allow them to function as **enzymes.** Enzymes are catalysts for the myriad chemical reactions that go on in a cell; that is, they facilitate reactions by participating in them but are not "used up" in the reactions—they are not substrates or products of the reactions. The hundreds of chemical reactions, collectively called **metabolism** or **metabolic reactions,** are each catalyzed by specific enzymes. These reactions would not occur, or would occur very slowly, if they were not mediated by enzymes. The reactions to derive energy from food molecules and synthesize cell structures and products, even the synthesis of DNA itself, require the participation of enzymes. In 1941 G.W. Beadle and E.L. Tatum suggested the one gene–one enzyme hypothesis: that a gene would constitute the genetic information necessary to synthesize one enzyme. The validity of the hypothesis, in a slightly modified form, is now widely accepted.

Since it is now known that a particular protein may be made of several chains of amino acids (polypeptides), the Beadle and Tatum hypothesis is expressed as **one gene–one polypeptide.** Thus, a mutation is a change in the order of the nitrogenous bases in the DNA, which codes for the order of amino acids in an enzyme, producing an enzyme with different properties. Mutations often involve a change in several nitrogenous bases in the gene but in some cases may result from the alteration of a single pair. When the properties of an enzyme are changed, the metabolic reaction it catalyzes is altered; therefore *metabolic reactions are under genic control* (Chapters 5 and 37).

_____ Growth, Life Cycle, and Differentiation

21. Growth is a fundamental characteristic of life. Its manifestation as the synthesis of protoplasm in every living organism has been referred to as the **growth law.** True growth is characterized by an increase in tissue or protoplasmic mass with cell division or cell enlargement or both. It thus depends on the incorporation of new materials from the environment and is subject to the availability of those materials (Chapters 6 and 36).

22. All organisms have a characteristic life cycle that they pass through as they grow. In the case of unicellular organisms, this life cycle may be as simple as growth and cell division, but the interspersion of resting stages, sexual reproduction, cyclical changes in body form, and other such events is common. In multicellular organ-

Figure 1-12

All organisms have a characteristic life cycle, which may be simple and direct, as in most unicellular organisms, or quite complex in advanced multicellular organisms such as these broad-tailed hummingbirds.
Photograph by L.L. Rue, III.

Figure 1-13

Wolf spider with egg case. All organisms develop a characteristic, genetically directed body plan.

Photograph by C.P. Hickman, Jr.

isms, development begins with a single cell, usually a fertilized egg, or **zygote.** This initially undergoes division (**cleavage**) into smaller and smaller cells with no increase in total mass and no true growth, but the preliminary cell division increases the total surface area of cell membranes, which facilitates the incorporation of nutrients required for actual growth. True developmental growth is accompanied by shaping of the embryo, called **morphogenesis,** and a progressive specialization of the cells, tissues, and structures into the organization of the whole organism, called **differentiation.** Thus begins the life cycle of the organism, which may be quite complex, including embryonic and juvenile development, adolescence, adult equilibrium, and senescence (Chapters 5, 6, 35, and 36).

23. All organisms develop a characteristic body plan. The patterns of growth are genetically directed and are usually constant for each stage of the life cycle from generation to generation. The inherited body plan may be described in terms of broadly inclusive characteristics, such as presence and type of internal body cavities, symmetry, and type of nervous system—all of which would be possessed by organisms with a common ancestor—or the plan may be described in terms of narrow characteristics possessed only by individuals of a certain species or population (Chapter 6).

24. Nuclear equivalence and cell differentiation are characteristics of cells in multicellular organisms. Since the body plan and all organization of the body are inherited, it is clear that *all* genetic information (the **genome**) for the attainment of that body plan must be present in the zygote, which replicates its DNA and confers that information on all its progeny cells. Thus, the cell nuclei of a multicellular organism, with few exceptions, are genetically alike. This is the **principle of nuclear equivalence.** However, it is also clear that *differentiated* cells are not all alike. Therefore only some of the information is transcribed and translated in a given cell. Cell differentiation results from the differential activity of the same set of genes in different cells. In the fully differentiated cell, most of the genome is fully repressed and silent. A muscle cell, for example, never translates the parts of its DNA instructions that would produce proteins unique to a nerve cell. During embryonic development, nuclei in different regions of the embryo provide different genetic information, resulting in regional differentiation of cells and tissue. The control of differentiation remains one of the great unsolved problems of biology. Whatever the molecular mechanisms, there is abundant evidence that differentiation is one of the responses to conditions or substances in the environment of a cell (Chapter 37).

Responses and Relations to the Environment of a Cell or Organism

25. Irritability is a characteristic of life. One of the fundamental characteristics of life is irritability, that is, the ability to react to an environmental stimulus. This is perhaps the most widely occurring of all adaptations. Broadly speaking, it can be interpreted as the ability to react to a stimulus in such a way as to promote the continued life of a cell or organism. The reaction may be, for example, to consume a food molecule or particle when such is present, to seek or avoid light, to pursue a prey organism, or to avoid a noxious substance. When such reactions can no longer be accomplished, the organism perishes. Throughout the life of an animal, matter and energy pass through the body, providing perturbations of the internal physiological state. Many physiological and metabolic mechanisms exist that function to compensate for such disturbances and to maintain conditions compatible with continued life within the organism. This tendency toward internal stabilization was recognized by Claude Bernard in the nineteenth century, and the concept was developed in the twentieth century by Walter B. Cannon, who called it the **principle of homeostasis.** Homeostasis is achieved at the cell, organ, and system levels by material and energy transport and in many instances is controlled by feedback mechanisms (Chapters 28 to 34).

26. Cells in a multicellular animal communicate with and affect each other. Reaction to stimuli and maintenance of homeostasis require mechanisms for communication between cells and organs in multicellular animals. Increasingly complex levels of organization in animals require correspondingly increasing complexities in communication between cells and organs. Communication between parts of an animal is by two primary means: **neural** and **hormonal.** Relatively rapid communication is by neural mechanisms and involves propagated electrochemical changes in cell membranes. Highly organized and complex nervous systems carry out this function in higher animals. Relatively less rapid or long-term adjustments in an animal are by hormonal or endocrine mechanisms. Hormones are substances produced by cells in one part of the body that regulate cell processes elsewhere in the organism when carried there by body fluids. Sometimes the hormones are produced by nerve cells, or cells derived from nerve cells, and in those cases the system is described as **neuroendocrine.** Many instances are now known in which substances produced by some individual animals reach other individuals in the population and function as hormones in the other individuals, producing adjustments in their physiological processes or behavior. Such substances are called **pheromones** (Chapters 32 to 34).

27. All animals interact with their environment. Whether able to react to a given environmental stimulus or not, all organisms in a given area interact with both the biological and physical factors in their environment. The earth's biomass is organized into a hierarchy of interacting units: the individual organism, the population, the community, and the ecosystem. Among the important generalizations in ecology are the concepts of **food chains** (producers, primary and secondary consumers, decomposers), **habitats,** and **niches.** The habitat is the spatial location where an animal lives. It is always physically circumscribed, although the space may be very large, such as an entire ocean, or tiny, such as the intestine of an insect. What the organism does—its role—in its habitat is its niche. The niche of an animal must be described in terms of the effects the organism has on other organisms in its habitat, and vice versa, as well as the effects on and by nonliving resources in the habitat. The possible effects on other animals include an array, such as whether the organism interacts with them as a predator, a prey, a mutual, a parasite, a competitor, or others. Insofar as individuals or populations compete for food, space, or other resources in a habitat, their niches overlap. If the competition is too strong, one of the individuals or populations will perish, be driven out of the habitat, or be forced to use other resources—to occupy a different niche. It has been found that no two species can occupy the same ecological niche at the same time and place (**principle of competitive exclusion; Gause's rule**) (Chapters 38 and 41).

Figure 1-14

Club-headed hydroids *Clava squamata* on seaweed. The concept of niche—the position or status or functional relationship of a species within a community—is an important ecological generalization. No two species can occupy precisely the same ecological niches at the same time and place.
Photograph by D.P. Wilson.

___ Summary

Zoology is the scientific study of animals and is part of biology, the scientific study of life. Animals and life can be defined only in terms of attributes that are associated with them. Characteristics of living organisms include organization, metabolism, growth, adaptability, irritability, reproduction, and interaction with the environment.

Science is characterized by a particular approach to the acquisition of human knowledge. It is guided by, and is explanatory with reference to, natural law, and it is testable, tentative, and falsifiable. The scientific method is the manner in which scientific knowledge is gained, and it has proved to be a powerful tool. Its essential constituents are observing events, forming a hypothesis on the basis of the observations, testing the hypothesis, and drawing a conclusion about the hypothesis on the basis of the tests. Tests may take the form of experiments. Every experiment must have two components: an experimental group and a control group. The control group is exactly like the experimental group and is treated exactly the same, except that the experimental variable is not applied to the control group. Results of the tests of the hypothesis are the data. A hypothesis for which there is a great deal of supporting data, particularly one that explains a very large number of observations, may be elevated to the status of a theory.

Evolution based primarily on the principle of natural selection is such a theory. The concept of natural selection was proposed by Charles Darwin and Alfred Russel Wallace, and Darwin developed a strong body of evidence to support it.

The principles given in this chapter illustrate the unity of biological science. All the cellular constituents, like the cells themselves, are governed by natural laws. Living organisms can come only from other living organisms, just as new cells can be produced only from preexisting cells. The nucleus of the cell carries the hereditary material, which confers a certain set of characteristics on its cellular progeny, which themselves may become new organisms on which natural selection may act. Living organisms have mechanisms that tend to compensate through internal and external changes to keep conditions within limits compatible with continued life.

Selected references

Beveridge, W.I.B. 1957. The art of scientific investigation. New York, W.W. Norton & Co., Inc.

Conant, J.B. 1952. Modern science and modern man. New York, Columbia University Press.

Medawar, P.B. 1957. A note on "the scientific method." In Medawar, P.B. The uniqueness of the individual. New York, Basic Books, Inc., Publishers.

Overton, W.R. 1982. Judgment, injunction, and memorandum opinion in the case of McLean vs. Arkansas Board of Education. Science 215:934-943. *Judge Overton's opinion is reprinted verbatim. It is highly recommended reading.*

Selected *Scientific American* articles

Butterfield, H. 1960. The scientific revolution. 203:173-192 (Sept.).

de Camp, L.S. 1969. The end of the monkey war. 220:15-21 (Feb.). *In 1968 the U.S. Supreme Court struck down the Arkansas statute that forbade the teaching of evolution in public schools and colleges. The conclusion that this marked the "end of the monkey war" was somewhat premature.*

CHAPTER 2

MATTER AND LIFE

Model of glucose, a hexose sugar manufactured in green plants from water and carbon dioxide.
All plant and animal tissues depend on the chemical energy stored within this
molecule, the most important carbohydrate in the living world.

Courtesy Biology Media.

Figure 2-1

Structure of carbon atom. A planetary system of 6 negatively charged electrons revolves around a dense nucleus of 6 positive protons and 6 uncharged neutrons.

BASIC STRUCTURE OF MATTER
Nature of Atoms

Although the ancient Greeks had certain conceptions of the composition of matter, such as the universe being composed of four elements—fire, air, earth, and water—our present concepts of the nature of matter have originated within the past two centuries. A.L. Lavoisier, a great French scientist of the eighteenth century, compiled the first list of elements, a total of 28 (1778). J. Dalton, an English chemist, conceived that matter is composed of atoms, which combine in definite proportions to form chemical compounds (1808). The Italian investigator A. Avogadro showed how many atoms of each kind make up each compounded atom and gave us the concept of the molecule (1811). By 1869 most of the 92 elements that occur in nature had been discovered, and the Russian chemist D.I. Mendeléev worked out his periodic table of the elements (Fig. 2-10). (Much more recently other elements have been synthesized in the laboratory; the total today for all natural and synthesized elements stands at 103.) Mendeléev arranged the elements into eight groups, relating the chemical elements on the basis of their properties, which are periodic functions of their atomic weights. If the elements are in a group of elements that have similar properties and relations, they follow a regular progression in the individual differences of their members.

For many years the atom was considered solid and indivisible. Then in 1911 Lord Rutherford showed that every atom consists of a positively charged nucleus surrounded by a negatively charged system of electrons (Fig. 2-1). An electron is a negatively charged particle with almost no mass. The nucleus, containing most of the atom's mass, is made up of two kinds of particles, **protons** and **neutrons**, clustered together in a very small volume. These two particles have about the same mass, each being about 2000 times heavier than an electron. The protons bear positive charges, and the neutrons are uncharged (neutral).

The positively charged protons, which would normally repel each other because they bear similar charges, are held together by powerful short-range nuclear forces. When an atomic nucleus is torn apart in a fission reaction, such as during the explosion of an atomic bomb, enormous amounts of energy are released. This energy stabilizes the structure of atoms, but it plays no part in the physical and chemical interactions that occur in the living body.

Although the number of protons in the nucleus is the same as the number of electrons revolving around the nucleus, the number of neutrons may vary. For every positively charged proton in the nucleus, there is a negatively charged electron. The total charge of the atom is thus neutral.

The number of protons in the nucleus is the **atomic number** of the atom. Thus, hydrogen, helium, and lithium, containing respectively 1, 2, and 3 protons in their nuclei, have atomic numbers of 1, 2, and 3, respectively. Since atoms are electrically neutral, the atomic number is also equal to the number of electrons revolving around the nucleus.

The **mass number** of an atom is the total number of protons and neutrons in its nucleus. The nucleus of an oxygen atom contains 8 protons and 8 neutrons. It therefore has a mass number of 16. The heaviest natural element, uranium, has a nucleus of 92 protons (its atomic number is thus 92) and 146 neutrons, and so its mass number is 238. The elements are designated by convenient symbols that show the atomic number as a subscript and the total number of protons and neutrons (mass number) as a superscript. Thus, oxygen is designated $^{16}_{8}O$, hydrogen $_1^1H$ (1 proton, no neutrons), helium $_2^4He$ (2 protons, 2 neutrons), and so on (Fig. 2-2).

The **atomic weight** of an atom is nearly the same as its mass number. However, a quick examination of a periodic table shows that none of the elements has an atomic weight of an exact integer. How are atomic weights derived? Obviously an atom weighs far too little to serve as a useful index for weight comparison. A hydrogen atom, for example, weighs 1.67×10^{-24} g. Consequently, physicists have assigned a set of meaningful relative weights to the elements, using carbon as a base for comparison. Carbon, $_6^{12}C$, with 6 protons and 6 neutrons, has been assigned the integral value 12. By this scale, protons and neutrons have masses of 1.0073 and 1.0087, respectively—masses close to, but not exactly, 1. (Electrons have an almost negligible mass of 0.00055.) No element, except carbon 12, has an atomic weight of an exact integer: hydrogen weighs 1.008; helium, 4.0026; lithium, 6.939; and so on.

The **gram atomic weight** of an element is its atomic weight expressed in grams. The number of atoms in a gram atomic weight is 6.02×10^{23} (Avogadro's number). This means that the gram atomic weight of all elements has the same number of atoms. One gram of hydrogen (its gram atomic weight) has the same number of atoms as does 16 g of oxygen or 12 g of carbon, their gram atomic weights.

The relative weight of a molecule, composed of 2 or more atoms, is known as the **gram molecular weight.** It is the sum of the gram atomic weights of all the atoms in a molecule. One gram molecular weight of carbon dioxide (CO_2) is 44 g (12 + 16 + 16); of water (H_2O), 18 g; and of oxygen (O_2), 32 g. As with gram atomic weight, defined previously, the gram molecular weight of any compound contains the same number of molecules (6.02×10^{23}) as the gram molecular weight of any other compound.

Still another expression of quantity of a substance is the **mole.** This unit combines the molecular weight and the number of molecules present. The number of moles of a compound present in a particular instance is equal to the weight of the compound present in that instance divided by its molecular weight:

$$\text{Moles} = \frac{\text{Weight in grams}}{\text{Molecular weight}}$$

For example, 18 g of water, having a molecular weight of 18, is 1 mole of water; 36 g of water is 2 moles. Since most compounds in living systems are present in much less than 1 mole quantities, the **millimole** (mmole, 0.001 mole) and the **micromole** (μmole, 0.000001 mole) are more commonly used in biology to express molecular quantities than is the mole.

Isotopes

It is possible for 2 atoms of the same element to have the same number or protons in their nuclei, but a different number of neutrons. For example, hydrogen exists in nature primarily as $_1^1H$; that is, it contains 1 proton but no neutron. However, there are also trace amounts of two other forms of hydrogen: $_1^2H$, which has 1 proton and 1 neutron and is called deuterium, and $_1^3H$, which has 1 proton and 2 neutrons and is called tritium. These three varieties differ only in the number of neutrons in the nucleus (Fig. 2-3). Such forms of an element, having the same charge but different atomic weights, are called **isotopes.**

Figure 2-2

Two lightest atoms. Since first shell closest to atomic nucleus can hold only 2 electrons, helium shell is closed so that helium is chemically inactive.

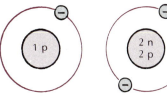

Hydrogen
Atomic number 1
Mass number 1

Helium
Atomic number 2
Mass number 4

Hydrogen 1

Deuterium
Hydrogen 2

Tritium
Hydrogen 3

Figure 2-3

Three isotopes of hydrogen. Of the three isotopes, hydrogen 1 makes up about 99.98% of all hydrogen, and deuterium (heavy hydrogen) makes up about 0.02%. Tritium is radioactive and is found only in traces in water. Numbers indicate approximate atomic weights. Most elements are mixtures of isotopes. Some elements (for example, tin) have as many as 10 isotopes.

Carbon

Oxygen

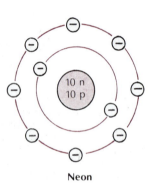

Neon

Figure 2-4

Electron shells of three common atoms. Since no atom can have more than 8 electrons in its outermost shell and 2 electrons in its innermost shell, neon is chemically inactive. However, the second shells of carbon and oxygen, with 4 and 6 electrons, respectively, are open so that these elements are electronically unstable and react chemically whenever appropriate atoms come into contact. Chemical properties of atoms are determined by their outermost electron shells.

Radioactive isotopes

Although most of the naturally occurring elements are stable, all elements have at least one radioactive isotope. These isotopes undergo spontaneous disintegration, with the emission of one or more of three types of particles, or rays: **gamma rays** (a form of electromagnetic radiation), **beta rays** (electrons), and **alpha rays** (positively charged helium nuclei stripped of their electrons). Most of the isotopes of greatest use in biological tracer studies are beta and gamma emitters. Virtually all are prepared synthetically in nuclear reactors and cyclotrons. Among the commonly used radioisotopes are carbon 14 ($^{14}_{6}C$), tritium ($^{3}_{1}H$), and phosphorus 32 ($^{32}_{15}P$). Using radioisotopes, biologists are able to trace movements of elements and tagged compounds through organisms. Our present understanding of metabolic pathways in animals and plants is in large part the result of this powerful analytical tool. Radioisotopes are also used to great advantage in the diagnosis of disease in humans, such as cancer of the thyroid gland.

Electron "shells" of atoms

According to Niels Bohr's planetary model of the atom, the electrons revolve around the nucleus of an atom in circular orbits of precise energy and size. All of the orbits of any one energy and size comprise an electron shell. This simplified picture of the atom has been greatly modified by recent experimental evidence; definite electron pathways are no longer hypothesized, and an electron shell is more vaguely understood as a thick region of space around the nucleus rather than a narrow shell of a particular radius out in space.

According to the quantum theory, the electrons surrounding the nucleus exist at discrete energy levels, called quantum levels. (This theory replaces the older idea that electrons revolve around the nucleus along definite paths or orbits, within definite, thin, spatial shells, and instead treats the location of electrons more vaguely.) A quantum level represents a discrete energy value. These energies, and hence the energies of electrons in these quantum levels, increase as the distance from the nucleus increases. The lowest quantum level corresponds to the lowest energy allowed for the electrons and the closest distance from the nucleus; it corresponds to the innermost shell of the atom. Higher quantum levels correspond to higher shells in the atom. Electrons tend to move as close to the nucleus as possible. However, there is a physical maximum to the number of electrons that can occupy each quantum level. Thus, as the inner level becomes filled, additional electrons are forced into more distant quantum levels. These outer electrons are more excited and have a higher energy content.

Although the picture of the atom described by the quantum theory provides a much better basis for understanding the atom, the old planetary model with the idea of electronic shells is useful in interpreting chemical phenomena. The number of concentric shells required to contain an element's electrons varies with the element. Each shell can hold a maximum number of electrons. The first shell next to the atomic nucleus can hold a maximum of 2 electrons, and the second shell can hold 8; other shells also have a maximum number, but no atom can have more than 8 electrons in its outermost shell. Inner shells are filled first, and if there are not enough electrons to fill all the shells, the outer shell is left incomplete. Hydrogen has 1 proton in its nucleus and 1 electron in its single orbit but no neutron. Since its shell can hold 2 electrons, it has an incomplete shell. Helium has 2 electrons in its single shell, and its nucleus is made up of 2 protons and 2 neutrons.

Since the 2-electron arrangement in helium's shell is the maximum number for this shell, the shell is closed and precludes all chemical activity. There is no known compound of helium. Neon is another inert (chemically inactive) gas because its outer shell contains 8 electrons, the maximum number (Fig. 2-4). However, stable compounds of xenon (an inert gas) with fluorine and oxygen are formed under special conditions. Oxygen has an atomic number of 8. Its 8 electrons are arranged with 2 in the first shell and 6 in the second shell (Fig. 2-4). It is active chemically, forming compounds with almost all elements except inert gases.

____ Molecules and Chemical Bonds

A molecule is a combination of 2 or more atoms joined by chemical bonds. A molecule may be composed of just one element, such as molecules of oxygen (O_2) and of hydrogen (H_2), or of different elements, such as carbon dioxide (CO_2) and methane (CH_4). The chemical bond joining 2 atoms in a molecule contains stored potential energy that is released when the bond is broken and is reestablished between atoms during chemical reactions. All chemical bonds involve the sharing of electrons by 2 atoms.

Ions and oxidation states

Elements react in such a way as to gain a stable configuration of electrons in their outer shells. The number of electrons in the outer shell varies from 0 to 8. With either 0 or 8 in this shell, the element is chemically inactive. When there are fewer than 8 electrons in the outer shell, the atom will tend to lose or gain electrons to have an outer shell of 8, which will result in a charged ion. Atoms with 1 to 3 electrons in the outer shell tend to lose them to other atoms and to become positively charged ions because of the excess protons in the nucleus. Atoms with 5 to 7 electrons in the outer orbit tend to gain electrons from other atoms and to become negatively charged ions because of the greater number of electrons than protons. Positive and negative ions tend to unite.

Every atom has a tendency to complete its outer shell to increase its stability in the presence of other atoms. Let us examine how 2 atoms with incomplete outer shells, sodium and chloride, can interact to fill their outer shells. Sodium, with 11 electrons, has 2 electrons in its first shell, 8 in its second shell, and only 1 in the third shell. The third shell is highly incomplete; if this third-shell electron were lost, the second shell would be the outermost shell and would produce a stable atom. Chlorine, with 17 electrons, has 2 in the first shell, 8 in the second, and 7 in the incomplete third shell. Chlorine must gain an electron to fill the outer shell and become a stable atom. Clearly, the transfer of the third-shell sodium electron to the incomplete chlorine third shell would yield simultaneous stability to both atoms.

Sodium, now with 11 protons but only 10 electrons, becomes electropositive (Na^+). In gaining an electron from sodium, chlorine contains 18 electrons but only 17 protons and thus becomes an electronegative chloride ion (Cl^-). Since unlike charges attract, a strong electrostatic force, called an **ionic bond** (Fig. 2-5), is formed. The ionic compound formed, sodium chloride, can be represented in electron dot notation ("fly-speck formulas") as:

$$Na\bullet + \bullet\overset{\bullet\bullet}{\underset{\bullet\bullet}{Cl}}\bullet \rightarrow Na^+ + (\overset{\bullet\bullet}{\underset{\bullet\bullet}{\bullet Cl \bullet}})^-$$

Figure 2-5

Ionic bond. When 1 atom of sodium and 1 of chlorine react to form a molecule, a single electron in the outer shell of sodium is transferred to the outer shell of chlorine. This causes the outer or second shell (third shell is empty) of sodium to have 8 electrons and also chlorine to have 8 electrons in its outer or third shell. The compound thus formed is sodium chloride (NaCl). By losing 1 electron, sodium becomes a positive ion, and by gaining 1 electron, chlorine (chloride) becomes a negative ion. This ionic bond is the strong electrostatic force acting between positively and negatively charged ions.

The number of dots shows the number of electrons present in the outer shell of the atom: 7 in the case of the neutral chlorine atom and 8 for the chloride ion; 1 in the case of the neutral sodium atom and none for the sodium ion.

Processes that involve the **loss of electrons** are called **oxidation** reactions; those that involve the **gain of electrons** are **reduction** reactions. Since oxidation and reduction always occur simultaneously, each of these processes is really a "half-reaction." The entire reaction is called an **oxidation-reduction** reaction, or simply a **redox** reaction. The terminology is confusing because oxidation-reduction reactions involve electron transfers, rather than (necessarily) any reaction with oxygen. However, it is easier to learn the system than to try to change accepted usage.

We now need to introduce the concept of **oxidation number.** This term refers to the charge an atom would have if the bonding electrons were arbitrarily assigned to the more electronegative of two interacting elements. For example, in the sodium chloride reaction, we consider that the bonding electron has been transferred to the chlorine atom. Consequently, sodium, having lost its electron, becomes electropositive and is said to have an oxidation number of $+1$. Chlorine, with its newly acquired electron, becomes electronegative and takes an oxidation number of -1. Some elements always exist in compounds in the same oxidation number. For example, oxygen in compounds almost always has an oxidation number of -2; sodium, $+1$; magnesium, $+2$; potassium, $+1$; and calcium, $+2$. However, most metals have two or more oxidation numbers. For example, iron may exist as $+2$ or $+3$, chromium as $+3$ or $+6$, and manganese as $+2$, $+4$, or $+7$. Other elements, such as hydrogen, can take either positive or negative oxidation numbers, depending on the character of the other element involved in the bonding.

Covalent bonds

Stability can also be achieved when 2 atoms share electrons. Let us again consider the chlorine atom, which, as we have seen, has an incomplete 7-electron outer shell. Stability is attained by gaining an electron. One way this can be done is for 2 chlorine atoms to *share* one pair of electrons (Fig. 2-6). To do this, the 2 chlorine atoms must *overlap* their third shells so that the electrons in these shells can now spread themselves over both atoms, thereby completing the filling of both shells. Many other elements can form covalent (or electron-pair) bonds. Examples are hydrogen (H_2)

$$H\bullet + H\bullet \rightarrow H \colon H$$

and oxygen (O_2)

$$\ddot{O} \colon + \colon \ddot{O} \rightarrow \ddot{O} \colon\colon \ddot{O}$$

In this case oxygen (which in compounds usually has an oxidation number of -2) must share two pairs of electrons to achieve stability. Each atom now has 8 electrons available to its outer shell, the stable number.

Covalent bonds are of great significance to living systems, since the major elements of living matter (carbon, oxygen, nitrogen, hydrogen) almost always share electrons in strong covalent bonds. The stability of these bonds is essential to the integrity of DNA and other macromolecules, which, if easily dissociated, would result in biological disorder.

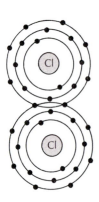

Figure 2-6

Covalent bond. Each chlorine atom has 7 electrons in its outer shell, and by sharing one pair of electrons, each atom acquires a complete outer shell of 8 electrons, thus forming a molecule of chlorine (Cl_2). Such a reaction is called a molecular reaction, and such bonds are called covalent bonds.

Carbon, which usually has an oxidation number of either $+4$ or -4 (its outer shell contains 4 electrons), is endowed with great potential for forming a variety of atomic configurations with itself and other molecules. It can, for example, share its electrons with hydrogen to form methane:

$$\cdot \overset{\displaystyle \cdot}{\underset{\displaystyle \cdot}{C}} \cdot + \; 4\,H\cdot \;\rightarrow\; H\overset{\displaystyle H}{\underset{\displaystyle H}{:\!\overset{\displaystyle \cdot\cdot}{\underset{\displaystyle \cdot\cdot}{C}}\!:}}H$$

Carbon now achieves stability with 8 electrons, and each hydrogen atom becomes stable with 2 electrons. Carbon can also bond with itself (and hydrogen) to form, for example, ethane:

$$H\overset{H\;\;H}{\underset{H\;\;H}{:\!C\!:\!C\!:}}H \quad \text{or} \quad H-\overset{\displaystyle H\;\;\;\;H}{\underset{\displaystyle H\;\;\;\;H}{C-C}}-H$$

Carbon also forms covalent bonds with oxygen:

$$\cdot \overset{\displaystyle \cdot}{\underset{\displaystyle \cdot}{C}}\cdot + \; 2\;\overset{\displaystyle \cdot\cdot}{\underset{\displaystyle \cdot\cdot}{O}}: \;\rightarrow\; \overset{\displaystyle \cdot\cdot}{\underset{\displaystyle \cdot\cdot}{O}}::C::\overset{\displaystyle \cdot\cdot}{\underset{\displaystyle \cdot\cdot}{O}}$$

This is a "double-bond" configuration usually written as $O{=}C{=}O$. Carbon can even form triple bonds as, for example, in acetylene:

$$H:C:::C:H \quad \text{or} \quad H-C{\equiv}C-H$$

The significant aspect of each of these molecules is that each carbon gains a share in 4 electrons from atoms nearby, thus attaining the stability of 8 electrons. The sharing may occur between carbon and other elements or other carbon atoms, and in many instances the 8-electron stability is achieved by means of multiple bonds.

These examples only begin to illustrate the amazing versatility of carbon. It is a part of virtually all compounds comprising living substance, and without carbon, life as we know it would not exist.

_____ Acids, Bases, and Salts

The hydrogen ion (H^+) is one of the most important ions in living organisms. The hydrogen atom contains a single electron. When this electron is completely transferred to another atom (not just shared with another atom as in the covalent bonds with carbon), only the hydrogen nucleus with its positive proton remains. Any molecule that dissociates in solution and gives rise to a hydrogen ion is an **acid**. An acid is classified as strong or weak, depending on the extent to which the acid molecule is dissociated in solution. Examples of strong acids that dissociate completely in water are hydrochloric acid ($HCl \rightarrow H^+ + Cl^-$) and nitric acid ($HNO_3 \rightarrow H^+ + NO_3^-$). Weak acids, such as carbonic acid ($H_2CO_3 \rightleftharpoons H^+ + HCO_3^-$), dissociate only slightly. A solution of carbonic acid is mostly undissociated carbonic acid molecules with only a small number of bicarbonate (HCO_3^-) and hydrogen ions (H^+) present.

A **base** contains negative ions called hydroxide ions and may be defined as a molecule or ion that will accept a proton (hydrogen ion). Bases are produced when compounds containing them are dissolved in water. Sodium hydroxide (NaOH) is a strong base because it will dissociate completely in water into sodium (Na^+) and hydroxide (OH^-) ions. Among the characteristics of bases is their ability to combine with hydrogen ions, thus decreasing their concentration. Like acids, bases vary in the extent to which they dissociate in aqueous solutions into hydroxide ions.

A **salt** is a compound resulting from the chemical interaction of an acid and a base. Common salt, sodium chloride (NaCl), is formed by the interaction of hydrochloric acid (HCl) and sodium hydroxide (NaOH). In water the HCl is dissociated into H^+ and Cl^- ions. The hydrogen and hydroxide ions combine to form water (H_2O), and the sodium and chloride ions remain as a dissolved form of salt (Na^+Cl^-):

$$H^+Cl^- + Na^+OH^- \rightarrow Na^+Cl^- + H_2O$$

     Acid   Base   Salt

Organic acids are usually characterized by having in their molecule the carboxyl group (—COOH). They are weak acids because a relatively small proportion of the H^+ reversibly dissociates from the carboxyl:

$$R{-}C{=}O \quad \rightleftharpoons \quad R{-}C{=}O \atop \ \ \ \ \ \ \ O^- \quad + H^+$$

R refers to an atomic grouping unique to the molecule. Some common organic acids are acetic, citric, formic, lactic, and oxalic. Many more of these will be encountered later in discussions of cellular metabolism.

Hydrogen ion concentration (pH)

Solutions are classified as acid, basic, or neutral according to the proportion of hydrogen (H^+) and hydroxide (OH^-) ions they possess. In acid solutions there is an excess of hydrogen ions; in alkaline, or basic, solutions the hydroxide ion is more common; and in neutral solutions both hydrogen and hydroxide ions are present in equal numbers.

To express the acidity or alkalinity of a substance, a logarithmic scale, a type of mathematical shorthand, is employed that uses the numbers 1 to 14. This is the pH, defined as:

$$pH = \log_{10} \frac{1}{[H^+]}$$

or

$$pH = -\log_{10}[H^+]$$

Thus, pH is the negative logarithm of the hydrogen ion concentration. In other words, when the hydrogen ion concentration is expressed exponentially, pH is the exponent, but with the *opposite* sign; if $H^+ = 10^{-2}$, then $pH = -(-2) = +2$. Unfortunately, pH can be a confusing concept because, as the H^+ decreases, the pH increases. Numbers below 7 indicate an acid range and numbers above 7 indicate alkalinity. The number 7 indicates neutrality, that is, the presence of equal numbers of H^+ and OH^- ions. According to this logarithmic scale, a pH of 3 is 10 times more acid than one of 4; a pH of 9 is 10 times more alkaline than one of 8.

In living systems pH plays an important role, for, in general, deviations from the normal usually result in severe damage. Most substances and fluids in the body are close to the point of neutrality, that is, pH of around 7. Blood, for instance, has a pH of about 7.35 in most terrestrial vertebrates, or just slightly on the alkaline side. Lymph is slightly more alkaline than blood. Saliva has a pH of 6.8, on the acid side. Gastric juice is the most acid substance in the body, about pH 1.6. The regulation of the pH in the body tissue fluids involves many physiological mechanisms; one of the most important is the buffer action of certain salts.

Buffer action

The hydrogen ion concentration in the extracellular fluids must be regulated so that metabolic reactions within the cell will not be adversely affected by a constantly changing hydrogen ion concentration, to which they are extremely sensitive. A change in pH of only 0.2 from the normal blood pH of about 7.35 can cause serious metabolic disturbances. To maintain pH within physiological limits, there are certain substances in cells and organisms that tend to compensate for any change in the pH when acids or alkalies are produced in metabolic reactions or are added to the body fluids. These are called **buffers.** A buffer is a mixture of slightly ionized weak acid and its completely ionized salt. In such a system, added H^+ combines with the anion of the salt to form undissociated acid, and added OH^- combines with H^+ to form water. The most important buffers in blood and other body fluids are the bicarbonates and phosphates. The bicarbonate buffer system consists of carbonic acid (H_2CO_3, a weak acid) and its salt, sodium bicarbonate ($NaHCO_3$). Sodium bicarbonate is strongly ionized into sodium ions (Na^+) and bicarbonate ions (HCO_3^-). When a strong acid (for example, HCl) is added to the fluid, the H^+ ions of the dissociated acid will react with the bicarbonate ion (HCO_3^-) to form a very weak acid, carbonic acid, which dissociates only slightly. Thus the H^+ ions from the HCl are removed and the pH is little altered. When a strong base (for example, NaOH) is added to the fluid, the OH^- ions of the strong base will react with the carbonic acid by removing H^+ ions from the H_2CO_3, to form water and bicarbonate ions. Again the H^+ ion concentration in solution is little altered and the pH remains nearly unchanged.

The cytoplasm within cells must also be buffered because CO_2 (which behaves as an acid when dissolved in water) and organic acid radicals, all end products of metabolic reactions, constantly appear and tend to increase the acidity of intracellular fluids. The pH is prevented from dropping too low, however, by organic buffers, especially amino acids and proteins, which can take up the H^+ and become undissociated weak acids.

——— Mixtures and Their Properties

Whenever masses of different kinds are thrown together, the result is called a mixture. All the different states of matter (solids, liquids, gases) may be involved in these mixtures. The mixtures we are mainly interested in here are those in which water or other fluid is one of the states of matter. When something is mixed with a liquid, any one of three kinds of mixtures is formed.

Molecular solutions

If crystals of salts or sugars are added to water, the molecules (or ions in the case of salts) are uniformly dispersed through the water, forming a **true solution.** Such solutions are transparent. In such a case the water is the **solvent** and the dissolved salt or sugar the **solute.** The freezing point of solutions is lower and the boiling point is higher than those of pure water.

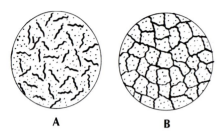

Figure 2-7

Sol and gel. **A,** Sol condition in which gelatin particles are the discontinuous phase and water the continuous phase. **B,** Gel condition in which gelatin particles form continuous phase (network), enclosing water as discontinuous phase.

Suspensions

If solids added to water remain in masses larger than molecules, the mixture is a suspension. Muddy water is a good example. When allowed to stand, the particles in suspension finally settle out to the bottom. Suspensions have a turbid appearance and have the same boiling and freezing points as pure water.

Colloidal solutions

Whenever the dispersed particles are intermediate in size between the molecular state and the suspension, a third mixture—the colloidal solution—is the result. The colloidal state is a condition in which one substance, such as a protein or other macromolecule, is dispersed in another substance to form many small phases suspended in one continuous phase. Thus, every colloid system consists of two phases: a discontinuous, or dispersed, phase and a continuous, or dispersion, phase (Fig. 2-7). Colloidal systems are common not only in living systems but in materials we encounter in our daily lives, as the following examples illustrate:

Colloidal system	Example
Solid dispersed in a liquid	Ink
Liquid dispersed in a liquid	Emulsions, such as cream
Liquid dispersed in a solid	Jellies, gelatin
Gas dispersed in a solid	Floating soap
Gas dispersed in a liquid	Foam, carbonated water
Liquid dispersed in a gas	Fog, clouds
Solid dispersed in a gas	Smoke, fine dust

Proteins are stable colloids because, first, they are charged ions in solution that repel each other, and second, each protein molecule attracts water molecules around it in definite layers. Immediately adjacent to the protein the water is closely oriented in a highly structured manner. This is referred to as "bound" water. Farther from the protein surface, the water molecules gradually lose their order, becoming completely random in the suspending fluid itself. Each protein molecule therefore becomes a much enlarged colloid particle as a result of surface forces that orient water in a regular structured form around it. The water forms the continuous phase of this colloidal system, as well as contributing to the discontinuous phase of hydrated protein particles. In fact, the protein more or less binds itself to the solvent, forming a rigid, stable system. Since the living cell is filled with proteins and other biopolymers, most of the cellular water becomes definitely oriented and structured by the presence of these colloids. This is an important characteristic that provides structure to the aqueous medium of the cell in which all metabolic activities proceed.

Many, although not all, colloidal systems show phase reversal. For example, when gelatin is poured into hot water, the gelatin particles (discontinuous phase) are dispersed through the water (continuous phase) in a thin consistency (Fig. 2-7). Such a condition is called a **sol.** When the solution cools, the gelatin becomes the continuous phase and the water is in the discontinuous phase. Moreover, the solution has stiffened and become semisolid and is called a **gel.** Heating the solution will cause it to become a sol again, and the phases are reversed.

Some proteins also exist in sol and gel states. The sol state is the normal fluid state of cellular proteins. The gel state occurs when proteins form numerous stronger linkages between molecules, producing a meshwork of intertwining fibers. The proteins then become the continuous phase that entraps water. The gelation of heated egg albumin and the formation of a blood fibrin clot in shed blood are examples of permanent phase reversals of protein caused by slight changes in their properties. Reversible gelation has been observed in the living cell and is believed to accompany several physiological processes in normal cellular activity.

Thus, colloids play important roles in the structure of cells by helping to preserve cell shape and providing stability to the cellular medium, by their tendency to hold water and resist desiccation, and by their capacity to show phase reversal in important physiological activities.

CHEMISTRY OF LIFE
Fitness of Earth for Life

In his classic book *Fitness of the Environment* (1913), the biochemist L.J. Henderson maintained that earth possesses "the best of all possible environments for life." Although we no longer maintain, as was once believed, that only the earth in all the universe harbors life, we do believe that only planets very similar to earth will have the special conditions that permit the evolution of life. Why is the earth so fit for life?

The earth is large enough to have a surface density that permits molecules to collect and align properly. As a colloid, material in cells is in an intermediate state between conditions too solid to allow change and conditions too fluid or gaseous to permit molecular organization. The earth's gravity is strong enough to hold an extensive gaseous atmosphere but not so strong that more than a trace of free hydrogen remains.

The temperature on earth is suitable for life, that is, within the range of $-50°$ to $+100°$ C. This is a narrow range of tolerance for life in a universe in which temperatures extend over millions of degrees. Above $100°$ C, life as we know it is impossible because biopolymers based on carbon and water would be rapidly hydrolyzed. Temperatures much below the freezing point prevent the growth of organisms by slowing chemical processes. Nevertheless, some bacteria and algae survive in and around hot springs at temperatures approaching $90°$ C. At the other extreme, many organisms flourish in the Arctic and Antarctic, where air temperatures may drop below $-70°$ C. Thus, life on earth presses against the limits imposed by the thermal requirements for life processes based on protoplasm.

There are other characteristics of the earth that make it an especially fit environment for life as we know it. The earth contains a suitable array of major and minor elements in the right proportions for the synthesis of organic compounds. And, finally, earth contains an abundance of water.

Water and Life

The evolution of complex biochemical systems based on carbon depended on the presence of water. Without water, life could not have evolved on earth, no matter how suitable the earth's environment might have been in other respects. Fanciful systems of life based on ammonia and silicates rather than on water and carbon have been suggested, but such speculations are totally hypothetical and in any case would require environmental conditions vastly different from those on earth.

Water is the most abundant of all compounds in cells, making up about 60% to 90% of most living organisms. The maintenance of a constant aqueous internal environment is a major physiological task for all organisms, both terrestrial and aquatic.

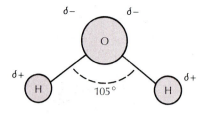

Figure 2-8

Molecular structure of water. The 2 hydrogen atoms bonded covalently to an oxygen atom are arranged at an angle of about 105 degrees. Since the electrical charge is not symmetrical, the molecule is polar with positively charged and negatively charged ends.

Water has several extraordinary properties that make it especially fit for its essential role in living systems. It is the most stable yet versatile of all solvents. Water is the only substance that occurs in nature in the three phases of solid, liquid, and vapor within the ordinary range of earth's temperatures. Water has a **high specific heat capacity:** 1 calorie is required to elevate the temperature of 1 g of water 1° C (such as from 15° to 16° C). Every other liquid but ammonia requires less heat to accomplish the same temperature increase. Water has twice the specific heat capacity of alcohol or oil, four times the specific heat capacity of aluminum, and 10 times the specific heat capacity of iron. Thus, the high thermal capacity of water has a great moderating effect on environmental temperature changes and is a great protective agent for all life.

Water also has a **high heat of vaporization.** More than 500 calories is required to change 1 g of liquid water into water vapor. This is twice as much heat as is required to vaporize methyl alcohol. For terrestrial animals (and plants), cooling produced by the evaporation of water is an important means of getting rid of excess heat.

Another important property of water from a biological standpoint is its **unique density behavior** during changes of temperature. Most liquids become denser with decreasing temperature. Water, however, reaches its maximum density at 4° C *while still a liquid,* and then becomes less dense with further cooling. Therefore ice *floats* rather than forming on the bottom of lakes and ponds. If it were not for this property, bodies of water would freeze solid from the bottom up in winter, and, except in warmer climates, would not necessarily completely melt in summer. Under these conditions, aquatic life would be severely limited.

Water has a **high surface tension,** greater than that of any other liquid but mercury. This property, caused by the great cohesiveness of water molecules, is important in the maintenance of protoplasmic form and movement. It also creates a unique ecological niche for insect forms, such as water striders and water boatmen, that skate on the surfaces of ponds. Despite its high surface tension, water has **low viscosity,** a property that favors the movement of blood through minute capillaries and of cytoplasm inside cellular boundaries.

From what we have said, clearly it is the stability of water that makes it such a fine medium for life. Actually, water's great resistance to changes in state is surprising because water is composed of oxygen and hydrogen, two of the most reactive elements known. We now know that the remarkable properties of water can be explained in large part on the basis of its structure. Water is a hydride of oxygen. The water molecule is shaped like an isosceles triangle: the legs of the triangle are two O—H bonds that subtend an angle of approximately 105 degrees (Fig. 2-8).

The water molecule is electrically neutral because it has an equal number of protons and electrons. However, the oxygen is so strongly electronegative that it tends to draw electrons away from the hydrogen nuclei. Consequently, each of the hydrogen atoms carries a net charge that is slightly positive ($\delta+$), and the oxygen atom carries a net charge that is slightly negative ($\delta-$) and twice as great as the hydrogen net charge. Thus, the water molecule is a permanent dipole with zones of negative and positive charge. Some sharing of the bonding pairs of electrons continues between the hydrogen and oxygen nuclei. Therefore these charges are not complete ionic charges (+ and −), but rather partial charges ($\delta+$ and $\delta-$) with the charge on each oxygen atom twice as great as that on each hydrogen atom.

In ice, water molecules tend to orient themselves so that the positively charged zone of one molecule faces the negatively charged zone of another. Each oxygen atom therefore becomes the center of a tetrahedron of other oxygen atoms (Fig. 2-9). The kind of linkage indicated in the diagram by a dashed line is a hydrogen bond. Although it is much weaker than the O—H bonds within each water molecule, it nevertheless requires substantial energy for breakage (approximately 5 kcal/mole). Hydrogen bonds are of great importance in the chemistry of life because they serve as atomic bridges that participate in the formation of macromolecules, especially proteins.

The tetrahedral arrays of water molecules in ice form an extensive, open, crystal-like network held together by hydrogen bonds. When ice melts, about 15% of the hydrogen bonds break, but in its usual liquid state, water is still thought to possess a fair degree of order. In fact, water molecules are more densely packed together in liquid water than in ice, and this is why ice floats rather than sinking to the bottom.

Hydrogen bonds give water most of its special properties. The attraction of water molecules to each other through hydrogen bonds is responsible for the high surface tension of water. The high specific heat capacity of water is a consequence of attractive forces between hydrogen bonds. When water is heated, much of the heat energy is used to rupture some of the hydrogen bonds, leaving a relatively small amount of heat to increase the kinetic energy (molecular movement), and thus the temperature, of the water. Similarly, the heat of vaporization of water is high because all of the hydrogen bonds between a water molecule and its neighbors must be ruptured before water can escape the surface and enter the air.

Finally, water is an excellent **solvent** for the ions of salts, which are so important to life processes. Salts dissolve to a much greater degree in water than they do in any other solvent. This results from the dipolar nature of water, which causes it to orient itself around charged particles dissolved in it. When, for example, NaCl is dissolved in water, the Na^+ and Cl^- ions present in the solid salt rapidly separate into independent Na^+ and Cl^- ions. The negative zones of the water dipoles align themselves around the Na^+ ions while the positive zones align themselves around the Cl^- ions. This keeps the ions separated, promoting a high degree of dissociation. Other solvents having less or no dipolar character are less able to align effectively around such ions and are therefore less able to dissolve the salt.

Water and life are part and parcel of each other. The special conditions on earth resulting from its ideal size, element composition, and nearly circular orbit at a perfect distance from a long-lived star, the sun, made possible the accumulation of water on the earth's surface. It is difficult even to imagine the origin of life without water.

_____ Chemical Elements of Life

Of the 92 naturally occurring elements, perhaps 46 are found in living substance. Twenty-four of these are considered essential for life, while others are present only because they exist in the environment with which the organism interacts. Of the 24 essential elements, six play especially important roles in living systems. These major elements, shown in red in Fig. 2-10, are carbon (C), hydrogen (H), nitrogen (N), oxygen (O), phosphorus (P), and sulfur (S). Most organic molecules are built with these six elements. Another five essential elements, found in less abundance in living systems and shown in light red in Fig. 2-10, are calcium (Ca), potassium (K), sodium (Na), chlorine (Cl), and magnesium (Mg). Several other elements, called trace elements, are found in minute amounts in animals and plants but are

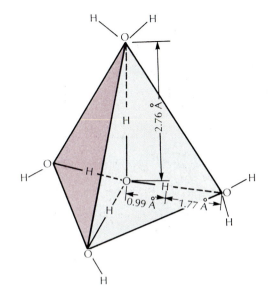

Figure 2-9

Geometry of water molecules. Each water molecule is linked by hydrogen bonds (*dashed lines*) to 4 other water molecules. If imaginary lines are used to connect the divergent oxygen atoms, a tetrahedron is obtained. In ice, the individual tetrahedrons associate to form an open lattice structure.

1 H 1.01																	2 He 4.00
3 Li 6.94	4 Be 9.01											5 B 10.8	6 C 12.0	7 N 14.0	8 O 16.0	9 F 19.0	10 Ne 20.2
11 Na 23.0	12 Mg 24.3											13 Al 27.0	14 Si 28.1	15 P 31.0	16 S 32.1	17 Cl 35.5	18 Ar 39.9
19 K 39.1	20 Ca 40.1	21 Sc 45.0	22 Ti 47.9	23 V 50.9	24 Cr 52.0	25 Mn 54.9	26 Fe 55.8	27 Co 58.9	28 Ni 58.7	29 Cu 63.5	30 Zn 65.4	31 Ga 69.7	32 Ge 72.6	33 As 74.9	34 Se 79.0	35 Br 79.9	36 Kr 83.8
37 Rb 85.5	38 Sr 87.6	39 Y 88.9	40 Zr 91.2	41 Nb 92.9	42 Mo 95.9	43 Tc 99	44 Ru 101.	45 Rh 103.	46 Pd 106.	47 Ag 108.	48 Cd 112.	49 In 115.	50 Sn 119.	51 Sb 122.	52 Te 128.	53 I 127.	54 Xe 131.
55 Cs 133.	56 Ba 137.	57 La 139.	72 Hf 178.	73 Ta 181.	74 W 184.	75 Re 186.	76 Os 190.	77 Ir 192.	78 Pt 195.	79 Au 197.	80 Hg 201.	81 Tl 204.	82 Pb 207.	83 Bi 209.	84 Po 210.	85 At 210.	86 Rn 222.
87 Fr 223.	88 Ra 226.	89 Ac 227.															

58 Ce 140.	59 Pr 141.	60 Nd 144.	61 Pm (147)	62 Sm 150.	63 Eu 152.	64 Gd 157.	65 Tb 159.	66 Dy 162.	67 Ho 165.	68 Er 167.	69 Tm 169.	70 Yb 173.	71 Lu 175.
90 Th 232.	91 Pa 231.	92 U 238.	93 Np 237.	94 Pu 242.	95 Am 243.	96 Cm 247.	97 Bk 247.	98 Cf 251.	99 Es 254.	100 Fm 253.	101 Md 256.	102 No 254.	103 Lr 257.

Figure 2-10

Periodic table of elements showing those essential to life. Six major elements in living systems are set in bright red; five essential minor elements are set in light red. Fifteen trace elements essential to life are set in boldface black. Other elements, notably aluminum, antimony, mercury, cadmium, lead, silver, and gold, are usually present in living systems in trace amounts but are not dietary essentials. The mass number is shown above, and the approximate atomic weight below, each element.

A curious period of mental disturbance in the brilliant career of Sir Isaac Newton, lasting about a year, has long puzzled historians. Now two researchers report that samples of Newton's hair, obtained from keepers of Newtonian relics, contained abnormally high concentrations of mercury and other heavy metals. Newton's symptoms suggest that he suffered from mercury poisoning. During this period Newton was immersed in alchemy, was constantly exposed to metals that he heated to volatile form, and had the habit of tasting the products of his experiments. He recovered from his madness, but his scientific genius never again equaled that of his prealchemy years.

nevertheless indispensable for life. These are manganese (Mn), iron (Fe), iodine (I), molybdenum (Mo), cobalt (Co), zinc (Zn), arsenic (As), selenium (Se), copper (Cu), chromium (Cr), tin (Sn), vanadium (V), silicon (Si), nickel (Ni), and fluorine (F). They are shown in black boldface type in Fig. 2-10.

Most trace elements are necessary components of enzyme systems. Some trace elements are also important constituents of organic compounds, such as the iron of hemoglobin and myoglobin. Iodine, the heaviest essential trace element, is a vital part of the thyroid hormones, thyroxine and triiodothyronine. Silicon is essential for normal bone calcification and probably also plays some functional role in connective tissue. The discovery of necessary trace elements requires ingenious and elaborate dietary studies to determine whether or not a particular element promotes growth or prevents deficiency diseases in test animals. In some cases the functional role of essential trace elements has yet to be defined.

Many elements are extremely toxic to life, even in small amounts. The most dangerous appear to be certain metals that are normally present in trace quantities in the environment but that may be concentrated by industrial activities. Trace pollutants of beryllium, nickel, and chromium have been linked with cancer, antimony and lead with heart disease, and cadmium and tungsten with enzyme impairment, leading to reduced life expectancy.

Mercury is being found with increasing frequency in both fresh and salt waters. Mercury from paper mills, which until recently used phenyl mercuric acetate as a fungicide to prevent cellulose rot, and from spillage and leakage from factories engaged in chlorine formation, settles to the bottom of freshwater streams, where it is converted by bacteria into soluble and highly toxic metalloorganic compounds. The half-life of these mercuric compounds in fish (which obtain it from the water and from invertebrate food organisms) may be as much as 1000 days. (The half-life is the time required for half of the material in a sample to disappear.) In humans who eat the fish, the half-life is only about 70 days.

Contamination from industrial lead, mainly from automobile exhaust but also from smelting, coal burning, and food in lead-soldered cans, appears to have occurred everywhere on earth. The amount of lead in the bones of an average American is about 500 times greater than the natural concentrations in the bones of Peruvians who lived in an unpolluted environment 1800 years ago (Settle and

Patterson, 1980). Lead levels today are thought to be high enough to cause subtle disturbances in biochemical systems. However, the harmful effects of lead are not exclusively a problem of our technological society. Poisoning from lead salts was known among the ancient Romans, who preferred lead utensils and drank water conducted through lead pipes. It has even been suggested (on rather thin evidence) that lead poisoning may account for the decline of Rome's ruling dynastic families.

It is not yet known just how our chemical milieu affects the structure of the animal body, or how necessary certain elements found in the body may be. Since living matter has come from the same elements that are found on this planet, it is evident that the composition of the earth restricts what elements go into the composition of the organism. But evolution has been very selective in choosing certain elements as the building blocks of life. Their interactions pose many problems about which little is known.

Chemical Complexity of Living Matter

The basis of biological activities is chemical reactions. These reactions involve chemical elements that are found in all organisms as well as in the nonliving world. Life must have had its beginning in combinations and reactions of chemicals. At first, only a small number of combinations and reactions were necessary for the initiation of life. As time went on, more complex substances or compounds with successively higher levels of organization and reactions appeared. Despite the incredible complexity of living matter, all biological phenomena operate according to the physical laws of chemistry and physics (Principle 1, p. 11).

Analysis of typical living matter reveals that it is composed of about 60% to 90% water (higher animals are usually about 60% to 70% water), 15% protein, 10% to 15% fats and other lipids, 1% carbohydrates, and 5% inorganic ions of various kinds (Na^+; K^+, Cl^-, $SO_4^=$, and others) (Fig. 2-11).

Many different categories of biomolecules are found in every cell of the organism. Most of them are dissolved or suspended in cellular water, in either ionized or nonionized form. Some organic substances (molecules containing carbon) form a part of the hard substances (horn, claws, hoofs, keratin, and others) of the body. Besides being in the cells and tissues of the body, organic components are also found in the environment, especially that of aquatic animals. Surprisingly, lake water may contain a far higher organic content than does ocean water. Some organic substances found in water are organic phosphorus and organic nitrogen compounds, amino acids, carotenoid substances, and vitamins.

Inorganic matter actually outweighs the organic part of living matter. The inorganic portion includes (1) water; (2) mineral solids consisting of crystals, secreted precipitates, bone, and shells; and (3) cellular minerals, either free or combined with organic compounds. Most of the cellular minerals are in the form of ions (H^+, Ca^{++}, Na^+, Mg^{++}, OH^-, $CO_3^=$, HCO_3^-, $PO_4^=$, Cl^-, and $SO_4^=$). Animals get these constituents from the water in which the minerals are dissolved from rocks and the soil.

Organic Molecules

The term "organic compounds" has been applied to substances derived from plants and animals. All organic compounds contain carbon, but many also contain hydrogen, oxygen, nitrogen, sulfur, phosphorus, salts, and other elements.

Figure 2-11

Relative composition of major constituents of cells of higher animals.

Organic compounds specifically are those carbon compounds in which the principal bonds are carbon-to-carbon and carbon-to-hydrogen.

Carbon with its valence of 4 has a great ability to bond with other carbon atoms in chains of varying lengths and configurations. More than a million organic compounds have been identified; more are being added daily. Carbon-to-carbon combinations introduce the possibility of enormous complexity and variety into molecular structure. A carbon chain can combine with hydrogen to form an **aliphatic** compound such as heptane or a ring structure (**aromatic** compound) such as benzene. Some other types of configurations are rings and chains joined to each other, multiple branches of chains, and helix arrangements. The diversity of carbon molecules has made possible the complex kinds of macromolecules that form the essence of life.

Heptane

Benzene

Carbohydrates: nature's most abundant organic substance

Carbohydrates are compounds of carbon, hydrogen, and oxygen. They are usually present in the ratio of 1 C:2 H:1 O and are grouped as H—C—OH. Familiar examples of carbohydrates are sugars, starches, and cellulose (the woody structure of plants). There is more cellulose on earth than all other organic materials combined. Carbohydrates are made synthetically from water and carbon dioxide by green plants, with the aid of the sun's energy. This process, called **photosynthesis,** is a reaction on which all life depends, for it is the starting point in the formation of food.

Carbohydrates are usually divided into the following three classes: (1) **monosaccharides,** or simple sugars; (2) **disaccharides,** or double sugars; and (3) **polysaccharides,** or complex sugars. Simple sugars are composed of carbon chains containing 4 carbons (tetroses), 5 carbons (pentoses), or 6 carbons (hexoses). Other simple sugars have up to 10 carbons, but these are not biologically important. Simple sugars, such as glucose, galactose, and fructose, all contain a free sugar group,

in which the double-bonded O may be attached to the terminal C of a chain (an aldehyde) or to a nonterminal C (a ketone). The hexose **glucose** (also called dextrose) is the most important carbohydrate in the living world. Glucose is often shown as a straight-chain aldehyde (Fig. 2-12, *A*), but in water it tends to form a cyclic compound (Fig. 2-12, *B*). This formula shows the ring structure of glucose, but it is misleading because it obscures the three-dimensional form of the mole-

Figure 2-12

Two ways of depicting the structural formula of the simple sugar glucose. In **A** the carbon atoms are shown in open-chain form. When dissolved in water, glucose tends to assume a ring form as in **B**. In this ring model the carbon atoms located at each turn in the ring are usually not shown.

cule. Rather than lying in a flat plane, the glucose molecule is "puckered" because the 4 atoms bonded to any single carbon molecule occupy the corners of a regular tetrahedron, four-cornered, pyramid-like figure. To better represent the structure of glucose than in the flat-plane ring structure, organic chemists have devised a "chair" model to show the configuration of glucose and other hexose molecules (Fig. 2-13). Although the three-dimensional chair conformation is the most accurate way to represent the simple sugars, we must remember that all forms of glucose, however represented, are the same molecule.

Other hexoses of biological significance are galactose and fructose. Their straight-chain structures are compared with that of glucose in Fig. 2-14.

Disaccharides are double sugars formed by the bonding of two simple sugars. An example is maltose (malt sugar), composed of 2 glucose molecules. As shown in Fig. 2-15, ==the 2 glucose molecules are condensed together by the removal of a molecule of water. This dehydration reaction, with the sharing of an oxygen atom by the two sugars, characterizes the formation of all disaccharides.== Two other common disaccharides are sucrose (ordinary cane, or table, sugar), formed by the linkage of glucose and fructose, and lactose (milk sugar), comprised of glucose and galactose.

Polysaccharides are made up of many molecules of simple sugars (usually glucose) linked together in long chains and are referred to by the chemist as polymers. Their empirical formula is usually written $(C_6H_{10}O_5)_n$, where n stands for the unknown number of simple sugar molecules of which they are composed.

Glucose

Galactose

Fructose

Figure 2-14

These three hexoses are the most common monosaccharides. Glucose and galactose are aldehyde sugars; fructose is a ketone sugar.

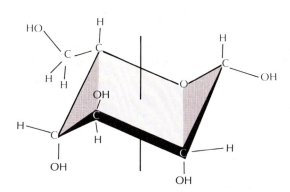

Figure 2-13

"Chair" representation of glucose molecule.

Maltose

Figure 2-15

Formation of a double sugar (disaccharide maltose) from 2 glucose molecules with the removal of 1 molecule of water.

←— α-1,6 linkage

α-1,4 linkages

Figure 2-16

Glycogen is a large, branched polysaccharide with a treelike structure. It is composed of linear chains of glucose molecules joined together by α-1,4 and α-1,6 linkages. A section of a glucose chain is shown enlarged at left.

Starch is the common storage form of sugar in most plants and is an important food constituent for animals. Glycogen (Fig. 2-16), or animal starch, is an important storage form for sugar in animals. It is found mainly in liver and muscle cells in vertebrates. When needed, glycogen is converted into glucose and is delivered by the blood to the tissues. Another polymer is cellulose, which is the principal structural carbohydrate of plants. It forms the fibrous part of the cell walls of plants (Fig. 2-17). Humans cannot digest cellulose, but some other animals, such as the herbivores, with the aid of bacteria, and termites, with the aid of flagellates (Fig. 8-11, p. 183), can do so.

The main role of carbohydrates in protoplasm is to serve as a source of chemical energy. Glucose is the most important of these energy carbohydrates. Some carbohydrates become basic components of protoplasmic structure, such as the pentoses that form constituent groups of nucleic acids and of nucleotides.

Lipids: fuel storage and building material

Lipids are fats and fatlike substances. They are composed of molecules of low polarity; consequently, they are virtually insoluble in water but are soluble in organic solvents such as acetone and ether. Three principal groups of lipids are neutral fats, phospholipids, and steroids.

Neutral fats

The neutral or "true" fats are the major fuels of animals. The average American man at age 25 contains 7.7 kg (17 pounds) of stored fat; women have even more: 10 kg (22 pounds). This represents approximately 40 days of stored fuel. Obese individuals may carry enough fat to supply the equivalent of a year of normal metabolism. Many species make much better use of this stored fat than do humans. When Atlantic salmon enter fresh water, they stop feeding and may remain active for as long as a year, utilizing stored fat exclusively.

Most fat in higher vertebrates is stored as adipose tissue, which accumulates especially under the skin and in the abdominal cavity. In fishes, lipids are stored principally in the liver and between the fibers of skeletal muscle. Stored fats represent food ingested in excess of the amount required to meet ongoing metabolic demands. Stored fat may be derived directly from dietary fat or indirectly from

Figure 2-17

Cellulose, the structural carbohydrate of plants and the most abundant of all organic compounds. Cellulose differs chemically from glycogen in two important ways. It lacks molecular branching and, as shown in **A,** the glucose molecules are joined together by β-1,4 linkages alternating with α-1,4 linkages. Glycogen and starch are composed entirely of α-1,4 linkages. **B,** Cellulose consists of bundles of long straight chains held together by hydrogen bonds between OH groups in neighboring chains.

Stearic acid   **Glycerol**   **Stearin**
(3 mol)   **(1 mol)**   **(1 mol)**

Figure 2-18

Neutral fats. **A,** Formation of a neutral fat from 3 molecules of stearic acid (a fatty acid) and glycerol. **B,** A neutral fat bearing three different fatty acids.

$$CH_3-(CH_2)_7-CH=CH-(CH_2)_7-COOH$$
Oleic acid

$$CH_3-(CH_2)_4-CH=CH-CH_2-CH=CH-(CH_2)_7-COOH$$
Linoleic acid

Figure 2-19

Unsaturated fatty acids: oleic acid having one double bond and linoleic acid having two double bonds. The remainder of the hydrocarbon chains of both acids is saturated.

dietary carbohydrates (especially glucose) that are converted to fat for storage. Fats are oxidized and released into the bloodstream as needed to meet tissue demands, especially for muscles.

Neutral fats are triglycerides, which are molecules consisting of glycerol and 3 molecules of fatty acids. Neutral fats are therefore esters, that is, a combination of an alcohol (glycerol) and an acid. Fatty acids in triglycerides are simply long-chain monocarboxylic acids; they vary in size but are commonly 14 to 24 carbons long. The production of a typical fat by the union of glycerol and stearic acid is shown in Fig. 2-18, *A.* In this reaction it can be seen that the 3 fatty acid molecules have united with the OH group of the glycerol to form stearin (a neutral fat), with the production of 3 molecules of water.

Most triglycerides contain two or three different fatty acids attached to glycerol, bearing ponderous names such as myristoyl palmitoyl stearoyl glycerol (Fig. 2-18, *B*). The fatty acids in this triglyceride are **saturated;** that is, every carbon within the chain holds 2 hydrogen atoms. Saturated fats, more common in animals than in plants, are usually solid at room temperature. **Unsaturated** fatty acids, typical of plant oils, have 2 or more carbon atoms joined by double bonds; that is, the carbons are not "saturated" with hydrogen atoms and are able to form additional bonds with other atoms. Two common unsaturated fatty acids are oleic acid and linoleic acid (Fig. 2-19). Plant fats such as peanut oil and corn oil tend to be liquid at room temperature.

CH₃
⊕|
H₃C—N—CH₃ **Choline group**
|
CH₂
|
CH₂
|
O   H
| |
O⁼.P—O—CH₂—C—CH₂—O
⊖:| | \
O   O   C=O
| /
O=C   H₂C
\   /
CH₂   CH₂
/   \
H₂C   H₂C
\   /
CH₂   CH₂
/   \
H₂C   H₂C
\   /
CH₂   CH₂
/   \
H₂C   H₂C   H
\   \   /
Palmitoyl CH₂   C **Oleoyl**
group H₂C   ‖ **group**
\   C
CH₂ / \
/ H₂C   H
H₂C
\
CH₂   CH₂
/   H₂C
H₂C   \
\   CH₂
CH₂   H₂C
/   \
H₂C   CH₂
\   H₂C
CH₃   \
H₂C   CH₂
\
CH₃

Figure 2-20

Lecithin (phosphatidyl choline), an important phospholipid of nerve membranes.

Phospholipids

Unlike the fats that are fuels and serve no structural roles in the cell, phospholipids are important components of the molecular organization of tissues, especially membranes. They resemble triglycerides in structure, except that one of the three fatty acids is replaced by phosphoric acid and an organic base. An example is lecithin, an important phospholipid of nerve membrane (Fig. 2-20).

Although phospholipids are related structurally to fats, they differ from them in one important respect: the phosphate group is charged and polar and therefore soluble in water. Since the remainder of the molecule is nonpolar, phospholipids can bridge two environments and serve to bind water-soluble molecules such as proteins to water-insoluble materials. In membranes, phospholipids tend to align themselves into bilayers with the insoluble fatty acid chains oriented toward the center of the "sandwich" and the polar phosphate groups directed toward the outer aqueous phases. The significance of this configuration is discussed in Chapter 5.

Steroids

Steroids are complex alcohols, structurally unlike fats but having fatlike properties. The steroids are a large group of biologically important molecules, including cholesterol (Fig. 2-21), vitamin D, many adrenocortical hormones, and the sex hormones.

Proteins: foundation substance of living matter

Proteins are large, complex molecules characterized by a high nitrogen content. They are the predominant type of macromolecule in cells, constituting more than 50% of the cell's dry weight.

Proteins serve as the chief structural material of protoplasm and play numerous other essential roles in living systems. They form enzymes: globular proteins specialized to serve as catalysts in virtually all biochemical activities of cells. Other proteins are antibodies, transport proteins, storage proteins, contractile proteins, and some hormones. In every living organism there are thousands of different proteins, each fitted to perform a specific functional or structural role.

A typical protein is composed of perhaps 200 amino acids arranged into a long, chainlike molecule. However, there is great variation in protein size, ranging from small proteins consisting of approximately 50 amino acids to complex enzymes containing more than 20,000 amino acids divided among several distinct chains.

Each of the numerous amino acids in a protein molecule could be any one of 20 different kinds of amino acids that commonly occur in living organisms (Fig. 2-22). There are many other amino acids in nature—more than 170 different amino acids are known to occur (usually rarely) in various animal and plant tissues—but only the standard 20 are coded in the cell's genes (Principle 18, p. 16). The remaining amino acids, when they occur, are derivatives produced by chemical modification of the standard 20 after the protein is synthesized.

Because the 20 amino acids may be arranged in all possible combinations, the number of different amino acid sequences even in the smallest proteins is incomprehensibly vast. Since proteins determine the biochemical uniqueness of each living organism, there is obviously no practical limit to biological variation. Yet proteins are anything but the products of random shuffling of amino acid building blocks. The sequence of amino acids in every protein is precisely deter-

Cholesterol

Figure 2-21

Cholesterol, a steroid. All steroids have a basic skeleton of four rings (three 6-carbon rings and one 5-carbon ring) with various side groups attached.

Glycine

Cysteine

Glutamine

Alanine

Methionine

Phenylalanine

Valine

Lysine

Tyrosine

Leucine

Arginine

Tryptophan

Isoleucine

Aspartic acid

Histidine

Serine

Asparagine

Proline

Threonine

Glutamic acid

Figure 2-22

The 20 naturally occurring amino acids.

Figure 2-23

Peptide bond is a covalent bond formed between the carboxyl carbon atom of one amino acid and the amino nitrogen atom of another amino acid, with the elimination of water.

Amino group Carboxyl group Amino group Carboxyl group Peptide bond

Figure 2-24

Polypeptide composed of five amino acids.

Terminal amino group   Terminal carboxyl group

Glycine Tyrosine Alanine Valine Tryptophan

mined by the genetic code in the cell's genes. Even a single alteration in the sequence may destroy its function.

Each of the 20 amino acids contains one amino group ($-NH_2$) and one carboxyl group ($-COOH$) attached to the same carbon atom. The remainder of the molecule is unique for each amino acid. The general formula for an amino acid is as follows:

The symbol R represents a "side group" unique for each acid. The amino acids range in complexity from glycine with a simple hydrogen atom as its side group to tryptophan with a complex aromatic ring side group.

In forming polypeptide chains, amino acids are linked by peptide bonds. In the formation of a peptide bond, the carboxyl group of one amino acid is linked by a covalent bond to the amino group of another, with the elimination of water (Fig. 2-23). The combination of two amino acids by a peptide bond forms a dipeptide, and, as is evident, there is still a free amino group on one and a free carboxyl group on the other. Addition of a third amino acid forms a tripeptide, and, by sequential addition of more amino acids, long **polypeptide** chains are built.

The polypeptide shown in Fig. 2-24 consists of five different amino acids linked by peptide bonds. When the chain exceeds about 50 amino acids, the molecule is called a **protein** rather than a polypeptide. Thus proteins are built up of a backbone involving the amino and carboxyl groups. The various side groups and the folding of the peptide chains determine the properties of the protein.

For convenience, biochemists have recognized four levels of protein organization: primary, secondary, tertiary, and quaternary. The **primary** structure of a protein is determined by the kind and sequence of amino acids making up the polypeptide chain. Because the bonds between the amino acids in the chain have a limited number of stable angles, the chain assumes certain recurrent structural patterns. This is called the **secondary** structure, and it is often that of an **alpha helix,** that is, helical turns in a clockwise direction like a screw (Fig. 2-25). The spirals of the chains are stabilized by weak **hydrogen bonds,** usually between a hydrogen atom of one amino acid and the peptide-bond oxygen of another amino acid in an adjacent turn of the helix. Hydrogen bonds provide definite spacing to the helix: there is 1 amino acid every 0.15 nm along the axis, and there is an average of 3.6 amino acids per turn. The properties of the alpha helix were worked out largely by Linus Pauling.

Not only does the polypeptide chain (primary structure) spiral into helical configurations (secondary structure), but also the helices themselves bend and fold, giving the protein its complex, yet stable, three-dimensional **tertiary** structure (Fig. 2-26). The folded chains are stabilized by the interactions between side groups of amino acids. The strongest of these interactions is the **disulfide bond,** a covalent bond between the sulfur atoms of pairs of cysteine (sis'tee-in) molecules that are brought together by folds in the polypeptide chain. Other kinds of bonds that help to stabilize the tertiary structure of proteins are hydrogen bonds, ionic (electrostatic) bonds, and hydrophobic bonds, in which nonpolar groups tend to be squeezed together by the surrounding water.

The term **quaternary** structure describes proteins that contain more than one polypeptide chain unit. For example, hemoglobin of higher vertebrates is composed of four polypeptide subunits nested together into a single protein molecule. Tertiary and quaternary structures of proteins are very important for the function of the proteins, for example, activity as enzymes (see the following discussion).

The complete structures of many proteins have now been thoroughly worked out. This has proved to be a monumental task, for not only must the correct amino acid sequence be determined, but also the complete three-dimensional configuration, that is, the exact way the polypeptide chains are folded and bonded together. Insulin, the pancreatic hormone that governs glucose metabolism, was the first protein to have its amino acid sequence determined. Insulin is a small protein (molecular weight 5700), consisting of two polypeptide chains containing 51 amino acids. The amino acid sequence was worked out by Frederick Sanger and his colleagues at Cambridge University in 1953. Sanger could not determine the three-dimensional configuration of insulin by the laborious techniques available at that time. By using x-ray crystallography and electron spin resonance (ESR) studies, subsequent workers have constructed what are believed to be fairly accurate pictures of the shape of many native proteins.

Figure 2-25

Alpha-helix pattern of a polypeptide chain. Hydrogen bonds *(dashed lines)* stabilize adjacent turns of the helix. *R,* Amino acid side chains.

Modified from Green, D. 1956. Currents of biochemical research. New York, Interscience Publishers, Inc.

Figure 2-26

Three-dimensional tertiary structure of the protein myoglobin. Adjacent folds of the polypeptide chain are held together by disulfide bonds that form between pairs of cysteine molecules. In the upper center of the molecule is the heme group, which combines with oxygen.

From Neurath, H. 1964. The proteins, vol. 2, ed. 2. New York, Academic Press, Inc.

Proteins as enzymes: the central role of enzymes in life

The life process involves thousands of chemical reactions occurring within cells. However, the chemical breakdown of large molecules and the release of energy by cellular activities would not proceed at any meaningful rate without catalysts. As every chemist knows, catalysts are chemical substances that accelerate reaction rates without affecting the products of the reaction and without being altered or destroyed as a result of the reaction. A catalyst cannot make an energetically impossible reaction happen; it simply accelerates a reaction that would proceed at a very slow rate in its absence.

Enzymes are the catalysts of the living world. Most of an animal's genome that has evolved over the ages codes for enzymes that control every aspect of life (Principle 20, p. 17). The literally thousands of different enzymes in an average cell regulate the release of energy used in respiration and promote the synthesis of materials for growth and for replacement of losses resulting from structural wear and tear. They are required for muscle contraction, determine molecular movement across membranes, and are involved in mental activities. Other enzymes accelerate the digestion and absorption of food. Enzymes bring order to the intricacy of life activities.

Nature of enzymes

Enzymes are complex molecules varying in size from small, simple proteins with a molecular weight of 10,000 to highly complex molecules with molecular weights up to 1 million. Many enzymes are pure proteins—delicately folded and interlinked chains of amino acids. Other enzymes require the participation of small nonprotein groups called **cofactors** to perform their enzymatic function. In some cases these cofactors are metallic ions (such as ions of iron, copper, zinc, magnesium, potassium, and calcium) that form a functional part of the enzyme. Examples are carbonic anhydrase, which contains zinc; the cytochromes, which contain iron; and troponin (a muscle contraction enzyme), which contains calcium. Another class of cofactors, called **coenzymes,** is organic. All coenzymes contain groups derived from vitamins, compounds that must be supplied in the diet. All of the B complex vitamins are coenzyme compounds. Since animals have lost the ability to synthesize the vitamin components of coenzymes, it is obvious that a vitamin deficiency can be serious. However, unlike dietary fuels and nutrients that must be replaced, once burned or assembled into structural materials, vitamins are recovered in their original form and used repeatedly. Examples of enzymes that contain vitamins are nicotinamide adenine dinucleotide (NAD), which contains nicotinic acid; coenzyme A, which contains pantothenic acid; and flavin adenine dinucleotide (FAD), which contains riboflavin. Other examples of the enzymatic roles of vitamins are given on pp. 755 and 756.

Action of enzymes

An enzyme functions by combining in a highly specific way with its **substrate,** the molecule on which it acts. The classical concept of this interaction, proposed by Emil Fisher in 1884, is that the enzyme contains an active site having a unique molecular configuration. This configuration, according to the hypothesis, is exactly complementary to at least a portion of the substrate molecule, which fits into it much as a key fits into a lock. The enzyme provides a unique chemical environment that increases the probability of a chemical reaction at specific sites on the substrate. The special catalytic talent of an enzyme resides in its power to reduce

How can biochemists be certain that an enzyme-substrate (ES) complex exists? The original evidence offered by Leonor Michaelis in 1913 is that, when the substrate concentration is increased while the enzyme concentration is held constant, the reaction rate reaches a maximum velocity (Fig. 2-28). This *saturation effect* is interpreted to mean that all catalytic sites become filled at high substrate concentration. It is not seen in uncatalyzed reactions. Other evidence includes the observation that the ES complex displays unique spectroscopic characteristics not displayed by either the enzyme or the substrate alone. Furthermore, some ES complexes can be isolated in pure form, and at least one kind (nucleic acids and their polymerase enzymes) has been directly visualized with the electron microscope.

Figure 2-27

Energy changes during enzyme catalysis of a substrate. The overall reaction proceeds with a net release of energy. In the absence of an enzyme, substrate is stable because of the large amount of activation energy needed to disrupt strong chemical bonds. The enzyme reduces the energy barrier by forming a chemical intermediate with a much lower internal energy state.

Figure 2-28

Effect of substrate concentration on the velocity of an enzyme-catalyzed reaction.

the high internal energy barrier through which substrate molecules must pass to be transformed into products. In effect, an enzyme steers the reaction through one or more intermediate steps, each of which requires much less activation energy than that required for a single-step reaction (Fig. 2-27). The enzyme combines with its substrate to form a precisely aligned **enzyme-substrate complex** in which the substrate is secured by covalent bonds to several points in the active site of the enzyme. The substrate is split, and its products are liberated from the enzyme, which is restored to its active form.

Emil Fisher's lock-and-key metaphor has proved to be a useful way of looking at enzyme-substrate interaction (Fig. 2-29, *A*). However, according to the contemporary view first suggested by D.E. Koshland (1973), the active site of the enzyme may be a flexible surface that enfolds, and conforms to, the substrate, rather than a fixed and nonyielding template, as the lock-and-key model held (Fig. 2-29, *B*). This newer **conformational hypothesis** has not altered a firmly held principle of enzyme action: the enzyme and substrate must combine so that active groups on the enzyme come into precise alignment with reactive sites on the substrate. Only then can the substrate be altered chemically. The necessity for correct alignment explains the high specificity of enzymes.

Enzymes that engage in important main-line sequences—such as the crucial energy-providing reactions of the cell that go on constantly—seem to operate in enzyme sets rather than in isolation. For example, the conversion of glucose to

Figure 2-29

Interaction of substrate and enzyme. **A,** Lock-and-key model. The enzyme's active site is exactly complementary in shape to that of the substrate. **B,** Conformational model. The enzyme changes shape when it binds the substrate, becoming complementary in shape only after the substrate is bound.

Figure 2-30

High specificity of trypsin. It splits only peptide bonds adjacent to lysine or arginine.

carbon dioxide and water proceeds through 19 reactions, each requiring a specific enzyme. Main-line enzymes are found in relatively high concentrations in the cell, and they may implement quite complex and highly integrated enzymatic sequences. One enzyme carries out one step, then passes the product to another enzyme that catalyzes another step, and so on. The reactions may be said to be coupled.

Specificity of enzymes

One of the most distinctive attributes of enzymes is their high specificity. This is a consequence of the exact molecular fit that is required between enzyme and substrate. Furthermore, an enzyme catalyzes only one reaction; unlike reactions carried out in the organic chemist's laboratory, no side reactions or by-products result. Specificity of both substrate and reaction is obviously essential to prevent a cell from being overwhelmed with useless by-products.

However, there is some variation in degree of specificity. Some enzymes catalyze the oxidation (dehydrogenation) of only one substrate; for example, succinic dehydrogenase catalyzes the oxidation of succinic acid only. Others, such as the proteolytic enzymes (for example, pepsin and trypsin), act only on certain bonds within the substrate molecule. Trypsin is quite specific in splitting peptide bonds on the carboxyl side of lysine and arginine only (Fig. 2-30). But since trypsin is undiscriminating about the shape and chemistry of the rest of the substrate, it can catalyze the breakdown of many different protein substrates having the trypsin-specific peptide bonds. Usually an enzyme will take on one substrate molecule at a time, catalyze its chemical change, release the product, and then repeat the process with another substrate molecule. The enzyme may repeat this process billions of times until it is finally worn out (after a few hours to several years) and is broken down by scavenger enzymes in the cell. Some enzymes are able to undergo successive catalytic cycles at dizzying speeds of up to a million cycles per minute, but most operate at slower rates.

Enzyme-catalyzed reactions

Enzyme-catalyzed reactions are theoretically reversible. This is signified by the double arrows between substrate and products. For example:

$$\text{Fumaric acid} + H_2O \rightleftharpoons \text{Malic acid}$$

However, for various reasons the reactions catalyzed by most enzymes tend to go only in one direction. For example, the proteolytic enzyme pepsin can degrade proteins into amino acids, but it cannot accelerate the rebuilding of amino acids into any significant amount of protein. The same is true of most enzymes that catalyze the hydrolysis of large molecules such as nucleic acids, polysaccharides, lipids, and proteins. There is usually one set of reactions and enzymes that break them down, but they must be resynthesized by a different set of reactions that are catalyzed by different enzymes. This apparent irreversibility exists because the chemical equilibrium usually favors the formation of the smaller degradation products.

The net **direction** of any chemical reaction is dependent on the relative energy contents of the substances involved. If there is little change in the chemical bond energy of the substrate and the products, the reaction is more easily reversible. However, if large quantities of energy are released as the reaction proceeds in one direction, more energy must be provided in some way to drive the reaction in the reverse direction. Thus, many if not most enzyme-catalyzed reactions are in practice irreversible unless the reaction is coupled to another that makes energy available. In the cell both reversible and irreversible reactions are combined in complex ways to make possible both synthesis and degradation.

Sensitivity of enzymes

Enzyme activity is sensitive to temperature and pH. As a general rule, enzymes work faster with increasing temperature, but only within certain limits. Moreover, this increase in velocity is not proportional to the rise in temperature. Usually the rate is doubled with each 10° C rise, but a change from 20° to 30° C has a greater effect than one from 30° to 40° C. The optimum temperature for enzymes of endothermic animals is about body temperature. Above 40° to 50° C most enzymes become unstable and may be inactivated altogether because the enzyme is denatured, or cooked.

Each enzyme usually works best within a certain range of acidity or alkalinity. Pepsin of the acid gastric juice is most active at about pH 1.8; trypsin of the alkaline pancreatic juice is most active at about pH 8.2. Most cellular enzymes work best when the pH is around neutral. In strong acid or alkaline solutions, most enzymes irreversibly lose their catalytic power.

Nucleic acids: genetic apparatus of the cell nucleus

Nucleic acids are complex substances of high molecular weight that represent a basic manifestation of life. The genetic information necessary for all aspects of biological inheritance is encoded in the sequence of these polymeric molecules (Principles 17 and 18, p. 16). Nucleic acids direct the synthesis of proteins, including all of the enzymes that in turn carry out the numerous routine synthetic and functional activities of the cell. Most important, nucleic acids are the only molecules that have the power (with the help of the right enzymes) to replicate themselves. This is the essential process that guarantees the accuracy of reproduction. To understand how nucleic acids perform these roles, we need to look closely at their chemical structures.

All cells contain two kinds of nucleic acids: deoxyribonucleic acid (DNA), which is the genetic material of the chromosomes of cells, and ribonucleic acid (RNA), which functions in protein synthesis. Both DNA and RNA are polymers built of repeated units called **nucleotides.** Each nucleotide contains three parts: a **sugar,** a **nitrogenous base,** and a **phosphate group.** The sugar is a pentose (5-carbon) sugar; in DNA it is **deoxyribose** and in RNA it is **ribose** (Fig. 2-31).

The nitrogenous bases of nucleotides are of two types: pyrimidines, which consist of a single, 6-membered ring, and purines, which are composed of two fused rings. Both of these types of compounds contain nitrogen as well as carbon in their rings, which is why they are called "nitrogenous" bases. Five bases in all occur in DNA and RNA (Fig. 2-32). The pyrimidines are thymine, cytosine, and

Figure 2-31

Ribose and deoxyribose, the pentose sugars of nucleic acids. A carbon atom lies in each of the four corners of the pentagon (labeled 1 to 4). Ribose has a hydroxyl group (−OH) and a hydrogen on the number 2 carbon; deoxyribose has 2 hydrogens at this position.

Figure 2-32

Purines and pyrimidines of DNA and RNA.

uracil, and the purines are adenine and guanine (Table 2-1). (Other bases are known to occur rarely in DNA and RNA.)

The sugar, phosphate group, and nitrogenous base are linked as shown in the generalized scheme for a nucleotide:

Phosphate   Sugar   Nitrogenous base

In DNA the backbone of the molecule is built of phosphoric acid and deoxyribose sugar; to this backbone are attached the nitrogenous bases (Fig. 2-33). However, one of the most interesting and important discoveries about the nucleic acids is that DNA is not a single polynucleotide chain but rather consists of *two* complementary chains that are precisely cross-linked by specific hydrogen bonding of purine and pyrimidine bases. It was found that the number of adenines is equal to the number of thymines, and the number of guanines equals the number of cytosines. This fact suggested a pairing of bases: adenine with thymine (AT) and guanine with cytosine (GC). The larger adenine (a purine) always attaches to the smaller thymine (a pyrimidine) by two hydrogen bonds, and the larger guanine (a purine) always attaches to the smaller cytosine (a pyrimidine) by three hydrogen bonds:

Thymine—adenine

Cytosine—guanine

Table 2-1 Chemical Components of DNA and RNA

	DNA	RNA
Purines	Adenine	Adenine
	Guanine	Guanine
Pyrimidines	Cytosine	Cytosine
	Thymine	Uracil
Sugar	2-Deoxyribose	Ribose
Phosphate	Phosphoric acid	Phosphoric acid

Figure 2-33

Section of DNA. Polynucleotide chain is built of a backbone of phosphoric acid and deoxyribose sugar molecules. Each sugar holds a nitrogenous base side arm. Shown from top to bottom are adenine, guanine, thymine, and cytosine.

The result is a ladder structure (Fig. 2-34). However, the ladder is twisted into a **double helix**, with about 10 base pairs for each complete turn of the helix (Fig. 2-35).

The determination of the structure of DNA has been widely acclaimed as the single most important biological discovery of this century. It was based on the x-ray diffraction studies of Maurice H.F. Wilkins and the ingenious proposals of Francis H.C. Crick and James D. Watson, published in 1953. Watson, Crick, and Wilkins were later awarded the Nobel Prize in medicine and physiology for their momentous work.

RNA is very similar to DNA in structure except that it consists of a *single* polynucleotide chain. In RNA one of the four bases, thymine (T), is replaced by uracil (U), and the sugar deoxyribose is replaced by ribose. In other respects the single RNA chain is joined together like each of the two DNA chains. RNA functions in the transcription and translation of genetic information (Principle 19, p. 16).

Figure 2-34

Double chain structure of DNA. The uprights of the "ladder" are the sugar-phosphate backbones of each DNA strand, and the connecting rungs are the paired nitrogenous bases, AT or GC.

Figure 2-35

DNA molecule.

After Etkin, W. 1973. BioScience 23:653.

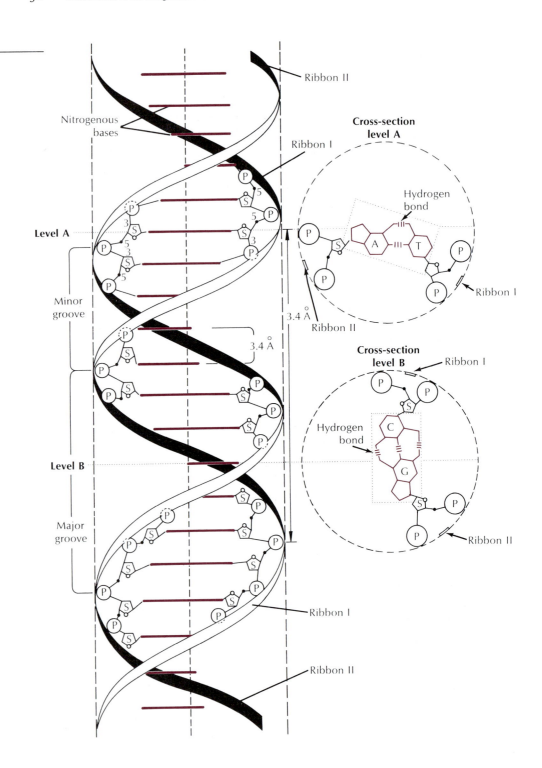

____ Summary

Atoms, the smallest units of chemical elements, consist of a positively charged nucleus of very small volume, surrounded by negatively charged electrons of almost no mass. The nucleus is made up of one or more positively charged protons (the atomic number, determining the chemical nature of the element) and uncharged neutrons. The total number of protons and neutrons is the mass number of the element. There may be more, less, or the same number of neutrons in the nucleus as protons, and these different forms of an element are called isotopes. The number of electrons, however, must equal the number of protons for the atom to have a total charge that is neutral.

According to Niels Bohr's planetary model of atoms, electrons orbit the nucleus at fixed distances, forming electron shells. Although this model remains useful in interpreting chemical phenomena, the newer quantum theory treats electron locations more vaguely as discrete energy levels that increase as electron distance from the nucleus increases. The innermost quantum level, or shell, can hold only 2 electrons, and each outer shell can hold a maximum of 8 electrons. Inner shells are filled first, and atoms tend to complete their shells by gaining or losing electrons or by sharing electrons with other atoms.

Transfers of electrons from one atom to another to increase stability are called oxidation-reduction reactions. The loss of electrons is an oxidation reaction; the gain of electrons is a reduction reaction.

Molecules are formed when 2 or more atoms are joined together by chemical bonds. Such bonds may be ionic bonds when 1 atom takes 1 or more electrons given up by another, or covalent bonds when 2 atoms share electrons. The carbon atom is especially versatile in bonding with itself or with other atoms and is the only element capable of forming the variety of molecules found in living things.

The acidity or alkalinity of solutions is expressed by the pH scale, defined as the negative logarithm of the hydrogen concentration. Buffers are substances that prevent large alterations in pH when acids or bases are introduced.

Colloidal systems, formed when one substance is dispersed within the continuous phase of another, play important roles in cellular activities. Proteins behave as stable colloidal systems.

The unique structure of water and its ability to form hydrogen bonds between adjacent water molecules are responsible for its special properties: solvency for ionic and polar substances; high heat capacity, boiling point, and surface tension; and less density as a solid than as a liquid. Life on earth could not have appeared without water.

Of the 92 naturally occurring elements, 24 are essential for life. Six of these—carbon, hydrogen, nitrogen, oxygen, phosphorus, and sulfur—are major elements, and the remaining 18 are found in small or trace quantities in living systems.

Living matter is composed of water, mineral salts, and organic molecules. Organic compounds are grouped into four main categories: carbohydrates, lipids, proteins, and nucleic acids.

Carbohydrates are composed entirely of carbon, hydrogen, and oxygen grouped as H—C—OH. Sugars serve as immediate sources of energy in living systems. Monosaccharides, or simple sugars, may bond together to form disaccharides or polysaccharides, which serve as storage forms of sugar or perform limited structural roles in cells.

Lipids exist principally as fats, phospholipids, and steroids. Fats stored in adipose tissue may be oxidized when needed to supply the energy demands of tissue. Phospholipids are essential components of membrane structure. Steroids are complex alcohols that form the basic structure of several sex and adrenocortical hormones.

Proteins are large molecules composed of amino acids linked together by peptide bonds. The amino acid chain, or primary structure of the protein, typically coils into a helix to form the secondary protein structure. The helix may itself fold into a stable three-dimensional tertiary structure, strengthened by interactions between amino acids in adjacent coils. Two or more peptide chains may interact to form a protein with quaternary structure. Proteins serve numerous informational, catalytic, and structural roles in living systems.

Enzymes are pure proteins or proteins associated with complex organic groups (coenzymes) that vastly accelerate reaction rates in living systems. An enzyme does this by temporarily binding its reactant (substrate) onto an active site. In this configuration, internal activation energy barriers are lowered enough to disrupt and split the substrate, and the enzyme is restored to its original form.

Nucleic acids are polymers of nucleotide units, each composed of a sugar, a nitrogenous base, and a phosphate group. Deoxyribonucleic acid (DNA) is the genetic material of nuclear chromosomes. Ribonucleic acid (RNA) functions in protein synthesis.

Selected references

Standard biochemistry and cellular biology texts are ideal sources of additional information on the topics in this chapter. The following selection is by no means exhaustive.

Bohinski, R.C. 1979. Modern concepts in biochemistry, ed. 3. Boston, Allyn & Bacon, Inc.

Dowben, R.M. 1969. General physiology. New York, Harper & Row, Publishers, Inc. *Advanced text focusing on physiochemical aspects of biological systems.*

Lehninger, A.L. 1982. Principles of biochemistry. New York, Worth Publishers, Inc. *Clearly presented advanced text.*

McGilvery, R.W. 1975. Biochemistry: a functional approach, ed. 2. Philadelphia, W.B. Saunders Co. *Advanced biomedical approach with fine summaries of general biochemical principles.*

Mertz, W. 1981. The essential trace elements. Science 213:1332-1338. *Effects of deficiencies in humans are described.*

Settle, D.M., and C.C. Patterson. 1980. Lead in albacore: guide to lead pollution in Americans. Science 207:1167-1176.

Sheeler, P., and D.E. Bianchi. 1980. Cell biology: structure, biochemistry, and function. New York, John Wiley & Sons, Inc. *Clear treatment of chemistry of macromolecules.*

Stryer, L. 1981. Biochemistry, ed. 2. San Francisco, W.H. Freeman & Co. Publishers.

Wolfe, S.L. 1981. Biology of the cell, ed. 2. Belmont, Calif., Wadsworth, Inc.

Yost, H.T. 1972. Cellular physiology. Englewood Cliffs, N.J., Prentice-Hall, Inc. *Advanced treatment of molecular physiology and biochemistry.*

Selected *Scientific American* articles

The collection of *Scientific American* readings edited by Hanawalt and Haynes (listed below) is an excellent source of articles on biochemical aspects of cell biology and should be consulted for articles that appeared before 1973. A selection of more recent articles appears here.

Capaldi, R. 1974. A dynamic model of cell membranes. 230:26-33 (Mar.). *Describes the membrane lipid bilayer and associated protein molecules.*

Hanawalt, P.C., and R.H. Haynes (eds.). 1973. The chemical basis of life: readings from *Scientific American.* San Francisco, W.H. Freeman & Co. Publishers.

Perutz, M.F. 1978. Hemoglobin structure and respiratory transport. 239:92-125 (Dec.).

Sharon, N. 1974. Glycoproteins. 230:78-86 (May). *These proteins with linked sugar side chains play several important functional roles.*

Sharon, N. 1980. Carbohydrates. 243:90-116 (Nov.). *Their structure and biological roles.*

Stroud, R.M. 1974. A family of protein-cutting proteins. 231:74-88 (July). *The serine proteases perform diverse functions despite their common descent from a single ancestral enzyme.*

CHAPTER 3

ORIGIN OF LIFE

Budding proteinoid microspheres. These lifeless creations of the prebiotic chemist's laboratory
possess certain properties of living cells: double-layered outer walls,
selective diffusion, and growth by budding.

Electron micrograph by S.W. Fox/Biology Media.

Where did life on earth come from? This is an ancient, intriguing question that we must suppose has aroused human curiosity since the dawn of cultural development. Although the great religions have sought to satisfy this curiosity, they have not provided nor were ever intended to provide a scientific explanation of the detailed sequence of events that culminated in the first appearance of life. To most biologists the question of life's beginnings is one of profound interest. The biologist is struck by the remarkable unity of nature (Principle 3, p. 11). As more concerning the identifiable components of life is learned, an evolutionary pattern in the structure and function of living things can be seen.

All organisms, from humans to the smallest microbes that transcend the rather arbitrary boundary between life and nonlife, share two kinds of basic biomolecules: nucleic acid and protein. As we have seen in the previous chapter, both molecules are large and complex in form. Except in some viruses, DNA is the material of inheritance; it provides the code by which inheritable traits are passed to the next generation of cells or organisms. RNA functions in several ways to translate the genetic code into materials characteristic of the cell. Proteins perform structural functions and, more important, catalyze or facilitate the myriad chemical reactions necessary to life. Yet despite the chemical complexity of these molecules and the diversity of functions they perform, in all organisms they are composed of relatively few main building blocks: 20 amino acids, five bases (adenine, guanine, cytosine, uracil, and thymine), two sugars (ribose and deoxyribose), and phosphate.

The remarkable uniformity of life extends also to cell function. Certain metabolic processes that convert foodstuffs into a usable form of energy consistently occur in a wide range of organisms, from the simplest to the most complex. This example, along with other examples of molecular and functional identity, suggests that all life must have had a common beginning.

Even though we acknowledge the kinship of living things, we must admit at the beginning that we do not know how life on earth originated. Until recently the study of life's origins was not considered worthy of serious speculation by biologists because, it was argued, the absence of a geological record made the course of events resulting in the appearance of life unknowable. This situation has changed.

Since 1950 several laboratories around the world have been devoting fulltime research to origin-of-life studies. It is a multidisciplinary effort that requires the contributions of scientists of several specialties: biologists, chemists, physicists, geologists, and astronomers. From such studies it has been possible to reconstruct a scenario of ancient events in which simple single-celled living organisms evolved more than 3.5 billion years BP (before the present) from inorganic constituents present on the surface of the earth. These studies are not attempts to prove or disprove any religious or philosophical belief, but rather they are endeavors to provide an intellectually satisfying account of how life on earth could have arisen by natural means.

▬ HISTORICAL PERSPECTIVE

People have always been awed and mystified by the question of how life originated on the earth. From ancient times it was commonly believed that life could arise by spontaneous generation from dead material, in addition to arising from parental organisms by reproduction (biogenesis). Frogs appeared to arise from damp earth, mice from putrefied matter, insects from dew, maggots from decaying meat, and so on. Warmth, moisture, sunlight, and even starlight were often mentioned as beneficial factors that encouraged spontaneous generation.

These ideas were developed into an elaborate theory by the Greeks and appeared frequently in the writings of Aristotle (384 to 322 BC). They became firmly entrenched in virtually all cultures, including those of the Far East, and were unquestioningly accepted by even relatively recent great figures such as Copernicus, Bacon, Galileo, Harvey, Descartes, Goethe, and Schelling. Spontaneous generation was also supported by Christian philosophers who pointed out that, according to the first chapter of Genesis, God did not create plants and animals directly but bade the waters to bring them forth.

Inevitably the question of spontaneous generation fell under the scrutiny of experimental science in the sixteenth, seventeenth, and eighteenth centuries. At first such studies were ill-conceived efforts to supplement natural observations of spontaneous generation by artificially producing various organisms in the laboratory.

The first attack on the doctrine of spontaneous generation occurred in 1668 when the Italian physician Francesco Redi exposed meat in jars, some uncovered and some covered with parchment or wire gauze. The meat in all the vessels spoiled, but only the open vessels had maggots, and he noticed that flies were constantly entering and leaving these vessels. He concluded that, if flies had no access to the meat, no worms would be found.

Although Redi's refutation of spontaneous generation became widely known, the doctrine was too firmly entrenched to be abandoned. In 1748 the English Jesuit priest John T. Needham boiled mutton broth and put it in corked containers. After a few days the medium was swarming with microscopic organisms. He concluded that spontaneous generation was real because he believed that he had killed all living organisms by boiling the broth and that he had excluded the access of others by sealing the tubes.

However, an Italian investigator, Abbé Lazzaro Spallanzani (1767), was critical of Needham's experiments and conducted experiments that dealt another blow against the theory of spontaneous generation. He thoroughly boiled extracts of vegetables and meat, placed these extracts in clean vessels, and sealed the necks of the flasks hermetically in flame. He then immersed the sealed flasks in boiling water for several minutes to make sure that all germs were destroyed. As controls, he left some tubes open to the air. At the end of 2 days, he found the open flasks swarming with organisms; the others contained none.

This experiment still did not settle the issue, for the advocates of spontaneous generation maintained either that air, which Spallanzani had excluded, was necessary for the production of new organisms or that the method he used had destroyed the vegetative power of the medium. When oxygen was discovered (1774), the opponents of Spallanzani seized on this as the vital element that he had destroyed in his experiments.

It remained for the great French scientist Louis Pasteur (Fig. 3-1) to silence all but the most stubborn proponents of spontaneous generation with an elegant series of experiments with his famous "swan-neck" flasks. Pasteur (1861) answered the objection to the lack of air by introducing fermentable material into a flask with a long S-shaped neck that was open to the air (Fig. 3-2). The flask and its contents were then boiled for a long time. Afterwards the flask was cooled and left undisturbed. No fermentation occurred because all organisms that entered the

Among the accounts of early efforts to produce organisms spontaneously in the laboratory is a recipe for making mice, given by the Belgian plant nutritionist Jean Baptiste van Helmont (1648). "If you press a piece of underwear soiled with sweat together with some wheat in an open jar, after about 21 days the odor changes and the ferment . . . changes the wheat into mice. But what is most remarkable is that the mice which came out of the wheat and underwear were not small mice, not even miniature adults or aborted mice, but adult mice emerge!"

Figure 3-1

Louis Pasteur, holding in his left hand one of the swan-necked flasks used to demonstrate the absence of spontaneous generation.
Courtesy Parke-Davis.

A

B

Figure 3-2

Louis Pasteur's swan-neck flask experiment. **A,** Sugared yeast water boiled in swan-neck flask remains sterile until neck is broken. **B,** Within 48 hours, flask is swarming with life.

open end were deposited on the floor of the neck and did not reach the flask contents. When the neck of the flask was cut off, the organisms in the air could fall directly on the fermentable mass and fermentation occurred within it in a short time. Pasteur concluded that, if suitable precautions were taken to keep out the germs and their reproductive elements, such as eggs and spores, no fermentation or putrefaction could take place.

Pasteur brought an end to the long and tenacious career of the concept of spontaneous generation. Pasteur's work showed that no living organisms come into existence except as descendants of similar organisms (Principle 9, p. 13). In announcing his results before the French Academy, Pasteur proclaimed, "Never will the doctrine of spontaneous generation arise from this mortal blow." Paradoxically, in showing that spontaneous generation did not occur as previously claimed (production of mice, maggots, frogs, and others), Pasteur also ended for a time further inquiry into the spontaneous origins of life. A lengthy period of philosophical speculation followed, but virtually no experimentation on life's origins was performed for 60 years.

Renewal of Inquiry: Oparin-Haldane Hypothesis

The rebirth of interest in the origins of life occurred in the 1920s. In that decade the Russian biochemist Alexander I. Oparin and the British biologist J.B.S. Haldane independently proposed that life originated on earth after an inconceivably long period of "abiogenic molecular evolution." Rather than arguing that the first living organisms miraculously originated all at once, a notion that had constrained fresh thinking for so long, Oparin and Haldane suggested that the simplest living units (for example, bacteria) came into being very gradually by the progressive assembly of inorganic molecules into more complex organic molecules. These molecules would react with each other to form living microorganisms.

Haldane proposed that the earth's primitive atmosphere consisted of water, carbon dioxide, and ammonia. When such a gas mixture is exposed to ultraviolet radiation, many organic substances such as sugars and amino acids are formed. Ultraviolet light must have been very intense on the primitive earth before the production of oxygen (by photosynthetic organisms), which reacted with ultraviolet rays to form ozone, a 3-atom form of oxygen. Today ozone serves as a protective screen to prevent such intense ultraviolet radiation from reaching the earth's surface. Haldane believed that the early organic molecules could accumulate in the primitive oceans to form a "hot dilute soup." In this primordial broth carbohydrates, fats, proteins, and nucleic acids might have been assembled to form the earliest microorganisms.

Oparin, too, suggested that the earth's primitive atmosphere lacked oxygen and instead contained hydrogen, methane, ammonia, and other reducing compounds. He proposed that the organic compounds required for life were formed spontaneously in such a reducing atmosphere under the influence of sunlight, lightning, and the intense heat of volcanoes.

The Oparin-Haldane hypothesis greatly influenced theoretical speculation on the origins of life during the 1930s and 1940s. Finally in 1953 Stanley Miller, working with Harold Urey in Chicago, made the first successful attempt to simulate with laboratory apparatus the conditions thought to prevail on the primitive earth. This experiment, described in more detail later in the chapter, demonstrated that important biomolecules are formed in surprisingly large amounts when an electrical discharge is passed through a reducing atmosphere of the kind proposed by Oparin. The realization that it was possible to simulate a prebiotic milieu in the laboratory ushered in a new era in origin-of-life studies. It coincided with the dawn of the space age and a new public interest in the question of life's origins.

PRIMITIVE EARTH
Formation of the Solar System

Most astronomers accept the "Big Bang" model, according to which the universe originated from a primeval fireball and has been expanding and cooling since its inception 10 to 20 billion years ago. The sun and the planets are believed to have been formed approximately 4.6 billion years ago out of a spherical cloud of cosmic dust and gases that had some angular momentum. The cloud collapsed under the influence of its own gravity into a rotating disc. As the material in the central part of the disc condensed to form the sun, a substantial amount of gravitational energy was released as radiation. The pressure of this outwardly directed radiation prevented the complete collapse of the nebula into the sun. The material left behind began to cool and eventually gave rise to the planets (Fig. 3-3).

The inner planets (Mercury, Venus, Earth, and Mars) are small and composed mostly of nonvolatile elements because the high temperatures of the cooling planets drove off the volatile elements. The outer planets are composed largely of volatile compounds, such as methane, ammonia, water, hydrogen, and helium, because these materials were blown outward into this region of the collapsing disc by the sun's radiation pressure. In the region occupied by the planets Jupiter and Saturn, massive bodies of hydrogen and helium condensed. The low temperatures and enormous gravitational fields of these bodies prevented their gases from escaping. It is believed that the condensation of the solar system was 95% complete within the relatively short time of 50,000 years.

Figure 3-3

Solar system showing narrow range of conditions suitable for life.

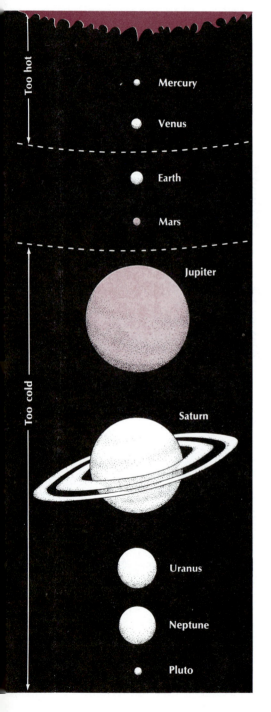

___ Origin of the Earth's Atmosphere

Evolution of the primeval reducing atmosphere

While the earth was condensing, the various atoms were sorted out according to weight. Heavy elements (silicon, aluminum, nickel, and iron) gravitated toward the center, whereas the lighter elements (hydrogen, oxygen, carbon, and nitrogen) remained in the surface gas. Hydrogen and helium, because of their volatility, continued to escape as the earth condensed, and these elements became severely depleted from the primeval atmosphere. Neon and argon were almost completely lost from the atmosphere. Oxygen, nitrogen, and water, which are the major constituents of our present oxidizing atmosphere, could not escape from the earth because they were present in nonvolatile, chemically combined forms trapped in dust particles. Later, as the earth condensed, water, carbon compounds, and nitrogen were released into the atmosphere from the earth's interior by volcanic activity, which was much more extensive then than it is now.

It is generally agreed that the earth's primeval atmosphere contained no more than a trace of oxygen. It was a **reducing atmosphere;** that is, it contained a predominance of molecules having less oxygen than hydrogen. Methane (CH_4) and ammonia (NH_3) are examples of fully reduced compounds. According to one view, such compounds, together with water, composed the early atmosphere of the earth. Carbon dioxide (CO_2), nitrogen (N_2), and traces of hydrogen (H_2) may also have been present. Another view, held chiefly by geochemists, is that the earth's early atmosphere was much like it is today except that it lacked oxygen: an atmosphere chiefly of nitrogen, carbon dioxide, and water vapor. According to this concept, the early atmosphere was only mildly reducing rather than strongly reducing as it would have been were methane and ammonia its principal components.

The character of the primeval atmosphere is very important in any discussion of the origins of life because the organic compounds of which living organisms are made are not stable in an oxidizing atmosphere. Organic compounds are not synthesized nonbiologically in our oxidizing atmosphere today, and they are not stable if they are introduced into it. According to Oparin, life could not have originated without the basic organic building blocks from which the first organisms were assembled. Consequently, modern origin-of-life hypotheses assume that the primeval atmosphere was reducing because the synthesis of compounds of biological importance occurs only under reducing conditions. Geochemical evidence tends to support the belief that the early atmosphere was a reducing one that arose by degassing of the earth's interior.

Appearance of oxygen

As water, nitrogen, and carbon dioxide continued to enter the atmosphere from volcanoes, the atmosphere became saturated with water vapor, and rain began to fall. Small lakes formed, enlarging into oceans. The oceans gradually became salted as rocks weathered. During this early period, which lasted 1.5 billion years, the atmosphere probably was still reducing well after the first living protocells such as algae and bacteria had evolved.

Our atmosphere today is strongly oxidizing. It contains 79% molecular nitrogen, approximately 21% free oxygen, 1% argon, and 0.03% carbon dioxide. Although the time course for its development is much disputed, at some point oxygen began to appear in significant amounts in the atmosphere. In the primitive reducing atmosphere, oxygen was formed by the decomposition of water in either of two ways.

The first is the photolytic action of ultraviolet light from the sun on water in the upper atmosphere.

$$2\ H_2O \xrightarrow{\text{UV light}} 2\ H_2 + O_2$$

The hydrogen produced escapes from the earth's gravitational field, leaving free oxygen to accumulate in the atmosphere. The amount produced by the photodissociation of water is now quite small, although it may have been significant over the immense span of time in which it has occurred.

The second and probably more important source of oxygen is photosynthesis. Almost all oxygen produced at the present time is produced by algae and land plants. Each day the earth's plants combine approximately 400 million tons of carbon with 70 million tons of hydrogen to set free 1.1 billion tons of oxygen. Oceans are a major source of oxygen. Almost all oxygen produced today is consumed by organisms oxidizing their food to carbon dioxide; if this did not occur, the amount of oxygen in the atmosphere would double in approximately 3000 years. Since Precambrian fossil algae resemble modern algae, and since algae today are the greatest producers of oxygen, it seems probable that most of the oxygen in the early atmosphere was produced by photosynthesis.

CHEMICAL EVOLUTION
Sources of Energy

According to the Oparin-Haldane hypothesis, a variety of carbon compounds gradually accumulated on the surface of the earth during a lengthy period of prebiotic chemical evolution. The primitive reducing atmosphere contained simple gaseous compounds of carbon, nitrogen, oxygen, and hydrogen, such as carbon dioxide, molecular nitrogen, water vapor, and perhaps methane and ammonia. These were the starting materials from which organic compounds were made. However, if these gaseous compounds are mixed together in a closed glass system and allowed to stand at room temperature, they never chemically react with each other. To promote a chemical reaction, a continuous source of **free energy** sufficient to overcome reaction-activation barriers must be supplied.

For example, one of the simplest and most important prebiotic chemical reactions is the formation of hydrogen cyanide (HCN) from nitrogen and methane. When an electrical discharge is passed through an atmosphere of nitrogen, some of the molecules absorb enough energy to dissociate into atoms.

$$N_2 \rightarrow 2\ N$$

Dissociated nitrogen atoms are highly reactive. If methane is present in the atmosphere, nitrogen atoms react to form hydrogen cyanide and hydrogen.

$$N + CH_4 \rightarrow HCN + \frac{3}{2}H_2$$

Other sources of energy such as ultraviolet light or heat could equally well cause the formation of hydrogen cyanide from nitrogen and methane. Once formed, hydrogen cyanide dissolves in rain and is carried into lakes and oceans where it and other reactive molecules can form organic compounds.

Table 3-1 Present Sources of Energy Averaged over the Earth

Source	Energy (cal/cm²/year)
Total radiation from sun	260,000
Infrared (above 700 nm)	143,000
Visible (350-700 nm)	113,600
Ultraviolet	
250-350 nm	2837
200-250 nm	522
150-200 nm	39
<150 nm	1.7
Electrical discharges	4
Shock waves	1.1
Radioactivity (to 1 km depth)	0.8
Volcanoes	0.13
Cosmic rays	0.0015

Modified from Miller, S.L., and L.E. Orgel. 1974. The origins of life on the earth. Englewood Cliffs, N.J., Prentice-Hall, Inc.

The sun is by far the most powerful source of free energy for the earth. Each year each square centimeter of the earth receives an average 260,000 calories of radiant energy. The way in which this energy is distributed over the infrared, visible, and ultraviolet regions of the spectrum is shown in Table 3-1. The gases present in the primitive atmosphere would not have absorbed visible or infrared energy. Since the solar energy available falls off rapidly in the ultraviolet region, only approximately 0.2% of the total energy is at wavelengths shorter than 200 nm, where it can be absorbed by molecules such as methane, water, and ammonia. Nevertheless, ultraviolet radiation must have been an important source of energy for photochemical reactions in the primitive atmosphere.

Electrical discharges must have provided another source of energy for chemical evolution. Although the total amount of electrical energy released by lightning is small compared to solar energy, nearly all of the energy of lightning is effective in synthesizing organic compounds in a reducing atmosphere. A single flash of lightning through a reducing atmosphere generates a large amount of organic matter. Thunderstorms may have been one of the most important sources of energy for organic synthesis.

Volcanoes and hot springs were available on the primitive earth as sources of energy, but it is doubtful that they were a major site of prebiotic organic synthesis. Cosmic rays, radioactivity, and sonic energy generated by ocean waves were also available sources of energy, but their contribution cannot be evaluated and was probably small in any case. Of the other sources of energy, only shock waves generated by meteorites passing through the primitive atmosphere may have produced a significant amount of organic matter. Meteorites generate intense temperatures as high as 20,000° C and pressures exceeding 15,000 atmospheres. A large meteorite could generate millions of tons of organic matter in its wake.

Figure 3-4

Dr. S.L. Miller and apparatus used in experiment on the synthesis of amino acids with an electric spark in a strongly reducing atmosphere.
Courtesy S.L. Miller.

Prebiotic Synthesis of Small Organic Molecules

The first steps leading toward life on earth happened when simple organic molecules were generated in the earth's reducing atmosphere by the action of lightning, ultraviolet radiation, and perhaps other kinds of available energy. These simple molecules were washed into lakes and oceans where they formed a "primordial soup." Our understanding of what happened to produce the first reactive organic molecules comes largely from a young branch of chemistry called prebiotic chemistry.

Earlier in this chapter we referred to Stanley Miller's pioneering simulation of primitive earth conditions in the laboratory. Miller built an apparatus designed to circulate a mixture of methane, hydrogen, ammonia, and water past an electric spark (Fig. 3-4). Water in the flask was boiled to produce steam that helped to circulate the gases. The products formed in the electrical discharge (representing lightning) were condensed in the condenser and collected in the U-tube and small flask (representing ocean).

After a week of continuous sparking, the water containing the products was analyzed. The results were surprising. Approximately 15% of the carbon that was originally in the reducing "atmosphere" had been converted into organic compounds that collected in the "ocean." The most striking finding was that many compounds related to life were synthesized. These included four amino acids commonly found in proteins, urea, and several simple fatty acids.

We can appreciate the astonishing nature of this synthesis when we consider that there are thousands of known organic compounds with structures no more complex than those of the amino acids formed. Yet in Miller's synthesis most of the relatively few substances formed were compounds found in living organisms. This was surely no coincidence, and it suggests that prebiotic synthesis on the primitive earth may have occurred under conditions that were not greatly different from those that Miller chose to simulate.

Miller's experiments recently have been criticized by geochemists who believe that the early atmosphere of the earth was quite different from Miller's strongly reducing simulated atmosphere. Nevertheless, Miller's work stimulated many other investigators to repeat and extend his experiment. It was soon found that amino acids could be synthesized in many different kinds of gas mixtures that were heated (volcanic heat), irradiated with ultraviolet light (solar radiation), or subjected to electrical discharge (lightning). All that was required to produce amino acids was that the gas mixture be reducing and that it be subjected violently to some energy source. In recent experiments, electrical discharges have been passed through mixtures of carbon monoxide, nitrogen, and water, yielding amino acids and nitrogenous bases. Although reaction rates were much slower than in atmospheres containing methane and ammonia, and yields were poor in comparison, these experiments support the hypothesis that the chemical beginnings of life can occur in atmospheres that are only mildly reducing. It has also been confirmed that no amino acids can be produced in an atmosphere containing oxygen.

Thus, the experiments of many scientists have shown that highly reactive intermediate molecules such as hydrogen cyanide, formaldehyde, and cyanoacetylene are formed when a reducing mixture of gases is subjected to a violent energy source. These react with water and ammonia or nitrogen to form more complex organic molecules, including amino acids, fatty acids, urea, aldehydes, sugars, purine and pyrimidine bases—indeed all the building blocks required for the synthesis of the most complex organic compounds of living matter.

___ Formation of Polymers
Need for concentration

The next stage in chemical evolution involved the condensation of amino acids, purines, pyrimidines, and sugars to yield larger molecules that resulted in proteins and nucleic acids. Such condensations do not occur easily in dilute solutions because the presence of excess water tends to drive reactions toward decomposition (hydrolysis). Although the primitive ocean has been called a primordial soup, it was probably a rather dilute one containing organic material that was approximately one tenth to one third as concentrated as chicken bouillon.

Prebiotic synthesis must have occurred in restricted regions where concentrations were higher. The primordial soup might have been concentrated by evaporation in lakes, ponds, or tide pools. Dilute aqueous solutions could also have been concentrated effectively by freezing. As ice freezes, organic solutes are concentrated in the solution that separates from the pure ice. This technique is employed to produce applejack from cider in the northern United States and Canada. When a barrel of cider is allowed to freeze, a liquid residue remains that contains most of the alcohol and flavoring materials.

The Oparin-Haldane hypothesis suggests that the primitive ocean was a *warm* primordial soup. However, there is increasing evidence that prebiotic synthesis may have occurred in a cold ocean rather than a warm one. In a cold ocean, not unlike the ocean today with an average temperature of $4°$ C, much of the polar

Figure 3-5

Electron micrograph of proteinoid micro-spheres. These proteinlike bodies can be produced in the laboratory from poly-amino acids and may represent precellular forms. They have definite internal ultrastructure. (×1700.)

Courtesy R.M. Syren and S.W. Fox, Institute of Molecular Evolution, University of Miami, Coral Gables, Fla.

water would be frozen. This would be favorable for prebiotic synthesis for two reasons: (1) freezing of the water would concentrate the organic molecules in the residue, and (2) the low temperatures would slow the spontaneous decomposition of organic compounds and polymers.

Another way prebiotic molecules might have been concentrated is by adsorption on the surface of clay and other minerals. Clay has the capacity to concentrate and condense large amounts of organic molecules from an aqueous solution.

Thermal condensations

Most biological polymerizations are dehydration reactions; that is, monomers are linked together by the removal of water. The peptide bond is a familiar example. In living systems dehydration reactions always take place in an aqueous (cellular) environment in the presence of the appropriate dehydrating enzymes. Without enzymes and energy supplied by ATP, the macromolecules (proteins and nucleic acids) of living systems soon break down into their constituent monomers.

One of the ways in which dehydration reactions could have occurred in primitive earth conditions without enzymes is by thermal condensation. The simplest dehydration is accomplished by driving off water from solids by direct heating. For example, if a mixture of all 20 amino acids is heated to 180° C, a good yield of polypeptides is obtained.

The thermal synthesis of polypeptides to form "proteinoids" has been studied extensively by the American scientist Sidney Fox. When proteinoids are boiled in water, they form enormous numbers of hard, minute spherules called microspheres. Proteinoid microspheres (Fig. 3-5) possess certain characteristics of living systems. Each is not more than 2 μm in diameter and is comparable in size and shape to spherical bacteria. Their outer walls appear to have a double layer, and they show osmotic and selective diffusion properties. They may grow by accretion or proliferate by budding like bacteria. There is no way to know whether proteinoids may have been the ancestors of the first cells or whether they are just interesting creations of the chemist's laboratory. They must be formed under conditions that would have been found only in volcanoes. Possibly organic polymers might have condensed on or in volcanoes and then, wetted by rain or dew, reacted further in solution to form polypeptides or polynucleotides.

ORIGIN OF LIVING SYSTEMS

The first living organisms were cells: autonomous membrane-bound units with a complex functional organization that permitted the essential activity of self-reproduction. The primitive chemical systems we have described lack this essential property. The principal problem in understanding the origin of life is explaining how primitive chemical systems could have become organized into living, autonomous, self-reproducing cells.

As we have seen, a lengthy chemical evolution on the primitive earth produced several molecular components of living forms. In a later stage of evolution, nucleic acids (DNA and RNA) began to behave as simple genetic systems that directed the synthesis of proteins, especially enzymes. However, this has led to a troublesome chicken-egg paradox: (1) How could nucleic acids have appeared without enzymes to synthesize them? (2) How could enzymes have evolved without nucleic acids to direct their synthesis? The most likely answer, as with the chicken and the egg, is that neither evolved first; they evolved together from a more primitive form. As suggested by Dickerson in 1978, the first protoorganisms were probably colloidal droplets containing nucleic acids that depended on activated monomers (bases, phosphate, and sugar) and inorganic coupling reagents for their construction rather than polymerase enzymes. If one or more proteins came together with the nucleic acid, they could have served as a protective "skin" to help stabilize the nucleic acid aggregate, giving this aggregate an advantage over less stable combinations. This would be particularly so if the nucleic acid could have served as a template to synthesize more protein, even with a random sequence of amino acids. It seems highly probable that many such combinations occurred and that some of the proteins, by the particular arrangement of positive and negative charges on their polypeptide chains, could have facilitated the synthesis of more nucleic acid. These proteins would have been the first enzymes, and there would have been a powerful selective pressure for production of more nucleic acid that favored the particular amino acid sequence in associated protein production. Thus, nucleic acids with the capacity to serve as templates for protein synthesis and proteins that behave as enzymes could have evolved together, and there may not have been a period of "naked genes" or "life without DNA."

Once this stage of organization was reached, natural selection began acting on these primitive self-replicating systems. This was a critical point. Before this stage, biogenesis was shaped by the favorable environmental conditions on the primitive earth and by the nature of the reacting elements themselves. When self-replicating systems became responsive to the forces of natural selection, they began to evolve. The more rapidly replicating and more successful systems were favored, and they replicated even faster. In short, the most efficient forms survived. From this evolved the genetic code and fully directed protein synthesis. The system was a protocell, and it could be called a living organism.

Origin of Metabolism

Living cells today are organized systems that possess complex and highly ordered sequences of enzyme-mediated reactions. Some cells trap solar energy and convert it into chemical bond energy, which is stored in glucose, ATP, and other molecules. Other cells are able to use these sources of bond energy to grow, divide, and maintain their internal integrity. Indeed, the attributes of life, involving energy conversion, assimilation, secretion, excretion, responsiveness to stimuli, and capacity to reproduce, all depend on the complex metabolic patterns characteristic of contemporary cells. How did such vastly complex metabolic schemes develop?

Organisms that depend on nutrient molecules they have not synthesized for their food supplies are known as **heterotrophs** (Gr., *heteros,* another, + *trophos,* feeder), whereas organisms that can synthesize their food from inorganic sources using light or another source of energy are called **autotrophs** (Gr., *autos,* self, + *trophos,* feeder) (Fig. 3-6). The earliest microorganisms are sometimes referred to as **primary heterotrophs** because they existed before there were any autotrophs. They were probably anaerobic, bacteria-like organisms similar to modern *Clostridium,* and they obtained all their nutrients directly from the environment. Chemical evolution had already supplied generous stores of nutrients in the prebiotic soup. There would be neither advantage nor need for the earliest organisms to synthesize their own compounds, as long as they were freely available from the

Figure 3-6

Koala, a heterotroph, feeding on a eucalyptus tree, an autotroph. All heterotrophs depend for their nutrients directly or indirectly on autotrophs that capture the sun's energy to synthesize their own nutrients.

Photograph by C.P. Hickman, Jr.

environment. But as soon as deficiencies of certain essential nutrients occurred, alternative sources had to be found. At that point, microorganisms that could synthesize these essential compounds from other accessible compounds would clearly have a greater advantage for surviving than those that could not.

For example, ATP is the immediate energy coinage of all living organisms. Since it has been formed experimentally in simulated prebiotic conditions, there is good reason to believe that it was present in the primitive environment and available to and used by protocells. Thus, early organisms would have depended on the environmental supply for their ATP requirements.

Once the supply was exhausted or became precarious, perhaps because of an increase in the numbers of organisms using it, protocells able to convert a precursor such as phosphoenolpyruvate to pyruvate and capture the energy released in the form of ATP would have had a tremendous advantage over those that lacked this capability. They would be selected for survival and would thrive. In the same way, when the supply of phosphoenolpyruvate became limiting, it would be necessary to synthesize it from another precursor (such as 2-phosphoglycerate) supplied by the environment. Again, the most successful organisms would have been those that chanced to develop this metabolic capability. Long sequences of reactions could have arisen in this manner.

An enzyme is required to catalyze each of these reactions. So, when we say that early protocells developed a reaction sequence as we have described (A made from B, B from C, and so on), we are really assuming that the appropriate enzymes appeared to catalyze these reactions. The numerous enzymes of cellular metabolism appeared when cells became able to utilize proteins for catalytic functions and thereby gained a selective advantage. No planning was required; the results were achieved through natural selection.

Appearance of Photosynthesis and Oxidative Metabolism

Eventually, almost all usable energy-rich nutrients of the prebiotic soup were consumed. This ushered in the next stage of biochemical evolution: the use of readily available solar radiation to provide metabolic energy. Photosynthesis, the production of organic compounds from sunlight and atmospheric carbon dioxide, is the only process that restores free energy to the biosphere. Plant photosynthesis makes possible the richness of life on earth as we know it today. The self-nourishing photoautotrophic organisms, mainly green plants, capture solar energy and use it to convert simple inorganic substances into organic materials. The energy-rich compounds they produce provide not only for their own functioning but for the secondary heterotrophic organisms, mainly animals, that feed on autotrophs. The heterotrophs in turn release important raw materials for autotrophs. This is the energy cycle of the biosphere that is powered by a steady supply of energy from the sun (Principle 2, p. 11).

The appearance of photosynthesis was of enormous consequence for evolution, but like other metabolic events it did not appear all at once. In plant photosynthesis, water is the source of the hydrogen that is used to reduce carbon dioxide to sugars. Oxygen is liberated into the atmosphere.

$$6\ CO_2 + 6\ H_2O \xrightarrow{\text{light}} C_6H_{12}O_6 + 6\ O_2$$

However, the first steps in the development of photosynthesis almost certainly did not involve the splitting of water because a large input of energy is required. Hydrogen sulfide is thought to have been abundant in the primitive earth and was probably the first reducing agent used in photosynthesis.

$$6 \text{ CO}_2 + 12 \text{ H}_2\text{S} \xrightarrow{\text{light}} \text{C}_6\text{H}_{12}\text{O}_6 + 12 \text{ S} + 6 \text{ H}_2\text{O}$$

Later, as hydrogen sulfide and other reducing agents except water were used up, oxygen-evolving photosynthesis appeared. This may have occurred as early as 3 billion years BP. Gradually oxygen began to accumulate in the atmosphere. When atmospheric oxygen reached approximately 1% of its present level, ozone began to accumulate and ultraviolet radiation was screened out. Now land and surface waters could be occupied, and oxygen production probably increased sharply.

But at this important juncture, accumulating atmospheric oxygen began to interfere with cellular metabolism, which up to this point had evolved under strictly reducing conditions. As the atmosphere slowly changed from a reducing to an oxidizing one, a new and highly efficient kind of energy metabolism appeared: **oxidative (aerobic) metabolism.** By using the available oxygen to oxidize glucose to carbon dioxide and water, much of the bond energy stored by photosynthesis could be recovered. Most living forms became wholly dependent on oxidative metabolism, and oxygen-evolving photosynthesis became essential for the continuation of life on earth.

The final phase in life's evolution followed. Although a vast span of time—more than 2 billion years—passed before multicellular organisms appeared, living cells, very much as we know them today, surrounded by semipermeable membranes and supporting an efficient oxygen-consuming form of metabolism, were flourishing on earth.

___ PRECAMBRIAN LIFE

As depicted on the inside back cover of this book, the Precambrian period spanned the geological time before the beginning of the Cambrian period 600 million years BP. At the beginning of the Cambrian period, most of the major phyla of invertebrate animals made their appearance within a few million years. This has been called the "Cambrian explosion" because before this time fossil deposits were rare and almost devoid of anything more complex than single-celled bacteria. We now recognize that the apparent rarity of Precambrian fossils was because they escaped notice owing to their microscopic size. What forms of life existed on earth before the burst of evolutionary activity in the early Cambrian world, and what organisms were responsible for the momentous change from a reducing to an oxidizing atmosphere?

___ Prokaryotes and the Age of Blue-Green Algae

The earliest bacteria-like organisms proliferated, giving rise to a great variety of bacterial forms, some of which were capable of photosynthesis. From these arose the oxygen-evolving **blue-green algae (cyanobacteria)** some 3 billion years ago.

Bacteria are called **prokaryotes,** meaning literally "before the nucleus." They contain a single chromosome comprised of a single, large molecule of DNA not

The name "algae" is misleading because it suggests a relationship to the eukaryotic green algae, and many scientists prefer the alternative name "cyanobacteria" for the group. These were the organisms responsible for producing oxygen released into the atmosphere. Study of the biochemical reactions in present cyanobacteria suggests that they evolved in a time of fluctuating oxygen concentration. For example, although they can tolerate atmospheric concentrations of oxygen (21%), the optimum concentration for many of their metabolic reactions is only 10%.

located in a membrane-bound nucleus, but found in a nuclear region, or **nucleoid.** The DNA is not complexed with histone proteins, and prokaryotes lack membranous organelles such as mitochondria, plastids, Golgi apparatus, and endoplasmic reticulum (Chapter 4). During cell division, the nucleoid divides without visible chromosomes, never by true chromosomal (mitotic) division.

Bacteria and especially blue-green algae ruled the earth's oceans unchallenged for some 1½ to 2 billion years. The blue-green algae reached the zenith of their success approximately 1 billion years BP, when filamentous forms produced great floating mats on the ocean surface. This long period of blue-green algae dominance, encompassing approximately two thirds of the history of life, has been called with justification the "age of blue-green algae" (Schopf, 1974). Bacteria and blue-green algae are so completely different from forms of life that evolved later that they have been placed in a separate kingdom, Monera (p. 158).

Within the last decade, however, Carl Woese and his colleagues at the University of Illinois have discovered that the prokaryotes actually comprise two distinct lines of descent: the eubacteria ("true" bacteria) and the archaebacteria. Although these two groups of bacteria look very much alike when viewed with the electron microscope, they are biochemically distinct. The cell walls of the archaebacteria do not contain muramic acid, as do those of all other bacteria, and there are fundamental differences in their metabolism. But the most compelling evidence for differentiating these two groups comes from the use of one of the newest and most powerful tools at the disposal of the evolutionist, the molecular sequencing technique (see marginal note). Woese found that the sequence of bases in one kind of RNA, ribosomal RNA, is sharply different from that of all other bacteria as well as from those found in the eukaryotes (see the following discussion). Woese believes that the archaebacteria are so distinctly different from the true bacteria that they should be considered as a separate kingdom, Archaebacteria. The Monera would then comprise only the true bacteria.

Appearance of the Eukaryotes

Approximately 1.5 billion years ago, after the accumulation of an oxygen-rich atmosphere, organisms with nuclei appeared. The **eukaryotes** ("true nucleus") have cells with membrane-bound nuclei containing **chromosomes** comprised of **chromatin.** In contrast to the prokaryote chromosome, constituents of chromatin include proteins called **histones** and RNA, in addition to the DNA. Both prokaryote and eukaryote chromosomes include some nonhistone proteins. Eukaryotes are generally larger than prokaryotes, contain much more DNA, and usually divide by some form of mitosis. Within their cells are numerous membranous organelles, including mitochondria in which the enzymes for oxidative metabolism are packaged. Protozoa, fungi, green and other algae, higher plants, and multicellular animals are composed of eukaryotic cells.

Prokaryotes and eukaryotes are profoundly different from each other (Fig. 3-7) and clearly represent a marked dichotomy in the evolution of life. The ascendancy of the eukaryotes resulted in a rapid decline in the dominance of blue-green algae as the eukaryotes proliferated and fed on them.

Why were the eukaryotes immediately so successful? Probably because they developed an important process facilitating rapid evolution: sex. Sex promotes great genetic variability in populations by mixing the genes of each two individ-

Molecular sequencing has emerged as the most successful approach to unraveling the genealogies of very ancient forms of life. An organism contains a living record of its past in the amino acid sequences of its proteins and in the nucleotide sequences of its nucleic acids, DNA and RNA. The sequences of nucleotides in the DNA of an organism's genes are an especially faithful record of evolutionary relationship because every gene that exists today is an evolved copy of a gene that existed millions, even billions, of years ago. Genes become altered by mutations through the course of time, but vestiges of the original gene usually persist. Using a technique that has become available only in the last few years, the sequence of nucleotides is determined in the entire molecule or in short segments of the molecule that have been cut apart with a specific enzyme. A catalog of the nucleotide sequences characteristic of each organism is then compiled. If genes for the same function in two different organisms are compared, the extent to which they differ is correlated with the time elapsed since the two organisms diverged from a common ancestor. Molecular phylogeny based on the sequencing technique has permitted biologists to move from speculation about relationships to the construction of actual phylogenies based on information locked within the cell.

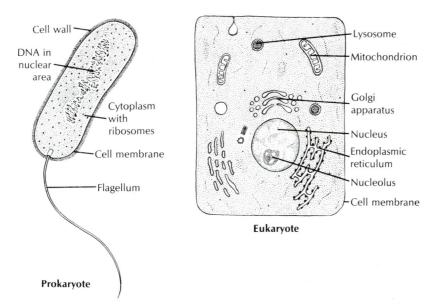

Cell wall

DNA in nuclear area

Cytoplasm with ribosomes

Cell membrane

Flagellum

Prokaryote

Lysosome

Mitochondrion

Golgi apparatus

Nucleus

Endoplasmic reticulum

Nucleolus

Cell membrane

Eukaryote

Figure 3-7

Comparison of prokaryote and eukaryote cells. The prokaryote cell is about one-tenth the size of the eukaryote cell.

uals that mate. By preserving favorable genetic variants, natural selection encourages rapid evolutionary change (Principle 4, p. 12). Prokaryotes propagate effectively and efficiently, but their mechanisms for interchange of genes, which does occur in some cases, lack the systematic genetic recombination characteristic of sexual reproduction.

The organizational complexity of the eukaryotes is so much greater than that of the prokaryotes that it is difficult to visualize how a eukaryote could have arisen from any known prokaryote. Margulis and others have proposed that eukaryotes did not in fact arise from any single prokaryote but were derived from a symbiosis ("life together") of two or more types. Mitochondria and plastids, for example, each contain their own complement of DNA (apart from the nucleus of the cell), which has some prokaryote characteristics. Mitochondria contain the enzymes of oxidative metabolism, and plastids (a plastid with chlorophyll is a chloroplast) carry out photosynthesis. It is easy to see how a host cell that was able to accommodate such guests in its cytoplasm would have had enormous competitive advantages.

Eukaryotes may have originated more than once. They were no doubt unicellular, and many were photosynthetic autotrophs. Some of these lost their photosynthetic ability and became heterotrophs, feeding on the autotrophs and the prokaryotes. As the blue-green algae were cropped, their dense filamentous mats began to thin, providing space for other species. Carnivores appeared and fed on the herbivores. Soon a balanced ecosystem of carnivores, herbivores, and primary producers appeared. This was ideal for evolutionary diversity. By freeing space, cropping herbivores encouraged a greater diversity of producers, which in turn promoted the evolution of new and more specialized croppers. An ecological pyramid developed with carnivores at the top.

The burst of evolutionary activity that followed at the end of the Precambrian period and beginning of the Cambrian period was unprecedented, and nothing approaching it has occurred since. Nearly all animal and plant phyla appeared and established themselves within a relatively brief period of a few million years. The eukaryotic cell made possible the richness and diversity of life on earth today.

___ Summary

A remarkable uniformity in the chemical constituents of living things and many of the reactions that go on in their cells suggests that life on earth may have had a common origin. Historically, it was believed that life could arise anytime, spontaneously, as long as the conditions were right. Some 60 years after Louis Pasteur disproved spontaneous generation, A.I. Oparin and J.B.S. Haldane proposed a long "abiogenic molecular evolution" on earth in which organic molecules slowly accumulated in a "primordial soup." The atmosphere of the primitive earth was reducing, and little or no free oxygen was present. Ultraviolet radiation reached the earth's surface with much greater intensity then because there was no ozone layer in the atmosphere. This, plus the electrical discharges of lightning, provided energy for the formation of organic molecules from hydrogen, methane, ammonia, water, and carbon dioxide. Some energy may have been provided by the shock waves of meteorites passing through the atmosphere. Stanley Miller and Harold Urey showed the plausibility of the Oparin-Haldane hypothesis by simple but ingenious experiments. Thus, amino acids, purines, fatty acids, sugars, and other molecules have been synthesized under conditions that may have prevailed on the primitive earth. One of the theoretical questions, namely, how dehydration reactions could have occurred in dilute solutions in water, has been answered by the preparation of model systems of coacervates and of thermal condensations to form protein microspheres. Enzymes and the genetic coding of nucleic acids probably arose together, rather than one before the other. When self-replicating systems became responsive to the forces of natural selection, evolution proceeded more rapidly.

The first organisms were the primary heterotrophs, living on the energy stored in molecules dissolved in the primordial soup. As such molecules were used up, autotrophs had a great selective advantage. Molecular oxygen began to accumulate in the atmosphere as an end product of photosynthesis, and finally the atmosphere became oxidizing. The organisms responsible for this were apparently blue-green algae (cyanobacteria). All bacteria are prokaryotes, organisms that lack a membrane-bound nucleus and other organelles in their cytoplasm. The prokaryotes consist of two genetically distinct groups that some believe should be considered separate kingdoms, Archaebacteria and Monera.

The eukaryotes originated after the atmosphere was oxidizing and apparently arose from symbiotic unions of two or more types of prokaryotes. Eukaryotes have most of their genetic material (DNA) borne in a membrane-bound nucleus and have mitochondria and other features. They include the eukaryotic algae, fungi, other plants, and all animals. Their evolutionary success is due in great degree to the variability conferred by sexual reproduction.

Selected references

Day, W. 1979. Genesis on planet earth: a search for life's beginning. East Lansing, Mich., The House of Talos Publishers. *Readable chronological account of life's origins, discussing recent experiments, and ending with thoughts on the future evolution of humans.*

Farley, J. 1974. The spontaneous generation controversy from Descartes to Oparin. Baltimore, The Johns Hopkins University Press.

Feinberg, G., and R. Shapiro. 1980. Life beyond earth: the intelligent earthling's guide to life in the universe. New York, William Morrow & Co., Inc. *Imaginative exploration of the possibilities of life in the universe.*

Folsome, C.E. 1979. The origin of life: a warm little pond. San Francisco, W.H. Freeman & Co. Publishers. *Concise account with a minimum of technical material.*

Fox, G.E., et al. 1980. The phylogeny of prokaryotes. Science **209**:457-463. *The results of studies by C. Woese and colleagues using 16S ribosomal RNA to determine relationships of bacteria, and showing a deep phylogenetic split indicating two major lines of descent, the archaebacteria and the true bacteria.*

Fox, S.W. 1980. New missing links. How did life begin? The Sciences **20**:18-21. *An up-to-date summary of the author's research on thermal proteinoids.*

Fox, S.W., and K. Dose. 1972. Molecular evolution and the origin of life. San Francisco, W.H. Freeman & Co. Publishers. *An advanced survey of wide scope. The authors' experiments with proteinoids are detailed.*

Frederick, J.F. (ed.). 1981. Origins and evolution of eukaryotic intracellular organelles. New York, New York Academy of Sciences. *Collection of conference papers representing two rival schools of thought (endosymbiotic versus autogenous) on the question of the origin of the eukaryotic cell. Advanced.*

Gribben, J.R. 1981. Genesis: the origins of man and the universe. New York, Delacorte Press/Eleanor Friede Books. *An astronomer's view of evolution from the "Big Bang" to the arrival of modern humans. Clearly written, wide-ranging explanation. Enjoyable and educational reading for all.*

Gutfreund, H. (ed.). 1981. Biochemical evolution. New York, Cambridge University Press. *Separately authored chapters having a selective coverage on evolution of biological systems. Advanced.*

Kenyon, D.H., and G. Steinman. 1969. Biochemical predestination. New York, McGraw-Hill Book Co. *One of the best books on the origin of life. Advanced and detailed but highly readable and with excellent summaries.*

Lemmon, R.M. 1970. Chemical evolution. Chemical Reviews **70**:95-109. *Excellent advanced review of this subject.*

Margulis, L. 1981. Symbiosis in cell evolution. San Francisco, W.H. Freeman & Co. Publishers. *Presents the case for the symbiotic origin of the eukaryotes.*

Margulis, L. 1982. Early life. Boston, Science Books International. *A simplified account of the development of life on earth. Well-illustrated; undergraduate level.*

Miller, S.L. 1953. A production of amino acids under possible primitive earth conditions. Science **117**:528. *The first report of the synthesis of amino acids in a reducing atmosphere.*

Miller, S.L., and L.E. Orgel. 1974. The origins of life. Englewood Cliffs, N.J., Prentice-Hall, Inc. *Advanced undergraduate level text emphasizing the chemical problems of life's origins.*

Oparin, A.I. 1953. The origin of life. New York, Dover Publications, Inc. *This is the paperback edition of Oparin's most important work, first published by Macmillan, Inc., in 1938. Later but in some ways less satisfactory versions have been published by Academic Press, Inc.*

Orgel, L.E. 1973. The origins of life: molecules and natural selection. New York, John Wiley & Sons, Inc. *Well-balanced treatment at the intermediate level.*

Ponnamperuma, C. 1972. The origins of life. New York, E.P. Dutton. *Popularized account. Well-illustrated.*

Schopf, J.W. 1974. Paleobiology of the Precambrian: the age of blue-green algae. Evolutionary Biology **7**:1-43.

Selected *Scientific American* articles

Barghoorn, E.S. 1971. The oldest fossils. **224**:30-42 (May). *Describes and illustrates fossils of algae and bacteria, some more than 3 billion years old.*

Cameron, A.G.W. 1975. The origin and evolution of the solar system. **233**:32-41 (Sept.).

Dickerson, R.E. 1978. Chemical evolution and the origin of life. **239**:70-86 (Sept.).

Eigen, M., W. Gardiner, P. Schuster, and R. Winkler-Oswatitsch. 1981. The origin of genetic information. **244**:88-118 (Apr.). *How the first genes and the genetic code may have developed.*

Glaessner, M.F. 1961. Precambrian animals. **204**:72-78 (Mar.).

Groves, D.I., J.S.R. Dunlop, and R. Buick. 1981. The early habitat of life. **245**:64-73 (Oct.). *Three and a half billion year old deposits in Western Australia may hold the first evidence of life on earth.*

Huang, S. 1960. Life outside the solar system. **202**:55-63 (Apr.).

Lawless, J.G., C.E. Folsome, and K.A. Kvenvolden. 1972. Organic matter in meteorites. **226**:38-46 (June). *Organic compounds found in meteorites appear not to be of biological origin.*

Margulis, L. 1971. Symbiosis and evolution. **225**:49-57 (Aug.).

Sagan, C., and F. Drake. 1975. The search for extraterrestrial life. **232**:80-89 (May). *There is little doubt that civilizations even more advanced than ours exist elsewhere in the universe, but locating them will require great effort.*

Wald, G. 1954. The origin of life. **191**:44-53 (Aug.). *A popular, concise account.*

Woese, C.R. 1981. Archaebacteria. **244**:98-122 (June). *Evidence that a group of bacteria, the methanogens and their relatives, represents a third ancient line of descent distinct from the true bacteria and the eukaryotes.*

CHAPTER 4

THE CELL AS THE UNIT OF LIFE

Liver cell, revealing the astonishing complexity of cellular internal organization. Surrounding the central nucleus is the cytoplasm, containing numerous organelles and inclusions suspended in a ground substance.

Electron micrograph by R. Rodewald, University of Virginia/BPS.

CELL CONCEPT

More than 300 years ago the English scientist and inventor Robert Hooke, using a primitive compound microscope, observed boxlike cavities in slices of cork and leaves. He called these compartments "little boxes or cells." In the years that followed Hooke's first demonstration of the remarkable powers of the microscope before the Royal Society of London in 1663, biologists gradually began to realize that cells were far more than simple containers filled with "juices."

Cells are the fabric of life. Even the most primitive cells are enormously complex structures that form the basic units of all living matter. All tissues and organs are composed of cells. In a human an estimated 40 trillion cells interact, each performing its specialized role in an organized community. In single-celled organisms all the functions of life are performed within the confines of one microscopic package. There is no life without cells. The idea that the cell represents the basic structural and functional unit of life is an important unifying concept of biology (Principle 11, p. 14).

With the exception of eggs, which are the largest cells (in volume) known, cells are small and mostly invisible to the unaided eye. Consequently, our understanding of cells paralleled technical advances in the resolving power of microscopes. The Dutch microscopist A. van Leeuwenhoek sent letters to the Royal Society of London containing detailed descriptions of the numerous organisms he had observed using high-quality single lenses that he had made (1673 to 1723). In the early nineteenth century, the improved design of the microscope permitted biologists to see separate objects only 1 μm apart. This advance was quickly followed by new discoveries that laid the groundwork for **modern cell theory**—a theory stating that all living organisms are composed of cells.

In 1838 Matthias Schleiden, a German botanist, announced that all plant tissue was composed of cells. A year later one of his countrymen, Theodor Schwann, described animal cells as being similar to plant cells, an understanding that had been long delayed because the animal cell is bounded only by a nearly invisible plasma membrane rather than the distinct cell wall characteristic of the plant cell. Schleiden and Schwann are thus credited with the unifying cell theory that ushered in a new era of productive exploration in cell biology.

In 1840 J. Purkinje introduced the term **protoplasm** to describe the cell contents. Protoplasm was at first thought to be a granular, gel-like mixture with special and elusive life properties of its own; the cell was viewed as a bag of thick soup containing a nucleus. Later the interior of the cell became increasingly visible as microscopes were improved and better tissue-sectioning and staining techniques were introduced. Rather than being a uniform granular soup, the cell interior is composed of numerous **cell organelles,** each performing a specific function in the life of the cell (Principle 12, p. 14). Today we realize that the components of a cell are so highly organized, structurally and functionally, that describing its contents as "protoplasm" is a bit like describing the contents of an automobile engine as "autoplasm."

How Cells Are Studied

Because cells are submicroscopic structures with complex and delicate internal organization, new technical approaches were required for the visual exploration of cell structure and function. The light microscope, with all its variations and modifications, has contributed more to biological investigation than any other

Units of measurement commonly used in microscopic study are micrometers, nanometers, and angstroms: 1 micrometer (μm) = 0.000001 meter (about $\frac{1}{25,000}$ inch); 1 nanometer (nm) = 0.000000001 meter; 1 angstrom (Å) = 0.0000000001 meter. Thus, 1 m = 10^3 mm = 10^6 μm = 10^9 nm = 10^{10} Å.

A   B

Figure 4-1

Liver cells of rat. **A,** Magnified about 700 times. Note prominently stained nucleus in each polyhedral cell. **B,** Portion of single liver cell, magnified about 6000 times. Single large nucleus dominates field; mitochondrion *(M),* rough endoplasmic reticulum *(RER),* and glycogen granules *(G)* are also seen.

From Morgan, C.R., and R.A. Jersild. 1970. Anat. Record **166:**575-586.

instrument developed by scientists. It has been a powerful exploratory tool for 300 years and continues to be so more than 50 years after the invention of the electron microscope. But, until the electron microscope was perfected, scientists' concept of the cell was limited to that which could be seen with magnifications of 1000 to 2000 diameters—the practical limit of the light microscope.

The electron microscope, invented in Germany in approximately 1931 and developed in the 1940s, employs high voltages to drive a beam of electrons through a vacuum to visualize an object. The wavelength of electrons is approximately 0.00001 that of ordinary white light, permitting far greater magnification (compare *A* and *B* of Fig. 4-1). Electron microscopes can detect objects only 0.001 the size of objects discernible with the best light microscope. Even large molecules such as DNA and proteins can actually be seen with the electron microscope.

Ordinary light as used with the light microscope is replaced in the electron microscope with a beam of electrons emitted from a tungsten filament; the glass lenses of the light microscope are replaced with magnets for focusing the electron beam; and the human eye is replaced with a fluorescent screen or a camera (Fig. 4-2). The system must be completely evacuated, and samples must be dry, nonvolatile, and cut into extremely thin sections. Image formation depends on differences in electron scattering, which in turn depend on the density of objects in the electron beam.

Since the atomic nuclei of such elements as oxygen, hydrogen, carbon, and phosphorus, of which the cell is largely composed, have "equivalent mass," the tissue must be treated with "electron stains" containing ions of elements such as osmium, lead, or uranium whose large nuclei block electrons more completely. These ions react with different chemical groups in the cell and are precipitated during these reactions. The electron micrograph shows these locations as dark, electron-opaque (electron-dense) parts of the cell.

Regions where these ions are not precipitated are seen as electron transparent (electron lucent). Because the electrons pass through the specimen to the photographic plate, the instrument is called a **transmission electron microscope.** In contrast, specimens prepared for the **scanning electron microscope** are not sec-

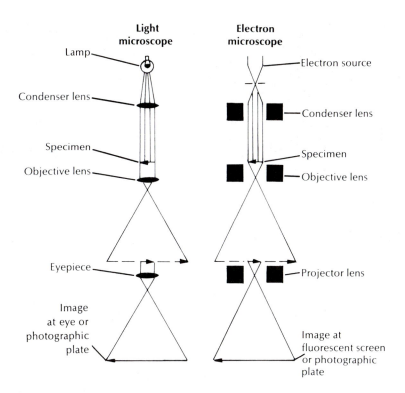

Figure 4-2

Comparison of optical paths of light and electron microscopes. To facilitate comparison, the scheme of the light microscope has been inverted from its usual orientation with light source below and image above.

tioned, and the electrons do not pass through them. Rather, the whole specimen is bombarded with electrons, causing secondary electrons to be emitted. Since the intensity of the secondary emissions varies with the angle of incidence of the primary beam, an apparent three-dimensional image is recorded in the photograph. Although the magnification capability of the scanning instrument is not nearly as great as that of the transmission microscope, the great depth of field has yielded much information about the surface features of many organisms and cells. An example of a scanning electron micrograph appears on p. 98.

Advances in the techniques of cell study have not been limited to improvements in microscopes but have included new methods of tissue preparation, staining for microscopic study, and the great contributions of modern biochemistry. For example, the various organelles of cells have differing, characteristic densities. Cells can be broken up with most of the organelles remaining intact, then centrifuged in a density gradient, and relatively pure preparations of each organelle may be recovered. Thus, the biochemical functions of the various organelles may be studied separately. The DNA and various types of RNA can be extracted and studied. Many enzymes can be purified and their characteristics determined. The use of radioactive isotopes has allowed elucidation of many metabolic reactions and pathways in the cell. Modern chromatographic techniques can separate chemically similar intermediates and products. Many more examples could be cited, and these have contributed enormously to our current understanding of cell structure and function.

ORGANIZATION OF CELLS

If we were to restrict our study of cells to fixed and sectioned tissues, we would be left with the erroneous impression that cells are static, quiescent, rigid structures. In fact, the cell interior is in a constant state of upheaval. Most cells are contin-

Table 4-1 Comparison of Prokaryotic and Eukaryotic Cells

Characteristic	Prokaryotic cell	Eukaryotic cell
Cell size	Mostly small (1-10 μm)	Mostly large (10-100 μm)
Genetic system	DNA with some nonhistone protein; simple, circular chromosome in nucleoid; nucleoid not membrane bound	DNA complexed with histone and nonhistone proteins in complex chromosomes within nucleus with membranous envelope
Cell division	Direct by binary fission or budding; no mitosis	Some form of mitosis; centrioles in many; mitotic spindle present
Sexual system	Absent in most; highly modified if present	Present in most; male and female partners; gametes that fuse
Nutrition	Absorption by most; photosynthesis by some	Absorption, ingestion, photosynthesis by some
Energy metabolism	Mitochondria absent; oxidative enzymes bound to cell membrane, not packaged separately; great variation in metabolic pattern	Mitochondria present; oxidative enzymes packaged therein; more unified pattern of oxidative metabolism
Intracellular movement	None	Cytoplasmic streaming, phagocytosis, pinocytosis

ually changing shape, pulsing, and heaving; their organelles twist and regroup in a cytoplasm teeming with starch granules, fat globules, and vesicles of various sorts. This description is derived from studies of living cell cultures with time-lapse photography. If we could see the swift shuttling of molecular traffic through gates in the cell membrane and the metabolic energy transformations within cell organelles, we would have an even stronger impression of internal turmoil. However, the cell is anything but a bundle of disorganized activity. There is order and harmony in the cell's functioning that represents the elusive phenomenon we call life. Studying this dynamic miracle of evolution through the microscope, we realize that, as we gradually comprehend more and more about this unit of life and how it operates, we are gaining a greater understanding of the nature of life itself.

___ Prokaryotic and Eukaryotic Cells

The radically different cell plan of prokaryotes and eukaryotes was described previously (p. 68). A fundamental distinction, expressed in their names, is that prokaryotes lack the membrane-bound nucleus present in all eukaryotic cells. Other major differences are summarized in Table 4-1.

Despite these differences, which are of paramount importance in cell studies, prokaryotes and eukaryotes have much in common. Both have DNA, use the same genetic code, and synthesize proteins. Many specific molecules such as ATP per-

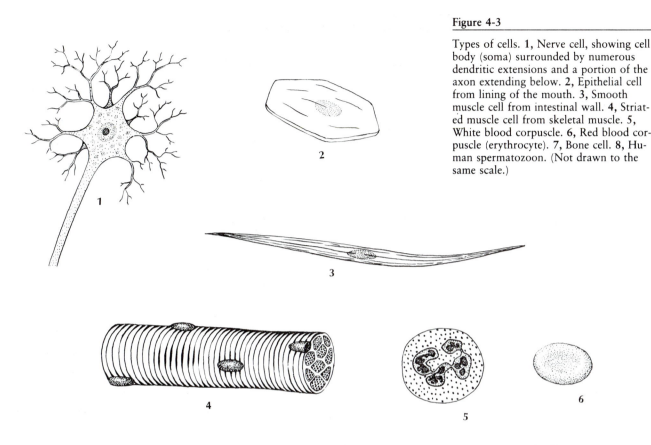

Figure 4-3

Types of cells. **1**, Nerve cell, showing cell body (soma) surrounded by numerous dendritic extensions and a portion of the axon extending below. **2**, Epithelial cell from lining of the mouth. **3**, Smooth muscle cell from intestinal wall. **4**, Striated muscle cell from skeletal muscle. **5**, White blood corpuscle. **6**, Red blood corpuscle (erythrocyte). **7**, Bone cell. **8**, Human spermatozoon. (Not drawn to the same scale.)

form similar roles in both. These fundamental similarities imply common ancestry (Principle 3, p. 11).

Prokaryotic organisms are bacteria separated into the kingdoms Archaebacteria and Monera. The most complex of these are the filamentous forms of cyanobacteria (blue-green algae) and certain other bacteria. All other organisms are eukaryotes distributed among four kingdoms: the unicellular kingdom Protista (protozoa and nucleated algae) and three multicellular kingdoms—Plantae (green plants), Fungi (true fungi), and Animalia (multicellular animals). The kingdom classifications are discussed in Chapter 7 (p. 157). The following discussion is restricted to eukaryotic cells, of which all animals are composed.

___ Components of Eukaryotic Cells and Their Functions

If the inside of the cheek is gently scraped with a blunt instrument and the scrapings are put on a slide in a drop of physiological salt solution and examined unstained with a microscope, living cells can be seen. The flat circular cells with small nuclei are the squamous epithelial cells that line much of the mouth.

Flat epithelial cells are only one of many different shapes assumed by cells. Although many cells, because of surface tension forces, assume a spherical shape when freed from restraining influences, others retain their shape under most conditions because of their characteristic cytoskeleton, or framework of microtubules (Fig. 4-3).

Figure 4-4

Generalized cell with principal organelles, as might be seen with the electron microscope. Each of the major organelles is shown enlarged. Membranes of organelles are believed to be continuous with, or derived from, the plasma membrane by an infolding process. Structure of other membranes (of nucleus, endoplasmic reticulum, mitochondria, and others) is probably similar to that of plasma membrane, shown enlarged at lower left.

Golgi complex

Centrioles

Microvilli

Smooth endoplasmic reticulum

Lysosome

Rough endoplasmic reticulum

Nucleus

Nucleolus

Mitochondrion

Plasma membrane

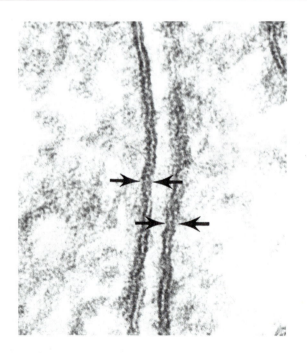

Figure 4-5

Plasma membranes of two adjacent cells. Each membrane *(between arrows)* shows a typical dark-light-dark staining pattern. (×325,000.)
Courtesy A. Wayne Vogl.

Figure 4-6

Microvilli of small intestine. (×85,000.)
Courtesy J.D. Berlin.

Nucleolus   Nucleus   Mitochondrion

Endoplasmic reticulum   Glycogen particles

Figure 4-7

Electron micrograph of part of hepatic cell of rat showing portion of nucleus *(left)* and surrounding cytoplasm. Endoplasmic reticulum and mitochondria are visible in cytoplasm, and pores *(arrows)* can be seen in nuclear membrane. ($\times14{,}000$.)
Courtesy G.E. Palade, The Rockefeller University, New York.

Figure 4-8

Electron micrograph of portion of pancreatic exocrine cell from guinea pig showing rough endoplasmic reticulum with ribosomes (small dark granules). Oval body *(bottom)* is mitochondrion. ($\times66{,}000$.)
Courtesy G.E. Palade.

Typically the eukaryotic cell is enclosed within a thin, sturdy, differentially permeable **plasma membrane** (Figs. 4-4 and 4-5). This structure regulates the flow of materials between the cell and its surroundings. In some cells, such as nerve cells, the plasma membrane also is involved in intercellular communication. In other cells, such as intestinal epithelium, the plasma membrane is modified into numerous, small, fingerlike projections called **microvilli** that increase the surface area of the cell (Fig. 4-6).

The most prominent organelle is the spherical or ovoid nucleus enclosed within *two* membranes to form the double-layered **nuclear envelope** (Fig. 4-7). At intervals the nuclear envelope is perforated by pores, permitting some continuity between the nuclear contents and the cytoplasm surrounding the nucleus. The nucleus contains chromatin and one or more dense, granular structures called **nucleoli** (sing., **nucleolus**) (Fig. 4-7). The chromatin is a complex of DNA and histone and nonhistone protein and carries the genetic information of the cell. Nucleoli are specialized parts of certain chromosomes that carry multiple copies of the DNA information to synthesize ribosomal RNA. After transcription from the nucleolar DNA, the ribosomal RNA combines with several different proteins to form a **ribosome** (Fig. 4-8), detaches from the nucleolus, and passes through nuclear pores to the cytoplasm.

The cytoplasm outside the nucleus contains many organelles such as mitochondria, Golgi complexes, centrioles, and endoplasmic reticulum. Plant cells typically contain **plastids,** the photosynthetic organelles, and bear a cell wall containing cellulose outside the plasma membrane. Animal cells lack plastids and are surrounded only by a plasma membrane.

The space between the membranes comprising the nuclear envelope connects at some points with the space (channels, or **cisternae**) within the membranes

Figure 4-9

Extensive smooth endoplasmic reticulum in a Sertoli cell from the testis of a ground squirrel. This kind of endoplasmic reticulum lacks ribosomes. (×22,800.)

Courtesy A. Wayne Vogl.

of the **endoplasmic reticulum (ER)** (Figs. 4-4, 4-7, and 4-8). The ER is a complex of membranes that separates some of the products of the cell from the synthetic machinery that produces them. The cisternae of the ER apparently function as routes for transport of certain substances within the cell. Often the membranes of the ER are lined on their outer surfaces with ribosomes and are thus designated **rough ER** (contrasted with **smooth ER,** without ribosomes) (Fig. 4-9). In some instances it has been shown that the protein synthesized by the ribosomes on the rough ER enters the cisternae and from there is transported to the Golgi apparatus or complex (Fig. 4-10). The **Golgi complex** is a stack of smooth, membranous cisternae (Fig. 4-11) that functions in the storage, modification, and packaging of protein products, especially secretory products. It does not synthesize protein but may add polysaccharide to the complex. As its products mature, the ends of the cisternae pinch off and become membrane-bound **vesicles** in the cytoplasm. The contents of some of these vesicles may be expelled to the outside of the cell as secretory products destined to be exported from a glandular cell. Others may contain digestive enzymes that remain in the cell that produces them. Such vesicles are called **lysosomes** (literally "loosening body," a body capable of causing lysis, or disintegration). The enzymes they contain are involved in the breakdown of foreign material, including bacteria engulfed by the cell. Lysosomes also are capable of breaking down injured or diseased cells and worn-out cellular components, since the enzymes they contain are so powerful that they kill the cell that formed them if the lysosome membrane ruptures. In normal cells the enzymes remain safely enclosed within the protective membrane.

Mitochondria (sing., **mitochondrion**) (Fig. 4-12) are conspicuous organelles present in nearly all eukaryotic cells. They are diverse in size, number, and shape; some are rodlike, and others are more or less spherical. They may be scattered uniformly through the cytoplasm, or they may be localized near cell surfaces and other regions where there is unusual metabolic activity. The mitochondrion is

Figure 4-10

System for assembling, isolating, and secreting proteins for export from, and use inside, a eukaryotic cell.

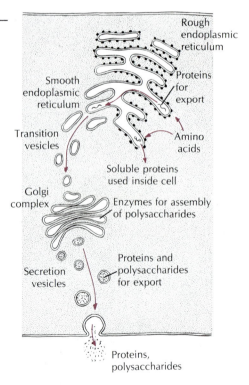

Rough endoplasmic reticulum

Proteins for export

Smooth endoplasmic reticulum

Transition vesicles

Amino acids

Soluble proteins used inside cell

Golgi complex

Enzymes for assembly of polysaccharides

Secretion vesicles

Proteins and polysaccharides for export

Proteins, polysaccharides

Golgi

Golgi

Figure 4-11

Golgi complexes in a Sertoli cell of ground squirrel testis. (×26,700.)

Courtesy A. Wayne Vogl.

composed of a double membrane. The outer membrane is smooth, whereas the inner membrane is folded into numerous platelike projections called **cristae** (Figs. 4-4 and 4-12). These characteristic features make mitochondria easy to identify among the organelles. Mitochondria are often called "powerhouses of the cell" because enzymes located on the cristae carry out the energy-yielding steps of aerobic metabolism. ATP, the most important energy storage molecule of all cells, is produced in this organelle. Mitochondria are self-replicating. They have a tiny, circular chromosome, resembling the chromosomes of prokaryotes but much smaller. The chromosome contains DNA that specifies some, but not all, of the proteins of the mitochondrion.

All of these cellular entities (except ribosomes) are composed of or enclosed within membranes. Eukaryotic cells also contain a variety of nonmembranous elements. **Microfilaments** are thin, linear structures, first observed distinctly in muscle cells, where they are responsible for the ability of the cell to contract. In

Figure 4-12

Electron micrograph of elongated mitochondrion in pancreatic exocrine cell of guinea pig. The mitochondrion has two membranes, an outer smooth membrane and an inner membrane that is folded inward into invaginations called cristae. These appear as incomplete transverse septa inside the mitochondrion. (×50,000.)
Courtesy G.E. Palade.

Microtubules   Intermediate filaments

Cortical filaments
(actin)

Figure 4-13

Cytoskeleton of a cell, showing its complex nature. Three visible cytoskeletal elements, in order of increasing diameter, are cortical filaments, intermediate filaments, and microtubules. (×66,600.)

Courtesy A. Wayne Vogl.

skeletal muscle, thin microfilaments composed of a protein called actin interdigitate with thicker myosin microfilaments. They are lined up in such a way as to give the muscle a striated appearance. Actin microfilaments have now been found in a wide variety of other kinds of cells, and they are apparently critical to certain mechanisms of movement of cells and substances within the cells. **Microtubules** (Fig. 4-21) are somewhat larger, tubular structures composed of the protein tubulin. They play a vital role in moving the chromosomes toward the daughter cells during cell division as will be seen later, and they form a supportive cytoskeleton in some cells; that is, they help the cell maintain its shape (Fig. 4-13). In addition, microtubules form essential parts of the structures of centrioles, cilia, and flagella. **Centrioles** (Fig. 4-21) determine the orientation of the plane of cell division. Although they do not occur in most cells of higher plants, they are an almost universal feature of animal cells. A centriole is a short cylinder formed from nine triplets of microtubules. Two centrioles are usually found close together, one at a right angle to the other, and they replicate before cell division.

Surfaces of Cells and Their Specializations

The free surface of epithelial cells (cells that cover the surface of a structure or line a tube or cavity) sometimes bears either **cilia** or **flagella.** These are vibratile, locomotory extensions of the cell surface that sweep materials past the cell. In single-celled animals (many of the protozoa) and some primitive multicellular forms, they propel the entire animal through a liquid medium. Flagella provide the means of locomotion for the male reproductive cells of most animals and many plants.

Cilia occur in large numbers on each cell and are relatively short (5 to 10 μm). Flagella typically, although not always, occur singly or in a small number per cell and are long, whiplike structures that may reach 150 μm in length. The distinction between cilia and flagella is that a cilium propels water parallel to the surface to which the cilium is attached, whereas a flagellum propels water parallel to the main axis of the flagellum (Fig. 28-8, p. 680). Their internal structure is the same. With few exceptions, the internal structures of locomotory cilia and flagella are composed of a long cylinder of nine pairs of microtubules enclosing a central pair. At the base of each cilium or flagellum is a **basal body (kinetosome)**, which is identical in structure to a centriole.

Cells covering the surface of a structure or cells packed together in a tissue may have specialized junctional complexes between them. Nearest the free surface, the two apposing cell membranes appear to fuse, forming a **tight junction** (Fig. 4-14). At various points small ellipsoid discs occur, just beneath the cell membrane in each cell. These appear to act as "spot-welds" and are called **desmosomes**. From each desmosome a tuft of microfilaments extends into the cytoplasm. **Gap junctions**, rather than serving as points of attachment, provide a means of intercellular communication. They are formed from tiny canals between cells so that the cytoplasm becomes continuous, and molecules can pass from one cell to the other.

Another specialization of the cell surface is the interdigitations of confronted cell surfaces where the plasma membranes of the cells infold and interdigitate very much like a zipper. They are especially common in the epithelium of kidney tubules. Microvilli, mentioned earlier, are another type of cell surface specialization (Figs. 4-6 and 4-14). With the electron microscope they can be seen clearly in the lining of the intestine where they greatly increase the absorptive and digestive surface. Such specializations appear as brush borders when viewed with the light microscope. The spaces between the microvilli are continuous with tubules of the ER, which may facilitate the movement of materials into the cells.

MEMBRANE STRUCTURE AND FUNCTION
Structure of the Cell Membrane

The incredibly thin, yet sturdy, plasma membrane that encloses every cell is vitally important in maintaining cellular integrity. Once believed to be a rather static entity that defined cell boundaries and kept cell contents from spilling out, the plasma membrane (also called the plasmalemma) has proved to be a dynamic structure having remarkable activity and selectivity. It is a permeability barrier that separates the interior from the external environment of the cell, regulates the vital flow of molecular traffic into and out of the cell, and provides many of the unique functional properties of specialized cells.

Membranes inside the cell surround the mitochondria, Golgi complex, ER, lysosomes, and other organelles. Indeed, the cell is a system of membranes that divide it into numerous compartments. Someone has estimated that if all the membranes present in 1 g of liver tissue were spread out flat, they would cover 30 square meters! Internal membranes share many of the structural features of the plasma membrane and are the site for many, perhaps most, of the cell's enzymatic reactions.

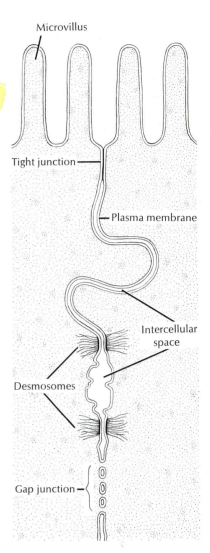

Figure 4-14

Two opposing plasma membranes forming the boundary between two epithelial cells. Various kinds of junctional complexes are found. The tight junction is a firm, adhesive band completely encircling the cell. Desmosomes are isolated "spot-welds" between cells. Gap junctions serve as sites of intercellular communication. Intercellular space may be greatly expanded in epithelial cells of some tissues.

Plasma membrane surrounding microvillus

Figure 4-15

Plasma membrane of microvilli. The membrane appears as a trilaminar structure consisting of two dense lines separated by a less dense intermediate layer. Courtesy J.D. Berlin.

The plasma membrane is composed almost entirely of proteins and lipids. The lipids that give the membrane its strength and provide other gross structural properties belong to a class of compounds called **phospholipids**. These are **amphipathic** ("both-experiencing") molecules with polar heads and nonpolar tails. The polar heads are electrically charged, consist of glycerol attached to phosphate and other groups, and are water soluble, or hydrophilic ("water-loving"). The nonpolar tails are uncharged hydrocarbon chains of fatty acids that are insoluble in water, or hydrophobic ("water-fearing").

The plasma membrane is so thin that it cannot be seen with the light microscope. Although some biologists of the nineteenth century doubted its existence, it soon became clear that there had to be a membrane surrounding cells that would account for the special permeability characteristics of the cell surface. Early chemical analyses showed the membrane to have a high lipid content, and this discovery led to the first meaningful speculations about membrane structure. In 1925 Gorter and Grendel discovered that lipids extracted from red blood cell membranes formed a monolayer on the surface of water that was approximately *double* the surface area of the red blood cells. They reasoned that the lipids had to be arranged in a double layer in the plasma membrane, with hydrophobic hydrocarbon chains facing each other in the center of the bilayer and the hydrophilic polar heads forming the membrane's surfaces. Later Danielli and Davson (1935) modified the model by adding layers of proteins to the membrane surface. These, they concluded, were necessary to reduce surface tension and make the membrane more stable.

High-resolution electron microscopy reveals a very thin (approximately 7.5 to 10 nm) double line at the cell surface (Figs. 4-5 and 4-15). The two narrow dark lines are believed to represent the polar ends of the phospholipids; the light middle interspace represents the fatty acid chain bilayer. This three-layered structure—two dark lines separated by a light interspace—is also characteristic of the membranes that surround the organelles within the cell.

Although all membranes are composed of lipids and proteins, the proteins are not found arranged in an orderly, static array on the lipid bilayer as proposed by the Danielli-Davson model. Some, called integral proteins, penetrate the lipid core of the membrane and may extend all the way through it. These may behave as channels through which small molecules such as sodium, potassium, and chloride are allowed to pass. Other proteins, called extrinsic proteins, float on the surface and can be easily removed by relatively mild experimental treatment of the membrane. Furthermore, the membrane appears to be remarkably restless and fluid, with proteins constantly moving and reorganizing their molecular configuration. These views of the plasma membrane are embodied in the **fluid-mosaic model** of membrane structure (Singer and Nicolson, 1972), which is now widely accepted (Fig. 4-16). Simply put, this model retains the lipid bilayer of earlier models and proposes that proteins, rather than forming a continuous layer on both surfaces, float about as units in the bilayer.

____ Function of the Cell Membrane

The plasma membrane acts as a gatekeeper for the entrance and exit of the many substances involved in cell metabolism. Some substances can pass through with ease, others enter slowly and with difficulty, and still others cannot enter at all. This is called the **selective behavior** of the cell membrane. Because conditions outside the cell are different from and more variable than conditions within the

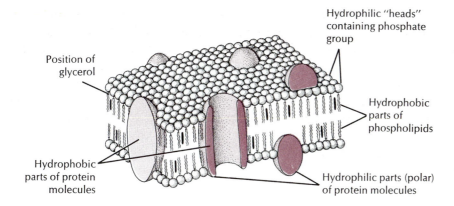

Position of glycerol

Hydrophilic "heads" containing phosphate group

Hydrophobic parts of phospholipids

Hydrophobic parts of protein molecules

Hydrophilic parts (polar) of protein molecules

Figure 4-16

Fluid-mosaic model of a cell membrane. Proteins are shown as solid blocks, but they consist of folded and coiled polypeptide chains. Some may be found on one or the other surface of the membrane, whereas others may extend the entire thickness. Some protein molecules may form pores through the membrane.

cell, it is necessary that the passage of substances across the membrane be rigorously controlled.

We recognize three principal ways that a substance may traverse the cell membrane: (1) by **free diffusion** along a concentration gradient; (2) by a **mediated transport system,** in which the substance binds to a specific site that in some way assists it across the membrane; and (3) by **endocytosis,** in which the substance is enclosed within a vesicle that forms on and detaches from the membrane surface to enter the cell.

Free diffusion and osmosis

If a living cell surrounded by a membrane is immersed in a solution having more solute molecules than the fluid inside the cell, a **concentration gradient** instantly exists between the two fluids. More solute molecules strike the membrane from the outside than from inside. Assuming that the membrane is **permeable** to the solute, there is a net movement of solute toward the inside, the side having the lower concentration. The solute diffuses "downhill" across the membrane until its concentrations on each side are equal.

Most cell membranes are **semipermeable,** that is, permeable to water but selectively permeable or impermeable to solutes. In free diffusion it is this selectiveness that regulates molecular traffic. As a rule, gases (such as oxygen and carbon dioxide), urea, and lipid-soluble solutes (such as hydrocarbons and alcohol) are the only solutes that can diffuse through biological membranes with any degree of freedom. This happens because of the lipid nature of membranes, which form a natural barrier to most biologically important molecules that are not lipid soluble. Since many water-soluble molecules readily pass through membranes, such movements cannot be explained by simple diffusion. Instead sugars, as well as many electrolytes and macromolecules, are moved across membranes by carrier-mediated processes, described in the next section.

If a membrane is placed between two unequal concentrations of solutes to which the membrane is impermeable or only weakly permeable, water flows through the membrane from the more dilute to the more concentrated solution. In effect the water molecules move down a concentration gradient from an area where the water molecules are more concentrated to an area where they are less concentrated. This is **osmosis.** To understand why this happens, we must view the system from the standpoint of the state of the water on each side.

Osmosis can be demonstrated by a simple experiment in which a selectively permeable membrane such as cellophane is tied tightly over the end of a funnel.

Figure 4-17

Simple membrane osmometer.

Water

Sugar
solution

Semipermeable
membrane

The funnel is filled with a sugar solution and placed in a beaker of pure water so that the water levels inside and outside the funnel are equal. In a short time the water level in the glass tube of the funnel rises, indicating that water is passing through the cellophane membrane into the sugar solution (Fig. 4-17).

Inside the funnel are sugar molecules, as well as water molecules. In the beaker outside the funnel are only water molecules. Thus the concentration of water is less on the inside because some of the available space is occupied by the larger, nondiffusible sugar molecules. A concentration gradient is said to exist for water molecules in the system. Water diffuses from the region of greater concentration of water (pure water outside) to the region of lesser concentration (sugar solution inside).

As water enters the sugar solution, the fluid level in the funnel rises, creating a hydrostatic pressure because of gravity inside the osmometer. Eventually the pressure produced by the increasing weight of solution in the funnel pushes water molecules out as fast as they enter. The level in the funnel becomes stationary and the system is in equilibrium. The **osmotic pressure** of the solution is equal to the hydrostatic pressure necessary to prevent further net entry of water.

The concept of osmotic pressure is not without problems. A solution reveals an osmotic "pressure" only when it is separated from solvent by a semipermeable membrane. It can be disconcerting to think of an isolated bottle of sugar solution as having osmotic "pressure" much as compressed gas in a bottle would have. Furthermore, the osmotic pressure is really the hydrostatic pressure that must be applied to a solution to keep it from gaining water. Consequently, biologists frequently use the term **osmotic potential** rather than osmotic pressure. However, since the term "osmotic pressure" is too firmly fixed in our vocabulary to be easily dislodged, it is necessary to understand the usage despite its potential confusion.

The *direct* measurement of osmotic pressure in biological solutions is seldom done today because the osmotic pressures of most biological solutions are so great that it would be impractical if not impossible to measure them with the simple membrane osmometer described. The osmotic pressure of human blood plasma would lift a fluid column more than 250 feet—if we could construct such a long, vertical tube and find a membrane that would not rupture from the pressure.

Indirect methods of measuring osmotic pressure are more practical. By far the most widely used measurement is the **freezing point depression.** This is a much faster and more accurate determination than is the direct measurement of osmotic pressure by the collodion membrane osmometer. Pure water freezes at exactly 0° C. As solutes are added, the freezing point is lowered; the greater the concentration of solutes, the lower the freezing point. Human blood plasma freezes at approximately −0.56° C; seawater freezes at approximately −1.80° C. Although the lowering of the freezing point of water by the presence of solutes is small, great accuracy of measurement is possible because the instruments used by biologists can detect differences of as little as 0.001° C.

Mediated transport

We have seen that the cell membrane is an effective barrier to the free diffusion of most molecules of biological significance. Yet it is essential that such materials enter and leave the cell. Nutrients such as sugars and materials for growth such as amino acids must enter the cell, and the wastes of metabolism must leave. Such molecules are moved across the membrane by special mechanisms built into the

A   B

Figure 4-18

A, Diffusion through membrane channels. **B,** Carrier-mediated transport. Simple diffusion through membrane channels differs from carrier-mediated transport in that the latter shows saturation at high concentration. Simple diffusion does not exhibit saturation at high concentration.

structure of the membrane. This is called **mediated transport,** meaning that a specific transport mechanism mediates, or facilitates, transfer across the membrane barrier.

Experimental evidence suggests that mediated transport of sugars, amino acids, and other solutes involves the reversible combination with membrane proteins. Such proteins are called **carriers**: protein molecules positioned within the membrane and capable of shuttling from one membrane surface to the other. It is assumed that the carrier molecule captures a solute molecule to be transported, forming a temporary carrier-solute complex, much as enzymes form a temporary enzyme-substrate complex (p. 45). The carrier molecule, with its fare, moves or rotates to the opposite surface, where the solute detaches and leaves the membrane. The carrier moves back, again presenting its attachment site for the pickup and transport of another solute molecule. Protein carriers are usually quite specific, recognizing and transporting only a limited group of chemical substances or perhaps even a single substance.

The carrier hypothesis is consistent with the observation that at high concentrations some solutes show a saturation effect. This means simply that the rate of influx reaches a plateau beyond which increasing the solute concentration has no further effect on influx rate (Fig. 4-18, *B*). This is evidence that the number of carriers available in the membrane is limited. When all become occupied by solutes, the rate of transport is at a maximum and cannot be increased. Simple diffusion shows no such limitation; the greater the difference in solute concentration on the two sides of the membrane, the faster the influx (Fig. 4-18, *A*).

At least two distinctly different kinds of carrier-mediated transport mechanisms are recognized: (1) **facilitated transport,** in which the carrier assists a molecule to diffuse through the membrane that it cannot otherwise penetrate, and (2) **active transport,** in which energy is supplied to the carrier systems to transport molecules in the direction opposite to the gradient. Facilitated transport therefore differs from active transport in that it sponsors movement in a downhill direction (in the direction of the concentration gradient) only and requires no metabolic energy to drive the carrier system.

In higher animals facilitated transport is important for the transport of glucose (blood sugar) into body cells that burn it as a principal energy source for the synthesis of ATP. The concentration of glucose is greater in the blood than in the cells that consume it, favoring inward diffusion, but glucose is a polar molecule that does not, by itself, penetrate the membrane rapidly enough to support the metabolism of many cells; the carrier system increases the inward flow of glucose.

In active transport, molecules are moved uphill against the forces of passive

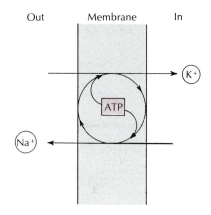

Out   Membrane   In

Figure 4-19

Sodium-potassium exchange pump, powered by bond energy of ATP, maintains the normal gradients of these ions across the cell membrane. Sodium is more concentrated outside the cell, and potassium is more concentrated inside.

diffusion. Active transport always involves the expenditure of energy (from ATP) because materials are pumped against a concentration gradient. Among the most important active transport systems in all animals are those that maintain sodium and potassium gradients between cells and the surrounding extracellular fluid or external environment. Most animal cells require a high internal concentration of potassium for protein synthesis at the ribosome and for certain enzymatic functions. The potassium concentration may be 20 to 50 times greater inside the cell than outside. Sodium, on the other hand, may be 10 times more concentrated outside the cell than inside. Both of these electrolyte gradients are maintained by the active transport of potassium into and sodium out of the cell. In many cells one kind of molecule or ion on one side of the membrane is exchanged for another kind of molecule or ion on the opposite side. The **sodium-potassium exchange pump** that maintains the sodium and potassium gradients across nerve cell membranes is an example (Fig. 4-19). There is evidence that 10% to 40% of all energy produced by some cells is used to power the sodium-potassium exchange pump.

Endocytosis

The ingestion of solid or fluid material by cells was observed by microscopists nearly 100 years before phrases such as "active transport" and "protein carrier mechanism" were a part of the biologist's vocabulary. Endocytosis is a collective term that describes two similar processes, **phagocytosis** and **pinocytosis**.

Phagocytosis, which literally means "cell eating," is a common method of feeding among the protozoa and lower metazoa. It is also the way in which white blood cells (leukocytes) engulf cellular debris and uninvited microbes in the blood. By phagocytosis, the cell membrane forms a pocket that engulfs the solid material. The membrane-enclosed vesicle then detaches from the cell surface and moves into the cytoplasm where its contents are digested by intracellular enzymes (Fig. 31-5, p. 744).

Pinocytosis, or "cell drinking," is similar to phagocytosis except that drops of fluid are sucked discontinuously through tubular channels into cells to form tiny vesicles. These may combine to form larger vacuoles. Both processes require metabolic energy, and in this respect they are forms of active transport.

MITOSIS AND CELL DIVISION

All cells of the body arise from the division of preexisting cells (Principle 11, p. 14). All the cells found in most multicellular organisms have originated from the division of a single cell, the **zygote,** which is formed from the union (fertilization) of an **egg** and a **sperm.** Cell division provides the basis for one form of growth, for both sexual and asexual reproduction, and for the transmission of hereditary qualities from one cell generation to another cell generation.

In the formation of **body cells** (somatic cells) the process of nuclear division is referred to as **mitosis.** By mitosis each "daughter cell" is assured of receiving a complete set of genetic instructions. Mitosis is a delivery system for distributing the chromosomes and the DNA they contain to continuing cell generations. Thus, all somatic cells, which number hundreds of billions in large animals, have the same genetic content, since all are descended by faithful reproduction of the original fertilized egg. As an animal grows, its somatic cells differentiate and assume different functions and appearances because of differential gene action. Even though most of the genes in specialized cells remain silent and unexpressed throughout the lives of those cells, every cell possesses a complete genetic complement. Mitosis ensures equality of genetic potential; later, other processes direct the orderly expression of genes during embryonic development by selecting from the genetic instructions that each cell contains. (These fundamental properties of cells of multicellular organisms are stated in Principles 21, 22, and 24, pp. 17 and 18, and are discussed further in Chapter 36.)

In animals that reproduce **asexually,** mitosis is the only mechanism for the faithful transfer of genetic information from parent to progeny. In animals that reproduce **sexually,** the parents must produce **sex cells** (gametes or germ cells) that contain only half the usual number of chromosomes, so that the offspring formed by the union of the gametes will not contain double the number of parental chromosomes. This requires a special type of *reductional* division called **meiosis,** described in Chapter 35.

_____ Structure of Chromosomes

As mentioned earlier, DNA in the eukaryotic cell occurs in chromatin, a complex of DNA with histone and nonhistone protein. The chromatin is organized into a number of discrete bodies called **chromosomes** (color bodies), so named because they stain deeply with certain biological dyes. In cells that are not dividing, the chromatin is loosely organized and dispersed, so that the individual chromosomes cannot be distinguished (Chapter 37, p. 912). Before division the chromatin condenses, and the chromosomes can be recognized and their individual morphological characteristics determined. They are of varied lengths and shapes, some bent and some rodlike. Their number is constant for the species, and every body cell (but not the germ cells) has the same number of chromosomes regardless of the cell's function. A human, for example, has 46 chromosomes in each body (somatic) cell.

During mitosis (nuclear division) the chromosomes shorten and become increasingly condensed and distinct, and each assumes a characteristic shape. At some point on the chromosome is a **centromere,** or constriction, to which are attached several spindle fibers that move the chromosome toward the pole during mitosis.

Chromosomes are always arranged in pairs, two of each kind. Of each pair, one comes from one parent and the other from the other parent. Thus, there are 23 pairs in the human species. Each pair usually has certain characteristics of shape and form that aid in identification. A biparental organism begins with the union of two gametes, each of which furnishes a **haploid** set of chromosomes (23 in humans) to produce a somatic or **diploid** number of chromosomes (46 in humans). The chromosomes of a haploid set are also called a **genome.** A fertilized egg consists of a paternal genome (chromosomes contributed by the father) and a maternal genome (chromosomes contributed by the mother).

The formidable problem of packaging the cell's DNA so that the genetic instructions are accessible for reading during the transcription process (the formation of messenger RNA from nuclear DNA) is described in Chapter 37, p. 911.

In 1974 it was discovered that the chromatin is composed of repeating subunits, called **nucleosomes.** Each nucleosome is a narrow "spool" or disc of histone proteins around which one and three fourths turns of double-helical DNA are wound to form a superhelix. The nucleosomes are linked together by the continuous DNA strand much like beads on a string. This arrangement is thought to explain the knobby appearance of chromatin fibers as revealed by high-resolution electron micrographs. Since the DNA is wound around the *outside* of the nucleosome beads, all base pairs of the molecule are accessible for transcription.

Interphase

Chromatin material appears granular; each chromosome reaches its maximum length and minimum thickness; duplication of chromosomes occurs at this stage

Figure 4-20

Stages of mitosis, showing division of a cell with two pairs of chromosomes. One chromosome of each pair is shown in red.

Early prophase

Each elongated chromosome now consists of 2 chromatids attached to single centromere; centrioles divide and spindle starts development

Late prophase

Double nature of short, thick chromosome more apparent; each chromosome made up of 2 sister chromatids; nucleolus usually disappears; nuclear envelope disintegrates

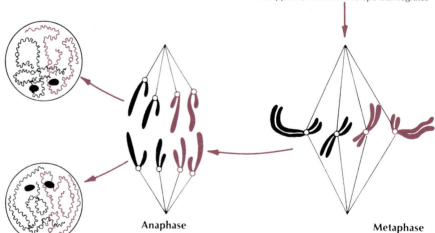

Telophase

Chromosomes become longer and thinner; chromosomes may lose identity; nuclear membrane reappears and spindle-astral fibers fade away; cell body divides into 2 daughter cells, each of which now enters interphase

Anaphase

Chromatids, now called daughter chromosomes, are in two distinct groups; daughter centromeres move apart and pull daughter chromosomes toward respective poles

Metaphase

Chromosomes arranged on equatorial plate; centromeres (not yet divided) anchored to equator of spindle

___ Stages in Mitosis

There are two distinct phases of cell division: the division of the nuclear chromosomes (**mitosis**) and the division of the cytoplasm (**cytokinesis**). Mitosis, the division of the nucleus (that is, chromosomal segregation), is certainly the most obvious and complex part of cell division and that of greatest interest to the cytologist. Cytokinesis normally immediately follows mitosis, although occasionally the nucleus may divide a number of times without a corresponding division of the cytoplasm. In such a case the resulting mass of protoplasm containing many nuclei is referred to as a **multinucleate cell.** An example is the giant resorptive cell type of bone (osteoclast), which may contain 15 to 20 nuclei. Sometimes a multinucleate mass is formed by cell fusion rather than nuclear proliferation. This arrangement is called a **syncytium.** An example is vertebrate skeletal muscle, which is composed of multinucleate fibers that have arisen by the fusion of numerous embryonic cells.

The process of mitosis is arbitrarily divided for convenience into four successive stages or phases, although one stage merges into the next without sharp lines of transition. These phases are prophase, metaphase, anaphase, and telophase (Fig. 4-20). When the cell is not actively dividing, it is in the "resting" stage or **interphase.** However, the cell may not be really "resting" at this stage because the DNA content of the nucleus is being duplicated between divisions. Thus when the cell begins "active" mitosis, it already has a double set of chromosomes.

Prophase

At the beginning of prophase, the centrioles migrate toward opposite sides of the nucleus. At the same time, fine fibers (microtubules) appear between the two pairs of centrioles to form a football-shaped **spindle,** so named because of its resemblance to nineteenth-century wooden spindles, used to twist thread together in spinning. Other fibers radiate outward from each centriole to form **asters.** The entire structure is the **mitotic apparatus,** and it increases in size and prominence as the centrioles move farther apart (Fig. 4-21).

At the same time, the diffuse nuclear chromatin condenses to form visible chromosomes. These actually consist of two identical sister **chromatids** formed during interphase. The sister chromatids are joined together at their centromere. At the end of prophase, the nuclear envelope quickly disappears.

Metaphase

During metaphase the condensed sister chromatids rapidly migrate to the middle of the nuclear region to form a **metaphasic plate** (Fig. 4-22). The centromeres line up precisely on the plate with the arms of the chromatids trailing off randomly in various directions. Spindle fibers now attach to each centromere.

Anaphase

The two chromatids of each double chromosome thicken and separate. The single centromere that has held the two chromatids together now splits so that two independent chromosomes, each with its own centromere, are formed. The chromosomes part more, evidently pulled by the spindle fibers attached to the centromeres. The arms of each chromosome trail along behind as though the chromo-

The spindle fibers are microtubules, long, hollow cylinders composed of the protein tubulin. Each tubulin molecule, actually a doublet composed of two globular proteins, is attached end to end to form a strand. Thirteen strands aggregate to form a microtubule. There is evidence that microtubules are able to shift their position in cells by a peculiar treadmill process; protein doublets are disassembled at one end of the tubule, are added again at the opposite end, then travel down the microtubule treadmill to be dropped off once again at the disassembly end. Energy for this process is provided by the nucleotide guanosine triphosphate (GTP). It is thought that the spindle fibers that attach the chromosome by its centromere to the centriole shorten by losing tubulin doublets at the polar end, while assembly at the chromosome end is blocked. Thus, the chromosomes are dragged toward their poles.

Figure 4-21

Fine structure of mitotic apparatus. At each pole of the spindles is a clear zone occupied by a pair of centrioles and surrounded by short microtubules. Other microtubules form spindle fibers, some of which extend from pole to pole while others attach to chromosomes.

From DuPraw, E.J. 1968. Cell and molecular biology. New York, Academic Press, Inc.

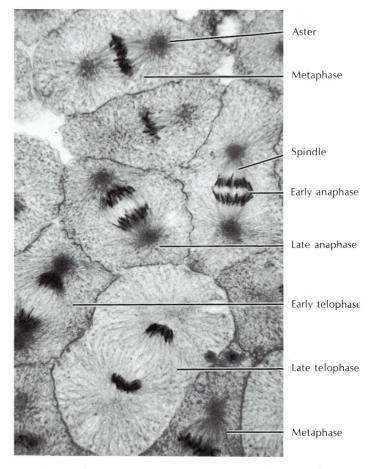

Aster

Metaphase

Spindle

Early anaphase

Late anaphase

Early telophase

Late telophase

Metaphase

Figure 4-22

Stages of mitosis in whitefish.
Courtesy General Biological Supply House, Inc., Chicago.

some were being dragged through a resisting medium. The spindle fibers are actually microtubules that somehow shorten to drag the chromosomes toward their respective poles. However, the fibers maintain the same thickness throughout anaphase, neither thickening nor thinning as the chromosomes separate.

Telophase

When the daughter chromosomes reach their respective poles, telophase has begun. The daughter chromosomes are crowded together and stain intensely with histological stains. The spindle fibers disappear and the chromosomes lose their identity, reverting to the diffuse chromatin network characteristic of the interphase nucleus. Finally, the nuclear membranes reappear around the two daughter nuclei.

___ Cytokinesis: Cell Division

During the final stages of nuclear division a **cleavage furrow** appears on the surface of the dividing cell and encircles it at the midline of the spindle. The cleavage furrow deepens and pinches the plasma membrane as though it were being tightened by an invisible rubber band. Microfilaments are present in the area of constriction, and it is speculated that actin and myosin filaments slide together to shorten the microfilaments in precisely the same manner that muscle cells contract (p. 683). Finally, the infolding edges of the plasma membrane meet and fuse, completing cell division.

___ Cell Cycle

Cycles are conspicuous attributes of life. The descent of a species through time is in a very real sense a sequence of life cycles (Principle 22, p. 17). Similarly, cells undergo cycles of growth and replication as they repeatedly divide. A cell cycle is a mitosis-to-mitosis cycle, that is, the interval between one cell generation and the next (Fig. 4-23).

Actual nuclear division occupies only about 5% of the cell cycle; the rest of the cell's time is spent in **interphase,** the stage between nuclear divisions. For many years it was thought that interphase was a period of rest because the nucleus appeared inactive as observed with the ordinary light microscope. In the early 1950s new techniques for revealing DNA replication in nuclei were introduced at the same time that biologists came to appreciate fully the significance of DNA as the genetic material. It was then discovered that DNA replication occurred during the interphase stage. Further studies revealed that many other protein and nucleic acid components essential to normal cell growth and division were synthesized during the seemingly quiescent interphase period.

The most vital event in the cell cycle—the replication of DNA—occurs during a phase called the S period (period of synthesis). In mammalian cells in tissue culture, the S period lasts about 6 of the 18 to 24 hours required to complete one cell cycle. In this period both strands of DNA must replicate; that is, new complementary partners are synthesized for both strands so that two identical molecules are produced from the original strand. In humans each chromosome contains approximately 175 million nucleotide pairs arranged in a double helix that makes one turn for every 10 nucleotide pairs (Fig. 2-35, p. 50). At an estimated rate of DNA synthesis of approximately 6000 base pairs per minute, it would take 486 hours to complete the replication of one DNA molecule. In fact, replication is completed in 6 hours. To explain how this could happen, it was suggested that DNA replication must proceed simultaneously at numerous points of origin along the molecule. Electron micrographs of replicating DNA isolated from chromosomes have confirmed this hypothesis. At multiple points of origin, DNA relocates bidirectionally, forming replicating loops (**replicons**) that eventually unite. The result of replication is two complete DNA molecules, each carrying the same coded message as the parent molecule.

The S period is preceded and succeeded by G_1 and G_2 periods respectively (G stands for "gap"), during which no DNA synthesis is occurring. For most cells, G_1 is an important preparatory stage for the replication of DNA that follows. During G_1, transfer RNA, ribosomes, messenger RNA, and several enzymes are synthesized. During G_2, spindle and aster proteins are synthesized in preparation for chromosome separation during mitosis. G_1 is typically of longer duration than G_2, although there is much variation in different cell types. Embryonic cells divide very rapidly because there is no cell growth between divisions, only subdivision of mass. DNA synthesis may proceed a hundred times more rapidly in embryonic cells than in adult cells, and the G_1 period is almost completely omitted.

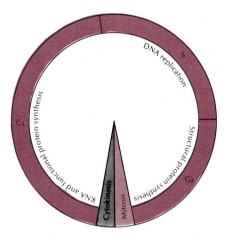

Figure 4-23

Cell cycle, showing relative duration of recognized periods. S, G_1, and G_2 are periods within interphase; S, synthesis of DNA; G_1, presynthetic period; G_2, postsynthetic period. Actual duration of the cycle and the different periods varies considerably in different cell types.

___ Flux of Cells

Cell division is important for growth, for replacement of cells lost to natural attrition and wear and tear, and for wound healing. Cell division is especially rapid during the early development of the organism. At birth the human infant has about 2 trillion cells from repeated division of a single fertilized egg. This immense number could be attained by just 42 cell divisions, with each generation dividing once every 6 to 7 days. With only five more cell divisions, the cell number would increase to approximately 60 trillion, the number of cells in a mature man weighing 75 kg. But of course no organism develops in this machinelike manner. Cell division is rapid during early embryonic development, then slows with age. Furthermore, different cell populations divide at widely different rates. In some the average period between divisions is measured in hours, whereas in others it is measured in days, months, or even years. Cells in the central nervous system stop dividing altogether after the early months of fetal development and persist without further division for the life of the individual. Muscle cells also stop dividing during the third month of fetal development, and future growth depends on enlargement of fibers already present.

In other tissues that are subject to wear and tear, lost cells must be constantly replaced. It has been estimated that in humans about 1% to 2% of all body cells—a total of 100 billion—are shed daily. Mechanical rubbing wears away the outer cells of the skin, and emotional stress can result in physical stress that affects many cells. Food in the alimentary canal rubs off lining cells, the restricted life cycle of blood corpuscles must involve enormous numbers of replacements, and during active sex life of males many millions of sperm are produced each day. Such losses of cells are made up by mitosis.

Cells undergo a senescence with aging. At some point in the life cycle of most cells, the cell substance breaks down, inert material is formed, metabolic processes slow down, and the synthetic power of enzymes decreases. These factors lead eventually to the death of the cell. In certain cases, products and secretions such as scales, feathers, and bony structures may persist after the death of the cell.

The usual constraints that operate to switch off normal cell division when tissue growth is complete are lacking in uncontrolled cancer cell growth. Whereas normal cells "know" when to stop dividing, cancer cells not only divide rapidly but also grow between divisions. Part of the current research on cancer is focused on how the cell division switch is controlled and why it becomes overridden by internal and external influences during tumor growth.

___ Summary

Cells are the basic structural and functional units of all living organisms. Cells and their highly organized components are studied by light and electron microscopy and by biochemical methods. The eukaryotic cells of animals and other higher organisms differ from the prokaryotic cells of bacteria in several respects, the most distinctive of which is the presence of a membrane-bound nucleus containing chromosomes that carry the hereditary material.

Cells are surrounded by a plasma membrane that regulates the flow of molecular traffic between the cell and its surroundings. The nucleus, enclosed by a double membrane, contains chromatin, which condenses into rodlike chromosomes during cell division, and one or more nucleoli. Outside the nuclear envelope is the cell cytoplasm, subdivided by a membranous network, the endoplasmic reticulum, which is often associated with ribosomes and probably functions in the transport of materials within the cell. Among the organelles within the cell is the Golgi complex, which functions in storage and packaging of proteins. The mitochondria are especially conspicuous organelles that contain the enzymes of oxi-

The electron microscope has contributed enormously to our understanding of cell structure and function. This electron micrograph reveals the fine structure of a vascular smooth muscle cell. (×60,000.)
Courtesy M.E. Todd.

dative energy metabolism. Lysosomes, other membrane-bound vesicles, microfilaments, and microtubules are often found in the cytoplasm. Centrioles are short cylinders of nine triplet microtubules that help organize the mitotic spindle. Cilia and flagella are hairlike, vibratile appendages associated with cell movement.

Substances can enter cells by diffusion, mediated transport, and endocytosis. Diffusion is the movement of molecules from an area of higher concentration to one of lower concentration, and osmosis is diffusion of water through a semipermeable membrane as a result of osmotic pressure. Osmotic pressure is not the same as hydrostatic pressure but is defined terms of equilibrium hydrostatic pressure. Solutes to which the membrane is impermeable require a carrier molecule to traverse it; carrier-mediated systems include facilitated transport (in the direction of a concentration gradient) and active transport (against a concentration gradient, which requires energy). Endocytosis includes bringing droplets (pinocytosis) or particles (phagocytosis) into the cell.

The capacity to grow by cell multiplication is a fundamental characteristic of living systems. Cell division includes mitosis, the division of the nuclear chromosomes, and cytokinesis, the division of the cytoplasm. Ordinary somatic cells, containing two of each kind of chromosome (and hence called diploid), replicate during mitosis and provide each daughter cell with a complete set of genetic instructions.

During interphase, before the beginning of mitosis, the chromosomal material (chromatin) divides, and the replicated chromosomes (sister chromatids) are held together by a centromere. In prophase, the first stage of mitosis, the replicated chromosomes condense into recognizable bodies. A spindle forms between the centrioles as they separate to opposite poles of the cell. At the end of prophase the nuclear envelope disintegrates. At metaphase the sister chromatids migrate to the center of the cell. At anaphase the centromeres divide and one of each kind of chromosome is pulled toward the centriole by the attached spindle fiber. At telophase the chromosomes gather in the position of the nucleus in each cell and revert to a diffuse chromatin network. The nuclear membranes reappear. Cell division is completed by separation of the cytoplasm between the daughter cells (cytokinesis). Mitosis itself is only a small part of the total cell cycle. In interphase, G_1, S, and G_2 periods are recognized, and the S period is the time when DNA is synthesized (the chromosomes are replicated).

Cells divide rapidly during embryonic development, then more slowly with age. Some cells continue to divide throughout the life of the animal to replace cells lost by attrition and wear, whereas others, such as nerve and muscle cells, complete their division during early development and never divide again.

Selected references

Avers, C.J. 1976. Cell biology. New York, D. Van Nostrand Co. *Textbook of cell structure and function; strong on organelle genetics and cytogenetics.*

DeWitt, W. 1977. Biology of the cell: an evolutionary approach. Philadelphia, W.B. Saunders Co. *An unusual cell biology text with an evolutionary perspective, dealing with life's origins and development.*

Dyson, R.D. 1978. Cell biology: a molecular approach, ed. 2. Boston, Allyn & Bacon, Inc. *Comprehensive introductory text.*

Finean, J.B., R. Coleman, and R.H. Michell. 1978. Membranes and their cellular functions. New York, John Wiley & Sons, Inc. *Primer on membrane structure and function, clearly written and imaginatively illustrated.*

Kennedy, D. 1974. Cellular and organismal biology: readings from *Scientific American.* San Francisco, W.H. Freeman & Co. Publishers. *An anthology of* Scientific American *articles on cell structure, regulation, and functional roles.*

Margolis, R.L., and L. Wilson. 1981. Microtubule treadmills: possible molecular machinery. Nature **293**:705-711. *Microtubules, the fibrous skeletal framework of eukaryotic cells, are labile structures serving several functions, including movement of chromosomes.*

Nilsson, L., and J. Linberg. 1973. Behold man. Boston, Little, Brown & Co. *Collection of superb photographs and scanning electron micrographs of organs, tissues, and embryos by an internationally recognized scientific photographer. Excellent explanatory legends accompany illustrations.*

Novikoff, A.B., and E. Holtzman. 1976. Cells and organelles, ed. 2. New York, Holt, Rinehart & Winston. *Clearly written and well-illustrated description of structure of cells and cell components and their function.*

Pfeiffer, J. 1972. The cell. New York, Time-Life Books, Inc. *Structure and function of cells with excellent picture essays.*

Sheeler, P., and D.E. Bianchi. 1980. Cell biology: structure, biochemistry, and function. New York, John Wiley & Sons, Inc. *Well-written, well-illustrated introductory cell biology textbook.*

Wolfe, S.L. 1981. Biology of the cell, ed. 2. Belmont, Calif., Wadsworth, Inc. *Attractive, up-to-date introductory textbook.*

Selected *Scientific American* articles

Albrecht-Buehler, G. 1978. The tracks of moving cells. **238**:68-76 (Apr.). *Many biological phenomena involve cell movements. A method for following cell migration in culture is described.*

Capaldi, R.A. 1974. A dynamic model of cell membranes. **230**:26-33 (Mar.). *Structure and function of the cell membrane are described.*

de Duve, C. 1963. The lysosome. **208**:64-72 (May).

Dustin, P. 1980. Microtubules. **243**:66-76 (Aug.).

Fox, C.F. 1972. The structure of cell membranes. **226**:30-38 (Feb.).

Kornberg, R.D., and A. Klug. 1981. The nucleosome. **244**:52-64 (Feb.).

Koshland, D.E., Jr. 1973. Protein shape and biological control. **229**:52-64 (Oct.). *The ability of enzymes to bend under external influences can explain how they control life processes.*

Lake, J.A. 1981. The ribosome. **245**:84-97 (Aug.). *This intracellular machine that synthesizes proteins is surprisingly complex.*

Margulis, L. 1971. Symbiosis and evolution. **225**:48-53 (Aug.). *The author offers evidence suggesting that mitochondria and chloroplasts were once independent organisms.*

Mazia, D. 1974. The cell cycle. **230**:54-64 (Jan.).

Neutra, M., and C.P. Leblond. 1969. The Golgi apparatus. **220**:100-107 (Feb.).

Porter, K.R., and J.B. Tucker. 1981. The ground substance of the living cell. **244**:56-67 (Mar.). *High-resolution electron microscopy elucidates the structure and function of microtubules in the cell.*

Racker, E. 1968. The membrane of the mitochondrion. **218**:32-39 (Feb.).

Staehelin, L.A., and B.E. Hull. 1978. Junctions between living cells. **238**:140-152 (May).

Stent, G.S. 1972. Cellular communication. **227**:42-51 (Sept.). *Cells communicate by means of hormones and nerve impulses.*

Wessells, N.K. 1971. How living cells change shape. **225**:76-82 (Oct.). *Microtubules and microfilaments act as a skeleton and muscle for the cell.*

CHAPTER 5

PHYSIOLOGY OF THE CELL

Vascular smooth muscle cell, showing the nucleus surrounded by mitochondria.
Each mitochondrion, containing the enzymes of the Krebs cycle and the
electron carriers of the respiratory chain, is the site of ATP
synthesis by oxidative phosphorylation. Mitochondria
are the powerhouses of the cell. (×30,000.)

Electron micrograph courtesy M.E. Todd.

In the protozoa all life processes occur within the borders of a single cell. In metazoans they are distributed among groups of specialized cells that have specific functions, such as nervous system coordination, digestion, and excretion, that benefit the whole organism—a "division of labor" that has contributed to the evolutionary success of multicellular animals. Nevertheless, certain activities are performed by every animal cell, whether a liver cell, a nerve cell, or a muscle cell. All cells must produce energy, synthesize their own internal structure, control much of their own activity, and guard their boundaries. In this chapter we consider these shared activities.

We start with the laws of thermodynamics and show how they apply to living systems. Then we examine ATP, the principal energy carrier in living organisms, and describe how it enables cells to perform biochemical work. Finally we introduce and trace in some detail the biochemical processes known collectively as cellular metabolism. These processes may appear intimidating at first, but there are many common themes in metabolism that are shared by all animals. The biochemical unity of living systems is an important biological principle (Principle 3, p. 11) that underscores the evolutionary kinship of life on earth.

—ENERGY AND THE LAWS OF THERMODYNAMICS

The purpose of this section is to introduce some general principles that apply to all energy exchanges in cells (Principle 2, p. 11).

The first law of thermodynamics states that energy cannot be created or destroyed. It can change from one form to another, but the total amount of energy in a system remains the same. In short, energy is conserved. Thus, if we burn gasoline in an engine, we do not create new energy but merely convert chemical energy in the gasoline to another form, in this example mechanical energy and thermal energy. The first law explains why perpetual motion machines could never work, no matter how ingeniously constructed. In such a machine energy is always transformed into heat because of friction between its parts. Measurements have shown that the amount of energy required to start the machine is precisely matched by an equivalent amount of heat lost from the machine up to the moment it stops.

Heat can be made to do work, of course, as it does in steam engines and numerous industrial applications. Living systems, however, find heat of limited application as a form of energy, although the endothermic mammals and birds use it to elevate and maintain a constant body temperature. But for the most part, heat is a useless commodity to cells because it is a nonspecific form of energy that cannot be recaptured and redistributed to power metabolic processes. Heat can do work only when there is a temperature gradient, and since all cells in an organism are at virtually the same temperature, there is no heat flow and no chance of accomplishing work.

Instead cells rely on chemical energy stored in chemical bonds. Bond energy is a form of potential energy, or energy of position, as opposed to kinetic energy, or energy of motion. Chemical bonds in organic molecules are storehouses of chemical potential energy that the cell gradually liberates and couples to a variety of energy-consuming processes.

As living oranisms convert stored energy into other forms, and eventually

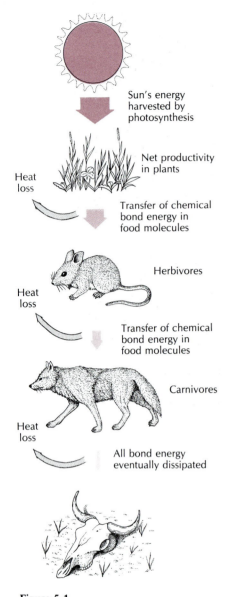

Sun's energy harvested by photosynthesis

Heat loss

Net productivity in plants

Transfer of chemical bond energy in food molecules

Herbivores

Heat loss

Transfer of chemical bond energy in food molecules

Carnivores

Heat loss

All bond energy eventually dissipated

Figure 5-1

Solar energy sustains virtually all life on earth. With each energy transfer, however, much energy is lost as heat.

into heat, less and less remains in reserve. How is it replenished? Our common experience tells us that the ultimate source of energy for life on earth is the sun. Sunlight is captured by chlorophyll molecules in green plants, which transform a portion of this energy into chemical bond energy (food energy). The energy accumulated by plants is called net productivity, and it supports all the rest of life on earth. Herbivorous animals eat plants and convert a small part of the potential chemical energy into animal tissue and a large part into heat that is invisibly dissipated into space from the earth's surface. Carnivorous animals eat the herbivores, and they in turn are eaten by other carnivores. At each step in the transfer of energy in such a food chain, a large part of the energy is lost as heat (Fig. 5-1).

At the cellular level, animals and plants use chemical energy stored in food to carry out hundreds of activities requiring energy. Thus animals are totally dependent on plants, which fortunately accumulate enough energy to sustain both themselves and the animals that feed on them. Plant photosynthesis and animal respiration are inextricably woven together in a vast cycle that is driven by the constant flux of energy from the sun.

There is yet another reason why living organisms require constant replenishment of energy from the outside, and this reason is expressed in the second law of thermodynamics: all energy of the universe is steadily moving toward increasing disorder and randomness. In effect, all forms of energy will inevitably be degraded to heat. In thermodynamics, disorder or randomness is termed entropy and is given the symbol S. Since entropy (disorder) increases in any given system (Fig. 5-2), the change in entropy (ΔS) is positive.

If this is true, do not living systems disobey the second law by increasing the molecular orderliness of their structure? Certainly an organism becomes vastly more complex during its development from fertilized egg to adult. But the process of growth and maintenance is achieved by breaking down complex food molecules into simple inorganic waste products. In other words, an animal increases the entropy of its food while growing or maintaining a constant body weight. If we balance the increase in complexity of the adult against the increase in entropy of waste products, we find that the total yield is greater disorder as predicted by the second law. Even the orderly structure of the individual is not permanent but will be dissipated when the animal dies.

The evolution of life forms seems at first to present a more difficult problem. Has not evolution over the ages seen the appearance of life forms of ever-increasing complexity and order and requiring ever more energy for their sustenance? Does evolution disprove the second law of thermodynamics? Or does the second law disprove evolution? (The argument that all forms of evolution violate the second law is a favorite of creationists. Evolution proceeds from randomness to order; entropy proceeds from order to randomness. How, ask the creationists, can evolution defy the randomizing force of the second law?)

There is an answer to this conundrum. The second law of thermodynamics applies to closed systems that no new energy can enter. The sun–earth–outer space system as a whole is closed in this sense and is trending toward increasing entropy in accordance with the second law. But the biosphere is an open system. Life on earth, by capturing the continuous flow of solar energy within the system, remains as a steady-state system of high internal order that opposes the tendency for entropic decay, at least for the period of time that life exists on earth. Hence evolution is possible and, of course, has been and is occurring. But life on earth is

Figure 5-2

Diffusion of solute through a solution, an example of entropy.

on borrowed time. In the end, and happily at a point in time far beyond our brief walk upon this flowering earth, the sun will die and so will life on earth.

In thermodynamic terms, what we have just said can be summarized as

$$\Delta S_{system} + \Delta S_{surroundings} > 0$$

Note that it is possible for the entropy of a system (such as living systems on earth) to *decrease* provided that it is more than offset by an *increase* in entropy of the surroundings (such as the sun and outer space). This also applies to biological reactions within cells.

Rather than trying to measure entropy changes in biochemical reactions, biochemists use the concept of **free energy**, contributed by the nineteenth-century American physicist Josiah W. Gibbs. **Gibbs free energy change** is a combination of the first and second laws of thermodynamics. The symbol for free energy is G, and change in free energy is designated ΔG. Changes in free energy are related by the equation

$$\Delta G = \Delta H - T\Delta S$$

where H is heat (also called enthalpy) taken up or given off by a reaction, T is absolute temperature ($-273.16°$ C), and S is entropy. T is introduced in the equation because entropy increases with increasing temperature. Free energy is the energy available for doing work. If we rearrange the equation as

$$\Delta H = \Delta G + T\Delta S$$

it becomes easier to relate to living systems. If T is held constant and the reaction produces no change in temperature (ΔH = 0), we see that in any **spontaneous** (downhill) reaction, ΔS is always positive and ΔG is always negative. Thus, free energy, the energy available in a system to do work, always declines. The great majority of reactions in cells result in a loss of free energy and are said to be **exergonic** (ΔG < 0). Such reactions proceed downhill and are spontaneous. However, some important reactions in cells can proceed toward a condition of decreasing entropy (ΔS > 0; increasing order) and require the addition of free energy. Such "uphill" reactions are termed **endergonic.** Thus, chemical reactions in cells may be either exergonic processes that proceed spontaneously with loss of free energy, or endergonic processes that have to be pushed uphill because the reactants end up with more free energy than they started with. Such reactions are important because many biosynthetic and active transport processes require the input of energy to proceed. However, in uphill reactions there is still an *overall* loss of free energy (increase in entropy) even though the reactant gains energy. If you carry a stone up a hill, you have performed an endergonic "reaction" because the stone contains more energy (potential energy of position) at the top of the hill than at the bottom. In this case, where did the energy to move the stone come from and in what form was it?

We have seen that the laws of thermodynamics do apply to living systems. The first law informs us that energy can be stored and that it is never "lost," although it may change form. The second law reminds us that all energy must eventually become totally randomized. But in becoming more random it may be made to perform work. Living systems gather energy from the environment, use it to do cellular work of metabolism, active transport, and motion, and then return it to the environment in less useful form. ATP is the ubiquitous energy-rich intermediate used by life forms to power "uphill" reactions of cellular synthesis.

CHEMICAL ENERGY TRANSFER BY ATP

As a rule, endergonic reactions in the cell are **coupled reactions** in which the nucleotide ATP transfers chemical energy from a molecule of relatively high energy content to a molecule of lower energy content. ATP is the intermediate in coupled reactions.

The ATP molecule consists of adenosine (the purine adenine and the 5-carbon sugar ribose) and a triphosphate group (Fig. 5-3). Most of the free energy in ATP resides in the triphosphate group, especially in two **phosphoanhydride bonds** between the three phosphate groups. These two bonds are called **high-energy bonds** because a great deal of free energy in the bonds is liberated when ATP is hydrolyzed to adenosine diphosphate (ADP) and inorganic phosphate. The high-energy groups in ATP are designated by the "tilde" symbol $\sim$. A high-energy phosphate bond is shown as $\sim$P and a low-energy bond (such as the bond linking the triphosphate group to adenosine) as —P. ATP may be symbolized as A—P $\sim$ P $\sim$ P and ADP as A—P $\sim$ P.

The hydrolysis of ATP to ADP liberates about 7.3 kcal of free energy per mole of ATP. Where does this energy go? Suppose that two compounds, X and Y, are condensed in an endergonic reaction that requires 2.5 kcal per mole; that is, the product XY contains 2.5 kcal more energy than did the compounds X and Y. Such a reaction could never occur spontaneously. However, ATP can drive this reaction as follows:

$$X + ATP \rightleftharpoons X{-}P + ADP \quad \Delta G = -3.0 \text{ kcal/mole}$$

The free energy loss in this phosphate transfer is 3.0 kcal, but X—P is now a "charged" molecule that is able to condense with Y as

$$X{-}P + Y \rightleftharpoons XY + P \quad \Delta G = -1.8 \text{ kcal/mole}$$

Again there has been a free energy loss in the reaction, this time 1.8 kcal. The total free energy loss of both reactions is 4.8 kcal. But ATP contributed more energy than this—7.3 kcal—at the start of the reaction sequence. If we balance the total reaction, we find that the sum of the free energy changes of the parent reactions is equal to the total free energy loss required to condense X and Y.

$$
\begin{array}{ll}
ATP + H_2O \rightleftharpoons ADP + P & \Delta G = -7.3 \text{ kcal/mole} \\
X + Y \rightleftharpoons XY & \underline{\Delta G = +2.5 \text{ kcal/mole}} \\
& \text{Total} = -4.8 \text{ kcal/mole}
\end{array}
$$

An endergonic reaction has occurred. In making this condensation happen, ATP has given up energy (becoming ADP), and compound X has received enough energy to enable the condensation reaction to proceed.

Next we must determine where ATP got its bond energy in the first place. When ATP donates its phosphate to a phosphate acceptor, ADP is formed. ADP is reconverted to ATP when it accepts a phosphate from a high-energy compound. The cycle between ADP and ATP can be shown as

$$ATP + H_2O \rightleftharpoons ADP + P + H^+$$

with a free energy change of 7.3 kcal. The reaction is reversible as symbolized by the bidirectional arrows. In the cell the shuttle between ADP and ATP participates in almost all phosphate transfers. Now we are in a position to understand how ATP couples reactions. It begins when ADP accepts a phosphate from a higher-energy phosphate compound and is converted to ATP. This higher-energy compound is commonly called a **fuel**, and it is significant that the phosphate bonds of

A calorie (cal) is the amount of heat required to heat 1 g of water from 14.5° to 15.5° C. One kilocalorie (kcal) = 1000 cal. Although the calorie is almost universally used in books and tables, it is no longer a part of the recently adopted International System of Units (SI system). The unit of energy in the SI system is the joule (J), defined as 4.184 J = 1 cal.

Figure 5-3

Adenosine triphosphate (ATP).

Adenine

Triphosphate

Ribose

several phosphorylated fuels contain more bond energy than ATP. Once ATP is formed, it delivers its terminal phosphate group to a phosphate acceptor. In the example above, the acceptor was compound X. Thus ATP couples the condensation reaction of $X + Y \rightleftharpoons XY$ with the dephosphorylation of the fuel substrate. If we call the fuel W, we can show the reaction as

$$W \sim P \quad ADP \quad X - P$$
$$W \quad ATP \quad X$$

X—P now has sufficient energy to complete the condensation reaction.

It should be emphasized that ATP is an energy-coupling molecule, *not a fuel*. The amount of ATP produced in respiration is totally dependent on its rate of utilization. In other words, ATP is produced by one set of reactions and immediately consumed by another. For example, ATP formed from the oxidation of glucose is used to synthesize proteins or lipids or to provide power for some other process, such as the contraction of skeletal muscles (Fig. 5-4). Living organisms do not produce and put aside vast amounts of ATP, hoarded against some future energy need. What they store is the fuel itself, in the form of carbohydrate and lipids especially. The turnover of ATP is so rapid, even in the "resting" cell, that the ATP molecule is consumed within a minute of its formation. The average human uses up about 40 kg of ATP each day, and much more during strenuous activity. ATP is formed as it is needed, primarily by oxidative processes in the mitochondria. Oxygen is not consumed unless ADP and phosphate molecules are available, and do not become available until ATP is hydrolyzed by some energy-consuming process. *Metabolism is therefore mostly self-regulating.*

Although ATP is crucial as an energy-coupling agent, certain other phosphorylated compounds have even higher bond energy, as mentioned previously. One of particular interest is creatine phosphate (Fig. 5-5). Creatine phosphate contains more available bond energy than ATP (about 10.3 kcal/mole as compared with 7.3 kcal/mole for ATP) and, unlike ATP, it is especially adapted for storage. Creatine phosphate is found in muscle and nerve cells; in muscle it can provide instant power for the rapid phosphorylation of ADP to form ATP to meet sudden energy needs. There is enough creatine phosphate in muscle for several minutes of muscle contraction. Creatine phosphate is found in all chordates and a few invertebrate groups (notably annelids and ophiuroid echinoderms). Most other invertebrates have a different phosphate storage compound, arginine phosphate.

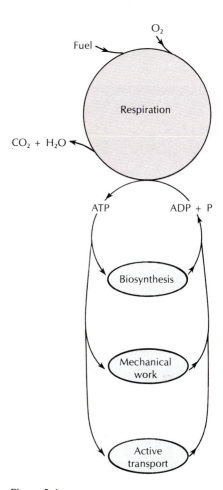

Figure 5-4

Production, use, and recycling of ATP in living systems.

Figure 5-5

Creatine phosphate.

___CELLULAR METABOLISM

Cellular metabolism refers to the collective total of chemical processes that occur within living cells. It is often called **intermediary metabolism** because the exchange of matter and energy between the cell and its environment proceeds in a stepwise manner through chemical pathways composed of numerous intermediates, or **metabolites.** Although intermediary metabolism appears hopelessly complex as depicted in detailed metabolic charts that often grace the walls of biochemists' laboratories, the central metabolic routes through which matter and energy are channeled are not difficult to understand. Biochemists are vastly furthered in their research by the fact that the same kinds of reaction sequences in metabolism occur in a great variety of life forms, from bacteria to humans.

Animal cells tap the stored energy of organic fuels (for example, simple sugars, fatty acids, and amino acids) through a series of controlled degradative steps. This process commonly makes use of molecular oxygen from the atmosphere. In return animal cells give off carbon dioxide as an end product, which is used by plant cells in making glucose and the more complex molecules. In this way the cellular energy cycle of life involves the harnessing of sunlight energy by green plants directly and by animal cells indirectly.

___Respiration: Generating ATP in the Presence of Oxygen

How electron transport is used to trap chemical bond energy

Having seen that ATP is the one common energy denominator by which all cellular machines are powered, we are in a position to ask how this energy is captured from fuel substrates. This question directs us to an important generalization: *all cells obtain their chemical energy requirements from oxidation-reduction reactions.* This means simply that in the degradation of fuel molecules, hydrogen atoms (electrons and protons) are passed from reducing agents to oxidizing agents with a release of energy. A portion of this energy is trapped and used to form the high-energy bonds of ATP. The release of energy during electron transfer and its conservation as ATP is the mainspring of cell activity and was a crucial evolutionary achievement.

Before we consider the important oxidation-reduction reactions in more detail, let us see what happens when a fuel molecule is degraded to liberate its free (chemical bond) energy. If we completely burn 1 mole (180 g) of glucose in a bomb calorimeter to carbon dioxide and water, we can show the combustion as

$$C_6H_{12}O_6 + 6\ O_2 \rightarrow 6\ CO_2 + 6\ H_2O \quad \Delta G = -686\ kcal$$

Burned in this way, all of the 686 kcal (686,000 calories) of free energy locked up in the structure of the glucose molecule is released as 686 kcal of heat. But in cell respiration a significant portion of this free energy is channeled into useful chemical energy as ATP. Thus, in the cell the reaction can be summarized as

$$C_6H_{12}O_6 + 38\ P + 38\ ADP + 6\ O_2 \rightarrow$$
$$6\ CO_2 + 6\ H_2O + 38\ ATP \quad \Delta G = -409\ kcal\ (as\ heat)$$

The difference between the 409 kcal lost as heat and the original 686 kcal of free energy in glucose is 277 kcal in 38 moles of ATP (about 7.3 kcal/mole). The passing of this free energy to ATP is accomplished, as we have already suggested, by electron transfer. Chemical energy is liberated when electrons are transferred from one compound to another.

Because they are so important, and to avoid later confusion, let us consider what we mean by oxidation-reduction ("redox") reactions. In these reactions there is a transfer of electrons from an electron donor (the reducing agent) to an electron acceptor (the oxidizing agent). As soon as the electron donor loses its electrons, it becomes oxidized. As soon as the electron acceptor accepts electrons, it becomes reduced. In other words, a reducing agent becomes oxidized when it reduces another compound, and an oxidizing agent becomes reduced when it oxidizes another compound. Thus, for every oxidation there must be a corresponding reduction.

In an oxidation-reduction reaction the electron donor and electron acceptor form a redox pair:

$$\text{Electron donor} \rightleftharpoons e^- + \text{Electron acceptor}$$
$$\text{(reducing agent)} \qquad \text{(oxidizing agent)}$$

When electrons are accepted by the oxidizing agent, energy is liberated because the electrons move to a more stable position. The *amount* of free energy liberated depends on the difference in tendency of the two compounds to donate electrons. This is termed their **electron pressure.** In the cell, electrons move from compounds of high electron pressure to compounds of lower electron pressure. By transferring electrons stepwise in this manner, energy is gradually released, and a maximum yield of ATP is realized.

Aerobic versus anaerobic metabolism

Ultimately, the electrons are transferred to a **final electron acceptor.** The nature of this final acceptor is the key that determines the overall efficiency of cellular metabolism. The heterotrophs can be divided into two great groups: **aerobes,** those that use molecular oxygen as the final electron acceptor, and **anaerobes,** those that employ some other molecule as the final electron acceptor.

Because humans and all of the other animals with which we are most familiar depend on oxygen, it may seem surprising that many primitive organisms live successfully under oxygen-free conditions. But we must recall that life on earth had its origins under reducing conditions; there was no oxygen in the primitive atmosphere for perhaps the first billion years of life on the primeval earth. During this formative period, the basic pattern of cellular metabolism evolved under strictly anaerobic conditions. Only later, as evolving photosynthetic organisms began to produce oxygen, did metabolic reactions appear in which the generation of ATP was coupled to the use of oxygen.

Today most animals use oxygen to generate high-energy phosphate. Strictly anaerobic organisms still exist and indeed occupy some important ecological niches. These organisms for the most part are bacteria that are restricted to the relatively few oxygen-free environments that remain on earth. Although some organisms are facultatively anaerobic, for the majority of animals oxygen is a necessity of life. Evolution has favored aerobic metabolism, not only because oxygen became available, but also because aerobic metabolism is vastly more efficient than anaerobic metabolism. In the absence of oxygen, only a very small fraction of the bond energy present in foodstuffs can be released. For example, when an anaerobic microorganism degrades glucose, the final electron acceptor (such as pyruvic acid) still contains most of the energy of the original glucose

Figure 5-6

Overview of respiration, showing the three stages in the complete oxidation of food molecules to carbon dioxide and water.

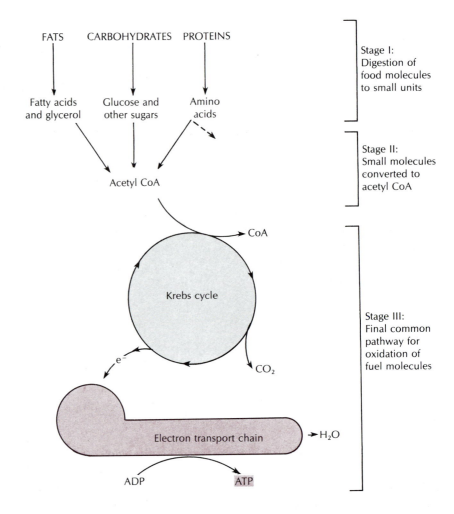

molecule. On the other hand, an aerobic organism, using oxygen as the final electron acceptor, can completely oxidize glucose to carbon dioxide and water. Almost 20 times as much energy is released when glucose is completely oxidized as when it is degraded only to the stage of lactic acid. An obvious advantage of aerobic metabolism is that a much smaller quantity of foodstuff is required to maintain a given rate of metabolism.

General description of respiration

Aerobic metabolism is more familiarly known as true **cellular respiration, defined as the oxidation of fuel molecules with molecular oxygen as the final electron acceptor.** As mentioned previously, the oxidation of fuel molecules describes the *removal of electrons* and *not* the direct combination of molecular oxygen with fuel molecules. Let us look at this process in general before considering it in more detail.

Hans Krebs, the British biochemist who contributed so much to our understanding of respiration, described three stages in the complete oxidation of fuel molecules to carbon dioxide and water (Fig. 5-6). In stage I, foodstuffs are digested into small molecules that can be absorbed into the circulation. There is no useful energy yield during digestion, which is discussed in Chapter 31. In stage II, most of the degraded foodstuffs are converted into a 2-carbon acetyl group, acetyl coenzyme A. This stage occurs in the cytosol. Some ATP is generated in stage II,

Figure 5-7

Phosphorylation of glucose.

but the yield is small compared with that obtained in the final stage of respiration. In stage III the final oxidation of fuel molecules occurs, with a large yield of ATP. This stage takes place in the mitochondria. Acetyl coenzyme A is channeled into the Krebs cycle where the acetyl group is completely oxidized to carbon dioxide. Electrons released from the acetyl groups are transferred to special carriers that pass them to electron acceptor compounds in the electron transport chain. At the end of the chain the electrons (and the protons accompanying them) are accepted by molecular oxygen to form water.

Glycolysis

We begin our journey through the stages of respiration with glycolysis, a nearly universal pathway in living organisms that converts glucose into pyruvic acid. In a series of reactions, glucose and other 6-carbon monosaccharides are split into 3-carbon fragments, pyruvic acid. Pyruvic acid is then enzymatically stripped of carbon dioxide to form acetyl coenzyme A. A single oxidation occurs during glycolysis, and each molecule of glucose yields 2 molecules of ATP.

The metabolism of glucose begins with its phosphorylation by ATP to form **glucose-6-phosphate.** Glucose-6-phosphate is an important intermediate because it is a stem compound that can lead into any of several metabolic pathways. However, the predominant metabolic fate for glucose-6-phosphate is entry into the glycolytic sequence. The glucose-6-phosphate is then rearranged at the expense of another molecule of ATP to form **fructose-1,6-diphosphate** (Fig. 5-7). The fuel has now been "primed" with phosphate groups and is sufficiently reactive to enable subsequent reactions to proceed. Obviously, the fuel molecule must release more energy—it eventually provides *much* more energy—than is loaned to it by ATP at the start. This is a kind of deficit financing that is required for an ultimate energy return many times greater than the original energy investment.

Fructose-1,6-diphosphate is next cleaved into two 3-carbon sugars, called **triose phosphates** (Fig. 5-8). These high-energy derivatives of glucose are then oxidized (the electrons are removed) in an important energy-yielding step. The electrons removed are accepted by **nicotinamide adenine dinucleotide** (NAD), a derivative of the vitamin niacin. NAD serves as a carrier molecule to convey high-energy electrons to the final electron transport chain. NAD and its reduced form NADH exist as a redox pair:

$$\text{Reduced substrate} + NAD^+ \rightleftharpoons NADH + H^+ + \text{Oxidized substrate}$$

In this oxidation, NAD^+ accepts a hydrogen ion and two electrons to form NADH. The remaining proton is released as free H^+ in the medium. This transfer produces a structural change in NAD having a free energy change of about -52 kcal/mole. This is a very large proportion of the total free energy available from the oxidation of glucose (686 kcal). As we shall see, several more molecules of

Figure 5-8

Glycolysis. Glucose is phosphorylated in two steps and raised to a
higher energy level. High-energy
fructose-1,6-diphosphate is split into
triose phosphates that are oxidized
exergonically to pyruvic acid, yielding ATP and NADH.

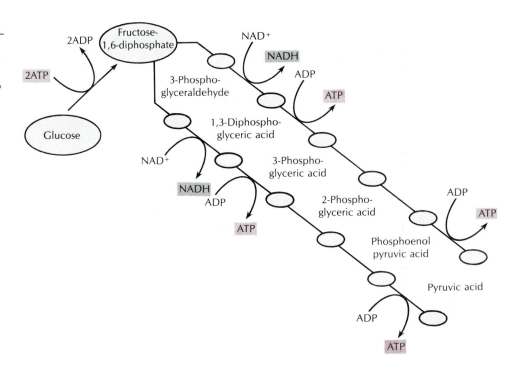

reduced NAD are formed as glucose oxidation proceeds. Altogether about 75% of
the free energy in glucose is transferred to NAD. This reduced NAD and the free
energy it contains are eventually used to synthesize ATP in the electron transport
chain.

The two triose phosphates next enter a four-step reaction sequence ending
with the formation of 2 molecules of pyruvic acid (Fig. 5-8). In two of these steps,
each molecule of triose phosphate yields a molecule of ATP. In other words, each
triose phosphate yields 2 ATP molecules, and since there are 2 triose phosphate
molecules, 4 ATP molecules are generated. Recalling that 2 ATP molecules were
used to prime the glucose initially, the net yield up to this point is 2 ATP molecules.

Acetyl coenzyme A: strategic intermediate in respiration

In aerobic metabolism the 2 molecules of pyruvic acid formed during glycolysis
enter the mitochondrion. Once inside, each pyruvic acid molecule is oxidized and
the 2 electrons are accepted by NAD^+ to form NADH. In the same reaction the
third carbon of pyruvic acid is released as carbon dioxide. This allows the 2-
carbon residue from pyruvic acid to condense with coenzyme A to form acetyl
coenzyme A (Fig. 5-9).

Acetyl coenzyme A is a critically important compound. Some two thirds of
all the carbon atoms in foods eaten by animals appear as acetyl coenzyme A at
some stage. It is the final oxidation of acetyl coenzyme A that provides energized
electrons used to generate ATP. Acetyl coenzyme A is also the source of nearly all
the carbon atoms found in the body's fats. A part of the molecule is a coenzyme
containing the vitamin **pantothenic acid,** another example of how vitamins play
important structural roles in critical cellular functions.

Figure 5-9

Formation of acetyl coenzyme A from
pyruvic acid.

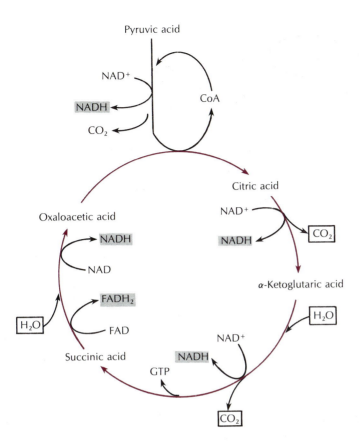

Figure 5-10

Krebs cycle in outline form showing the production of reduced NAD, reduced FAD, guanosine triphosphate (GTP), and carbon dioxide.

Krebs cycle: oxidation of acetyl coenzyme A

The degradation (oxidation) of the 2-carbon acetyl group of acetyl coenzyme A occurs in a cyclic sequence called the Krebs cycle (Fig. 5-10) in honor of Sir Hans A. Krebs, who worked out the sequence in the 1930s. The cycle is also often referred to as the tricarboxylic acid (TCA) cycle or the citric acid cycle. The reactions in this final common pathway for the oxidation of fuel molecules occur in the matrix of the mitochondrion (see Fig. 5-13). Fuel molecules that enter the cycle as acetyl coenzyme A are first condensed with 4-carbon oxaloacetic acid to form 6-carbon citric acid. Coenzyme A then recycles to pick up another acetyl group, thus repeatedly transferring acetyl groups from pyruvic acid to oxaloacetic acid. Citric acid is then degraded through a series of reactions that end in the regeneration of oxaloacetic acid. The 2 carbon atoms that enter the cycle as acetyl coenzyme A leave the cycle as 2 molecules of carbon dioxide.

As the acetyl group is oxidized, carbon atom by carbon atom, three pairs of electrons are transferred to NAD^+ and one pair to flavine adenine dinucleotide (FAD), an electron carrier that functions like NAD. Thus, with each completion of the Krebs cycle, 8 hydrogen atoms are removed in pairs by the electron carriers NAD and FAD. These reduced electron carriers are subsequently oxidized by the electron transport chain, where the electron energy is used to generate ATP. The 2 molecules of carbon dioxide diffuse out of the mitochondrion and into the circulation to be finally eliminated via the respiratory system. At another point in the cycle a molecule of guanosine triphosphate (GTP) is formed; its high-energy phosphate is readily transferred to ADP to form ATP. It is noteworthy that this is the only place in the Krebs cycle where ATP is formed *directly*. All the remaining energy is transferred to the electron transport chain.

Figure 5-11

Representation of a section of mitochondrion as seen through a high-resolution electron microscope, showing the inner membrane spheres where ATP is generated. The density of the spheres is actually many times greater than depicted.

A prosthetic group is a nonpolypeptide unit, tightly bound to a protein, that is essential to the protein's activity. Many enzymes have prosthetic groups.

Electron transport chain

The transfer of electrons from reduced NAD and FAD to the final electron acceptor, molecular oxygen, is accomplished in an elaborate electron transport chain. The function of this chain is to permit the controlled release of free energy to drive the synthesis of ATP. At three points along the chain, ATP production occurs by the phosphorylation of ADP. This method of energy capture is called oxidative phosphorylation because the formation of high-energy phosphate is coupled to oxygen consumption, and this depends on the demand for ATP by other metabolic activities within the cell. The actual *mechanism* of ATP formation by oxidative phosphorylation is not known with certainty; we can only say that the transfer of electrons does something that is translated into the production of high-energy phosphate bonds. Currently, the most widely accepted explanation of this mechanism is the chemiosmotic coupling theory (Hinkle and McCarty, 1978), described later in the chapter.

Localization and function of electron carriers

Oxidative phosphorylation, a complex process, would be unable to function efficiently, if at all, were the enzymes just floating freely in the cytoplasm of the cell. There is now abundant evidence that the oxidative enzymes and electron carriers are arranged in a highly ordered state on the inner membranes of the mitochondria.

Remember that mitochondria are composed of two membranes. The outside membrane forms a smooth sac enclosing the inner membrane, which is turned into numerous ridges called **cristae.** The inner membrane is studded with enormous numbers of minute, stalked particles called **inner membrane spheres.** The electron carriers of the respiratory chain are restricted to the inner membrane where, presumably, they are located on the inner membrane spheres. An artist's rendering of a section of mitochondrion as it might appear under the high-resolution electron microscope is shown in Fig. 5-11.

Electrons are transported from NADH to oxygen through a series of electron carriers (Fig. 5-12). These are, in their order in the chain, **flavin mononucleotide** (FMN), the prosthetic group of a protein (flavoprotein); **coenzyme Q,** a nonprotein chemically related to vitamin K; and a series of **cytochromes,** all proteins containing a heme prosthetic group and similar in structure to hemoglobin of vertebrate red blood cells. The step-by-step transfer of electrons down this chain happens because each successive enzyme has a lower electron pressure than its predecessor. With each step a portion of the energy is lost as heat, but the rest of the energy is conserved in the molecules of ATP formed during the electron transfer. Only the last member of the chain, cytochrome a-a$_3$ (also called cytochrome oxidase) can transfer its electrons to oxygen. Thus, the 2 electrons from NADH pass through an electron cascade, a series of discrete steps that permits the gradual harvesting of electron energy.

The advantage of an electron cascade becomes apparent when we compare the free energy present in NADH (53 kcal/mole) with the energy required to synthesize ATP from ADP. The formation of ATP requires at least 7.3 kcal/mole, the energy necessary for the hydrolysis of ATP. Clearly, there is enough energy in NADH to form several molecules of ATP. Since all exergonic energy transfers are accompanied by loss of free energy, it would be impossible to realize the theoret-

Figure 5-12

Electron transport chain. Electrons are transferred from one carrier to the next, terminating with molecular oxygen to form water. A carrier is reduced by accepting electrons and then is reoxidized by donating electrons to the next carrier. ATP is generated at three points in the chain. These electron carriers are located in the inner membrane of mitochondria.

Hydrogen ions are pumped across inner membrane as electrons flow down electron transport chain

Figure 5-13

Mitchell's hypothesis for pumping hydrogen ions from matrix to intermembrane space of mitochondrion.
Modified from Stryer, L. 1981. Biochemistry, ed. 2. San Francisco, W.H. Freeman & Co. Publishers.

ical ATP harvest of 7 ATP molecules (52 divided by 7.3). In fact there are three sites along the respiratory chain where there is enough free energy *change* (9 to 10 kcal/mole) to make ATP synthesis possible. These sites are shown in Fig. 5-12. Thus, the oxidation of NADH yields 3 ATP molecules. The other electron carrier bringing energy from the Krebs cycle is $FADH_2$. It enters the electron transport chain at coenzyme Q, which is at a lower energy level in the sequence and so yields only 2 ATP molecules.

Coupling mechanisms for ATP synthesis

How is the oxidation of NADH coupled to ATP synthesis? This question has been intensively investigated. The currently favored hypothesis, now supported by a wealth of evidence, is the **chemiosmotic mechanism** first proposed by the British biochemist Peter Mitchell in 1961. The model states that ATP synthesis is driven by a gradient of hydrogen ions created by the energy released during electron transport. The mechanism is easiest to understand if it is divided into two broad parts: (1) establishing the hydrogen ion gradient, and (2) synthesis of ATP.

There is abundant evidence that the transport of electrons through the respiratory chain results in the pumping of hydrogen ions from the mitochondrial matrix to the intermembrane space between the outer and inner mitochondrial membranes (Fig. 5-13). The electron transport carriers are located *in* the inner

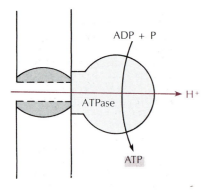

Figure 5-14

Tentative mechanism for generating ATP in mitochondrion inner membrane spheres.

Modified from Hinkle, P.C., and R.E. McCarty. 1978. Sci. Am. **238:**104-123.

membrane. Each pair of electrons donated to the respiratory chain by NADH produces three pairs of hydrogen ions, which are ejected to the intermembrane space by enzymatic transfer. Because NADH carries only 1 hydrogen, the additional hydrogen ions are absorbed from the matrix as the electrons flow down the respiratory chain. At the end of the chain an additional 2 hydrogen ions are removed from the matrix and combined with one half of an oxygen molecule to form H_2O. Thus the hydrogen ion concentration increases in the intermembrane compartment and a membrane potential is created, with the intermembrane side positive. The model also postulates that the electron carriers are very precisely positioned in the inner membrane so that hydrogen ions can move in *only* one direction, from inside to outside. Furthermore, the inner membrane must be impermeable to hydrogen ions to prevent the hydrogen gradient from running down as fast as it is created.

The hydrogen gradient is believed to drive the synthesis of ATP in an **ATP synthesis complex** that consists of two parts. High-resolution electron micrographs of the inner mitochondrial membrane show it to be studded on the matrix side with numerous spherical projections (Fig. 5-14). These contain **adenosine triphosphatase** (ATPase), an enzyme capable of catalyzing the formation of ATP from ADP and inorganic phosphate. The other portion of the complex consists of a channel in the inner membrane lying directly beneath the spherical projections. Through these channels hydrogen ions can approach from the intermembrane compartment to the active enzyme site in the spheres. The hydrogen ions flowing into this channel, following an osmotic gradient, interact with ATPase and its substrates at the active site, resulting in the synthesis of ATP. These are the major features of the hypothesis for which Mitchell received the Nobel Prize in 1978. As with any hypothesis of such complexity, and dealing with elements that cannot be seen but must be measured indirectly by ingenious experiments, certain details remain controversial. At first largely rejected by the scientific community that now embraces it, the model is a brilliant example of deductive biochemistry.

Efficiency of oxidative phosphorylation

We are now in a position to calculate the ATP yield from the complete oxidation of glucose (Fig. 5-15). The overall reaction is:

$$\text{Glucose} + 36\ \text{ADP} + 36\ \text{P} + 6\ O_2 \rightarrow 6\ CO_2 + 36\ \text{ATP} + 6\ H_2O$$

ATP has been generated at several points along the way. First of all, 2 ATP molecules were used to phosphorylate glucose in the initial priming reaction. Then 4 ATP molecules were produced during glycolysis. Two more high-energy bonds were formed directly in the Krebs cycle as GTP. The greatest harvest of ATP occurred during oxidative phosphorylation when NADH and $FADH_2$ yielded their electrons to the respiratory chain. Two NADH molecules were formed during glycolysis; each yields 2 ATP for a total of 4 ATP. Two more NADH appeared when pyruvic acid was decarboxylated to acetyl coenzyme A; each yields 3 ATP for a total of 6 ATP. Two $FADH_2$ formed in the Krebs cycle yield 2 ATP each, a total of 4 ATP. And finally, 6 NADH formed in the Krebs cycle yield 3 ATP each for a total of 18 ATP. The net yield is 36 ATP. (Note that 38 ATP were produced but that 2 ATP were used up in the initial glucose phosphorylation.)

The free energy yield from glucose is 686 kcal/mole. The free energy stored in the net yield of 36 ATP is 263 kcal/mole. Thus, the thermodynamic efficiency of ATP formation is $^{263}/_{686}$, or 38.3%.

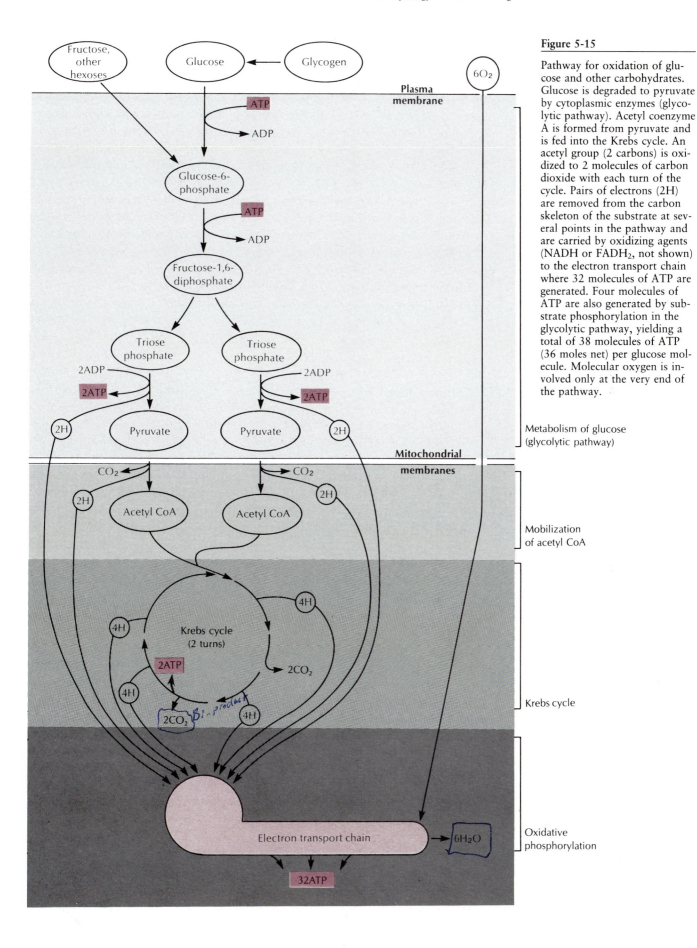

Figure 5-15

Pathway for oxidation of glucose and other carbohydrates. Glucose is degraded to pyruvate by cytoplasmic enzymes (glycolytic pathway). Acetyl coenzyme A is formed from pyruvate and is fed into the Krebs cycle. An acetyl group (2 carbons) is oxidized to 2 molecules of carbon dioxide with each turn of the cycle. Pairs of electrons (2H) are removed from the carbon skeleton of the substrate at several points in the pathway and are carried by oxidizing agents (NADH or FADH$_2$, not shown) to the electron transport chain where 32 molecules of ATP are generated. Four molecules of ATP are also generated by substrate phosphorylation in the glycolytic pathway, yielding a total of 38 molecules of ATP (36 moles net) per glucose molecule. Molecular oxygen is involved only at the very end of the pathway.

Metabolism of glucose (glycolytic pathway)

Mobilization of acetyl CoA

Krebs cycle

Oxidative phosphorylation

We must note, however, that energy yield calculations are not nearly as precise as our neat figures suggest. The free energy change for the hydrolysis of ATP rises as the concentration of reactants and products is reduced. So the efficiency for the total oxidation of glucose could be higher than 38%. On the other hand, the stated yield of 3 ATP molecules for every NADH molecule entering the electron transport chain was never better than an approximation because it was difficult to measure the true energy cost of making the process work. Recent studies (Hinkle and McCarty, 1978) suggest that only about 2 ATP molecules are synthesized per electron pair. The energy loss is believed to be due to the cost of concentrating ADP in the mitochondria and of moving ATP back out of the mitochondria as it is formed. If these values are correct, the ATP yield for the complete oxidation of glucose should be revised sharply downward from 36 molecules of ATP per molecule of glucose to about 25. Still, the overall efficiency of glucose oxidation would be about 27%, comparing favorably with human-designed energy conversion systems, which seldom exceed 5% to 10% efficiency.

Anaerobic Glycolysis: Generating ATP without Oxygen

Up to this point we have been describing aerobic metabolism, or respiration. The complete oxidation of glucose involves the formation of pyruvate by cytoplasmic enzymes followed by the oxidation of pyruvate in the mitochondria. It is in the latter, mitochondrial stage of respiration that the energies of electrons are tapped and used to generate ATP by oxidative phosphorylation. The important feature of aerobic metabolism is that oxygen is the final electron acceptor, and the complete oxidation of fuel substrates is possible only in the presence of oxygen.

We will now consider how animals generate ATP without oxygen, that is, anaerobically. Anaerobic organisms break down carbon compounds by **fermentation,** an ancient metabolic device for obtaining energy in an atmosphere devoid of oxygen. The term "fermentation," meaning "cause to rise," was originally used to describe the action of yeasts that break down glucose into alcohol (ethanol) and carbon dioxide, end products that long ago created occupations for both brewers and bakers. Alcohol (or in animals, lactic acid) is the major end product of **glycolytic fermentation,** or simply **anaerobic glycolysis,** defined as the anaerobic degradation of glucose to yield a reduced end product not requiring molecular oxygen.

In anaerobic glycolysis, glucose and other 6-carbon sugars are first broken down stepwise to a pair of 3-carbon pyruvic acid molecules, yielding 2 molecules of ATP and 2 atoms of hydrogen. This pathway, shown in Fig. 5-16, is precisely the same glycolytic pathway that in aerobic metabolism directs glucose into the Krebs cycle (compare Fig. 5-15 with Fig. 5-16). But in the absence of molecular oxygen, further oxidation of pyruvic acid cannot occur. Both pyruvic acid and carrier-bound hydrogen accumulate in the cytoplasm because neither can proceed in oxidative channels without oxygen. The problem is neatly solved by the formation of lactic acid from pyruvic acid. Pyruvate becomes the final electron acceptor and lactate the end product of anaerobic glycolysis.

Anaerobic glycolysis is a primitive and inefficient metabolic pathway that yields only 2 moles of ATP per mole of glucose; by comparison oxidative phosphorylation nets 36 moles. Despite its inefficiency, it has not been discarded by evolution—its key virtue being that it provides *some* high-energy phosphate in

The term "glycolysis" ("sweet releasing") was coined to describe the anaerobic conversion of glucose to lactic acid. However, many biochemists today use "glycolysis" to refer to the breakdown of sugar to pyruvate, the initial sequence of reactions leading into the Krebs cycle. This is the sense in which we use the term here. The anaerobic breakdown of sugar to lactic acid is referred to as anaerobic glycolysis. The distinction between "glycolysis" and "anaerobic glycolysis" is one of convenience, because the enzyme sequence from glucose to pyruvate is the same under both aerobic and anaerobic conditions.

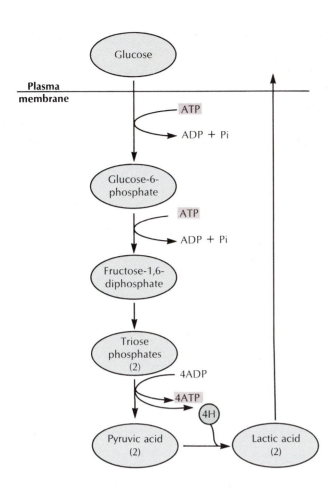

Figure 5-16

Anaerobic glycolysis, a process that proceeds in the absence of oxygen. Glucose is broken down to 2 molecules of pyruvic acid, generating 4 molecules of ATP and yielding 2, since 2 molecules of ATP are used to produce fructose-1,6-diphosphate. Pyruvic acid, the final electron acceptor for the hydrogen atoms and electrons released during pyruvic acid formation, is converted to lactic acid.

situations where oxygen is absent or in short supply. Many microorganisms have the opportunistic capacity to metabolize anaerobically when the oxygen supply is limited, then to switch to aerobic metabolism when oxygen is plentiful (facultative anaerobes). Most animals have retained the glycolytic pathway that serves as an important backup system capable of providing short-term generation of ATP during brief periods of heavy energy expenditure, when the slow rate of oxygen delivery would be a limiting factor. Vertebrate skeletal muscle may rely heavily on glycolysis during short bursts of activity when contraction is too rapid and too powerful to be sustained by oxidative phosphorylation. This may mean the difference between survival and death in emergency situations. The lactic acid that accumulates in muscle during anaerobic glycolysis diffuses out into the blood and is carried to the liver where it is oxidized.

Some animals rely heavily on anaerobic glycolysis during normal activities. For example, diving birds and mammals fall back on glycolysis almost entirely to give them the energy needed to sustain a long dive. And salmon would never reach their spawning grounds were it not for anaerobic glycolysis providing almost all the ATP used in the powerful muscular bursts needed to carry them up rapids and falls. Many parasitic animals have dispensed with oxidative phosphorylation entirely. They secrete relatively reduced end products of their energy metabolism, such as succinic acid, acetic acid, and propionic acid. These compounds are produced in mitochondrial reactions that derive several more molecules of ATP than does the cycle from glycolysis to lactic acid, although these sequences are still far less efficient than the classical electron transport system.

Goldfish are remarkably tolerant of oxygen-poor water and, in winter, can survive for days without any oxygen at all. Under such conditions they rely on glycolysis for their energy requirements. To avoid excessive buildup of lactic acid, the end product of glycolysis, they convert much of the lactic acid into alcohol, which diffuses out of the body. The Canadian team that recently made the discovery points out that the novel pathway prevents lactic acid from making the fish acidotic by swamping the fish's limited blood buffering system. Ethanol is neutral, and excessive acid accumulation is avoided. Could goldfish be more content than other fishes that presumably lack the ability to generate their own alcohol?

Figure 5-17

Hydrolysis of a triglyceride (neutral fat) by intracellular lipase. The R groups of each fatty acid represent a hydrocarbon chain.

___ Metabolism of Lipids

Animal fats are **triglycerides** (neutral fats), molecules composed of glycerol and 3 molecules of fatty acids. These fuels are important sources of energy for many metabolic processes in most animals. There is far more fat than glycogen in a mammalian body.

The first step in the breakdown of a triglyceride is the splitting of glycerol from the 3 fatty acid molecules (Fig. 5-17). Glycerol and the fatty acids then proceed through separate pathways. Glycerol, a 3-carbon carbohydrate, is phosphorylated and enters the glycolytic pathway as a triose phosphate. From that point it is oxidized in the aerobic pathway like any other carbohydrate.

The remainder of the triglyceride molecule is fatty acids, carboxylic acids with long hydrocarbon chains. One of the abundant naturally occurring fatty acids is **stearic acid.**

Stearic acid

We know that fats enter the mitochondrial processes through acetyl coenzyme A. What happens in brief is that the long hydrocarbon chain of a fatty acid is sliced up by oxidation, 2 carbons at a time; these are released from the end of the molecule as acetyl coenzyme A. The process is repeated until the entire chain has been reduced to several 2-carbon acetyl units. The first two cycles of the oxidation of a 10-carbon fatty acid are diagrammed in Fig. 5-18. The oxidation begins with the linking of coenzyme A to the end of the fatty acid. This activation, or "priming," requires 2 high-energy phosphate bonds from ATP—deficit financing again. Then the third carbon from the end is stripped of its hydrogens; these are accepted by NAD and FAD and transferred to the electron transport chain to form ATP. In the next step a molecule of acetyl coenzyme A is sliced off the end and another molecule of coenzyme A adds itself to the chain, now 2 carbons shorter. These steps are repeated until the entire chain has been converted to acetyl coenzyme A. In the example shown in Fig. 5-18, two more cycles are required to complete the oxidation. (In the final cycle a 4-carbon chain is split into 2 acetyl coenzyme A molecules.) All of the acetyl coenzyme A molecules are fed into the Krebs cycle (Fig. 5-19).

How much ATP is gained by fatty acid oxidation? ATP is generated in the electron transport chain by the hydrogens stripped from the carbon chain during fatty acid breakdown, as well as by metabolism of the acetyl coenzyme A units. With allowance for the 2 high-energy phosphate bonds expended to attach the first acetyl coenzyme A molecule, it has been calculated that the complete oxidation of 18-carbon stearic acid will net 146 ATP molecules. By comparison, 3 molecules of glucose (also totaling 18 carbons) yield 108 ATP molecules. Since there are three fatty acids in each triglyceride molecule, a total of 440 ATP molecules is formed. An additional 22 molecules of ATP are generated in the breakdown of glycerol, giving a grand total of 462 molecules of ATP. Little wonder that fat is considered the king of animal fuels! Fats are more concentrated fuels than carbohydrates because fats are almost pure hydrocarbons; they contain more

$$CH_2 \quad CH_2 \quad CH_2 \quad \mathbf{CH_2} \quad \mathbf{CH_2} \quad O$$

$$CH_2 \quad CH_2 \quad \mathbf{CH_2} \quad \mathbf{CH_2} \quad C$$

$$OH$$

10-C fatty acid

ATP, CoA

PP + AMP

$$CH_2 \quad CH_2 \quad CH_2 \quad \mathbf{CH_2} \quad \mathbf{CH_2} \quad O$$

$$CH_2 \quad CH_2 \quad \mathbf{CH_2} \quad \mathbf{CH_2} \quad C$$

$$CoA$$

10-C acyl CoA

NAD⁺

NADH

FAD   two oxidations

FADH₂

$$CH_2 \quad CH_2 \quad CH_2 \quad \mathbf{CH_2} \overset{O}{\underset{\|}{}} \mathbf{CH_2} \quad O$$

$$CH_2 \quad CH_2 \quad \mathbf{CH_2} \quad C \quad C$$

$$CoA$$

10-C ketoacyl CoA

CoA

$$CH_2 \quad CH_2 \quad CH_2 \quad \mathbf{CH_2} \overset{O}{\underset{\|}{}} \qquad\qquad O$$

$$CH_2 \quad CH_2 \quad \mathbf{CH_2} \quad C—CoA + H_3C—C—CoA$$

8-C acyl CoA   Acetyl CoA

NAD⁺

NADH

FAD

FADH₂

$$CH_2 \quad CH_2 \quad \mathbf{CH_2} \overset{O}{\underset{\|}{}} \mathbf{CH_2} \quad O$$

$$CH_2 \quad CH_2 \quad \mathbf{C} \qquad C$$

$$CoA$$

8-C ketoacyl CoA

CoA

$$CH_2 \quad CH_2 \quad \mathbf{CH_2} \overset{O}{\underset{\|}{}} \qquad\qquad O$$

$$CH_2 \quad CH_2 \quad \mathbf{C}—CoA + H_3C—\overset{O}{\underset{\|}{C}}—CoA$$

6-C acyl CoA   Acetyl CoA

Figure 5-18

First two removals of 2-carbon fragments in the oxidation of a low-carbon fatty acid.

Figure 5-19

Oxidation of a fatty acid.

Stearic acid

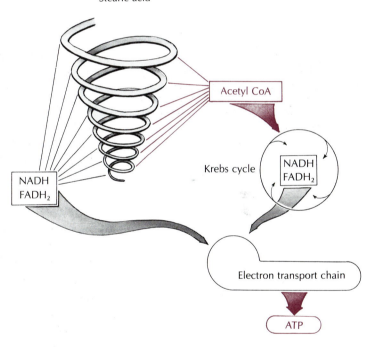

Stored fats are the greatest reserve fuel in the body. Most of the usable fat resides in adipose tissue that is composed of specialized cells packed with globules of triglycerides. Adipose tissue is widely distributed in the abdominal cavity, in muscles, around deep blood vessels, and especially under the skin. Women average about 30% more fat than men, and this is responsible in no small measure for the curved contours of the female figure. However, its aesthetic contribution is strictly subsidiary to its principal function as an internal fuel depot. Indeed, humans can only too easily deposit large quantities of fat, generating personal unhappiness and hazards to health.

The physiological and psychological aspects of obesity are now being investigated by many researchers. There is increasing evidence that body fat deposition is regulated by a feeding control center located in the lateral and ventral regions of the hypothalamus, an area in the floor of the forebrain. The set point of this regulator determines the normal weight for the individual, which may be rather persistently maintained above or below what is considered normal for the human population. Thus, obesity is not always due to overindulgence and lack of self-control, despite popular notions to the contrary.

hydrogen per carbon atom than sugars do, and it is the energized electrons of hydrogen that generate high-energy bonds, when they are carried through the mitochondrial electron transport system.

Fat stores are derived principally from surplus fats and carbohydrates in the diet. Acetyl coenzyme A is the source of carbon atoms used to build fatty acids. Since all major classes of organic molecules (carbohydrates, fats, and proteins) can be degraded to acetyl coenzyme A, all can be converted into stored fat. The biosynthetic pathway for fatty acids resembles a reversal of the catabolic pathway already described but requires an entirely different set of enzymes. From acetyl coenzyme A, the fatty acid chain is assembled 2 carbons at a time. Because fatty acids release energy when they are oxidized, they obviously require an input of energy for their synthesis. This is provided principally by electron energy from glucose degradation. Thus the total ATP derived from oxidation of a molecule of triglyceride is not as great as previously calculated, because varying amounts of energy are required for synthesis and storage.

Metabolism of Proteins

Because proteins are composed of amino acids, 20 in all (Fig. 2-22, p. 41), the central topic of our consideration is amino acid metabolism. Amino acid metabolism is complex. For one thing each of the 20 amino acids requires a separate pathway of biosynthesis and degradation. For another, amino acids are precursors to tissue proteins, enzymes, nucleic acids, and other nitrogenous constituents that form the very fabric of the cell. The central purpose of carbohydrate and fat oxidation is to provide energy to construct and maintain these vital macromolecules.

Let us begin with the **amino acid pool** in the blood and extracellular fluid from which the tissues draw their requirements. When animals eat proteins, these are digested in the gut, releasing the constituent amino acids, which are then absorbed (Fig. 5-20). Tissue proteins also are hydrolyzed during normal growth, repair, and tissue restructuring; their amino acids join those derived from protein foodstuffs to enter the amino acid pool. A portion of the amino acid pool is used to rebuild tissue proteins, but most animals ingest a protein surplus. Since amino acids are not excreted as such in any significant amounts, they must be disposed of in some way. In fact, amino acids can be and are metabolized through oxidative pathways to yield high-energy phosphate. In short, excess proteins serve as fuel as do carbohydrates and fats. Their importance as fuel obviously depends on the nature of the diet. In carnivores that ingest a diet of almost pure protein and fat, nearly half of their high-energy phosphate is derived from amino acid oxidation.

Before entering the fuel depot, nitrogen must be removed from the amino acid molecule. This is done in either of two ways. Some amino acids are **deaminated** (their amino group splits off) to yield ammonia and a keto acid:

$$R\text{—}\underset{\underset{NH_2}{|}}{CH}\text{—}COOH + H_2O \rightarrow R\text{—}\overset{\overset{O}{\|}}{C}\text{—}COOH + NH_3 + H_2$$

Amino acid   Keto acid Ammonia

Most amino acids, however, undergo **transamination** in which the amino group is transferred to a keto acid to yield a new amino acid, often glutamic acid:

$$R—CH—COOH + HOOC—CH_2—CH_2—\overset{\overset{O}{\|}}{C}—COOH \rightleftharpoons R—\overset{\overset{O}{\|}}{C}—COOH + HOOC—CH_2—CH_2—CH—COOH$$

Amino acid   α-Ketoglutaric acid   Keto acid   Glutamic acid

(with NH₂ shown below the first CH, and NH₂ below the final CH)

Glutamic acid can then be oxidized to liberate ammonia. Thus, amino acid degradation yields two main products, ammonia and carbon skeletons, which are handled in different ways.

Once the nitrogen atoms are removed, the carbon skeletons of amino acids can be completely oxidized, usually by way of pyruvate or acetate. These residues then enter regular routes used by carbohydrate and fat metabolism. This brings us finally to the disposal of ammonia, a complicated story both biochemically and evolutionarily that we can examine only in a general way in this chapter.

Ammonia is a highly toxic waste product. Its disposal offers little problem to aquatic animals because it is soluble and readily diffuses through the respiratory surfaces into the surrounding medium. Terrestrial forms cannot get rid of ammonia so conveniently and must detoxify it by converting it to a relatively nontoxic compound. The two principal compounds formed are **urea** and **uric acid**, although a variety of other detoxified forms of ammonia are excreted by different invertebrate and vertebrate groups. Among the vertebrates, amphibians and especially mammals produce urea. Reptiles and birds, as well as many terrestrial invertebrates, produce uric acid.

The key feature that seems to determine the choice of nitrogenous waste is the availability of water in the environment. When water is abundant, the chief nitrogenous waste is ammonia. When water is restricted, it is urea. For animals living in truly arid habitats (for example, insects, pulmonate snails, many birds, and lizards) it is uric acid. The distinguishing attribute of uric acid is that it is highly insoluble and easily precipitates from solution, allowing its removal in solid form. It is not so much the adults that benefit from uric acid's insolubility (since many forms excreting urea also live successfully in dry habitats) as it is their embryos. Birds and reptiles lay eggs enclosed in water-impermeable shells containing not only the embryo but also all the supportive supplies that it will require for its development: nutrients, fuel, and a small amount of water that must be used with the greatest economy. Furthermore, the embryo has no way to jettison its wastes. As the embryo develops, amino acids are metabolized, yielding ammonia that must be immediately detoxified. Urea is an unsuitable product because it requires too much water for its storage. The solution is uric acid, which is retained in harmless, solid form in the allantois, one of the embryonic membranes (p. 874). When the hatchling emerges into its new world, the accumulated uric acid, along with the shell and membranes that supported development, is discarded.

___ Management of Metabolism

The complex pattern of enzyme reactions that constitutes metabolism cannot be explained entirely in terms of physicochemical laws or chance happenings. Although some enzymes do indeed "flow with the tide," the activity of others is rigidly controlled. In the former case, suppose the purpose of an enzyme is to convert A to B. If B is removed by conversion into another compound, the enzyme will tend to restore the original ratio of B to A. Since many enzymes act reversibly, this can result, according to the metabolic situation prevailing, in synthesis or

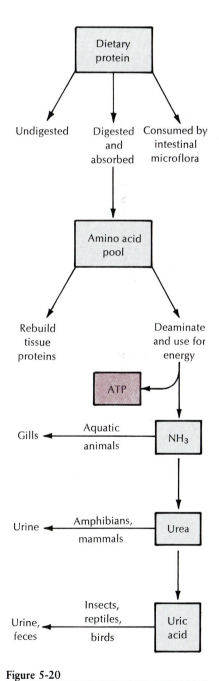

Figure 5-20

Fate of dietary protein.

Figure 5-21

Regulation by ATP of the activity of phosphofructokinase as measured by reaction velocity. A high ATP level depresses enzyme activity by binding to a regulatory site on the enzyme molecule.

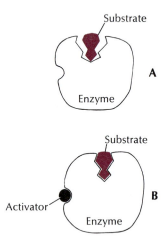

Figure 5-22

Enzyme regulation. **A,** The active site of an enzyme may only loosely fit its substrate in the absence of an activator. **B,** With the regulatory site of the enzyme occupied by an activator, the enzyme binds the substrate, and the site becomes catalytically active.

degradation. For example, an excess of a Krebs cycle intermediate would result in its contribution to glycogen synthesis; a depletion of such a metabolite would lead to glycogen breakdown. This automatic compensation (equilibration) is not, however, sufficient to explain all that actually takes place in an organism, as for example, what happens at branch points in a metabolic pathway.

It has been found that there are mechanisms for critically regulating enzymes in both *quantity* and *activity*. Certain molecules can switch off (or sometimes on) the synthesis of enzymes. It has been found that the presence of a particular amino acid in the medium in which a bacterium is growing may serve as a signal to switch off production of the enzymes involved in its synthesis, since the bacterium has no need for this. Normally enzyme synthesis is controlled by genetic mechanisms. **Structural genes** that code for the amino acid sequence of an enzyme can be turned off by **repressor proteins,** which are coded by a **regulator gene.** This scheme, known as the **operon model** of gene expression, and detailed on p. 925, can explain **enzyme induction** in which cells begin to synthesize a certain enzyme only after the substrate for that enzyme appears in the cell. In this way the *amount* of an enzyme can be controlled. It is a relatively slow process.

There are also more subtle mechanisms of control that operate by affecting the *activity* of already existing enzymes. The systems producing ATP must not be excessively active when the organism is at rest but must be called into action when needed. Several enzymes, occurring at certain critical positions on the pathway from glycogen to carbon dioxide, can be "switched on or off." A good example of this is the enzyme phosphofructokinase, which acts between glucose-6-phosphate and fructose-1,6-diphosphate (Fig. 5-7). The activity of this enzyme is depressed by high concentrations of ATP (Fig. 5-21) or citric acid, because their presence means that a sufficient amount of precursors has reached the Krebs cycle and additional glucose is not needed. Alternatively, the activity of the enzyme is *enhanced* by AMP because its presence means that ATP is rapidly being consumed for some cellular activity. This common form of enzyme regulation is characteristically brought about by signal molecules that are normal metabolites (in contrast to hormones that are solely for communication). They act by altering the shape (or conformation) of the enzyme protein and thus improve or diminish the effectiveness of the enzyme as a catalyst (Fig. 5-22).

As well as being subject to alteration in physical shape, some enzymes exist in two forms. These may be chemically different. Glycogen phosphorylase, which breaks glucose-6-phosphate units off a glycogen molecule, can exist as a relatively inert *b* form, but the *b* form can be converted reversibly to a more active *a* form. The hormone epinephrine, reaching a liver cell by way of the blood, affects the cell membrane in such a way that a complicated train of events is set in motion, resulting in a phosphate group being attached to a serine in the enzyme. This phosphorylated enzyme is extremely active and enables a rapid flow of sugar toward the Krebs cycle to take place. Epinephrine also has the reverse effect on the enzymes that work in the other direction, such as glycogen synthase, leading to the synthesis of glycogen, and it switches the synthase off at the critical time when glucose is needed. The messenger for this kind of activation/inactivation can be either a hormone or a particular metabolite.

Many cases of enzyme regulation are known, but these selected examples must suffice to illustrate the importance of enzyme regulation in the integration of metabolism.

____ Summary

Living systems are subject to the same laws of thermodynamics that govern non-living systems. The first law states that energy cannot be destroyed, although it may change form. The second law states that all energy proceeds toward total randomness, or increasing entropy. Solar energy trapped by photosynthesis as chemical bond energy is passed through the food chain where it is used for biosynthesis, active transport, and motion, before finally being degraded to heat energy. Living organisms are able to decrease their entropy and maintain high internal order because the biosphere is an open system from which energy can be captured and used. Energy available for use in biochemical reactions is termed free energy.

The coupling of biochemical reactions is achieved primarily by adenosine triphosphate (ATP). Free energy held in chemical bonds can be transferred through the high-energy phosphate bonds of ATP to molecules having lower bond energy. ATP is formed as it is needed from fuels such as glucose and is used to power various cellular processes.

Animals liberate the stored energy of fuels (sugars, fatty acids, amino acids) through a series of discrete degradative steps. Energy is released as electrons, which are transferred by oxidation-reduction reactions that end in the generation of ATP.

Most animals are aerobic, meaning that oxygen from the environment is used as the final electron acceptor in cellular metabolism. Organisms that can survive without oxygen, and that use some other molecule (such as pyruvic acid) as the final electron acceptor, are termed anaerobic. Aerobic metabolism is much more efficient than anaerobic metabolism.

Glycolysis, the first stage in the oxidation of fuel molecules, is a sequence of reactions that converts glucose to pyruvic acid. The net yield is 2 molecules of ATP and 2 molecules of reduced NAD, an electron acceptor that, in aerobic organisms, transfers its electrons to the electron transport chain.

In aerobic metabolism, pyruvic acid is decarboxylated to form acetyl coenzyme A, which enters the Krebs cycle. The Krebs cycle is a series of reactions occurring inside the mitochondria where acetyl coenzyme A is broken down to carbon dioxide. In the course of the reactions, energized electrons are passed to electron acceptors NAD and FAD. A molecule of ATP also is formed.

The final stage in respiration is the electron transport chain, composed of a complex series of enzymes located in the inner membrane of the mitochondrion. ATP is formed at three sites as electrons are passed along this chain of electron carriers from reduced NAD and FAD to oxygen. This is called oxidative phosphorylation. The currently favored hypothesis to explain the coupling of electron flow to ATP synthesis is the Mitchell chemiosmotic theory. It proposes that ATP synthesis is driven by a gradient of hydrogen ions across the inner mitochondrial membrane. The complete degradation of a molecule of glucose by oxidative phosphorylation yields 36 molecules of ATP. However, recent calculations suggest that the yield of ATP available for cellular work may be less than this.

Triglycerides (neutral fats) are especially rich depots of metabolic energy because the fatty acids of which they are composed are highly reduced and anhydrous. Fatty acids are degraded by sequential removal of 2-carbon units, which enter the Krebs cycle through acetyl coenzyme A.

Amino acids in excess of requirements for synthesis of proteins and other biomolecules are used as fuel. They are degraded by deamination or transamination to yield ammonia and carbon skeletons. The latter enter the Krebs cycle to be oxidized. Ammonia is a highly toxic waste product that aquatic animals quickly dispose of through respiratory surfaces. Terrestrial animals, however, convert ammonia into much less toxic compounds, urea or uric acid, for disposal.

The integration of metabolic pathways is rigidly regulated by mechanisms that control both the amount and activity of enzymes. The quantity of many enzymes is regulated by certain molecules that switch on or off enzyme synthesis in the nucleus. Enzyme activity may be altered by the presence or absence of metabolites that cause conformational changes in enzymes and thus improve or diminish their effectiveness as catalysts. Certain hormones may activate inactive enzymes.

Selected references

Avers, C.J. 1976. Cell biology. New York, D. Van Nostrand Co. *Energy transfer is clearly presented in Chapter 7.*

Hochachka, P.W. 1980. Living without oxygen. Cambridge, Mass., Harvard University Press.

Klotz, I.M. 1967. Energy changes in biochemical reactions. New York, Academic Press, Inc. *Concise introduction to thermodynamics in metabolism.*

Lehninger, A.L. 1982. Principles of biochemistry. New York, Worth Publishers. *Lucidly written and amply illustrated undergraduate biochemistry text.*

McGilvery, R.W. 1979. Biochemistry: a functional approach, ed. 2. Philadelphia, W.B. Saunders Co. *Well-written mammalian biochemistry text.*

Mitchell, P. 1979. Keilin's respiratory chain concept and its chemiosmotic consequences. Science **206:** 1148-1159. *Nobel lecture review of the chemiosmotic theory.*

Stryer, L. 1981. Biochemistry, ed. 2. San Francisco, W.H. Freeman & Co. Publishers. *Clear explanations and good diagrams.*

Wolfe, S.L. 1981. Biology of the cell, ed. 2. Belmont, Calif., Wadsworth, Inc. *Well-written and up-to-date.*

Selected *Scientific American* articles

Changeux, J.-P. 1965. The control of biochemical reactions. **212:**36-45 (Apr.). *How metabolism is regulated.*

Dickerson, R.E. 1980. Cytochrome c and the evolution of energy metabolism. **242:**136-153 (Mar.). *How a molecular pedigree of organic evolution is constructed from a family of electron-transferring proteins.*

Green, D.E. 1960. The synthesis of fat. **202:**46-51 (Feb.).

Hinkle, P.C., and R.E. McCarty. 1978. How cells make ATP. **238:**104-123 (Mar.). *Describes the chemiosmotic theory of ATP formation.*

Lehninger, A.L. 1960. Energy transformations in the cell. **202:**104-114 (May).

Lehninger, A.L. 1961. How cells transform energy. **205:**62-73 (Sept.).

Meyerhof, O. 1950. Biochemistry. **183:**62-68 (Sept.). *A famous biochemist recounts key discoveries in a young science.*

Neurath, H. 1964. Protein-digesting enzymes. **211:**68-79 (Dec.). *Structure and function of the proteolytic digestive enzymes.*

Racker, E. 1968. The membrane of the mitochondrion. **218:**32-39 (Feb.). *Its secrets are unlocked by disassembling it and attempting to reassemble it.*

Shulman, R.G. 1983. NMR spectroscopy of living cells. **248:**86-93 (Jan.). *This technique allows metabolic reactions to be observed in living tissue.*

CHAPTER 6

ARCHITECTURAL PATTERN
OF AN ANIMAL

Gonionemus murbachi, an organism exhibiting radial symmetry. (×6.)

Photograph by D.P. Wilson.

The architecture of most animals conforms to a well-defined plan. The basic uniformity of biological organization derives from the supposed common ancestry of animals and from their basic cellular construction. Despite the vast differences in structural complexity of animals ranging from the simplest protozoa to humans, all share an intrinsic material design and fundamental functional plan. In the last analysis, whatever unity we see among animal organization is explained by just one fact: all animals live on Earth, a planet bearing a unique set of physical properties that has molded the nature of life on it. Yet even as the biologist takes some comfort from the belief in the basic unity of life—and many areas of biological endeavor, such as general physiology and molecular biology, are grounded on this faith—we must admit that animals exhibit an incredible diversity of specific structural and functional adaptations.

Animals are shaped by their particular habitat: its physical nature and its biotic community. Such adaptations are not *caused* by the environment; rather they arise when, by natural selection, beneficial variations are preserved. This concept will be clearer when evolution is discussed in Chapter 38. In this chapter we deal with the fundamental uniformity of animal structure that is recognizable despite the numerous specializations, both subtle and prominent, that have modified the basic plan.

GRADES OF ORGANIZATION IN ANIMAL COMPLEXITY

How has increased animal complexity, so evident in animal phylogeny, arisen? The unicellular forms are complete organisms that carry on all the basic functions of higher forms. Within the confines of their cell, they often show remarkable organization and division of labor, such as skeletal elements, locomotor devices, fibrils, and beginnings of sense organs. The metazoa, or multicellular animals, on the other hand, have differentiated into tissues and organs that are specialized for specific functions. The metazoan cell is not the equivalent of a protozoan cell; it is only a specialized part of the whole organism and is incapable of independent existence.

We can recognize five grades of organization. Each grade is more complex than the one before, and, as a general rule, it is a more advanced and more recent evolutionary product.

1. *Protoplasmic grade of organization.* Protoplasmic organization is found in protozoa and other unicellular organisms. All life functions are confined within the boundaries of a single cell, the fundamental unit of life. Within the cell, protoplasm is differentiated into organelles capable of carrying on specialized functions.

2. *Cellular grade of organization.* Cellular organization is an aggregation of cells that are functionally differentiated. A division of labor is evident, so that some cells are concerned with, for example, reproduction, others with nutrition. Such cells have little tendency to become organized into tissues. Some protozoan colonial forms having somatic and reproductive cells might be placed in this category. Many authorities also place the sponges at this level.

3. *Cell-tissue grade of organization.* A step beyond the preceding is the aggregation of similar cells into definite patterns or layers, thus becoming a tissue. Sponges are considered by some authorities to belong to this grade, although the

jellyfish and their relatives (Cnidaria) are usually referred to as the beginning of the tissue plan. Both groups are still largely of the cellular grade of organization because most of the cells are scattered and not organized into tissues. An excellent example of a tissue in cnidarians is the **nerve net,** in which the nerve cells and their processes form a definite tissue structure, with the function of coordination.

4. *Tissue-organ grade of organization.* The aggregation of tissues into organs is a further step in advancement. Organs are usually made up of more than one kind of tissue and have a more specialized function than tissues. The first appearance of this level is in the flatworms (Platyhelminthes), in which there are a number of well-defined organs such as eyespots, proboscis, and reproductive organs. In fact, the reproductive organs are well organized into a reproductive system.

5. *Organ-system grade of organization.* When organs work together to perform some function, we have the highest level of organization—the organ system. The systems are associated with the basic body functions—circulation, respiration, digestion, and the others. Typical of all the higher forms, this type of organization is first seen in the nemertean worms, which have a complete digestive system distinct from the circulatory system.

___ Size and Complexity

It is probably evident from the preceding list that, as animals become more complex, they tend to become larger. One reason is that increasing complexity is the result of specialization and division of labor within body tissues. An ameba can be small because it can move without muscles, digest food without a gut, excrete its wastes without a kidney, coordinate its activities without a brain, and breathe without gills. More advanced animals have specialized organs for these functions, and this means they are usually larger.

Large body size offers other advantages. Perhaps the most obvious is that in the predator-prey contest, predators are almost always larger than their prey. Exceptions are few and usually are related to an especially aggressive behavior that compensates for small size. Larger animals prey on smaller ones not only because they have bigger mouths and appetites, but also because they usually are faster. Since the predator must first catch its prey, while the prey must escape its predator if it is to survive, the advantage of larger size is clear.

Another advantage of large body size that is usually overlooked is that large animals can move themselves about at a lesser energy cost than small animals. This becomes clear when we look at the cost of running for a given group of animals (for example, mammals) of various body sizes (Fig. 6-1). A large mammal consumes more oxygen than a small mammal, of course, but the cost of moving 1 g of its body over a given distance is much less for the large animal than for a small one. This makes sense when we compare the relative ease with which a horse can run a mile with the herculean task that running the same distance would present to a mouse!

Still another advantage that accompanies large size is greater internal stability, that is, the capacity to regulate the internal environment of the body. (This is known in physiological language as **homeostasis** and is discussed in Chapter 30.) The ability to maintain internal stability despite changes in the external environment allows organisms to invade otherwise hostile habitats. For example, only the homeotherms (warm-blooded animals such as birds and mammals) can remain active through all seasons in regions with severe winter climates.

Figure 6-1

Net cost of running for mammals of various sizes. Each point represents the cost (measured in rate of oxygen consumption) of moving 1 g of body over 1 km. The cost decreases with increasing body size.

Modified from Schmidt-Nielsen, K. 1972. How animals work. New York, Cambridge University Press.

Although being big confers certain advantages to an animal, it is obvious that large animals have not displaced small ones; indeed, small animals are probably as numerous today as they ever were. Small organisms long ago occupied all the available small ecological niches, and the only way a new species could succeed was to displace an organism from an existing niche or adapt to a new and larger one. This has certainly been one of the factors promoting the evolutionary trend toward increasing body size. Nevertheless, every animal, whether large or small, is a success in its ecological niche. In fact, the most abundant groups of animals on earth today are those with short generation times and, consequently, small size. To these countless creatures, "small is beautiful."

CONCEPT OF INDIVIDUALITY

The question, "What is an individual animal?" may seem trifling and obvious. We have little difficulty recognizing a worm, a bird, or a dog as an individual, and certainly all humans are individuals. But in unicellular animals that reproduce by asexual fission or budding or fragmentation, the distinction of individuality begins to blur. Where is the "individual" in an organism that merely divides generation after generation? Is a flatworm an individual when it can be cut into numerous pieces, each of which will grow into a new organism? Are colonial forms individuals? We can appreciate that these questions are difficult to answer. Individualization also includes death, since the individual must have a limited existence. Clearly, the concept of individuality does not apply readily to many primitive forms that divide repeatedly and are, in a sense, imperishable.

An individual is traditionally identified as an adult. When we refer to a worm, a bird, or a dog, we instantly and automatically picture an adult worm, bird, or dog. But a dog is a dog, genetically at least, from fertilized egg to death—as zygote, embryo, fetus, puppy, adolescent, and adult. Zoologists feel more comfortable considering an individual to be a brief time-slice out of a **life cycle** of an organism (Principle 22, p. 17). The idea that the whole life cycle is the central unit of biology on which evolution acts is finding increasing favor among zoologists (Bonner, 1965).

PRELIMINARY SURVEY OF ANIMAL EMBRYOLOGY

Embryology is the study of the progressive growth and differentiation that occurs during the early development of an organism. A brief summary of embryology is necessary for understanding the pattern of an animal and also for understanding some of the basic concepts used in describing animal groups and their classification. The developmental process and its control are discussed in greater detail in Chapter 36.

General Pattern of Development

Let us begin by restating Principle 22 (p. 17) introduced in the preceding section. All animals have a characteristic life cycle. Admittedly the life cycle is somewhat indistinct in many protozoa (such as the ameba) that are potentially immortal because they are part of ancestral lines that have never experienced natural senescence and death. The parental organism reproduces by simply dividing into two daughter cells, each essentially a continuation of the parent. In these forms there is no true individual, only progressive individualization that "ends" with division.

Early in the life history of all metazoans, however, there occurs a differentiation of the germ cell from the body or soma cells. It is the uniting of the germ cells (male sperm and female ova) that gives rise to a new generation (sexual reproduction), while the body (soma) cells die. The real life cycle of a metazoan starts with the union of an ovum (egg) with a spermatozoon, a process called fertilization.

The fertilized egg, called a **zygote**, is really a one-celled organism, and from it develops a complete animal by the process of **differentiation.** How this occurs is only partly known. All the information necessary for development is contained within the fertilized egg, principally in the genes of the egg's nucleus. The actual blueprint for differentiation is coded within the DNA molecules of the genes. The heredity of the organism stabilizes the pattern of development; the variation that makes evolutionary changes possible is contributed by the gene segregation that occurs during the formation of gametes and recombination of maternal and paternal genes at fertilization.

Every species develops a characteristic body plan (Principle 23, p. 18). As the body plan takes shape during development, certain basic characteristics of the phylum appear before the specific qualities of the species appear. Such basic qualities may be symmetry, a longitudinal axis, and (if a vertebrate) a notochord, dorsal tubular nerve cord, three major pairs of sensory organs, paired pharyngeal pouches, a chambered heart, a liver, paired kidneys, paired pectoral and pelvic appendages, and others. There are overlappings of some of these characteristics in both vertebrates and invertebrates. As development continues, the individual acquires the morphological characters of its lower taxa (class, order, family, and genus) and finally of its own species. This indicates that development proceeds from the general to the specific in gross morphological characteristics.

The stages of embryogenesis are as follows:

1. *Fertilization.* The activation of the egg by a sperm in biparental reproduction; the union of these male and female gametes forms a zygote, which is the starting point for development
2. *Cleavage and blastulation.* The division of the zygote into smaller and smaller cells (cleavage) to form a hollow ball of tiny cells (blastula)
3. *Gastrulation.* The sorting out of cells of the blastula into germ layers (ectoderm, mesoderm, endoderm) that become committed to the formation of future body organs (the role of the germ layers in differentiation is described below)
4. *Differentiation.* The formation of body organs and tissues, which take on their specialized functions; the basic body plan of the animal becomes established
5. *Growth.* Increase in size of the animal by cell division or cell enlargement; growth depends on the intake of food to supply material for the synthesis of protoplasm

Types of eggs

Eggs may be classified as follows with respect to yolk distribution (Fig. 6-2).

The **isolecithal egg** (also called homolecithal) is small, and the small amount of yolk (deutoplasm) and cytoplasm is uniformly distributed through the egg, with the nucleus near the center. Cleavage is typically **holoblastic** (that is, the cleavage planes pass completely through the embryo), and the cells are completely separated by cell membranes at each division. The cells (blastomeres) are nearly equal in size. Such eggs are found in the protochordates (such as sea squirts and amphioxus) and the echinoderms (sea stars and sea urchins).

In the **telolecithal egg** the large amount of yolk (50% to 90%) tends to be concentrated toward one pole (the vegetal pole) where metabolism is lower. The protoplasm and nucleus are found mainly at the opposite (animal) pole, where metabolic activity is greater. There are two classes of telolecithal eggs. The first is yolked eggs with holoblastic cleavage, in which the later cleavages produce unequal cells—small cells, or micromeres, at the animal pole and large cells, or macromeres, at the vegetal pole. Amphibians and bony fish have this kind of egg. The second is yolked eggs (megalecithal) with **meroblastic** (partial or discoidal) cleavage, in which the small amount of protoplasm is concentrated at the animal

Isolecithal   Centrolecithal

Telolecithal-holoblastic

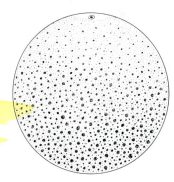

Telolecithal-meroblastic

Figure 6-2

Types of eggs. Isolecithal (echinoderms and amphioxus) have small yolk evenly distributed. Centrolecithal (insects and other arthropods) have cytoplasm centered but migrating out at cleavage, leaving yolk centered. Telolecithal with holoblastic cleavage (amphibians and bony fishes) have yolk concentrated at vegetal pole. Telolecithal with meroblastic cleavage (birds and reptiles) have cytoplasm concentrated in germinal disc at animal pole.

Figure 6-3

Cell division in developing embryos of *Echinus esculentus,* a common sea urchin. Cells become progressively smaller with no growth between divisions. Present are four- and eight-cell stages, many-celled stage, and early blastula. (×165.)
Photograph by D.P. Wilson.

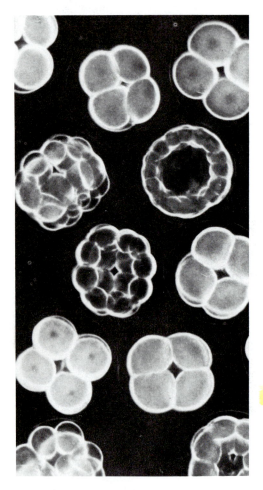

pole in the germinal disc, or blastoderm, where cleavage occurs. These eggs are usually large, contain a great deal of albumin (egg white) derived from the oviducts, and have a hard or soft shell. Bird and reptile eggs are good examples (Fig. 6-7).

In the **centrolecithal egg** the nucleus and the surrounding layer of protoplasm are at first in the center of the egg, but as cleavage occurs, most of the nucleated masses of cytoplasm migrate to the periphery and form a cellular layer (blastoderm), leaving the yolk in the center of the egg. From the blastoderm the embryo develops. These eggs are characteristic of advanced arthropods such as insects.

In addition to the plasma membrane universally present in eggs, there are in the various animal groups many kinds of protective membranes or envelopes around the eggs. These include the **vitelline membrane,** or fertilization membrane, secreted by the egg, the **zona pellucida** formed by ovarian follicle cells of mammals, the **egg jelly** from the oviducts of bony fish and amphibians, and the **chitinous shell** (chorion) from the ovarian tubules of insects.

Fertilization and formation of the zygote

The fusion of the pronuclei of sperm and egg to form a zygote restores the diploid number of chromosomes, combines the maternal and paternal genetic traits, and activates the egg to develop. This process is discussed in more detail in Chapter 36.

Cleavage and blastulation

The unicellular zygote now begins to divide, first into two cells, those two into four cells, those four into eight. Repeated again and again, these cell divisions soon convert the zygote into a ball of cells. This process, called **cleavage,** occurs by mitosis. But unlike ordinary body-cell mitosis, there is no true growth (that is, increase in protoplasmic mass) (Fig. 6-3). With each subsequent division, the cells are reduced in size by one half. The cleavage process converts a single, very large, unwieldy egg into many small, more maneuverable, ordinary-sized cells called blastomeres.

Cleavage patterns are greatly affected by the amount of yolk in the egg. In eggs with very little yolk, such as those of mammals, the cytoplasm is uniformly distributed through the egg, and the nucleus is in or near the egg center. In such eggs, cleavage is complete (holoblastic), and the daughter cells formed at each division are of approximately equal size. The eggs of frogs and other amphibians are richly supplied with yolk that tends to be massed in the so-called vegetal pole of the egg. The opposite, or animal, pole contains the egg cytoplasm and the nucleus. The early cleavage divisions tend to be displaced toward the animal pole because the mass of relatively inactive yolk in the vegetal pole retards the rate of cleavage in that region (Fig. 6-6). Birds and reptiles produce the largest eggs of all animals. Nearly all of this comparatively enormous size is storage food—the part of the egg we commonly call yolk and the investment of albumin, or egg white. The active cytoplasm, containing the nucleus, is but a tiny disc (the blastodisc) resting on top of the ball of yolk. Cleavage (meroblastic) is confined to this area of cytoplasm, since the cell divisions cannot possibly cut through the vast bulk of inert yolk (Fig. 6-7).

Radial and spiral cleavage

Holoblastic cleavage is also classified on the basis of cleavage pattern. In **radial cleavage,** the cleavage planes are symmetrical to the polar axis and produce tiers, or layers, of cells on top of each other (Fig. 6-4). Radial cleavage is **indeterminate** in the sense that there is no definite relation between the position of any of the *early* blastomeres and the specific tissue it will form in the embryo. Blastomeres are said to be equipotential and each, if separated from the others, may be capable of giving rise to a complete embryo. Radial cleavage is found among the **Deuterostomia,** an assemblage of animals that includes the Echinodermata, the Chordata, and two minor phyla.

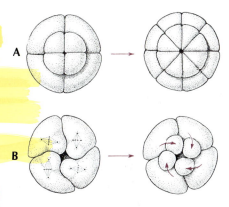

Figure 6-4

Radial and spiral cleavage. **A,** Radial cleavage shown at eight- and 16-cell stages. **B,** Spiral cleavage, showing the transition from four- to eight-cell stage. Arrows indicate clockwise movement of small cells (micromeres) following division from large cells (macromeres).

Spiral cleavage is a different pattern of cleavage typical of a different group of animals. The cleavage planes are oblique to the polar axis and typically produce quartets of unequal cells that come to lie, not on top of each other, but in the furrows between adjacent cells. Although there are many variations of spiral cleavage, the classical pattern is shown in Fig. 6-4. Spiral cleavage is characteristically **determinate** because the fate of each blastomere is fixed as soon as cleavage begins. All blastomeres must be present to form a whole embryo, and if one is separated from the rest, it will develop abnormally. With determinate cleavage, twins from a single zygote (identical twins) cannot develop. One of the curious features of spiral cleavage is that at the 29-cell stage a blastomere called the 4d cell is formed that will give rise to all of the mesoderm of the embryo. With few exceptions, spiral cleavage is found in the Platyhelminthes, Mollusca, Annelida, Arthropoda, and many smaller phyla (see illustration inside the front cover of this book). We shall pursue this distinction in Chapter 36.

Cleavage, however modified by the presence of varying amounts of yolk and different cleavage patterns, results in a cluster of cells, called a **blastula** (Figs. 6-5 to 6-7). In many animals, such as the amphibian and mammalian embryos, the cells rearrange themselves around a central fluid-filled cavity called the **blastocoel.**

We have seen that cleavage has resulted in the proliferation of several thousand maneuverable cells poised for further development. There has been a great increase in total DNA content, since each of the many daughter cell nuclei, by chromosomal replication at mitosis, contains as much DNA as the original zygote nucleus.

Figure 6-5

Early embryology of amphioxus.

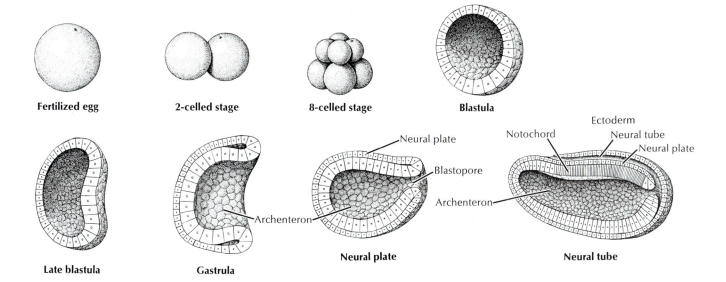

Fertilized egg   **2-celled stage**   **8-celled stage**   **Blastula**

Late blastula   **Gastrula**   Neural plate — Blastopore — Archenteron   **Neural plate**   Notochord — Archenteron — Ectoderm — Neural tube — Neural plate   **Neural tube**

Cleavage

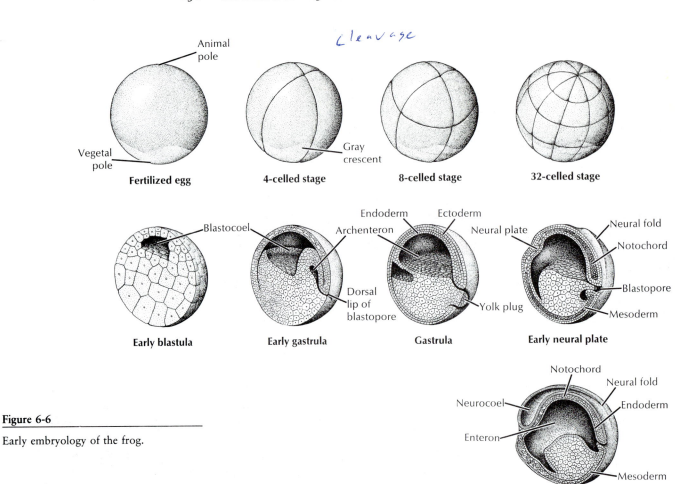

Figure 6-6

Early embryology of the frog.

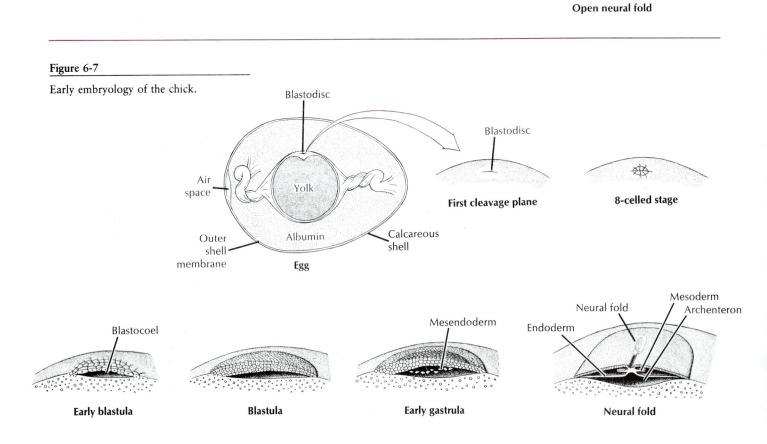

Figure 6-7

Early embryology of the chick.

Gastrulation

Gastrulation is a regrouping process in which new and important cell associations are formed. Up to this point the embryo has divided itself up into a multicellular complex; the cytoplasm of these numerous cells is nearly in the same position as in the original undivided egg. In other words, there has been no significant movement or displacement of the cells from their place of origin. As gastrulation begins, the cells become rearranged in an orderly way by morphogenetic movements.

In the **amphioxus** (Fig. 6-5) the blastoderm of the vegetal pole bends inward so that the whole embryo becomes converted into a double-walled, cup-shaped structure. The structure lining the new cavity thus formed is the **archenteron** (primitive gut), and its opening to the outside is the **blastopore**. In amphibians (Fig. 6-6) the type of gastrulation that occurs in the amphioxus is impossible. The cleavage divisions at the lower or vegetal pole are slowed by the inert yolk so that the resulting blastula consists of many small cells at the animal pole and a few large cells at the vegetal pole. Cells on the surface begin to sink inward (invaginate) at one point, the blastopore. Through the curved groove of the blastopore, surface cells move as a sheet to the interior to form an embryo of two **germ layers, ectoderm** and **endoderm.** As invagination proceeds, a platelike area of cells rolls over the dorsal lip of the blastopore and becomes stretched along the roof of the archenteron; this is the future notochord. The third germ layer, the **mesoderm,** rolls over the lateral and ventral lip of the blastopore and, once inside, penetrates between the endoderm on the inside and the ectoderm on the outside. The three germ layers now formed are the primary structural layers that play crucial roles in the further differentiation of the embryo. The outer layer, or ectoderm, will give rise to the nervous system and outer epithelium of the body. The middle layer, or mesoderm, will give rise to the circulatory, skeletal, and muscular structures. The inner layer, or endoderm (also called entoderm), will develop into the digestive tube and its associated structures.

In certain simple metazoans, only two germ layers are formed, the endoderm and ectoderm. These animals are called **diploblastic.** In all higher forms, the mesoderm also appears, either from pouches of the archenteron or from other cells. This three-layered condition is called **triploblastic.**

Formation of the coelom

The coelom, or true body cavity that contains the viscera, may be formed by one of two methods—**schizocoelous** or **enterocoelous** (Fig. 6-8)—or by modification of these methods. (The two terms are descriptive, for *schizo* comes from the Greek *schizein*, to split; *entero* is a Greek form from *enteron*, gut; *coelous* comes from the Greek *koilos*, hollow or cavity.) In schizocoelous formation the coelom arises, as the word implies, from the splitting of mesodermal bands that originate from the blastopore region and grow between the ectoderm and endoderm; in enterocoelous formation the coelom comes from pouches of the archenteron, or primitive gut.

Since coelom formation occurs very early in embryonic development, the appearance of two quite different methods of formation among animals is believed to signal a fundamental division in metazoan evolution. The **deuterostome** division of the metazoa mostly follows the enterocoelous method of coelom formation. The **protostome** division follows the schizocoelous method. Advanced chordates are exceptions to this distinction because their coelom is formed by

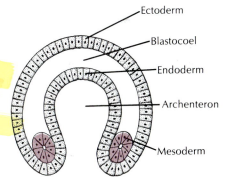

Ectoderm

Blastocoel

Endoderm

Archenteron

Mesoderm

**Mollusc
Schizocoelous**

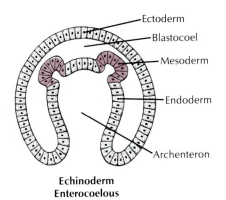

Ectoderm

Blastocoel

Mesoderm

Endoderm

Archenteron

**Echinoderm
Enterocoelous**

Figure 6-8

Two types of mesoderm and coelom formation: schizocoelous, in which mesoderm originates from wall of archenteron near lips of blastopore, and enterocoelous, in which mesoderm and coelom develop from endodermal pouches.

mesodermal splitting (schizocoelous), although in other respects they develop as deuterostomes, the division to which they are assigned. Other characteristics that distinguish these two phylogenetic divisions of bilateral animals are radial, indeterminate cleavage and spiral, determinate cleavage, mentioned before.

Differentiation

With formation of the three primary germ layers, cells continue to regroup and rearrange themselves into primordial cell masses. As masses develop, they become increasingly committed to specific directions of differentiation. Cells that previously had the potential to develop into a variety of structures now lose this diverse potential and assume commitments to become, for example, kidney cells, intestinal cells, or brain cells. Differentiation is discussed in more detail in Chapter 36.

Fate of Germ Layers

The following are some of the vertebrate structures that normally arise from the three germ layers:

Ectoderm
Epidermis of skin
Lining of mouth, anus, nostrils
Sweat and sebaceous glands
Epidermal coverings such as hair, nails, feathers, horns, epidermal scales, enamel of teeth
Nervous system, including sensory parts of eye, nose, ear

Endoderm
Lining of alimentary canal
Lining of respiratory passages and lungs
Secretory parts of liver and pancreas
Thyroid, parathyroid, thymus
Urinary bladder
Lining of urethra

Mesoderm
Skeleton and muscles
Dermis of skin
Dermal scales and dentin
Excretory and reproductive systems
Connective tissue
Blood and blood vessels
Mesenteries
Lining of coelomic cavity

The assignment of early embryonic layers to specific "germ layers" (a somewhat unfortunate term that is not to be confused with "germ cells," which are the eggs and sperm) is for the convenience of embryologists and of no concern to the embryo. The idea that each germ layer can give rise to certain tissues and organs only, and to no others, is no longer held. It is now known that the interactions of cells play a part in determining their differentiation in vertebrate animals. The precise position of a cell with relation to other cells and tissues during early development often controls the real fate of that cell. Under some conditions a certain germ layer may give rise to structures normally arising from a different germ layer. Experiments have demonstrated that a presumptive ectodermal structure, when grafted into appropriate regions, may form organs that normally come from a different germ layer. Therefore the topographic position of cells in their development must play a significant role in their final fate and destiny.

Embryological development must be considered quite flexible. The biological system cannot be restricted to a definite pattern even though normally it appears to be. Are there any organs or structures that do not come from any germ layer? In a strict sense the germ cells do not originate from any of the three germ layers because they come directly from cells that were segregated in the early cleavage stages of the fertilized egg.

ORGANIZATION OF THE BODY

The body consists of three elements: (1) cells (discussed earlier), (2) body fluids, and (3) extracellular structural elements.

Body Fluids

Water permeates all tissues and spaces in the body, but it is naturally separated into certain fluid "compartments." In all metazoa, the two major body fluid compartments are the **intracellular space,** within the body's cells, and the **extracellular space,** outside the cells. In animals with closed vascular systems (such as the vertebrates), the extracellular space can be further subdivided into the **blood plasma** (the fluid portion of the blood outside the cells; blood cells are really part of the intracellular compartment) and **interstitial fluid.** The interstitial fluid, or tissue fluid, occupies the spaces surrounding the cells. Body fluid compartmentalization varies among the invertebrates, but all share with the vertebrates the basic subdivision of fluid between the intracellular and extracellular compartments.

Extracellular Structural Elements

The extracellular, or intercellular,* substance is the supporting material of the organism such as connective tissue, cartilage, and bone. It provides mechanical stability, protection, and a depot of materials for exchange and serves as a medium for extracellular reactions. It is responsible for tissue firmness and cellular support. Two types of extracellular tissue are recognized: **formed** and **amorphous.** The formed type includes collagen (white fibrous tissue). Collagen is the most abundant protein in the animal kingdom and makes up the major part of the fibrous constituent of the skin, tendon, ligaments, cartilage, and bone. Elastin, which gives elasticity to the tissues, also belongs to the formed type. Amorphous intercellular substance (ground substance) is composed of mucopolysaccharides arranged in long-chain polymers.

Tissues

A **tissue** is a group of similar cells (together with associated cell products) specialized for the performance of a common function. The study of tissues is called histology. All cells in metazoan animals take part in the formation of tissues. Sometimes the cells of a tissue may be of several kinds, and some tissues have a great many intercellular materials.

---

*The term "intercellular," meaning "between cells," should not be confused with the term "intracellular," meaning "within cells."

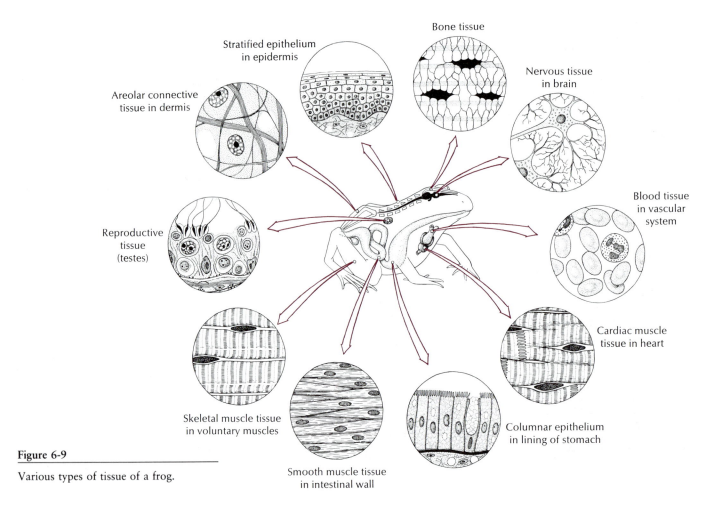

Figure 6-9

Various types of tissue of a frog.

The different types of tissues originate from the basic properties of living cells. These properties, and the tissues that are the manifestations of these properties, are irritability and conductivity (nervous tissue), contractility (muscle tissue), support and adhesion (connective tissue), absorption and secretion (epithelial tissue), and fluidity and conductivity (vascular tissue) (Fig. 6-9). This is a surprisingly short list of basic tissue types that are able to meet the requirements of the diverse morphological patterns of all animals. Each of the basic tissues can be subdivided into several types that are specialized for many different functions. Some of these are depicted in Fig. 6-9.

During embryonic development, the germ layers differentiate by a process called **histogenesis** into the five major tissues: epithelial tissue, connective or supporting tissue, muscular or contractile tissue, nervous tissue, and vascular tissue.

Epithelial tissue

An **epithelium** is a sheet of cells that covers an external or internal surface. On the outside of the body, the epithelium forms a protective covering. Inside, the epithelium lines all the organs of the body cavity, as well as ducts and passageways through which various materials and secretions move. On many surfaces the epithelial cells are often modified into glands that produce lubricating mucus or specialized products such as hormones or enzymes.

Simple columnar   Simple squamous   Simple cuboidal

Figure 6-10

Types of simple epithelium.

Pseudostratified   Transitional (relaxed)

Transitional (stretched)

Stratified columnar

Figure 6-11

Types of stratified and transitional epithelial tissue.

Epithelia are classified on the basis of cell form and number of cell layers. A **simple epithelium** is one layer thick (Fig. 6-10), and its cells may be **squamous** (flat), as in endothelium of blood vessels; **cuboidal** (short prisms), as in glands and ducts; or **columnar** (tall), as in the stomach and intestine. Any of these three forms of cells may occur in several layers as a **stratified epithelium** (as in skin, sweat glands, and urethra) (Fig. 6-11). Some stratified epithelia can change the number of their cell layers by being stretched out (**transitional,** such as the urinary bladder). Others have cells of different heights and give the appearance of stratified epithelia (**pseudostratified,** such as the trachea). Many epithelia may be **ciliated** at their free surfaces (such as the oviduct).

Connective tissue

Connective tissues bind together and support all other structures. They are so common that the removal of all other tissues from the body would still leave the complete form of the body clearly apparent. Connective tissue is made up of relatively few **cells** and a great deal of formed material such as **fibers** and ground substance (**matrix**) in which the fibers are embedded. There are three types of fibers: white or collagenous (the most common type), yellow or elastic, and branching or reticular. Connective tissue may be classified in various ways, but all the types fall under either **loose connective tissue** (reticular, areolar, adipose) or **dense connective tissue** (sheaths, ligaments, tendons, cartilage, bone) (Figs. 6-12 and 6-13).

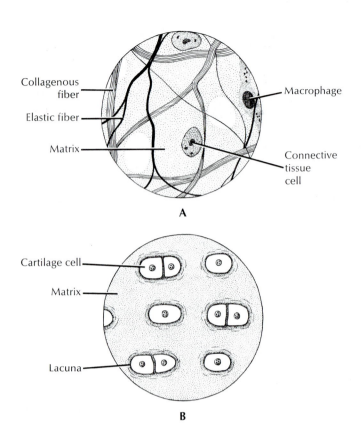

Collagenous fiber

Elastic fiber

Matrix

Macrophage

Connective tissue cell

A

Cartilage cell

Matrix

Lacuna

B

Figure 6-12

A, Areolar, a type of loose connective tissue. **B,** Hyaline cartilage, most common form of cartilage in body and a type of dense connective tissue.

Figure 6-13

Section of bone, a type of dense connective tissue, showing several cylindrical osteons typical of bone. (×180.)

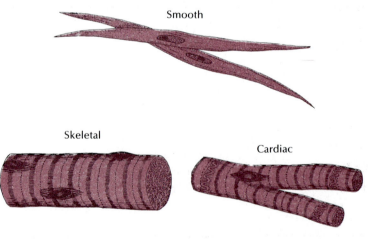

Smooth

Skeletal

Cardiac

Figure 6-14

Three kinds of vertebrate muscle fibers, as they appear when viewed with the light microscope.

Figure 6-15

Photomicrograph of skeletal muscle showing several striated fibers lying side by side. (×600.)
Courtesy J.W. Bamberger.

Figure 6-16

Two myoepithelial basket cells surrounding salivary secretory cells. Each myoepithelial cell is made up of a central body with long cytoplasmic processes, and myoepithelial cells may be considered a fourth type of muscular tissue. They resemble smooth muscle cells.

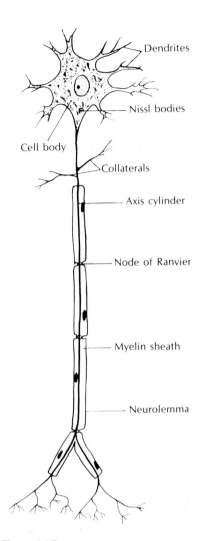

Figure 6-17

Neuron.

Muscular tissue

Muscle is the most common tissue in the body of most animals. It is made up of elongated cells or fibers specialized for contraction. It originates (with few exceptions) from the mesoderm, and its unit is the cell or **muscle fiber.** The unspecialized cytoplasm of muscles is called **sarcoplasm,** and the contractile elements within the fiber are the **myofibrils.** Structurally, muscles are either **smooth** (fibers unstriped) or **striated** (fibers cross-striped) (Fig. 6-14).

 Smooth muscle lines the walls of blood vessels and surrounds internal organs such as the intestine and uterus. It is sometimes called involuntary muscle, since it generally cannot be controlled at will. **Skeletal muscle** (Fig. 6-15) is striated muscle that moves the skeleton. It is voluntary muscle. **Cardiac muscle,** the muscle of the heart, is also striated muscle but is involuntary.

 Another type of muscular tissue is made up of **myoepithelial** cells (Fig. 6-16) found in sweat, salivary, and mammary glands between the epithelium and connective tissue. They extend branching processes around the secretory cells of the glands. Their function may be to squeeze secretions from the acini toward the surface openings of the larger ducts.

Nervous tissue

Nervous tissue is specialized for the reception of stimuli and the conduction of impulses. The structural and functional unit of the nervous system is the **neuron** (Fig. 6-17), a nerve cell made up of a body containing the nucleus and its processes or fibers. In most animals the bodies of nerve cells are restricted to the central nervous system and ganglia, but the fibers may extend long distances through the body. Neurons are arranged in chains, and the point of contact between neurons is a **synapse.** Some fibers are wrapped with an insulating sheath (medullated, or myelinated); in others the sheath is absent (nonmedullated).

 Sensory neurons are concerned with conducting impulses from sensory **receptors** in the skin or sense organs to nerve centers (brain or spinal cord). **Motor neurons** carry impulses from the nerve centers to muscles or glands (**effectors**) that are thus stimulated to respond. **Association neurons** form various connections between other neurons.

Figure 6-18

Heart showing various types of tissue in its structure.

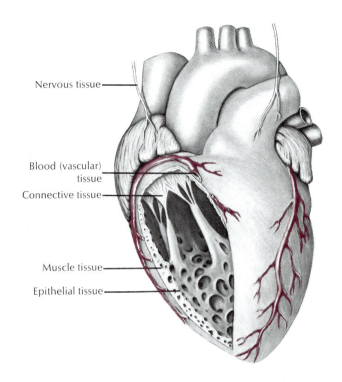

Nervous tissue

Blood (vascular) tissue
Connective tissue

Muscle tissue
Epithelial tissue

Vascular tissue

Blood, lymph, and tissue fluids are types of vascular tissues. Blood is a fluid tissue composed of **white blood cells, red blood cells, platelets,** and a liquid: **plasma.** Traveling through blood vessels, the blood carries to the tissue cells the materials necessary for their life processes. **Lymph** and **tissue fluids** arise from blood by filtration and serve in the exchange between cells and blood.

___ Organs and Systems

An organ is a group of tissues organized into a larger functional unit. In higher forms an organ may have most or all of the five basic tissue types. For example, the heart (Fig. 6-18) has epithelial tissue for covering and lining, connective tissue for framework, muscular walls for contraction, nervous elements for coordination, and vascular tissue for transportation.

All organs have a characteristic structural plan. Usually one tissue carries the burden of the organ's chief function, as muscle does in the heart; the other tissues perform supportive roles. The chief functional cells of an organ are called its **parenchyma;** the supporting tissues are its **stroma.** For instance, in the pancreas the secreting cells are the parenchyma; the capsule and connective tissue framework represent the stroma.

Organs are, in turn, associated in groups to form **systems,** with each system concerned with one of the basic functions. The higher metazoa have 11 organ systems: skeletal, muscular, integumentary, digestive, respiratory, circulatory, excretory, nervous, special sensory, endocrine, and reproductive. However, all living organisms perform the same basic functions. The need for procuring and using food and for movement, protection, perception, and reproduction are equally basic to an ameba, a clam, an insect, or a human. Obviously, because of differences in size, structure, and environment, each must meet these problems in a different manner.

ANIMAL BODY PLANS

Thus far in this chapter we have considered the characteristics of body design that animals share. We are ready now to consider the various architectural plans that distinguish major groups of animals. These appear enormously diverse, as even a cursory examination of the different invertebrate and vertebrate groups will reveal. However, it is possible to resolve them into four "master plans" (Gardiner, 1972): the unicellular plan, cell-aggregate plan, blind-sac plan, and tube-within-a-tube plan. These, together with some of their most important modifications, are shown in Fig. 6-19. All but the first are multicellular plans. Four of the most important determinants of multicellular body plans are symmetry, presence or absence of a body cavity, presence or absence of segmentation, and cephalization.

Animal Symmetry

Symmetry refers to balanced proportions, or the correspondence in size and shape of parts on opposite sides of a median plane. **Spherical symmetry** means that any plane passing through the center divides the body into equivalent, or mirrored, halves. This type of symmetry is found chiefly among some of the protozoa and is rare in other groups of animals. Spherical forms are best suited for floating and rolling.

Radial symmetry applies to forms that can be divided into similar halves by two or more planes passing through the longitudinal axis. These are the tubular, vase, or bowl shapes found in some sponges and in the hydras, jellyfish, sea urchins, and the like, in which one end of the longitudinal axis is usually the mouth. A variant form is **biradial symmetry** in which, because of some part that is single or paired rather than radial, only one or two planes passing through the longitudinal axis produce mirrored halves. Sea walnuts, which are more or less globular in form but have a pair of tentacles, are an example. Radial and biradial animals are usually sessile, freely floating, or weakly swimming. The two phyla that are primarily radial, Cnidaria and Ctenophora, are called the **Radiata.**

In **bilateral symmetry** only a sagittal plane can divide the animal into two mirrored portions—right and left halves (Fig. 6-20). Bilateral animals make up all of the higher phyla and are collectively called the **Bilateria.** They are better fitted for directional movement (forward) than radially symmetrical animals.

Let us review some of the convenient terms used for locating regions of animal bodies (Fig. 6-20). **Anterior** is used to designate the head end; **posterior,** the opposite or tail end; **dorsal,** the back side; and **ventral,** the front or belly side. **Medial** refers to the midline of the body, **lateral** to the sides. **Distal** parts are farther from the middle of the body than some point of reference; **proximal** parts are nearer. **Pectoral** refers to the chest region or the area supported by the forelegs, and **pelvic** refers to the hip region or the area supported by the hindlegs. A **frontal plane** divides a bilateral body into dorsal and ventral halves by running through the anteroposterior axis and the right-left axis at right angles to the **sagittal plane,** the plane dividing an animal into right and left halves. A **transverse plane** would cut through a dorsoventral and a right-left axis at right angles to both the sagittal and frontal planes and would result in anterior and posterior portions.

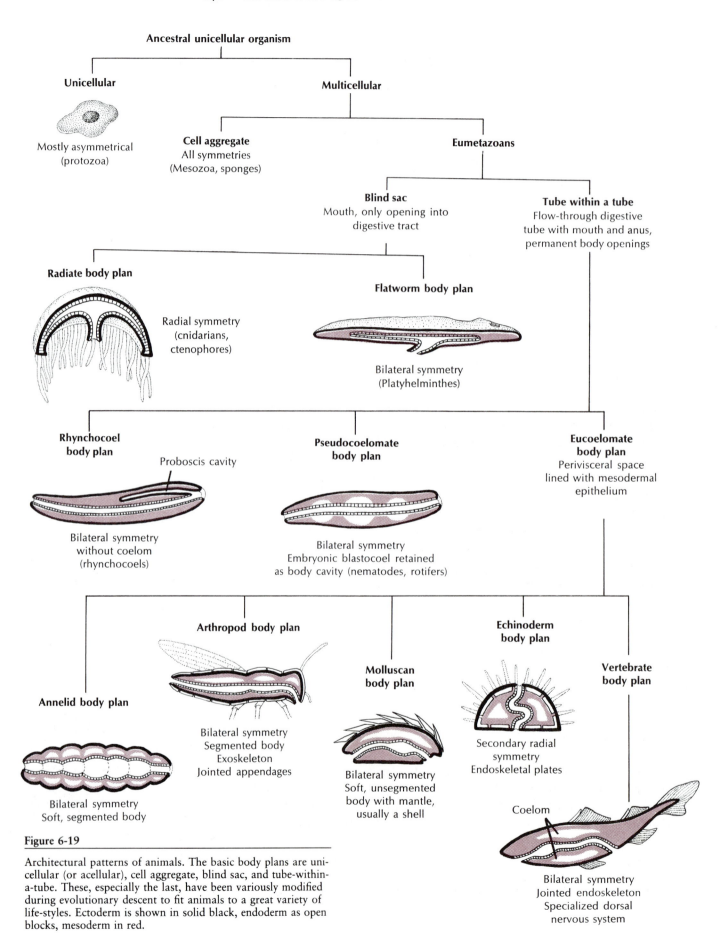

Figure 6-19

Architectural patterns of animals. The basic body plans are uni-cellular (or acellular), cell aggregate, blind sac, and tube-within-a-tube. These, especially the last, have been variously modified during evolutionary descent to fit animals to a great variety of life-styles. Ectoderm is shown in solid black, endoderm as open blocks, mesoderm in red.

Figure 6-20

The planes of symmetry as illustrated by a bilateral animal.

___ Body Cavities

The bilateral animals can be grouped according to their body-cavity type or lack of body cavity (Fig. 6-19). In higher animals the main body cavity is the **coelom,** a fluid-filled space that surrounds the gut. The two methods of coelom formation— schizocoelous and enterocoelous—were described on p. 131. The coelom provides coelomic animals with a "tube-within-a-tube" arrangement (Fig. 6-21). The true coelom develops within the mesoderm and is thus lined with mesodermal epithelium called the **peritoneum.** The coelom is of great significance in animal evolution. It provides increased body flexibility and space for visceral organs and permits greater size and complexity by exposing more cells to surface exchange. The fluid-filled space also serves as a hydrostatic skeleton in some forms, aiding them in such functions as movement and burrowing.

Acoelomate Bilateria

The more primitive bilateral animals do not have a true coelom. In fact, the flatworms and a few others have *no body cavity* surrounding the gut. The region between the ectodermal epidermis and the endodermal digestive tract is completely filled with mesoderm in the form of parenchyma.

Pseudocoelomate Bilateria

Nematodes and several other phyla have a cavity surrounding the gut, but it is not lined with mesodermal peritoneum. It is derived from the blastocoel of the embryo and represents a persistent blastocoel. This type of body cavity is called a **pseudocoel,** and its possessors also have a "tube-within-a-tube" arrangement.

Eucoelomate Bilateria

The remainder of the bilateral animals possess a **true coelom** lined with mesodermal peritoneum.

Figure 6-21

Tube-within-a-tube arrangement.

Chordata

Figure 6-22

Segmented phyla. These three phyla have all made use of an important principle in nature—metamerism, or repetition of structural units. Annelids and arthropods are definitely related, but chordates have derived their segmentation independently. Segmentation brings more varied specialization because segments, especially in arthropods, have become modified for different functions.

Metamerism (Segmentation)

Metamerism is the serial repetition of similar body segments along the longitudinal axis of the body. Each segment is called a **metamere, or somite.** In forms such as the earthworm and other annelids, in which metamerism is most clearly represented, the segmental arrangement includes both external and internal structures of several systems. There is repetition of muscles, blood vessels, nerves, and the setae of locomotion. Some other organs, such as those of sex, are repeated in only a few somites. In higher animals much of the segmental arrangement has become obscure.

True metamerism is found in only three phyla—Annelida, Arthropoda, and Chordata (Fig. 6-22)—although superficial segmentation of the ectoderm and the body wall may be found among many diverse groups of animals.

Cephalization

The differentiation of a head end is called **cephalization** and is found chiefly in bilaterally symmetrical animals. The concentration of nervous tissue and sense organs in the head bestows obvious advantages to an animal moving through its environment head first. This is the most efficient positioning of instruments for sensing the environment and responding to it. Usually the mouth of the animal is located on the head as well, since so much of an animal's activity is concerned with procuring food. Cephalization is always accompanied by differentiation along an anteroposterior axis (**polarity**). Polarity usually involves gradients of activities between limits, such as between the anterior and posterior ends.

HOMOLOGY AND ANALOGY

In comparative studies of animals the concepts of **homology** (similarity in origin) and **analogy** (similarity in function or appearance, but not in origin) are frequently used to express the mechanisms responsible for similar patterns of morphology or function in different animals. For example, the bones in a whale flipper are homologous to the bones of a human arm and of a bat wing (Fig. 38-10, p. 946), although in appearance and function they are quite different. They are homologous because all share a common ancestry and embryonic origin. All develop similarly from a limb bud within which forms a single proximal bone (humerus), two parallel bones located more distally (radius and ulna), and several small bones more distal to the latter (wrist bones and phalanges). Later in development, significant modifications appear that shape the limb for the totally different function each will perform in these three different mammals.

Analogy denotes similarity of function and often of appearance as well. Just as different functions make homologous structures dissimilar in form, similar functions can make nonhomologous structures resemble each other. The wings of a bird and a butterfly obviously perform similar flight functions, but they are not homologous because they have totally different origins. Their resemblance is only superficial. The skeletal framework of the bird's wing with its feathered surface corresponds to the basic vertebrate pentadactyl limb plan. The wing of a butterfly is supported by cuticular thickenings ("veins"), and the surface is a cuticular membrane composed of two cell layers. They are analogous structures.

Homology is a relative term. If one always insists on similarity of structure *and* development for strict homology, as is sometimes done, then many structures that might be considered homologous do not meet these requirements. For instance, the wing of a bird and the wing of a bat are homologous only insofar as both are derived from pentadactyl forelimbs. They are analogous, however, for they have the same function. In examining homologous structures it is best to keep in mind the following question: to what extent or degree do they share a common origin? Of course, even this question contains a nebulous element, since all animals are related, having presumably descended from a common ancestor in the distant past. Homology implies a close evolutionary kinship. Convergent evolution, or the independent origin of two similar structures, is caused by independent mutations that are favored under similar environments. Horns have appeared independently many times in mammals, but should they be considered homologous? Perhaps the best criterion for homology would be homologous genes, but this is impossibly strict at our present state of knowledge, although recent advances in molecular sequencing suggest that this criterion of homology may soon be successfully applied.

The principle of homology, although difficult to define strictly, has a wide application in zoology. It is used as an argument for evolution because it is based on the idea of inheritance from common ancestors. Homology is also important in classifying animals. As more is known about animals, chemical identity may become an important aspect of homology among organisms. A plan of archetypes with which the structures of animals are compared may thus be formulated, not only from gross morphological structures but also from their biochemical resemblances.

___ Summary

From the relatively simple organisms that made up the beginnings of life on earth, animal evolution has progressed through a history of ever more intricately organized forms. Organelles became integrated into cells, cells into tissues, tissues into organs, and organs into systems. Whereas a unicellular animal carries out all life functions within the confines of a single cell, an advanced multicellular animal is an organization of subordinate units that are united at successive levels.

All metazoa pass through a characteristic life cycle that usually begins with the union of male and female germ cells in fertilization. This fusion of sperm and egg pronuclei is followed by a series of developmental stages—cleavage, blastulation, gastrulation, differentiation of tissues and organs, and growth—that adheres to a predictable pattern within a species and among related species within a taxon.

The animal body consists of cells, body fluids, and extracellular structural elements. The cells of metazoans develop into various tissues made up similar cells performing common functions. The basic tissue types are nervous, connective, epithelial, muscular, and vascular. Tissues are organized into larger functional units called organs, and organs are associated to form systems.

Every organism has an inherited body plan that may be described in terms of broadly inclusive characteristics, such as symmetry, presence or absence of body cavities, partitioning of body fluids, presence or absence of segmentation, degree of cephalization, and type of nervous system.

The concept of homology expresses the idea of similarity resulting from common embryological origin and evolutionary ancestry. Analogy means similarity of function and/or appearance, but without common origin. Homologous structures and behaviors are accepted as evidence for evolution and are used in animal classification.

Selected references

Bloom, W., and D.W. Fawcett. 1975. A textbook of histology, ed. 10. Philadelphia, W.B. Saunders Co. *Authoritative and superbly illustrated advanced treatise on human histology.*

Bonner, J.T. 1965. Size and cycle. Princeton, N.J., Princeton University Press. *An essay on the significance of size of the organism in the life cycle.*

Eyre, D.R. 1980. Collagen: molecular diversity in the body's protein scaffold. Science 207:1315-1322. *Biosynthesis, structure, and function of the most abundant animal protein.*

Gardiner, M.S. 1972. The biology of invertebrates. New York, McGraw-Hill Book Co.

Guttman, B.S. 1976. Is "levels of organization" a useful biological concept? BioScience 26:112-113.

Hancox, N.M. 1972. Biology of bone. London, Cambridge University Press. *Well-illustrated monograph dealing with bone structure, deposition, and resorption.*

Hertel, H. 1963. Structure-form-movement. New York, Reinhold Publishing Corp. *An unconventional but interesting attempt to interrelate biology and engineering.*

Karp, G., and N.J. Berrill. 1981. Development. New York, McGraw-Hill Book Co. *One of the best contemporary developmental biology texts.*

Kessel, R.G., and R.H. Kardon. 1979. Tissues and organs: a text-atlas of scanning electron microscopy. San Francisco, W.H. Freeman & Co. Publishers. *Vivid collection of scanning electron micrographs.*

Krommenhock, W., J. Sebus, and G.J. van Esch. 1979. Biological structures. Baltimore, University Park Press. *Includes fine color photographs of mammalian cells and tissues.*

MacMahon, J.A., D.L. Phillips, J.V. Robinson, and D.J. Schimpf. 1978. Levels of biological organization: an organism-centered approach. BioScience 28:700-704. *Presents a hierarchy of organization from subatomic particles through separate supraorganismic levels.*

Romer, A.S., and T.S. Parsons. 1977. The vertebrate body. Philadelphia, W.B. Saunders Co. *Excellent comparative anatomy text with good descriptions of body tissues and organs.*

Saunders, J.W., Jr. 1982. Developmental biology: patterns, problems, principles. New York, Macmillan, Inc.

von Bertalanffy, L. 1952. Problems of life. London, Watts & Co. *Levels of organization are among several topics discussed in this classic book dealing with biological concepts.*

Wainwright, S.A., W.D. Biggs, J.D. Currey, and J.M. Gosline. 1976. Mechanical design in organisms. New York, John Wiley & Sons, Inc. *Deals with the materials with which animals are constructed and how they are adapted to specific life habitats. Technical.*

Selected *Scientific American* articles

Fraser, R.D.B. 1969. Keratins. 221:86-96 (Aug.). *Studies are unveiling the chemical architecture of this remarkable protein.*

Gross, J. 1961. Collagen. 204:120-130 (May). *Chemical and physical characteristics of the most abundant protein on earth.*

McLean, F.C. 1955. Bone. 192:84-91 (Feb.). *Briefly describes the role of bone in maintaining the blood calcium level.*

Ross, R., and P. Bornstein. 1971. Elastic fibers in the body. 224:44-52 (June). *Elastic fibers in skin, arteries, and ligaments permit stretch and rebound.*

CHAPTER 7

CLASSIFICATION AND PHYLOGENY OF ANIMALS

Carolus Linnaeus, the great Swedish naturalist who founded our modern system of classification in the mid-eighteenth century. This statue of a youthful Linnaeus stands before his home in the old university town of Uppsala, Sweden.

Photograph by C.P. Hickman, Jr.

ANIMAL CLASSIFICATION

Zoologists have named more than 1.5 million species of animals, and thousands more are added to the list each year. Yet some zoologists believe that species named so far make up less than 20% of all living animals and less than 1% of all those that have existed in the past.

To communicate with each other about the diversity of life, biologists have found it a practical necessity not only to name living organisms but to classify them. It is not just that the desire to put things into some kind of order is a fundamental activity of the human mind. A system of classification is a storage, retrieval, and communication mechanism for biological information. This is the science of **taxonomy.** It is concerned with the naming of each kind of organism by a uniformly adopted system that best expresses the degree of similarity of organisms. The science of **systematics** is somewhat broader in that it embraces taxonomy, which is concerned with classification, and evolutionary biology, which is the study of organismic diversity and orderliness of nature. Systematics is really comparative biology, because it uses everything that is known about animals to understand their relationships and evolutionary history.

Linnaeus and the Development of Classification

Although the history of human efforts to distinguish and name plants and animals must have been rooted in the beginnings of language, the great Greek philosopher and biologist Aristotle was the first to attempt seriously the classification of organisms on the basis of structural similarities. Following the Dark Ages in Europe, the English naturalist John Ray (1627-1705) introduced a more comprehensive classification system and a modern concept of species. The flowering of systematics in the eighteenth century culminated in the work of Carolus Linnaeus (1707-1778) (Fig. 7-1), who gave us our modern scheme of classification.

Linnaeus was a Swedish botanist at the University of Uppsala. He had a great talent for collecting and classifying objects, especially flowers. Linnaeus worked out a fairly extensive system of classification for both plants and animals. His scheme of classification, published in his great work *Systema Naturae,* emphasized morphological characters as a basis for arranging specimens in collections. Actually his classification was largely arbitrary and artificial, and he believed strongly in the constancy of species. He divided the animal kingdom down to species, and according to his scheme each species was given a distinctive name. He recognized four classes of vertebrates and two classes of invertebrates. These classes were divided into orders, the orders into genera, and the genera into species. Since his knowledge of animals was limited, his lower groups, such as the genera, were very broad and included animals that we now realize are only distantly related. As a result, much of his classification has been drastically altered, yet the basic principle of his scheme is followed at the present time.

Linnaeus's scheme of arranging organisms into an ascending series of groups of ever-increasing inclusiveness is the **hierarchical system** of classification. Species were grouped into genera, genera into orders, and orders into classes. This taxonomic hierarchy has been considerably expanded since Linnaeus's time. The major categories, or **taxa** (sing., **taxon**), now used are as follows, in descending series: kingdom, phylum, class, order, family, genus, and species. This hierarchy of seven ranks can be subdivided into finer categories, such as superclass, subclass, infraclass, superorder, and suborder. In all, more than 30 taxa are recognized. For

Figure 7-1

Carolus Linnaeus (1707-1778). This portrait was made of Linnaeus at age 68, 3 years before his death.

Courtesy British Museum (Natural History), London.

Linnaeus wrote, "The Author of Nature, when He created species, imposed on His Creations an eternal law of reproduction and multiplication within the limits of their proper kinds. He did indeed in many instances allow them the power of sporting in their outward appearances, but never that of passing from one species to another."

Table 7-1 Examples of Classification of Animals

	Human	Gorilla	Southern leopard frog	Katydid
Phylum	Chordata	Chordata	Chordata	Arthropoda
Subphylum	Vertebrata	Vertebrata	Vertebrata	
Class	Mammalia	Mammalia	Amphibia	Insecta
Subclass	Eutheria	Eutheria		
Order	Primates	Primates	Salientia	Orthoptera
Suborder	Anthropoidea	Anthropoidea		
Family	Hominidae	Pongidae	Ranidae	Tettigoniidae
Subfamily			Raninae	
Genus	*Homo*	*Gorilla*	*Rana*	*Scudderia*
Species	*Homo sapiens*	*Gorilla gorilla*	*Rana pipiens*	*Scudderia furcata*
Subspecies			*Rana pipiens sphenocephala*	*Scudderia furcata furcata*

very large and complex groups, such as the fishes and insects, these additional ranks are required to express recognized degrees of evolutionary divergence. Unfortunately, they also contribute complexity to the system.

Linnaeus's system for naming species is known as **binomial nomenclature.** Each species has a latinized name composed of two words (hence binomial). The first word is the genus, written with a capital initial letter; the second word is the specific name that is peculiar to the species and is written with a small initial letter (Table 7-1). The genus name is always a noun, and the specific name is usually an adjective that must agree in gender with the genus. For instance, the scientific name of the common robin is *Turdus migratorius* (L., *turdus*, thrush; *migratorius*, of the migratory habit).

There are times when a species is divided into subspecies, in which case a **trinomial nomenclature is employed** (see katydid example, Table 7-1). Thus to distinguish the southern form of the robin from the eastern robin, the scientific term *Turdus migratorius achrustera* (duller color) is employed for the southern type. The trinomial nomenclature is really an addition to the Linnaean system, which is basically binomial. The generic, specific, and subspecific names are printed in italics (underlined if handwritten or typed).

It is important to recognize that *only* the species is binomial. All ranks above the species are uninomial nouns, written with a capital initial letter. We must also note that the second word of a species is an epithet that has no meaning by itself. The scientific name of the white-breasted nuthatch is *Sitta carolinensis*. The "carolinensis" may be and is used in combination with other genera to mean "of Carolina," as for instance *Parus carolinensis* (Carolina chickadee) and *Anolis carolinensis* (green anole, a lizard). The genus name, on the other hand, may stand alone to designate a taxon that may include several species.

Figure 7-2

Type specimens of crustaceans in the Smithsonian Institution's Natural History Museum in Washington, D.C.
Photograph by C.P. Hickman, Jr.

___ Species

Despite the central importance of the species concept in biology, biologists do not agree on a single rigid definition that applies to all cases. Before Darwin's time, the species was considered a primeval pattern, or archetype, divinely created. With gradual acceptance of the concept of organic evolution, scientists realized that species were not fixed, immutable units but have evolved one from another. Sometimes the gaps between species are so subtle that they can be distinguished only by the most careful examination. In other instances, a species is so distinctive in every way that it is clearly unique and only remotely related to other species. Consequently, the criteria of taxonomy have undergone gradual changes.

At first each species was supposed to have been represented by a **type** that was used as a fixed standard. The **typological specimen** was duly labeled and deposited in some prestigious center such as a museum (Fig. 7-2). Anyone classifying a particular group would always take the pains to compare specimens with the available typological specimens. Since variations from the type specimen nearly always occurred, these differences were supposed to be attributable to imperfections during embryonic development and were considered of minor significance.

The **typological** (or **morphological**) **species concept** of classifying persisted for a long period (and still does to some extent). During this time, though, the idea that species represent lineages in evolutionary descent was becoming more firmly established. Gradually taxonomists began to think of species as *groups of interbreeding natural populations that are reproductively isolated from other such groups* (Mayr, 1969). This concept of **genetic incompatibility** between different species therefore replaced the earlier idea of **character discontinuity** for species separation. Taxonomists began to think of species as populations in which every individual is unique and in which every individual may change to a greater or lesser extent when placed in a different environment. This is the **biological species** concept. It is still important, nevertheless, for a person who describes a species to deposit a specimen in a museum so that later taxonomists can examine an actual specimen that the original author believed was a member of that species (Fig. 7-2).

The modern concept of species is of course the antithesis of that of the typologist, to whom variations from the type specimen are illusions caused by small mistakes during embryonic development. In population studies the type is considered an abstract average of *real* variations that occur within the interbreeding population. Thus, the species must be regarded as an **interbreeding population** made up of individuals of common descent and sharing intergrading characteristics.

The biological species concept is not without difficulties. For one thing, it does not apply to organisms that reproduce asexually because there is no way to test the interbreeding criterion in uniparental species. For another, it is a "static" concept that does not flex easily with the slow, usually unmeasurable, changes that occur in a species through time. Furthermore, even in species that reproduce sexually, reproductive isolation may be only partial. Not infrequently, populations are found that are in an intermediate stage of differentiation between races, which can interbreed, and species, which cannot. They cannot be classed as definite races or as definite species, and so are sometimes called semispecies.

Despite these problems, the biological species concept works satisfactorily most of the time. Reproductive barriers do exist. Sometimes pairs of species can be made to hybridize, but then produce sterile offspring. A well-known example is the sterile mule, the offspring of a mare and a male ass. Even when fertile hybrids are possible, they are normally prevented by various external barriers, such as anatomical incompatibilities and, especially, behavioral patterns that create aversions to mating with the wrong species.

Basis for Formation of Taxa

Classification emphasizes the natural relationships of animals. Descent from a common ancestor explains similarity in character; the more recent the descent, the more closely the animals are grouped in taxonomic units. The genera of a particular family show less diversity than do the families of an order. This is because the common ancestor of families within an order is more remote than the common ancestor of different genera within a family. The same applies to higher categories. The common ancestor of the various vertebrate classes, for example, must be much older than the common ancestor of orders of mammals within the class Mammalia.

It is apparent that this criterion of evolutionary ancestry is not a very definite one for use in setting up taxa. There is no way to define a class that does not apply equally well to an order or a family. The genera of certain ancient groups, such as the molluscs, may actually be much older than orders and classes of other groups. The taxonomist must arrange the classifications so that all members of a taxon, as far as can be determined, are related to one another more than they are to the members of any other taxon of the same rank. Obviously, the assignment of taxonomic rank depends on the opinion of the taxonomist making the study, and this is one reason classification has been called as much an art as a science (G.G. Simpson, 1961). As more is learned about animals and their relationships, changes in classification are required. This brings instability to biological nomenclature and reduces its efficiency as a reference system.

To avoid problems with the biological species concept, the evolutionary species concept has been proposed. *An evolutionary species is a single lineage of ancestor-descendant populations that maintains its identity from other such lineages and that has its own evolutionary tendencies and historical fate* (Wiley, 1981). In this definition, "identity" means any quality a species uses to keep its line separated from other species. Each species "knows" its identity and has recognition systems in appearance and behavior and ecological roles to maintain reproductive isolation. The evolutionary species concept has the advantage of embracing both asexual and sexual organisms.

The **law of priority** also brings about frequent changes. The first name proposed for a taxonomic unit that is published and meets other proper specifications has priority over all subsequent names proposed. The rejected duplicate names are called **synonyms.** It is disturbing sometimes to find that a species that has been well established for years must undergo a change in terminology when some industrious systematist discovers that on the basis of priority or for some other reason the species is, according to this "law," misnamed.

Despite such difficulties, the hierarchical system of classification is the accepted system, and it is a very useful one. To reduce confusion in the field of taxonomy and to lay down a uniform code of rules for the classification of animals, the International Commission on Zoological Nomenclature was established in 1898. This commission meets from time to time to formulate rules and make decisions in connection with taxonomic work.

____ Recent Trends in Taxonomy

Since Darwin's time, biological units have been classified on the basis of common descent, using morphological characters. But it is not always clear just what this evolutionary relationship is. Only the fossil record can supply convincing evidence, and this is often lacking. There is an inherent danger of circular reasoning in taxonomic work: hypotheses about taxonomic relationships are used as evidence of phylogenetic relationships, and these in turn are used to make judgments about taxonomic relationships. Clearly, there is a duality to the science of systematics. On the one hand, it is charged with naming organisms and placing them in some kind of order. On the other, systematics is supposed to help unravel the course of evolution. It is an unsteady mix of the practical and the theoretical. Most biologists firmly believe that systematics should legitimately concern itself with both these functions, but the difficulty of doing so has placed stresses on established taxonomic procedures.

There are today three major schools of taxonomy. These competing methodologies, which we describe below, grew out of dissatisfaction with the arbitrary way in which classification schemes were being applied. Some taxonomists relied heavily on the fossil record, some on outward appearance of living forms, and others on the embryological record and "recapitulation" (defined later in this chapter), and still others attempted to meld together these approaches. These problems stimulated the search for new approaches.

Numerical taxonomy

In all taxonomic work it is first necessary to recognize **characters** that can be used to describe an organism adequately and place it in the proper taxon. A character is any feature or attribute that can be described, measured, weighed, pictured, counted, scored, or otherwise defined about an organism.

In 1763 the Frenchman M. Adanson proposed a scheme of classification that involved the grouping of individuals into a particular species according to the number of shared characters. Thus, each member of a species would have a majority of the total characteristics of the taxon, even though some of its characters were not shared with others of the same taxon. Such a classification has quantitative rather than qualitative significance. The classification lacks the phyletic relationship of evolutionary taxonomy (Adanson lived long before Darwin's time). However, this scheme has been revived (especially by plant taxonomists) in

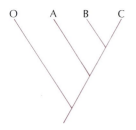

Figure 7-3

Simple cladogram. *O* represents the out-group, and *A, B,* and *C* the more closely related groups. In this cladogram, *B* and *C* are shown as most closely related and would have the largest number of syn-apomorphies. *A* would have a smaller number of synapomorphies with *B* and *C,* and we could estimate that it had branched off from the common ancestral line of all three at an earlier stage. All characteristics shared by *O, A, B,* and *C* would be considered primitive and thus would have been possessed by the common ancestor of all four. A cladogram is meant to show only relative degree of relationship and not actual historical events. Therefore, unlike traditional "phylogenetic trees," cladograms carry no time scale (compare with Fig. 23-1, pp. 522 and 523).

recent years and has given rise to **phenetics** (Gr., *phainein,* to show) or **numerical taxonomy,** which makes use of the computer method to determine similarities among organisms. As many arbitrarily chosen characters as possible are selected and fed into a computer, and an analysis is made of the calculations. Species or groups are then clustered by similarity.

Numerical taxonomy (or numerical phenetics) is perhaps the most standardized in methodological approach of the three schools of taxonomy. This approach aims simply at producing meaningful groupings of organisms and makes no attempt to reconstruct the evolutionary history of groups. Numerical taxonomy has been criticized by evolutionary biologists, who point out that groups of organisms *are* the products of evolution and that any satisfactory taxonomy must fully account for evolutionary history.

Cladistics

An alternative to phenetics in the study of taxonomic relationships is the method of **cladistics** (Gr., *cladus,* branch), first elaborated by W. Henning (1950). This method does purport to yield significant phylogenetic information. With it one can set up a kind of phylogenetic tree, called a **cladogram** (Fig. 7-3), that represents the branching off of related groups of animals from their common ancestors, with closer branch points indicating closer phylogenetic relationships.

Although the theory of cladistics may seem complicated, its rationale is fairly simple. In practice the investigator is interested in studying the evolutionary relationships of certain groups of animals, for example, species within a genus or genera within a family. Another genus or species is selected, which the worker believes is only distantly related to the groups of interest; this distantly related taxon is called the **outgroup.** Then a variety of characteristics are chosen that will be used to compare among the more closely related groups and the outgroup. These characteristics may be morphological, physiological, biochemical, behavioral, or any others that may have been subject to change during the course of evolution. If the outgroup has been correctly selected, all characteristics it has in common with the related groups may be considered *primitive,* that is, they are characteristics possessed by the common ancestor of both the outgroup and the related groups. Characteristics shared by the related groups, but not possessed by the outgroup, are *derived.* Shared derived characters are called **synapomorphies.** The more synapomorphies that two groups have in common, the more closely they are related, and the more closely their branching from a common ancestor must be placed on a phylogenetic tree. If a synapomorphy is found between the outgroup and one of the more lately evolved groups, then according to cladistic theory only one of two conclusions is possible: the synapomorphy is the product of convergent evolution, or there has been some mistake, such as in the choice of the outgroup. Cladistics is a valuable method of distinguishing primitive and derived characteristics and of estimating the relative degree of evolutionary relationship between groups of organisms.

Evolutionary systematics

Evolutionary taxonomy has been considered the traditional approach to classification, at least since Darwin, because it bases taxonomy on evolutionary theory. Its goal is to reconstruct evolutionary history as closely as possible. In its modern form it applies many of the same approaches used in cladistics, but it includes

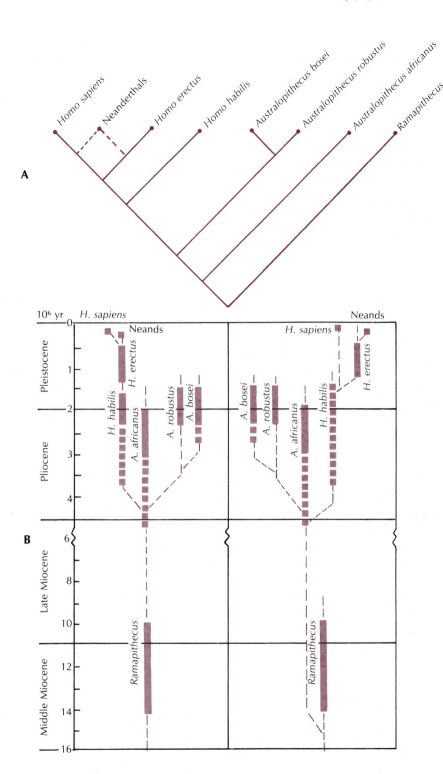

Figure 7-4

Comparison of a cladogram and phylogenetic trees of hominids. **A,** Cladogram of hominid relationships constructed from the analysis of primitive and specialized (derived) characters. **B,** Two phylogenetic trees consistent with the cladogram. Solid lines represent known African hominids, broken solid lines represent tentative fossil assignments, and broken thin lines are inferred lines of descent without direct fossil evidence. These schemes are based on fossil finds as of 1977; for an updated hominid evolution based on more recent fossil finds, see Chapter 39.

From Tattershall, I., and N. Eldredge. 1977. Am. Sci. 65:204-211.

more information, especially ancestor-descendant relationships that are lacking in phenetics and strict cladistic classification. Phylogenetic trees are used to depict patterns of evolutionary descent. The difference between a cladogram and a phylogenetic tree is illustrated in Fig. 7-4. In phylogenetic trees, the lines portray evolutionary species and the branches represent speciation events. A geological time scale is usually included, and sometimes the number of species in a group at any time is indicated by the widening and thinning of the branch lines (see Fig. 23-1, pp. 522 and 523, for example).

___ANIMAL PHYLOGENY

The different approaches to classification that we have just described tend to obscure a basic agreement: order in the biological world derives from evolution. Hierarchical classification schemes are possible because relationships between species are due to descent with modification from ancestral species. Reconstructing lines of descent leading to living animals is not unlike attempts to ferret out the ancestral history (genealogy) of one's own family. Neither plant or animal species nor members of one's family arose spontaneously, but rather they represent branching of ancestral forms. The phylogeny of an animal group, then, represents our concept of the path its evolution has taken. It is the evolutionary history of the group.

Unfortunately, the evolutionary origin of most animal phyla is shrouded in the obscurity of Precambrian times. Because fossil records are fragmentary, our reconstructions of patterns of evolutionary relationships must have relied to a large extent on evidence from comparative morphology and embryology. Relationships are naturally more easily established within the smaller taxonomic units (such as species, genera, orders) than in the classes and phyla.

Other techniques are now in use in systematics that offer great promise in solving problems of phylogenetic relationships and evolution. Research is being carried out in animal behavior, comparative biochemistry, serology, cytology, genetic homology, and comparative physiology with this aim in view.

For example, it has been shown that there are certain homologies among polynucleotide sequences in the DNA molecules of such different forms as fish and humans. These sequences appear to be genes that have been retained with little change throughout vertebrate evolution. Possible phenotypical expressions of these homologous sequences are bilateral symmetry, notochord, and hemoglobin, as well as others. By using a single strand of DNA from one species and short radioactive pieces of a DNA strand from another species and mixing the strands together, it was found that some of the smaller strands paired with similar regions on the large strand, indicating that the paired parts had common genes.

Another recent technique involves the recognition of RNA codons by transfer RNA of another species. These new biochemical methods of classification are used to complement, rather than replace, the older, more established methods. In general, molecular evidences have not agreed very well with the fossil evidence. Nevertheless, the new molecular approach provides a potentially powerful tool for the systematist.

Although the representation of ancestral relationships of animals in the form of a "family tree" seems obvious today, it was not apparent to biologists before classification became founded on evolutionary theory. Even Darwin never attempted a pictorial diagram of animal relationships. Yet, despite all the shortcomings that any phylogenetic tree must possess, especially the danger of depicting and accepting highly tentative relationships as dogmatic certainty, such a scheme is a valuable tool. A family tree ties the taxa together in an evolutionary blueprint. Constructing a family tree is a creative activity based on judgment and experience and as such is always subject to modification as new information becomes available.

In each of the following chapters on animal phyla, we include a summary of that group's origins and the relationships within the group. The student is encouraged to make frequent reference to the geological time scale on the inside back cover of this book and to the phylogenetic tree of multicellular animals on the inside front cover. We have based conclusions about group histories on recent informed opinion. Although we recognize that family trees can give false impressions, we have nonetheless used them in the absence of a better alternative. They may be viewed as educated speculations and as such with a certain measure of skepticism; at the same time they are not science fiction. They are derived from close studies of morphology and a thorough understanding of general biological principles by scientists who have devoted their lives to this form of detective work. Evolution, with its idea of life transforming itself through the ages, is supported by a vast wealth of fossil and living evidence. It is after all the framework of biology.

Some Helpful Definitions

In the discussions on evolutionary relationships in ensuing chapters, terms such as lower, higher, primitive, advanced, specialized, generalized, adaptation, and fitness will be used frequently, and an understanding of their meaning may be critical to an understanding of the discussion to follow.

The terms **lower** and **higher** usually refer to a group's relative position on a phylogenetic tree; that is, the level at which it is believed to have branched off a main stem of evolution. For example, sponges and jellyfish are usually considered to belong to "lower" phyla because they are believed to have been among the earliest metazoa. In other words, they originated near the base of the family tree of the animal kingdom.

The terms **primitive** and **advanced** are often used when discussing relationships within a particular group. A primitive species is one that possesses a great many of the same characteristics believed to have belonged to the ancestral stock from which it evolved. An advanced species is one that has undergone considerable change from the primitive condition, usually because of adaptation to a changed environment or to a different mode of living. Among the molluscs, for example, the caudofoveates are considered to be more primitive (that is, more like the hypothetical mollusc ancestor) than the snails, clams, or octopuses. A primitive species is not "less perfect" than an advanced species, since it may be as well adapted to its own type of environment as the advanced one is to the environment for which it has become especially adapted. Also, a species or group may be primitive in some respects and advanced in others.

Specialized might refer either to an organism or to one or more of its parts that has become adapted to a particular ecological niche or to a particular function. A more **generalized** species or structure may share the characteristics of two or more distinct groups or structures. For example, many of the small aquatic crustaceans have a number of similar feathery trunk appendages, all serving several functions, such as swimming, respiration, filter feeding, or egg bearing. Such multipurpose appendages would be considered generalized in comparison with the highly specialized defensive chelipeds or sensory antennae of the crayfish, the pollen-collecting legs of the honeybee, or the digging forelegs of the mole cricket. Each of these specialized appendages is adapted for one primary function.

An **adaptation** is any characteristic of an organism taken in the context of how the characteristic helps the organism survive and reproduce. Many adaptations are possessed in common by a wide variety of animals, but the word is most often used in reference to special adaptations for a particular habitat or environment. Indeed, the more *special adaptations* the animal has, the more *specialized* the animal is. Any characteristic or any change in a characteristic is said to have **adaptive value**, if it tends toward greater fitness of the organism for a particular niche or habitat.

An organism is **fitted** to its environment when it is adjusted or adapted to it. Its **fitness** for any particular place or mode of living is the degree of its adjustment, suitability, or adaptation to that particular environment or niche.

ONTOGENY, PHYLOGENY, AND RECAPITULATION

Phylogeny, as we have seen, represents the evolutionary history of any taxon. **Ontogeny,** on the other hand, refers to the history of the development of an individual through its entire life. All metazoans pass through certain common developmental stages. The stages, in succession, are the zygote, cleavage, blastulation, and gastrulation. Haeckel believed that each of these successive stages in the development of an individual represented one of the adult forms that appeared in its evolutionary history. As he phrased it, "Ontogeny is the short and rapid recapitulation of phylogeny. During its own development . . . an individual repeats the most important changes in form evolved by its ancestors during their long and slow paleontological development." According to this theory, the zygote of a developing individual represented the protozoan or protistan stage of its evolutionary history; the blastula represented the hollow colonial protozoa; and the gastrula, the adult cnidarians. The human embryo with gill depressions in the neck was believed to represent the stage when our adult ancestors were aquatic. On this basis he gave his generalization: *ontogeny (individual development) recapitulates (repeats) phylogeny (evolutionary descent).* This notion later became known as the **biogenetic law** (Principle 7, p. 12).

Haeckel's hypothesis of **recapitulation** was based on the flawed premise that evolutionary change occurs by the successive addition of stages to the end of an unaltered ancestral ontogeny. This was an outgrowth of his belief in Lamarck's concept of the inheritance of acquired characters (p. 937).

K.E. von Baer, a nineteenth-century embryologist, had noticed long before Haeckel the general similarity between the embryonic stages and the adults of certain animals, but von Baer had arrived at a different and sounder interpretation. According to his view, the earlier stages of all embryos tend to look alike, but as development proceeds, the embryos become more dissimilar. In other words, he believed that the embryos of higher and lower forms resemble each other more the earlier in their development that they are compared and *not* that embryos of higher forms resemble the adults of lower forms.

The fascination with and debates over recapitulation gradually waned as scientists became more absorbed in Mendelian genetics, experimental embryology, and cell and molecular biology, and the whole question fell into a mild state of disrepute. S.J. Gould (1977) has brought the matter again into the limelight. He contends that there *are* parallels between the stages of ontogeny and phylogeny but that features appearing at one stage of an ancestral ontogeny may be shifted to earlier or later stages in descendants. If a feature that appears at a specific point in the ontogeny of an ancestor arises earlier and earlier in descendants, we have one parallel producing recapitulation (the descendant's ontogeny repeats an evolutionary sequence of stages that characterized its ancestors at that specific point). If a feature that appears at a specific point in the ontogeny of an ancestor arises later and later in the descendants, we have an inverse parallel producing **paedomorphosis** (the retention of ancestral juvenile characters by later stages in the ontogeny of descendants). In other words, the rate of development of a feature in a descendant's ontogeny may be faster or slower than the rate of development of that same feature in an ancestor's ontogeny. This phyletic change in timing of development Gould calls **heterochrony.**

▬ KINGDOMS OF LIFE

Since Aristotle's time, it has been traditional to assign every living organism to one of two kingdoms: plant or animal. However, the two-kingdom system has outlived its usefulness. Although it is easy to place rooted, photosynthetic organisms such as trees, flowers, mosses, and ferns among the plants and to place food-ingesting, motile forms such as worms, fishes, and mammals among the animals, unicellular organisms present difficulties (Chapter 1). Some forms are claimed both for the plant kingdom by botanists and for the animal kingdom by zoologists. An example is *Euglena* (p. 180) and its phytoflagellate kin, which are motile, like animals, but have chlorophyll and photosynthesize, like plants. Other groups such as the bacteria were rather arbitrarily assigned to the plant kingdom.

It was inevitable that biologists would try to resolve these problems by separating problem groups into new kingdoms. This was first done in 1866 by Haeckel, who proposed the new kingdom Protista to include all single-celled organisms. At first the bacteria and blue-green algae, forms that lack nuclei bounded by a membrane, were included with nucleated unicellular organisms. Finally the important differences between the anucleate bacteria and blue-green algae (prokaryotes) and all other organisms that have cells with membrane-bound nuclei (eukaryotes) were recognized. The prokaryote-eukaryote distinction is actually much more profound than the plant-animal distinction of the traditional system. The many differences between prokaryotes and eukaryotes are summarized on p. 76.

In 1969 R.H. Whittaker proposed a five-kingdom system that incorporated the basic prokaryote-eukaryote distinction (Fig. 7-5). The kingdom Monera contains the prokaryotes; the eukaryotes are divided among the remaining four kingdoms. The kingdom Protista contains the unicellular eukaryotic organisms (protozoa and unicellular eukaryotic algae). The multicellular organisms are split into three kingdoms on the basis of mode of nutrition and other fundamental differences in organization. The kingdom Plantae includes multicellular photosynthesizing organisms, higher plants, and multicellular algae. Kingdom Fungi contains the molds, yeasts, and fungi that obtain their food by absorption. The invertebrates (except the protozoa) and the vertebrates comprise the kingdom Animalia. Most of these forms ingest their food and digest it internally, although some parasitic forms are absorptive. The supposed evolutionary relationships of the five kingdoms are shown in Fig. 7-5. The Protista are believed to have given rise to all three multicellular kingdoms, which therefore have evolved independently.

Exclusion of the unicellular protozoa from the animal kingdom, in which

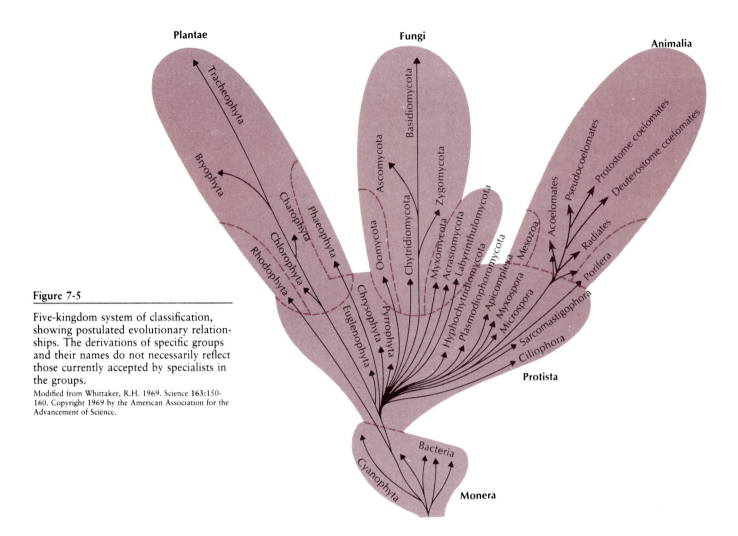

Figure 7-5

Five-kingdom system of classification, showing postulated evolutionary relationships. The derivations of specific groups and their names do not necessarily reflect those currently accepted by specialists in the groups.

Modified from Whittaker, R.H. 1969. Science **163**:150-160. Copyright 1969 by the American Association for the Advancement of Science.

they have been traditionally included, presents a didactic problem for the zoologist. In the five-kingdom system, the classical phylum Protozoa was divided into seven groups that were each elevated to phylum status. This change emphasizes the fluid nature of the hierarchical system of classification pointed out earlier in this chapter. The latest classification adopted by the Society of Protozoologists organized the protozoa into seven other phyla on the basis of fundamental differences between groups (Chapter 8). On the other hand, the protozoa share many animal-like characteristics. Most ingest their food; many have specialized organelles and advanced locomotory systems, portending tissue differentiation in multicellular forms; many reproduce sexually; and some flagellate forms are colonial with division of labor among cell types, again suggestive of a metazoan pattern. For the purposes of this book, we will consider the protozoa as animals.

ORIGIN OF METAZOA

Unraveling the origin of the multicellular animals (metazoans) has presented many problems for zoologists. It is generally believed that they evolved from unicellular organisms, but there is much disagreement over which group of unicellular organisms gave rise to them, and how. The three prevalent hypotheses in current use are (1) that the metazoans arose from a syncytial (multinucleate) ciliate in which cell boundaries later evolved, (2) that they arose from a colonial flagellate in which the cells gradually became more specialized and interdependent, and (3) that the origin of metazoans was polyphyletic, or derived from more than one group of unicellular organisms.

Proponents of the **syncytial ciliate hypothesis** believe that metazoans arose from primitive single-celled ciliates, which at first were multinucleated (having more than one nucleus) but later, by acquiring cell membranes around the nuclei, became compartmentalized into the multicellular condition. The ancestral ciliates, like many modern ones, tended toward bilateral symmetry, so that the earliest metazoans were bilateral and similar to the present primitive flatworms. There are several objections to this hypothesis. It ignores the embryology of the flatworms in which nothing similar to cellularization occurs; it does not explain the presence of flagellated sperm in the metazoans; and, perhaps more important, it infers that the radially symmetrical cnidarians are derived from the flatworms, thus making bilateral symmetry more primitive than radial symmetry.

The **colonial flagellate hypothesis**—first proposed by Haeckel in 1874—is the classical scheme, which, with various revisions, still has many followers. According to this hypothesis, the metazoans are derived from a hollow, spherical, colonial flagellate (protozoan). The individual cells within the colony became differentiated for specific functional roles (reproductive cells, nerve cells, somatic cells, and so on), thus subordinating cellular independence to the welfare of the colony as a whole. The colonial ancestral form was at first radially symmetrical, similar perhaps to the free-swimming planula larvae of the cnidarians (jellyfishes and others). This larva is radially symmetrical and has no mouth. The cnidarians with their radial symmetry could have evolved from this form.

Bilateral symmetry could have evolved later when some of these planula-like ancestors became adapted for a creeping form of locomotion on the ocean floor. Dorsal and ventral surfaces would have differentiated, a ventral mouth would have appeared, and a start would have been made toward cephalization (a concentration of neurons and sensory structures at the anterior). This would have led to bilateral symmetry and the evolution of the primitive flatworms, which later gave rise to all other bilateral forms.

Some zoologists prefer the idea that the metazoans had a **polyphyletic origin** and suggest that the sponges, cnidarians, ctenophores, and flatworms each evolved independently—the sponges and cnidarians probably evolving from colonial flagellates, and the ctenophores and flatworms from ciliates. This is of course a compromise between the other two hypotheses.

In any case, by whatever route, the primitive flatworms (acoel) are believed to be the most primitive of the bilateral animals.

Table 7-2 Basis for Distinction between Divisions of Bilateral Animals*

Protostomes	Deuterostomes
Mouth from, at, or near blastopore	New mouth from stomodeum
Anus new formation	Anus from or near blastopore
Cleavage mostly spiral and involving all organ systems	Cleavage mostly radial and involving only dorsal myotomes
Embryology mostly determinate (mosaic)	Embryology usually indeterminate
In coelomate protostomes coelom forms as split in mesodermal bands; schizocoelous	All coelomate, coelom from fusion of enterocoelous pouches (except chordates, which are schizocoelous)
Endomesoderm usually from a particular blastomere designated 4d	Endomesoderm from enterocoelous pouching (except chordates)
Includes phyla Platyhelminthes, Rhynchocoela, Annelida, Mollusca, Arthropoda, minor phyla	Includes phyla Echinodermata, Hemichordata, Chaetognatha, and Chordata

*Embryos of many of the advanced members of each group may have some or all of these characteristics obscured or lost.

LARGER DIVISIONS OF THE ANIMAL KINGDOM

Although the phylum is often considered to be the largest and most distinctive taxonomic unit, zoologists often find it convenient to combine phyla under a few large groups because of certain common embryological and anatomical features. Such large divisions may have a logical basis, because not only are the members of some of these arbitrary groups united by common traits, but evidence also indicates some relationship in phylogenetic descent.

Subkingdom Protozoa (unicellular)—protozoan phyla
Subkingdom Metazoa (multicellular)—all other phyla
  Branch A (Mesozoa)—phylum Mesozoa, the mesozoa
  Branch B (Parazoa)—phylum Porifera, the sponges
  Branch C (Eumetazoa)—all other phyla
    Grade I (Radiata)—phyla Cnidaria, Ctenophora
    Grade II (Bilateria)—all other phyla
      Division A (Protostomia)—characteristics in Table 7-2
        Acoelomates—phyla Platyhelminthes, Rhynchocoela (Nemertina)
        Pseudocoelomates—phyla Rotifera, Gastrotricha, Kinorhyncha, Gnathostomulida, Nematoda, Nematomorpha, Acanthocephala, Entoprocta
        Eucoelomates—phyla Mollusca, Annelida, Arthropoda, Priapulida, Echiurida, Sipunculida, Tardigrada, Pentastomida, Onychophora, Pogonophora, Phoronida, Ectoprocta, Brachiopoda
      Division B (Deuterostomia)—characteristics in Table 7-2
        Phyla Echinodermata, Chaetognatha, Hemichordata, Chordata

As in the outline, the bilateral animals are customarily divided into protostomes and deuterostomes on the basis of their embryological development (Table 7-2). However, some of the phyla are difficult to place into one of these two categories because they possess some of the characteristics of each group (Chapter 19).

____ Summary

Systematics is concerned with the speciation, classification, and phylogeny of animals. It includes a system of uniform naming of kinds of animals and the erection of a classification scheme that reflects evolutionary relationships. The scheme is hierarchical, and the most widely used groupings (taxa) are as follows, in order of increasing inclusiveness: species, genus, family, order, class, phylum, and kingdom. Subdivisions of all of these are commonly used as necessary. The basic binomial system of nomenclature, giving each kind of organism a generic and a specific name, originated with Carolus Linnaeus and is still in use today. The biological species concept has replaced the older typological concept of a species. A biological species is an interbreeding (or potentially interbreeding) population that is reproductively isolated from other such groups. It is not immutable through time but changes during the course of evolution. If a species is given more than one name, the earliest name published with an appropriate description of the organism is considered the correct name, and other, later names become synonyms.

There are today three schools of taxonomy having different approaches to classification of organisms. Numerical taxonomy (phenetics) groups taxa according to a statistical analysis of their total similarities and dissimilarities. A phenetic arrangement does not infer evolutionary relationships. A second approach is cladistics, which uses primitive and derived characters to arrive at a branching pattern of relationships called a cladogram. The third approach is evolutionary systematics, which bases classification on inferred evolutionary history.

Although morphology, embryology, and the fossil record are still used as criteria for assessing evolutionary relationships, other characteristics such as behavioral, serological, biochemical, cytological, and physiological characteristics are increasingly used in modern systematics. A highly useful device for visualizing evolutionary relationships and derivations from ancestral groups is the phylogenetic tree.

The following terms have specific meanings in evolutionary biology, each of which should be carefully distinguished and understood: higher, lower, primitive, advanced, specialized, generalized, adaptation, and fitness.

The earlier view that embryonic stages of an animal were similar to adult stages of its ancestor (recapitulation) has been replaced by the idea that animal embryos often tend to resemble the embryos of their ancestors.

Three hypotheses have been advanced to explain the origin of the metazoa (multicellular animals): (1) that they arose from a multinucleate ciliate that later became multicellular, (2) that they arose from a colonial flagellate in which cells became specialized and interdependent, or (3) that they arose from more than one group of unicellular organisms (polyphyletic).

The broadest, most inclusive categories of living organisms have been traditionally considered the plant and animal kingdoms. However, most biologists now prefer the five-kingdom scheme: Monera (prokaryotes), Protista (protozoa and eukaryotic algae), Fungi, Plantae, and Animalia. As considered in this book, the Animalia contains the subkingdoms Protozoa (unicellular phyla) and Metazoa (multicellular phyla). Among the metazoa, important groupings are the radial and the bilateral animals, and among the bilateral, the Protostomia and the Deuterostomia.

Selected references

Clifford, H.T., and W. Stephenson. 1975. An introduction to numerical classification. New York, Academic Press, Inc. *Methods of numerical approaches to classification are clearly described and compared to classical taxonomy. Less detailed than the Sneath and Sokal book.*

Crowson, R.A. 1970. Classification and biology. New York, Atherton Press. *A thorough treatment of the methods and problems of zoological, botanical, and paleontological classification.*

Eldridge, N., and J. Cracraft. 1980. Phylogenetic patterns and the evolutionary process. New York, Columbia University Press. *Cladistics explained and evaluated.*

Gould, S.J. 1977. Ontogeny and phylogeny. Cambridge, Mass., The Belknap Press of Harvard University Press. *A review of the historical development and collapse of the theory of recapitulation, and a discussion of modern concepts, such as heterochrony—changes in developmental timing, producing parallels between ontogeny and phylogeny—and neoteny, which Gould terms the most important determinant of human evolution.*

Hennig, W. 1950. Phylogenetic systematics. (1966 translation by D.D. Davis and R. Zangerl. Urbana, University of Illinois Press.)

Hyman, L.H. 1940-1967. The invertebrates, 6 vols. New York, McGraw-Hill Book Co. *Informative discussions on the phylogenies of most of the invertebrates are treated in this outstanding series of monographs. Vol. 1 contains a discussion of the colonial hypothesis of the origin of metazoa, and vol. 2 contains a discussion of the origin of bilateral animals, body cavities, and metamerism.*

Ivanov, A.V. 1976. Correlation between the Protostomia and the Deuterostomia and the classification of the animal kingdom. Zool. Zh. 55(8):1125-1137. *In Russian with Russian and English summaries.*

Jeffrey, C. 1973. Biological nomenclature. London, Edward Arnold, Ltd. *A concise, practical guide to the principles and practice of biological nomenclature and a useful interpretation of the Codes of Nomenclature.*

Levine, N.D., and others. 1980. A newly revised classification of the Protozoa. J. Protozool. 27:37-58.

Margulis, L. 1974. Five-kingdom classification and the origin and evolution of cells. Evol. Biol. 7:45-78. *Describes a modified version of the Whittaker five-kingdom system.*

Margulis, L., and K.V. Schwartz. 1982. Five kingdoms: an illustrated guide to the phyla of life on earth. San Francisco, W.H. Freeman & Co. Publishers. *Illustrated catalog and descriptions of all major groups with bibliography and glossary.*

Mayr, E. 1969. The biological meaning of species. Biol. J. Linn. Soc. **1**:311-320.

Mayr, E. 1981. Biological classification: toward a synthesis of opposing methodologies. Science **214**:510-516. *Three competing methodologies are compared. An important article full of insights.*

Nelson, G., and N. Platnick. 1981. Systematics and biogeography: cladistics and vicariance. New York, Columbia University Press. *Advanced.*

Parker, S.P. (ed.). 1982. Synopsis and classification of living organisms, 2 vols. New York, McGraw-Hill Book Co. *Monumental collection of more than 8000 articles on descriptions and systematic positions of all taxa, excluding fossil groups, down to the family level. Accurate text. The appendix contains an article on biological classification.*

Raven, P.H., B. Berlin, and D.E. Breedlove. 1971. The origins of taxonomy. Science **174**:1210-1213.

Ross, H.H. 1974. Biological systematics. Reading, Mass., Addison-Wesley Publishing Co., Inc. *Theory and practice of systematics are presented and exemplified from animals, plants, and microorganisms. Very comprehensive and useful.*

Simpson, G.G. 1961. Principles of animal taxonomy. New York, Columbia University Press. *An outstanding contribution of the basic principles of systematics and morphological diversity.*

Sneath, P.H.A., and R.R. Sokal. 1973. Numerical taxonomy. San Francisco, W.H. Freeman & Co. Publishers. *Extensive treatment of taxonomic theory, methods of classification, and the implications and application of numerical taxonomy.*

Whittaker, R.H. 1969. New concepts of the kingdoms of organisms. Science **163**:150-160. *The author's five-kingdom system.*

Wiley, E.O. 1981. Phylogenetics: the theory and practice of phylogenetic systematics. New York, John Wiley & Sons, Inc. *Excellent, thorough presentation of cladistic theory.*

Selected *Scientific American* articles

Dayhoff, M.O. 1969. Computer analysis of protein evolution. **221**:87-95 (July).

Kimura, M. 1979. The neutral theory of molecular evolution. **241**:98-126 (Nov.). *Exemplifies how molecular studies may be used in systematics.*

Sokal, R.R. 1966. Numerical taxonomy. **215**:106-116 (Dec.).

PART TWO

Marine invertebrates in a subtidal community.

THE DIVERSITY
OF ANIMAL LIFE

The 1.5 million named species of animals are witness to the enormous diversity of animal life believed to have descended from a common ancestor through evolutionary processes (discussed in Part Four). Classification of animals is based on evolutionary relationships—the only way, biologically, that the diversity of life can be understood. Through progressive adaptation to varied and changing environmental opportunities, animals have expanded into practically every environmental niche that can support life.

The following chapters deal with the adaptive radiation that has occurred among animals, the relationships of the various groups to each other, the evolutionary advances that have pointed the way toward higher phyla, and the distinctive characteristics of each of the types that make up the varied fauna of our earth.

CHAPTER 8

THE UNICELLULAR ANIMALS
Protozoan Phyla

Peritromus, a marine member of the phylum Ciliophora, has prominent buccal membranelles curving around its anterior end *(at right).* These membranelles are formed from fused cells.

Photograph by P.W. Johnson.

Position in Animal Kingdom

The protozoan is a complete organism in which all life activities are carried on within the limits of a single plasma membrane. Because their protoplasmic mass is not subdivided into cells, protozoa are sometimes termed "acellular," but many people prefer "unicellular" to emphasize the many structural similarities to the cells of multicellular animals (see Principle 11, p. 14).

The term "Protista" is used by some biologists to refer to all unicellular organisms, whether they are plant or animal. When applied in this way, the category includes the unicellular algae, protozoa, bacteria, yeasts, and so on. Most biologists prefer to use "Protista" to denote only those unicellular organisms whose nucleus is bounded by a nuclear membrane (eukaryotic) and the term "Monera" to include those unicellular organisms without a nuclear membrane (prokaryotic), such as the bacteria and the blue-green algae (see p. 157).

The protozoa are eukaryotic protistans. The eukaryote-prokaryote distinction was summarized in Chapter 4 (p. 76) and mentioned again in Chapter 7 (p. 157).

Biological Contributions

1. **Intracellular specialization** (division of labor within the cell) involves the organization of functional organelles in the cell.
2. The earliest indication of **division of labor between cells** is seen in certain colonial protozoa that have both somatic and reproductive zooids (individuals) in the colony.
3. **Asexual reproduction** by mitotic division is first developed in the protists.
4. **True sexual reproduction** with zygote formation is found in some protozoa.
5. The responses (taxes) of protozoa to stimuli represent the **beginning of reflexes and instincts** as we know them in metazoans.
6. The most primitive animals with an **exoskeleton** are certain shelled protozoa.
7. **All types of nutrition** are developed in the protozoa: autotrophic, saprozoic, and holozoic.

THE PROTOZOAN PHYLA

The organisms referred to as protozoa are united only on the basis of a single, negative characteristic: they are not multicellular. This concept was recognized, in a way, by the American zoologist Libbie Hyman (1940), who preferred the term "acellular" rather than the traditional "unicellular" to describe protozoa. She distinguished them as "animals whose body substance is not partitioned into cells." Although most zoologists have returned to describing protozoa as unicellular because of electron microscope studies subsequent to Hyman's book, the concept of acellularity is still a valuable one. It reminds us that the traditionally recognized phylum Protozoa was not a natural phylogenetic grouping. An enormous amount of information on protozoan structure, life histories, and physiology has accumulated in recent years, and the Society of Protozoologists published a new classification of protozoa in 1980, recognizing *seven* separate phyla. We will adopt the new classification because it comes closer to reflecting real evolutionary relationships than the older, simpler systems, but there is no way to give adequate treatment to all groups, even all phyla, of protozoa in a book of this size.

We can say, nevertheless, that the protozoan phyla demonstrate a basic body plan—the single eukaryotic cell—and that they amply demonstrate the enormous adaptive potential of that plan. Over 64,000 species have been named, and over half of these are fossil. Although they are unicellular, protozoa are not simple. They are functionally complete organisms with many complicated structures. Their various organelles tend to be more specialized than those of the average cell in a multicellular animal. Particular organelles may perform as skeletons, sensory systems, conducting mechanisms, and so on.

Protozoa are found wherever life exists. They are highly adaptable and easily distributed from place to place. They require moisture, whether they live in marine or freshwater habitats, soil, decaying organic matter, or plants and animals. They may be sessile or free swimming, and they form a large part of the floating plankton. The same species are often found widely separated in time as well as space. Some species may have spanned geological eras of over 100 million years.

Despite their wide distribution, many protozoa can live successfully only within narrow environmental ranges. Species adaptations vary greatly, and successions of species frequently occur as environmental conditions change. These changes may be brought about by physical factors, such as the drying up of a pond or seasonal changes in temperature, or by biological changes, such as predator pressure.

Protozoa play an enormous role in the economy of nature. Their fantastic numbers are attested by the gigantic ocean and soil deposits formed by their skeletons. About 10,000 species of protozoa are symbiotic in or on other animals or plants, sometimes even other protozoa. (See the discussion of population interactions in Chapter 41.) The relationship may be mutualistic, commensalistic, or parasitic, depending on the species involved. Some of the most important diseases of humans and domestic animals are caused by parasitic protozoa.

A number of species are colonial and some have multicellular stages in their life cycles, which may lead one to wonder why such protozoa are not considered multicellular organisms. The reasons are that they usually have clearly recognizable, noncolonial relatives and, more arbitrarily, that they do not have more than one kind of nonreproductive cell and they do not undergo embryonic development. By definition, multicellular animals have more than one kind of nonreproductive cell in their bodies and undergo embryogenesis.

CHARACTERISTICS

1. Unicellular; some colonial, and some with multicellular stages in their life cycles
2. Mostly microscopic, although some large enough to be seen with the unaided eye
3. All symmetries represented in the group; shape variable or constant (oval, spherical, or other)
4. No germ layer present
5. No organs or tissues, but specialized organelles found; nucleus single or multiple — *protoplasmic level*
6. Free living, mutualism, commensalism, parasitism all represented in the group
7. Locomotion by pseudopodia, flagella, cilia, and direct cell movements; some sessile
8. Some provided with a simple endoskeleton or exoskeleton, but mostly naked *w/o shell*
9. Nutrition of all types: autotrophic (manufacturing own nutrients by photosynthesis), heterotrophic (depending on other plants or animals for food), saprozoic (using nutrients dissolved in the surrounding medium)
10. Habitat: aquatic, terrestrial, or symbiotic
11. Reproduction asexually by fission, budding, and cysts and sexually by conjugation or by syngamy (union of male and female gametes to form a zygote)

CLASSIFICATION

The four main groups of protozoa traditionally recognized were the flagellates, amebas, spore formers, and ciliates. The system that follows reflects a much more phylogenetic arrangement, including the recognition that amebas and flagellates are more closely related to each other than they are to other groups, and that the "spore formers" represent several completely unrelated forms.

Phylum Sarcomastigophora (sar'ko-mas-ti-gof'o-ra) (Gr., *sarkos,* flesh, + *mastix,* whip, + *phora,* bearing). Flagella, pseudopodia, or both types of locomotory organelles; usually with only one type of nucleus; typically no spore formation; sexuality, when present, essentially syngamy.

Subphylum Mastigophora (mas-ti-gof'o-ra) (Gr., *mastix,* whip, + *phora,* bearing). One or more flagella typically present in adult stages; autotrophic or hererotrophic or both; reproduction usually asexual by fission.

Class Phytomastigophorea (fi'to-mas-ti-go-for'e-a) (Gr., *phyton,* plant, + *mastix,* whip, + *phora,* bearing). Plantlike flagellates, usually bearing chromoplasts, which contain chlorophyll. Examples: *Chilomonas, Euglena, Volvox, Ceratium, Peranema, Noctiluca.*

Class Zoomastigophorea (zo'o-mas-ti-go-for'e-a) (Gr., *zōon,* animal, + *mastix,* whip, + *phora,* bearing). Flagellates without chromoplasts; one to many flagella; ameboid forms with or without flagella in some groups; species predominantly symbiotic. Examples: *Trichomonas, Trichonympha, Trypanosoma, Leishmania, Dientamoeba.*

Subphylum Opalinata (o'pa-lin-a'ta) (N.F., *opaline,* like opal in appearance, + +*ata,* group suffix). Body covered with longitudinal rows of cilium-like organelles; parasitic; cytostome (cell mouth) lacking; two to many nuclei of one type. Examples: *Opalina, Protoopalina.*

Subphylum Sarcodina (sar-ko-di'na) (Gr., *sarkos,* flesh, + *ina,* belonging to). Pseudopodia typically present; flagella present in developmental stages of some; cortical zone of cytoplasm relatively undifferentiated compared with other major taxa; body naked or with external or internal skeleton; free living or parasitic.

Superclass Rhizopoda (ri-zop'o-da) (Gr., *rhiza,* root, + *pous, podos,* foot). Locomotion by lobopodia, filopodia, or reticulopodia, or by cytoplasmic flow without production of discrete pseudopodia. Comprised of eight classes, some of which are listed below.

Class Lobosea (lo-bo'se-a) (Gr., *lobos,* lobe). Pseudopodia lobose or more or less filiform but produced from broader lobe; usually uninucleate; no fruiting bodies. Examples: *Amoeba, Entamoeba, Acanthamoeba, Naegleria, Pelomyxa, Arcella, Difflugia.*

Class Eumycetozoea (yu'mi-set-o-zo'e-a) (Gr., *eu,* good, true, + *mykes,* fungus, + *zōon,* animal). Ameboid feeding stage, flagellated stage present or absent; produce aerial fruiting bodies with one to thousands of spores. Examples: *Dictyostelium, Physarum.*

Class Filosea (fi-los'e-a) (L., *filum,* thread). Hyaline, filiform pseudopodia, often branching, sometimes rejoining; no spores or flagellated stages known. Examples: *Vampyrella, Euglypha, Gromia.*

Class Granuloreticulosea (gran'yu-lo-re-tik'yu-los'e-a) (L., *granulum,* dim. of *granum,* grain, + *reticulum,* dim. of *rete,* net). Delicate, finely granular or hyaline reticulopodia or, rarely, finely pointed, granular but nonrejoining pseudopodia. Examples: *Allogromia, Fusulina, Textularia, Elphidium, Globigerina.*

Superclass Actinopoda (ak'ti-nop'o-da) (Gr., *aktis, aktinos,* ray, + *pous, podos,* foot). Often spherical, usually planktonic; pseudopodia in form of axopodia, with microtubular supporting structure.

Class Acantharea (a'kan-thar'e-a) (Gr., *akantha,* spine or thorn). Strontium sulfate skeleton comprised of 20 or more radiating spines more or less joined in cell center; extracellular outer (cortex) and inner envelopes usually present; inner envelope often closely lining central cell mass; marine, usually planktonic. Examples: *Acanthometra, Lithoptera.*

Class Polycystinea (pol'e-sis-tin'e-a) (Gr., *polys,* many, + *kystis,* bladder). Siliceous skeleton in most species, usually of solid elements, consisting of one or more latticed shells with or without radial spines, or of spicules; capsular membrane usually of grossly polygonal plates with many more than three pores; marine, planktonic. Example: *Thalassicolla.*

Class Phaeodarea (fe'o-dar'e-a) (Gr., *phaios,* dusky, + *daria,* suffix). Skeleton of mixed silica and organic matter, consisting of usually hollow spines and shells; very thick capsular membrane with three pores; marine, planktonic. Examples: *Aulacantha, Challengeron.*

Class Heliozoea (he′le-o-zo′e-a) (Gr., *helios*, sun, + *zōon*, animal). Without central capsule; skeletal structures, if present, siliceous or organic; axopodia radiating on all sides; most species freshwater. Examples: *Clathrulina, Actinophrys, Actinosphaerium.*

Phylum Labyrinthomorpha (la′bi-rinth-o-morf′a) (Gr., *labyrinth*, maze, labyrinth, + *morph*, form, + *a*, suffix). Small group living on algae; mostly marine or estuarine. Example: *Labyrinthula.*

Phylum Apicomplexa (a′pi-com-plex′a) (L., *apex*, tip or summit, + *complex*, twisted around, + *a*, suffix). Characteristic set of organelles (apical complex) associated with anterior end present in some developmental stages; cilia and flagella absent except for flagellated microgametes in some groups; cysts often present; all species parasitic.

Class Perkinsea (per-kin′se-a). Small group parasitic in oysters.

Class Sporozoea (spor′o-zo′e-a) (Gr., *sporos*, seed, + *zōon*, animal). Spores or oocysts typically present that contain infective sporozoites; locomotion of mature organisms by body flexion, gliding, or undulation of longitudinal ridges; flagella present only in microgametes of some groups; pseudopods ordinarily absent, if present they are used for feeding, not locomotion; one or two host life cycles. Examples: *Monocystis, Gregarina, Eimeria, Plasmodium, Toxoplasma, Babesia.*

Phylum Myxozoa (mix-o-zo′a) (Gr., *myxa*, slime, mucus, + *zōon*, animal). Parasites of lower vertebrates, especially fishes, and invertebrates.

Phylum Microspora (mi-cros′por-a) (Gr., *micro*, small, + *sporos*, seed). Parasites of invertebrates, especially arthropods, and lower vertebrates.

Phylum Ascetospora (as-e-tos′por-a) (Gr., *asketos*, curiously wrought, + *sporos*, seed). Small group that is parasitic in invertebrates and a few vertebrates.

Phylum Ciliophora (sil-i-of′or-a) (L., *cilium*, eyelash, + Gr., *phora*, bearing). Cilia or ciliary organelles in at least one stage of life cycle; two types of nuclei, with rare exception; binary fission across rows of cilia, budding and multiple fission also occur; sexuality involving conjugation, autogamy, and cytogamy; nutrition heterotrophic; contractile vacuole typically present; most species free living, but many commensal, some parasitic. (This is a very large group, now divided by the Society of Protozoologists classification into three classes and numerous orders and suborders. The classes are separated on the basis of technical characteristics of the ciliary patterns, especially around the cytostome, the development of the cystostome, and other characteristics.) Examples: *Paramecium, Colpoda, Tetrahymena, Balantidium, Stentor, Blepharisma, Epidinium, Euplotes, Vorticella, Carchesium, Trichodina, Podophrya, Ephelota.*

——— Form and Function

Inasmuch as protozoa are cells, in many aspects their structure and physiology are the same as those of cells of multicellular animals. However, because they must carry on all the functions of life as individual organisms, and because they show such enormous diversity in form, habitat, feeding, and so on, many features are unique to various protozoan cells.

Nucleus and cytoplasm

As in other eukaryotes, the nucleus is a membrane-bound structure whose interior communicates with the cytoplasm by small pores (Fig. 4-5, p. 78). Within the nucleus the genetic material (DNA) is borne on chromosomes. Except during cell division, the chromosomes are not usually condensed in a form that can be distinguished, although during fixation of the cells for light microscopy, the chromosome material (chromatin) often clumps together irregularly, leaving some areas within the nucleus relatively clear. The appearance is described as **vesicular** and is characteristic of many protozoan nuclei (Fig. 8-1). Condensations of chro-

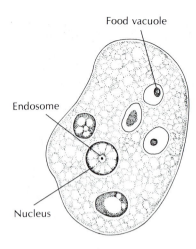

Food vacuole

Endosome

Nucleus

Nucleus

Chromatoida body

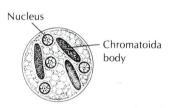

Figure 8-1

Entamoeba histolytica, the cause of amebic dysentery in humans. The trophozoite *(above)* is the actively moving and feeding form. It contains a single nucleus and several food vacuoles. The cyst *(below)* can tolerate conditions outside the body and is infective to the new host. It contains four nuclei and several chromatoidal bodies. The chromatoidal bodies are an organized form of RNA. On excystment in the small intestine of the host, the nuclei will divide again, and the cytoplasm divides to produce eight small amebas. The nuclei of both the trophozoite and the cyst are vesicular and have a central endosome (see text).

Drawing by Jeanne Robertson. From Schmidt, G.D., and L.S. Roberts. 1981. Foundations of parasitology, ed. 2. St. Louis, The C.V. Mosby Co.

matin may be distributed around the periphery of the nucleus or internally in distinct patterns. In some flagellates the chromosomes are visible through the interphase as they would appear during prophase of mitosis.

Also within the nucleus, one or more **nucleoli** are often present. **Endosomes** are nucleoli that remain as discrete bodies during mitosis; they are characteristic of phytoflagellates, parasitic amebas, and trypanosomes (Figs. 8-1, 8-8, and 8-11).

The **macronuclei** of ciliates are described as **compact** or **condensed** because the chromatin material is more finely dispersed and clear areas cannot be observed with the light microscope (Fig. 8-21).

Cellular organelles like those in the cells of multicellular animals can be distinguished in the cytoplasm of many protozoa. These include mitochondria, endoplasmic reticulum, Golgi apparatus, and various vesicles. Chloroplasts, the membrane-bound organelles in which photosynthesis takes place, are found in most phytoflagellates (Fig. 8-9).

Sometimes the peripheral and the central areas of the cytoplasm can be distinguished as **ectoplasm** and **endoplasm** (Fig. 8-3). The endoplasm appears more granular and contains the nucleus and cytoplasmic organelles. The ectoplasm appears more transparent (hyaline) under the light microscope, and it bears the bases of the cilia or flagella. The ectoplasm is often more rigid and is in the gel state of a colloid, whereas the more fluid endoplasm is in the sol state.

Locomotor organelles

The chief means by which protozoa move are by cilia and flagella and by pseudopodial movement. Both of these mechanisms are extremely important in the biology of higher animals as well.

Cilia and flagella

Many small metazoans use cilia not only for locomotion but also to create water currents for their feeding and respiration. Ciliary movement is vital to many species in such functions as handling food, reproduction, excretion, and osmoregulation.

It is now known that the distinction between cilia and flagella is purely arbitrary. A cilium propels water parallel to the surface to which the cilium is attached, whereas a flagellum propels water parallel to the main axis of the flagellum (Fig. 28-8, p. 680). Electron microscopy has shown that they are structurally the same. Each contains nine pairs of longitudinal fibrils arranged in a circle around a central pair (Fig. 8-2), and this is true for all flagella and cilia in the animal kingdom, with a few notable exceptions. This "9 + 2" tube of fibrils in the flagellum or cilium is its **axoneme;** the axoneme is covered by a membrane continuous with the cell membrane covering the rest of the organism. At about the point where the axoneme enters the cell proper, the central pair of fibrils ends at a small plate within the circle of nine pairs (Fig. 8-2, *A*). Also at about that point, another fibril joins each of the nine pairs, so that these form a short tube extending from the base of the flagellum into the cell and consisting of nine *triplets* of fibrils. The short tube of nine triplets is the **kinetosome** and is exactly the same in structure as the **centriole** (see p. 82). The centrioles of some flagellates may give rise to the kinetosomes, or the kinetosomes may function as centrioles. All typical flagella and cilia have a kinetosome at their base, regardless of whether they are borne by a

A

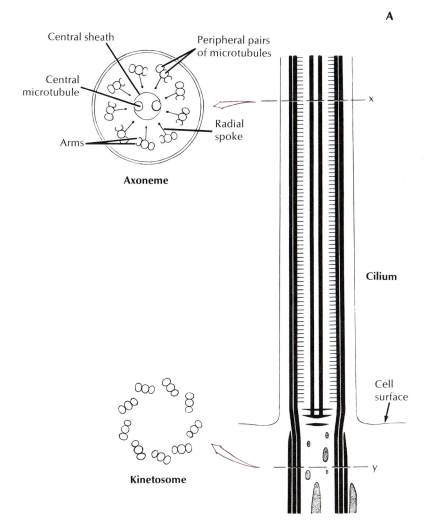

Central sheath

Peripheral pairs
of microtubules

Central
microtubule

Radial
spoke

Arms

Axoneme

x

Cilium

Cell
surface

y

Kinetosome

B

Figure 8-2

A, The axoneme is comprised of nine
pairs of fibrils plus a central pair, and it
is enclosed within the cell membrane.
The central pair ends at about the level
of the cell surface in a basal plate (axo-
some). The peripheral fibrils continue inward for a short distance to comprise
two of each of the triplets in the kinetosome (at level *y* in **A**). **B,** Electron micrograph of section through several flagella,
corresponding to section at *x* in **A**.
(×133,000.)

Electron micrograph courtesy I.R. Gibbons, Harvard University.

protozoan or metazoan cell. The kinetosomes of protozoa have older, traditional
names (**blepharoplast, basal body, basal granule**) that are still in common
usage.

The current explanation for ciliary and flagellar movement is the **sliding
microtubule hypothesis.** The movement is powered by the release of chemical
bond energy in ATP (p. 102). Two little arms are visible in electron micrographs
on each of the pairs of peripheral tubules in the axoneme (Fig. 8-2), and these bear
the enzyme adenosine triphosphatase (ATPase), which cleaves the ATP. When the
bond energy in ATP is released, the arms "walk along" one of the filaments in the
adjacent pair, causing it to slide relative to the other filament in the pair. Shear
resistance, causing the axoneme to bend when the filaments slide past each other,
is provided by "spokes" from each doublet to the central pair of fibrils. These are
also visible in electron micrographs.

Pseudopodia

Although pseudopodia are the chief means of locomotion in the Sarcodina, they
can be formed by a variety of flagellate protozoa, as well as by ameboid cells of
many invertebrates. In fact, much of the defense against disease in the human
body depends on ameboid white blood cells, and ameboid cells in many other
animals, vertebrate and invertebrate, play similar roles.

Figure 8-3

Ameba in active locomotion. Arrows indicate the direction of streaming protoplasm. The first sign of new pseudopodium is thickening of the ectoplasm to form a clear hyaline cap, into which the fluid endoplasm flows. As the endoplasm reaches the forward tip, it fountains out and is converted into ectoplasm, forming a stiff outer tube that lengthens as the forward flow continues. Posteriorly the ectoplasm is converted into fluid endoplasm, replenishing the flow. Substratum is necessary for ameboid movement.

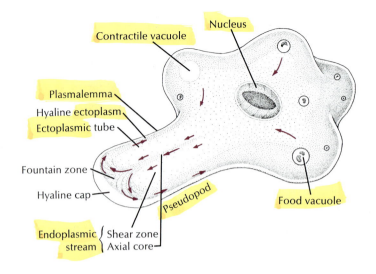

Figure 8-4

Ameboid movement. Series photographed at intervals of about half a minute. *Right*, Pseudopodium is extending toward escaping rotifer.

Photographs by F.M. Hickman.

In the protozoa, pseudopodia exist in several forms. The most familiar are the **lobopodia** (Fig. 8-3), which are rather large, blunt extensions of the cell body containing both endoplasm and ectoplasm. Some amebas characteristically do not extend individual pseudopodia, but the whole body moves with pseudopodial movement; this is known as the **limax** form (for a genus of slugs, *Limax*). **Filipodia** are thin extensions, usually branching, and containing only ectoplasm. They are found in members of the sarcodine class Filosea, such as *Euglypha* (Fig. 8-7, *B*). **Reticulopodia** (Fig. 8-13) are distinguished from filipodia in that reticulopodia repeatedly rejoin to form a netlike mesh, although some protozoologists believe that the distinction between filipodia and reticulopodia is artificial. Members of the superclass Actinopoda have **axopodia** (Fig. 8-13), which are long, thin pseudopodia supported by axial rods of microtubules (Fig. 8-5). The microtubules are arranged in a definite spiral or geometrical array, depending on the species, and constitute the axoneme of the axopod. Axopodia can be extended or retracted, apparently by addition or removal of microtubular material. Since the tips can adhere to the substrate, the animal can progress by a rolling motion, shortening the axonemes in front and extending those in the rear. Cytoplasm can flow along

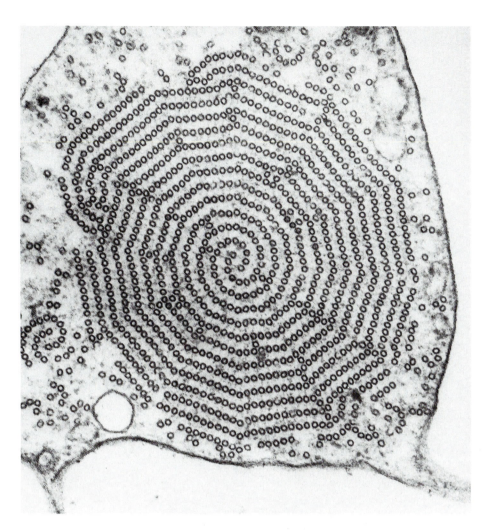

Figure 8-5

Electron micrograph of a section through an axopodium of *Actinosphaerium nucleofilum*. The axoneme of the axopodium is comprised of an array of microtubules, which may vary from three to many in number depending on the species. Some species can extend or retract their axopodia quite rapidly. (×99,000.)
Courtesy L. Evans Roth.

the axonemes, toward the body on one side and in the reverse direction on the other.

How pseudopodia work has long attracted the interest of zoologists, but we have only recently gained some insight into the phenomenon. When a typical lobopodium begins to form, an extension of ectoplasm called the hyaline cap appears, and endoplasm begins to flow toward and into the hyaline cap (Fig. 8-3). As the endoplasmic material flows into the hyaline cap, it fountains out to the periphery and changes from the sol to the gel state; that is, it becomes ectoplasm. Thus, the ectoplasm is a tube through which the endoplasm flows as the pseudopodium extends. On the trailing (uroid) side of the animal, ectoplasm becomes endoplasm. At some point the pseudopodium becomes anchored to the substrate, and the animal is drawn forward. Although these events can be easily observed under the light microscope, the force that causes the endoplasm to flow through the ectoplasmic tube is obscure. Several hypotheses have been proposed but have been wholly or partially discarded. It now appears that ameboid movement, like that of muscle, and somewhat similar to that of cilia, involves tiny filaments sliding past each other. Extracts of amebas have been treated with ATP, producing gelation, contractility, streaming of particles, and extrusion of water. Oriented fibrils have been shown in the gel phase by electron microscopy, and myosin filaments have been identified in *Amoeba proteus*. Similar mechanisms apparently account for cytoplasmic streaming in all types of pseudopodia.

Podophrya

Didinium

Leidyopsis

Amoeba

Figure 8-6

Some feeding methods among protozoa. *Amoeba* surrounds a small flagellate with pseudopodia. *Leidyopsis*, a flagellate living in the intestine of termites, forms pseudopodia and ingests wood chips. *Didinium*, a ciliate, feeds only on *Paramecium*, which it swallows through a temporary cytostome in its anterior end. Sometimes more than one *Didinium* feed on the same *Paramecium*. *Podophrya* is a suctorian ciliophoran. Its tentacles attach to its prey and suck prey cytoplasm into the body of the *Podophrya*, where it is pinched off to form food vacuoles. Technically, all of these methods are types of phagocytosis.

Excretion and osmoregulation

Vacuoles can be seen in the cytoplasm of many protozoa under the light microscope, and some of these vacuoles periodically fill with a fluid substance that is then expelled. Evidence is strong that these **contractile vacuoles** (Figs. 8-3, 8-9, and 8-21) function principally in osmoregulation. They are more prevalent and fill and empty more frequently in freshwater protozoa than in marine and endosymbiotic species, where the surrounding medium would be more nearly isosmotic to the cytoplasm. Smaller species, which have a greater surface-to-volume ratio, generally have more rapid filling and expulsion rates in their contractile vacuoles. Excretion of metabolic wastes, on the other hand, is almost entirely by diffusion. The main end product of nitrogen metabolism is ammonia, which readily diffuses out of the small bodies of protozoa.

The contractile vacuoles, sometimes called water expulsion vesicles, differ considerably in complexity among the various types of protozoa. In amebas the contractile vacuoles are not usually found at any particular site, being passively carried around in the endoplasm. Small vesicles join the contractile vacuole, emptying their contents into it as the vacuole fills. The vacuole finally joins its membrane to the surface membrane and empties its contents to the outside.

Some ciliates, such as *Blepharisma,* have contractile vacuoles with filling mechanisms similar to that described for amebas. Others, such as *Paramecium,* have more complex contractile vacuoles. In these the contractile vacuoles are located in a specific position beneath the cell membrane, with an "excretory" pore leading to the outside, and surrounded by the ampullae of about six feeder canals (Fig. 8-21). The feeder canals, in turn, are surrounded by fine tubules about 20 nm in diameter, which connect with the canals during filling of the ampullae and at their lower ends connect with the tubular system of the endoplasmic reticulum. The ampullae and the contractile vacuole are surrounded by bundles of fibrils, which may play a role in the contraction of these structures. Contraction of the ampullae fills the vacuole. When the vacuole contracts to discharge its contents to the outside, the ampullae become disconnected from the vacuole, so that backflow is prevented.

Nutrition

Protozoa can be categorized broadly into autotrophs and heterotrophs (see p. 65) according to whether they can synthesize their own organic constituents from inorganic substrates or must have organic molecules synthesized by other organisms. Another kind of classification, usually applied to heterotrophs, involves those that ingest visible particles of food (**phagotrophs,** or **holozoic** feeders) as contrasted with those ingesting food in a soluble form (**osmotrophs,** or **saprozoic** feeders). However, reality is not so simple, even among the one-celled animals. Autotrophic protozoa use light energy to synthesize their organic molecules (phototrophs), but they often practice phagotrophy and osmotrophy as well. Even among the heterotrophs, few are exclusively either phagotrophic or osmotrophic. The single order Euglenida (class Phytomastigophorea) contains some forms that are mainly phototrophs, some that are mainly osmotrophs, and some that are primarily phagotrophs. The species of *Euglena* show considerable variety in nutritional capability. Some require certain preformed organic molecules, even though they are autotrophs, and some lose their chloroplasts if maintained in darkness, thus becoming permanent osmotrophs.

Holozoic nutrition implies phagocytosis (Fig. 8-6), in which there is an infolding or invagination of the cell membrane around the food particle. As the invagination extends farther into the cell, it is pinched off at the surface (p. 744). The food particle is thus contained in an intracellular, membrane-bound vesicle, the **food vacuole** or **phagosome.** Small vesicles containing digestive enzymes, the lysosomes, fuse with the phagosome and pour their contents into it, where digestion begins. As the digested products are absorbed across the vacuole membrane, the phagosome becomes smaller. Any undigestible material may be released to the outside by a reversal of the phagocytic process, the vacuole again fusing with the cell surface membrane. In most ciliates, many flagellates, and many apicomplexans, the site of phagocytosis is a definite mouth structure, the **cytostome** (Figs. 8-6, 8-16, and 8-21). In amebas, phagocytosis can occur at almost any point by envelopment of the particle with pseudopodia. Particles must be ingested through the opening of the test, or shell, in amebas that have tests. Flagellates may form a temporary cytostome, usually in a characteristic position, or they may have a permanent cytostome with specialized structure. Many ciliates have a characteristic structure for expulsion of waste matter, the **cytopyge** or **cytoproct,** found in a characteristic location. In some the cytopyge also serves as the site for expulsion of the contents of the contractile vacuole.

Saprozoic feeding may be by pinocytosis or by transport of solutes directly across the outer cell membrane. Pinocytosis and transport across the cell membrane are discussed on p. 88. Direct transport across the membrane may be by diffusion, facilitated transport, or active transport. Diffusion is probably of little or no importance in the nutrition of protozoa, except possibly in some endosymbiotic species. Some important food molecules, such as glucose and amino acids, may be brought into the cell by facilitated diffusion and active transport.

Reproduction

Strictly speaking, reproduction among the protozoa is asexual. Sexual reproduction, in the sense that sex cells unite and then embryonate to form a new individual, does not occur; protozoa do not have embryos. Nevertheless, sexual phenomena do occur widely among the protozoa, and sexual processes may precede certain phases of asexual reproduction. The essential features of sexual processes include a reduction division of the chromosome number to half (diploid number to haploid number), the development of sex cells (gametes) or at least gamete nuclei, and usually a fusion of the gamete nuclei.

Fission

The cell multiplication process that results in more individuals in the protozoa is referred to as fission. The most common type of fission is **binary,** in which two essentially identical individuals result (Fig. 8-7). When the progeny cell is considerably smaller than the parent and then grows to adult size, the process is called **budding.** This occurs in some ciliates. In **multiple fission,** division of the cytoplasm (cytokinesis) is preceded by several nuclear divisions, so that a number of individuals are produced almost simultaneously (Figs. 8-1 and 8-17). Multiple fission, or **schizogony,** is common among the Sporozoea and some Sarcodina. If the multiple fission is preceded by or associated with union of gametes, it is referred to as **sporogony.**

All of the foregoing types of division are accompanied by some form of mitosis (p. 88). However, the process is often somewhat unlike that found in

It has been shown that a stimulatory substance, or "inducer," must be present in the surrounding medium for many protozoa to initiate pinocytosis. Several proteins act as inducers, but some salts and other substances can also stimulate pinocytosis; it appears that the inducer must be a positively charged molecule. Pinocytosis takes place at the inner end of the cytopharynx in the protozoa possessing that structure.

Figure 8-7

Binary fission in some sarcodines and flagellates. **A,** The two nuclei of *Arcella* divide as some of its cytoplasm is extruded and begins to secrete a new test for the daughter cell. **B,** The test of another sarcodine, *Euglypha*, is constructed of secreted platelets. Secretion of the platelets for the daughter cell is begun before the cytoplasm begins to move out the aperture. As these are used to construct the test of the daughter cell, the nucleus divides. **C,** *Trypanosoma* has a kinetoplast (part of the mitochondrion) near the kinetosome of its flagellum close to its posterior end in the stage shown. All of these parts must be replicated before the cell divides. **D,** Division of *Euglena*.

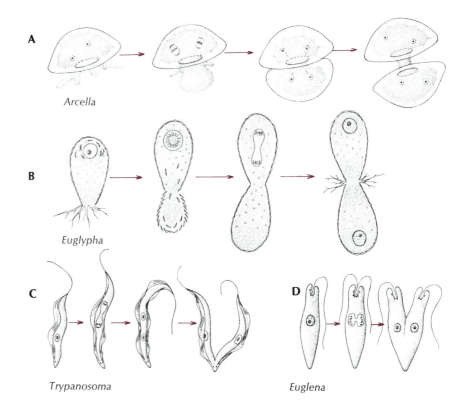

Arcella

Euglypha

Trypanosoma

Euglena

higher animals. For example, the nuclear membrane often persists through mitosis, and the microtubular spindle may be formed within the nuclear membrane. Centrioles have not been observed in nuclear division of ciliates; the nuclear membrane persists in micronuclear mitosis, with the spindle within the nucleus. The macronucleus of ciliates seems simply to elongate, constrict, and divide without any recognizable mitotic phenomena (amitosis).

Sexual processes

Although all protozoa reproduce asexually, and some are apparently exclusively asexual, the widespread occurrence of sex among the protozoa testifies to its selective value as a means of genetic recombination. The gamete nuclei, or pronuclei, which fuse in fertilization to restore the diploid number of chromosomes, are usually borne in special gamete cells. When the gametes all look alike, they are called **isogametes,** but most species have two dissimilar types, or **anisogametes.**

We are accustomed to thinking of the timing of meiosis as it occurs in metazoa, during or just before gamete formation: **gametic meiosis.** This is indeed the case in some flagellates, the Heliozoea, and the Ciliophora. However, in other flagellates and in the Sporozoea, the first divisions *after* fertilization are meiotic (**zygotic meiosis**) (Fig. 8-17), and all the individuals produced asexually (mitotically) in the life cycle up to the next zygote are haploid. It is believed that most protozoa that do not reproduce sexually are haploid, but this is difficult to show since there is no meiosis. In some of the Granuloreticulosa (foraminiferans), there is an alternation of haploid and diploid generations (**intermediary meiosis**), a phenomenon widespread among plants.

The fertilization of one individual gamete by another is called **syngamy,** but some sexual phenomena in protozoa do not involve that process. Examples are **autogamy,** in which gametic nuclei arise by meiosis and fuse to form a zygote within the same organism that produced them, and **conjugation,** in which there is an exchange of gametic nuclei between paired organisms (conjugants). Conjugation will be described further in the discussion of the paramecium.

Encystment and excystment

Separated as they are from their external environment only by their delicate external cell membrane, it seems astonishing that protozoa could be so successful in habitats frequently subjected to extremely harsh conditions. This is surely related to their ability to form cysts: dormant forms marked by the possession of resistant external coverings and a more or less complete shutdown of metabolic machinery. Cyst formation is also important to many parasitic forms that must survive a harsh environment between hosts (Fig. 8-1). However, some parasites do not form cysts, apparently depending on direct transfer from one host to another. Reproductive phases such as fission, budding, and syngamy may occur in the cysts of some species (Fig. 8-1). Encystment has not been found in *Paramecium*, and it is rare or absent in marine forms.

The conditions stimulating encystment are incompletely understood, although in some cases cyst formation is cyclic, occurring at a certain stage in the life cycle. In most free-living forms, adverse change in the environment favors encystment. Such conditions may include food deficiency, desiccation, increased tonicity of the environment, decreased oxygen concentration, or pH or temperature change.

During encystment a number of organelles, such as cilia or flagella, are resorbed, and the Golgi apparatus secretes the cyst wall material, which is carried to the surface in vesicles and extruded.

Although the exact stimulus for excystation (escape from cysts) is usually unknown, a return of favorable conditions initiates excystment in those protozoa in which the cysts are a resistant stage. In parasitic forms the excystment stimulus may be more specific, requiring conditions similar to those found in the host.

Cysts of some soil-inhabiting and freshwater protozoa have amazing durability. The cysts of the soil ciliate *Colpoda* can survive 7 days in liquid air and 3 hours at 100° C. Survival of *Colpoda* cysts in dried soil has been shown for up to 38 years, and those of a certain small flagellate *(Podo)* can survive up to 49 years! Not all cysts are so sturdy, however. Those of *Entamoeba histolytica* will tolerate gastric acidity but not desiccation, temperature above 50° C, or sunlight.

___ Representative Types

This section describes some representatives of each large group of protozoa to give the student a basis for comparing the groups and an idea of the diversity of protozoa. Forms such as *Amoeba* and *Paramecium*, although large and easy to obtain for study, are not wholly representative because their life histories are somewhat simpler than those of other members of the respective groups.

Phylum Sarcomastigophora

The Sarcomastigophora includes both protozoa that move by flagella (Mastigophora) and those that move by pseudopodia (Sarcodina). These characteristics are not mutually exclusive; some mastigophorans (flagellates) can form and use pseudopodia, and a number of sarcodines have flagellated stages in their life cycles.

Subphylum Mastigophora—the flagellated protozoa

Although some flagellates can form pseudopodia, their primary means of locomotion is by one or more flagella. What are probably the most primitive protozoa are found in this subphylum. The group is divided into the phytoflagellates (class Phytomastigophorea), which usually have chlorophyll and are thus plantlike, and the zooflagellates (class Zoomastigophorea), which do not have chlorophyll, are either holozoic or saprozoic, and thus are animal like.

Consideration of the phytoflagellates as animals by the zoologists and as plants by the botanists has led to a curious taxonomic anomaly. According to the zoologists (Society of Protozoologists classification), they comprise a class of one phylum, but according to the botanists they should be placed in several different divisions (a division is a taxon of plants equivalent in rank to a phylum of animals) and classes within the divisions. In our acceptance of the Sarcomastigophora as including the plantlike flagellates, we tend to concur with Dodson (1971) that "the blurred areas then remain, not as a defect, but as evidence that evolution from common ancestors is one of the basic facts of life, that all eukaryotes are in fact related."

Phytoflagellates

Phytoflagellates usually have one or two (sometimes four) flagella and chromatophores (also called chromoplasts or chloroplasts), which contain the pigments used in photosynthesis. They are mostly free living and include such familiar forms as *Euglena, Chlamydomonas, Peranema, Volvox,* and the dinoflagellates. *Peranema* (Fig. 8-8) is related to *Euglena* but is a colorless phytoflagellate with holozoic nutrition. *Chilomonas* is another common form that is an important food item for amebas. Some of the flagellates are colonial, living in groups of individuals (zooids), and in some species the number of zooids per colony is characteristic (Fig. 8-8).

Among the most interesting of all the phytoflagellates are the dinoflagellates. They have a longitudinal and an equatorial flagellum, each borne at least partly in grooves on the body. The body may be naked or covered by cellulose plates or valves or by a cellulose membrane. Most dinoflagellates have brown or yellow chromatophores, although some are colorless. Many species, both colorless and pigmented, can ingest prey through a mouth region between the plates near the posterior area of the body. *Ceratium* (Fig. 8-8), for example, has a thick covering with long spines, into which the body extends, but it can catch food with posterior pseudopodia and ingest it between the flexible plates in the posterior groove. *Noctiluca* (Fig. 8-8), a colorless dinoflagellate, is a voracious predator and has a long, motile tentacle, near the base of which its only, short flagellum emerges. *Noctiluca* is one of many marine organisms that can produce light (bioluminescence). Several groups of phytoflagellates are planktonic primary producers (Chapter 41) in freshwater and marine environments; however, dinoflagellates are the most important, particularly in the sea. The dinoflagellates referred to as zooxanthellae live in mutualistic association in the tissues of certain invertebrates, including other protozoa, sea anemones, horny and stony corals, and clams. The association with stony corals is of ecological and economic importance because only corals with symbiotic zooxanthellae can form coral reefs (Chapter 10).

Euglena viridis

Euglena viridis (Fig. 8-9) is a flagellate commonly studied in introductory zoology courses. Its natural habitat is freshwater streams and ponds where there is considerable vegetation. The organisms are spindle shaped and about 60 μm long, but some species of *Euglena* are smaller and some larger (*E. oxyuris* is 500 μm long). Just beneath the outer membrane of *Euglena* are proteinaceous strips and microtubules that form the **pellicle**. In *Euglena* the pellicle is flexible enough to permit bending, but in other euglenids it may be more rigid. A **flagellum** extends from a flask-shaped **reservoir** at the anterior end, and another, short flagellum ends within the reservoir. A **kinetosome** is found at the base of each flagellum, and a **contractile vacuole** empties into the reservoir. A red eyespot, or **stigma**, apparently functions in orientation to light. Within the cytoplasm are oval **chloroplasts** that bear chlorophyll (a chromoplast that bears chlorophyll is a chloroplast) and give the organism its greenish color. **Paramylum bodies** of various shapes are masses of a starchlike food storage material.

The nutrition of *Euglena* is normally autotrophic (holophytic), but if kept in the dark the organism makes use of saprozoic nutrition, absorbing nutrients through its body surface. Mutants of *Euglena* can be produced that have permanently lost their photosynthetic ability. Although *Euglena* does not ingest solid food, some euglenids are phagotrophic. *Peranema* has a cytostome that opens alongside the flagellar reservoir.

The role of dinoflagellates may not be a positive one in some instances, such as when they produce a "red tide." Although this name was originally applied to situations in which the organisms reproduced in such profusion (producing a "bloom") under particular physical conditions that the water turned red from their color, any instance of a dinoflagellate or algal bloom producing detectable levels of toxic substances is now called a red tide. The water may be red, brown, yellow, or not remarkably colored at all. The toxic substances are apparently not harmful to the organisms that produce them, but they may be highly poisonous to fish and other marine life. Red tides in Florida have been associated with *Ptychodiscus brevis*, in California and New England with species of *Gonyaulax,* and in the Indian Ocean with a blue-green alga, *Trichodesmium.* There may be little overt effect on sea life, particularly in *Gonyaulax* red tides, but clams and other bivalve molluscs feed on the dinoflagellates, concentrating the toxin, and become quite poisonous to humans. Red tides have resulted in considerable economic losses to the shellfish industry. Another dinoflagellate, *Gambierdiscus toxicus,* produces a toxin that is concentrated in the food chain (Chapter 41). Humans can be severely poisoned and even die after eating fish containing the toxin. The illness, known as ciguatera, is especially associated with consumption of large, coral reef fishes, such as large barracudas, jacks, snappers, moray eels, and groupers.

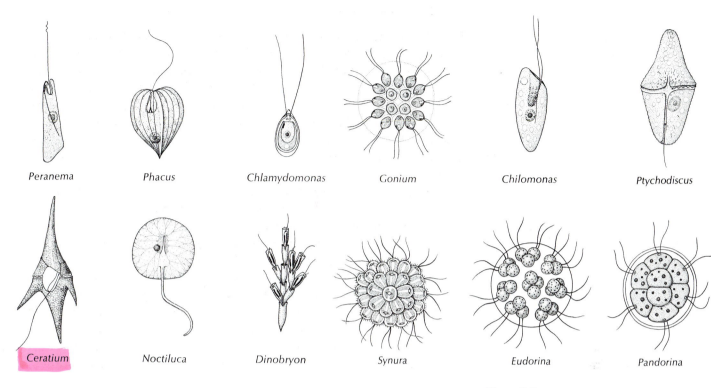

Peranema   Phacus   Chlamydomonas   Gonium   Chilomonas   Ptychodiscus

Ceratium   Noctiluca   Dinobryon   Synura   Eudorina   Pandorina

Figure 8-8

Diversity among the Phytomastigophorea. *Pandorina, Eudorina, Synura, Gonium,* and *Dinobryon* are colonial. *Ptychodiscus, Ceratium,* and *Noctiluca* are dinoflagellates.

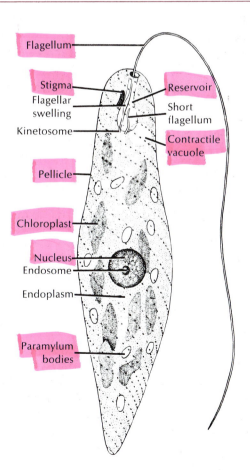

Flagellum
Stigma
Flagellar swelling
Kinetosome
Reservoir
Short flagellum
Contractile vacuole
Pellicle
Chloroplast
Nucleus
Endosome
Endoplasm
Paramylum bodies

Figure 8-9

Euglena. Features shown are a combination of those visible in living and stained preparations.

Figure 8-10

Life cycle of *Volvox*. Asexual reproduction occurs in spring and summer when specialized diploid reproductive cells divide to form young colonies that remain in the mother colony until large enough to escape. Sexual reproduction occurs largely in autumn when haploid sex cells develop. The fertilized ova may encyst and so survive the winter, developing into mature asexual colonies in the spring. In some species the colonies have separate sexes; in others both eggs and sperm are produced in the same colony.

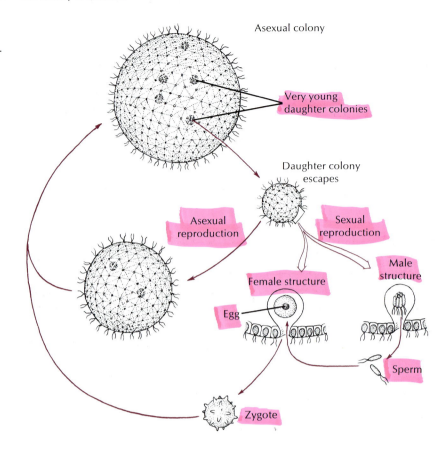

The original polarity of the zooids in the colony is such that the flagella are protruding into the interior cavity. To end up with the flagella on the outside, so that locomotion is possible, the entire colony must turn itself inside out. This process, called inversion, is *very unusual.* Of all other living organisms, only the sponges (phylum Porifera) have a comparable developmental process.

Euglena reproduces by binary fission and can encyst to survive adverse environmental conditions.

Volvox globator

Volvox (Fig. 8-10) is a colonial phytoflagellate often studied in introductory courses because its mode of colony formation is somewhat similar to embryonic development of some metazoa. The order to which *Volvox* belongs (Volvocida) includes many freshwater flagellates, mostly green, with a cellulose cell wall through which two short flagella project. Many are colonial forms (Fig. 8-8, *Pandorina, Eudorina, Gonium*).

Volvox (Fig. 8-10) is a green hollow sphere that may reach a diameter of 0.5 to 1 mm. It is a colony of many thousands of zooids (up to 50,000) embedded in the gelatinous surface of a jelly ball. Each cell is much like a euglenid, with a nucleus, a pair of flagella, a large chromoplast, and a red stigma. Adjacent cells are connected with each other by cytoplasmic strands. At one pole (usually in front as the colony moves), the stigmata are a little larger. Coordinated action of the flagella causes the colony to move by rolling over and over.

In *Volvox* we have a division of labor to the extent that most of the zooids are somatic cells concerned with nutrition and locomotion, and a few germ cells located in the posterior half are responsible for reproduction. Reproduction is asexual or sexual. In either case only certain zooids located around the equator or in the posterior half take part.

Asexual reproduction in *Volvox* occurs by the repeated mitotic division of one of the germ cells to form a hollow sphere of cells, with the flagellated ends of the cells inside. The sphere then turns itself inside out to form a daughter colony similar to the parent colony. Several daughter colonies are formed inside the parent colony before they escape by rupture of the parent (Fig. 8-10).

Codosiga   Trypanosoma   Trichonympha   Spirotrichonympha   Trichomonas

Figure 8-11

In **sexual reproduction** some of the zooids differentiate into **macrogametes** or **microgametes** (Fig. 8-10). The macrogametes are fewer and larger and are loaded with food for nourishment of the young colony. The microgametes, by repeated division, form bundles or balls of small flagellated sperm that when mature leave the mother colony and swim about to find a mature ovum. When a sperm fertilizes an egg, the zygote so formed secretes a hard, spiny, protective shell around itself. When released by the breaking up of the parent colony, the zygote remains quiescent during the winter. Within the shell the zygote undergoes repeated division, producing a small colony that is released in the spring. A number of asexual generations may follow, during the summer, before sexual reproduction occurs again.

Zooflagellates

The zooflagellates are all colorless, lacking chromatophores, and have holozoic or saprozoic nutrition. Most are symbiotic.

Some of the most important protozoan parasites are zooflagellates. Many of them belong to the genus *Trypanosoma* (Fig. 8-11) and live in the blood of fish, amphibians, reptiles, birds, and mammals. Some are nonpathogenic, but others produce severe diseases in humans and domestic animals. *T. brucei gambiense* and *T. brucei rhodesiense* cause African sleeping sickness in humans, and *T. brucei brucei* causes a related disease in domestic animals. They are transmitted by the tsetse fly *(Glossina)*. *T. b. rhodesiense,* the more virulent of the sleeping sickness trypanosomes, and *T. b. brucei* have natural reservoirs (antelope and other wild mammals) that are apparently not harmed by the parasites. *T. cruzi* causes Chagas' disease in humans in Central America and South America. It is transmitted by the bite of the "kissing bug" *(Triatominae).* Three species of *Leishmania* cause disease in humans. One is a serious visceral disease affecting especially the liver and spleen, one causes lesions in the mucous membranes of the nose and throat, and the least serious causes a type of skin lesion. They are transmitted by sandflies. Visceral leishmaniasis and cutaneous leishmaniasis are common in parts of Africa and Asia, and the mucocutaneous form is found in Central America and South America.

Several species of *Trichomonas* (Fig. 8-11) are symbiotic. *T. hominis* is found in the cecum and colon of humans and apparently causes no disease. *T. vaginalis* inhabits the urogenital tract of humans, is transmitted venereally, and may cause vaginitis. Other species of *Trichomonas* are widely distributed through all classes of vertebrates and many invertebrates.

Giardia lamblia often causes no disease in the intestine of humans but may sometimes produce severe diarrhea. It is transmitted through fecal contamination.

Some Zoomastigophorea. *Codosiga* is a colonial flagellate with cells similar to those found in sponges (phylum Porifera). The others are all symbiotic. *Trichonympha, Spirotrichonympha,* and *Trichomonas* are commonly found in the gut of termites and wood roaches, where they help digest cellulose from the wood eaten by the insects. Species of *Trichomonas* are also found in humans. *Trypanosoma* is a parasite of various animals, and some species cause serious disease in humans and domestic animals.

Figure 8-12

Giant ameba *(Pelomyxa* sp.) is easily visible to the unassisted eye. At left is a normal-sized *Amoeba proteus;* above are several paramecia.

Courtesy Carolina Biological Supply Co., Burlington, N.C.

Figure 8-13

Diversity among the Sarcodina. *Difflugia, Arcella,* and *Amoeba* belong to the rhizopod class Lobosea and have lobopodia. The foraminiferan *Globigerina* belongs to the class Granuloreticulosea and shows reticulopodia. *Actinophrys* and *Clathrulina* are actinopod heliozoeans. They have axopodia.

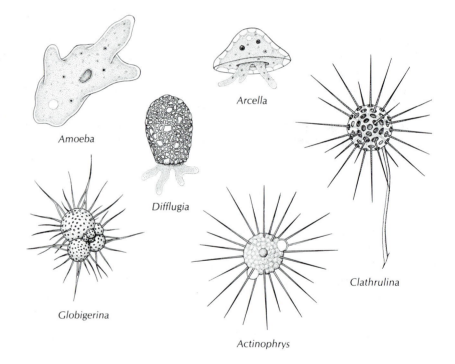

Amoeba

Arcella

Difflugia

Clathrulina

Globigerina

Actinophrys

Subphylum Sarcodina
Superclass Rhizopoda

Amoeba proteus. Of the amebas, the most commonly studied species is *Amoeba proteus.* They live in slow streams and ponds of clear water, often in shallow water on aquatic vegetation or on the sides of ledges. They are rarely found free in water, for they require a substratum on which to crawl. They have an irregular shape because of their power to thrust out lobopodia at any point on their bodies. They are colorless and about 250 to 600 µm in greatest diameter. Unlike *Euglena,* the **pellicle** consists only of the cell membrane. **Ectoplasm** and **endoplasm** are prominent. Organelles such as **nucleus, contractile vacuole, food vacuoles,** and small **vesicles** can be observed easily with the light microscope. Amebas live on algae, protozoa, rotifers, and even other amebas, upon which they

A
B

feed by phagocytosis. An ameba can live for many days without food but decreases in volume during this process. The time necessary for the digestion by a food vacuole varies with the kind of food but is usually around 15 to 30 hours. When the ameba reaches full size, it divides by binary fission with typical mitosis.

Other Rhizopoda. There are many species of amebas; for example, *A. verrucosa* has short pseudopodia; *Pelomyxa carolinensis (Chaos chaos)* (Fig. 8-12) is several times as large as *A. proteus;* and *A. radiosa* has many slender pseudopodia.

There are many entozoic amebas, most of which live in the intestines of humans or other animals. Two common genera are *Endamoeba* and *Entamoeba*. *Endamoeba blattae* is the endocommensal in the intestine of cockroaches, and related species are found in termites. *Entamoeba histolytica* (Fig. 8-1) is the most important rhizopod parasite of humans. It lives in the large intestine and on occasion can invade the intestinal wall by secreting enzymes that attack the intestinal lining. If this occurs, a serious and sometimes fatal amebic dysentery may result. The organisms may be carried by the blood to the liver and other organs and cause abscesses there. Many infected persons show few or no symptoms but are carriers, passing cysts in their feces. Infection is spread by contaminated water or food containing the cysts.

Other species of *Entamoeba* found in humans are *E. coli* in the intestine and *E. gingivalis* in the mouth. Neither of these species is known to cause disease.

Not all rhizopods are "naked" as are the amebas. Some have their delicate plasma membrane covered with a protective **test** or shell. *Arcella* and *Difflugia* (Fig. 8-13) are common sarcodines. They have a test of secreted siliceous or chitinoid material that may be reinforced with grains of sand. They move by means of pseudopodia that project from openings in the shell.

The **foraminiferans** (class Granuloreticulosea) are an ancient group of shelled rhizopods found in all oceans, with a few in fresh and brackish water. They are mostly bottom living, but a few live in open water. Their tests are of numerous types (Figs. 8-13 and 8-14). Most tests are many chambered and are made of calcium carbonate, although silica, silt, and other foreign materials are sometimes

Figure 8-14

A, Living foraminiferans. **B,** Glass model of *Globigerina bulloides.* Foraminiferans (class Granuloreticulosea) are ameboid marine protozoans that secrete a calcareous, many-chambered test in which to live and then extrude protoplasm through pores to form a layer over the outside. The animal begins with one chamber, and as it grows, it secretes a succession of new and larger chambers, continuing this process throughout life. Foraminiferans are planktonic animals, and when they die, their shells are added to the ooze on the ocean's bottom.

A, Courtesy R. Vishniac; B, courtesy American Museum of Natural History.

Figure 8-15

Types of radiolarian tests. In his study of these beautiful forms collected on the famous *Challenger* expedition, Haeckel worked out our present concepts of symmetry.

Courtesy General Biological Supply House, Inc., Chicago.

used. Slender pseudopodia extend through openings in the test, then branch and run together to form a protoplasmic net (**reticulopodia**) in which they ensnare their prey. Here the captured prey is digested, and the digested products are carried into the interior by the flowing protoplasm. The life cycles of foraminiferans are complex, for they have multiple division and alternation of haploid and diploid generations (intermediary meiosis).

Some of the slime molds (class Eumycetozoa), especially *Dictyostelium discoideum*, have been studied intensively because of their fascinating developmental cycle. Under natural conditions this species lives in forest detritus throughout the world. It feeds on bacteria and reproduces by binary fission as long as the food supply is plentiful. When food runs short, however, the amebas are attracted to each other, streaming toward a central point to form a **pseudoplasmodium** (large mass of discrete cells). Under the same conditions, some species actually fuse to become a large multinucleate individual (**plasmodium**). The pseudoplasmodium of *Dictyostelium* may migrate some distance to a favorable location, where it forms a stalk with a fruiting body on top. Within the fruiting body are formed resistant cysts, which are widely dispersed upon rupture of the fruiting body. Many details about the development, genetics, and biochemistry of these organisms are known.

Superclass Actinopoda

The Actinopoda is comprised of the mostly freshwater class Heliozoea and the three marine classes Acantharea, Phaeodarea, and Polycystinea. Members of the marine classes are commonly known as radiolarians. All have axopodia, and except for some of the heliozoeans, they have tests. These protozoa are beautiful little animals.

The biological characteristics of the freshwater Heliozoea are somewhat better known than those of the other actinopods. Examples are *Actinosphaerium*, which is about 1 mm in diameter and can be seen with the unassisted eye, and *Actinophrys* (Fig. 8-13), only 50 μm in diameter; neither has a test. *Clathrulina* (Fig. 8-13) secretes a latticed test.

The oldest known animals are found among the radiolarians. Radiolarians are nearly all pelagic (live in open water). Most of them are planktonic in shallow water, although some live in deep water. Their highly specialized skeletons are intricate in form and of great beauty (Fig. 8-15). The body is divided by a central capsule that separates inner and outer zones of cytoplasm. The central capsule, which may be spherical, ovoid, or branched, is perforated to allow cytoplasmic continuity. The skeleton is made of silica, strontium sulfate, or a combination of silica and organic matter and usually has a radial arrangement of spines that extend through the capsule from the center of the body. At the surface a shell may be fused with the spines. Around the capsule is a frothy mass of cytoplasm from which axopodia arise (p. 174). These are sticky to catch the prey, which are carried by the streaming protoplasm to the central capsule to be digested. The ectoplasm on one side of the axial rod moves outward, or toward the tip, while on the other side it moves inward, or toward the test.

Radiolarians may have one or many nuclei. Their life history is not completely known, but binary fission, budding, and sporulation have been observed in them.

Role of Sarcodina in building earth deposits

The foraminiferans and the radiolarians have existed since Precambrian times and have left excellent fossil records. In many instances their hard shells have been preserved unaltered. Many of the extinct species closely resemble present-day ones. They were especially abundant during the Cretaceous and Tertiary periods. Some of them were among the largest protozoa that have ever existed, measuring up to 100 mm or more in diameter.

For untold millions of years the tests of dead foraminiferans have been sinking to the bottom of the ocean, building up a characteristic ooze rich in lime and silica. Much of this ooze is made up of the shells of the genus *Globigerina* (Fig. 8-14, B). About one third of the sea bottom is covered with *Globigerina* ooze. This ooze is especially abundant in the Atlantic Ocean.

The radiolarians (Figs. 8-13 and 8-15), with their less soluble siliceous shells, are usually found at greater depths (15,000 to 20,000 feet), mainly in the Pacific and Indian oceans. Radiolarian ooze probably covers about 2 to 3 million square miles. Under certain conditions, radiolarian ooze forms rocks (chert). Many fossil radiolarians are found in the Tertiary rocks of California.

The thickness of these deep-sea sediments has been estimated at 700 to 4000 m. Although the average rate of sedimentation must vary greatly, it is always very slow. *Globigerina* ooze has probably increased 1 to 12.5 mm in 1000 years. As many as 50,000 shells of foraminiferans may be found in a single gram of sediment, which gives some idea of the magnitude of numbers of these microorganisms and the length of time it has taken them to form the sediment carpet on the ocean floor.

Of equal interest and of greater practical importance are the limestone and chalk deposits that were laid down by the accumulation of these microorganisms when sea covered what is now land. Later, through a rise in the ocean floor and other geological changes, this sedimentary rock emerged as dry land. The chalk

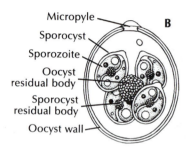

Figure 8-16

A, Diagram of an apicomplexan sporozo-ite or merozoite at the electron micro-scope level, illustrating the apical com-plex. The polar ring, conoid, micro-nemes, rhoptries, subpellicular microtu-bules, and micropore (cytostome) are all considered components of the apical complex. B, Infective oocyst of *Eimeria*. The oocyst is the resistant stage and has undergone multiple fission after zygote formation (sporogony).

deposits of many areas of England, including the White Cliffs of Dover, were formed in this way. The great pyramids of Egypt were made from stone quarried from limestone beds that were formed by a very large foraminiferan that flour-ished during the early Tertiary period.

Since fossil foraminiferans and radiolarians can be brought up in well drill-ings, their identification is often important to oil geologists for correlation of rock strata.

Phylum Apicomplexa

All apicomplexans are endoparasites, and their hosts are found in many animal phyla. The presence of a certain combination of organelles, the **apical complex,** distinguishes this subphylum (Fig. 8-16, *A*). The apical complex is usually present only in certain developmental stages of the organisms; for example, **merozoites** and **sporozoites** (Fig. 8-17). Some of the structures, especially the **rhoptries** and **micronemes,** apparently aid in penetrating the host's cells or tissues.

Locomotor organelles are less obvious in this group than in other protozoa. Pseudopodia occur in some intracellular stages, and gametes of some species are flagellated. Tiny contractile fibrils can form waves of contraction across the body surfaces to propel the organism through a liquid medium.

The life cycle usually includes both asexual and sexual reproduction, and there is sometimes an invertebrate intermediate host. At some point in the life cycle, the organisms develop a **spore** (**oocyst**), which is infective for the next host and is often protected by a resistant coat.

Class Sporozoea

The most important class of the phylum Apicomplexa, the Sporozoea, contains three subclasses: the Gregarinia, the Coccidia, and the Piroplasmia. The grega-rines are common parasites of invertebrates, but they are of little economic sig-nificance. Piroplasms are of some veterinary importance; for example, *Babesia bigemina* causes Texas red-water fever in cattle.

Subclass Coccidia

The Coccidia are intracellular parasites in invertebrates and vertebrates, and the group includes species of very great medical and veterinary importance.

Eimeria. The name "coccidiosis" is generally applied only to infections with *Eimeria* or *Isospora.* Humans are occasionally infected with species of *Isospora,* but apparently there is little disease. Some species of *Eimeria* may cause serious disease in some domestic animals. The symptom is usually severe diarrhea or dysentery.

E. tenella is often fatal to young fowl, producing severe pathogenesis in the intestine. The organisms undergo schizogony (p. 177) in the intestinal cells, finally producing gametes. After fertilization the zygote forms an oocyst that passes out of the host in the feces (Fig. 8-16, *B*). Sporogony occurs within the oocyst outside the host, producing eight sporozoites in each oocyst. Infection occurs when a new host accidentally ingests a sporulated oocyst and the sporozoites are released by digestive enzymes.

Toxoplasma. A similar life cycle occurs in *Toxoplasma gondii,* a parasite of cats, but this species produces extraintestinal stages as well. The extraintestinal stages can develop in a wide variety of animals other than cats—for example,

A

Male gamete
Female gamete
Fertilization
Ookinete
Oocyst beneath stomach lining
Sporogony occurs
Sporozoites develop in oocyst
Sporozoites released and migrate to salivary gland

Female *Anopheles* bites human and ingests gametocytes
Salivary gland
Mosquito infects human by injecting salivary juice

Blood vessel
In human
sporozoites

Sporozoites enter liver cells, undergo schizogony

Macrogametocyte
Microgametocyte
sweat

Stages in liver cells

B

Merozoites released, infect other red blood cells; some become gametocytes

Stages in red blood cells
chill

Merozoites enter red blood cells and undergo schizogony

Merozoites released, infect other liver cells or enter red blood cells

Figure 8-17

Life cycle of *Plasmodium vivax*, one of the protozoa (class Sporozoea) that causes malaria in humans. **A,** Sexual cycle produces sporozoites in body of mosquito. Meiosis occurs just after zygote formation (zygotic meiosis). **B,** Sporozoites infect human and reproduce asexually, first in liver cells and then in red blood cells. Malaria is spread by *Anopheles* mosquito, which sucks up gametocytes along with human blood, then, when biting another victim, leaves sporozoites in new wound.

rodents, cattle, and humans. Gametes and oocysts are not produced by the extraintestinal forms, but they can initiate the intestinal cycle in a cat that eats infected prey. In humans *Toxoplasma* causes little or no ill effects except in a woman infected during pregnancy, particularly in the first trimester. Such infection greatly increases the chances of a birth defect in the baby; it is now believed that 2% of all mental retardation in the United States is the result of congenital toxoplasmosis. The normal route of infection for humans is apparently the consumption of infected beef that is insufficiently cooked.

Plasmodium—the malarial organism. The best known of the coccidians is *Plasmodium,* the causative organism of the most important infectious disease of humans: **malaria.** Malaria is a very serious disease, difficult to control and widespread, particularly in tropical and subtropical countries. Four species of *Plasmodium* infect humans. Although each produces its own peculiar clinical picture, all four have similar cycles of development in their hosts (Fig. 8-17).

The parasite is carried by mosquitoes *(Anopheles),* and sporozoites are injected into the human with the insect's saliva during its bite. The sporozoites penetrate liver cells and initiate schizogony. The products of this division then enter other liver cells to repeat the schizogonous cycle, or in *P. falciparum* they

Figure 8-18

Some representative ciliates. *Euplotes* have stiff cirri used for crawling about. Contractile myonemes in ectoplasm of *Stentor* and in stalks of *Vorticella* allow great expansion and contraction. Note the macronuclei, long and curved in *Euplotes* and *Vorticella*, shaped like a string of beads in *Stentor*.

Vorticella   Stentor

Euplotes

Dileptus

Acineta

Zoothamnium

Epistylis

Tetrahymena

penetrate the red blood cells after only one cycle in the liver. The period when the parasites are in the liver is the **incubation period,** and it lasts from 6 to 15 days, depending on the species of *Plasmodium*.

Merozoites released as a result of the liver schizogony enter red blood cells, where they begin a series of schizogonous cycles. When they enter the cells, they become ameboid **trophozoites,** feeding on hemoglobin. The end product of the parasite's digestion of hemoglobin is a dark, insoluble pigment: **hemozoin.** The hemozoin accumulates in the host cell, is released when the next generation of merozoites is produced, and eventually accumulates in the liver, spleen, or other organs. The trophozoite within the cell grows and undergoes schizogony, producing six to 36 merozoites, depending on the species, which burst forth to infect new red cells. When the red blood cell containing the merozoites bursts, it releases the parasite's metabolic products, which have accumulated there. The release of these foreign substances into the patient's circulation causes the chills and fever characteristic of malaria.

Since the populations of schizonts maturing in the red blood cells are synchronized to some degree, the episodes of chills and fever have a periodicity characteristic of the particular species of *Plasmodium*. In *P. vivax* (benign tertian) malaria, the episodes occur every 48 hours; in *P. malariae* (quartan) malaria, every 72 hours; in *P. ovale* malaria, every 48 hours; and in *P. falciparum* (malignant tertian) malaria, about every 48 hours, although the synchrony is less well defined in this species. People usually recover from infections with the first three species, but mortality may be high in untreated cases of *P. falciparum* infection. Unfortunately, *P. falciparum* is the most common species, accounting for 50% of all malaria in the world.

After some cycles of schizogony in the red blood cells, infection of new cells by some of the merozoites results in the production of **microgametocytes** and **macrogametocytes** rather than another generation of merozoites. When the gametocytes are ingested by a mosquito feeding on the patient's blood, they mature into **gametes,** and fertilization occurs. The zygote becomes a motile **ookinete,** which penetrates the stomach wall of the mosquito and becomes the **oocyst.** Within the oocyst sporogony occurs, and thousands of **sporozoites** are produced. The oocyst ruptures, and the sporozoites migrate to the salivary glands, from which they are transferred to a human by the bite of the mosquito. Development in the mosquito requires 7 to 18 days but may be longer in cool weather.

The elimination of mosquitoes and their breeding places by insecticides, drainage, and other methods has been effective in controlling malaria in some areas. However, the difficulties in carrying out such activities in remote areas and

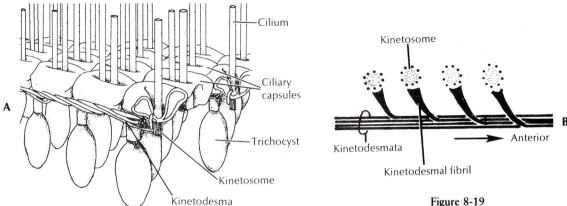

Figure 8-19

Infraciliature of a ciliate. **A,** Structure of
the pellicle and its relation to the neuro-
motor system. **B,** Portion of a kinety,
made up of the kinetosomes (basal bodies
of the cilia) and their kinetodesmata (fibrils).

the acquisition of resistance to insecticides by mosquitoes and to antimalarial
drugs by *Plasmodium* (especially *P. falciparum*) mean that malaria will be a serious disease of humans for a long time to come.

Other species of *Plasmodium* parasitize birds, reptiles, and mammals. Those
of birds are transmitted chiefly by the *Culex* mosquito.

Phylum Ciliophora

The ciliates are a large and interesting group, with a great variety of forms living in
all types of freshwater and marine habitats. They are the most structurally complex and diversely specialized of all the protozoa. The majority are free living, but
some are commensal or parasitic. They are usually solitary and motile, but some
are sessile and some colonial. There is great diversity of shape and size. In general,
they are larger than most other protozoa, but they range from very small (10 to 12
µm) up to 3 mm long. All have cilia that beat in a coordinated rhythmical manner,
although the arrangement of the cilia may vary and some lack cilia as adults.

Ciliates are always multinucleate, possessing at least one **macronucleus** and
one **micronucleus,** but varying from one to many of either type. The macronuclei
are apparently responsible for metabolic and developmental functions and for
maintaining all the visible traits, such as the pellicular apparatus. Macronuclei
vary in shape among the different species (Figs. 8-18 and 8-21). The micronuclei
participate in sexual reproduction and give rise to macronuclei after exchange of
micronuclear material between individuals. The micronuclei divide mitotically,
and the macronuclei divide amitotically.

The **pellicle** of ciliates may consist only of the cell membrane or in some
species may form a thickened armor. The cilia are short and usually arranged in
longitudinal or diagonal rows. Their structure is comparable to that of flagella,
with axoneme and kinetosome, except that cilia are shorter (Fig. 8-2). Cilia may
cover the surface of the animal or may be restricted to the oral region or to certain
bands.

In some forms the cilia are fused into a sheet called an **undulating membrane**
or into smaller **membranelles,** both used to propel food into the **cytopharynx**
(gullet). In other forms there may be fused cilia forming stiffened tufts called **cirri,**
often used in locomotion by the creeping ciliates (Fig. 8-18).

An apparently structural system of fibers, in addition to the kinetosomes,
makes up the **infraciliature,** just beneath the pellicle (Fig. 8-19). Each cilium terminates beneath the pellicle in its kinetosome, and from each kinetosome a **kineto-
desmal fibril** arises and passes along beneath the row of cilia, joining with the

other fibrils of that row. The kinetosomes and fibrils (**kinetodesmata**) of that row make up what is known as a **kinety** (Fig. 8-19). All ciliates seem to have kinety systems, even those that lack cilia at some stage. The infraciliature apparently does not coordinate the ciliary beat, as formerly thought. Coordination of the ciliary movement seems to be by waves of depolarization of the cell membrane moving down the animal, similar to the phenomenon in a nerve impulse (p. 761).

Many ciliates have contractile fibrils that early investigators called **myonemes.** With the aid of the light microscope, these can be seen to run in rows parallel with the rows of kinetosomes. The electron microscope reveals that there are actually two systems of fibrils, the **km fibers** (composed of stacks of microtubules) and the **M bands** (bundles of tubular microfilaments lying beneath the km fibers). Both km fibers and M bands are attached to the kinetosomes. Recent studies indicate that the M bands may be the ones responsible for contraction. In *Stentor,* mechanical stimuli cause waves of contractions to spread in both oral and aboral directions; an electric stimulus, however, causes contraction simultaneously in all areas of the body.

Most ciliates are holozoic. Most of them possess a cytostome (mouth) that in some forms is a simple opening and in others is connected to a gullet or ciliated groove. The mouth in some is strengthened with stiff, rodlike trichites for swallowing larger prey; in others, such as the paramecia, ciliary water currents carry microscopic food particles toward the mouth. *Didinium* has a proboscis for engulfing the paramecia on which it feeds (Fig. 8-6). Suctorians paralyze their prey and then ingest the contents through tubelike tentacles by a complex feeding mechanism that apparently combines phagocytosis with a sliding filament action of microtubules in the tentacles (Fig. 8-6).

Some ciliates have curious small bodies in their ectoplasm between the bases of the cilia. Examples are **trichocysts** (Figs. 8-19 and 8-21) and **toxicysts.** Upon mechanical or chemical stimulation, these bodies explosively expel a long, threadlike structure. The mechanism of expulsion is unknown. The function of trichocysts is thought to be defensive, although this is unclear. When a paramecium is attacked by a *Didinium,* it expels its trichocysts but to no avail. Toxicysts, however, release a poison that paralyzes the prey of carnivorous ciliates. Toxicysts are structurally quite distinct from trichocysts. Many dinoflagellates have structures very similar to trichocysts.

Among the more striking and familiar of the ciliates are *Stentor* (Gr., herald with a loud voice), trumpet shaped and solitary, with a bead-shaped macronucleus (Fig. 8-18); *Vorticella* (L., dim. of *vortex,* a whirlpool), bell shaped and attached by a contractile stalk (Fig. 8-18); *Euplotes* (Gr., *eu,* true, good, + *ploter,* swimmer) and *Stylonychia,* with flattened bodies and groups of fused cilia (cirri) that function as legs (Fig. 8-18); *Blepharisma,* slender and pink; and *Spirostomum,* very long and wormlike in appearance.

Paramecium—a representative ciliate

Paramecia are usually abundant in ponds or sluggish streams containing aquatic plants and decaying organic matter.

Form and function

The paramecium is often described as slipper shaped. *Paramecium caudatum* is 150 to 300 μm in length and is blunt anteriorly and somewhat pointed posteriorly (Fig. 8-20). The animal has an asymmetrical appearance because of the **oral groove,** a depression that runs obliquely backward on the ventral side.

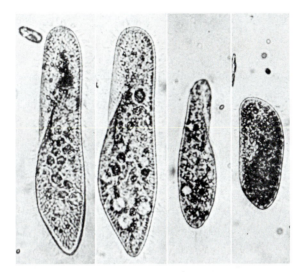

Figure 8-20

Comparison of four common species of *Paramecium* photographed at the same magnification. *Left to right: P. multimicronucleatum, P. caudatum, P. aurelia,* and *P. bursaria.*

Courtesy Carolina Biological Supply House Co., Burlington, N.C.

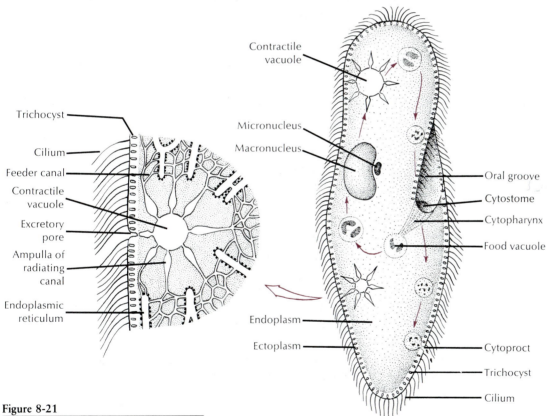

Trichocyst

Cilium

Feeder canal

Contractile vacuole

Excretory pore

Ampulla of radiating canal

Endoplasmic reticulum

Contractile vacuole

Micronucleus

Macronucleus

Oral groove

Cytostome

Cytopharynx

Food vacuole

Endoplasm

Ectoplasm

Cytoproct

Trichocyst

Cilium

Figure 8-21

Left, enlarged section of a contractile vacuole (water expulsion vesicle) of *Paramecium.* Water is believed to be collected by endoplasmic reticulum, emptied into feeder canals and then into the vesicle. The vesicle contracts to empty its contents to the outside, thus serving as an osmoregulatory organelle. *Right, Paramecium,* showing gullet, food vacuoles, and nuclei.

The **pellicle** is a clear, elastic membrane divided into hexagonal areas by tiny elevated ridges (Fig. 8-19), and its entire surface is covered with cilia arranged in lengthwise rows. Just below the pellicle is the thin clear **ectoplasm** that surrounds the larger mass of granular **endoplasm** (Fig. 8-21). Embedded in the ectoplasm just below the surface are the spindle-shaped **trichocysts**, which alternate with the bases of the cilia. The infraciliature can be seen only with special fixing and staining methods.

The **cytostome** at the end of the oral groove leads into a tubular **cytopharynx**, or **gullet**. Along the gullet an undulating membrane of modified cilia keeps food moving. Fecal material is discharged through a **cytoproct** posterior to the oral groove (Fig. 8-21). Within the endoplasm are food vacuoles containing food in various stages of digestion. There are two **contractile vacuoles**, each consisting of a central space surrounded by several **radiating canals** that collect fluid and empty it into the central vacuole. Excretion and osmoregulation were described on p. 176.

P. caudatum has two nuclei: a large kidney-shaped **macronucleus** and a smaller **micronucleus** fitted into the depression of the former. These can usually be seen only in stained specimens. The number of micronuclei varies in different species. *P. multimicronucleatum* may have as many as seven.

Paramecia are holozoic, living on bacteria, algae, and other small organisms. The cilia in the oral groove sweep food particles in the water into the cytostome, from which point they are carried into the cytopharynx by the undulating membrane. From the cytopharynx the food is collected into a food vacuole that is constricted into the endoplasm. The food vacuoles circulate in a definite course through the protoplasm (cyclosis) while the food is being digested by enzymes from the endoplasm. The indigestible part of the food is ejected through the cytoproct.

The body of the paramecium is elastic, allowing it to bend and squeeze its way through narrow places. Its cilia can beat either forward or backward, so that the animal can swim in either direction. The cilia beat obliquely, causing the animal to rotate on its long axis. In the oral groove the cilia are longer and beat more vigorously than the others so that the anterior end swerves aborally. As a result of these factors, the animal moves forward in a spiral path (Fig. 8-22, *B*).

When a ciliate, such as a paramecium, comes in contact with a barrier or a disturbing chemical stimulus, it reverses its cilia, backs up a short distance, and swerves the anterior end as it pivots on its posterior end. This is called an **avoiding reaction** (Fig. 8-22, *A*). It may continue to change its direction to keep itself some distance away from the noxious stimulus, and it may react in a similar fashion to keep itself within the zone of an attractant. The paramecium may also change its swimming speed. How does the paramecium "know" when to change directions or swimming speed? Interestingly, the reactions of the organism depend on the effects of the stimulus on the electrical potential difference across its cell membrane (see p. 763). The paramecia slightly hyperpolarize in attractants and depolarize in repellents that depend on the avoiding reaction, and they more strongly hyperpolarize in repellents and depolarize in attractants that depend on changes in swimming speed.

Reproduction

Paramecia reproduce only by binary fission across kineties but have certain forms of sexual phenomena called conjugation and autogamy.

Locomotor responses, by which an animal more or less continuously orients itself with respect to a stimulus, are called taxes (sing., taxis). Movement toward the stimulus is a positive taxis; movement away is a negative taxis. Some examples are thermotaxis, response to heat; phototaxis, response to light; thigmotaxis, response to contact; chemotaxis, response to chemical substances; rheotaxis, response to currents of air or water; galvanotaxis, response to constant electric current; and geotaxis, response to gravity. Some stimuli do not cause an orienting response but simply a change in movement: more rapid movement, more frequent random turning, or slowing or cessation of movement. Such responses are known as kineses. Is the avoiding reaction of a paramecium a taxis or a kinesis?

In **binary fission** the micronucleus divides mitotically into two daughter micronuclei, which move to opposite ends of the cell (Fig. 8-23). The macronucleus elongates and divides amitotically.

Conjugation occurs at intervals in ciliates. Conjugation is the temporary union of two individuals to exchange chromosomal material (Fig. 8-24). During the union the macronucleus disintegrates and the micronucleus of each individual

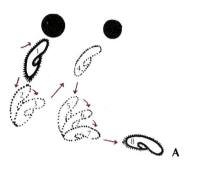

Figure 8-22

A, Avoidance reaction of *Paramecium.*
B, Spiral path of swimming *Paramecium.*

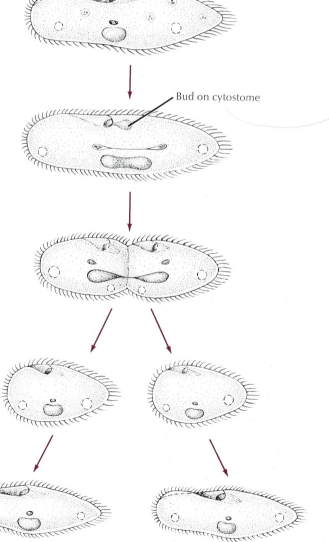

Micronucleus begins
mitosis

1. Micronucleus in mitosis
2. Macronucleus begins elongation
3. Bud appears on cytostome

Bud on cytostome

1. Micronucleus divides
2. Macronucleus pulls in two
3. New gullet forms
4. Two new contractile vacuoles appear

Division of cell
body completed

Two daughter
paramecia

Figure 8-23

Binary fission in a ciliophoran *(Paramecium).* Division is across rows of cilia.

Figure 8-24

Sexual reproduction, or conjugation, in *Paramecium caudatum*. **A,** Similar individuals come in contact on oral surface; micronuclei prepare to divide. **B** and **C,** Micronuclei divide twice (meiosis), resulting in four haploid nuclei in each partner. **D,** Three nuclei degenerate; remaining one divides to form "male" and "female" pronuclei. **E,** Male pronuclei are exchanged between conjugants. **F,** In each conjugant, male and female pronuclei fuse to form synkaryon pronucleus (diploid); conjugants now separate. **G to I,** In each exconjugant the synkaryon divides three times to form eight micronuclei; the old macronucleus is gradually resorbed. **J,** Four of the micronuclei become macronuclei; three are resorbed; one prepares to divide as the cytosome divides. **K** and **L,** Micronucleus divides twice as the cytosome divides twice; each of the four resulting daughter cells receives a micronucleus and one of the four macronuclei.

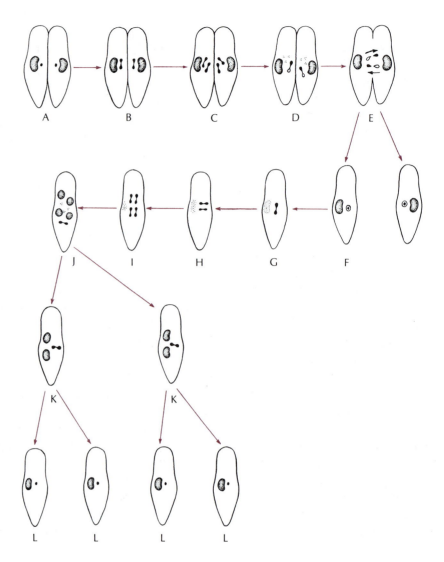

undergoes meiosis, giving rise to four haploid micronuclei, three of which degenerate (Fig. 8-24, *A* to *D*). The remaining micronucleus then divides into two haploid pronuclei, one of which crosses over into the conjugant partner. When the exchanged pronucleus unites with the pronucleus of the partner, the diploid number of chromosomes is restored (Fig. 8-24, *E* and *F*).

The two paramecia next separate, and in each paramecium the fused micronucleus, which is comparable to a zygote in higher forms, divides by mitosis into two, four, and eight micronuclei. Four of these micronuclei enlarge and become macronuclei, and three of the other four micronuclei disappear (Fig. 8-24, *G* and *J*). Then the paramecium itself divides twice, resulting in four paramecia, each with one micronucleus and one macronucleus. Following this complicated process, the animals may continue to reproduce by binary fission without the necessity of conjugation.

The result of conjugation is similar to that of zygote formation, for each exconjugant contains hereditary material from two individuals. The advantage of sexual reproduction is that it permits gene recombinations, thus increasing genetic variation in the population. Although ciliates in clone cultures can apparently reproduce repeatedly and indefinitely without conjugation, the stock seems even-

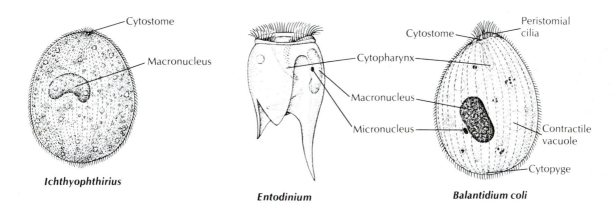

Ichthyophthirius

Entodinium

Balantidium coli

Figure 8-25

Some symbiotic ciliates. *Balantidium coli* is a parasite of humans and other mammals. This ciliate is common in pigs, in which it does little damage. In humans it may produce intestinal ulcers and severe chronic dysentery. Infections are common in parts of Europe, Asia, and Africa but are rare in the United States. *Ichthyophthirius* causes a common disease in aquarium and wild freshwater fish, known as "ick" to many fish culturists. Untreated, it can cause much loss of exotic fish. *Entodinium* is a complex ciliate found in the rumen of cows and sheep.

tually to lose vigor. Conjugation restores vitality to a stock. Seasonal changes or a deteriorating environment will usually stimulate sexual reproduction.

In 1937 it was discovered that not every paramecium would conjugate with any other paramecium of the same species. T.M. Sonneborn (1957) found that there were physiological differences between individuals that set them off into **mating types.** Ordinarily conjugation will not occur between individuals of the same mating type but only with an individual of another (complementary) mating type. It was also found that within a single species there are a number of varieties, each of which has mating types that conjugate among themselves but not with the mating types of other varieties. In *Paramecium aurelia,* for instance, each of six varieties has two mating types; conjugation, however, will occur only between members of opposite or complementary mating types within their own variety. With few exceptions, each variety has only two interbreeding mating types. There is no morphological basis for distinguishing mating types within a variety; such differences that exist must be physiological. Some varieties, however, can be distinguished from each other morphologically.

Mating types are also found in other species of paramecia and in other ciliates.

Autogamy is a process of self-fertilization that is similar to conjugation except that there is no exchange of nuclei. After the disintegration of the macronucleus and the meiotic divisions of the micronucleus, the two haploid pronuclei fuse to form a synkaryon that is homozygous (rather than heterozygous as in the case of exconjugants).

Within each species of *Paramecium* the individuals exhibit morphological and physiological differences. Since these differences are usually more minor and more superficial than those that distinguish species, the groups within a species are referred to as strains, biotypes, or varieties. Most species of protozoa can be divided into a number of these groups.

Symbiotic ciliates

Many symbiotic ciliates live as commensals, but some can be harmful to their hosts. *Balantidium coli* lives in the large intestine of humans, pigs, rats, and many other mammals (Fig. 8-25). There seem to be host-specific strains, and the organism is not easily transmitted from one species to another. Transmission is by fecal contamination of food or water. Usually the organisms are not pathogenic, but in humans they sometimes invade the intestinal lining and cause a dysentery similar to that caused by *Entamoeba histolytica.* The disease can be serious and even fatal.

Other species of ciliates live in other hosts. *Entodinium* (Fig. 8-25) is a commensal in the rumen of cattle, and *Nyctotherus* occurs in the colon of frogs and toads. In aquarium and wild freshwater fish, *Ichthyophthirius* causes a disease known to many fish culturists as "ick."

Suctorians

Suctorians are ciliates in which the young possess cilia and are free swimming, and the adults grow a stalk for attachment, become sessile, and lose their cilia. They have no cytostome but feed by long, slender, tubelike tentacles. The suctorian captures living prey, usually a ciliate, by the tip of one or more tentacles and paralyzes it. The cytoplasm of the prey then flows through the attached tentacles, forming food vacuoles in the feeding suctorian (Fig. 8-6).

One of the best places to find freshwater suctorians is in the algae that grow on the carapace of turtles. Common genera of suctorians found there are *Anarma* (without stalk or test) and *Squalorophrya* (with stalk and test). Other freshwater representatives are *Podophrya* (Fig. 8-6) and *Dendrosoma*. *Acinetopsis* and *Ephelota* are saltwater forms.

Suctorian parasites include the *Trichophrya*, which is parasitic on the gills of the small-mouthed black bass and may cause serious damage to the fish; *Allantosoma*, which occurs in the intestine of certain mammals; and *Sphaerophrya*, which is found in *Stentor*.

___ Phylogeny and Adaptive Radiation

Phylogeny

Protozoa are usually placed at the base of the phylogenetic tree of animals. Doubtless, multicellular animals were derived from a protozoan or protozoan-like ancestor, perhaps more than once. Sponges, for example, may well have been derived separately from other metazoa. Colonial protozoa, particularly among flagellates (Fig. 8-10), show various degrees of cell aggregation and some differentiation that suggest the body plans of early metazoa.

The mechanism of ciliary coordination and kineses shown by ciliates, depending on establishment of a membrane potential, polarization, and depolarization, suggests the antecedent among the protozoa of the mechanism of neural transmission, coordination, and cell-to-cell communication among the metazoa.

With the exception of certain shell-bearing Sarcodina, such as foraminiferans and radiolarians, protozoa have left no fossil records. Mastigophorans may be the oldest of all protozoa, perhaps having arisen from bacteria and spirochetes, but the group is probably polyphyletic. Most of the phytoflagellates are more closely related to the green algae than they are to zooflagellates. Some colorless phytoflagellates have chlorophyll-bearing relatives, and some autotrophic forms are facultatively saprophytic in darkness. Hence, the common origin of animals and plants may lie in the Phytomastigophorea. That the amebas were derived from the flagellates is indicated by the pseudopodia of some flagellates and the flagellated states of some amebas. However, the different classes of Sarcodina may have arisen independently from different kinds of flagellates. Some heliozoans are flagellated.

Sporozoea, which are all specialized parasites, probably came from flagellated ancestors: they often have ameboid feeding stages and flagellated gametes. Aggregation and fruiting body formation in the Eumycetozoa suggest affinities to the fungi, as is indicated by their common name, slime molds, and some scientists do consider them fungi. The origin of the ciliates is somewhat obscure, but the basic structural similarity of the flagellum to the cilium is undeniable.

Ciliophrys marina is a small marine heliozoan (subphylum Sarcodina, superclass Actinopoda) that can change *rapidly* and *reversibly* from a rapidly swimming flagellate with no axopodia to a more typical heliozoan with axopodia and slowly beating flagellum. Davidson (1982) suggested that the structure of *C. marina* shows derivation from the chrysomonad phytoflagellates.

Adaptive radiation

Some of the wide range of adaptations of protozoa have been described in the preceding pages. The Sarcodina range from bottom-dwelling, naked species to planktonic forms such as the foraminiferans and radiolarians with beautiful, intricate tests. There are many symbiotic species of amebas. Flagellates likewise show adaptations for a similarly wide range of habitats, with the added variation of photosynthetic ability in many species of Phytomastigophorea. The fine line between plants and animals at this level is shown by our ability to turn a "plant" into an "animal" by experimentally destroying the chloroplasts of *Euglena*.

Within a single-cell body plan, the division of labor and specialization of organelles are carried furthest in the ciliates. These have become the most complex of all protozoa. Specializations for intracellular parasitism have been adopted by the Sporozoea, Microspora, and Myxozoa.

___ Summary

The assemblage of animals known as protozoa is a large, heterogeneous group now recognized as being comprised of seven phyla. The largest and most important of the phyla are the Sarcomastigophora (flagellates and amebas), the Apicomplexa (coccidians, malaria-causing organisms, and others), and the Ciliophora (ciliates). They demonstrate the great adaptive potential of the basic body plan, the single eukaryotic cell. They occupy a vast array of niches and habitats, and many species have complex and specialized organelles.

All protozoa have one or more nuclei, and these often appear vesicular under the light microscope. Macronuclei of ciliates are compact. Endosomes are often present in the nuclei. Many protozoa have organelles similar to those found in metazoan cells.

Pseudopodial or ameboid movement is a locomotory and food-gathering mechanism in protozoa and plays a vital role as a defense mechanism in metazoa. It is accomplished by an incompletely known process of microfilaments moving past each other, and it requires expenditure of energy from ATP. Ciliary movement is likewise important in both protozoa and metazoa. Currently, the most widely accepted mechanism to account for ciliary movement is the sliding microtubule hypothesis.

Various protozoa feed by holophytic, holozoic, or saprozoic means. The excess water that enters their bodies is expelled by contractile vacuoles (water-expulsion vesicles). Respiration and waste elimination are through the body surface. Protozoa reproduce asexually by binary fission, multiple fission, and budding: sexual processes are common. Cyst formation to withstand adverse environmental conditions is an important adaptation in many protozoa.

Most phytoflagellates are photosynthetic, and many zooflagellates are important parasites. They move by beating one or more flagella. Sarcodines move by pseudopodia; many are important members of planktonic communities, and some are parasites. Many have a test, or shell. All apicomplexans are parasitic, and they include *Plasmodium,* which causes malaria. The Ciliophora move by means of cilia or ciliary organelles. They are a large and diverse group, and many are complex in structure.

Selected references

Barnes, R.D. 1980. Invertebrate zoology, ed. 4. Philadelphia, Saunders College/Holt, Rinehart & Winston.

Corliss, J.D. 1979. The ciliated protozoa: characterization, classification, and guide to the literature, ed. 2. New York, Pergamon Press, Inc.

Davidson, L.A. 1982. Ultrastructure, behavior, and algal flagellate affinities of the helioflagellate *Ciliophrys marina*, and the classification of the helioflagellates (Protista, Actinopoda, Heliozoea). J. Protozool. 29:19-29.

Dodson, E.O. 1971. The kingdoms of organisms. Syst. Zool. 20:265-281.

Edds, K.T. 1981. Cytoplasmic streaming in a heliozoan. BioSystems 14:371-376.

Farmer, J.N. 1980. The Protozoa: introduction to protozoology. St. Louis, The C.V. Mosby Co.

Grell, K.G. 1973. Protozoology. Heidelberg, Springer-Verlag.

Harrison, G. 1978. Mosquitoes, malaria and man: a history of the hostilities since 1880. New York, E.P. Dutton. *A fascinating story, well told.*

Hyman, L.H. 1940. The invertebrates: Protozoa through Ctenophora, vol. 1. New York, McGraw-Hill Book Co. *An extensive and exhaustive section is devoted to the morphology and physiology of protozoa.*

Jahn, T.L., and F.F. Jahn. 1949. How to know the Protozoa. Dubuque, Iowa, William C. Brown Co., Publishers. *A manual on the identification and description of protozoan forms.*

Kudo, R.R. 1966. Protozoology, ed. 5. Springfield, Ill., Charles C Thomas, Publisher.

Lee, C. 1980. Fish poisoning with particular reference to ciguatera. J. Trop. Med. Hyg. 83:93-97.

Leedale, G.F. 1967. Euglenoid flagellates. Englewood Cliffs, N.J., Prentice-Hall, Inc.

Levine, N.D. 1973. Protozoan parasites of domestic animals and man. Minneapolis, Burgess Publishing Co.

Levine, N.D., and others. 1980. A newly revised classification of the protozoa. J. Protozool. 27:37-58. *This classification is a revision of that published in 1964 by the Committee on Systematics and Evolution of the Society of Protozoologists. It is the most authoritative classification currently available.*

Pennak, R.W. 1978. Freshwater invertebrates of the United States, ed. 2. New York, John Wiley & Sons, Inc. *A reference work with considerable attention devoted to protozoa.*

Pettersson, H. 1954. The ocean floor, New Haven, Conn., Yale University Press. *The role foraminiferans and radiolarians have played in building up the sediment carpet of the ocean floor is vividly described in this little book.*

Pitelka, D.R. 1963. Electron-microscopic structure of Protozoa. New York, Macmillan, Inc. *A fine account of the ultrastructure of protozoa.*

Rudzinska, M.A. 1973. Do suctoria really feed by suction? BioScience 23(2):87-94.

Sarjeant, W.A.S. 1974. Fossil and living dinoflagellates. New York, Academic Press, Inc.

Satir, P. 1968. Studies on cilia. III. Further studies on the cilia tip and a "sliding filament" model of ciliary motility. J. Cell. Biol. 39:77-94.

Schmidt, G.D., and L.S. Roberts. 1981. Foundations of parasitology, ed. 2. St. Louis, The C.V. Mosby Co. *A parasitology text containing a good account of protozoan parasites.*

Sleigh, M.A. 1962. The biology of cilia and flagella. New York, Macmillan, Inc. *An excellent summary.*

Sleigh, M.A. 1973. The biology of protozoa. New York, American Elsevier Publishers, Inc. *Well-written text, integrated form and function with many micrographs and diagrams of cell cycles.*

Sonneborn, T.M. 1957. Breeding systems, reproductive methods, and species problems in Protozoa. In Mayr, E. (ed.). The species problem. Washington, D.C., American Association for the Advancement of Science, pp. 155-324. *A good analysis of mating types of protozoa.*

Van Houten, J. 1979. Membrane potential changes during chemokinesis in *Paramecium*. Science 204:1100-1103.

Vickerman, K., and F.E.G. Cox. 1967. The Protozoa. Boston, Houghton Mifflin Co.

Wichterman, R. 1953. The biology of *Paramecium*. New York, McGraw-Hill Book Co. *A well-written treatise on one genus of protozoans.*

Selected *Scientific American* articles

Alvarado, C.A., and L.J. Bruce-Chevatt. 1962. Malaria. 206:86-98 (May).

Bonner, J.T. 1950. *Volvox:* a colony of cells. 182:52-55 (May).

Bonner, J.T. 1969. Hormones in social amoebae and mammals. 220:78-91 (June).

Hawking, F. 1970. The clock of the malaria parasite. 222:123-131 (June).

Hutner, S.H., and J.A. McLaughlin. 1958. Poisonous tides. 199:92-98 (Aug.).

Lazarides, E., and J.P. Revel. 1979. The molecular basis of cell movement. 240:100-113 (May).

Satir, P. 1974. How cilia move. 231:45-52 (Nov.).

C H A P T E R   9

T H E   L O W E S T   M E T A Z O A N S

Phylum Mesozoa

Phylum Placozoa

Phylum Porifera—Sponges Start p 204

A small fish (*Gobiosoma* sp.) lies perched atop a tube sponge
(*Verongia* sp.) on a Caribbean coral reef.

Photograph by S.K. Webster, Monterey Bay Aquarium/BPS.

Position in Animal Kingdom

The multicellular animals, or Metazoa, are typically divided into three branches: Mesozoa (a single phylum), Parazoa (phylum Porifera, the sponges; and phylum Placozoa), and Eumetazoa (all other phyla).

Although Mesozoa and Parazoa are multicellular, neither fits into the general plan of organization of the other phyla. Such cellular layers as they possess are not homologous to the germ layers of the Eumetazoa, and neither group has developmental patterns in line with the other metazoans. The poriferans are considered to be aberrant, that is, deviating widely from standard patterns. This is the reason for the name Parazoa, which means the "beside-animals." Placozoans may be the most primitive free-living animals. They show relationships to the Porifera.

Biological Contributions

1. Although the simplest in organization of all the metazoans, the mesozoans and sponges do comprise a higher level of morphological and physiological integration than that found in protozoan colonies. Both groups may be said to belong to a **cellular level of organization.**

2. The mesozoans, although composed simply of an outer layer of somatic cells and an inner layer of reproductive cells, nevertheless have a very complex reproductive cycle somewhat suggestive of that of the trematodes (flukes). Mesozoans are entirely parasitic.

3. Placozoans are essentially comprised of two epithelia with fluid and some fibrous cells between them.

4. The poriferans are more complex, with several types of cells differentiated for various functions, some of which are organized into **incipient tissues** of a low level of integration.

5. The developmental patterns of the phyla are different from those of other phyla, and their embryonic layers are not homologous to the germ layers of other phyla.

6. The sponges have developed a unique system of **water currents** on which they depend for food and oxygen.

___PHYLUM MESOZOA

The name Mesozoa (mes-o-zo′a) (Gr., *mesos*, in the middle, + *zōon*, animal) was coined by an early investigator (van Beneden, 1876) who believed the group to be a "missing link" between protozoa and metazoa. These minute, ciliated, wormlike animals represent an extremely simple level of organization. All mesozoans live as parasites in marine invertebrates, and the majority of them are only 0.5 to 7 mm in length. Most are made up of only 20 to 30 cells arranged basically in two layers. The layers are not homologous to the germ layers of higher metazoans.

There are two classes of mesozoans, the Rhombozoa and the Orthonectida, but they differ so much from each other that some authorities believe they should be placed in separate phyla.

___ Class Rhombozoa

The rhombozoans (Gr., *rhombos,* a spinning top, + *zōon,* animal) live in the kidneys of benthic cephalopods (bottom-dwelling octopuses, cuttlefishes, and squids). Two orders are recognized: Dicyemida (Gr., *di,* two, + *kyēma,* embryo) and Heterocyemida (Gr., *heteros,* another, + *kyēma,* embryo). The adults, called **vermiforms** (or nematogens), are long and slender. They have an outer layer of 20 to 30 ciliated somatic cells (the number is constant within a species) surrounding a long, slender axial cell in which there are a number of small reproductive cells (Fig. 9-1, *A*). The reproductive cells by repeated division give rise to

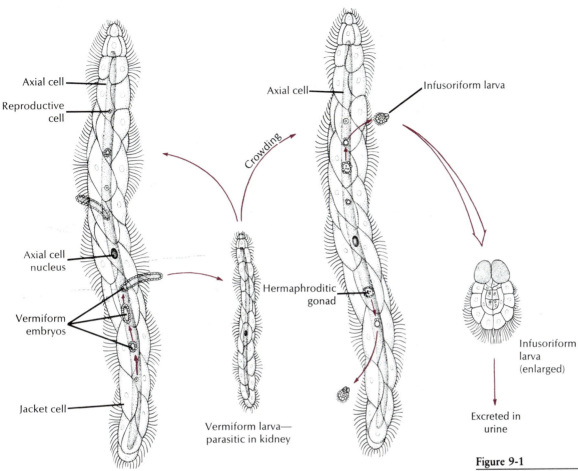

Axial cell
Reproductive cell
Axial cell
Infusoriform larva
Axial cell nucleus
Crowding
Hermaphroditic gonad
Vermiform embryos
Jacket cell
Vermiform larva— parasitic in kidney

Infusoriform larva (enlarged)

Excreted in urine

A   **B**

Figure 9-1

Two methods of reproduction by mesozoans. **A,** Asexual development of vermiform larvae from reproductive cells in the axial cell of the adult. **B,** Under crowded conditions in the host kidney, reproductive cells develop into gonads with gametes that produce infusoriform dispersal larvae that are shed in the host urine.

Modified from Lapan, E.A., and H. Morowitz. 1972. Sci. Am. **227:**94-101 (Dec.).

vermiform embryos (also called **primary nematogens**) similar to the parent. These are released from the parent's body into the urine of the host, where they grow and eventually attach to the spongy tissue of the kidney and begin to reproduce. The inner kidney lining may eventually be covered with thousands of these wormlike parasites.

As the population in the kidney becomes overcrowded, some of the adult members begin another type of reproduction by which dispersal of the species can occur. Instead of developing into vermiform embryos, the reproductive cells develop into a gonadlike structure producing male and female gametes that fuse in fertilization. The zygotes develop into minute (0.04 mm) ciliated **infusoriform larvae** (Fig. 9-1, *B*) quite unlike the parent. These are shed with the urine into the seawater and sink to the bottom. The infusoriforms are not immediately infective to a new host; therefore some development must occur outside the host, or possibly an intermediate host is necessary. This part of the life cycle is still unknown. When a new host is infected, the first stage that develops in its kidney is the **stem vermiform** (stem nematogen), which develops into an adult vermiform that produces vermiform larvae. This starts a new population, which is increased by more vermiform larvae until overpopulation again brings about the development of the infusoriform dispersion larvae.

Class Orthonectida

Orthonectids (Gr., *orthos*, straight, + *nektōs*, swimming) parasitize a variety of invertebrates, such as brittle stars, bivalve molluscs, polychaetes, and nemerteans. The best-known orthonectid is *Rhopalura*, a parasite of brittle stars. The life cycles involve sexual and asexual phases. The asexual stage is quite different from that of the dicyemids. It consists of a multinucleated mass of protoplasm called a **plasmodium**, which by division ultimately gives rise to males and females. These are composed of an outer layer of ciliated somatic cells surrounding an inner mass of germ cells (Fig. 9-2). Large numbers of the adults are shed into the seawater, where fertilization occurs.

Phylogeny of Mesozoans

There is still much to learn about these mysterious little parasites, but probably one of the most intriguing questions is the place of mesozoans in the evolutionary picture. Some investigators believe them to be primitive or degenerate flatworms and even believe that they should be classed with the Platyhelminthes. Others place them close to protozoa as truly primitive forms, possibly related to the ciliates. Whether metazoans and mesozoans derived independently from protozoan beginnings or whether mesozoans are indeed degenerate flatworms is still an enigma.

PHYLUM PLACOZOA

The phylum Placozoa (Gr., *plax, plakos,* tablet, plate, + *zōon,* animal) was proposed in 1971 by K.G. Grell to contain a single species, *Trichoplax adhaerens* (Fig. 9-3, *A*), a tiny (2 to 3 mm) marine form that had been considered to be either a mesozoan or a cnidarian larva by various workers in the past. The body is platelike and has no symmetry, no organs, and no muscular or nervous system. It is comprised of a dorsal epithelium of flagellated cover cells and shiny spheres, a thick ventral epithelium containing flagellated cells and nonflagellated gland cells, and a space between the epithelia containing fluid and fibrous cells (Fig. 9-3, *B*). The organisms glide over their food, secrete digestive enzymes upon it, and then absorb the products. Grell considers *Trichoplax* diploblastic (see p. 131), with the dorsal epithelium representing ectoderm and the ventral epithelium representing endoderm because of its nutritive function. The phylogenetic position of placozoans is uncertain, although they are certainly very primitive. They seem to be closest to the Porifera.

PHYLUM PORIFERA—SPONGES

Sponges belong to phylum Porifera (po-rif'-er-a) (L., *porus*, pore, + *fera*, bearing). The bodies of sponges bear myriads of tiny pores and canals that comprise a filter-feeding system adequate for their inactive life-style, for they are sessile animals. They depend on the water currents carried through their unique canal systems to bring them food and oxygen and to carry away their body wastes. Their bodies are little more than masses of cells embedded in a gelatinous matrix and stiffened by a skeleton of minute **spicules** of calcium or silica or by "spongy" fibers

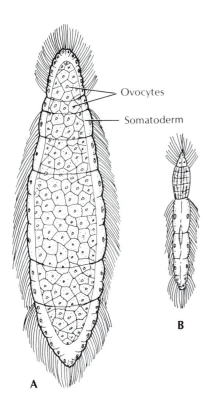

Figure 9-2

A, Female and, **B,** male orthonectid *(Rhopalura).* This mesozoan parasitizes such forms as flatworms, molluscs, annelids, and brittle stars. The structure consists of a single layer of ciliated epithelial cells surrounding an inner mass of sex cells.

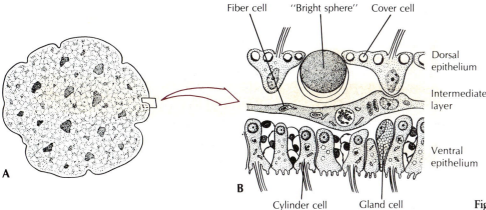

Fiber cell   "Bright sphere"   Cover cell

Dorsal epithelium

Intermediate layer

Ventral epithelium

A

B

Cylinder cell   Gland cell

Figure 9-3

A, *Trichoplax adhaerens* is a marine, platelike animal only 2 to 3 mm in diameter. The only member of the phylum Placozoa, it is one of the most primitive multicellular animals known. **B,** Section through *Trichoplax adhaerens*, showing histological structure.

Redrawn from Grell, K.G. 1972. Z. Morph. Tiere 73:297-314.

of a keratose substance called spongin. They have no organs or true tissues, and even their cells show a certain degree of independence. As sessile animals with only negligible body movement, they have not evolved a nervous system or sense organs and have only the simplest of contractile elements.

So, although they are multicellular, sponges share few of the characteristics of other metazoan phyla. They seem to be outside the line of evolution leading from the protozoa to the other metazoans: a dead-end branch. It is for this reason that they are often called the Parazoa (Gr., *para,* beside or alongside of, + *zōon,* animal).

Most sponges are colonial, and they vary in size from a few millimeters to the great loggerhead sponges, which may reach 2 m or more across. Many sponge species are brightly colored because of pigments in the dermal cells. Red, yellow, orange, green, and purple sponges are not uncommon. However, the color fades quickly when the sponges are removed from the water. Some sponges, including the simplest and most primitive, are radially symmetrical, but many are quite irregular in shape. Some stand erect, some are branched or lobed, and others are low, even encrusting, in form. Some bore holes into shells or rocks.

Most of the 5000 or more sponge species are marine, although some 150 species live in fresh water. Marine sponges are abundant in all seas and at all depths, and a few even exist in brackish water. Although the embryos are free swimming, the adults are always attached, usually to rocks, shells, corals, or other submerged objects. Some benthic forms even grow on sand or mud bottoms. Their growth patterns often depend on the shape of the substratum, the direction and speed of the water currents, and the availability of space, so that the same species may differ markedly in appearance under different environmental circumstances. Sponges in calm waters may grow taller and straighter than those in rapidly moving waters.

Many animals (crabs, nudibranchs, mites, bryozoans, and fish) live as commensals or parasites in or on sponges. The larger sponges particularly tend to harbor a large variety of invertebrate commensals. On the other hand, sponges grow on many other living animals, such as molluscs, barnacles, brachiopods, corals, or hydroids. Some crabs attach pieces of sponge to their carapaces for camouflage and for protection, since most predators seem to find sponges distasteful. Some reef fishes, however, are known to graze on shallow-water sponges.

The sponges are an ancient group, with an abundant fossil record extending back to the Cambrian period and even, according to some claims, the Precambrian.

CHARACTERISTICS

1. Multicellular; body a loose aggregation of cells of mesenchymal origin
2. Body with pores (ostia), canals, and chambers that serve for passage of water
3. Mostly marine; all aquatic
4. Radial symmetry or none
5. Epidermis of flat pinacocytes; most interior surfaces lined with flagellated collar cells (choanocytes) that create water currents; a gelatinous protein matrix called mesohyl (mesoglea) contains amebocytes of various types and skeletal elements
6. Skeleton of calcareous or siliceous crystalline spicules, protein spongin, or a combination
7. No organs or true tissues; digestion intracellular; excretion and respiration by diffusion
8. Reactions to stimuli apparently local and independent; nervous system probably absent
9. All adults sessile and attached to substratum
10. Asexual reproduction by buds or gemmules and sexual reproduction by eggs and sperm; free-swimming ciliated larvae

CLASSIFICATION

Class Calcispongiae (cal-si-spun′je-e) (L., *calcis*, lime, + Gr., *spongos*, sponge) (**Calcarea**). Have spicules of calcium carbonate that often form a fringe around the osculum (main water outlet); spicules needle shaped or three or four rayed; all three types of canal systems (asconoid, syconoid, leuconoid) represented; all marine. Examples: *Scypha, Leucosolenia.*

Class Hyalospongiae (hy′a-lo-spun′je-e) (Gr., *hyalos*, glass, + *spongos*, sponge) (**Hexactinellida**). Have six-rayed, siliceous spicules extending at right angles from a central point; spicules often united to form network; body often cylindrical or funnel shaped; flagellated chambers in simple syconoid or leuconoid arrangement; habitat mostly deep water; all marine. Examples: Venus's flower basket (*Euplectella*), *Hyalonema.*

Class Demospongiae (de-mo-spun′je-e) (Gr., *demos*, people, + *spongos*, sponge). Have siliceous spicules that are not six rayed, or spongin, or both; leuconoid-type canal systems; one family found in fresh water; all others marine. Examples: *Thenea, Cliona, Spongilla, Myenia,* and all bath sponges.

Class Sclerospongiae (skler′o-spun′je-e) (Gr., *skleros*, hard, + *spongos*, sponge). Secrete massive basal skeleton of calcium carbonate, with living tissue extending into the skeleton from 1 mm to 3 cm or more, extending above skeleton less than 1 mm; have siliceous spicules similar to Demospongiae (sometimes absent), and spongin fibers; leuconoid organization; inhabit caves, crevices, tunnels, and deep water on coral reefs. Examples: *Astrosclera, Calcifibrospongia, Ceratoporella, Merlia.*

___ Form and Function

The only body openings of these unusual animals are pores, usually many tiny ones called **ostia** for incoming water, and a few large ones called **oscula** (sing., **osculum**) for water outlet. These openings are connected by a system of canals, some of which are lined with peculiar flagellated collar cells called **choanocytes**, whose flagella maintain a current of environmental water through the canals. Water enters the canals through a multitude of tiny incurrent pores (**dermal ostia**) and leaves by way of one or more large oscula. The choanocytes not only keep the water moving but also trap and phagocytize food particles that are carried in the water. The cells lining the passageways are very loosely organized. Collapse of the canals is prevented by the skeleton, which, depending on the species, may be made up of needlelike calcareous or siliceous spicules, a meshwork of organic spongin fibers, or a combination of the two.

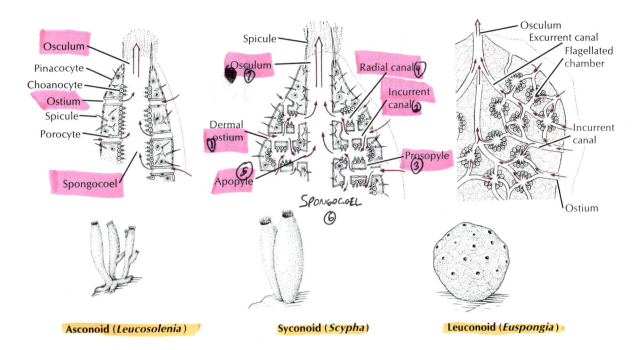

Asconoid (*Leucosolenia*)   Syconoid (*Scypha*)   Leuconoid (*Euspongia*)

Sessile animals make few movements and therefore need little in the way of nervous, sensory, or locomotor parts. Sponges apparently have lived as sessile animals from their earliest appearance and have never acquired specialized nervous or sensory structures, and they have only the very simplest of contractile systems.

Types of canal systems

Most sponges fall into one of three types of canal systems: asconoid, syconoid, or leuconoid (Fig. 9-4).

Asconoids—flagellated spongocoels

The asconoid sponges have the simplest type of organization. They are small and tube shaped. Water enters through microscopic dermal pores into a large cavity called the **spongocoel, which is lined with choanocytes.** The choanocyte flagella pull the water through the pores and expel it through a single large osculum (Fig. 9-4). *Leucosolenia* (Gr., *leukos*, white, + *sōlen*, pipe) is an asconoid type of sponge. Its slender, tubular individuals grow in groups attached by a common stolon, or stem, to objects in shallow seawater (Fig. 9-5). Asconoids are found only in class Calcispongiae.

Syconoids—flagellated canals

Synconoid sponges look somewhat like larger editions of asconoids, from which they were derived. They have the tubular body and single osculum, but the body wall, which is thicker and more complex than that of asconoids, contains choanocyte-lined radial canals that empty into the spongocoel (Fig. 9-4). The spongocoel in syconoids is lined with epithelial-type cells rather than flagellated cells as in asconoids. Water enters through a large number of dermal ostia into **incurrent canals** and then filters through tiny openings called **prosopyles** into the choanocyte-lined **radial canals** (Fig. 9-6). There food is ingested by the choanocytes,

Figure 9-4

Three types of sponge structure. The degree of complexity from simple asconoid to complex leuconoid type has involved mainly the water-canal and skeletal systems, accompanied by outfolding and branching of the collar cell layer. The leuconoid type is considered the major plan for sponges, for it permits greater size and more efficient water circulation.

Figure 9-5

A cluster of sponges removed from a
dock where it was attached by a slender
stalk, perhaps a bit of algae. Around the
stalk (above) is a bit of breadcrumb
sponge *Halichondria*, a leuconoid-type
sponge. To the right is a mass of branching *Leucosolenia*, an asconoid sponge,
and at left are three large and two small
Scypha, syconoid sponges.
Photograph by D.P. Wilson.

whose flagella force the water on through internal pores (**apopyles**) into the spongocoel. From there it emerges through the osculum. Syconoids do not usually form highly branched colonies as do the asconoids. During development, syconoid sponges pass through an asconoid stage; the flagellated canals form by evagination of the body wall. This is one evidence that syconoid sponges were derived from asconoid ancestral stock. Syconoids are found in classes Calcispongiae and Hyalospongiae. *Scypha* (Gr., *skyphos*, cup) is a commonly studied example of the syconoid type of sponge (Fig. 9-5).

Leuconoids—flagellated chambers

Leuconoid organization is the most complex of the sponge types and the best adapted for increase in sponge size. Most leuconoids form large colonial masses, each member of the mass having its own osculum, but individual members are poorly defined and often impossible to distinguish (Fig. 9-7). Clusters of flagellated chambers are filled from incurrent canals and discharge water into excurrent canals that eventually lead to the osculum (Fig. 9-4). Most sponges are of the leuconoid type, which occurs in both class Calcispongiae and class Demospongiae.

These three types of canal systems—asconoid, syconoid, and leuconoid—are correlated with the evolution of sponges from simple to complex forms. Evolutionary changes involved increasing the flagellated surfaces in proportion to the volume, thus providing more collar cells to meet the food demands. This was achieved by the outpushing of the spongocoel of a simple sponge such as the asconoid type to form the radial canals (lined with flagellated cells) of the sycon-

Dermal epithelium

Dermal ostium

Incurrent canal

Radial canal

Amebocyte

Choanocytes

Amphiblastula larva

Mesohyl

Gastral epithelium

Spongocoel

oid type. Further folding of the body wall produced the complex canals and chambers of the leuconoid type.

Types of cells

Sponge cells are loosely arranged in a gelatinous matrix called **mesohyl** (mesoglea, mesenchyme) (Figs. 9-6 and 9-8). The mesohyl is the "connective tissue" of the sponges; in it are found various ameboid cells, fibrils, and skeletal elements. There are several types of cells in sponges.

Figure 9-8

Small section through sponge wall, showing four types of sponge cells. Pinacocytes are protective and contractile; choanocytes create water currents and engulf food particles; amebocytes have a variety of functions; collencytes appear to have a contractile function.

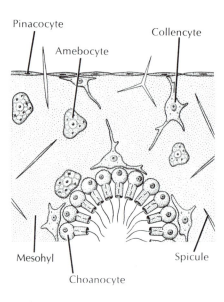

Pinacocyte

Amebocyte

Collencyte

Mesohyl

Choanocyte

Spicule

Pinacocytes

The nearest approach to a true tissue in sponges is found in the arrangement of the **pinacocyte** cells of the epidermis (Fig. 9-8). These are thin, flat, epithelial-type cells that cover the exterior surface and some interior surfaces. Pinacocytes are somewhat contractile and help regulate the surface area of the sponge. Some of the pinacocytes are modified as contractile **myocytes,** which are usually arranged in circular bands around the oscula or pores, where they help regulate the rate of water flow.

Choanocytes

The choanocytes, which line the flagellated canals and chambers, are ovoid cells with one end embedded in the mesohyl and the other exposed. The exposed end bears a flagellum surrounded by a collar (Figs. 9-8 and 9-9). The electron microscope shows the collar to be made up of adjacent microvilli, connected to each other by delicate microfibrils, so that the collar forms a fine filtering device for straining food particles from the water (Fig. 9-9, *B* and *C*). The beat of the flagellum pulls water through the sievelike collar and forces it out through the open top of the collar. Particles too large to enter the collar become trapped in secreted mucus and slide down the collar to the base where they are phagocytized by the cell body. Larger particles have already been screened out by the small size of the dermal pores and prosopyles. The food engulfed by the cells may be digested in food vacuoles within the choanocyte or passed on to a neighboring amebocyte for digestion.

Amebocytes

Various ameboid cells, called amebocytes, move about in the mesohyl (Fig. 9-8) and carry out a number of functions. Some are filled with food reserves, aid in digestion, or carry pigments; others, called **archaeocytes,** form reproductive cells. Some, called **scleroblasts,** secrete the spicules, and others, called **spongioblasts,** secrete the spongin fibers of the skeleton. Some star-shaped cells called **collencytes** appear to be contractile and to secrete collagenous fibrils into the mesohyl. **Lophocytes** are a highly motile type of amebocyte and function in secretion of

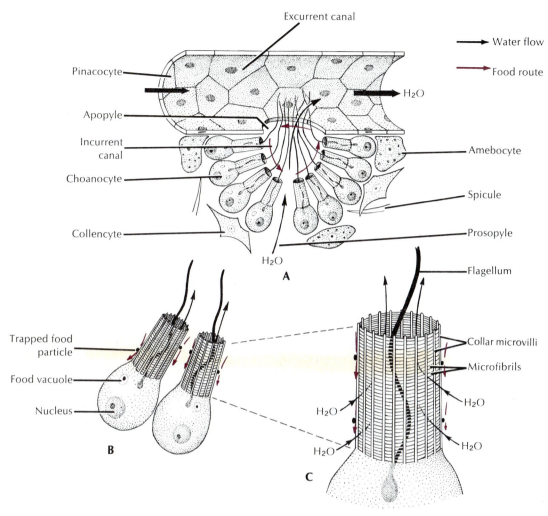

Excurrent canal

Water flow

Food route

Pinacocyte

H_2O

Apopyle

Incurrent canal

Amebocyte

Choanocyte

Spicule

Collencyte

Prosopyle

H_2O

Flagellum

A

Trapped food particle

Collar microvilli

Food vacuole

Microfibrils

Nucleus

H_2O

H_2O

H_2O

H_2O

B

C

Figure 9-9

Food trapping by sponge cells. **A,** Cutaway section of canals showing cellular structure and direction of water flow. **B,** Two choanocytes and, **C,** structure of the collar. Small red arrows indicate movement of food particles.

bundles of fibrils. Some authorities have suggested a nervous function for the collencytes or lophocytes, but as yet there is no conclusive evidence to support this claim.

Types of skeletons

The skeleton gives support to the sponge, preventing collapse of the canals and chambers. In calcareous sponges the spicules are composed mostly of crystalline calcium carbonate and have one, three, or four rays (Fig. 9-10). The Demospongiae have siliceous spicules (with one, two, or four rays), spongin fibers, or both spicules and spongin. Glass sponges have siliceous spicules with six rays arranged in three planes at right angles to each other. In *Monorhaphis* (Gr., *mono,* alone, + *rhaphis,* needle), a glass sponge, the spicules are composed of an axial fiber of a protein called spiculin, surrounded by cylindrical layers of noncrystalline hydrated silica, and finally by another layer of spiculin. There are many variations in the shape of spicules, and these structural variations are of taxonomic importance.

The protein spongin forms a tough, branching, fibrous network that supports the soft lining tissues alone or in combination with spicules.

Siliceous spicules
(Hexactinellida)

Siliceous spicules
(Demospongiae)

Spongin

Calcareous

Figure 9-10

A, Types of spicules found in sponges. There are amazing diversity, complexity, and beauty of form among the many types of spicules. **B,** Some sponge body forms.

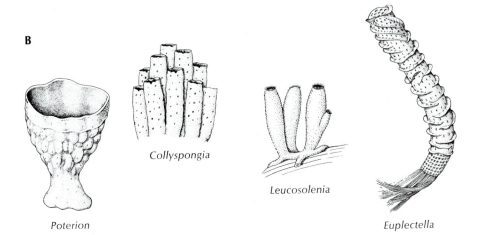

Poterion

Collyspongia

Leucosolenia

Euplectella

Sponge physiology

Sponges apparently feed on fine detritus particles, planktonic organisms, and bacteria that are screened by the dermal pores and prosopyles and again by the choanocyte collars. Choanocytes ingest the smallest particles, and pinacocytes and amebocytes phagocytize larger food particles. Food is often passed from cell to cell. Digestion, which is **intracellular** (occurs within the cells), may be started in a collar cell and completed in an amebocyte or transferred to a third cell for the final stage. Thus, the wandering amebocytes perform a carrier service, act as digesters, and serve as storage warehouses. Although the choanocyte-lined chambers are the chief areas for feeding activity, they are not in any sense comparable to the digestive tracts of other metazoans.

There are no respiratory or excretory organs; both functions are apparently carried out by diffusion in individual cells. Contractile vacuoles have been found in amebocytes and choanocytes of freshwater sponges.

All the life activities of the sponge depend on the current of water flowing through the body. A sponge pumps a remarkable amount of water. *Leuconia* (Gr., *leukos,* white), for example, is a small leuconoid sponge about 10 cm tall and 1 cm in diameter. It is estimated that water enters through some 81,000 incurrent canals at a velocity of 0.1 cm/second. However, *Leuconia* has more than 2 million flagellated chambers whose combined diameter is much greater than that of the canals, so that in the chambers the water slows down to 0.001 cm/second, allowing ample opportunity for food capture by the collar cells. All of the water is expelled through a single osculum at a velocity of 8.5 cm/second: a jet force capable of carrying waste products some distance away from the sponge. Some large sponges have been found to filter 1500 liters of water a day.

Because of the screening action of the ostia, the prosopyles, and collars, only the finest food particles reach the choanocytes. Ostia average 50 μm in diameter and prosopyles about 5 μm. The tiny spaces between the microvilli that make up a collar are only about 0.1 μm wide. Thus, the choanocytes capture the smallest particles, and slightly larger bits are engulfed by amebocytes or pinacocytes.

The only visible activities and responses in sponges, other than the propulsion of water, are slight alterations in shape and the closing and opening of the incurrent and excurrent pores, and these movements are very slow. The most common response is closure of the oscula. Apparently excitation spreads from cell to cell, although some zoologists point to the possibility of coordination by means of substances carried in the water currents, and some have tried, not very successfully, to demonstrate the presence of nerve cells.

Reproduction

Sponges reproduce both asexually and sexually. **Asexual reproduction** occurs by means of bud formation. **External buds,** after reaching a certain size, may become detached from the parent and float away to form new sponges, or they may remain to form colonies. **Internal buds,** or **gemmules,** are formed in freshwater sponges and some marine sponges. Here, archaeocytes are collected together in the mesohyl and become surrounded by a siliceous shell or by a cluster of spicules. When the parent animal dies, the gemmules survive and remain dormant, preserving the life of the species during periods of freezing or severe drought. Later the cells in the gemmules escape through a special opening, the **micropyle,** and develop into new sponges. Gemmulation in freshwater sponges (Spongillidae) is thus an adaptation to the changing seasons. Gemmules are also a means of colonizing new habitats, since they can be spread by streams or by animal carriers. What prevents the gemmules from hatching during the season of formation rather than remaining dormant? It has been shown that some species secrete a substance that inhibits early germination of the gemmules. Gemmule formation is apparently influenced by both light and temperature, although sponges have no known photoreceptors.

It is interesting to note that investigators studying *Ephydatia fluviatilis* (Gr., *ephydatios,* of the water), a freshwater sponge, have discovered that there are several strains of the species and that sponges hatched from gemmules of one strain can fuse with others of the same strain, but not with products of gemmules of any other strain. The differences in strains are assumed to be genetic.

In **sexual reproduction** ova and sperm develop from archaeocytes or from choanocytes. The ova are fertilized in the mesohyl, and the embryos develop there and finally break out into the canals and spongocoel to be carried out the osculum. Embryogenesis follows a very unusual path, which is found in no other metazoan group. In the Calcispongiae and primitive Demospongiae a hollow blastula develops, with flagellated cells toward the interior. The blastula then turns *inside out* (**inversion**), the flagellated ends of the cells becoming directed to the outside! The larva is now called an **amphiblastula** (Figs. 9-6 and 9-11). Its flagellated cells (**micromeres**) are at one end, and the larger, nonflagellated cells (**macromeres**) are at the other. In contrast to other metazoan embryos, the micromeres invaginate into or are overgrown by the macromeres. The flagellated micromeres become the choanocytes of the new sponge (Fig. 9-11). The free-swimming larva of other sponges is a solid-bodied **parenchymula.** The outwardly directed, flagellated cells migrate to the interior after the larva settles and become the choanocytes in the flagellated chambers.

Some sponges are **monoecious** (have both male and female sex cells in one individual), and others are **dioecious** (have separate sexes).

Regeneration and somatic embryogenesis

Sponges have a tremendous ability to repair injuries and to restore lost parts, a process called **regeneration.** Regeneration does not imply a reorganization of the entire animal, but only of the wounded portion.

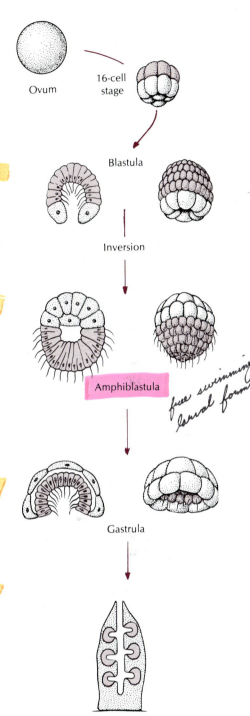

Ovum

16-cell stage

Blastula

Inversion

Amphiblastula   *free swimming larval form*

Gastrula

Figure 9-11

Development of the sponge *Scypha.*

On the other hand, if a sponge is cut into small fragments, or if the cells of a sponge are entirely dissociated and are allowed to fall into small groups, or aggregates, entire new sponges can develop from these fragments or aggregates of cells. This process has been termed **somatic embryogenesis.** Somatic embryogenesis involves a complete reorganization of the structure and functions of the participating cells or bits of tissue. Isolated from the influence of adjoining cells, they can realize their own potential to change in shape or function as they develop into a new organism.

A great deal of experimental work has been done in this field. The process of reorganization appears to differ in sponges of differing complexity. There is still some controversy concerning just what mechanisms lead to the adhesion of the cells and the share that each type of cell plays in the formative process.

___ Class Calcispongiae (Calcarea)

The Calcispongiae (called Calcarea in earlier classifications) are the calcareous sponges, so called because their spicules are composed of calcium carbonate. The spicules are straight (monaxons) or have three or four rays. These sponges tend to be small—10 cm or less in height—and tubular or vase shaped. They may be asconoid, syconoid, or leuconoid in structure. Though many are drab in color, some are bright yellow, red, green, or lavender. *Leucosolenia* and *Scypha* are marine shallow-water forms commonly studied in the laboratory. *Leucosolenia* is a small asconoid sponge that grows in branching colonies, usually arising from a network of horizontal, stolonlike tubes (Fig. 9-5). *Scypha* is a solitary sponge that may live singly or form clusters by budding (Fig. 9-5). The vase-shaped, typically syconoid animal is 1 to 3 cm long, with a fringe of straight spicules around the osculum that discourages small animals from entering.

___ Class Hyalospongiae (Hexactinellida)—Glass Sponges

The glass sponges make up the class Hyalospongiae (formerly Hexactinellida). They are nearly all deep-sea forms that are collected by dredging. Most of them are radially symmetrical, with vase- or funnel-shaped bodies that are usually attached by stalks of root spicules to a substratum (Fig. 9-10, *Euplectella*) (N.L. from Gr., *euplektos,* well plaited). They range from 7.5 cm to more than 1.3 m in length. Their distinguishing features are the skeleton of six-rayed siliceous spicules that are commonly bound together into a network forming a glasslike structure and the **trabecular net** of living tissue produced by the fusion of the pseudopodia of many types of amebocytes. Within the trabecular net are elongated, finger-shaped chambers lined with choanocytes and opening into the spongocoel. The osculum is unusually large and may be covered over by a sievelike plate of silica. There is no epidermis or gelatinous mesohyl, and both the external surface and the spongocoel are lined with the trabecular net. The skeleton is rigid, and muscular elements (myocytes) appear to be absent. The general arrangement of the chambers fits glass sponges into both syconoid and leuconoid types. Their structure is adapted to the slow, constant currents of sea bottoms, for the channels and pores of the sponge wall are relatively large and uncomplicated and permit an easy flow of water. Little, however, is known about their physiology.

The latticelike network of spicules found in many glass sponges is of exquisite beauty, such as that of *Euplectella,* or Venus's flower basket (Fig. 9-10), a classic example of the Hyalospongiae.

A   B   C

Figure 9-12

Marine Demospongiae. **A,** *Dasychalina cyathina* is a vaselike sponge that reaches 30 cm in height. The large opening at the top is not an osculum; rather, the oscula open into the interior cavity. **B,** *Tethya aurantia* is orange and shaped like a flattened sphere. **C,** *Callispongia plicifera* is another vasiform species. Dull purple, it may show a light blue fluorescence. This is a view of a colony from above, looking into the "vase."

A and **C,** Photographs by L.S. Roberts; **B,** photograph by D.W. Gotshall.

Class Demospongiae

Class Demospongiae contains more than 80% of the sponge species, including most of the larger sponges. The spicules are siliceous but are not six rayed, and they may be bound together by spongin or may be absent altogether. All members of the class are leuconoid, and all are marine except one family, the Spongillidae, or freshwater sponges.

Freshwater sponges are widely distributed in well-oxygenated ponds and streams, where they encrust plant stems and old pieces of submerged wood. They may resemble a bit of wrinkled scum, be pitted with pores, and be brownish or greenish in color. Common genera are *Spongilla* (L., *spongia,* from Gr., *spongos,* sponge) and *Myenia.* Freshwater sponges are most common in midsummer, although some are more easily found in the fall. They die and disintegrate in late autumn, leaving the gemmules (already described) to produce the next year's population. They also reproduce sexually. When examined closely, freshwater sponges reveal a thin dermis overlying large subdermal spaces (separated by columns of spicules) with many water channels in the interior. There are usually several oscula, each of which (at least in *Myenia*) is mounted on a small chimneylike tube. Their spiculation also includes a spongin network.

The marine Demospongiae are quite varied in both color and shape (Fig. 9-12). Some are encrusting; some are tall and fingerlike; some are low and spreading; some bore into shells; and some are shaped like fans, vases, cushions, or balls (Fig. 9-12). Loggerhead sponges may grow several meters in diameter.

The so-called bath sponges *(Spongia, Hippospongia)* belong to the group called horny sponges, which have spongin skeletons and lack spicules entirely.

Class Sclerospongiae

The Sclerospongiae are a small group of sponges that secrete a massive calcareous skeleton and are thus often called coralline sponges. Living tissue extends from 1 mm to 3 cm or more into the skeleton but only 1 mm above it. Their organization is leuconoid, as in the Demospongiae, and siliceous spicules and spongin are present in three of the four orders. Sclerosponges live in cryptic habitats (deeply shaded or completely dark locations) on coral reefs, such as crevices, caves, undersurfaces of overhangs, and deep water. They are believed to be relict representatives of ancient groups with a geological history extending from the Cambrian period. When modern corals and their symbiosis with algal cells (see p. 244) arose in the Mesozoic era, they were very successful and came to dominate the reefs. However, because the corals depend physiologically on the algal cells growing in their tissues, they must have adequate light. Thus, sclerosponges and certain other organisms were able to exploit the unoccupied cryptic habitats.

___ Phylogeny and Adaptive Radiation
Phylogeny

The sponges originated before the Cambrian period. Two groups of calcareous spongelike organisms occupied early Paleozoic reefs. The Devonian period saw the rapid development of many glass sponges. That sponges are related to protozoa is shown by their phagocytic method of nutrition and the resemblance of their flagellated larvae to colonial protozoa. The possibility that sponges arose from choanoflagellates (protozoa that bear collars and flagella) earned support for a time. However, many zoologists object to the hypothesis because sponges do not acquire collars until late in their embryological development. The outer cells of the larvae are flagellated but not collared, and they do not become collar cells until they become internal. Also, collar cells are found in certain corals and echinoderms, so they are not unique to the sponges.

Another hypothesis is that sponges derived from a hollow, free-swimming colonial flagellate, such as gave rise to the ancestral stocks of other metazoans. Certainly the sponge larvae resemble such flagellate colonies. The curious process of inversion occurs in the colonial phytoflagellate *Volvox*. The development of the water canals and the movement of the flagellated cells to the interior to become choanocytes may have occurred as the sponges began to assume a sessile existence. Whatever the origin, it is obvious that the sponges diverged early from the main line leading to other metazoans. Their phylogenetic remoteness from other metazoans is shown by their low level of organization, the independent nature of their cells, the absence of organs, and their body structure built around a system of water canals. They became a "dead-end" phylum.

Adaptive radiation

The Porifera have been a highly successful group that has branched out into several thousand species and a variety of marine and freshwater habitats. Their diversification centers largely on their unique water-current system and its various degrees of complexity. The proliferation of the flagellated chambers in the leuconoid sponges was more favorable to an increase in body size than that of the asconoid and syconoid sponges because facilities for feeding and gaseous exchange were greatly enlarged.

___ Summary

Members of the phylum Mesozoa are very simply organized animals that are parasitic in the kidneys of cephalopod molluscs (class Rhombozoa) and in several other invertebrate groups (class Orthonectida). They have only two cell layers, but these are not homologous to the germ layers of higher metazoans. They have a complicated life history that is still incompletely known. Whether their simple organization is primitive or derived from a more advanced group is unknown.

The phylum Placozoa has only one member, a small platelike marine organism. It too has only two cell layers, but some workers believe that these layers are homologous to ectoderm and endoderm of higher metazoans. The closest relatives of the placozoans seem to be the sponges.

The sponges (phylum Porifera) are an abundant marine group with some freshwater representatives. They have various specialized cells, but these are not organized into tissues or organs. They depend on the flagellar beat of their choanocytes to circulate water through their bodies for food gathering and respiratory gas exchange. They are supported by secreted skeletons of calcareous or siliceous spicules, spongin fibers, or a combination of spicules and spongin in most species. The canal systems through which water circulates in sponges can be described as asconoid, syconoid, and leuconoid, in order of increasing complexity. Sponges are efficient filter feeders on particles less than 50 μm in diameter, which are admitted by the ostia. Particles are phagocytized along the canals and prosopyles by pinacocytes and amebocytes, and the microvillar sieve of the choanocytes filters out particles down to 0.1 μm.

Sponges reproduce asexually by budding and gemmules (internal buds). Some sponges are monoecious and some dioecious. Embryogenesis is unusual and includes inversion, amphiblastula formation, and growth of the macromeres over the micromeres. Some sponges have a parenchymula larva. Sponges have great regenerative abilities.

Calcispongiae have calcareous spicules of monaxons or are three or four rayed. They are usually small and may be asconoid, syconoid, or leuconoid in structure.

Hyalospongiae are mostly deep-sea forms and have a skeleton of six-rayed siliceous spicules bound together in a trabecular net. The arrangement of their flagellated chambers shows both syconoid and leuconoid types.

Demospongiae are the largest and most abundant class of sponges. One family occurs in fresh water. Their spicules are siliceous (but not six rayed) but may be absent in some species. A protein called spongin may be present. All species are leuconoid, and some may reach great size (up to several meters). They show great diversity in size, color, form, and habitat.

Sclerospongiae are a small group of sponges with a massive, basal calcareous skeleton, of which they inhabit the outer few millimeters or centimeters. Siliceous spicules and spongin may be present. They occupy cryptic habitats on coral reefs.

Sponges are an ancient group, remote phylogenetically from other metazoans. They have been successful, and their adaptive radiation is centered on elaboration of the water circulation and filter feeding system.

Selected references

Barnes, R.D. 1980. Invertebrate zoology, ed. 4. Philadelphia, Saunders College/Holt, Rinehart & Winston.

Berguist, P.R. 1978. Sponges. Berkeley, University of California Press. *Excellent monograph on sponge structure, classification, evolution, and general biology.*

Brown, C.H. 1975. Structural materials in animals. New York, John Wiley & Sons, Inc.

Florkin, M., and B.T. Scheer. 1968. Chemical zoology, vol. 2. New York, Academic Press, Inc. *Section I contains six papers on Porifera.*

Fry, W.G. 1970. Biology of the Porifera. New York, Academic Press, Inc. *A collection of papers presented at a symposium of the Zoological Society of London.*

Giese, A.C., and S.S. Pearse (eds.). 1974. Reproduction of marine invertebrates, vol. 1. New York, Academic Press. Inc.

Gilbert, J.J., and T.L. Simpson. 1976. Gemmule polymorphism in the freshwater sponge *Spongilla lacustris*. Arch. Hydrobiol. 78(2):268-277. *Describes two types of gemmules and discusses their adaptive significance.*

Gosner, K.L. 1971. Guide to identification of marine and estuarine invertebrates: Cape Hatteras to the Bay of Fundy. New York, John Wiley & Sons, Inc., pp. 51-65.

Grell, K.G. 1971. *Trichoplax adhaerens* F.E. Schulze und die Entstehung der Metazoen. Naturwiss. Rundschau 24:160-161.

Grell, K.G. 1982. Placozoa. In S.P. Parker (ed.). Synopsis and classification of living organisms, vol. 1. New York, McGraw-Hill Book Co.

Hartman, W.D. 1982. Porifera. In S.P. Parker (ed.). Synopsis and classification of living organisms, vol. 1. New York, McGraw-Hill Book Co.

Hyman, L.H. 1940. The invertebrates: Protozoa through Ctenophora, vol. 1. New York, McGraw-Hill Book Co. *Contains chapters on Mesozoa and Porifera.*

Jackson, J.B.C., T.F. Goreau, and W.D. Hartman. 1971. Recent brachiopod-coralline sponge communities and their paleoecological significance. Science 173:623-625.

Kaestner, A. 1967. Invertebrate zoology, vol. 1. New York, John Wiley & Sons, Inc.

Light, S.R., R.I. Smith, F.A. Pitelka, D.P. Abbott, and F.M. Weesner. 1967. Intertidal invertebrates of the central California coast. Berkeley, University of California Press. *Contains keys to common West Coast sponges.*

Long, M.E., and D. Doubelet. 1977. Consider the sponge. Nat. Geogr. 151(3):392-407. *Beautiful color photographs of sponges.*

McConnaughey, B.H. 1963. The Mesozoa. In E.C. Dougherty (ed.). The lower Metazoa: comparative biology and phylogeny. Berkeley, University of California Press. *The author stresses the resemblance between the Mesozoa and the parasitic flatworms.*

McConnaughey, B.H. 1968. The Mesozoa. In M. Florkin and B.T. Scheer (eds.). Chemical zoology, vol. 2. New York, Academic Press, Inc.

Pennak, R.W. 1978. Fresh-water invertebrates of the United States, ed. 2. New York, John Wiley & Sons, Inc. *A reference work with considerable attention devoted to Porifera.*

Rasmont, R. 1970. Some new aspects of the physiology of freshwater sponges. In W.G. Fry (ed.). Biology of the Porifera. New York, Academic Press, Inc. *He believes that the gemmules of some species, or at least of some strains of sponges, undergo a true diapause, similar to that of insects.*

Schmidt, G.D., and L.S. Roberts. 1981. Foundations of parasitology, ed. 2. St. Louis, The C.V. Mosby Co. *Has a chapter on the Mesozoa.*

Stunkard, H.W. 1972. Clarification of taxonomy in Mesozoa. Syst. Zool. 21:210-214. *Contains a good review of the literature.*

Stunkard, H.W. 1982. Mesozoa. In S.P. Parker (ed.). Synopsis and classification of living organisms, vol. 1. New York, McGraw-Hill Book Co.

van Beneden, E. 1876. Recerches sur les dicyémides. Bruxelles Acad. Roy. Belg. Bull. Cl. Sci. 41:1160-1205, 42:35-97. *One of the first investigations on the group that was discovered in 1839. He considered them intermediate between the Protozoa and the Metazoa.*

Selected *Scientific American* articles

Lapan, E.A., and H.J. Morowitz. 1972. The Mesozoa. 227:94-101 (Dec.). *The author presents evidence that the Dicyemida (the Orthonectida may represent a different group because of their complexity) are not simplified flatworms but are at the simplest known level of multicellular organization and may help in understanding the processes of cell differentiation.*

Newell, N.D. 1972. The evolution of reefs. 226(6):54-65.

CHAPTER 10

THE RADIATE ANIMALS

Phylum Cnidaria
Phylum Ctenophora

Coral expanse on the Great Barrier Reef of Australia, showing numerous species of reef-building (hermatypic) corals.

Photograph by K. Sandved.

Position in Animal Kingdom

The two phyla Cnidaria and Ctenophora make up the radiate animals, which are characterized by **primary radial** or **biradial symmetry** and which represent the most primitive of the eumetazoans. Radial symmetry, in which the body parts are arranged concentrically around the oral-aboral axis, is particularly suitable for **sessile** or sedentary animals. Biradial symmetry is basically a type of radial symmetry in which only two planes through the oral-aboral axis divide the animal into mirror images because of the presence of some part that is single or paired. All other eumetazoans have a primary bilateral symmetry; that is, they are bilateral or were derived from an ancestor that was bilateral.

Neither phylum has advanced generally beyond the **tissue level of organization,** although a few organs occur. In general, the ctenophores have a more complex structure than that of the cnidarians.

Biological Contributions

1. Both phyla have developed two well-defined **germ layers,** ectoderm and endoderm; a third, or mesodermal, layer, which is derived embryologically from the ectoderm, is present in some. The body plan is saclike, and the body wall is composed of two distinct layers, epidermis and gastrodermis, derived from the ectoderm and endoderm, respectively. The gelatinous matrix, mesoglea, between these layers may be structureless, may contain a few cells and fibers, or may be composed largely of mesodermal connective tissue and muscle fibers.

2. An internal body cavity, the **gastrovascular cavity,** is lined by the gastrodermis and has a single opening, the mouth, which also serves as the anus.

3. **Extracellular digestion** occurs in the gastrovascular cavity, and intracellular digestion takes place in the gastrodermal cells.

4. Most radiates have **tentacles,** or extensible projections around the oral end, that aid in food capture.

5. The first true **nerve cells** (protoneurons) occur in the radiates, but the nerves are arranged as a nerve net, with no central nervous system.

6. **Sense organs** appear first in the radiates and include well-developed statocysts (organs of equilibrium) and ocelli (photosensitive organs).

7. Locomotion in the free-moving forms is achieved by either **muscular contractions** (cnidarians) or **ciliary comb plates** (ctenophores). However, both groups are still better adapted to floating or being carried by currents than to strong swimming.

8. **Polymorphism** in the cnidarians has widened their ecological possibilities. In many species the presence of both a polyp (sessile and attached) stage and a medusa (free-swimming) stage permits occupation of a benthic (bottom) and a pelagic (open-water) habitat by the same species.

9. Some unique features are found in these phyla, such as **nematocysts** (stinging organoids) in cnidarians and **colloblasts** (adhesive organoids) and **ciliary comb plates** in ctenophores.

▬PHYLUM CNIDARIA

The phylum Cnidaria (ny-dar′e-a) (Gr., *knide,* nettle, + L., *aria* [pl. suffix], like or connected with) is an interesting group of more than 9000 species. It takes its name from the cells called **cnidocytes,** which contain the stinging organoids (**nematocysts**) characteristic of the phylum. Nematocysts are *formed and used* only by cnidarians and by one species of ctenophore. Another name for the phylum, Coelenterata (se-len′te-ra′ta) (Gr., *koilos,* hollow, + *enteron,* gut, + L., *ata* [pl. suffix], characterized by), is used less frequently than formerly, and it sometimes is now employed to refer to both radiate phyla, since its meaning is equally applicable to both.

The cnidarians are generally regarded as being close to the basic stock of the metazoan line. Although their organization has a structural and functional simplicity not found in other Metazoa, they are a rather successful phylum, forming a significant proportion of the biomass in some locations. They are widespread in marine habitats, and there are a few in fresh water. Although they are sessile or, at best, fairly slow moving or slow swimming, they are quite efficient predators of organisms that are much swifter and more complex. The phylum includes some of nature's strangest and loveliest creatures: the branching, plantlike hydroids; the flowerlike sea anemones; the jellyfishes; and those architects of the ocean floor, the horny corals (sea whips, sea fans, and others), and all the hard corals whose thousands of years of calcareous house-building have produced great reefs and coral islands (p. 219).

Cnidarians are found most abundantly in shallow marine habitats, especially in warm temperate and tropical regions. There are no terrestrial species. Colonial hydroids are usually found attached to mollusc shells, rocks, wharves, and other animals in shallow coastal water, but some species are found at great depths. Floating and free-swimming medusae are found in open seas and lakes, often far from the shore. Floating colonies such as the Portuguese man-of-war and *Velella* (L., *velum,* veil, + *ellus,* dim. suffix) have floats or sails by which the wind carries them.

Some molluscs and flatworms eat hydroids bearing nematocysts and use these stinging cells for their own defense. Some other animals feed on cnidarians, but cnidarians rarely serve as food for humans.

Cnidarians sometimes live symbiotically with other animals, often as commensals on the shell or other surface of their host. Algae frequently live as mutuals in the tissues of cnidarians, notably in some freshwater hydras and in reef-building corals. The presence of the algae in reef-building corals limits the occurrence of coral reefs to relatively shallow, clear water where there is sufficient light for the photosynthetic requirements of the algae. These kinds of corals are an essential component of coral reefs, and reefs are extremely important habitats in tropical waters. Coral reefs are discussed further later in the chapter.

Although many cnidarians have little economic importance, reef-building corals are an important exception. Fish and other animals associated with reefs provide substantial amounts of food for humans, and reefs are of economic value as tourist attractions. Precious coral is used for jewelry and ornaments, and coral rock serves for building purposes.

Planktonic medusae may be of some importance as food for fish that are of commercial value; the reverse is also true—the young of the fish fall prey to cnidarians.

CHARACTERISTICS

1. Entirely aquatic, some in fresh water but mostly marine
2. **Radial symmetry** or biradial symmetry around a longitudinal axis with **oral and aboral** ends; no definite head
3. Two basic types of individuals: **polyps** and **medusae**
4. Exoskeleton or endoskeleton of chitinous, calcareous, or protein components in some
5. Body with two layers, epidermis and gastrodermis, with mesoglea (**diploblastic**); mesoglea with cells and connective tissue (ectomesoderm) in some (**triploblastic**)
6. **Gastrovascular cavity** (often branched or divided with septa) with a single opening that serves as both mouth and anus; extensible tenacles usually encircling the mouth or oral region
7. Special stinging cell organoids called **nematocysts** in either epidermis or gastrodermis or in both; nematocysts abundant on tentacles, where they may form batteries or rings

Polyp type

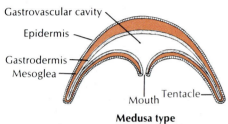

Medusa type

Figure 10-1

Comparison between the polyp and medusa types of individuals.

8. **Nerve net** with symmetrical and asymmetrical synapses; with some sensory organs; diffuse conduction
9. Muscular system (epitheliomuscular type) of an outer layer of longitudinal fibers at base of epidermis and an inner one of circular fibers at base of gastrodermis; modifications of this plan in higher cnidarians, such as separate bundles of independent fibers in the mesoglea
10. Asexual reproduction by budding (in polyps) or sexual reproduction by gametes (in all medusae and some polyps); sexual forms monoecious or dioecious; **planula larva**; holoblastic indeterminate cleavage
11. No excretory or respiratory system
12. No coelomic cavity

CLASSIFICATION

Class Hydrozoa (hy-dro-zo'a) (Gr., *hydra*, water serpent, + *zōon*, animal). Solitary or colonial; asexual polyps and sexual medusae, although one type may be suppressed; hydranths with no mesenteries; medusae (when present) with a velum; both freshwater and marine. Examples: *Hydra, Obelia, Physalia, Tubularia*.

Class Scyphozoa (sy-fo-zo'a) (Gr., *skyphos*, cup, + *zōon*, animal). Solitary; polyp stage reduced or absent; bell-shaped medusae without velum; gelatinous mesoglea much enlarged; margin of bell or umbrella typically with eight notches that are provided with sense organs; all marine. Examples: *Aurelia, Cassiopeia, Rhizostoma*.

Class Cubozoa (ku'bo-zo'a) (Gr., *kybos*, a cube, + *zōon*, animal). Solitary; polyp stage reduced; bell-shaped medusae square in cross section, with tentacle or group of tentacles hanging from a bladelike pedalium at each corner of the umbrella; margin of umbrella entire, without velum but with velarium; all marine. Examples: *Tripedalia, Carybdea, Chironex, Chiropsalmus*.

Class Anthozoa (an-tho-zo'a) (Gr., *anthos*, flower, + *zōon*, animal). All polyps; no medusae; solitary or colonial; enteron subdivided by at least eight mesenteries or septa bearing nematocysts; gonads endodermal; all marine.

  Subclass Zoantharia (zo'an-tha'ri-a) (N.L., from Gr., *zōon*, animal, + *anthos*, flower, + L., *aria*, like or connected with). With simple unbranched tentacles; mesenteries in pairs; sea anemones, hard corals, and others. Examples: *Metridium, Anthopleura, Tealia, Astrangia, Acropora*.

  Subclass Ceriantipatharia (se-ri-ant'i-pa-tha'ri-a) (N.L., combination of Ceriantharia and Antipatharia). With simple unbranched tentacles; mesenteries unpaired; tube anemones and black or thorny corals. Examples: *Cerianthus, Antipathes, Stichopathes*.

  Subclass Alcyonaria (al'cy-o-na'ri-a) (Gr., *alkonion*, kind of sponge resembling nest of kingfisher [*alkyōn*, kingfisher], + L., *aria*, like or connected with). With eight pinnate tentacles; eight complete, unpaired mesenteries; soft and horny corals. Examples: *Tubipora, Alcyonium, Gorgonia, Plexaura, Renilla*.

──── Form and Function
Polymorphism in cnidarians

One of the most interesting—and sometimes puzzling—aspects of this phylum is the dimorphism and often polymorphism displayed by many of its members. In general, all cnidarian forms fit into one of two morphological types: the **polyp**, or hydroid form, which is adapted to a sedentary or sessile life, and the **medusa**, or jellyfish form, which is adapted for a floating or free-swimming existence (Fig. 10-1).

Most polyps have tubular bodies with a mouth at one end surrounded by tentacles. The aboral end is usually attached to a substratum by a pedal disc or other device. Polyps may live singly or in colonies. Colonies of some species include more than one kind of individual, each specialized for a certain function, such as feeding, reproduction, or defense (Fig. 10-2).

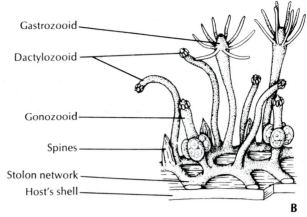

Gastrozooid

Dactylozooid

Gonozooid

Spines

Stolon network

Host's shell

B

A

Figure 10-2

A, A hermit crab with its cnidarian commensals. The shell is blanketed with polyps of the hydrozoan *Hydractinia milleri.* **B,** Portion of a colony of *Hydractinia*, showing the types of zooids and the stolon (hydrorhiza) from which they grow. The crab is camouflaged by the cnidarians, and the cnidarians get a free ride and bits of food from their host's meals. **A,** Photograph by R. Harbo.

Medusae are free swimming and have bell-shaped or umbrella-shaped bodies and tetramerous symmetry (body parts arranged in fours). The mouth is usually centered on the concave side, and tentacles extend from the rim of the umbrella.

The sea anemones and corals (class Anthozoa) are all polyps, and the true jellyfishes (class Scyphozoa) are all medusae but may have a polypoid larval stage. The colonial hydroids of class Hydrozoa, however, sometimes have life histories that featured both the polyp, or hydroid, stage and the free-swimming medusa stage—rather like a Jeckyll-and-Hyde existence. A species that has both the attached polyp and the floating medusa within its life history can take advantage of the feeding and distribution possibilities of both the pelagic (open-water) and the benthic (bottom) types of environment.

Superficially the polyp and medusa seem very different. But actually each has retained the saclike body plan that is basic to the phylum (Fig. 10-1). The medusa is essentially an unattached polyp with the tubular portion widened and flattened into the bell shape.

Both the polyp and the medusa possess the three body wall layers typical of the cnidarians, but the jellylike layer of mesoglea is much thicker in the medusa, constituting the bulk of the animal and making it more buoyant. It is because of this mass of mesogleal "jelly" that the medusae are commonly called jellyfishes.

Nematocysts—the stinging organoids

One of the most characteristic structures in the entire cnidarian group is the stinging organoid called the **nematocyst** (Fig. 10-3). Over 20 different types of nematocysts have been described in the cnidarians so far; they are important in taxonomic determinations. The nematocyst is a tiny capsule composed of material similar to chitin and containing a coiled tubular "thread" or filament, which is a continuation of the narrowed end of the capsule. This end of the capsule is covered by a little lid, or **operculum.** The inside of the undischarged thread may bear tiny barbs, or spines.

The nematocyst is enclosed in the cell that has secreted it, the **cnidocyte** (during its development, the cnidocyte is properly called the **cnidoblast**). Most

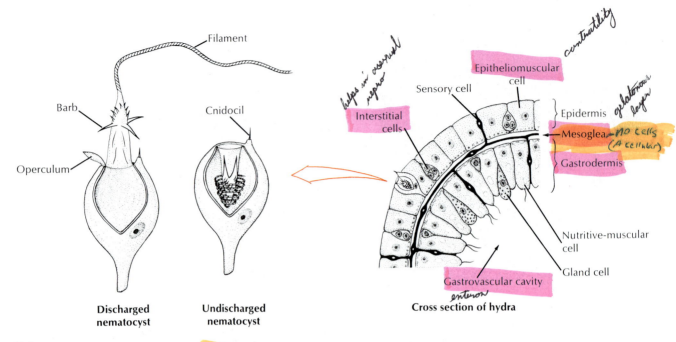

Discharged
nematocyst

Undischarged
nematocyst

Cross section of hydra

Handwritten annotations on figure: helps in asexual repro · Interstitial cells · Sensory cell · contractility · Epitheliomuscular cell · Epidermis · gelatinous layer · Mesoglea — no cells (Acellular) · Gastrodermis · Nutritive-muscular cell · Gland cell · Gastrovascular cavity · enteron

Labels on left figures: Filament · Barb · Cnidocil · Operculum

Figure 10-3

At left, structure of a stinging cell. At right, portion of the body wall of a hydra. Cnidocytes, which contain the nematocysts, arise in the epidermis from interstitial cells.

Note again the distinction between osmotic and hydrostatic pressure (p. 86). The nematocyst is never required actually to contain 140 atmospheres of hydrostatic pressure within itself; such a hydrostatic pressure would doubtless cause it to explode. As the water rushes in during discharge, the osmotic pressure falls rapidly, while the hydrostatic pressure rapidly increases.

   Not all nematocysts have barbs or inject poison. Some, for example, do not penetrate the prey but rapidly recoil like a spring after discharge, grasping and holding any part of the prey caught in the coil.

cnidocytes are provided with a triggerlike **cnidocil,** which is a modified flagellum with a kinetosome at its base. Contact of the cnidocil with an object such as prey provides tactile stimulation for the nematocyst to discharge. Cnidocytes with their nematocysts are borne in invaginations of ectodermal cells and, in some forms, in gastrodermal cells, and they are especially abundant on the tentacles. When a nematocyst is discharged, its cnidocyte is absorbed and a new one replaces it. Nematocysts used in defense and food capture require chemical stimulation (presence of organic compounds from other animals) to discharge, as well as tactile stimulation. Adhesive nematocysts usually do not discharge in food capture.

   The mechanism of nematocyst discharge is remarkable. Inside the capsule the osmotic pressure is 140 atmospheres. When stimulated to discharge, the nematocyst membrane becomes permeable to water, and the high internal osmotic pressure causes water to rush into the capsule. The operculum opens, the increase in *hydrostatic pressure* within the capsule pushes the thread out with great force, and the thread turns inside out as it goes. At the everting end of the thread, the barbs flick to the outside like tiny switchblades. This minute but awesome weapon then injects poison when it penetrates the prey.

   The nematocysts of most cnidarians are not harmful to humans, but the stings of the Portuguese man-of-war (Fig. 10-15) and certain jellyfish are quite painful and in some cases may be dangerous.

Nerve net

The nerve net of the cnidarians is one of the best examples of a diffuse nervous system in the animal kingdom. This plexus of nerve cells is found both at the base of the epidermis and at the base of the gastrodermis, forming two interconnected nerve nets. Nerve processes (axons) end on other nerve cells at synapses or at junctions with sensory cells or effector organs (nematocysts or epitheliomuscular cells). Nerve impulses are transmitted from one cell to another by release of a neurotransmitter from small vesicles on one side of the synapse or junction (p. 765). One-way transmission between nerve cells in higher animals is ensured because the vesicles are located on only one side of the synapse. However, cnidarian nerve nets are peculiar in that many of the synapses have vesicles of neu-

Nerve cell

Neuromuscular junction

Interneuronal synapse

Epitheliomuscular cell

Nerve cell

Figure 10-4

Transmission electron micrograph of neuronal synapse and neuromuscular junction in the scyphistoma of the jellyfish *Aurelia*. Contrast the symmetrical two-way interneuronal synapse (vesicles on both sides) to the asymmetrical junction of the nerve with the epitheliomuscular cell. (×67,300.)

From Westfall, J.A. 1973. Am. Zool. 13:237.

rotransmitters on both sides, allowing transmission across the synapse in either direction (Fig. 10-4). Another peculiarity of cnidarian nerves is the absence of any sheathing material (myelin) on the axons.

There is no concentrated grouping of nerve cells to suggest a "central nervous system." Nerves are grouped, however, in the "ring nerves" of hydrozoan medusae and in the marginal sense organs of scyphozoan medusae. In some cnidarians the nerve nets form two or more systems: in Scyphozoa there is a fast conducting system to coordinate swimming movements and a slower one to coordinate movements of tentacles.

The nerve cells of the net have synapses with slender sensory cells that receive external stimuli, and the nerve cells have junctions with epitheliomuscular cells and nematocysts. Together with the contractile fibers of the epitheliomuscular cells, the sensory-nerve cell net combination is often referred to as a **neuromuscular system,** an important landmark in the evolution of the nervous system. The nerve net is never completely lost from higher forms. Annelids have it in their digestive systems. In the human digestive system it is represented by nerve plexuses in the musculature. The rhythmical peristaltic movements of the stomach and intestine are coordinated by this counterpart of the cnidarian nerve net.

Class Hydrozoa

The majority of hydrozoans are marine and colonial in form, and the typical life cycle includes both the asexual polyp and the sexual medusa stages. Some, however, such as the freshwater hydra, have no medusa stage. Some marine hydroids do not have free medusae (Fig. 10-5), whereas some hydrozoans occur only as medusae and have no polyp.

The hydra, although not a typical hydrozoan, has become a favorite as an introduction to Cnidaria because of its size and ready availability. Combining its study with that of a representative colonial marine hydroid such as *Obelia* (Gr., *obelias,* round cake) gives an excellent idea of the class Hydrozoa.

Figure 10-5

A colony of *Tubularia crocea*. Medusa buds do not detach from *Tubularia* polyps, but instead shed their gametes in place.

Photograph by R. Harbo.

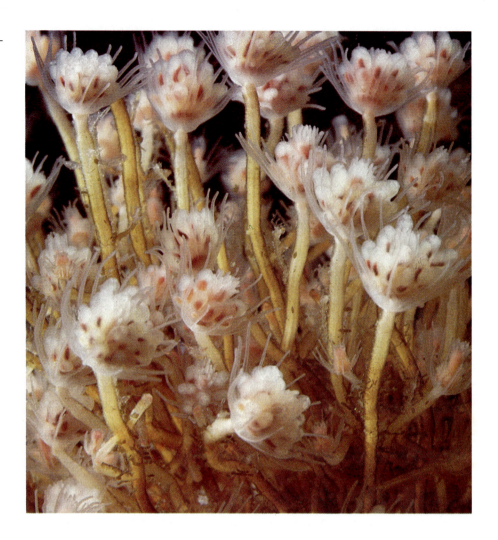

Hydra—a freshwater hydrozoan

The common freshwater hydra (Fig. 10-6) is a solitary polyp and one of the few cnidarians found in fresh water. Its normal habitat is the underside of aquatic leaves and lily pads in cool, clean fresh water of pools and streams. The hydra family is found throughout the world, with 10 species occurring in the United States.

Body plan

The body of the hydra can extend to a length of 25 to 30 mm or can contract to a tiny, jellylike mass. It is a cylindrical tube with the lower (aboral) end drawn out into a slender stalk, ending in a basal or **pedal disc** for attachment. This pedal disc is provided with gland cells to enable the hydra to adhere to a substratum and also to secrete a gas bubble for floating. In the center of the disc there may be an excretory pore. The **mouth,** located on a conical elevation called the **hypostome,** is encircled by six to 10 hollow tentacles that, like the body, can be greatly extended when the animal is hungry.

The mouth opens into the **gastrovascular cavity,** which communicates with the cavities in the tentacles. In some individuals **buds** may project from the sides, each with a mouth and tentacles like the parent. Testes or ovaries, when present, appear as rounded projections on the surface of the body (Fig. 10-6).

Body wall

The body wall surrounding the gastrovascular cavity consists of an outer **epidermis** (ectodermal) and an inner **gastrodermis** (endodermal) with **mesoglea** between them (Fig. 10-3).

Epidermis

The epidermis is made up of small cubical cells and is covered with a delicate cuticle. This layer contains several types of cells: epitheliomuscular, interstitial, gland, cnidocyte, and sensory and nerve cells.

Epitheliomuscular cells make up most of the epidermis and serve both for covering and for muscular contraction. The bases of most of these cells are extended parallel to the tentacle or body axis and contain myofibrils (myonemes), thus forming a layer of longitudinal muscle next to the mesoglea. Contraction of these fibrils shortens the body or tentacles.

Interstitial cells are the undifferentiated stem cells found among the bases of the epitheliomuscular cells. Differentiation of the interstitial cells gives rise to cnidoblasts, sex cells, buds, nerve cells, and others, but generally not to epitheliomuscular cells (which reproduce themselves).

Gland cells are tall cells around the pedal disc and mouth that secrete an adhesive substance for attachment and sometimes a gas bubble for floating.

Cnidocytes containing nematocysts are found throughout the epidermis. Three functional types of nematocysts are found in the hydra: those that penetrate the prey and inject poison (penetrants, Fig. 10-3); those that recoil and entangle the prey (volvents); and those that secrete an adhesive substance used in locomotion and attachment (glutinants).

Sensory cells are scattered among the other epidermal cells, especially around the mouth and the tentacles and on the pedal disc. The free end of each sensory cell bears a flagellum, which is the sensory receptor for chemical and tactile stimuli. The other end branches into fine processes, which synapse with the nerve cells.

Nerve cells of the epidermis are generally multipolar (have many processes), although in more highly organized cnidarians the cells may be bipolar (with two processes). Their processes (axons) form synapses with sensory cells and other nerve cells and junctions with epitheliomuscular cells and cnidocytes. There are both one-way (morphologically asymmetrical) and two-way synapses with other nerve cells (Fig. 10-4).

Gastrodermis

The gastrodermis, a layer of cells lining the gastrovascular cavity, is made up chiefly of large, flagellated, columnar epithelial cells with irregular flat bases. The cells of the gastrodermis include nutritive-muscular, interstitial, and gland cells.

Nutritive-muscular cells are usually tall columnar cells and have laterally extended bases containing myonemes. The myofibrils run at right angles to the body or tentacle axis and so form a circular muscle layer. However, this muscle layer in hydras is very weak, and longitudinal extension of the body and tentacles is brought about mostly by increasing the volume of water in the gastrovascular cavity. The water is brought in through the mouth by the beating of the flagella on the nutritive-muscular cells. Thus, the water in the gastrovascular cavity serves as a **hydrostatic skeleton.** The two flagella on the free end of each cell also serve to circulate food and fluids in the digestive cavity. The cells often contain large

Figure 10-6

Hydra with developing bud and ovary.
Courtesy Carolina Biological Supply Co., Burlington, N.C.

Over 230 years ago, Abraham Trembley was astonished to discover that isolated sections of the stalk of hydra could regenerate and each become a complete animal. Since then, over 2000 investigations of hydra have been published, and the organism has become a classic model for the study of morphological differentiation. The mechanisms governing morphogenesis have great practical importance, and the simplicity of hydra lends itself to these investigations. Substances controlling development (morphogens), such as those determining which end of a cut stalk will develop a mouth and tentacles, have been discovered, and they may be present in the cells in extremely low concentrations (10^{-10} M).

Figure 10-7

A, Hungry hydra catches an unwary water flea with the nematocysts of its tentacles and, B, swallows it whole. C, Hydra is full, but not too full to capture a protozoan for dessert.

Photographs by F.M. Hickman.

numbers of food vacuoles. Gastrodermal cells in the green hydra (*Chlorohydra* [Gr., *chloros,* green, + *hydra,* a mythical nine-headed monster slain by Hercules]) bear green algae (zoochlorella), which give the hydras their color. This is probably a case of symbiotic mutualism, since the algae use the respiratory carbon dioxide from the hydra to form organic compounds useful to the host and secrete oxygen as a by-product of their photosynthesis. They receive shelter and probably other physiological requirements in return.

Interstitial cells are scattered among the bases of the nutritive cells. They may transform into other types of cells when the need arises.

Gland cells in the hypostome and in the column secrete digestive enzymes. Mucous glands about the mouth aid in ingestion.

Cnidocytes are not found in the gastrodermis because nematocysts are lacking in this layer.

Mesoglea

The mesoglea lies between the epidermis and gastrodermis and is attached to both layers. It is gelatinous, or jellylike, and has no fibers or cellular elements. It is a continuous layer that extends over both body and tentacles, thickest in the stalk portion and thinnest in the tentacles. This arrangement allows the pedal region to withstand great mechanical strain and gives the tentacles more flexibility. The mesoglea helps to support the body and acts as a type of elastic skeleton.

Locomotion

Unlike colonial polyps, which are permanently attached, the hydra can move about freely by gliding on its basal disc, aided by mucus secretions. Or using a "measuring worm" movement, it can loop along by bending over and attaching its tentacles to the substratum. It may even turn end over end or detach itself and, by forming a gas bubble on its basal disc, float to the surface.

Feeding and digestion

Hydras feed on a variety of small crustacea, insect larvae, and annelid worms. The hydra awaits its prey with tentacles extended (Fig. 10-7). The food organism that brushes against its tentacles may find itself harpooned by scores of nematocysts that render it helpless, even though it may be larger than the hydra. The tentacles move toward the mouth, which slowly widens. Well moistened with mucus secretions, the mouth glides over and around the prey, totally engulfing it.

The activator that actually causes the mouth to open is the reduced form of glutathione, which is found to some extent in all living cells. Glutathione is released from the prey through the wounds made by the nematocysts, but only animals releasing enough of the chemical to activate the feeding response are eaten by the hydra. This explains how a hydra distinguishes between *Daphnia,* which it relishes, and some other forms that it refuses. When glutathione is placed in water containing hydras, each hydra will go through the motions of feeding even though no prey is present.

Inside the gastrovascular cavity, gland cells discharge enzymes on the food. The digestion is started in the gastrovascular cavity (extracellular digestion), but many of the food particles are drawn by pseudopodia into the nutritive-muscular cells of the gastrodermis, where intracellular digestion occurs. Ameboid cells may carry undigested particles to the gastrovascular cavity, where they are eventually expelled with other indigestible matter.

Asexual

Sexual

Polyp
Stage

Figure 10-8

Life cycle of *Obelia*, showing alternation of polyp (asexual) and medusa (sexual) stages. *Obelia* is a calyptoblastic hydroid; that is, its polyps as well as its stems are protected by continuations of the perisarc. Contrast with *Eudendrium* (Fig. 10-9).

Reproduction

The hydra reproduces sexually and asexually. In asexual reproduction, buds appear as outpocketings of the body wall and develop into young hydras that eventually detach from the parent. Most species are dioecious. Temporary gonads (Fig. 10-6) usually appear in the autumn, stimulated by the lower temperatures and perhaps also by the reduced aeration of stagnant waters. Eggs in the ovary usually mature one at a time and are fertilized by sperm shed into the water.

The zygotes undergo holoblastic cleavage to form a hollow blastula. The inner part of the blastula delaminates to form the endoderm (gastrodermis), and the mesoglea is laid down between the ectoderm and endoderm. A cyst forms around the embryo before it breaks loose from the parent, enabling it to survive the winter. Young hydras hatch out in spring when the weather is favorable.

Hydroid colonies

Far more representative of class Hydrozoa than the hydras are hydroids that have a medusa stage in their life cycle. *Obelia* is often used in laboratory exercises for beginning students to illustrate the hydroid type (Fig. 10-8).

A typical hydroid has a base, a stalk, and one or more terminal zooids. The base by which the colonial hydroids are attached to the substratum is a rootlike stolon, or **hydrorhiza**, which gives rise to one or more stalks called **hydrocauli**. The living cellular part of the hydrocaulus is the tubular **coenosarc**, composed of the three typical cnidarian layers surrounding the coelenteron (gastrovascular cavity). The protective covering of the hydrocaulus is a nonliving chitinous sheath, or

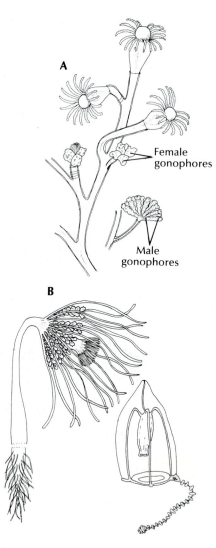

A

Female
gonophores

Male
gonophores

B

Figure 10-9

Gymnoblastean hydroids. **A,** *Eudendrium*
forms a bushy colony with naked hydranths and gonophores. There are no
free medusae. **B,** *Corymorpha* is a solitary hydroid. Its gonophores produce
free-swimming medusae, each with a single trailing tentacle.

perisarc. Attached to the hydrocaulus are the individual polyp animals, or zooids.
Most of the zooids are feeding polyps called **hydranths,** or **gastrozooids.** They may
be tubular, bottle shaped, or vaselike, but all have a terminal mouth and a circlet
of tentacles. In some forms, such as *Obelia,* the perisarc continues as a protective
cup around the polyp into which it can withdraw for protection (Fig. 10-8). In
others the polyp is naked (Fig. 10-9). In some forms the perisarc is an inconspicuous, thin film.

The hydranths, much like miniature hydras, capture and ingest prey, such as
tiny crustaceans, worms, and larvae, thus providing nutrition for the entire colony. After partial digestion in the hydranth, the digestive broth passes into the
common coelenteron where intracellular digestion occurs.

Circulation within the coelenteron is a function of the flagellated gastrodermis but is also aided by rhythmical contractions and pulsations of the body, which
occur in many hydroids.

Just as hydras reproduce asexually by budding, the colonial hydroids bud off
new individuals, thus increasing the size of the colony. New feeding polyps arise
by budding, and medusoid buds also arise on the colony. In *Obelia* these medusae
are budded from a reproductive polyp called a **gonangium.** The young medusae
leave the colony as free-swimming individuals that mature and produce gametes
(eggs and sperm) (Fig. 10-8). In some species the medusae remain attached to the
colony and shed their gametes there. In other species the medusae never develop
and the gametes are shed by male and female gonophores (Fig. 10-9). Embryonation of the zygote results in a ciliated planula larva that swims about for a time.
Then it settles down to a substratum to develop into a minute polyp that gives rise,
by asexual budding, to the hydroid colony, thus completing the life cycle.

Hydroid medusae are usually smaller than scyphozoan medusae, ranging
from 2 or 3 mm to several centimeters in diameter (Figs. 10-10 and 10-11). The
margin of the bell projects inward as a shelflike **velum,** which partly closes the
open side of the bell and is used in swimming (Fig. 10-12). Muscular pulsations
that alternately fill and empty the bell propel the animal forward, aboral side first,
with a sort of "jet propulsion." The tentacles attached to the bell margin are richly
supplied with nematocysts.

The mouth opening at the end of a suspended **manubrium** leads to a stomach
and four radial canals that connect with a ring canal around the margin. This in
turn connects with the hollow tentacles. Thus, the coelenteron is continuous from
mouth to tentacles, and the entire system is lined with gastrodermis. Nutrition is
similar to that of the hydranths.

The nerve net is usually concentrated into two nerve rings at the base of the
velum. The bell margin is liberally supplied with sensory cells. It usually also bears
two kinds of specialized sense organs: **statocysts,** which are small organs of equilibrium (Fig. 10-12, *B*), and **ocelli,** which are light-sensitive organs.

Freshwater medusae

The freshwater medusa *Craspedacusta sowerbyi* (Fig. 10-13) (order Hydroida)
may have evolved from marine ancestors in the Yangtze River of China. Probably
introduced with shipments of aquatic plants, this interesting form has now been
found in many parts of Europe, all over the United States, and in parts of Canada.
The medusa may attain a diameter of 20 mm.

The polyp phase of this animal is tiny (2 mm) and appears to be more or less
degenerate, for it has no perisarc and no tentacles. It occurs in colonies of a few

Figure 10-10

Hydrozoan medusa, *Gonionemus vertens*. This small medusa, 2 to 3 cm in diameter, is the dominant stage in the life cycle of this species. The attached polyp stage is tiny and solitary.
Photograph by R. Harbo.

Figure 10-11

Bell medusa, *Polyorchis penicillatus*, medusa stage of an unknown attached polyp.
Photograph by D.W. Gotshall.

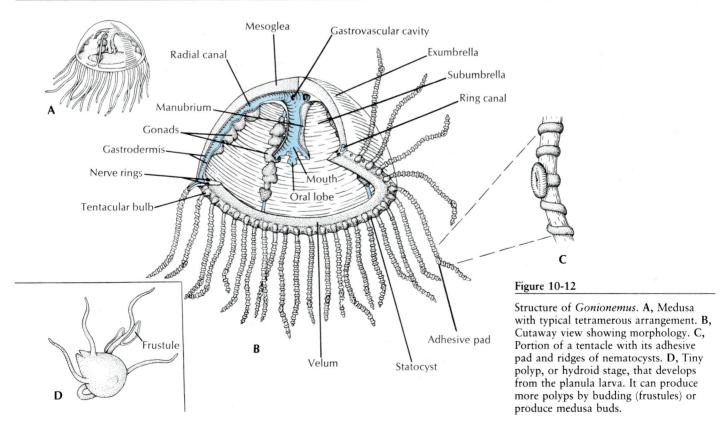

Figure 10-12

Structure of *Gonionemus*. **A,** Medusa with typical tetramerous arrangement. **B,** Cutaway view showing morphology. **C,** Portion of a tentacle with its adhesive pad and ridges of nematocysts. **D,** Tiny polyp, or hydroid stage, that develops from the planula larva. It can produce more polyps by budding (frustules) or produce medusa buds.

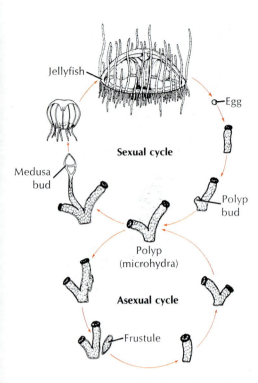

Sexual cycle

Asexual cycle

Jellyfish

Egg

Medusa
bud

Polyp
bud

Polyp
(microhydra)

Frustule

Figure 10-13

Life cycle of *Craspedacusta,* a freshwater hydrozoan. The polyp has three methods of sexual reproduction: by budding off new individuals, which may remain attached to the parent (colony formation); by constricting off nonciliated planula-like larvae (frustules), which can move around and give rise to new polyps; and by producing medusa buds, which develop into sexual jellyfish.

A

B

Figure 10-14

These hydrozoans form calcareous skeletons that resemble true coral. **A,** California hydrocoral, *Allopora californica* (order Stylasterina). **B,** *Millepora alcicornis* (order Milleporina) commonly forms platelike colonies, but it often grows over the horny skeleton of gorgonians (see p. 243), as is shown here. The thin, tentacle-like processes seen in this photograph are dactylozooids. They are generously supplied with powerful nematocysts that produce a burning sensation on human skin, accounting for the common name of fire coral.

A, Photograph by D.W. Gotshall; B, photograph by L.S. Roberts.

A

B

Figure 10-15

A, Three Portuguese man-of-war colonies, *Physalia physalis* (order Siphonophora, class Hydrozoa), lie stranded in shallow water. Colonies often drift onto southern ocean beaches, where they are a hazard to bathers. Each colony of medusa and polyp types is integrated to act as one individual. As many as a thousand zooids may be found in one colony. The nematocysts secrete a powerful neurotoxin. **B,** Several different types of zooids can be seen suspended from the pneumatophore (float).

A, Photograph by C. Lane; B, photograph by L.S. Roberts.

polyps. For a long time its relation to the medusa was not recognized, and thus the polyp was given a name of its own, *Microhydra ryderi*. On the basis of its relationship to the jellyfish and the law of priority, both the polyp and the medusa should be called *Craspedacusta* (N.L., *craspedon,* velum, + Gr., *kystis,* bladder).

The polyp has three methods of asexual reproduction, as shown in Fig. 10-13.

Floating colonies

Members of the orders Siphonophora and Chondrophora are among the most specialized of the Hydrozoa. They form polymorphic swimming or floating colonies made up of several types of modified medusae and polyps.

Physalia (Gr., *physallis,* bladder), or the Portuguese man-of-war (Fig. 10-15), is one such colony with a rainbow-hued float of blues and pinks that carries it along on the surface waters of tropical seas. Many are blown to shore on the eastern coast of the United States. The long, graceful tentacles, actually zooids, are laden with nematocysts and are capable of inflicting painful stings. The float, called a **pneumatophore,** is believed to have expanded from the original larval polyp. It contains an air sac arising from the body wall and filled with a gas similar to air. The float acts as a type of nurse-carrier for future generations of individuals that bud from it and hang suspended in the water. Some of the siphonophores, such as *Stephalia* and *Nectalia,* possess swimming bells as well as a float.

There are several types of polyp individuals (Fig. 10-15, *B*). The **gastrozooids** are feeding polyps with a single long tentacle arising from the base of each. Some of these long stinging tentacles become separated from the feeding polyp and are called **dactylozooids,** or fishing tentacles. These sting the prey and lift them to the lips of the feeding polyps. Among the modified medusoid individuals are the **gonophores,** which are little more than sacs containing either ovaries or testes.

An interesting mutualistic relationship exists between *Physalia* and a small fish called *Nomeus* (Gr., herdsman) that swims among the tentacles with perfect safety. Other larger fish trying to catch *Nomeus* are caught by the deadly tentacles. *Nomeus* probably feeds on bits of *Physalia*'s prey and certainly gains a measure of protection from predation by its refuge among the *Physalia* tentacles. Why the fish is not stung to death by its host's nematocysts is unclear, but like the anemone fish to be discussed later, *Nomeus* is probably protected by a skin mucus that does not stimulate nematocyst discharge.

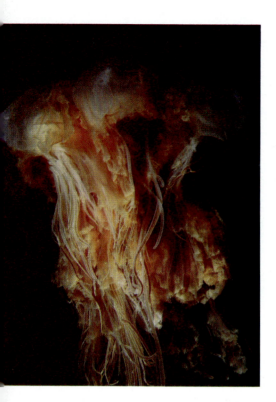

Figure 10-16

Giant jellyfish, *Cyanea capillata* (order Semaeostomeae, class Scyphozoa). A North Atlantic species of *Cyanea* reaches a bell diameter exceeding 2 m. It is known as the "sea blubber" by fishermen.

Photograph by R. Harbo.

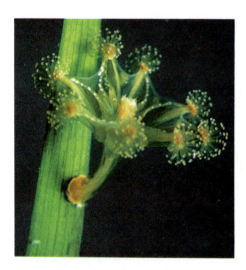

Figure 10-17

Haliclystus auricula (order Stauromedusae, class Scyphozoa). Members of this order are unusual scyphozoans in that the medusae are sessile and attached to seaweed or other objects.

Photograph by K. Sandved.

___ Class Scyphozoa

Class Scyphozoa (si-fo-zo′a) (Gr., *skyphos*, cup) includes most of the larger jellyfishes, or "cup animals." A few, such as *Cyanea* (Gr., *kyanos*, dark-blue substance), may attain a bell diameter exceeding 2 m and tentacles 60 to 70 m long (Fig. 10-16). Most scyphozoans, however, range from 2 to 40 cm in diameter. Most are found floating in the open sea, some even at depths of 3000 m, but one unusual order is sessile and attaches by a stalk to seaweeds and other objects on the sea bottom (Fig. 10-17). Their coloring may range from colorless to striking orange and pink hues.

The bells of different species vary in depth from a shallow saucer shape to a deep helmet or goblet shape. The jelly (mesoglea) layers are unusually thick, giving the bell a fairly firm consistency. The jelly is 95% to 96% water. Unlike the hydromedusae, this layer in the scyphomedusae also contains ameboid cells and fibers, so that it is called a **collenchyme.** Movement is by rhythmical pulsations of the umbrella. There is no velum as in the hydromedusae. There may be many tentacles or few, and they may be short as in *Aurelia* (L., *aurum*, gold) or long as in *Cyanea. Aurelia* (Fig. 10-18) is a familiar species 7 to 10 cm in diameter, commonly found in the waters off both the east and west coasts of the United States, and widely used for the study of Scyphozoa.

The margin of the umbrella is scalloped, usually with each indentation bearing a pair of **lappets,** and between them is a sense organ called a **rhopalium** (tentaculocyst). *Aurelia* has eight such notches. Some scyphozoans have four, others 16. Each rhopalium is club shaped and contains a hollow statocyst for equilibrium and one or two pits lined with sensory epithelium. In some species the rhopalia also bear **ocelli.**

The mouth is centered on the subumbrella side. The manubrium is usually drawn out to form four frilly **oral arms** that are used in capturing and ingesting prey.

The tentacles, the manubrium, and often the entire body surface are well supplied with nematocysts that can give painful stings. However, the primary function of scyphozoan nematocysts is not to attack humans but to paralyze prey animals, which are conveyed to the mouth lobes with the help of the other tentacles or by the bending of the umbrella margin.

Aurelia, which has comparatively short tentacles, feeds on small planktonic animals. These are caught in the mucus of the umbrella surface, are carried to "food pockets" on the umbrella margin by cilia, and are picked up from the pockets by the oral lobes whose cilia carry the food to the gastrovascular cavity. Flagella in the gastrodermis layer keep a current of water moving to bring food and oxygen into the stomach and carry out wastes.

Cassiopeia (L., mythology, queen of Ethiopia), a jellyfish common to Florida waters, and *Rhizostoma* (Gr., *rhiza*, root, + *stoma*, mouth), which can be found in colder waters, belong to a group differing from that of *Aurelia* both in their lack of tentacles on the umbrella margin and in the structure of the oral arms. During development, the edges of the oral lobes fold over and fuse, forming canals (**arms** or **brachial canals**) that become highly branched. These open to the surface at frequent intervals by pores called "mouths"; the original mouth is obliterated in the fusion of the oral lobes. Planktonic organisms caught in the mucus of the frilly oral arms are transported to the mouths and then up the brachial canals to the gastric cavity by cilia. In contrast to the usual swimming habit of medusae, *Cassiopeia* is usually found lying on its "back" in shallow lagoons. Its umbrella mar-

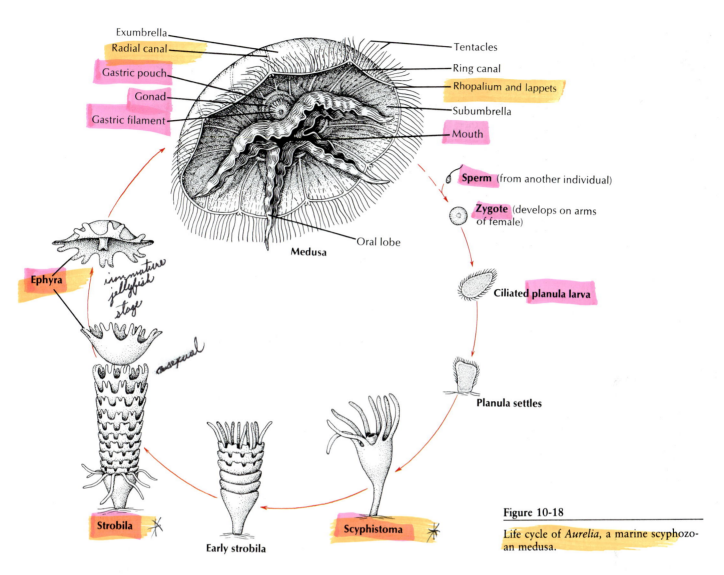

Exumbrella
Radial canal
Gastric pouch
Gonad
Gastric filament

Tentacles
Ring canal
Rhopalium and lappets
Subumbrella
Mouth

Sperm (from another individual)
Zygote (develops on arms of female)
Ciliated planula larva

Oral lobe

Medusa

Ephyra

immature jellyfish stage

asexual

Planula settles

Strobila

Early strobila

Scyphistoma

Figure 10-18

Life cycle of *Aurelia,* a marine scyphozoan medusa.

gin contracts about 20 times a minute, creating water currents to bring plankton into contact with the mucus and nematocysts of its oral lobes. Its tissues are abundantly supplied with symbiotic algal cells (zooxanthellae).

Internally, extending out from the stomach of scyphozoans are four **gastric pouches** in which gastrodermis extends down in little tentacle-like projections called **gastric filaments.** These are covered with nematocysts to further quiet any prey that may still be struggling. Gastric filaments are lacking in the hydromedusae. A complex system of **radial canals** branches out from the pouches to a **ring canal** in the margin and makes up a part of the gastrovascular cavity.

The **nervous system** in scyphozoans seems to be of a synaptic nerve net type, with a subumbrella net that controls bell pulsations and another, more diffuse net that controls local reactions such as feeding.

The sexes are separate, with the gonads located in the gastric pouches. Fertilization is internal, with the sperm being carried by ciliary currents into the gastric pouch of the female. The zygotes may develop in the seawater or may be brooded in folds of the oral arms. The ciliated planula larva becomes attached and develops into a **scyphistoma,** a hydralike form (Fig. 10-19). By a process of **strobilation** the scyphistoma of *Aurelia* forms a series of saucerlike buds, **ephyrae,** and

A

B

Figure 10-19

A, Scyphistoma (polyp stage) of the large jellyfish *Cassiopeia*. The individual at left shows the mouth. To the left of the bell are two buds that will detach and develop into new scyphistomas. In the spring young ephyrae bud off, one at a time, from the oral side to become medusae. **B,** Scyphistoma *(right)* and strobilas *(left)* of *Aurelia aurita* hanging down from a rock. The strobila at left has an ephyra nearly ready to separate.

A, Photograph by F.M. Hickman; B, photograph by D.P. Wilson.

is now called a **strobila** (Figs. 10-18 and 10-19, *B*). When the ephyrae break loose, they grow into mature jellyfish.

In *Cassiopeia* the scyphistoma does not form a strobila, as in *Aurelia*, but buds off young medusae one at a time (monodisc strobilation) (Fig. 10-19, *A*). The scyphistoma can also constrict off small planula-like ciliated buds that swim about and then settle down to become other scyphistomas.

Class Cubozoa

The Cubozoa were until recently considered an order (Cubomedusae) of Scyphozoa. The medusoid is the predominant form (Fig. 10-20); the polypoid is inconspicuous and in most cases unknown. Some cubozoan medusae may range up to 25 cm tall, but most are about 2 to 3 cm. In transverse section the bells are almost square. A tentacle or group of tentacles is found at each corner of the square at the umbrella margin. The base of each tentacle is differentiated into a flattened, tough blade called a **pedalium** (Fig. 10-20). Rhopalia are present. The umbrella margin is not scalloped, and the subumbrella edge turns inward to form a **velarium**. The velarium functions as a velum does in the hydrozoan medusae, increasing swimming efficiency, but it differs structurally. Cubomedusae are strong swimmers and voracious predators, feeding mostly on fish. Stings of some species can be fatal to humans.

The complete life cycle is known for only one species, *Tripedalia cystophora* (L., *tri*, three, + Gr., *pedalion*, rudder). The polyp is tiny (1 mm tall), solitary, and sessile. It buds off new polyps laterally, which detach and creep away. The polyps do not produce ephyrae but metamorphose directly into medusae.

Chironex fleckeri (Gr., *cheir*, hand, + *nĕxis*, swimming) is a cubomedusa known as the sea wasp. Its stings are quite dangerous and sometimes fatal. Most of the fatal stings have been reported from tropical Australian waters. *Chironex* is a large cubomedusa, and fatalities usually follow quite massive stings. Witnesses have described victims as being covered with "yards and yards of sticky wet string." The stings are very painful, and death, if it is to occur, ensues within a matter of minutes. If death does not occur within 20 minutes after stinging, complete recovery is likely.

Figure 10-20

Carybdea, a cubozoan medusa.

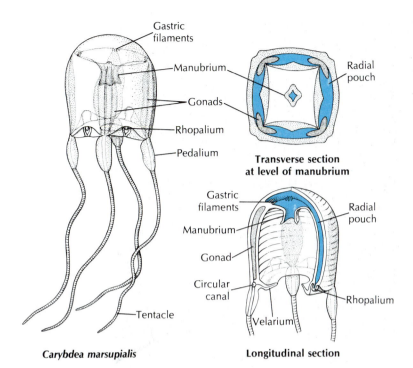

Carybdea marsupialis

Transverse section at level of manubrium

Longitudinal section

Class Anthozoa

The anthozoans, or "flower animals," are polyps with a flowerlike appearance (Fig. 10-21). There is no medusa stage. Anthozoans are all marine and are found in both deep and shallow water and in polar seas as well as tropical seas. They vary greatly in size and may be solitary or colonial. Many of the forms are supported by skeletons.

The class has three subclasses: **Zoantharia**, made up of the sea anemones, hard corals, and others; the **Ceriantipatharia**, which includes only the tube anemones and thorny corals; and the **Alcyonaria**, containing the soft and horny corals, such as sea fans, sea pens, sea pansies, and others. The zoantharians and ceriantipatharians have a **hexamerous** plan (of six or multiples of six) or polymerous symmetry and have simple tubular tentacles arranged in one or more circlets on the oral disc. The alcyonarians are **octamerous** (built on a plan of eight) and always have eight pinnate (featherlike) tentacles arranged around the margin of the oral disc (Fig. 10-22).

The gastrovascular cavity is large and partitioned by mesenteries, or septa, that are inward extensions of the body wall. Where one mesentery extends into the gastrovascular cavity from the body wall, another extends from the diametrically opposite side; thus, they are said to be **coupled**. In the Zoantharia, the mesenteries are not only coupled, they are also **paired** (Fig. 10-23). The muscular arrangement varies among the different groups, but there are usually circular muscles in the body wall and longitudinal and transverse muscles in the mesenteries.

The mesoglea is a mesenchyme containing ameboid cells. There is a general tendency toward biradial symmetry in the septal arrangement and in the shape of the mouth and pharynx. There are no special organs for respiration or excretion.

Figure 10-21

Sea anemones are the familiar and colorful "flower animals" of tide pools, rocks, and pilings of the intertidal zone. Most, however, are subtidal, their beauty seldom revealed to human eyes. These are rose anemones, *Tealia piscivora*.
Photograph by D.W. Gotshall.

A

B

Figure 10-22

Orange sea pen *Ptilosarcus gurneyi* (order Pennatulacea, class Anthozoa). Sea pens are colonial forms that inhabit soft bottoms. **A,** Entire colony. The base of the fleshy body of the primary polyp is buried in the bottom. It gives rise to numerous secondary, branching polyps, shown enlarged in **B.** The pinnate tentacles characteristic of the subclass Alcyonaria are apparent.

A, Photograph by J.L. Rotman; **B,** photograph by R. Harbo.

Sea anemones

Sea anemone (order Actiniaria) polyps are larger and heavier than hydrozoan polyps (Figs. 10-21 and 10-24). Most of them range from 5 mm or less to 100 mm in diameter, and from 5 mm to 200 mm long, but some grow much larger. Some of them are quite colorful. Anemones are found in coastal areas all over the world, especially in the warmer waters. They attach by means of their pedal discs to shells, rocks, timber, or whatever submerged substrata they can find. Some burrow in the bottom mud or sand.

Sea anemones are cylindrical in form with a crown of tentacles arranged in one or more circles around the mouth on the flat **oral disc** (Fig. 10-23). The slit-shaped mouth leads into a **pharynx.** At one or both ends of the mouth is a ciliated groove called a **siphonoglyph,** which extends into the pharynx. The siphonoglyph creates a water current directed into the pharynx. The cilia elsewhere on the pharynx direct water outward. The currents thus created carry in oxygen and remove wastes. They also help maintain an internal fluid pressure or a hydrostatic skeleton that serves in lieu of a true skeleton as a support for opposing muscles.

The pharynx leads into a large **gastrovascular cavity** that is divided into six radial chambers by means of six pairs of **primary (complete) septa,** or **mesenteries,** extending vertically from the body wall to the pharynx (Fig. 10-23). These chambers communicate with each other and are open below the pharynx. Smaller (**incomplete**) mesenteries partially subdivide the larger chambers and provide a means of increasing the surface area of the gastrovascular cavity. The free edge of each incomplete septum forms a type of sinuous cord called a **septal filament** that is provided with nematocysts and with gland cells for digestion. In many anemones the lower ends of the septal filaments are prolonged into **acontia threads,** also

Figure 10-23

Structure of a sea anemone. The free edges of the septa and the acontia threads are equipped with nematocysts to complete the paralyzation of prey begun by the tentacles.

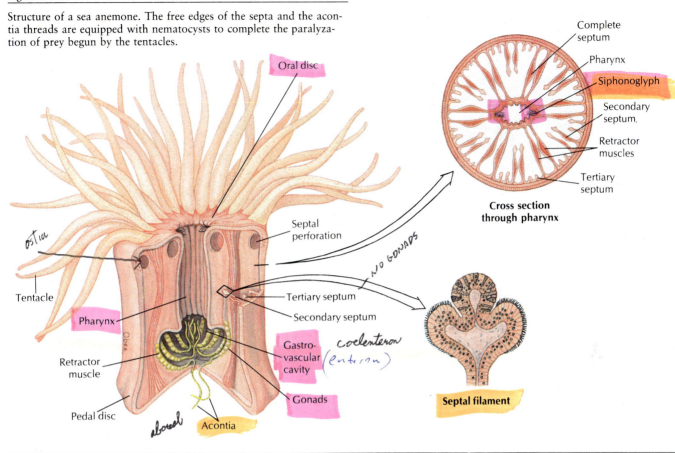

Oral disc

Complete septum

Pharynx

Siphonoglyph

Secondary septum

Retractor muscles

Tertiary septum

Cross section through pharynx

Ostia

Septal perforation

NO GONADS

Tentacle

Tertiary septum

Secondary septum

Pharynx

Gastro-vascular cavity

coelenteron (enteron)

Retractor muscle

Septal filament

Pedal disc

Gonads

aboral

Acontia

Figure 10-24

Anthozoan "flower animals." Several white sea anemones *(Metridium senile)* are surrounded by branching masses of crimson soft corals *(Gersemia rubiformis)*.

Photograph by R. Harbo.

Figure 10-25

A sea anemone that swims. When attacked by a predatory sea star *Dermasterias*, the anemone *Stomphia didemon* detaches from the bottom and rolls or swims spasmodically to a safer location. Photograph by R. Harbo.

provided with nematocysts and gland cells, that can be protruded through the mouth or through pores in the body wall to help overcome prey or provide defense. The pores also aid in the rapid discharge of water from the body when the animal is endangered and contracts to a small size.

Sea anemones are carnivorous, feeding on fish or almost any live animals of suitable size. Some species live on minute forms caught by ciliary currents.

Feeding behavior in many zoantharians is under chemical control. Some respond to reduced glutathione. In certain others two compounds are involved: asparagine, the feeding activator, causes a bending of the tentacles toward the mouth; then reduced glutathione induces swallowing of the food.

Sea anemones are muscular, having muscle fibers not only in the epidermis and gastrodermis but also in the collenchyme. There are definite muscle bands in the mesenteries. Most anemones can glide along slowly on their pedal discs. They can expand and stretch out their tentacles in search of small vertebrates and invertebrates, which they overpower with tentacles and nematocysts and carry to the mouth.

When disturbed, sea anemones contract and draw in their tentacles and oral discs. Some anemones are able to swim, to a limited extent, by rhythmical bending movements, which may be a mechanism for escape from enemies such as sea stars and nudibranchs. *Stomphia,* for example, at the touch of a predatory sea star, will detach its pedal disc and make creeping or swimming movements to escape (Fig. 10-25). This escape reaction is caused not only by the touch of the star but also by exposure to drippings exuded by the star or to crude extracts made from its tissues. The sea star drippings contain steroid saponins that are toxic and irritating to most invertebrates. Extracts given off by nudibranchs can also provoke this reaction in sea anemones.

Anemones form some interesting mutualistic relationships with other organisms. Many species harbor symbiotic algae (zooxanthellae) within their tissues, similar to the hard coral–zooxanthellae association (described later in the chapter), and the anemones profit from the products of algal photosynthesis (p. 251). Some anemones habitually attach to the shells occupied by certain hermit crabs. The hermit encourages the relationship and, finding its favorite species, which it recognizes by touch, it massages the anemone until it detaches. The hermit crab holds the anemone against its own shell until the anemone is firmly attached. The crab probably derives some protection and camouflage from the anemone. The anemone gets free transportation and particles of food dropped by the hermit crab.

Certain damselfishes (clown fishes) (family Pomacentridae) form associations with large anemones, especially in tropical Indo-Pacific waters. An unknown property of the skin mucus of the fish causes the anemone's nematocysts not to discharge, but if some other fish is so unfortunate as to brush the anemone's tentacles, it is likely to become a meal. The anemone obviously provides shelter for the anemone fish, and the fish may help ventilate the anemone by its movements, keep the anemone free of sediment, and even lure an unwary victim to seek the same shelter.

The sexes are separate in sea anemones, and the gonads are arranged on the margins of the mesenteries. The zygote develops into a ciliated larva. Asexual reproduction commonly occurs by **pedal laceration** or by longitudinal fission, occasionally by transverse fission or by budding. In pedal laceration, small pieces of the pedal disc break off as the animal moves, and each of these regenerates a small anemone.

Zoantharian corals

The zoantharian corals belong to the order Scleractinia, sometimes known as the true or stony corals. The stony corals might be described as miniature sea anemones that live in calcareous cups they themselves have secreted (Fig. 10-26 and p. 219). Like that of the anemones, the coral polyp's gastrovascular cavity is subdivided by mesenteries arranged in multiples of six (hexamerous) and its hollow tentacles surround the mouth, but there is no siphonoglyph.

Instead of a pedal disc, the epidermis at the base of the column secretes the limy skeletal cup, including the sclerosepta, which project up into the polyp between the true mesenterial septa (Fig. 10-26, *F*). The living polyp can retract into the safety of the cup when not feeding. Since the skeleton is secreted below the living tissue rather than within it, the calcareous material is an exoskeleton. In the colonial corals, the skeleton may become massive, building up over many years, with the living coral forming a sheet of tissue over the surface. The gastrovascular cavities of the polyps are all connected through this sheet of tissue.

Three other small orders of Zoantharia are recognized.

Tube anemones and thorny corals

Members of the subclass Ceriantipatharia have coupled but unpaired mesenteries. The tube anemones (order Ceriantharia) are solitary and live in soft bottom sediments, buried to the level of the oral disc. They occupy tubes constructed of secreted mucus and threads of nematocyst-like organoids, into which they can withdraw. The thorny or black corals (order Antipatharia) (Fig. 10-27) are colonial and attached to a firm substratum. Their skeleton is of a horny material and has thorns. Both of these orders are small in numbers of species and are limited to warmer waters of the sea.

Alcyonarian corals

Alcyonarians are often referred to as octocorals because of their strict octomerous symmetry, with eight pinnate tentacles and eight unpaired, complete mesenteries (Fig. 10-22). They are all colonial, and the gastrovascular cavities of the polyps

Figure 10-26

A, Cup coral *Tubastrea* sp. The polyps form clumps resembling groups of sea anemones. Although often found on coral reefs, *Tubastrea* is not a reef-building coral (ahermatypic) and has no symbiotic zooxanthellae in its tissues. **B,** *Acropora palmata*, the elkhorn coral. The *A. palmata* zone is characteristic of Caribbean reefs in the upper part of the fore reef slope. Hermatypic corals, such as *A. palmata*, tend to be shades of brown, green, and yellow, reflecting the presence of the zooxanthellae in their tissues. **C,** The polyps of *Montastrea cavernosa* are tightly withdrawn in the daytime but open to feed at night, as in **D. E,** *Porites porites* is common on Caribbean reefs in shallow water. **F,** Mushroom coral *Fungia* sp. This is a common, unattached species of the Great Barrier Reef.

A and **F,** Photographs by C.P. Hickman, Jr.; **B** to **E,** photographs by L.S. Roberts.

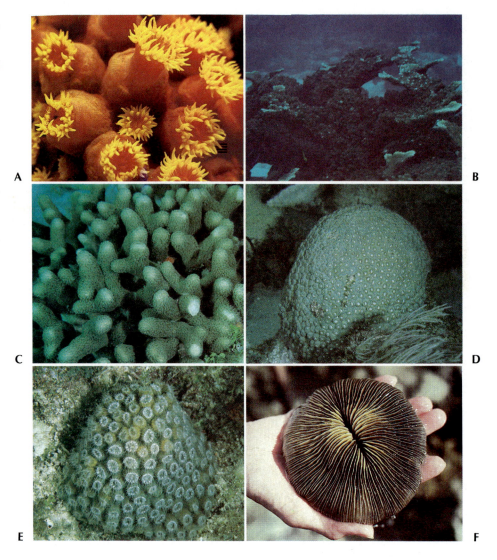

Figure 10-27

A, Colony of *Antipathes*, a black or thorny coral (order Antipatharia, class Anthozoa). Most abundant in deep waters in the tropics, black corals secrete a tough, proteinaceous skeleton that can be worked into jewelry. **B,** The polyps of Antipatharia have six simple, nonretractile tentacles. The spiny processes on the skeleton are the origin of the common name thorny corals.

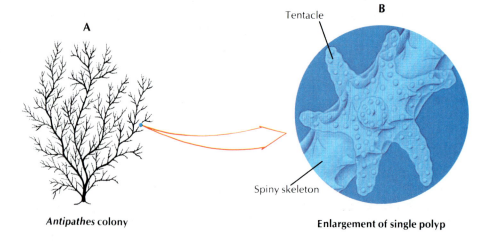

Tentacle

Spiny skeleton

Antipathes colony

Enlargement of single polyp

A

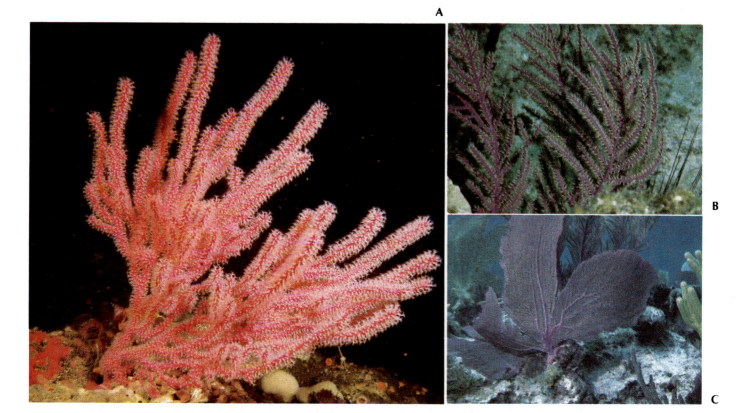

B

C

Figure 10-28

Colonial gorgonian, or horny, corals (order Gorgonacea, class Anthozoa) are conspicuous components of reef faunas, especially of the West Indies. **A,** Red gorgonian *Lophogorgia chilensis.* **B,** A sea plume, *Pseudopterogorgia* sp. **C,** A sea fan *Gorgonia ventalina.*

A, Photograph by D.W. Gotshall; **B,** photograph by L.S. Roberts; **C,** photograph by W.C. Ober.

communicate through a system of gastrodermal tubes called **solenia.** The solenia run through an extensive mesoglea (**coenenchyme**) in most alcyonarians, and the surface of the colony is covered by epidermis. The skeleton is secreted in the coenenchyme and consists of limy spicules, fused spicules, or a horny protein, often in combination. Thus, the skeletal support of most alcyonarians is an endoskeleton. The variation in pattern among the species of alcyonarians lends great variety to the form of the colonies: from the soft coral *Gersemia* (Fig. 10-24), with its spicules scattered through the coenenchyme, to the tough, axial supports of the sea fans and other gorgonian corals (Fig. 10-28), to the fused spicules of the organ-pipe coral. *Renilla* (L., *ren,* kidney, + *illa,* suffix), the sea pansy, is a colony reminiscent of a pansy flower. Its polyps are embedded in the fleshy upper side and a short stalk that supports the colony is embedded in the sea floor (Fig. 10-29). *Ptilosarcus* (Gr., *ptilon,* feather, + *sarkos,* flesh), a sea pen, is a member of the same order and may reach a length of 50 cm (Fig. 10-22).

The graceful beauty of the alcyonarians—in hues of yellow, red, orange, and purple—helps create the "submarine gardens" of the coral reefs.

Coral reefs

Most students will have seen photographs or movies giving a glimpse of the vibrant color and life found on coral reefs, and some may have been fortunate enough to visit a reef. Coral reefs are among the most productive of the ecosytems and they have a diversity of life forms rivaled only by the tropical rain forest. They are large formations of calcium carbonate (limestone) in shallow tropical seas laid down by living organisms over thousands of years; living plants and animals are confined to the top layer of reefs where they add more and more calcium carbon-

Figure 10-29

Sea pansy *Renilla reniformis* (order Pennatulacea, class Anthozoa). The eight pinnate tentacles characteristic of the subclass Alcyonaria can be distinguished. Photograph by K. Sandved.

ate to that deposited by their predecessors. The most important organisms that precipitate calcium carbonate from seawater to form reefs are the scleractinian, **hermatypic** (reef-building) **corals** (Fig. 10-26, *B* to *E*) and **coralline algae.** Not only do the coralline algae contribute to the total mass of calcium carbonate, but their precipitation of the substance helps to hold the reef together. Some alcyonarians and hydrozoans (especially *Millepora* [L., *mille*, thousand, + *porus*, pore] spp., the "fire coral," Fig. 10-14, *B*) contribute in some measure to the calcareous material, and an enormous variety of other organisms contribute small amounts. However, hermatypic (Gr., *herma*, support, mound, + *typos*, type) corals seem essential to the formation of large reefs, since such reefs do not occur where these corals cannot live.

Hermatypic corals require warmth, light, and the salinity of undiluted seawater. This limits coral reefs to shallow waters between 30 degrees north and 30 degrees south latitude and excludes them from areas with upwelling of cold water or areas near major river outflows with attendant low salinity and high turbidity. These corals require light because they have mutualistic algae (zooxanthellae) living in their tissues. The microscopic zooxanthellae are very important to the corals: their photosynthesis and fixation of carbon dioxide furnish food molecules for their hosts, they recycle phosphorus and nitrogenous waste compounds that otherwise would be lost, and they enhance the ability of the coral to deposit calcium carbonate.

Several types of reefs are commonly recognized. The **fringing reef** is close to a land mass with either no lagoon or a narrow lagoon between it and the shore. A **barrier reef** runs roughly parallel to shore and has a wider and deeper lagoon than does a fringing reef. **Atolls** are reefs that encircle a lagoon but not an island. These types of reefs typically slope rather steeply into deep water at their seaward edge. **Patch** or **bank reefs** occur some distance back from the steep, seaward slope in the lagoons of barrier reefs or atolls. The so-called Great Barrier Reef, extending 1260 miles long and up to 90 miles from the shore off the northeast coast of Australia, is actually a complex of reef types.

Fringing, barrier, and atoll reefs all have distinguishable zones that are characterized by different groups of corals and other animals. The side of the reef facing the sea is the **reef front** or **fore reef slope** (Fig. 10-30). The reef front is more or less parallel to the shore and perpendicular to the predominant direction of wave travel. It slopes downward into deeper water, sometimes gently at first, then precipitously. Characteristic assemblages of scleratinian corals grow deep on the slope, high near the crest, and in zones between. In shallow water or slightly emergent at the top of the reef front is the **reef crest.** The upper front and the crest bear the greatest force of the waves and must absorb great energy during storms. Pieces of coral and other organisms are broken off at such times and thrown shoreward onto the **reef flat,** which slopes down into the lagoon. The reef flat thus receives a supply of calcareous material that is eventually broken down into coral sand. The sand is stabilized by the growth of plants such as turtle grass and coralline algae and is ultimately cemented into the mass of the reef by precipitation of carbonates. A reef is not an unbroken wall facing the sea but is highly irregular, with grooves, caves, crevices, channels through from the flat to the front, and deep, cup-shaped holes ("blue holes"). Alcyonarians tend to grow in these areas that are more protected from the full force of the waves, as well as on the flat and the deeper areas of the fore reef slope. Many other kinds of organisms inhabit the cryptic locations such as caves and crevices.

Enormous numbers of species and individuals of invertebrate groups and

Figure 10-30

A, Profile of a barrier reef. **B,** Portion of an atoll from the air. Reef slope plunges into deep water at left (dark blue), lagoon at right.

B, Photograph by C.P. Hickman, Jr.

fishes populate the reef ecosystem. For example, there are 300 *common* species of fishes on Caribbean reefs. It is marvelous that such diversity and productivity can be maintained, since the reefs are washed by the nutrient-poor waves of the open ocean. Although relatively little nutrient enters the ecosystem, little is lost because the interacting organisms of the reef are so efficient in recycling. Even the feces released by the fish are fed upon by the corals!

PHYLUM CTENOPHORA

Ctenophora (te-nof'o-ra) (Gr., *kteis, ktenos,* comb, + *phora,* pl. of bearing) is comprised of fewer than 100 species. All are marine forms. They take their name from the eight rows of comblike plates they bear for locomotion. Common names for ctenophores are "sea walnuts" and "comb jellies." Ctenophores, along with cnidarians, represent the only two phyla having primary radial symmetry, in contrast to other metazoans, which have primary bilateral symmetry.

Ctenophores do not have nematocysts, except in one species (*Haeckelia rubra,* after Ernst Haeckel, nineteenth-century German zoologist) that is provided with nematocysts on certain regions of its tentacles but lacks colloblasts. These nematocysts are apparently a part of this ctenophore and are not "appropriated" by eating a cnidarian.

In common with the cnidarians, ctenophores have not advanced beyond the tissue grade of organization. There are no definite organ systems in the strict meaning of the term.

The ctenophores are strictly marine animals and are all free swimming

Figure 10-31

A, Comb jelly *Pleurobrachia* sp. (order Cydippida, class Tentaculata). Its fragile beauty is especially evident at night when it luminesces from its comb rows. **B,** *Mnemiopsis* sp. (order Lobata, class Tentaculata).

A, Photograph by J.L. Rotman; **B,** photograph by K. Sandved.

except for a few creeping and sessile forms. They occur in all seas but especially in warm waters.

Although feeble swimmers and more common in surface waters, ctenophores are sometimes found at considerable depths. They are often at the mercy of tides and strong currents, but they avoid storms by swimming downward in the water. In calm water they may rest vertically with little movement, but when moving they use their ciliated comb plates to propel themselves mouth-end forward. Highly modified forms such as *Cestum* (L., *cestus,* girdle) use sinuous body movements as well as their comb plates in locomotion.

The fragile, transparent bodies of ctenophores are easily seen at night when they emit light (luminesce).

CHARACTERISTICS

1. Symmetry **biradial;** arrangement of internal canals and the position of the paired tentacles change the radial symmetry into a combination of the two (**radial + bilateral**)
2. Usually ellipsoidal or spherical in shape, **with radially arranged rows of comb plates for swimming**
3. Ectoderm, endoderm, and a mesoglea (ectomesoderm) with scattered cells and muscle fibers; may be considered **triploblastic**
4. Nematocysts absent (except in one species), but **adhesive cells (colloblasts)** present
5. Digestive system consisting of mouth, pharynx, stomach, a series of canals, and anal pores
6. Nervous system consisting of a subepidermal plexus concentrated around the mouth and beneath the comb plate rows; an **aboral sense organ** (statocyst)
7. No polymorphism
8. Reproduction monoecious; gonads (endodermal origin) on the walls of the digestive canals, which are under the rows of comb plates; determinate cleavage; cydippid larva
9. Luminescence common

COMPARISON WITH CNIDARIA

Ctenophores resemble the cnidarians in the following ways:
1. Form of radial symmetry; together with the cnidarians, they form the group Radiata
2. Aboral-oral axis around which the parts are arranged
3. Well-developed gelatinous ectomesoderm (collenchyme)
4. No coelomic cavity
5. Diffuse nerve plexus
6. Lack of organ systems
They differ from the cnidarians in the following ways:
1. No nematocysts except in *Haeckelia*
2. Development of muscle cells from mesenchyme
3. Presence of comb plates and colloblasts
4. Mosaic, or determinate type of development
5. Presence of pharynx generally
6. No polymorphism
7. Never colonial
8. Presence of anal openings

CLASSIFICATION

Class Tentaculata (ten-tak-yu-la′ta) (L., *tentaculum,* feeler, + *ata,* group suffix). With tentacles; tentacles may or may not have sheaths into which they retract; some types flattened in oral-aboral axis for creeping; others compressed in tentacular plane to a bandlike form; in some the comb plates may be confined to the larval form. Examples: *Pleurobrachia, Cestum.*

Class Nuda (nu′da) (L., *nudus,* naked). Without tentacles, but flattened in tentacular plane; wide mouth and pharynx; gastrovascular canals much branched. Example: *Beroe.*

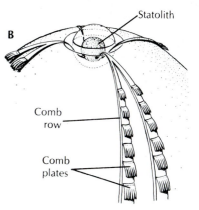

Figure 10-32

The comb jelly *Pleurobrachia*, a ctenophore. **A**, Hemisection. **B**, External view.

—— Class Tentaculata

Representative type—Pleurobrachia

Pleurobrachia (Gr., *pleuron*, side, + L., *brachia*, arms) is often used as a representative of this group of ctenophores. Its transparent body is about 1.5 to 2 cm in diameter (Fig. 10-31, *A*). The oral pole bears the mouth opening, and the aboral pole has a sensory organ, the **statocyst.**

Comb plates

On the surface are eight equally spaced bands called **comb rows** that extend as meridians from the aboral pole and end before reaching the oral pole (Fig. 10-32). Each band is made up of transverse plates of long fused cilia called **comb plates** (Fig. 10-33, *B*). Ctenophores are propelled by the beating of the cilia on the comb plates. The beat in each row starts at the aboral end and proceeds successively along the combs to the oral end. All eight rows normally beat in unison. The animal is thus driven forward with the mouth in advance. The animal can swim backward by reversing the direction of the wave.

Tentacles

The two **tentacles** are long and solid and very extensible, and they can be retracted into a pair of **tentacle sheaths.** When completely extended, they may be 15 cm long. The surface of the tentacles bears **colloblasts,** or glue cells (Fig. 10-33, *A*), which secrete a sticky substance for catching and holding small animals.

Body wall

The cellular layers of ctenophores are similar to those of the cnidarians. Between the epidermis and gastrodermis is a jellylike **collenchyme,** which makes up most of the interior of the body and contains muscle fibers and ameboid cells.

Digestive system and feeding

The **gastrovascular system** consists of a mouth, a pharynx, a stomach, and a system of gastrovascular canals that branch through the jelly to run to the comb plates, tentacular sheaths, and elsewhere (Fig. 10-32). Two blind canals terminate near the mouth, and an aboral canal passes near the statocyst and divides into two small **anal canals** through which undigested material is expelled.

Figure 10-33

A, Colloblast, an adhesive cell characteristic of ctenophores. **B,** Portion of comb rows showing comb plates, each composed of transverse rows of long fused cilia.

Ctenophores live on small planktonic organisms such as copepods. The glue cells on the tentacles enable the ctenophore to adhere to the small prey and carry it to the mouth. Digestion is both extracellular and intracellular.

Respiration and excretion

Respiration and excretion occur through the body surface.

Nervous and sensory systems

Ctenophores have a nervous system similar to that of the cnidarians. It is made up of a subepidermal plexus, which is concentrated under each comb plate, but there is no central control as is found in higher animals.

The **sense organ** at the aboral pole is a statocyst. Tufts of cilia support a calcareous statolith, with the whole being enclosed in a bell-like container. Alterations in the position of the animal change the pressure of the statolith on the tufts of cilia. The sense organ is also concerned in coordinating the beating of the comb rows but does not trigger their beat.

The epidermis of ctenophores is abundantly supplied with sensory cells, so the animals are sensitive to chemical and other forms of stimuli. When a ctenophore comes in contact with an unfavorable stimulus, it often reverses the beat of its comb plates and backs up. The comb plates are very sensitive to touch, which often causes them to be withdrawn into the jelly. Neuroid conduction is present in the epithelial cells.

Reproduction

Pleurobrachia, like other ctenophores, is monoecious. The gonads are located on the lining of the gastrovascular canals under the comb plates. Fertilized eggs are discharged through the epidermis into the water.

Cleavage in the ctenophores is determinate (mosaic), since the various parts of the animal that will be formed by each cleavage cell are determined early in embryogenesis. If one of the cells is removed in the early stages, the resulting embryo will be deficient. This type of development differs from that of cnidarians, which is indeterminate. The free-swimming cydippid larva is superficially similar to the adult ctenophore and develops directly into an adult.

____ Other Ctenophores

Ctenophores are fragile and beautiful creatures. Their transparent bodies glisten like fine glass, brilliantly iridescent during the day and luminescent at night.

One of the most striking ctenophores is *Beroe* (L., a nymph), which may be more than 100 mm in length and 50 mm in breadth (Fig. 10-34, *A*). It is conical or thimble shaped and is flattened in the tentacular plane. The tentacular plane in *Beroe* is defined as where the tentacles would have been, because it has a large mouth but no tentacles. It is pink. The body wall is covered with an extensive network of canals formed by the union of the paragastric and meridional canals. Venus's girdle *(Cestum,* Fig. 10-34, *B)* is highly compressed in the tentacular plane. Bandlike, it may be more than 1 m long and presents a graceful appearance as it swims in the oral direction. The highly modified *Ctenoplana* (Gr., *ktenos,* comb, + L., *planus,* flat) and *Coeloplana* (Gr., *koilos,* hollow, + L., *planus,* flat) (Fig. 10-34, *C)* are rare but are interesting because they have disc-shaped bodies flattened in the oral-aboral axis and are adapted for creeping rather than swimming. A common ctenophore along the Atlantic and Gulf coasts is *Mnemiopsis*

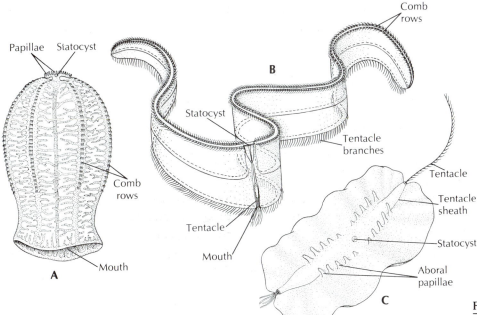

Figure 10-34

Diversity among the phylum Ctenophora. **A,** *Beroe* sp. (order Beroida, class Nuda). **B,** *Cestum* sp. (order Cestida, class Tentaculata). **C,** *Coeloplana* sp. (order Platyctenea, class Tentaculata).

(Gr., *mnēmē,* memory, + *opsis,* appearance) (Fig. 10-31, *B*), which has a laterally compressed body with two large oral lobes and unsheathed tentacles.

Nearly all ctenophores give off flashes of luminescence at night, especially such forms as *Mnemiopsis* (Fig. 10-31, *B*). The vivid flashes of light seen at night in southern seas are often caused by members of this phylum.

PHYLOGENY AND ADAPTIVE RADIATION
Phylogeny

The origin of the cnidarians and ctenophores is obscure, although the most widely supported theory today is that the radiate phyla arose from a radially symmetrical, planula-like ancestor. Such an ancestor could have been common to the radiates and to the higher metazoa, the latter having been derived from a branch whose members habitually crept about on the sea bottom. Such a habit would select for bilateral symmetry. Others became sessile or free floating, conditions for which radial symmetry is a selective advantage. A planula larva in which an invagination formed to become the gastrovascular cavity would correspond roughly to a cnidarian with an ectoderm and an endoderm.

The trachyline medusae (an order of class Hydrozoa) are sometimes considered the most primitive of modern cnidarians because of their direct development from the planula and actinula larvae to the medusa. Such a group could have given rise to the three classes of cnidarians, with further development of the polyp and subsequent loss of the medusa occurring in the anthozoan line. Some zoologists now believe that the Scyphozoa are the most primitive of the cnidarian classes, with the Cubozoa providing a link between the Scyphozoa and the Hydrozoa. Colonial hydrozoans could then have arisen from an ancestor like *Tripedalia* whose polyp buds failed to separate.

In light of their many resemblances to the cnidarians, the ctenophores may have originated from the same ancestral stock, such as the trachyline or scyphozoan medusae, but conclusive evidence is not available.

___ Adaptive Radiation

In their evolution neither phylum has deviated far from its basic plan of structure. In the Cnidaria, both the polyp and medusa are constructed on the same scheme. Likewise, the ctenophores have adhered to the arrangement of the comb plates and their biradial symmetry.

Nonetheless, the cnidarians are a successful phylum in terms of numbers of individuals and species, demonstrating a surprising degree of diversity considering the simplicity of their basic body plan. They are efficient predators, many feeding on prey quite large compared to themselves. Some are adapted for feeding on small particles. The colonial form of life is well explored, with some colonies growing to great size among the corals, and others, such as the siphonophores, showing astonishing polymorphism and specialization of individuals within the colony.

___ Summary

The phyla Cnidaria and Ctenophora have a primary radial symmetry; radial symmetry is an advantage for sessile or free-floating organisms. The Cnidaria are surprisingly efficient predators because they possess stinging organoids called nematocysts. Both phyla are essentially diploblastic, with a body wall comprised of epidermis and gastrodermis and a mesoglea between. The digestive-respiratory (gastrovascular) cavity has a mouth and no anus. Cnidarians are at the tissue level of organization. They have two basic body types (polypoid and medusoid), and in many hydrozoans and scyphozoans the life cycle involves both the asexually reproducing polyp and the sexually reproducing medusa.

That unique organoid, the nematocyst, is secreted by a cnidoblast (which becomes the cnidocyte) and is contained coiled within a capsule. On discharge, some types of nematocysts penetrate the prey and inject poison. Discharge is effected by a change in permeability of the capsule and an increase in internal hydrostatic pressure owing to high osmotic pressure within the capsule.

There is no concentrated central nervous system in cnidarians; the nerves are spread throughout the body in a netlike arrangement. Some synapses can transmit impulses in either direction. Neuroid conduction is present.

Most hydrozoans are colonial and marine, but the freshwater hydras are commonly demonstrated in class laboratories and have the typical polypoid structure. The body is approximately cylindrical in shape, with the mouth surrounded by nematocyst-bearing tentacles at one end. The various cell types are also typical: epitheliomuscular, interstitial, gland, sensory, nerve, and nutritive-muscular cells. Hydras reproduce asexually by budding and sexually after formation of gonads in the cylinder wall; they have no medusoid stage. The more typical form, found in most marine hydrozoans, is that of a branching colony containing many polyps (hydranths), and a free-swimming medusa stage. An example of a floating, colonial hydrozoan with numerous body forms (both polypoid and medusoid) in the colony is the Portuguese man-of-war, *Physalia*.

The scyphozoans are the typical jellyfish, in which the medusoid is the dominant body form. Many scyphozoans have an inconspicuous polypoid stage that reproduces asexually (scyphistoma). Scyphozoan medusae differ from hydrozoan medusae in that scyphozoans have complex sensory structures called rhopalia and do not have a velum.

Sea anemones *Metridium senile* attached to clams in a tide pool.
Photograph by H.W. Pratt/BPS.

The cubozoans are a small class of cnidarians that are predominantly medusoid. They include the dangerous sea wasps. Cubomedusae have rhopalia and a velarium, which is a velumlike structure.

The anthozoans are all marine and are polypoid; there is no medusoid stage. They include two large and important subclasses: Zoantharia (with hexamerous or polymerous symmetry and paired mesenteries) and Alcyonaria (with octomerous symmetry). A small subclass of the Anthozoa is the Ceriantipatharia (with symmetry as in Zoantharia but with unpaired mesenteries). The largest zoantharian orders contain the sea anemones, which are mostly solitary and do not have a secreted skeleton, and the stony corals, which are mostly colonial and secrete a calcareous exoskeleton. Stony corals are the critical component in coral reefs, habitats of great beauty, productivity, and ecological and economic value. The Alcyonaria contain the soft and horny corals, many of which are important and beautiful components of coral reefs.

The Ctenophora are biradial organisms that swim by means of eight comb rows. The combs are modified from cilia. Only one species has nematocysts, but adhesive cells (colloblasts) are characteristic of the phylum. These weakly swimming animals capture small prey with the aid of the colloblasts.

Cnidaria and Ctenophora are probably derived from an ancestor that resembled the planula larva of the cnidarians. In spite of their relatively simple level of organization, the cnidarians are a successful and important phylum.

Selected references

Barnes, D.J. 1970. Coral skeletons: an explanation of their growth and structure. Science 170:1305-1308.

Barnes, J.H. 1966. Studies on three venomous cubomedusae. In W.J. Rees (ed.). The Cnidaria and their evolution. Symposia of the Zoological Society of London, no. 16. London, Academic Press, Inc., Ltd. *Presents morphological studies of cubomedusae producing significant human injury along the Australian coast, clinical details, treatment, and evidence that fatal stingings have been due to* Chironex fleckeri.

Barnes, R.D. 1980. Invertebrate zoology, ed. 4. Philadelphia, Saunders College/Holt, Rinehart & Winston.

Bayer, F.M. 1961. The shallow-water Octocorallia of the West Indian region. The Hague, Martinus Nijhoff Publishers.

Bayer, F.M., and H.B. Owre. 1968. The free-living lower invertebrates. New York, Macmillan, Inc.

Burnett, A.L. 1973. Biology of *Hydra*. New York, Academic Press, Inc.

Colin, P.I. 1978. Caribbean reef invertebrates and plants. Neptune City, N.J., T.F.H. Publications, Inc. *Many color photographs, very good for sight recognition of Caribbean reef corals and other invertebrates.*

Dougherty, E.C. (ed.). 1963. The lower Metazoa. Berkeley, University of California Press. *Deals with comparative biology and phylogeny of the lower metazoan phyla.*

Dunn, D.F. 1982. Cnidaria. In S.P. Parker (ed.). Synopsis and classification of living organisms, vol. 1. New York, McGraw-Hill Book Co.

Faulkner, D., and R. Chesher. 1979. Living corals. New York, Clarkson N. Potter, Inc. *A volume of color photographs of Pacific corals, including considerable information about them; a beautiful book and a feast for the eyes.*

Fraser, C.M. 1937. Hydroids of the Pacific coast of Canada and the United States. Toronto, University of Toronto Press. *This monograph and a similar one on the hydroids of the Atlantic coast are the most comprehensive taxonomic studies yet made on the group in North America.*

Goreau, T.F., and L.S. Land. 1974. Fore-reef morphology and depositional processes, North Jamaica. In L.F. Laporte (ed.). Reefs in time and space. Special publication no. 18. Tulsa, Society of Economic Paleontologists and Mineralogists.

Gosner, K.L. 1971. Guide to identification of marine and estuarine invertebrates. New York, Interscience. *An essential aid for students of the invertebrates found along the northeastern coast of the United States.*

Harbison, G.R., and L.P. Madin. 1982. Ctenophora. In S.P. Parker (ed.). Synopsis and classification of living organisms, vol. 1. New York, McGraw-Hill Book. Co.

Hyman, L.H. 1940. The invertebrates: Protozoa through Ctenophora. New York, McGraw-Hill Book Co. *Extensive accounts are given of the Cnidaria and the ctenophores in the last two chapters of this authoritative work.*

Kaestner, A. 1967. Invertebrate zoology, vol. 1. New York, Interscience.

Mackie, G.O. 1970. Neuroid conduction and the evolution of conducting tissues. Q. Rev. Biol. 45:319-332.

Macklin, M., T. Roma, and K. Drake. 1972. Water excretion by hydra. Science 179:194-195.

Mariscal, R.N. 1971. Experimental studies on the protection of anemone fishes from sea anemones. In T.C. Cheng (ed.). Aspects of the biology of symbiosis. Baltimore, University Park Press.

Muscatine, L., and H.M. Lenhoff (eds.). 1974. Coelenterate biology: reviews and new perspectives. New York, Academic Press, Inc. *Highly recommended for further reading; it has chapters on histology, nematocysts, neurobiology, development, symbioses, bioluminescence, and Ctenophora.*

Muscatine, L., R.R. Pool, and R.K. Trench. 1975. Symbiosis of algae and invertebrates: aspects of the symbiont surface and the host-symbiont interface. Trans. Am. Microsc. Soc. 94:450-469.

Pennak, R.W. 1978. Freshwater invertebrates of the United States, ed. 2. New York, John Wiley & Sons, Inc. *Chapter 4 is devoted to the freshwater cnidarians.*

Rees, W.J. (ed.). 1966. The Cnidaria and their evolution. New York, Academic Press, Inc. *A symposium on various aspects of cnidarian evolution, plus articles on other topics.*

Schaller, H.C. 1976. Action of the head activator as a growth hormone in hydra. Cell Differ. 5:1-11.

Smith, F.G.W. 1948. Atlantic reef corals. Miami, University of Miami Press. *This is a valuable aid for identification of Atlantic reef-building corals.*

Stearn, C.W., T.P. Scoffin, and W. Martindale. 1977. Calcium carbonate budget of a fringing reef on the west coast of Barbados. I. Zonation and productivity. Bull. Mar. Sci. 27:479-510. *The zonation of the small reef studied by these authors resembles in many respects that of many Caribbean reefs.*

Totton, A.K., and G.O. Mackie. 1960. Studies on *Physalia physalis* (L.). Discovery Reports 30:301-407. Cambridge, Eng., Cambridge University Press. *Monograph on the natural history and morphology (Totton) and the behavior and histology (Mackie) of the Portuguese man-of-war.*

Webster, G. 1971. Morphogenesis and pattern formation in hydroids. Biol. Rev. 46(1):1-46.

Westfall, J.A. 1973. Ultrastructural evidence for neuromuscular systems in coelenterates. Am. Zool. 13:237-246.

Selected *Scientific American* articles

Berrill, N.J. 1957. The indestructible hydra. 197:118-125 (Dec.). *Describes the remarkable regenerative powers of the hydra.*

Feder, H.A. 1972. Escape responses in marine invertebrates. 227:92-100 (July).

Gierer, A. 1974. Hydra as a model for the development of biological form. 231:44-54 (Dec.).

Goreau, T.F., N.I. Goreau, and T.J. Goreau. 1979. Corals and coral reefs. 241:124-135 (Aug.). *A good summary of the biology, ecology, and physiology of reef corals.*

Lane, C.E. 1960. The Portuguese man-of-war. 202:158-168 (Mar.). *This beautiful but dangerous hydrozoan represents a remarkable colonial development.*

Loomis, W.F. 1959. The sex gas of hydra. 200:145-156 (Apr.). *The carbon dioxide tension of the water appears to play an important role in controlling sexual reproduction in hydras.*

Newell, N.D. 1972. The evolution of reefs. 226:54-65 (June).

CHAPTER 11

THE ACOELOMATE ANIMALS

Phylum Platyhelminthes
Phylum Rhynchocoela
Phylum Gnathostomulida

Tubulanus annulatus, a nemertine worm.

Photograph by D.P. Wilson.

Position in Animal Kingdom

1. The Platyhelminthes, or flatworms, the Rhynchocoela, or ribbon worms, and the Gnathostomulida, or jaw worms, are the most primitive groups of animals to have **primary bilateral symmetry,** the type of symmetry assumed by all higher animals.
2. These phyla have only one internal space, the digestive cavity, with the region between the ectoderm and endoderm filled with mesoderm in the form of muscle fibers and mesenchyme (parenchyma). Since they lack a coelom or a pseudocoelom, they are termed **acoelomate animals,** and because they have three well-defined germ layers, they are termed triploblastic.
3. Acoelomates show more specialization and division of labor among their organs than do the radiate animals because the mesoderm makes more elaborate organs possible. Thus, the acoelomates are said to have reached the **organ-system level of organization.**
4. They belong to the protostome division of the Bilateria and have spiral cleavage, and at least the platyhelminths and rhynchocoels have determinate cleavage.

Biological Contributions

1. The acoelomates have developed the basic **bilateral** plan of organization that has been widely exploited in the animal kingdom.
2. The **mesoderm** is now developed into a well-defined embryonic germ layer (**triploblastic**), making available a great source of tissues, organs, and systems.
3. Along with bilateral symmetry, **cephalization** has been established. There is some centralization of the nervous system evident in the **ladder type of system** found in flatworms.
4. Along with the subepidermal musculature, there is also a mesenchymal system of muscle fibers.
5. They are the most primitive animals with an **excretory system.**
6. The rhynchocoels are the most primitive animals to have a **circulatory system** with blood and a **one-way alimentary canal.** Although not stressed by zoologists, the rhynchocoel cavity in ribbon worms is technically a true coelom, but as it is merely a part of the proboscis mechanism, it is not of evolutionary significance.
7. Unique and specialized structures occur in all three phyla. The parasitic habit of many flatworms has led to many specialized adaptations, such as organs of adhesion.

The Platyhelminthes (Gr., *platys,* flat, + *helmins,* worm), or flatworms, the Rhynchocoela (Gr., *rhynchos,* beak, + *koilos,* hollow), or ribbon worms, and the Gnathostomulida (Gr., *gnathos,* jaw, + *stoma,* mouth, + L., *ulus,* dim.), or jaw worms, are the most primitive groups of animals to have primary bilateral symmetry, the type of symmetry assumed by all higher animals. Bilateral symmetry is much more suitable for active movement than is radial symmetry. Active crawling or swimming is itself a selective pressure for better sensory organs and nervous control and coordination. It is clearly more efficient to have such organs and centers concentrated in an area of the body that meets the environment first: the anterior end. Selection for an anterior end with its concentrated sensory and nervous organs creates bilateral symmetry and, concurrently, the evolution of a head, or cephalization. All animal groups higher in the evolutionary tree than the Platyhelminthes are bilaterally symmetrical or have been derived from bilateral ancestors.

These phyla have only one internal space, the digestive cavity, with the region between the ectoderm and endoderm filled with mesoderm in the form of muscle fibers and mesenchyme (parenchyma). Since they lack a coelom or a pseudocoel, they are termed **acoelomate** animals, and because they have three well-defined germ layers, they are **triploblastic.** Acoelomates show more specialization and division of labor among their organs than do the radiate animals because the mesoderm makes more elaborate organs possible; thus, the acoelomates are said to have reached the organ-system level of organization.

These phyla belong to the protostome division of the Bilateria and have spiral cleavage. They have some centralization of the nervous system, with a concentration of nerves anteriorly and a ladder-type arrangement of trunks and connectives down the body. They have an excretory (or osmoregulatory) system, and the rhynchocoels are the most primitive phylum with a circulatory system. They also have a one-way digestive system, with an anus as well as a mouth.

PHYLUM PLATYHELMINTHES

The term "worm" has been loosely applied to elongated, bilateral invertebrate animals without appendages. At one time zoologists considered worms (Vermes) to be a group in their own right. Such a group included a highly diverse assortment of forms. This unnatural assemblage has been reclassified into various phyla. By tradition, however, zoologists still refer to the various groups of these animals as flatworms, ribbon worms, roundworms, segmented worms, and the like.

The Platyhelminthes were derived from an ancestor that probably had many cnidarian-like characteristics, perhaps an ancestor shared by the cnidarians. Nonetheless, replacement of the jellylike mesoglea of cnidarians with a cellular, mesodermal parenchyma laid the basis for a more complex organization. Parenchyma is a form of "packing" tissue containing more cells and fibers than the mesoglea of the cnidarians. In at least some platyhelminths, the parenchyma is comprised of the noncontractile cell bodies of muscle cells.

Flatworms range in size from a millimeter or less to some of the tapeworms that are many meters in length. Their flattened bodies may be slender, broadly leaflike, or long and ribbonlike.

The flatworms include both free-living and parasitic forms, but the free-living members are found exclusively in the class Turbellaria. A few turbellarians are symbiotic or parasitic, but the majority are adapted as bottom dwellers in marine or fresh water or live in moist places on land. Many, especially of the larger species, are found on the underside of stones and other hard objects in freshwater streams or in the littoral zones of the ocean.

Relatively few turbellarians live in fresh water. Planarians (Fig. 11-1) and some others frequent streams and spring pools; others prefer flowing water of mountain streams. Some species occur in fairly hot springs. Terrestrial turbellarians are found in fairly moist places under stones and logs.

All members of the classes Monogenea and Trematoda (the flukes) and the class Cestoda (the tapeworms) are parasitic. Most of the Monogenea are ectoparasites, but all the trematodes and cestodes are endoparasitic. Many species have indirect life cycles with more than one host; the first host is often an invertebrate, and the final host is usually a vertebrate. Humans serve as hosts for a number of species. Certain larval stages may be free living.

CHARACTERISTICS

1. Three germ layers (**triploblastic**)   *cephalic (head)*
2. **Bilateral symmetry;** definite polarity of <u>anterior</u> and <u>posterior</u> ends   *caudal (tail)*
3. **Body flattened dorsoventrally;** oral and genital apertures mostly on ventral surface
4. Epidermis may be cellular or syncytial (ciliated in some); **rhabdites** in epidermis of most Turbellaria; epidermis a syncytial **tegument** in Monogenea, Trematoda, and Cestoda

Figure 11-1

Stained planarian.
Courtesy Carolina Biological Supply Co., Burlington, N.C.

Eyespot
Auricle
Anterior trunk of enteron
Pharynx
Posterior trunks of enteron

5. Muscular system primarily of a sheath form and of mesodermal origin; layers of circular, longitudinal, and sometimes oblique fibers beneath the epidermis
6. No internal body space other than digestive tube (acoelomate); spaces between organs filled with parenchyma, a form of connective tissue or mesenchyme
7. Digestive system incomplete (gastrovascular type); absent in some — Cestoda
8. **Nervous system consisting of a pair of anterior ganglia with longitudinal nerve cords connected by transverse nerves and located in the mesenchyme in most forms;** similar to cnidarians in primitive forms
9. Simple sense organs; eyespots in some
10. Excretory system of two lateral canals with branches bearing **flame cells (protonephridia)**; lacking in some primitive forms   H₂O balance
11. Respiratory, circulatory, and skeletal systems lacking; lymph channels with free cells in some trematodes
12. Most forms monoecious; reproductive system complex, usually with well-developed gonads, ducts, and accessory organs; internal fertilization; development direct in free-swimming forms and those with a single host in the life cycle; usually indirect in internal parasites in which there may be a complicated life cycle often involving several hosts
13. Class Turbellaria mostly free living; classes Monogenea, Trematoda, and Cestoda entirely parasitic

CLASSIFICATION

Class Turbellaria (tur′bel-lar′e-a) (L., *turbellae* [pl.], stir, bustle, + *aria*, like or connected with)—the turbellarians. Usually free-living forms with soft flattened bodies; covered with ciliated epidermis containing secreting cells and rodlike bodies (rhabdites); mouth usually on ventral surface sometimes near center of body; no body cavity except intercellular lacunae in parenchyma; mostly hermaphroditic, but some have asexual fission. Examples: *Dugesia* (planaria), *Microstomum, Planocera.*
Class Monogenea (mon′o-gen′e-a) (Gr., *mono,* single, + *gene,* origin, birth)—the monogenetic flukes. Body covered with a syncytial tegument without cilia; body usually leaflike to cylindrical in shape; posterior attachment organ with hooks, suckers, or clamps, usually in combination; monoecious; development direct, with single host and usually with free-swimming, ciliated larva; all parasitic, mostly on skin or gills of fish. Examples: *Dactylogyrus, Polystoma, Gyrodactylus.*
Class Trematoda (trem′a-to′da) (Gr., *trematodes,* with holes, + *eidos,* form)—the digenetic flukes. Body covered with a syncytial tegument without cilia; leaflike or cylindrical in shape; usually with oral and ventral suckers, no hooks; alimentary canal usually with two main branches; mostly monoecious; development indirect, with first host a mollusc, final host usually a vertebrate; parasitic in all classes of vertebrates. Examples: *Fasciola, Clonorchis, Schistosoma.*
Class Cestoda (ses-to′da) (Gr., *kestos,* girdle, + *eidos,* form)—the tapeworms. Body covered with nonciliated, syncytial tegument; general form of body tapelike; scolex with suckers or hooks, sometimes both, for attachment; body usually divided into series of proglottids; no digestive organs; usually monoecious; parasitic in digestive tract of all classes of vertebrates; development indirect with two or more hosts; first host may be vertebrate or invertebrate. Examples: *Diphyllobothrium, Hymenolepis, Taenia.*

___ Class Turbellaria

Turbellarians are mostly free-living worms that range in length from 5 mm or less to 50 cm. Usually covered with ciliated epidermis, these are mostly creeping worms that combine muscular with ciliary movements to achieve locomotion. The mouth is on the ventral side. Unlike the trematodes and cestodes, they have simple life cycles.

The orders of Turbellaria can be divided into two groups based on specialization of the female reproductive system and embryogenesis. In the more prim-

Figure 11-2

Cross section of planarian through pharyngeal region, showing relationships of body structures.

itive group, the yolk for nutrition of the developing embryo is contained in the egg cell itself (**endolecithal**), and the embryogenesis shows the spiral determinate cleavage typical of protostomes (p. 129). In the more advanced group, the egg cell contains little or no yolk, and the yolk is contributed by cells released from organs called **vitellaria** (**ectolecithal**). Usually a number of yolk cells are combined with the zygote within the eggshell, affecting cleavage in such a way that the spiral pattern cannot be distinguished.

Of the several orders in the more primitive group, the order Acoela (Gr., *a*, without, + *koilos*, hollow) is often regarded as having changed least from the ancestral form. Its members are small and have a mouth but no gastrovascular cavity or excretory system. Food is merely passed through the mouth or pharynx into temporary spaces that are surrounded by a syncytial mesenchyme where gastrodermal phagocytic cells digest the food intracellularly. The order has a syncytial epidermis and a diffuse nervous system.

Form and function

The freshwater planarians, such as *Dugesia* (formerly called *Euplanaria* but changed by priority to *Dugesia* after Dugès, who first described the form in 1830), belong to one of the more advanced orders and are used extensively in introductory laboratories. The outer covering is a ciliated epidermis resting on a basement membrane. It contains rod-shaped **rhabdites** that, when discharged with water, swell and form a protective mucous sheath around the body. Single-cell mucous glands open on the surface of the epidermis (Fig. 11-2). Tyler (1976) described dual-gland adhesive organs in the epidermis of most turbellarian orders. These consist of three cell types: viscid and releasing gland cells and anchor cells (Fig. 11-3). Secretions of the viscid gland cells apparently fasten the microvilli of the anchor cells to the substrate, and the secretions of the releasing gland cells provide a quick, chemical detaching mechanism.

In the body wall below the basement membrane of tubellarians are layers of **muscle fibers** that run circularly, longitudinally, and diagonally. A meshwork of **parenchyma** cells, developed from mesoderm, fills the spaces between muscles and visceral organs. Parenchyma cells in some, perhaps all, flatworms are not a separate cell type but are the noncontractile portions of muscle cells (Lumsden and Specian, 1980).

Freshwater planarians move by gliding, head slightly raised, over a slime track secreted by the marginal adhesive glands. The beating of the epidermal cilia in the slime track drives the animal along. Rhythmical muscular waves can also be seen passing backward from the head as it glides. A less common method is crawling.

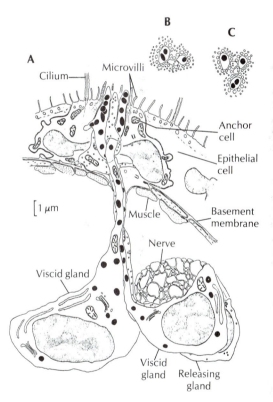

Figure 11-3

A, Reconstruction of dual-gland adhesive organ of the turbellarian *Haplopharynx* sp. There are two viscid glands and one releasing gland, which lie beneath the body wall. The anchor cell lies within the epidermis, and one of the viscid glands and the releasing gland are in contact with a nerve. **B** and **C,** Arrangement, as seen in transverse section, of microvilli and neck tips in an organ with two viscid glands and one releasing gland, **B,** and in an organ with three viscid glands and two releasing glands, **C.**

From Tyler, S. 1976. Zoomorphologie **84**:1-76.

Figure 11-4

A, Reproductive and osmoregulatory systems in planaria. Portions of male and female organs omitted to show part of osmoregulatory system. Inset at left is enlargement of flame cell. B, Diagrammatic view of digestive system and ladder-type nervous system of planaria. Cut section shows relation of pharynx, in resting position, to digestive system and mouth on ventral surface. C, Pharynx extended through ventral mouth.

Nutrition and digestion

The digestive system includes a mouth, a pharynx, and an intestine. The pharynx, enclosed in a **pharyngeal sheath** (Fig. 11-4), opens posteriorly just inside the mouth, through which it can extend (Fig. 11-4). The intestine has three many-branched trunks, one anterior and two posterior. The whole forms a **gastrovascular cavity** lined with columnar epithelium (Fig. 11-4).

Planarians are mainly carnivorous, feeding largely on small crustaceans, nematodes, rotifers, and insects. They can detect food from some distance by means of chemoreceptors. They entangle their prey in mucus secretions from the mucous glands and rhabdites. The planarian grips its prey with its anterior end, wraps its body around the prey, extends its proboscis, and sucks up minute bits of the food. Intestinal secretions contain proteolytic enzymes for some **extracellular digestion.** Bits of food are sucked up into the intestine, where the phagocytic cells of the gastrodermis complete the digestion (**intracellular**). The gastrovascular cavity ramifies to most parts of the body, and food is absorbed through its walls into the body cells. Undigested food is egested through the pharynx.

Excretion and osmoregulation

Except in the Acoela the osmoregulatory system of turbellarians consists of canals with tubules that end in **flame cells (protonephridia)** (Fig. 11-4, A). The flame cell surrounds a small space into which a tuft of cilia projects. The space is continuous with the tubule complex, and the beat of the cilia (resembling a flickering flame) provides force to drive fluids through the system. The tubules lead into collecting ducts that finally open to the outside by pores. Among the various flatworms, there may be a single protonephridium or from one to four pairs. In planarians they anastomose into a network along each side of the animal (Fig. 11-4) and may empty through many nephridiopores. That this system is mainly osmoregulatory is indicated by the observation that it is reduced or absent in marine turbellarians, which do not have to expel excess water.

Metabolic wastes are removed largely by diffusion through the body wall.

Respiration

There are no respiratory organs. Exchange of gases takes place through the body surface.

Nervous system

The most primitive flatworm nervous system, found in some of the acoels, is a **subepidermal nerve plexus** resembling the nerve net of the cnidarians. Other flatworms have, in addition to a nerve plexus, one to five pairs of **longitudinal nerve cords** lying under the muscle layer. The more advanced flatworms tend to have the lesser number of nerve cords. Freshwater planarians have one ventral pair (Fig. 11-4, *B*). Connecting nerves form a "ladder-type" pattern. The brain is a bilobed mass of ganglion cells arising anteriorly from the ventral nerve cords. Except in the acoels, which have a diffuse system, the neurons are organized into sensory, motor, and association types—an important advance in the evolution of the nervous system.

Sense organs

Active locomotion in flatworms has favored not only cephalization in the nervous system but also advancements in the development of sense organs. Ocelli, or light-sensitive eyespots, are common in the turbellarians (Fig. 11-1).

Tactile cells and chemoreceptive cells are abundant over the body, and in planarians they form definite organs on the auricles (the earlike lobes on the sides of the head). Some also have statocysts for equilibrium and rheoreceptors for sensing water current direction.

Reproduction

Many turbellarians reproduce both asexually (by fission) and sexually. Asexually, the freshwater planarian merely constricts behind the pharynx and separates into two animals, each of which regenerates the missing parts—a quick means of population increase. There is evidence that a reduced population density results in an increase in the rate of fissioning. In some forms, such as *Stenostomum* (Gr., *stenos*, narrow, + *stoma*, mouth) and *Microstomum* (Gr., *mikros*, small, + *stoma*, mouth), in which fissioning occurs, the individuals do not separate at once but remain attached, forming chains of zooids (Fig. 11-5, *B* and *C*).

Turbellarians are monoecious (hermaphroditic) but practice cross-fertilization. During the breeding season each individual develops both male and female organs, which usually open through a common genital pore (Fig. 11-4, *A*). After copulation one or more fertilized eggs and some yolk cells become enclosed in a small cocoon. The cocoons are attached by little stalks to the underside of stones or plants. Embryos emerge as juveniles that resemble mature adults. In some marine forms the egg develops into a ciliated free-swimming larva.

____ Class Monogenea

The monogenetic flukes traditionally have been placed as an order of the Trematoda, but they are sufficiently different to deserve a separate class. They are all parasites, primarily of the gills and external surfaces of fish. A few are found in the urinary bladders of frogs and turtles, and one has been reported from the eye of a hippopotamus. Although widespread and common, monogeneans seem to cause little damage to their hosts under natural conditions. However, like numerous

Phagocata

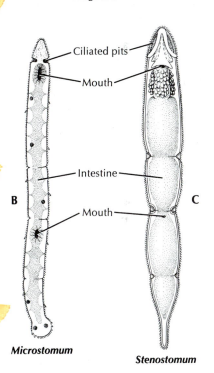

Microstomum

Stenostomum

Figure 11-5

Some small freshwater turbellarians. **A,** *Phagocata* has numerous pharynges. **B** and **C,** Incomplete fission results for a time in a series of attached zooids.

Figure 11-6

Gyrodactylus cylindriformis, ventral view.

From Mueller, J.F., and H.J. Van Cleave. 1932. Roosevelt Wildlife Annals.

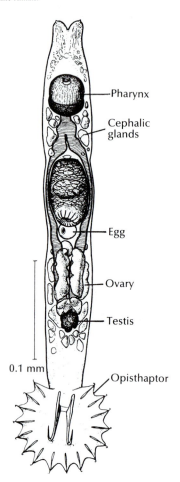

- Pharynx
- Cephalic glands
- Egg
- Ovary
- Testis
- Opisthaptor

0.1 mm

other fish pathogens, they become a serious threat when their hosts are crowded together, as in fish farming.

The life cycles of monogeneans are direct, with a single host. The egg hatches a ciliated larva, the **oncomiracidium,** that attaches to the host or swims around awhile before attachment. The oncomiracidium bears hooks on its posterior, which in many species become the hooks on the large posterior attachment organ (**opisthaptor**) of the adult. Because the monogenean must cling to the host and withstand the force of water flow over the gills or skin, adaptive radiation has produced a wide array of opisthaptors in different species. Opisthaptors may bear large and small hooks, suckers, and clamps, often in combination with each other.

Common genera are *Gyrodactylus* (L., *gyro*, a circle, + Gr., *daktylos*, toe, finger) (Fig. 11-6) and *Dactylogyrus* (Gr., *daktylos,* toe, finger, + L., *gyro*, a circle), both of economic importance to fish culturists, and *Polystoma* (Gr., *polys*, many, + *stoma*, mouth), found in the urinary bladder of frogs.

____ Class Trematoda

Trematodes are all parasitic flukes, and as adults they are almost all found as endoparasites of vertebrates. They are chiefly leaflike in form and are structurally similar in many respects to the more advanced Turbellaria. A major difference is found in the body covering, or **tegument,** which does not bear cilia in the adult. Furthermore, in common with Monogenea and Cestoda, cell bodies are sunk beneath the outer layer (Fig. 11-7) and superficial muscle layers and communicate with the outer layer (distal cytoplasm) by processes extending between the muscles. Because the distal cytoplasm is continuous, with no intervening cell membranes, the tegument is **syncytial.** This peculiar epidermal arrangement is probably related to adaptations for parasitism in ways that are still unclear.

Other structural adaptations for parasitism are more apparent: various penetration glands or glands to produce cyst material; organs for adhesion such as suckers and hooks; and increased reproductive capacity. Otherwise, trematodes retain several turbellarian characteristics, such as a well-developed alimentary canal (but with the mouth at the anterior, or cephalic, end) and similar reproductive, excretory, and nervous systems, as well as a musculature and parenchyma that are only slightly modified from those of the Turbellaria. Sense organs are poorly developed.

Of the subclasses of Trematoda, Aspidogastrea and Didymozoidea are small and poorly known groups, but Digenea (Gr., *dis*, double, + *genos*, race) is a large group with many species of medical and economic importance.

Subclass Digenea

With rare exceptions, digenetic trematodes have an indirect life cycle, the first (**intermediate**) host being a mollusc and the final (**definitive**) host being a vertebrate. In some species a second, and sometimes even a third, intermediate host intervenes. The group has been very successful and they inhabit, according to species, a wide variety of sites in their hosts: all parts of the digestive tract, respiratory tract, circulatory system, urinary tract, and reproductive tract.

One of the world's most amazing biological phenomena is the digenean life cycle. Although the cycles of different species vary widely in detail, a typical example would include the adult, egg, miracidium, sporocyst, redia, cercaria, and

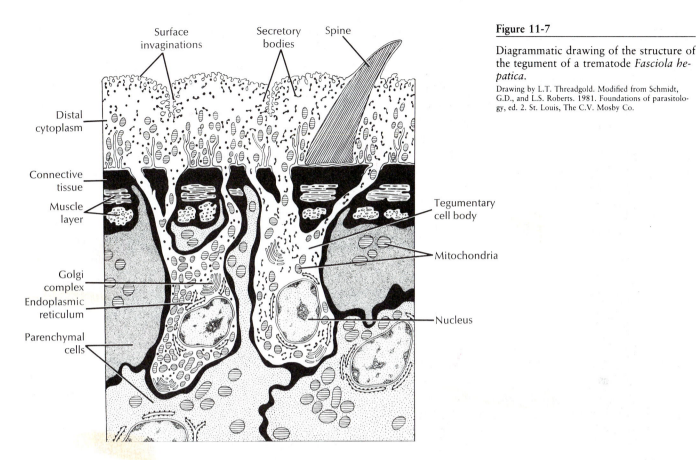

Figure 11-7

Diagrammatic drawing of the structure of the tegument of a trematode *Fasciola hepatica.*

Drawing by L.T. Threadgold. Modified from Schmidt, G.D., and L.S. Roberts. 1981. Foundations of parasitology, ed. 2. St. Louis, The C.V. Mosby Co.

metacercaria stages (Fig. 11-8). The **egg** usually passes from the definitive host in the excreta and must reach water to develop further. There, it hatches to a free-swimming, ciliated larva, the **miracidium.** The miracidium penetrates the tissues of a snail, where it transforms into a **sporocyst.** The sporocyst reproduces asexually to yield either more sporocysts or a number of **rediae.** The rediae, in turn, reproduce asexually to produce more rediae or to produce **cercariae.** In this way a single egg can give rise to an enormous number of progeny. The cercariae emerge from the snail and penetrate a second intermediate host or encyst on vegetation or other objects to become **metacercariae,** which are juvenile flukes. The adult grows from the metacercaria when that stage is eaten by the definitive host.

Some of the most serious parasites of humans and domestic animals belong to the Digenea. The first digenetic life cycle to be worked out was that of *Fasciola hepatica* (L., *fasciola,* a small bundle, band), which causes "liver rot" in sheep and other ruminants. The adult fluke lives in the bile passage of the liver, and the eggs are passed in the feces. After hatching, the miracidium penetrates a snail to become a sporocyst. There are two generations of rediae, and the cercaria encysts on vegetation. When the infested vegetation is eaten by the sheep or other ruminant (or sometimes humans), the metacercariae excyst and grow into young flukes.

Clonorchis sinensis—liver fluke of humans

Clonorchis (Gr., *clon,* branch, + *orchis,* testis) (Fig. 11-8) is the most important liver fluke of humans and is common in many regions of the Orient, especially in China, southern Asia, and Japan. Cats, dogs, and pigs are also often infected.

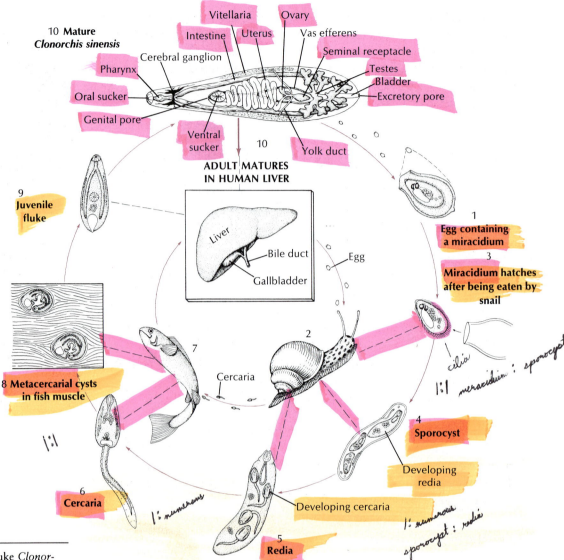

10 **Mature**
Clonorchis sinensis

Vitellaria   Ovary
Intestine   Uterus   Vas efferens
Seminal receptacle
Cerebral ganglion   Testes
Pharynx   Bladder
Oral sucker   Excretory pore
Genital pore
Ventral sucker   Yolk duct
ADULT MATURES IN HUMAN LIVER
10

9 **Juvenile fluke**

Liver
Bile duct
Gallblader

Egg

1 **Egg containing a miracidium**

3 **Miracidium hatches after being eaten by snail**

cilia

1:1 miracidium : sporocyst

4 **Sporocyst**

Developing redia

8 **Metacercarial cysts in fish muscle**

7
Cercaria

2

6 **Cercaria**

Developing cercaria

1: numerous

5 **Redia**

1: numerous sporocyst : redia

Figure 11-8

Life cycle of human liver fluke *Clonorchis sinensis*. Egg, *1*, shed from adult trematode, *10*, in bile ducts of human, is carried out of body in feces and is ingested by snail *(Parafossarulus)*, *2*, in which miracidium, *3*, hatches and becomes mother sporocyst. *4*, Young rediae are produced in sporocyst, grow, *5*, and in turn produce young cercariae. Cercariae then leave snail, *6*, find a fish host, *7*, and burrow under scales to encyst in muscle, *8*. When raw or improperly cooked fish containing cysts is eaten by a human, metacercaria is released, *9*, and enters bile duct, where it matures, *10*, to shed eggs into feces, *1*, thus starting another cycle.

Structure

The worms vary from 10 to 20 mm in length (Fig. 11-8). Their structure is typical of many trematodes in most respects. They have an **oral sucker** and a **ventral sucker**. The **digestive system** consists of a pharynx, a muscular esophagus, and two long, unbranched intestinal ceca. The **excretory system** consists of two protonephridial tubules, with branches provided with flame cells or bulbs. The two tubules unite to form a single median tubule that opens to the outside. The **nervous system**, like that of turbellarians, is made up of two cerebral ganglia connected to longitudinal cords that have transverse connectives.

The **reproductive system** is hermaphroditic and complex. The **male system** is made up of two branched **testes** and two **vasa efferentia** that unite to form a single **vas deferens**, which widens into a **seminal vesicle**. The seminal vesicle leads into an **ejaculatory duct**, which terminates at the genital opening. Unlike most trematodes, *Clonorchis* does *not* have a protrusible copulatory organ, the cirrus. The female system contains a branched **ovary** with a short **oviduct**, which is joined by ducts from the **seminal receptacle** and the **vitellaria** at the ootype. The ootype is surrounded by a glandular mass, **Mehlis' gland**, of uncertain function. From Mehlis' gland the much-convoluted **uterus** runs to the genital pore. Cross-fertilization between individuals is usual, and sperm are stored in the seminal receptacle. When an ovum is released from the ovary, it is joined by a sperm and a group of vitelline cells and is fertilized. The vitelline cells release a proteinaceous shell material, which is stabilized by a chemical reaction; the Mehlis' gland secretions are added; and the egg passes into the uterus.

Life cycle

The normal habitat of the adults is in the bile passageways of humans and other fish-eating mammals (Fig. 11-8). The eggs, each containing a complete **miracidium,** are shed into the water with the feces but do not hatch until they are ingested by the snail *Parofossarulus* or related genera. The eggs, however, may live for some weeks in water. In the snail the miracidium enters the tissues and transforms into the **sporocyst** (a baglike structure with embryonic germ cells), which produces one generation of **rediae.** The redia is elongated, with an alimentary canal, a nervous system, an excretory system, and many germ cells in the process of development. The rediae pass into the liver of the snail where the germ cells continue embryonation and give rise to the tadpolelike **cercariae.**

The cercariae escape into the water, swim about until they meet with fish of the family Cyprinidae, and then bore into the muscles or under the scales. Here the cercariae lose their tails and encyst as **metacercariae.** If a mammal eats raw infected fish, the metacercarial cyst dissolves in the intestine, and the young flukes apparently migrate up the bile duct, where they become adults. There the flukes may live for 15 to 30 years.

The effect of the flukes on humans depends mainly on the extent of the infection. A heavy infection may cause a pronounced cirrhosis of the liver and may result in death. Cases are diagnosed through fecal examinations. To avoid infection, all fish used as food should be thoroughly cooked. Destruction of the snails that carry larval stages would be a method of control.

Schistosoma—blood flukes

Schistosomiasis, infection with blood flukes of the genus *Schistosoma* (Gr., *schistos,* divided, + *soma,* body), ranks as one of the major infectious diseases in the world, with 200 million people infected. The disease is widely prevalent over much of Africa and parts of South America, the West Indies, the Middle East, and the Far East. The old generic name for the worms was *Bilharzia* (from Theodor Bilharz, German parasitologist who discovered *Schistosoma haematobium*), and the infection was called bilharziasis, a name still used in many areas.

The blood flukes differ from most other flukes in being dioecious and having the two branches of the digestive tube united into a single tube in the posterior part of the body. The male is broader and heavier and has a large, ventral groove, the **gynecophoric canal,** posterior to the ventral sucker. The gynecophoric canal embraces the long, slender female (Fig. 11-9).

Three species account for most of the schistosomiasis in humans: *S. mansoni,* which lives primarily in the venules draining the large intestine; *S. japonicum,* which is found mostly in the venules of the small intestine; and *S. haematobium,* which lives in the venules of the urinary bladder. *S. mansoni* is common in parts of Africa, Brazil, northern South America, and the West Indies; species of *Biomphalaria* are the principal snail intermediate hosts. *S. haematobium* is widely prevalent in Africa, using snails of the genera *Bulinus* and *Physopsis* as the main

Figure 11-9

Adult male and female *Schistosoma mansoni* in copulation. Male has long gynecophoric canal that holds female (the darkly stained individual) during insemination and oviposition. Humans are usually hosts of adult parasites, found mainly in Africa but also in South America and elsewhere. Humans become infected by wading or bathing in cercaria-infested waters.
AFIP No. 56-3334.

Figure 11-10

Human abdomen, showing schistosome dermatitis caused by penetration of schistosome cercariae that are unable to complete development in humans. Sensitization to allergenic substances released by cercariae results in rash and itching.

Original photograph courtesy R.E. Kuntz. From H. Zaiman (ed.), A pictorial presentation of parasites.

Unfortunately, some projects intended to raise the standard of living in some tropical countries, such as the Aswan High Dam in Egypt, have increased the prevalence of schistosomiasis by creating more habitats for the snail intermediate hosts. Before the dam was constructed, the 500 miles of the Nile River between Aswan and Cairo was subjected to annual floods; alternate flooding and drying killed many snails. Four years after dam completion, the prevalence of schistosomiasis had increased sevenfold along that segment of the river. The prevalence in fishermen around the lake above the dam increased from a very low level to 76%.

intermediate hosts. *S. japonicum* is confined to the Far East, and its hosts are several species of *Oncomelania*.

The plan of the life history of blood flukes is similar in all species. Eggs are discharged in human feces or urine; if they get into water, they hatch out as ciliated **miracidia,** which must contact the required kind of snail within a few hours to survive. In the snail, they transform into **sporocysts,** which produce another generation of sporocysts. The daughter sporocysts give rise to **cercariae** directly, without the formation of rediae. The cercariae escape from the snail and swim about until they come in contact with the bare skin of a human. They penetrate the skin, shedding their tails in the process, and reach a blood vessel where they enter the circulatory system. There is no metacercarial stage. The young schistosomes make their way to the hepatic portal system of blood vessels and undergo a period of development in the liver before migrating to their characteristic sites. As eggs are released by the adult female, they are somehow extruded through the wall of the venule and through the gut or bladder lining, to be voided with the feces or urine, according to species. Many eggs do not make this difficult transit and are swept by the blood flow back to the liver or other areas, where they become centers of inflammation and tissue reaction.

The main ill effects of schistosomiasis result from the eggs. With *S. mansoni* and *S. japonicum*, eggs in the intestinal wall cause ulceration, abscesses, and bloody diarrhea with abdominal pain. Similarly, *S. haematobium* causes ulceration of the bladder wall with bloody urine and pain on urination. Eggs swept to the liver or other sites cause symptoms associated with the organs where they lodge. When they are caught in the capillary bed of the liver, they impede circulation and cause cirrhosis, a fibrotic reaction that interferes with liver function. Of the three species, *S. haematobium* is considered the least serious and *S. japonicum* the most severe. The prognosis is poor in heavy infections of *S. japonicum* without early treatment.

Control is best carried out by educating people to dispose of their body wastes hygienically, a difficult problem with poor people under primitive conditions.

Schistosome dermatitis (swimmer's itch)

Various species of schistosomes in several genera are known to cause a rash or dermatitis when their cercariae penetrate hosts that are unsuitable for further development (Fig. 11-10). The cercariae of several genera whose normal hosts are North American birds cause dermatitis in bathers in northern lakes. The severity of the rash increases with an increasing number of contacts with the organisms, or sensitization. After penetration, the cercariae are attacked and killed by the host's immune mechanisms, and they release allergenic substances, causing itching. The condition is more an annoyance than a serious threat to health, but there may be economic losses to persons depending on vacation trade around infested lakes.

Paragonimus—lung flukes

Several species of *Paragonimus* (Gr., *para*, beside, + *gonimos*, generative), a fluke that lives in the lungs of its host, are known from a variety of mammals. *Paragonimus westermani* (Fig. 11-11), found in the Orient, Southwest Pacific, and some parts of South America, parasitizes a number of wild carnivores, humans, pigs, and rodents. Its eggs are coughed up in the sputum, swallowed, then eliminated with the feces. The metacercariae are found in freshwater crabs, and the infection is acquired by eating uncooked crab meat. The infection causes respiratory symptoms, with breathing difficulties and chronic cough. Fatal cases are common. A closely related species, *P. kellicotti,* is found in mink and similar animals in North America, but only one human case has been recorded. Its metacercariae are in crayfish.

Some other trematodes

Fasciolopsis buski (L., *fasciola,* small bundle, + Gr., *opsis,* appearance) (intestinal fluke of humans) parasitizes humans and pigs in India and China. Larval stages occur in several species of planorbid snails, and the cercariae encyst on water chestnuts, an aquatic vegetation eaten raw by humans and pigs.

Leucochloridium is noted for its remarkable sporocysts. Snails (*Succinea*) eat vegetation infected with eggs from bird droppings. The sporocysts become much enlarged and branched, and the cercariae encyst within the sporocyst. The sporocysts enter the snail's head and tentacles, become brightly striped with orange and green bands, and pulsate at frequent intervals. Birds are attracted by the enlarged and pulsating tentacles, eat the snails, and so complete the life cycle.

___ Class Cestoda

Cestoda, or tapeworms, differ in many respects from the preceding classes. They usually have long, flat bodies in which there is a linear series of sets of reproductive organs. Each set is called a proglottid and is usually set off at its anterior and posterior ends by zones of muscle weakness, marked externally by grooves. There is a complete lack of a digestive system. As in Monogenea and Trematoda, there are no external, motile cilia in the adult, and the tegument is of a distal cytoplasm with sunken cell bodies beneath the superficial muscle layer (Fig. 11-7). In contrast to the monogenes and trematodes, however, their entire surface is covered with minute projections called **microtriches**. The microtriches greatly enlarge the surface area of the tegument, which is a vital adaptation of the tapeworm since it must absorb all its nutrients across the tegument.

Tapeworms are nearly all monoecious. They have well-developed muscles, and their excretory system and nervous system are somewhat similar to those of other flatworms. They have no special sense organs but do have sensory endings in the tegument that are modified cilia. One of their most specialized structures is the **scolex**, or holdfast, which is the organ of attachment. It is usually provided with suckers or suckerlike organs and often with hooks or spiny tentacles (Fig. 11-12).

With rare exceptions, all cestodes require at least two hosts, and the adult is a parasite in the digestive tract of vertebrates. Often one of the intermediate hosts is an invertebrate.

The class Cestoda is divided into two subclasses: Cestodaria and Eucestoda. The Cestodaria is a small group found in a few lower vertebrates. Their bodies are not divided into separate proglottids and have only one set of reproductive organs (**monozoic**). Their larvae have 10 hooks.

The Eucestoda contains the great majority of species in the class. With the exception of two small orders, the members of this subclass have the body divided into a series of proglottids and are thus referred to as **polyzoic**. Their larval forms all have six hooks, rather than 10 as in the Cestodaria. The main body of the

Oral sucker
Vitellaria
Intestine
Ovary
Ventral sucker
Uterus
Vitelline ducts
Testes
Excretory bladder

Figure 11-11

Pulmonary fluke *Paragonimus westermani* infects human lung, producing paragonimiasis. Adults are up to 2 cm long. Eggs discharged in sputum or feces hatch into free-swimming miracidia that enter snails. Cercariae from snails enter freshwater crabs and encyst in soft tissues. Humans are infected by eating poorly cooked crabs or by drinking water containing larvae freed from dead crabs.

Photograph by R.E. Kuntz and J.A. Moore. From Schmidt, G.D., and L.S. Roberts. 1981. Foundations of parasitology, ed. 2. St. Louis, The C.V. Mosby Co.

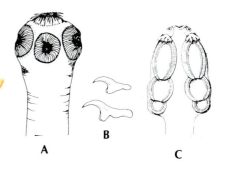

A   B   C

Figure 11-12

Two tapeworm scolices. **A,** Scolex of *Taenia solium* (pork tapeworm) with apical hooks and suckers. (Scolex of *Taeniarhynchus saginatus* is similar, but without hooks.) **B,** Hooks of *T. solium.* **C,** Scolex of *Acanthobothrium coronatum,* a tapeworm of sharks. This species has large leaflike sucker organs divided into chambers with apical suckers and hooks.

Table 11-1 Common Cestodes of Humans

Common and scientific name	Means of infection; prevalence in humans
Beef tapeworm (*Taeniarhynchus saginatus*)	Eating rare beef; most common of all tapeworms in humans
Pork tapeworm (*Taenia solium*)	Eating rare pork
Fish tapeworm (*Diphyllobothrium latum*)	Eating rare or poorly cooked fish; fairly common in Great Lakes region of United States, and other areas of world where raw fish is eaten
Dog tapeworm (*Dipylidium caninum*)	Unhygienic habits of children (juveniles in flea and louse); moderate frequency
Dwarf tapeworm (*Vampirolepis nana*)	Juveniles in flour beetles; common
Unilocular hydatid (*Echinococcus granulosus*)	Cysts of juveniles in humans; infection by contact with dogs; common wherever humans are in close relationship with dogs and ruminants
Multilocular hydatid (*Echinococcus multilocularis*)	Cysts of juveniles in humans; less common than unilocular hydatid

worms, the chain of proglottids, is called the **strobila**. Typically, there is a **germinative zone** just behind the scolex where new proglottids are formed. As new proglottids are differentiated in front of it, each individual segment moves posteriorly in the strobila, and its gonads mature. The proglottid is usually fertilized by another proglottid in the same or a different strobila. The shelled embryos form in the uterus of the proglottid, and either they are expelled through a uterine pore or the entire proglottid is shed from the worm as it reaches the posterior end.

Some zoologists have maintained that the proglottid formation of cestodes represents "true" segmentation (metamerism), but we do not support this view. Segmentation of tapeworms is best considered a replication of sex organs to increase reproductive capacity and is not related to the metamerism found in Annelida, Arthropoda, and Chordata (p. 142).

More than 1000 species of tapeworms are known to parasitologists. Almost all vertebrate species are infected. Normally, adult tapeworms do little harm to their hosts. The most common tapeworms found in humans are given in Table 11-1.

Taeniarhynchus saginatus—beef tapeworm
Structure

Taeniarhynchus saginatus (Gr., *tainia,* band, ribbon, + *rhynchos,* beak, snout) is referred to as the beef tapeworm, but it lives as an adult in the alimentary canal of humans. The juvenile form is found primarily in the intermuscular tissue of cattle. The mature adult may reach a length of 10 m or more. Its scolex has four suckers for attachment to the intestinal wall, but no hooks. A short neck connects the scolex to the **strobila,** which may be made up of as many as 2000 **proglottids.** The terminal **gravid proglottids** bear shelled, infective larvae (Fig. 11-13) and are detached and shed in the feces.

The tapeworm shows some unity in its organization, for **excretory canals** in the scolex are also connected to the canals, two on each side, in the proglottids,

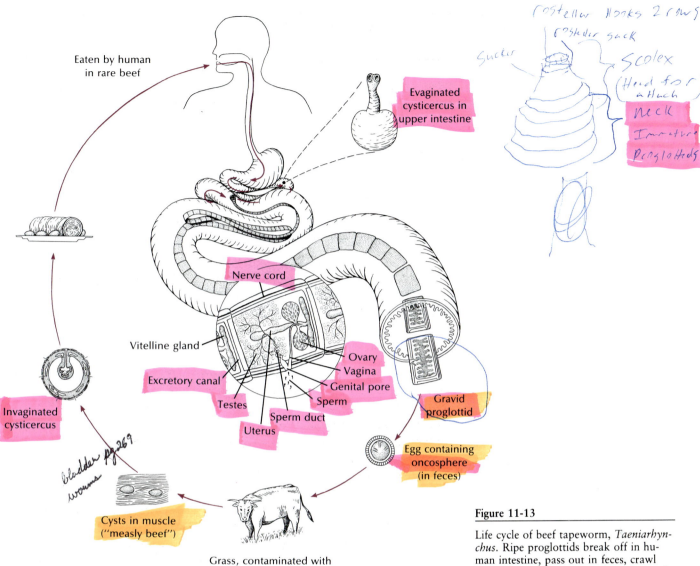

Handwritten notes (top right):
rostellar Hooks 2 rows
rostellar sack
Sucker
Scolex
(Head for a Hech)
neck
Immature
Proglottids

Eaten by human
in rare beef

Evaginated
cysticercus in
upper intestine

Nerve cord

Vitelline gland

Excretory canal

Testes

Ovary
Vagina
Genital pore
Sperm
Sperm duct

Uterus

Invaginated
cysticercus

Gravid
proglottid

Egg containing
oncosphere
(in feces)

bladder pg 269
worms

Cysts in muscle
("measly beef")

Grass, contaminated with
eggs, ingested by cow

Figure 11-13

Life cycle of beef tapeworm, *Taeniarhynchus*. Ripe proglottids break off in human intestine, pass out in feces, crawl out of feces onto grass, and are ingested by cattle. Eggs hatch in cow's intestine, freeing oncospheres, which penetrate into muscles and encyst, developing into "bladder worms." Human eats infected rare beef, and cysticercus is freed in intestine where it attaches to the intestine wall, forms a strobila, and matures.

and two longitudinal **nerve cords** from a **nerve ring** in the scolex run back into the proglottids also (Fig. 11-14). Attached to the excretory ducts are the **flame cells.** Each mature proglottid also contains **muscles** and **parenchyma** as well as a complete set of **male** and **female organs** similar to those of a trematode.

In the order to which this species belongs, however, the vitellaria are typically a single, compact **vitelline gland** located just posterior to the ovaries. When the gravid proglottids break off and pass out with the feces, they usually crawl out of the fecal mass and onto vegetation nearby. There they may be picked up by grazing cattle. The proglottid ruptures as it dries up, further scattering the embryos on soil and grass. The embryos may remain viable on grass for as long as 5 months.

Life cycle

When cattle swallow the eggs, the eggs hatch, and the six-hooked larvae (**oncospheres**) burrow through the intestinal wall into the blood or lymph vessels and finally reach voluntary muscle, where they encyst to become **bladder worms** (juveniles called **cysticerci**). There the juveniles develop an invaginated scolex but

Figure 11-14

Photomicrograph of mature proglottid of *Taenia pisiformis*, dog tapeworm. Portions of two other proglottids also shown.

Courtesy General Biological Supply House, Inc., Chicago.

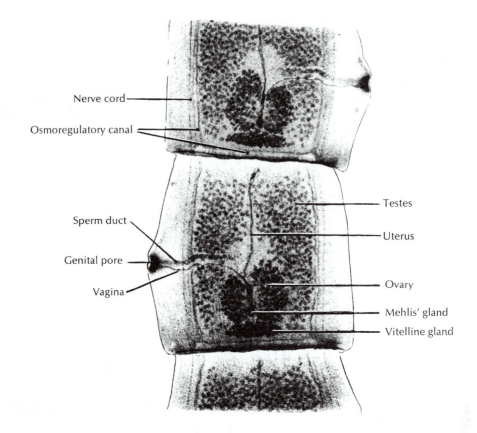

remain quiescent. When infected "measly" meat (Fig. 11-15) is eaten by a suitable host, the cyst wall dissolves, the scolex evaginates and attaches to the intestinal mucosa, and new proglottids begin to develop. It takes 2 to 3 weeks for a mature worm to form. When a person is infected with one of these tapeworms, numerous gravid proglottids are expelled daily, sometimes crawling out the anus by themselves. Humans become infected by eating rare roast beef, steaks, and barbecues. Considering that about 1% of American cattle are infected, that 20% of all cattle slaughtered are not federally inspected, and that even in inspected meat one fourth of infections are missed, it is not surprising that tapeworm infection is fairly common. Infection is precluded when meat is thoroughly cooked.

Some other tapeworms
Taenia solium—pork tapeworm

The adult *Taenia solium* (Gr., *tainia*, band, ribbon) lives in the small intestine of humans, whereas the juveniles live in the muscles of pigs. Adults may be 7 m or longer. The scolex has both suckers and hooks arranged on its tip (Fig. 11-12, *A* and *B*), the **rostellum**. The life history of this tapeworm is similar to that of the beef tapeworm. Humans become infected by eating improperly cooked pork. The incidence of infection is much lower than that of the beef tapeworm, probably because rare pork is less popular.

The pork tapeworm (*T. solium*) is considered more dangerous than *T. saginatus* because the cysticerci, as well as the adults, can develop in humans. If eggs or proglottids are accidentally ingested by a human, or proglottids shed from an adult worm are carried back to the stomach by reverse peristalsis, the liberated embryos migrate to any of several organs and form cysticerci. The condition is

Figure 11-15

"Measly" pork showing cysts of bladder worms, *Taenia solium.* Beef heavily infected with beef tapeworm has a similar appearance, but lighter infections may be much less obvious.
Photograph by F.M. Hickman.

called **cysticercosis.** Common sites are the eye or brain, and infection in such locations results in blindness or serious neurological symptoms.

Diphyllobothrium latum—fish tapeworm

The adult *Diphyllobothrium* (Gr., *dis,* double, + *phyllon,* leaf, + *bothrion,* hole, trench) is found in the intestine of humans, dogs, cats, and other mammals; the immature stages are in crustaceans and fish. This tapeworm, often called the broad tapeworm, is the largest of the cestodes that infect humans. It sometimes reaches a length of 20 m and may have more than 3000 proglottids. Eggs discharged in water by the human host hatch and may be swallowed by the first intermediate host, a tiny crustacean *(Cyclops).* When the crustacean is eaten by a fish, the young juvenile migrates to the muscles where it may grow to as much as 25 mm long. Usually it encysts in the muscle. When raw or poorly cooked fish is eaten by a suitable host, the juvenile is liberated and grows into adult form. It has been known to live in a person for many years. Broad tapeworm infections are found all over the world; in the United States infections are most common in the Great Lakes region. In Finland, but apparently not other areas, the worm may cause a serious anemia.

Dipylidium caninum—dog tapeworm

Dipylidium (Gr., *dis,* double, + *pylē,* gate, entrance, + *eidos,* form) is common in pet dogs and cats and sometimes in children. It may be 30 cm or more in length and may have about 200 proglottids. The juvenile is found in the louse and flea. The dog or cat becomes infected by licking or biting these ectoparasites. It takes about 2 weeks for the worm to mature.

Vampirolepis nana—dwarf tapeworm

The dwarf tapeworm (Serb., *vampira,* blood-sucking demon, + *lepis,* a scale) is the smallest and perhaps the most common human tapeworm in the world. Its life cycle is unique in that an intermediate host is optional. The adults are 20 to 40 mm long and have 100 to 200 proglottids. The same species, although perhaps a different strain, is very common in mice. When eaten by a human or rodent, the

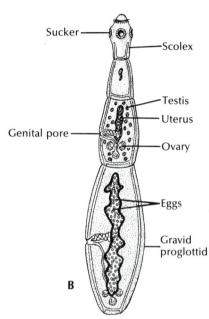

Figure 11-16

Echinococcus granulosus, dog tapeworm, which may be dangerous to humans. **A,** Early hydatid cyst or bladder-worm stage found in cattle, sheep, hogs, and sometimes humans produces hydatid disease. Humans acquire disease by unsanitary habits in association with dogs. When eggs are ingested, liberated larvae usually encyst in the liver, lungs, or other organs. Brood capsules containing scolices are formed from the inner layer of each cyst. The cyst enlarges, developing other cysts with brood pouches. It may grow for years, to the size of a basketball, necessitating surgery. **B,** Adult tapeworm lives in intestine of dog or other carnivore.

oncospheres are liberated and penetrate the intestinal mucosa, where they grow into a **cysticercoid** juvenile. After a few days they reenter the lumen of the intestine and mature into adult worms. Alternatively, if a grain beetle or any one of numerous other insects eats the eggs along with rodent feces, the larva penetrates to the insect's hemocoel and forms the cysticercoid there. The human or rodent becomes infected by ingesting the grain beetle.

The common tapeworm of rats, *Hymenolepis diminuta* (Gr., *hymēn,* membrane, + *lepis,* scale), is occasionally found in humans, but it is important for other reasons. Because its hosts are easily maintained in the laboratory, and because the worms are moderately large (up to 1 m long), *H. diminuta* is a very convenient form for experimental parasitology. Consequently, parasitologists know more about this species than any other cestode.

Echinococcus granulosus—unilocular hydatid

The adult *E. granulosus* (Gr., *echinos,* hedgehog, + *kokkos,* kernel) (Fig. 11-16, *A*) is found in dogs and other canines; the juveniles are found in more than 40 species of mammals, including humans, monkeys, sheep, reindeer, and cattle. Thus, humans serve as an intermediate host in the case of this tapeworm. The adults are only 5 to 10 mm long and have just three or four proglottids. When ingested by a suitable intermediate host, the oncosphere migrates to the liver, lung, or some other organ and slowly begins to form a special kind of cysticercus called a **hydatid cyst** (Gr., *hydatis,* watery vesicle). The hydatid grows very slowly, taking 5 months to reach a size of 1 cm, but it can grow for a very long time—up to 20 years—reaching the size of a basketball in an unrestricted site such as the liver. If the hydatid grows in a critical site such as the heart or central nervous system, serious symptoms may be felt in a much shorter time. The main cyst maintains a single or unilocular chamber, but within the main cyst, daughter cysts bud off, and each contains thousands of scolices. Each scolex will produce a worm when eaten by a canine. The only treatment is surgical removal of the hydatid.

Echinococcus multilocularis—multilocular hydatid

Echinococcus multilocularis is closely related to *E. granulosus,* except that the main definitive hosts are foxes and the main intermediate hosts are rodents. Humans can also serve as intermediate hosts. Instead of developing a thick, laminated layer and growing into a large, single cyst, like *E. granulosus, E. multilocularis* has a thin outer wall that grows and infiltrates processes into the surrounding host tissues like a cancer. Each process may have several small, fluid-filled pockets containing scolices; thus, the hydatid is **multilocular.** *E. multilocularis* is more rare in humans than is *E. granulosus,* and that is fortunate, since surgery is much more difficult because of the invasive nature of the cyst.

Moniezia expansa—sheep tapeworm

The adult is found in sheep and goats (Fig. 11-17); the juvenile grows in a small mite (family Oribatidae).

Taenia pisiformis—dog tapeworm

Taenia pisiformis is widely used as a type for study in the laboratory (Fig. 11-14). The cysticerci occur in the mesenteries and liver of rabbits; the adults are found in cats and dogs. Its occurrence in humans is rare.

PHYLUM RHYNCHOCOELA (NEMERTINA)

Rhynchocoela (ring′ko-se′la) (Gr., *rhynchos,* beak, + *koilos,* hollow) are often called the ribbon worms. Their name refers to the proboscis, a long muscular tube that can be thrust out swiftly to grasp the prey. The phylum was formerly called Nemertea or Nemertina (nem′er-ti′na) (Gr., *Nemertes,* one of the Nereids, unerring one, + *ina,* belonging to), with both names referring to the unerring aim of the proboscis. These worms are still often spoken of as the nemertean or nemertine worms. They are thread-shaped or ribbon-shaped worms; nearly all of them are marine. Some live in secreted gelatinous tubes. There are about 650 species in the group.

Nemertine worms are usually less than 20 cm long, although a few are several meters in length. *Lineus longissimus* (L., *linea,* line) is said to reach 30 m. Their colors are often bright, although most are dull or pallid. In the odd genus *Gorgonorhynchus* (Gr., *Gorgo,* name of a female monster of terrible aspect, + *rhynchos,* beak, snout) the proboscis is divided into many proboscides, which appear as a mass of wormlike structures when everted.

With few exceptions, the general body plan of the nemertines is similar to that of Turbellaria. Like the latter, their epidermis is ciliated and has many gland cells. Another striking similarity is the presence of flame cells in the excretory system. Recently rhabdites have been found in several nemertines, including *Lineus.* However, nemertines differ from flatworms in their reproductive system. They are mostly dioecious. In the marine forms there is a ciliated **pilidium larva.** This helmet-shaped larva has a ventral mouth but no anus—another flatworm characteristic. It also has some resemblance to the trochophore larva that is found in annelids and molluscs. Other flatworm characteristics are the presence of bilateral symmetry and a mesoderm and the lack of a coelom. All in all, the present evidence seems to indicate that the nemertines came from an ancestral form closely related to Platyhelminthes.

The nemertines show some advances over the flatworms. One of these is the eversible **proboscis** and its sheath, for which there are no counterparts among Platyhelminthes. Another difference is the presence of an **anus** in the adult. These forms have a **complete digestive system,** the first to be found in the animal kingdom. They are also the simplest animals to have a **blood-vascular** system.

A few of the nemertines are found in moist soil and fresh water, but by far the larger number are marine. At low tide they are often coiled up under stones. It seems probable that they are active at high tide and quiescent at low tide. Some nemertines such as *Cerebratulus* (L., *cerebrum,* brain, + *ulus,* dim. suffix) often live in empty mollusc shells. The small species live among seaweed, or they may be found swimming near the surface of the water. Nemertines are often secured by dredging at depths of 5 to 8 m or deeper. A few are commensals or parasites. *Prostoma rubrum* (Gr., *pro,* before, in front of, + *stoma,* month) which is 20 mm or less in length, is a well-known freshwater species.

CHARACTERISTICS
1. Bilateral symmetry; highly contractile body that is cylindrical anteriorly and flattened posteriorly
2. Three germ layers
3. Epidermis with cilia and gland cells; rhabdites in some
4. Body spaces with parenchyma, which is partly gelatinous
5. An **eversible proboscis,** which lies free in a cavity (rhynchocoel) above the alimentary canal

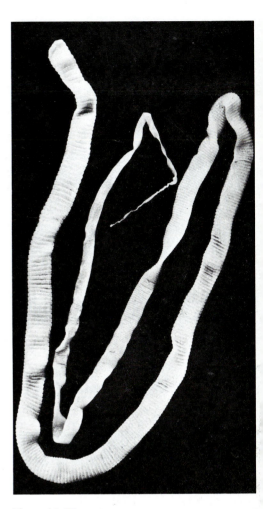

Figure 11-17

Sheep tapeworm *Moniezia expansa.* Note progressive increase in size from young proglottids budded from neck *(center)* to oldest (gravid) proglottids, shown at upper left.
Photograph by F.M. Hickman.

Figure 11-18

Ribbon worm *Tubulanus annulatus* (phylum Rhynchocoela) may be several feet long. The anterior end has the enlarged, rounded cephalic lobe.

From *Adaptive radiation—the mollusks,* an Encyclopaedia Brittanica film.

6. **Complete digestive system** (mouth to anus)
7. Body-wall musculature of outer circular and inner longitudinal layers with diagonal fibers between the two; sometimes another circular layer inside the longitudinal layer
8. **Blood-vascular system with two or three longitudinal trunks**
9. Acoelomate, although the rhynchocoel technically may be considered a true coelom
10. Nervous system usually a four-lobed brain connected to paired longitudinal nerve trunks or, in some, middorsal and midventral trunks
11. Excretory system of two coiled canals, which are branched with **flame cells**
12. Sexes separate with simple gonads; asexual reproduction by fragmentation; few hermaphrodites; **pilidium larva** in some
13. No respiratory system
14. Sensory **ciliated pits** or **head slits** on each side of head, which communicate between the outside and the brain; tactile organs and ocelli (in some)
15. In contrast to Platyhelminthes, few parasitic nemertines

CLASSIFICATION

Class Enopla (en′o-pla) (Gr., *enoplos,* armed). Proboscis usually armed with stylets; mouth opens in front of brain. Examples: *Amphiporus, Prostoma.*

Class Anopla (an′o-pla) (Gr., *anoplos,* unarmed). Proboscis lacks stylets; mouth opens below or posterior to brain. Examples: *Cerebratulus, Tubulanus, Lineus.*

_____ Class Enopla

Most nemertines have a close resemblance to each other, although some are very long and difficult to study in the laboratory because their internal organs are not easily seen. Nemertines are slender worms and very fragile (Fig. 11-18) with a great diversity in size. *Amphiporus,* which is taken here as a representative type, is one of the smaller ones.

Form and function

Amphiporus (Gr., *amphi,* both sides of, + *porus,* pore) (Fig. 11-19) is from 20 to 80 mm long and about 2.5 mm wide. It is dorsoventrally flattened and has rounded ends. The body wall comprises an epidermis of ciliated columnar cells and layers of circular and longitudinal muscles (Fig. 11-20, *A*). A partly gelatinous parenchyma fills the space around the visceral organs. Ocelli are located at the anterior end. The thick-lipped mouth is anteroventral, with the opening of the proboscis just above it.

The **proboscis** is not connected with the digestive tract but is an eversible organ that can be protruded from its cavity, the **rhynchocoel,** and used for defense and catching prey (Fig. 11-19). It lies within a sheath to which it is attached by muscles. The rhynchocoel is filled with fluid, and by muscular pressure on this fluid the anterior part of the tubular proboscis is everted, or turned inside out. The proboscis apparatus is an invagination of the anterior body wall, and its structure therefore duplicates that of the body wall. The retractor muscles attached at the end are used to retract the everted proboscis, much like inverting the tip of a finger of a glove by a string attached inside at its tip. The proboscis is armed with a sharp-pointed stylet. A frontal gland also opens at the anterior end by a pore.

Locomotion

Nemertines can move with considerable rapidity by the combined action of their well-developed musculature and its cilia. They glide mainly against a substratum;

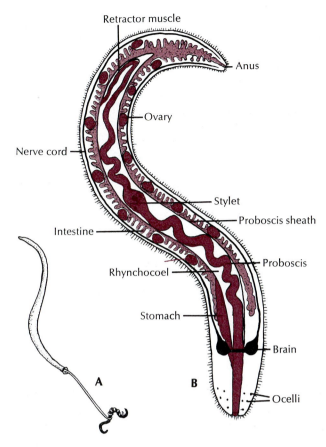

Figure 11-19

A, *Amphiporus*, with proboscis extended to catch prey. **B,** Structure of female nemertine worm *Amphiporus* (diagrammatic). Dorsal view to show proboscis.

Figure 11-20

A, Diagrammatic cross section of female nemertine worm. **B,** Excretory and circulatory systems of anterior region of nemertine worm. Flame bulbs along nephridial canal are closely associated with lateral blood vessels.

some species make use of muscular waves in crawling. Some nemertines have the interesting method of protruding the proboscis, attaching themselves by means of the stylet, and then drawing the body up to the attached position.

Feeding and digestion

The nemertines are carnivorous and voracious, eating either dead or living prey. In seizing their prey they thrust out the slime-covered proboscis, which quickly ensnares the prey by wrapping around it (Fig. 11-19, *A*). The stylet also pierces and holds the prey. Then retracting the proboscis, the nemertine draws the prey near the mouth, where it is engulfed by the esophagus that is thrust out to meet it.

The **digestive system** is complete and extends straight through the length of the body to the terminal **anus,** lying ventral to the proboscis sheath. The **esophagus** is straight and opens into a dilated part of the tract, the **stomach.** The blind anterior end of the intestine as well as the main intestine is provided with paired **lateral ceca.** The alimentary tract is lined with ciliated epithelium, and in the wall of the esophagus there are glandular cells.

Digestion is largely extracellular in the intestinal tube, and when the food is ready for absorption, it passes through the cellular lining of the intestinal tract into the blood-vascular system. The indigestible material passes out the anus (Fig. 11-19, *B*), in contrast to Platyhelminthes in which it leaves by the mouth.

Circulation

The blood-vascular system is simple and enclosed with a single dorsal vessel and two lateral vessels (Fig. 11-20, *B*) connected by transverse vessels. All three longitudinal vessels join together anteriorly to form a type of collar. The blood is usually colorless, containing nucleated corpuscles. However, in some nemertines the blood is red, green, yellow, or orange from the presence of pigments whose function in unknown. There is no heart, and the blood is propelled by the muscular walls of the blood vessels and by bodily movements.

Excretion and respiration

The excretory system contains a pair of lateral tubes with many branches and flame cells (Fig. 11-20, *B*). Each lateral tube opens to the outside by one or more pores. Waste is picked up from the parenchymal spaces and blood by the flame cells and carried by the excretory ducts to the outside. Many of the protonephridia are so closely associated with the circulatory system that their function appears truly excretory, in contrast to their apparently osmoregulatory function in Platyhelminthes. Respiration occurs through the body surface.

Nervous system

The nervous system includes a brain composed of four fused ganglia, one pair dorsal and one pair ventral, united by commissures (connecting nerves). Five longitudinal nerves extend from the brain posteriorly—a large lateral trunk on each side of the body, paired dorsolateral trunks, and one middorsal trunk. These are connected by a network of nerve fibers. From the brain, nerves run to the proboscis, to the ocelli and other sense organs, and to the mouth and esophagus. In addition to the ocelli, there are other sense organs, such as tactile papillae, sensory pits and grooves, and probably auditory organs.

Reproduction and development

The reproductive system in *Amphiporus* is dioecious. The gonads in either sex lie between the intestinal ceca (Fig. 11-19). From each gonad a short duct (gonopore) runs to the dorsolateral body surface. Eggs and sperm are discharged into the water, where fertilization occurs. Egg production in the females is usually accompanied by degeneration of the other visceral organs.

Nemertines have a spiral, determinate cleavage. The mesoderm is partly from the endoderm and partly from the ectoderm. The rhyncocoel develops as a cavity in the mesoderm and is, therefore, technically a coelomic cavity, but it is not homologous to the coelom in higher forms.

A pilidium larva develops, which is helmet shaped and bears a dorsal spike of fused cilia and a pair of lateral lobes. The entire larva is covered with cilia and has a mouth and alimentary canal but no anus. In some nemertines the zygote develops directly without undergoing metamorphosis. The freshwater species, *Prostoma rubrum*, is hermaphroditic. A few nemertines are viviparous.

Regeneration

Nemertines have great powers of regeneration. At certain seasons some of them fragment by autotomy, and from each fragment a new individual develops. This is especially noteworthy in the genus *Lineus*. Fragments from the anterior region will produce a new individual more quickly than will one from the posterior part. Sometimes the proboscis is shot out with such force that it is broken off from the body. In such a case a new proboscis is developed within a short time.

PHYLUM GNATHOSTOMULIDA

The first species of the Gnathostomulida (nath'o-sto-myu'lid-a) (Gr., *gnathos*, jaw, + *stoma*, mouth, + L., *ulus*, dim. suffix) was observed in 1928 in the Baltic, but its description was not published until 1956. Since then jaw worms have been found in many parts of the world, including the Atlantic coast of the United States, and over 80 species in 18 genera have been described.

Gnathostomulids are delicate wormlike animals and are 0.5 to 1 mm long (Fig. 11-21). They live in the interstitial spaces of very fine sandy coastal sediments and silt and can endure conditions of very low oxygen. They are often found in large numbers and frequently in association with gastrotrichs, nematodes, ciliates, tardigrades, and other small forms.

Lacking a pseudocoel, a circulatory system, and an anus, the gnathostomulids show some similarities to the turbellarians and were at first included in that group. However, their parenchyma is poorly developed, and their pharynx is reminiscent of the rotifer mastax. The pharynx is armed with a pair of lateral jaws used to scrape fungi and bacteria off the substratum. And, although the epidermis is ciliated, each epidermal cell has but one cilium, a condition rarely found in the lower bilateral animals except in some gastrotrichs.

Gnathostomulids can glide, swim in loops and spirals, and bend the head from side to side. Sexual stages may include males, females, and hermaphrodites. Fertilization is internal.

The phyletic relationships of the Gnathostomulida are still obscure, but they seem to be intermediate between the Platyhelminthes and the pseudocoelomate phyla.

PHYLOGENY AND ADAPTIVE RADIATION
Phylogeny

Platyhelminthes and Rhynchocoela are apparently closely related, with the flatworms being the more primitive. There can be little doubt that the bilaterally symmetrical flatworms were derived from a radial ancestor, perhaps one very similar to the planula larva of the cnidarians. Some investigators believe that this **planuloid ancestor** may have given rise to one branch of descendants that were sessile or free floating and radial, which became the Cnidaria, and another branch that acquired a creeping habit and bilateral symmetry, which became the Platyhelminthes. Bilateral symmetry is a selective advantage for creeping or swimming animals because sensory structures are concentrated on the anterior, the end that first encounters environmental stimuli (cephalization).

The transformation from a planuloid ancestor to an early platyhelminth involved a number of body modifications, such as an oral-aboral flattening, with the oral end becoming the ventral surface and the ventral surface adapting for locomotion with the aid of cilia and muscles. The small flatworms of the order Acoela seem to meet many of the requirements of an early ancestor of Platyhelminthes. They have several characteristics in common with the planula larva of

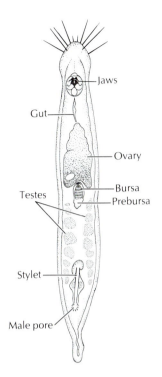

Figure 11-21

Gnathostomula jenneri (phylum Gnathostomulida) is a tiny member of the interstitial fauna between grains of sand or mud. Species in this family are among the most commonly encountered jaw worms, found in shallow water and down to depths of several hundred meters.
From Sterrer, W.E. 1972. Syst. Zool. 21:151.

the cnidarians, such as no epidermal basement membrane, no digestive system, a nerve plexus under the epidermis, and no distinct gonads. The acoeloid ancestor gave rise to the other orders of Turbellaria and the other classes in the phylum. It may be that the ancestral cestodes never had a digestive tract and therefore did not lose it in their adaptation to parasitism.

The Rhynchocoela probably arose from flatworm stock: the body construction of ciliated epidermis, muscles, and mesenchyme-filled spaces is similar in both groups. The rhynchocoels are more advanced than the flatworms in having a complete digestive system, a vascular system, and a more highly organized nervous system.

The Gnathostomulida occupy a position intermediate between the Platyhelminthes and the pseudocoelomate phyla (Chapter 12). Monociliated cells are found in some gastrotrichs, and their protonephridial system is similar to that of gastrotrichs. Their jaws show similarities to the rotifer mastax. However, their complete ciliation, arrangement of body wall muscles, cleavage pattern, and reproductive system strongly suggest a relationship to the primitive Turbellaria.

_____ Adaptive Radiation

The flatworm body plan, with its creeping adaptation, placed a selective advantage on bilateral symmetry and further development of cephalization, ventrodorsal regions, and caudal differentiation. Because of their body shape and metabolic requirements, early flatworms must have been well preadapted for parasitism and gave rise to symbiotic lines on numerous occasions. These lines produced descendants that were extremely successful as parasites, and many flatworms became very highly specialized for that mode of existence.

The ribbon worms have stressed the proboscis apparatus in their evolutionary diversity. Its use in capturing prey may have been secondarily evolved from its original function as a highly sensitive organ for exploring the environment. Although the ribbon worms have advanced beyond the flatworms in their complexity of organization, they have been dramatically less successful as a group. Perhaps the possession of a proboscis was a deterrent to a parasitic habit but highly efficient as a predator tool, or perhaps some critical preadaptations were simply not present.

Likewise, the jaw worms have not radiated nor been nearly as successful as the flatworms. However, they have exploited the marine interstitial environment, particularly zones of very low oxygen concentration.

_____ Summary

The Platyhelminthes, the Rhynchocoela, and the Gnathostomulida are the most primitive phyla that are bilaterally symmetrical, a condition of adaptive value for actively crawling or swimming animals. They have neither a coelom nor a pseudocoel and are thus acoelomate. They are triploblastic and at the organ-system level of organization.

Of the classes of Platyhelminthes, the Turbellaria are mostly free living, and the Monogenea, Trematoda, and Cestoda are all parasitic. The more primitive orders of Turbellaria are endolecithal, but the more advanced Turbellaria and the other classes of flatworms are ectolecithal; that is, the yolk for embryonic development is not incorporated into the ovum but is contributed by separate vitelline cells.

The outer surface of turbellarians is covered by a ciliated epidermis containing mucous cells and rod-shaped rhabdites, which function together in locomotion. Many have a dual-gland system that helps them adhere to the substratum. Planarians are mostly carnivorous and take in food through their eversible pharynx on their ventral side. Digestion is extracellular and intracellular. Osmoregulation is by flame cell protonephridia, and removal of metabolic wastes and respiration are across the body wall. Except for the most primitive turbellarians, flatworms have a ladder-type nervous system with motor, sensory, and association neurons. Various types of sensory receptors are found in the planarians, including photosensitive ocelli. Turbellarians are hermaphroditic, and many also reproduce asexually by fission.

Members of all the other classes of flatworms are covered by a nonciliated, syncytial tegument with a vesicular distal cytoplasm and cell bodies beneath superficial muscle layers. The Monogenea are important ectoparasites of fishes and have a direct life cycle (without intermediate hosts). These contrast with the digenetic trematodes, which have a mollusc intermediate host and almost always a vertebrate definitive host. The great amount of asexual reproduction that occurs in the intermediate host helps to increase the chances that some of the offspring will reach a definitive host. Aside from their tegument, digeneans share many basic structural characteristics with the Turbellaria.

The Digenea includes a number of important parasites of humans and domestic animals. *Clonorchis sinensis* is a liver fluke, and some species of *Schistosoma*, a trematode living in blood vessels, are important pathogens.

The cestodes, or tapeworms, generally have a scolex (holdfast) organ at their anterior end, followed by a long chain of proglottids. They live as adults in the digestive tract of vertebrates. Their tegument is similar in basic structure to that of trematodes, except that it is covered by minute projections called microtriches. This is an adaptation to aid in absorption of nutrients, because the cestodes do not have a digestive tract. Tapeworms are almost all monoecious, and each proglottid contains a complete set of reproductive organs of both sexes. New proglottids form at the anterior end, just behind the scolex, and move posteriorly as they mature and are fertilized and the embryos develop. The shelled larva is passed in the feces, sometimes within a shed proglottid, and the juvenile develops in a vertebrate or invertebrate intermediate host. Some tapeworms are common in humans.

Members of the Rhynchocoela have not been nearly as successful as a group, compared to the Platyhelminthes, but they are structurally more advanced than the flatworms. They have a complete digestive system with an anus and a true circulatory system. They are free living, mostly marine, and they capture their prey by ensnaring it with their long, eversible proboscis.

Members of the Gnathostomulida are tiny worms that live between sediment grains in the sea bottom in zones of low oxygen concentration. They have jaws similar to a rotifer mastax, an epidermis with a single cilium on each cell, and a digestive tract with no anus.

The flatworms and the cnidarians both probably evolved from a common ancestor (planuloid), of whose descendants some became sessile or free floating and radial, and some became creeping and bilateral. The more advanced flatworms were probably derived from an ancestor resembling the turbellarian order Acoela, whereas the rhynchocoelans arose from platyhelminth stock.

Although they are acoelomate, the gnathostomulids show affinities with the pseudocoelomate phyla. They were probably derived from a primitive turbellarian.

Selected references

Barnes, R.D. 1980. Invertebrate zoology, ed. 4. Philadelphia, Saunders College/Holt, Rinehart & Winston.

Cable, R.M. 1965. Thereby hangs a tail. J. Parasitol. 51:3-12. *This reference and the following one have interesting discussions on the nature of the trematode life cycle.*

Cable, R.M. 1971. Parthenogenesis in parasitic helminths. Am. Zool. 11:267-272.

Coe, W.R. 1943. Biology of the nemerteans of the Atlantic Coast of North America. Trans. Conn. Acad. Arts Sci. 35:129-328. *This is only one of many valuable papers on Rhynchocoela by this author.*

Hunter, G.W., J.C. Swartzwelder, and D.F. Clyde. 1976. Tropical medicine, ed. 5. Philadelphia, W.B. Saunders Co. *A valuable source of information on parasites of medical importance.*

Hyman, L.H. 1951. The invertebrates: Platyhelminthes and Rhynchocoela, vol. 2. New York, McGraw-Hill Book Co. *A comprehensive account of this group, with excellent illustrations and bibliography.*

Lumsden, R.D. 1975. Surface ultrastructure and cytochemistry of parasitic helminths. Exp. Parasitol. 37:267-339.

Lumsden, R.D., and R. Specian. 1980. The morphology, histology, and fine structure of the adult stage of the cyclophyllidean tapeworm *Hymenolepis diminuta*. In H.P. Arai (ed.). Biology of the tapeworm *Hymenolepis diminuta*. New York, Academic Press, Inc.

Pappas, P.W., and C.P. Read. 1975. Membrane transport in helminth parasites: a review. Exp. Parasitol. 37:469-530.

Pennak, R.W. 1978. Freshwater invertebrates of the United States, ed. 2. New York, John Wiley & Sons, Inc. *Includes an excellent description of the structure and life history of the freshwater nemertine Prostoma graecense.*

Rieger, R.M., and M. Mainitz. 1977. Comparative fine structure study of the body wall in Gnathostomulida and their phylogenetic position between Platyhelminthes and Aschelminthes. Zeitschr. Zool. Systematic Evolutionsforsch. 15:9-35.

Schell, S.C. 1970. How to know the trematodes. Dubuque, Iowa, William C. Brown Co., Publishers.

Schmidt, G.D. 1970. How to know the tapeworms. Dubuque, Iowa, William C. Brown Co., Publishers.

Schmidt, G.D., and L.S. Roberts. 1981. Foundations of parasitology, ed. 2. St. Louis, The C.V. Mosby Co. *Good accounts of the form and function of trematodes and cestodes; emphasizes species of medical and veterinary importance.*

Smyth, J.D. 1966. The physiology of trematodes. San Francisco, W.H. Freeman & Co. Publishers.

Smyth, J.D. 1969. The physiology of cestodes. San Francisco, W.H. Freeman & Co. Publishers.

Sterrer, W. 1972. Systematics and evolution within the Gnathostomulida. Syst. Zool. 21:151-173.

Thomas, A.P. 1883. The life history of the liver fluke (*Fasciola hepatica*). Q. J. Microsc. Sci. (ser. 2) 23:99-133. *This classic work represents the first life history of a digenetic trematode to be worked out. It gave a great impetus to work in the field of parasitology.*

Tyler, S. 1976. Comparative ultrastructure of adhesive systems in the Turbellaria. Zoomorphologie 84:1-76.

Van der Schalie, H. 1974. Aswan High Dam revisited. Environment 16(9):18-20, 25-26.

Wardle, R.A., and J.A. McLeod. 1952. The zoology of tapeworms. Minneapolis, University of Minnesota Press. *A comprehensive account invaluable to the serious student of cestodes.*

Wardle, R.A., J.A. McLeod, and S. Radinovsky. 1974. Advances in the zoology of tapeworms, 1950-1970. Minneapolis, University of Minnesota Press.

CHAPTER 12

THE PSEUDOCOELOMATE ANIMALS

Phylum Rotifera

Phylum Gastrotricha

Phylum Kinorhyncha

Phylum Nematoda

Phylum Nematomorpha

Phylum Acanthocephala

Phylum Entoprocta

Anterior end of a hookworm *Necator americanus*. The common name is derived from the characteristic dorsal flexure, shown here. A parasite of humans, the worm attaches itself to the host's intestinal wall and sucks blood, and the buccal capsule with its large teeth *(at right)* and the muscular esophagus *(running to left)* are very effective in this function.

Photograph by L.S. Roberts.

Position in Animal Kingdom

In the seven phyla covered in this chapter, the original blastocoel of the embryo persists as a space, or body cavity, between the enteron and the body wall. Because this cavity lacks the peritoneal lining found in the true coelomates, it is called a **pseudocoel**, and the animals possessing it are called **pseudocoelomates**. Pseudocoelomates belong to the Protostomia division of the bilateral animals.

Biological Contributions

The pseudocoel is a distinct advancement over the solid body structure of the acoelomates. It may be filled with fluid or may contain a gelatinous substance with some mesenchyme cells. In common with a true coelom, the pseudocoel presents certain adaptive potentials, although these are by no means realized in all members: (1) greater freedom of movement; (2) space for the development and differentiation of digestive, excretory, and reproductive systems; (3) a simple means of circulation or distribution of materials throughout the body; (4) a storage place for waste products to be discharged to the outside by excretory ducts; and (5) a hydrostatic organ. Since most pseudocoelomates are quite small, the most important functions of the pseudocoel are probably in circulation and as a means to maintain a high internal hydrostatic pressure.

The complete mouth-to-anus digestive tract is found in these phyla and in all higher phyla.

THE PSEUDOCOELOMATES

Vertebrates and higher invertebrates have a true **coelom,** or peritoneal cavity, which is formed in the mesoderm during embryonic development and is therefore lined with a layer of mesodermal epithelium, the **peritoneum.** The pseudocoelomate phyla have a pseudocoel rather than a true coelom. It is derived from the embryonic blastocoel rather than from a secondary cavity within the mesoderm. It is a space not lined with peritoneum, between the gut and the mesodermal and ectodermal components of the body wall.

Seven distinct groups of animals belong to the pseudocoelomate category: Rotifera, Gastrotricha, Kinorhyncha, Nematoda, Nematomorpha, Acanthocephala, and Entoprocta. The first five of these groups have certain similarities that have led some authorities to place them as classes in a phylum called Aschelminthes (as'kel-min'theez) (Gr., *askos*, bladder, + *helmins*, worm). However, they differ so much that any phyletic relationship is highly debatable, and other authorities perfer to consider them as separate phyla. Some group the five together loosely as individual phyla under a superphylum Aschelminthes. The Entoprocta have sometimes been grouped with the Ectoprocta, together called the Bryozoa (moss animals). However, because the ectoprocts have a true coelom, they are usually considered a separate phylum, and the term "bryozoans" is generally taken to exclude the entoprocts in current usage.

However one classifies them, the pseudocoelomates are a heterogeneous assemblage of animals. Most of them are small; some are microscopic; some are fairly large. Some, such as the nematodes, are found in freshwater, marine, terrestrial, and parasitic habitats; others, such as the Acanthocephala, are strictly parasitic. Some have unique characteristics, such as the lacunar system of the acanthocephalans, the ciliary corona of the rotifers, or the zonites of the kinorhynchs.

Even in such a diversified grouping, some characteristics are shared. All have a body wall of epidermis (often syncytial), a dermis, and muscles surrounding the pseudocoel. The digestive tract is complete (except in Acanthocephala), and it, along with the gonads and excretory organs, is within the pseudocoel and bathed in perivisceral fluid. The epidermis in many secretes a nonliving cuticle with some specializations such as bristles or spines.

A constant number of cells or nuclei in the individuals of a species, a condition known as **eutely,** is common to several of the groups, and in most of them there is an emphasis on the longitudinal muscle layer.

CHARACTERISTICS

1. Symmetry bilateral; unsegmented; triploblastic (three germ layers)
2. Body cavity an unlined **pseudocoel**
3. Size mostly small; some microscopic; a few a meter or more in length
4. Body vermiform; body wall a **syncytial** or cellular epidermis with thickened cuticle, sometimes molted; muscular layers mostly of **longitudinal fibers;** cilia absent in several phyla
5. Digestive system (lacking in acanthocephalans) complete with mouth, enteron, and anus; pharynx muscular and well developed: **tube-within-a-tube arrangement;** digestive tract usually only an epithelial tube with **no definite muscle layer**
6. Circulatory and respiratory organs lacking
7. Excretory system of canals and protonephridia in some; cloaca that receives excretory, reproductive, and digestive products may be present
8. Nervous system of cerebral ganglia or of a circumenteric nerve ring connected to anterior and posterior nerves; sense organs of ciliated pits, papillae, bristles, and some eyespots
9. Reproductive system of gonads and ducts that may be single or double; sexes nearly always separate, with the male usually smaller than the female; eggs microscopic with shell often containing chitin
10. Development may be direct or within a complicated life history; cleavage mostly mosaic; **cell or nuclear constancy common**

Phylum Rotifera

Rotifera (Ro-tif'e-ra) (L., *rota,* wheel, + *fera,* those that bear) derive their name from the characteristic ciliated crown, or **corona,** that, when beating, often gives the impression of rotating wheels. Rotifers range from 40 μm to 3 mm in length, but most are between 100 and 500 μm long. Some have beautiful colors, although most are transparent, and some have bizarre shapes (Fig. 12-1). Their shapes are often correlated with their mode of life. The floaters are usually globular and saclike; the creepers and swimmers are somewhat elongated and wormlike; and the sessile types are commonly vaselike, with a cuticular envelope (lorica). Some are colonial. One of the best-known genera is *Philodina* (Gr., *philos,* fond of, + *dinos,* whirling) (Fig. 12-2), which is often used for study.

Rotifers are a cosmopolitan group of about 1500 species, some of which are found throughout the world. Most of the species are freshwater inhabitants, a few are marine, some are terrestrial, and some are epizoic (live on the body of another animal) or parasitic.

Rotifers are adapted to many kinds of ecological conditions. Most species are benthic, living on the bottom or in vegetation of ponds or along the shores of freshwater lakes where they swim or creep about on the vegetation. A large proportion of the species that live in the water film between sand grains of beaches (meiofauna) are rotifers. Pelagic forms (Fig. 12-1, *B*) are common in the surface waters of freshwater lakes and ponds, and they may exhibit cyclomorphosis, that is, seasonal variations in body form.

Many species of rotifers can endure long periods of desiccation, during which they resemble grains of sand. While in a desiccated condition, rotifers are very tolerant of temperature variations, especially those rotifers that dwell in

A   B

Stephanoceros fimbriatus   *Asplanchna priodonta*

C   D

Squatinella rostrum   *Macrochaetus longipes*

Figure 12-1

Variety of body form in rotifers. **A,** *Stephanoceros* has five, long, fingerlike coronal lobes with whorls of short bristles. It catches its prey by closing its funnel when food organisms swim into it, and the bristly lobes prevent the prey from escaping. **B,** *Asplanchna* is a pelagic, predatory genus with no foot. **C,** *Squatinella* has a semicircular, nonretractable, transparent hoodlike extension covering the head. **D,** *Macrochaetus* is dorsoventrally flattened.

A, From Voigt, M., and W. Koste. 1978. Rotaria, die Radertiere Mitteleuropas, ed. 2. Berlin, Borntraeger; B, from Edmonson, W.T. (ed.). 1959. Ward and Whipple's freshwater biology, ed. 2. New York, John Wiley & Sons, Inc.; C and D, from Ruttner-Kolisko, A. 1974. Die Binnengewasser 26(suppl.):1.

Mouth

Corona

Flame bulb

Eyespot

Brain

Mastax

Salivary glands

Gastric gland

excretory canal

Germo-vitellarium

Stomach

Pulsating vesicle

Cloacal bladder

Intestine

Pedal glands

Anus

Bood

Toe (foot)

Figure 12-2

Structure of *Philodina* rotifer.

mosses. True encystment occurs in only a few rotifers. On addition of water, desiccated rotifers resume their activity.

Strictly marine species are rather few in number. Some of the littoral (intertidal) species of the sea may be freshwater ones that are able to adapt to seawater.

CLASSIFICATION

Class Seisonidea (sy'son-id'e-a) (Gr., *seisōn*, earthen vessel, + *eidos*, form). Marine; elongated form; corona vestigial; sexes similar in size and form; females with pair of ovaries and no vitellaria; single genus *(Seison)* with two species; epizoic on gills of a crustacean *(Nebalia)*.

Class Bdelloidea (del-oid'e-a) (Gr., *bdella*, leech, + *eidos*, form). Swimming or creeping forms; anterior end retractile; corona usually with pair of trochal discs; males unknown; parthenogenetic; two germovitellaria. Examples: *Philodina* (Fig. 12-2), *Rotaria*.

Class Monogononta (mon'o-go-non'ta) (Gr., *monos*, one, + *gonos*, primary sex gland). Swimming or sessile forms; single germovitellarium; males reduced in size; eggs of three types (amictic, mictic, dormant). Examples: *Asplanchna* (Fig. 12-1, *B*), *Epiphanes*.

Form and function
External features

The body of the rotifer is comprised of a head bearing a ciliated corona, a trunk, and a posterior tail, or foot. It is covered with a cuticle and is nonciliated except for the corona.

The ciliated **corona,** or crown, surrounds a nonciliated central area of the head called the **apical field,** which may bear sensory bristles or papillae. The appearance of the head end depends on which of the several types of corona it has—usually a circlet of some sort, or a pair of trochal (coronal) discs (the term "trochal" comes from a Greek word meaning wheel). The cilia on the corona beat in succession, giving the appearance of a revolving wheel or pair of wheels. The **mouth** is located in the corona on the midventral side. The coronal cilia are used in both locomotion and feeding.

The **trunk** may be elongated, as in *Philodina* (Fig. 12-2), or saccular in shape (Fig. 12-1). It contains the visceral organs and often bears sensory antennae. It is covered by a transparent cuticle that in *Philodina* and others is superficially ringed so as to simulate segmentation but in many other forms is much thickened to form an outer case or **lorica,** often arranged in plates or rings.

The **foot** is narrower and usually bears one to four toes. Its cuticle may be ringed so that it is telescopically retractile. It is tapered gradually in some forms (Fig. 12-2) and sharply set off in others (Fig. 12-1). The foot is an attachment organ and contains pedal glands that secrete an adhesive material used by both sessile and creeping forms. In swimming pelagic forms, the foot is usually reduced. Rotifers move by creeping with leechlike movements aided by the foot, or by swimming with the coronal cilia, or both.

Internal features

Underneath the cuticle is the **syncytial epidermis,** which secretes the cuticle, and bands of **subepidermal muscles,** some circular, some longitudinal, and some running through the pseudocoel to the visceral organs. The **pseudocoel** is large, occupying the space between the body wall and the viscera. It is filled with fluid, some of the muscle bands, and a network of mesenchymal ameboid cells.

The **digestive system** is complete. Some rotifers feed by sweeping minute organic particles or algae toward the mouth by the beating of the coronal cilia. The cilia are able to sort out and dispose of the larger unsuitable particles. The pharynx (**mastax**) is fitted with a muscular portion that is equipped with hard jaws (**trophi**) for sucking in and grinding up the food particles. The constantly chewing pharynx is often a distinguishing feature of these tiny animals. Carnivorous species feed on protozoa and small metazoans, which they capture by trapping or grasping. The trappers have a funnel-shaped area around the mouth. When small prey swim into the funnel, the lobes fold inward to capture and hold them until they are drawn into the mouth and pharynx. The hunters have trophi that can be projected and used like forceps to seize the prey, bring it back into the pharynx, and then pierce it or break it up so that the edible parts can be sucked out and the rest discarded. The salivary and gastric glands are believed to secrete enzymes for extracellular digestion. Absorption occurs in the stomach.

The **excretory system** typically consists of a pair of **protonephridial tubules,** each with several **flame cells,** that empty into a common bladder. The bladder, by pulsating, empties into the **cloaca**—into which the intestine and oviducts also empty. The fairly rapid rate of pulsation of the protonephridia—one to four times per minute—would indicate that the protonephridia are important osmoregulatory organs. The water apparently enters through the mouth rather than across the cuticle; even marine species empty their bladder at frequent intervals.

The **nervous system** consists of a bilobed brain, dorsal to the mastax, that sends paired nerves to the sense organs, mastax, muscles, and viscera. Sensory organs include paired eyespots (in some species such as *Philodina*), sensory bristles and papillae, and ciliated pits and dorsal antennae.

Reproduction

Rotifers are dioecious, but the males are usually smaller than the females. In the order Bdelloidea males are entirely unknown, and in Monogononta they seem to occur only for a few weeks of the year.

The female reproductive system in the Bdelloidea and Monogononta consists of combined ovaries and yolk glands (**germovitellaria**) and oviducts that open into the cloaca. Yolk is supplied to the developing ova by way of flow through cytoplasmic bridges, rather than as separate yolk cells as in many Platyhelminthes.

In the Bdelloidea (*Philodina,* for example), all females are parthenogenetic and produce diploid eggs that hatch into diploid females. These reach maturity in a few days. In the class Seisonidea the females produce haploid eggs that must be fertilized and that develop into either males or females. In the Monogononta, however, females produce two kinds of eggs. During most of the year diploid females produce thin-shelled, **diploid amictic eggs.** These develop parthenogenetically into diploid amictic females. However, such rotifers often live in temporary ponds or streams and are cyclic in their reproductive patterns. Any one of several environmental factors—for example, crowding, diet, or photoperiod (according to species)—may induce the amictic eggs to develop into diploid mictic females that will produce thin-shelled **haploid mictic eggs.** If these eggs are not fertilized, they develop into haploid males. But if fertilized, the eggs develop a thick, resistant shell and become dormant. They survive over winter ("winter eggs") or until environmental conditions are again suitable, at which time they hatch into diploid females. Dormant eggs are often dispersed by winds or birds, which may account for the peculiar distribution patterns of rotifers.

Figure 12-3

Chaetonotus, a gastrotrich. **A,** Dorsal surface. **B,** Internal structure, ventral view.

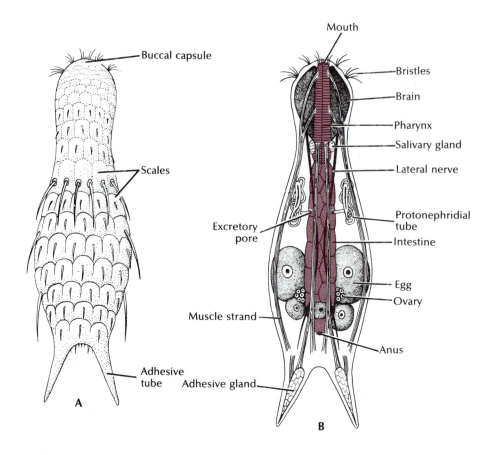

The male reproductive system includes a single testis and a ciliated sperm duct that runs to a genital pore (males usually lack a cloaca). The end of the sperm duct is specialized as a copulatory organ. Copulation is usually by hypodermic impregnation; that is, the penis can penetrate any part of the female body wall and inject the sperm directly into the pseudocoel.

Females hatch with adult features, needing only a few days' growth to reach maturity. Males often do not grow and are sexually mature at hatching.

Cell or nuclear constancy

Most structures in rotifers are syncytial, but the nuclei in the various organs are said to show a remarkable constancy in numbers in any given species (**eutely**). For example, E. Martini (1912) reported that in one species of rotifer he always found 183 nuclei in the brain, 39 in the stomach, 172 in the corona epithelium, and so on. Not all zoologists are convinced that cell or nuclear constancy is always that absolute.

Phylum Gastrotricha

Gastrotricha (gas-tro-tri′ka) (N.L., fr. Gr., *gaster, gastros,* stomach or belly, + *thrix, trichos,* hair) includes small, ventrally flattened animals about 65 to 500 μm long, somewhat like rotifers but lacking the corona and mastax and having a characteristically bristly or scaly body. They are usually found gliding on the bottom, or on an aquatic plant or animal substrate, by means of their ventral cilia, or they comprise part of the meiofauna in the interstitial spaces between bottom particles.

Gastrotrichs are found in both fresh and salt water. The 400 or so species are about equally divided between the two media. Many species are cosmopolitan, but only a few occur in both fresh water and the sea. Much is yet to be learned about their distribution.

CLASSIFICATION

Order Macrodasyida (mac′ro-das-e′i-da) (Gr., *makros*, long, large + *dasys*, hairy, shaggy). Several to many adhesive tubes borne anteriorly, posteriorly, and laterally; pharyngeal pores present. Examples: *Macrodasys, Urodasys, Turbanella.*

Order Chaetonotida (ke′to-not′i-da) (N.L., *chaeta*, bristle, from Gr., *chaité*, long hair, + *notum*, back) Fewer adhesive tubes than macrodasyids, usually restricted to two at posterior end; no pharyngeal pores. Examples: *Chaetonotus, Lepidodermella.*

Form and function

The gastrotrich (Figs. 12-3 and 12-4) is usually elongated, with a convex dorsal surface bearing a pattern of bristles, spines, or scales, and a flattened ciliated ventral surface. Cells on the ventral surface may be monociliated or multiciliated. The head is often lobed and ciliated, and the tail end may be forked.

A syncytial epidermis is found beneath the cuticle. Longitudinal muscles are better developed than are circular ones, and in most cases they are unstriated. Adhesive tubes secrete a substance for attachment. A dual-gland system for attachment and release is present, similar to that described for the Turbellaria (p. 257). The pseudocoel is somewhat reduced and contains no amebocytes.

The digestive system is complete and is made up of a mouth, a muscular pharynx, a stomach-intestine, and an anus (Fig. 12-3, *B*). The food is largely algae, protozoa, and detritus, which are directed to the mouth by the head cilia. Digestion appears to be extracellular. The protonephridia are equipped with cyrtocytes rather than flame bulbs or flame cells. Cyrtocytes have a single flagellum enclosed in a cylinder of cytoplasmic rods.

The nervous system includes a brain near the pharynx and a pair of lateral nerve trunks. Sensory structures are similar to those in rotifers, except that the eyespots are generally lacking.

Gastrotrichs are hermaphroditic, although the male system of the chaetonotids is so poorly developed that they are functionally parthenogenetic females. The female reproductive system consists of one or two ovaries, a uterus, an oviduct, and a gonopore, which may open anteriorly to, or in common with, the anus.

Like the rotifers, chaetonotid gastrotrichs produce thin-walled, rapidly developing eggs and thick-shelled, dormant eggs. The thick-shelled eggs can withstand harsh environmental conditions and may survive dormancy for some years. Development is direct, and the juveniles have the same form as adults.

_____ Phylum Kinorhyncha

Kinorhyncha (kin′o-ring′ka) (Gr., *kinein*, to move, + *rhynchos*, beak) are marine worms a little larger than rotifers and gastrotrichs but usually not more than 1 mm long. The phylum has also been called Echinodera, meaning spiny necked.

Kinorhynchs are cosmopolitan, living from pole to pole, from intertidal areas to 6000 m in depth. Most live in mud or sandy mud, but some have been found in algal holdfasts, sponges, or other invertebrates. They feed mainly on diatoms. About 100 species have been reported. Among the best-known genera of the Kinorhyncha are *Echinoderes, Pycnophyes,* and *Kinorhynchus.*

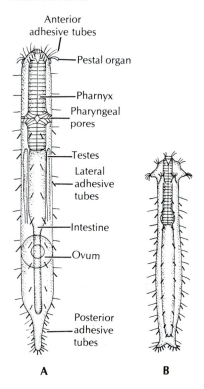

Figure 12-4

Gastrotrichs in the order Macrodasyida. **A,** *Macrodasys.* **B,** *Turbanella.*
From Hummon, W.D. 1982. In S.P. Parker (ed.). Synopsis and classification of living organisms, vol. 1. New York, McGraw-Hill Book Co.

Anterior adhesive tubes
— Pestal organ
— Pharnyx
Pharyngeal pores
— Testes
Lateral adhesive tubes
— Intestine
— Ovum
Posterior adhesive tubes

A   **B**

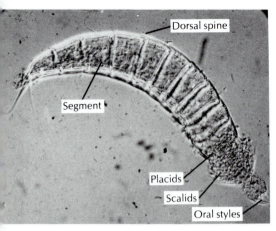

Figure 12-5

Echinoderes, a kinorhynch, is a minute marine worm. Segmentation is superficial. Head with its circle of spines is retractile.

Photograph by L.S. Roberts.

Form and function

The body of the kinorhynch is divided into 13 segments, which bear spines but have no cilia (Fig. 12-5). The retractile head has a circlet of spines with a small retractile proboscis. The body is flat underneath and arched above. The body wall is made up of a cuticle, a syncytial epidermis, and longitudinal epidermal cords, much like those of nematodes. The arrangement of the muscles is correlated with the segments, and circular, longitudinal, and diagonal muscle bands are all represented.

A kinorhynch cannot swim. In the silt and mud where it commonly lives, it burrows by extending the head into the mud and anchoring it with spines. It then draws the body forward until the head is retracted into the body. When disturbed, the kinorhynch draws in the head and protects it with a closing apparatus of cuticular plates (Fig. 12-5).

The digestive system is complete, with a mouth at the tip of the proboscis, a pharynx, an esophagus, a stomach-intestine, and an anus. Kinorhynchs feed on diatoms or on organic material in the mud where they burrow.

The pseudocoel is filled with amebocytes containing fluid. The excretory system is made up of a multinucleated **solenocyte** protonephridium on each side of the tenth and eleventh segments. Each solenocyte has one long and one short flagellum.

The nervous system is in contact with the epidermis, with a multilobed brain encircling the pharynx, and with a ventral ganglionated nerve cord extending throughout the body. Sense organs are represented by eyespots in some and by the sensory bristles.

Sexes are separate, with paired gonads and gonoducts. There is a series of about six juvenile stages and a definitive, nonmolting adult.

Phylum Nematoda—Roundworms

It has been said that, if the earth were to disappear, leaving only the nematode worms, the general contour of the earth's surface would be outlined by the worms, because they are present in nearly every conceivable kind of ecological niche. Approximately 10,000 species have been named, but it has been estimated that, if all species were known, the number would be nearer 500,000. They live in the sea, in fresh water, and in soil, from polar regions to the tropics, and from mountaintops to the depths of the sea. Good topsoil may contain billions of nematodes per acre. Nematodes also parasitize virtually every type of animal and many plants. The effects of nematode infestation on crops, domestic animals, and humans make this phylum one of the most important of all parasitic animal groups.

Free-living nematodes feed on bacteria, yeasts, fungal hyphae, and algae. They may be saprozoic, saprophytic, or coprozoic (live in fecal material). Predatory species may eat rotifers, tardigrades, small annelids, and other nematodes. Many species feed on plant juices from higher plants, which they penetrate, sometimes causing agricultural damage of great proportions. Nematodes themselves may be prey for mites, insect larvae, and even nematode-capturing fungi.

Virtually every species of vertebrate and many invertebrates serve as hosts for one or more types of parasitic nematodes. Nematode parasites in humans cause much discomfort, disease, and death, and in domestic animals they are the source of great economic loss.

CLASSIFICATION

Classification of the nematodes is somewhat more satisfactory at the order and superfamily level; the division into classes relies on characteristics that are not striking and that are difficult for the novice to distinguish. Two classes are usually recognized.

> **Class Phasmidia** (faz-mid′e-a) (Gr., *phasm*, phantom, + *idia*, dim. suffix) (Secernentea). Body with a pair of minute sensory pouches (phasmids) near posterior tip; similar pair of sense organs at anterior end (amphids) poorly developed; excretory system with one or two lateral canals, with or without associated glandular cells; both free-living and parasitic forms. Examples: *Rhabditis, Ascaris, Enterobius.*
>
> **Class Aphasmidia** (a′faz-mid′e-a) (Gr., *a*, without, + *phasm*, phantom, + *idia*, dim. suffix) (Adenophorea). Phasmids lacking, amphids usually well developed; excretory system of one or more renette cells (glandular); caudal and hypodermal glands common; mostly free living, but includes some parasites. Examples: *Dioctophyme, Trichinella, Trichuris.*

Form and function

Distinguishing characteristics of this large group of animals are their cylindrical shape; their flexible, nonliving cuticle; their lack of motile cilia or flagella; and the muscles of their body wall, which have several unusual features, such as the fact that the muscles run in a longitudinal direction only. Correlated with their lack of cilia, nematodes do not have protonephridia; their excretory system consists of one or more large gland cells opening by an excretory pore, or a canal system without gland cells, or both gland cells and canals together. Their pharynx is characteristically muscular with a triradiate lumen and resembles the pharynx of the gastrotrichs and of the kinorhynchs. Use of the pseudocoel as a hydrostatic organ is highly developed in the nematodes, and much of the functional morphology of the nematodes can be best understood in the context of the high **hydrostatic pressure** (turgor) in the pseudocoel.

Most nematode worms are less than 5 cm long, and many are microscopic, but some parasitic nematodes are more than 1 m in length.

The outer body covering is a relatively thick, noncellular **cuticle** secreted by the underlying epidermis. The cuticle is of great functional importance to the worm, serving to contain the high hydrostatic pressure exerted by the fluid in the pseudocoel. The several layers of the cuticle are primarily of **collagen**, a structural protein also abundant in vertebrate connective tissue. Three of the layers are comprised of crisscrossing fibers, which confer some longitudinal elasticity on the worm but severely limit its capacity for lateral expansion.

Beneath the epidermis is a layer of **longitudinal muscles**. There are no circular muscles in the body wall. The muscles are arranged in four bands, or quadrants, marked off by four epidermal cords that project inward to the pseudocoel.

The fluid-filled pseudocoel, in which the internal organs lie, constitutes a hydrostatic skeleton. Hydrostatic skeletons, found in many invertebrates, lend support by transmitting the force of muscle contraction to the enclosed, noncompressible fluid. Normally, muscles are arranged antagonistically, so that movement is effected by contraction of one group of muscles and relaxation of the other. However, nematodes do not have circular body wall muscles to antagonize the longitudinal muscles; therefore the cuticle must serve that function. Compression of the cuticle on the side of the muscular contraction and stretching on the

Figure 12-6

Rhabditis, a common free-living nematode that feeds on decaying plant and animal matter. Some species that feed on manure undergo a developmental arrest at the third-stage juvenile until they "hitchhike" to a new food supply on a dung beetle. In this drawing of a female, the intestine overlies and hides the germinal zone of the posterior ovary. As in most nematodes, the proximal end of the oviduct serves as a sperm storage area; the oocytes are penetrated by ameboid sperm as they pass through and then complete meiosis.

After Hirschmann, H., modified from Sasser, J.N., and W.R. Jenkins. 1960. Nematology. Chapel Hill, University of North Carolina Press.

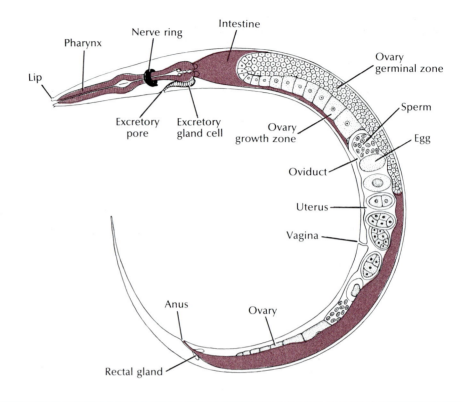

Figure 12-7

Scale diagram of part of the tip of the head of *Meloidogyne* sp. cut open to reveal one of the two amphids.

From Bird, A.F. 1971. The structure of nematodes. New York, Academic Press, Inc.

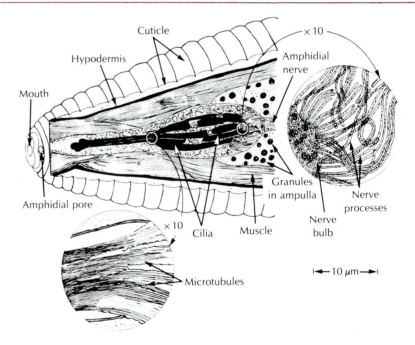

opposite side are the forces that return the body to resting position when the muscles relax; this produces the characteristic thrashing motion seen in nematode movement. An increase in efficiency of this system can be achieved only by an increase in hydrostatic pressure. Consequently, the hydrostatic pressure in the nematode pseudocoel is much higher than is usually found in other kinds of animals that have hydrostatic skeletons but also have antagonistic muscle groups.

Table 12-1 Common Parasitic Nematodes of Humans in North America

Common and scientific names	Mode of infection; prevalence
Hookworm (*Ancylostoma duodenale* and *Necator americanus*)	Contact with juveniles in soil that burrow into skin; common in southern states
Pinworm (*Enterobius vermicularis*)	Inhalation of dust with ova and by contamination with fingers; most common parasite in United States
Intestinal roundworm (*Ascaris lumbricoides*)	Ingestion of embryonated ova in contaminated food; common in rural areas of Appalachia and southeastern states
Trichina worm (*Trichinella spiralis*)	Ingestion of infected pork muscle; occasional in humans throughout North America
Whipworm (*Trichuris trichiura*)	Ingestion of contaminated food or by unhygienic habits; usually common wherever *Ascaris* is found

The alimentary canal of the nematode consists of a **mouth** (Fig. 12-6), a muscular **pharynx**, a long nonmuscular **intestine**, a short **rectum**, and a terminal **anus**. Food material is sucked into the pharynx when the muscles in its anterior portion contract rapidly and open the lumen. Relaxation of the muscles anterior to the food mass closes the lumen of the pharynx, forcing the food posteriorly toward the intestine. The intestine is one cell layer thick. Food matter is moved posteriorly by body movements and by additional food being passed into the intestine from the pharynx. Defecation is accomplished by muscles that simply pull the anus open, and the expulsive force is provided by the pseudocoelomic pressure.

The adults of many parasitic nematodes have an anaerobic energy metabolism; thus, a Krebs cycle and cytochrome system characteristic of aerobic metabolism are absent. Energy is derived through glycolysis and probably through some incompletely known electron transport sequences. Interestingly, some free-living nematodes and free-living stages of parasitic nematodes are obligate aerobes and have a Krebs cycle and cytochrome system.

A **ring of nerve tissue** and ganglia around the pharynx gives rise to small nerves to the anterior end and to two **nerve cords**, one dorsal and one ventral. **Sensory papillae** are concentrated around the head and tail. The **amphids** are a pair of somewhat more complex sensory organs that open on each side of the head at about the same level as the cephalic circle of papillae (Fig. 12-7). The amphidial opening leads into a deep cuticular pit with sensory endings of modified cilia. The amphids are usually reduced in nematode parasites of animals, but most parasitic nematodes bear a bilateral pair of **phasmids** near the posterior end. They are similar in structure to the amphids.

Most nematodes are dioecious. The male is smaller than the female, and its posterior end usually bears a pair of **copulatory spicules.** Fertilization is internal, and eggs are usually stored in the uterus until deposition. After embryonation a juvenile worm hatches from the egg. The four juvenile stages are separated by a molt, or shedding, of the cuticle. Many parasitic nematodes have free-living juvenile stages. Others require an intermediate host to complete their life cycles.

The copulatory spicules of male nematodes are not true intromittent organs, since they do not conduct the sperm, but are another adaptation to cope with the high internal hydrostatic pressure. The spicules must hold the vulva of the female open while the ejaculatory muscles overcome the hydrostatic pressure in the female and rapidly inject sperm into her reproductive tract. Furthermore, nematode spermatozoa are unique among those studied in the animal kingdom in that they lack a flagellum and acrosome. Within the female reproductive tract, the sperm become ameboid and move by pseudopodial movement. Could this be another adaptation to the high hydrostatic pressure in the pseudocoel?

Figure 12-8

Ascaris suum of pigs, which is very similar morphologically to *Ascaris lumbricoides* of humans. **A,** Male and female. Male *(right)* has characteristic sharp kink in end of tail. **B,** Intestine of pig, nearly completely blocked by *A. suum* (threads were inserted to hold worms in place). Such heavy infections are also fairly common with *A. lumbricoides* in humans.

A, Photograph by F.M. Hickman; **B,** photograph by L.S. Roberts. From Schmidt, G.D., and L.S. Roberts. 1981. Foundations of parasitology, ed. 2. St. Louis, The C.V. Mosby Co.

Nematode parasites of humans

As mentioned previously, nearly all vertebrates and many invertebrates are parasitized by nematodes. A number of these are very important pathogens of humans and domestic animals. A few nematodes are common in humans in North America (Table 12-1), but they and many others usually abound in tropical countries. Only a few will be mentioned in this discussion.

Ascaris lumbricoides—the large roundworm of humans

Because of its size and availability, *Ascaris* (Gr., *askaris*, intestinal worm) is usually selected as a type for study in zoology, as well as in experimental work. Thus, it is probable that more is known about the structure, physiology, and biochemistry of *Ascaris* than of any other nematode. This genus includes several species. One of the most common, *A. megalocephala*, is found in the intestine of horses. *A. lumbricoides* (Fig. 12-8) is one of the most common parasites found in humans; recent surveys have shown a prevalence of up to 64% in some areas of the southeastern United States. The large roundworm of pigs, *A. suum,* is morphologically close to *A. lumbricoides,* and they were long considered the same species.

A female *Ascaris* may lay 200,000 eggs a day; they are passed out in the host's feces. Given suitable soil conditions, embryonation is complete within 2 weeks. Direct sunlight and high temperatures are rapidly lethal, but the eggs have an amazing tolerance to other adverse conditions, such as desiccation or lack of oxygen. The eggs can remain viable for many months or even years in the soil. Infection usually occurs when eggs are ingested with uncooked vegetables or when children put soiled fingers or toys in their mouths. Unsanitary defecation habits "seed" the soil, and viable eggs remain long after all signs of the fecal matter have disappeared.

When embryonated eggs are swallowed by a host, the tiny juveniles hatch. They burrow through the intestinal wall into the veins or lymph vessels and are carried through the heart to the lungs. There they break out into the alveoli and are carried up the bronchi to the trachea. If the infection is large, they may cause a serious pneumonia at this stage. On reaching the pharynx, the juveniles are swallowed, pass through the stomach, and finally mature about 2 months after the eggs were ingested. In the intestine the worms cause abdominal symptoms and allergic reactions, and in large numbers they may cause intestinal blockage. Perforation of the intestine with resultant peritonitis is not uncommon, and wandering worms may occasionally emerge from the anus or throat or may enter the trachea or eustachian tubes and middle ears.

Toxocara

Infection of dogs and cats with species of the genus *Toxocara* is extremely common in the United States. Surveys indicate that 20% of adult dogs and 98% of puppies are infected. The life cycles of these species are quite similar to that of *Ascaris lumbricoides,* with soil being seeded with eggs from dog and cat feces. Humans, especially children, may become infected, but in this abnormal host the worms do not mature in the intestine. Their development is arrested, and the juvenile worms continue to wander in the tissues, causing a condition called **visceral larva migrans.** Visceral larva migrans is much more common than the number of reported cases suggests because most cases go undetected unless the juveniles wander into some vital spot, such as the eye, where they may cause blindness in the affected eye.

Hookworms

The hookworms commonly found in humans are *Necator americanus* (L., *necator*, killer) and *Ancylostoma duodenale* (Gr., *ankylos*, crooked, + *stoma*, mouth). Their common name refers to the fact that their anterior end curves dorsally, suggesting a hook (p. 279). *N. americanus* was discovered in the New World, but it was probably introduced there through the slave trade. It is the more common of the two in humans and accounts for 95% of hookworm infection in the United States. Formerly, this parasite was a major disease agent in the southeastern United States, but through sanitation efforts and control campaigns, the prevalence there was reduced from more than 40% in 1910 to around 4% in 1963.

Hookworms have a large buccal cavity armed with cutting plates or teeth (Fig. 12-9). They attach to the wall of the small intestine and feed on blood. For reasons that are not clear, they suck much more blood from the gut wall than they use for food, simply passing it through their alimentary tract, mostly unchanged. Hence, **hookworm disease** is a disease of **blood loss** and is largely manifested by symptoms of **anemia** (low hemoglobin and red cells in the blood). The severity of the disease, or even whether any disease at all is produced, is determined by several factors, the most important of which are the number of worms present and the general nutritional state of the host. Larger numbers of worms can produce disease in a person who has a diet deficient in protein.

The life cycle differs from that of *Ascaris*, although as with *Ascaris*, only one host is involved. The eggs pass out with the feces of the host, embryonate in the soil, and hatch spontaneously. The juveniles are free living, feeding on microorganisms and fecal matter. They grow and molt their cuticle twice to become infective third-stage juveniles. Development is then arrested until they reach a new host. When a host comes in contact with the third-stage juvenile, the worm penetrates the host skin, is carried by the blood to the lungs, breaks through the alveoli, goes up the trachea to the pharynx, is swallowed, and finally reaches the small intestine. Since the eggs and juveniles require shade, moisture, and warmth for survival, hookworms occur mainly in tropical and subtropical areas.

Trichina worms

Trichinella spiralis (Gr., *trichinos,* of hair, + *ella,* dim. suffix) is the tiny nematode responsible for the potentially lethal disease **trichinosis**. Adult worms burrow in the mucosa of the small intestine where the female produces living juveniles. The

Figure 12-9

Section through anterior end of hookworm attached to human intestine. The cutting plates of the mouth pinch off a bit of mucosa from which the thick muscular pharynx sucks blood. Esophageal glands secrete an anticoagulant to prevent blood clotting.
AFIP No. 33810.

Figure 12-10

Muscle infected with trichina worm *Trichinella spiralis.* Juveniles may live 10 to 20 years in these cysts. If eaten in poorly cooked meat, the juveniles are liberated in the intestine. They quickly mature and release many juveniles into the blood of the host.

A   B

Figure 12-11

Pinworms, *Enterobius vermicularis*. **A,** Adult pinworms; the male is much smaller. **B,** Group of pinworm eggs, which are usually discharged at night around the anus of the host, who, by scratching during sleep, may contaminate fingernails and clothing. This may be the most common and widespread of all human helminth parasites.

Courtesy Indiana University School of Medicine, Indianapolis.

juveniles penetrate blood vessels and are carried to the skeletal muscles where they coil up and form a cyst that eventually becomes calcified (Fig. 12-10). The worms may live in the cysts for years. When meat containing live cysts is swallowed, the juveniles are liberated into the intestine where they mature and produce living young.

In addition to humans, *T. spiralis* can infect many other mammals, including hogs, rats, cats, and dogs. Humans most often acquire the parasite by eating improperly cooked pork. Hogs become infected by eating garbage containing pork scraps with cysts or by eating infected rats.

Heavy infections are very serious; about 20 deaths have been caused by *T. spiralis* in the United States during the last 10 years. Lighter infections are much more common, and about 2.4% of the population of the United States is infected. The simplest preventive measure is the thorough cooking of all pork.

Pinworms

The pinworm, *Enterobius vermicularis* (Gr., *enteron*, intestine, + *bios*, life), is the most common helminth parasite of humans in the United States. Its prevalence is estimated conservatively at 30% in children and 16% in adults, and it is found among people in all socioeconomic groups, from the deep South to Alaska. Fortunately, it is relatively nonpathogenic. The adults (Fig. 12-11, *A*) live in the large intestine and cecum. The females, up to about 12 mm in length, migrate to the anal region at night to lay their eggs (Fig. 12-11, *B*). Scratching the resultant itch effectively contaminates the hands and bed clothes. Eggs embryonate rapidly and become infective within 6 hours at body temperature. When they are swallowed, they hatch in the duodenum and mature in the large intestine. The diagnosis is made by applying the sticky side of cellulose tape around the anus to collect eggs and then examining the tape under the microscope. Several drugs are very effective against pinworm, but all members of a family should be treated at the same time, since the worm easily spreads through a household. Small numbers of pinworms do not usually produce symptoms, but larger numbers may cause intestinal disturbance, perianal itching, and even nervousness and irritability in children.

Whipworms

Trichuris trichiura (Gr., *thrix*, hair, + *ura*, tail) is probably the most common nematode of humans after *Enterobius* and *Ascaris*, especially in children in warmer locales. The eggs are passed in the feces and embryonate in the soil. Adults live in the lower ileum and cecum, where damage to the intestinal mucosa in heavy infections can result in serious disease, and occasionally even death.

Filarial worms

At least eight different species of filarial nematodes infect humans, and some of these worms are major causes of disease. Some 250 million people in tropical countries are infected with *Wuchereria bancrofti* (named for Otto Wucherer) or *Brugia malayi* (named for S.L. Brug), which places these species among the scourges of humanity. The worms live in the lymphatic system, and the females are as long as 100 mm. The disease symptoms are associated with inflammation and obstruction of the lymphatic system. The females release live young, the tiny **microfilariae,** into the blood and lymph. When the microfilariae are ingested by the appropriate species of mosquito, along with its blood meal, they penetrate the mosquito's gut and develop to third-stage, infective juveniles. They escape from the proboscis sheath of the mosquito when it is feeding again on a human and penetrate the wound made by the mosquito bite. Although the infection may be asymptomatic, various inflammatory responses usually occur, and the dramatic manifestations of **elephantiasis** are occasionally produced. This condition is associated with long and repeated exposure to the worms and is marked by an excessive growth of connective tissue and enormous swelling of affected parts, such as the scrotum, legs, arms, and more rarely, the vulva and breasts (Fig. 12-12).

Another filarial worm, *Oncocerca volvulus* (Gr., *onkos*, barb, hook, + *kerkos*, tail) infects more than 30 million people in parts of Africa, Arabia, Central America, and South America. It causes **river blindness** and is carried by the blackfly, *Simulium* sp.

Guinea worms

Dracunculus medinensis (L., *draco*, dragon, + *unculus*, small), the guinea worm, is found in certain areas of Africa, India, and the Middle East. The male is small, but the female is up to 80 cm long and lies just under the surface of the skin of its host, where it appears much like a varicose vein. The worm causes an ulcer in the skin through which it discharges living larvae on contact with water. The larvae are picked up by the small aquatic crustacean *Cyclops*, in which they undergo further development (Fig. 12-13, *B*). Infections occur from drinking water containing the *Cyclops*. The worms can be removed surgically, but the time-honored method of removing the adult worm has been to wind it out on a small stick, a little each day (Fig. 12-13, *A*). It is interesting to note that the "fiery serpent" of biblical times was probably the guinea worm.

Figure 12-12

Elephantiasis of leg caused by adult filarial worms of *Wuchereria bancrofti,* which live in lymph passages and block the flow of lymph. Tiny juveniles, called microfilariae, are picked up with blood meal of mosquitoes, where they develop to infective stage and are transmitted to a new host.

AFIP No. 44430-1.

A

Figure 12-13

A, Guinea worm *Dracunculus* being extracted from host by winding one turn of the stick each day to prevent rupturing the worm and causing infection. Surgery is a more modern method. **B,** *Cyclops,* a copepod, containing *Dracunculus* larvae in body cavity.

A, Courtesy J. Donges. From H. Zaiman (ed.). A pictorial presentation of parasites.

Figure 12-14

Structure of *Paragordius*, a nematomorph. **A,** Longitudinal section through the anterior end. **B,** Transverse section. **C,** Posterior end of male and female worms. Nematomorphs, or "horsehair worms," are very long and very thin. Their pharynx is usually a solid cord of cells and is nonfunctional. *Paragordius*, whose pharynx opens through to the intestine, is unusual in this respect and also in the possession of a photosensory organ ("eye").

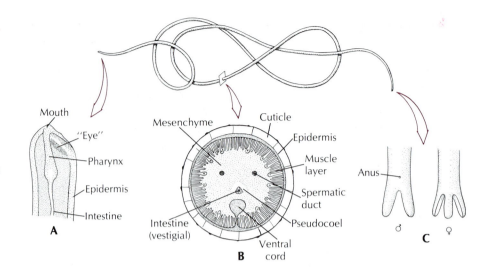

Phylum Nematomorpha

The popular name for the Nematomorpha (nem'a-to-mor'fa) (Gr. *nēma, nēmatos,* thread, + *morphe,* form) is "horsehair worms," based on an old superstition that the worms arise from horsehairs that happen to fall into the water. They were long included with the nematodes, with which they share the structure of the cuticle, presence of epidermal cords, longitudinal muscles only, and pattern of nervous system. However, since the early larval form of some species has a striking resemblance to the Priapulida, it is impossible to say to what group the nematomorphs are most closely related.

The horsehair worms are free living as adults and parasitic in arthropods as juveniles. As a group they have worldwide distribution and a variety of aquatic habitats and may be found in both running and standing water. Adults do not feed but will live almost anywhere in wet or moist surroundings if the oxygen is adequate. Juveniles do not emerge from the arthropod host unless there is water nearby. Adults are often seen wriggling slowly about in ponds or streams, with males being more active than females. The female discharges her eggs in water in long strings. Some juveniles, such as *Gordius* (named for an ancient king who tied an intricate knot), a cosmopolitan genus, are believed to encyst on vegetation that may later serve as food for a grasshopper or other arthropod. In the marine form *Nectonema* (Gr., *nēktos,* swimming, + *nēma,* thread), juveniles occur in hermit crabs and other crabs.

Form and function

Horsehair worms are extremely long and slender, with a cylindrical body. They may reach a length of 1.5 m with a diameter of only 3 mm, but most are smaller with a diameter of 1 to 2 mm. The anterior ends are usually rounded, and the posterior ends are rounded or have two or three caudal lobes (Fig. 12-14).

The body wall is much like that of nematodes: a secreted **cuticle,** an **epidermis,** and musculature of **longitudinal muscles** only. Ventral or dorsal and ventral, but not lateral, **epidermal cords** are present. The **pseudocoel** in many species is largely filled with parenchymal cells.

The **digestive system** is vestigial. The pharynx is a solid cord of cells, and the intestine does not open to the cloaca. The larval forms absorb food from their arthropod hosts through the body wall, and the adults apparently live on stored nutrients.

Circulatory, respiratory, and excretory systems are lacking. There are a nerve ring around the pharynx and a midventral nerve cord. Each sex has a pair of gonads and a pair of gonoducts that empty into the cloaca. The young hatch from the eggs and somehow gain entry into the arthropod host. After several months in the hemocoel of the host, the matured worm emerges into the water. Curiously, if the host is a terrestrial insect, it is stimulated by an unknown mechanism to seek water.

___ Phylum Acanthocephala

The members of the phylum Acanthocephala (a-kan'tho-sef'a-la) (Gr., *akantha,* spine or thorn, + *kephalē,* head) are commonly known as "spiny-headed worms." The phylum derives its name from one of its most distinctive features, a cylindrical invaginable proboscis bearing rows of recurved spines, by which it attaches itself to the intestine of its host. All acanthocephalans are endoparasitic, living as adults in the intestines of vertebrates.

Various species range in size from less than 2 mm to more than 1 m in length, with the females of a species usually larger than the males. In life the body is usually bilaterally flattened, with numerous transverse wrinkles. The worms are usually cream color but may be yellowish or brown as a result of absorption of pigments from the intestinal contents.

Acanthocephalans inflict traumatic damage by penetrating the intestinal wall with the spiny proboscis. In many cases there is remarkably little inflammation, but in some species the inflammatory response of the host is intense. Great pain can be produced, particularly if the gut wall is completely perforated.

More than 500 species are known, most of which parasitize fish, birds, and mammals, and the phylum is worldwide in distribution. However, no species is normally a parasite of humans, although rarely humans are infected with species that usually occur in other hosts. *Macracanthorhynchus hirudinaceus* (Gr., *makros,* long, large, + *akantha,* spine, thorn, + *rhynchos,* beak) occurs throughout the world in the small intestine of pigs and occasionally in other mammals.

Larvae of spiny-headed worms develop in arthropods, either crustaceans or insects, depending on the species.

CHARACTERISTICS

1. Body cylindrical (often flattened in life); anterior end with **spiny retractile proboscis** and sheath
2. **Tegument** syncytial, containing fluid-filled channels (lacunae); body wall with circular and longitudinal muscles
3. Fluid-filled pseudocoel
4. No digestive, respiratory, or circulatory systems
5. Excretory system, when present, with two branched ciliated protonephridia connected to a common excretory duct
6. Nervous system with a central ganglion within the proboscis receptacle and nerves to proboscis and body; sensory endings on proboscis and genital bursa
7. Sexes separate; shelled larvae embryonate in pseudocoel of female; special selector apparatus in female system
8. Adults parasitic in intestine of vertebrates; juveniles develop in arthropods; other animals may serve as transport hosts

---

Figure 12-15

Structure of a spiny-headed worm (phylum Acanthocephala). **A** and **B**, Eversible spiny proboscis by which the parasite attaches to the intestine of the host, often doing great damage. Since they lack a digestive tract, food is absorbed through the tegument. **C**, Male is typically smaller than female.

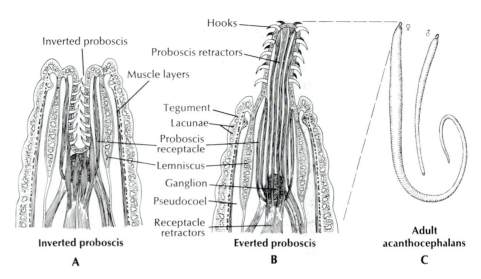

Inverted proboscis — Muscle layers — Tegument — Lacunae — Proboscis receptacle — Lemniscus — Ganglion — Pseudocoel — Receptacle retractors — Hooks — Proboscis retractors

Inverted proboscis / **A**   **Everted proboscis** / **B**   **Adult acanthocephalans** / **C**

Form and function

In life the body is somewhat flattened, although it is usual for specimens to be treated with tap water before fixation so that fixed specimens are turgid and cylindrical (Fig. 12-15, C).

The body wall is syncytial, and its surface is punctured by minute crypts 4 to 6 μm deep, which greatly increase the surface area of the tegument. About 80% of the thickness of the tegument is the radial fiber zone, which contains a **lacunar system** of ramifying fluid-filled canals (Fig. 12-15, A and B). The function of the lacunar system is unclear, but it may serve in distribution of nutrients. Attached to the neck region are two elongated **lemnisci** (extensions of the epidermis and lacunar system) that may serve as reservoirs of the lacunar fluid from the proboscis when that organ is invaginated.

The **proboscis,** bearing rows of recurved hooks, is attached to the neck region (Fig. 12-15) and can be inverted into a **proboscis receptacle** by retractor muscles. The proboscis is a forbidding organ and can cause serious damage to the intestine of its host.

There are a pair of **protonephridia** with flame cells that unite to form a common tube opening into the sperm duct or uterus.

Since acanthocephalans have no digestive tract, they must absorb all nutrients through their tegument. They can absorb various molecules by specific membrane transport mechanisms, and their tegument can carry out pinocytosis. The tegument bears some enzymes, such as peptidases, which can cleave several dipeptides, and the amino acids are then absorbed by the worm. Like cestodes, acanthocephalans require host dietary carbohydrate, but their mechanism for absorption of glucose is different. As glucose is absorbed, it is rapidly phosphorylated and compartmentalized, so that a metabolic "sink" is created into which glucose in the surrounding medium can flow. Glucose can diffuse down a concentration gradient into the worm because it is constantly removed as soon as it enters.

A pair of tubular **genital ligaments,** or **ligament sacs,** extends posteriorly from the end of the proboscis receptacle. The male has a pair of **testes,** each with a **vas deferens,** and a common **ejaculatory duct** that ends in a small **penis.** During copulation sperm are ejected into the vagina, travel up the genital duct, and escape into the pseudocoel.

In the female the ovarian tissue in the ligament sac breaks up into **ovarian balls** that rupture the ligament sacs and float free in the pseudocoel. One of the ligament sacs leads to a funnel-shaped **uterine bell** that receives the developing shelled embryos and passes them on to the uterus (Fig. 12-16). An interesting and unique **selective apparatus** operates here. Fully developed embryos are slightly longer than immature ones, and they are passed on into the uterus, while immature eggs are retained for further maturation.

The shelled embryos, which are discharged in the feces of the vertebrate host, do not hatch until eaten by the intermediate host. For *M. hirudinaceus* this is any of several species of soil-inhabiting beetle larvae, especially scarabeids. Grubs of the June beetle *(Phyllophaga)* are frequent hosts. Here the larva (**acanthor**) burrows through the intestine and develops into the juvenile (**cystacanth**). Pigs are infected by eating the grubs. Multiple infections may do considerable damage to the pig's intestine, and perforations may occur.

Phylum Entoprocta

Entoprocta (en'to-prok'ta) (Gr., *entos*, within, + *proktos*, anus) is a small phylum of fewer than 100 species of tiny, sessile animals that superficially resemble hydroid cnidarians but have ciliated tentacles that tend to roll inward (Fig. 12-17). Most entoprocts are microscopic, and none is more than 5 mm long. They are all stalked and sessile forms; some are colonial, and some are solitary. All are ciliary feeders.

With the exception of the genus *Urnatella* (L., *urna*, urn, + *ellus*, dim. suffix), all entoprocts are marine forms that have a wide distribution from the polar regions to the tropics. Most marine species are restricted to coastal and brackish waters and often grow on shells and algae. Some are commensals on marine annelid worms. Freshwater entoprocts occur on the underside of rocks in running

Figure 12-16

Scheme of the genital selective apparatus of a female acanthocephalan. It is a unique device for separating immature from mature fertilized eggs. Eggs containing larvae enter the uterine bell and pass on to the uterus and exterior. Immature eggs are shunted into the ventral ligament sac or into the pseudocoel to undergo further development.

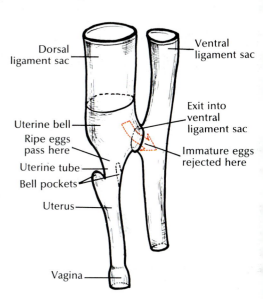

Figure 12-17

A, *Loxosomella*, a solitary entoproct. **B**, *Urnatella*, a freshwater entoproct, forms small colonies of two or three stalks from a basal plate. Both solitary and colonial entoprocts can reproduce asexually by budding, as well as sexually.

A, Photograph by L.S. Roberts; **B**, modified from Con, C. 1936. Kamptozoa. In H.G. Bronn (ed.). Klassen and Ordnungen des Tier-Reichs, vol. 4, part 2. Leipzig, Akademische Verlagsgesselschaft.

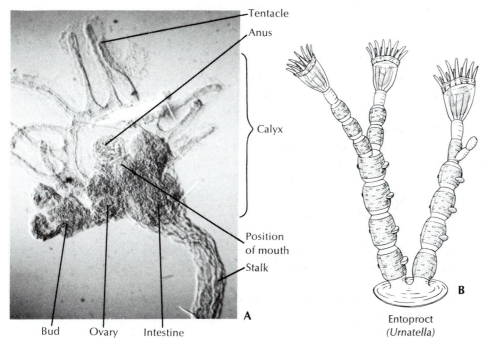

Entoproct
(Urnatella)

water. *U. gracilis* is the only common freshwater species in North America (Fig. 12-17, *B*).

Form and function

The body, or **calyx,** of the entoproct is cup shaped, bears a **crown,** or circle, of ciliated **tentacles,** and may be attached to a substratum by a single **stalk** and an attachment disc with adhesive glands, as in the solitary *Loxosomella* (Gr., *loxos,* crooked, + *soma,* body, + *ellus,* dim. suffix) (Fig. 12-17, *A*), or by two or more stalks in colonial forms. Both tentacles and stalk are continuations of the body wall. The eight to 30 tentacles making up the crown are ciliated on their lateral and inner surfaces, and each can move individually. The tentacles can roll inward to cover and protect the mouth and anus but cannot be retracted into the calyx.

Movement is usually restricted in entoprocts, but *Loxosoma,* which lives in the tubes of marine annelids, is described as quite active, moving over the annelid and its tube freely.

The gut is ∪ shaped and ciliated, and both the mouth and the anus open within the circle of tentacles. Entoprocts are **ciliary filter feeders.** Long cilia on the sides of the tentacles keep a current of water containing protozoa, diatoms, and particles of detritus moving in between the tentacles. Short cilia on the inner surfaces of the tentacles capture the food and direct it downward toward the mouth.

The **body wall** consists of a cuticle, cellular epidermis, and longitudinal muscles. The **pseudocoel** is largely filled with a gelatinous parenchyma in which is embedded a pair of **protonephridia** and their ducts, which unite and empty near the mouth. There is a well-developed **nerve ganglion** on the ventral side of the stomach, and the body surface bears sensory bristles and pits. Circulatory and respiratory organs are absent. Exchange of gases occurs through the body surface, probably much of it through the tentacles.

Some species are monoecious, some dioecious, and some appear to be **protandric;** that is, the gonad at first produces sperm and later eggs. The gonoducts open within the circle of tentacles.

Fertilized eggs develop in a depression, or brood pouch, between the gonopore and the anus. Entoprocts have a modified spiral cleavage pattern with mosaic blastomeres. The coeloblastula is formed by invagination. The trochophore-like larva is ciliated and free swimming. It has an apical tuft of cilia at the anterior end and a ciliated girdle around the ventral margin of the body. Eventually the larva settles to the substratum and inverts to form the adult.

____ Phylogeny and Adaptive Radiation
Phylogeny

Hyman (1951) grouped the Rotifera, Gastrotricha, Kinorhyncha, Nematoda, and Nematomorpha into a single phylum (Aschelminthes). All of these phyla share a certain combination of characteristics, including the fact that they are usually wormlike, have a cuticle secreted by an epidermis that is underlain by muscles not arranged in regular circular and longitudinal layers, have a brain that is a circumenteric nerve ring, have determinate cleavage and eutely, and lack a muscle layer in the intestine. Hyman contended that the evidences of relationships were so concrete and specific that they could not be disregarded. Nevertheless, most authors now consider that differences between the groups are sufficient to merit phylum status for each, although some accept the concept of the Aschelminthes as a superphylum. These phyla may well have been derived originally from the protostome line via an acoelomate common ancestor resembling the rhabdocoel flatworms. The possible relationship of the Gnathostomulida to the Gastrotricha and Rotifera was mentioned in Chapter 11.

Acanthocephalans are highly specialized parasites with a unique structure and have doubtless been so for millions of years. Any ancestral or other related group that would shed a clue to the phyletic relationships of the Acanthocephala is probably long since extinct. Like the cestodes, acanthocephalans have no digestive tract and must absorb all nutrients across the tegument, but the tegument of the two groups is quite different in structure. Also, acanthocephalans are pseudocoelomate and show eutely, as in the nematodes, although here, too, the structural and developmental differences are great. Thus, the Acanthocephala are an isolated phylum, not closely related to any known form.

The entoprocts were once included with the phylum Ectoprocta in a phylum called Bryozoa, but the ectoprocts are true coelomate animals, and many zoologists prefer to place them in a separate group. Ectoprocts are still often referred to as bryozoans. The Entoprocta may be distantly related to the Ectoprocta, but there is little evidence of close relationship. The entoprocts may have arisen as an early offshoot of the same line that led to the ectoprocts.

Adaptive radiation

Certainly the most impressive adaptive radiation in this group of phyla is shown by the nematodes. They are by far the most numerous in terms of both individuals and species, and they have been able to adapt to almost every habitat available to animal life. Their basic pseudocoelomate body plan, with the cuticle, hydrostatic skeleton, and longitudinal muscles, has proved generalized and plastic enough to adapt to an enormous variety of physical conditions. Free-living lines gave rise to parasitic forms on at least several occasions, and virtually all potential hosts have been exploited. All types of life cycle occur: from the simple and direct to the complex, with intermediate hosts; from normal dioecious reproduction to parthenogenesis, hermaphroditism, and alteration of free-living and parasitic generations. A major factor contributing to the evolutionary opportunism of the nematodes has been their extraordinary capacity to survive conditions suboptimal for viability, for example, the developmental arrests in many free-living and animal parasitic species and the ability to undergo cryptobiosis in many free-living and plant parasitic species.

___ Summary

The phyla covered in this chapter possess a body cavity called a pseudocoel, which is derived from the embryonic blastocoel, rather than a secondary cavity in the mesoderm (coelom). Several of the groups exhibit eutely, a constant number of cells or nuclei in adult individuals of a given species.

The phylum Rotifera is comprised of small, mostly freshwater organisms with a ciliated corona, which creates currents of water to draw planktonic food toward the mouth. The mouth opens into a muscular pharynx, or mastax, that is equipped with jaws.

Many rotifers can produce both amictic and mictic eggs. Amictic eggs are diploid and develop parthenogenetically into females. Mictic eggs are haploid and, if unfertilized, develop parthenogenetically into males. Fertilized mictic eggs develop into resistant, dormant eggs that can overwinter and give rise to females.

The Gastrotricha and Kinorhyncha are small phyla of tiny, aquatic pseudocoelomates. Gastrotrichs move by cilia or adhesive glands, and kinorhynchs anchor and then pull themselves forward by the spines of their first segment.

By far the largest and most important of this group of phyla are the nematodes, of which there may be as many as 500,000 species in the world. They are more or less cylindrical, tapering at the ends, and covered with a tough, secreted cuticle. The body wall muscles are longitudinal only, and to function well in locomotion, such an arrangement must enclose a volume of fluid in the pseudocoel at high hydrostatic pressure. This has a profound effect on most of nematodes' other physiological functions, such as ingestion of food, egestion of feces, excretion, and copulation. Most nematodes are dioecious, and there are four juvenile stages, each separated by a molt of the cuticle. Almost all animals and many plants have nematode parasites, and many other nematodes are free living in soil and aquatic habitats. Some nematode parasites of humans are the large roundworm (*Ascaris lumbricoides*), hookworms (for example, *Necator americanus*), trichina worm (*Trichinella spiralis*), pinworm (*Enterobius vermicularis*), and various filarial worms (for example, *Wuchereria bancrofti*). Some parasitic nematodes have part of their life cycle free living, some undergo a tissue migration in their host, and some have an intermediate host in their life cycle.

The Nematomorpha or horsehair worms are related to the nematodes and have parasitic juvenile stages in arthropods, followed by a free-living, aquatic, nonfeeding adult stage.

All Acanthocephalans are parasitic in the intestines of vertebrates as adults, and their juvenile stages develop in arthropods. They have an anterior, invaginable proboscis armed with spines, which they embed in the intestinal wall of their host. They do not have a digestive tract and so must absorb all nutrients across their tegument. Their tegument also bears a system of channels (lacunar system) of uncertain function.

The Entoprocta are small, sessile, aquatic animals with a crown of ciliated tentacles encircling both the mouth and anus.

The Rotifera, Gastrotricha, Kinorhyncha, Nematoda, and Nematomorpha have been included by some workers in a phylum Aschelminthes, but most biologists believe that the groups are not sufficiently related to be encompassed by a single phylum. It is possible that they were derived from a common ancestor in the protostome line. Phylogenetic relationships of the Acanthocephala and Entoprocta are even more obscure. Of all these phyla, the Nematoda have achieved enormous evolutionary success and undergone great adaptive radiation.

Selected references

Barnes, R.D. 1980. Invertebrate zoology, ed. 4. Philadelphia, Saunders College/Holt, Rinehart & Winston.

Bird, A.F. 1971. The structure of nematodes. New York, Academic Press, Inc.

Croll, N.A., and B.E. Matthews. 1977. Biology of nematodes. New York, John Wiley & Sons, Inc.

Donner, J. 1966. Rotifers. New York, Frederick Warne & Co., Inc.

Giese, A.C., and J.S. Pearse. 1974. Reproduction of marine invertebrates, vol. 1. New York, Academic Press, Inc. *Includes chapters on Nematoda, Rotifera, Gastrotricha, Kinorhyncha, and Gnathostomulida.*

Higgins, R.P. 1982. Kinorhyncha. In S.P. Parker (ed.). Synopsis and classification of living organisms, vol. 1. New York, McGraw-Hill Book Co.

Hummon, W.D. 1982. Gastrotricha. In S.P. Parker (ed.). Synopsis and classification of living organisms, vol. 1. New York, McGraw-Hill Book Co.

Hunter, G.W., J.C. Swartzwelder, and D.F. Clyde. 1976. Tropical medicine, ed. 5. Philadelphia, W.B. Saunders Co.

Hyman, L.H. 1951. The invertebrates: Acanthocephala, Aschelminthes, and Entoprocta, vol. 3. New York, McGraw-Hill Book Co. *Describes with great accuracy the many types of these phyla.*

Jenkins, W.R., and D.P. Taylor. 1967. Plant nematology. New York, Van Nostrand Reinhold Co.

Kaestner, A. 1967. Invertebrate zoology, vol. 1. New York, Interscience.

Lee, D.L., and H.J. Atkinson. 1977. The physiology of nematodes, ed. 2. New York, Columbia University Press.

Levine, N.D. 1980. Nematode parasites of domestic animals and of man, ed. 2. Minneapolis, Burgess Publishing Co.

Martini, E. 1912. Studien über die Konstang histologischer Elemente. III. Hydatina Senta. Zeitsch. Wiss. Zool. **102**:425-645.

Nogrady, T. 1982. Rotifera. In S.P. Parker (ed.). Synopsis and classification of living organisms, vol. 1. New York, McGraw-Hill Book Co.

Pennak, R.W. 1978. Freshwater invertebrates of the United States, ed. 2. New York, Interscience.

Reidl, R.I. 1969. Gnathostomulida from America. Science **163**:445-452.

Schmidt, G.D., and L.S. Roberts. 1981. Foundations of parasitology, ed. 2. St. Louis, The C.V. Mosby Co.

Van Cleave, H.J. 1953. Acanthocephala of North American mammals. Ill. Biol. Monographs, vol. 23, nos. 1 and 2. Urbana, University of Illinois Press.

Warren, K.S. 1974. Helminthic diseases endemic in the United States. Am. J. Trop. Med. Hyg. **23**:723-730.

Woollacott, R.M., and R.L. Zimmer (eds.). 1977. Biology of the bryozoans. New York, Academic Press, Inc. *A technical volume with several authors, at least one of whom contends that the ectoprocts are related to the entoprocts and evolved from them.*

CHAPTER 13

THE MOLLUSCS

Phylum Mollusca

The flamingo tongue, *Cyphoma gibbosum,* is a showy inhabitant of Caribbean coral reefs, where it is associated with gorgonians. This snail has a smooth, creamy orange to pink shell that is normally covered by the brightly marked mantle.

Photograph by L.S. Roberts.

Position in Animal Kingdom

1. The molluscs are one of the major groups of true **coelomate** animals.
2. They belong to the **protostome** branch, or schizocoelomous coelomates, and have spiral and determinate cleavage.
3. All the **organ systems** are present and well developed.
4. Many molluscs have a **trochophore larva** similar to the trochophore larva of marine annelids, marine turbellarians, and some others.

Biological Contributions

1. In molluscs gaseous exchange occurs not only through the body surface as in lower invertebrates, but also in specialized **respiratory organs** in the form of **gills** or **lungs**.
2. They have an open **circulatory system** in most classes, with pumping **heart**, vessels, and blood sinuses. In most cephalopods the circulatory system is closed.
3. The efficiency of the respiratory and circulatory systems in the cephalopods has made greater body size possible. Invertebrates reach their largest size in some of the cephalopods.
4. They have a fleshy **mantle** that in most cases secretes a shell and is variously modified for a number of functions.
5. Features unique to the phylum are the **radula** and the muscular **foot**.
6. The highly developed direct **eye** of higher molluscs is similar to the indirect eye of the vertebrates but arises as a skin derivative in contrast to the brain eye of vertebrates (convergent evolution, Principle no. 6, p. 12).

▬ THE MOLLUSCS

The Mollusca (mol-lus′ka) (L., *molluscus,* soft) is one of the largest animal phyla after the Arthropoda. There are nearly 50,000 living species (Boss, 1971) and some 35,000 fossil species. The name Mollusca indicates one of their distinctive characteristics, a soft body.

This very diverse group includes the chitons, tooth shells, snails, slugs, nudibranchs, sea butterflies, clams, mussels, oysters, squids, octopuses, and nautiluses. The group ranges from fairly simple organisms to some of the most complex of invertebrates, and in size from almost microscopic to the giant squid *Architeuthis.* These huge molluscs may grow to 18 m long, including their tentacles. They may weigh 450 kg (1000 pounds). The shells of some of the giant clams, *Tridacna gigas,* which inhabit the Indo-Pacific coral reefs, reach 1.5 m in length and weigh more than 225 kg. These are extremes, however, for probably 80% of all molluscs are less than 5 cm in maximum shell size. The phylum includes some of the most sluggish and some of the swiftest and most active of the invertebrates. It includes herbivorous grazers, predaceous carnivores, filter feeders, detritus feeders, and parasites.

Molluscs are found in a great range of habitats, from the tropics to polar seas, at altitudes exceeding 7000 m, in ponds, lakes, and streams, on mud flats, in pounding surf, and in open ocean from the surface to the abyssal depths. Most of them live in the sea, and they represent a variety of life-styles, including bottom feeders, burrowers, borers, and pelagic forms.

According to the fossil evidence, the molluscs originated in the sea, and most of them have remained there. Much of their evolution occurred along the shores, where food was abundant and habitats were varied. Only the bivalves and gastropods moved on to brackish and freshwater habitats. As filter feeders, the bivalves were unable to leave aquatic surroundings. Only the snails (gastropods) actually invaded the land. Terrestrial snails are limited in their range by their need for humidity, shelter, and the presence of calcium in the soil.

A

Figure 13-1

Molluscs: a diversity of life forms. The basic body plan of this ancient group has become variously adapted for different habitats. **A,** Marine snail *(Calliostoma annulata),* class Gastropoda, subclass Prosobranchia. **B,** Nudibranch *(Hermissenda crassicornis),* class Gastropoda, subclass Opisthobranchia. **C,** Chiton *(Tonicella lineata),* class Polyplacophora. **D,** Octopus *(Octopus* sp.), class Cephalopoda. **E,** Marine clam *(Donax denticulatus)* with siphons and foot extended, class Bivalvia.

A to D, Photographs by R. Harbo; E, photograph by K. Sandved.

A wide variety of molluscs are used as food. Pearl buttons are obtained from shells of bivalves. The Mississippi and Missouri river basins have furnished material for most of this industry in the United States; however, supplies are becoming so depleted that attempts are being made to propagate bivalves artificially. Pearls, both natural and cultured, are produced in the shells of clams and oysters, most of them in a marine oyster, *Meleagrina,* found around eastern Asia (Fig. 13-3, *B).*

Some molluscs are destructive. The burrowing shipworms, which are bivalves of several species (Fig. 13-24), do great damage to wooden ships and wharves. To prevent the ravages of shipworms, wharves must be either creosoted or built of concrete. Snails and slugs frequently damage garden and other vegetation. In addition, snails often serve as intermediate hosts for serious parasites. The boring snail *Urosalpinx* rivals the sea star in destroying oysters.

In this chapter we explore the various major groups of molluscs, those that apparently met with little evolutionary success and those that have been enormously successful. All are based on the basic body plan of the Mollusca, which is described later in the chapter. Before proceeding, however, we must turn our attention briefly to a major anatomical feature that makes its appearance in the molluscs: the coelom.

___ Significance of the Coelom

Heretofore we have been studying animals that lack a true coelom. These follow several patterns. In the radiates with gelatinous mesoglea between the body surface and the enteron, diffusion of substances is a simple matter. In flatworms body spaces are filled with cellular parenchyma of endomesoderm; here the need for a better transport method is met by the extensive branching of the gastrovascular cavity and of the protonephridial system throughout the body. In the nemertines this is aided by a system of blood vessels.

In the pseudocoelomates the parenchyma is replaced by spongy or open spaces: the pseudocoel. Fluid in the pseudocoel bathes the organs, providing a means of internal transport serviceable enough for small animals. Lacking mesenteries, the organs lie loose in the body cavity. The pseudocoelomates are all small; obviously such an arrangement would be unsuitable for larger forms.

In the coelomates the coelom develops as a secondary cavity within the mesoderm. The coelomic cavity is completely surrounded by mesodermal epithelium, called **parietal peritoneum.** There is ample room in the coelom not only for organs but also for **mesenteries,** continuations of the peritoneum that hold the organs in place. The organs are themselves covered with **visceral peritoneum.** This ensures a more stable arrangement of organs with less crowding. The alimentary canal can become more muscular, more highly specialized, and more diversified without interfering with other organs, such as the heart, liver, or lungs.

The coelom performs other important functions. It is filled with **coelomic fluid,** and its lining is often ciliated to keep the fluid moving. Thus, it aids in the movement of materials, such as absorbed foods and metabolic wastes, from one place to another. In many smaller coelomates no other transport system is necessary. In animals with a vascular system, the mesenteries provide an ideal location for the network of blood vessels necessary to deliver blood to every body organ.

The coelom can also serve as a hydrostatic skeleton. Circular and longitudinal body wall muscles, acting as antagonists, can contract or relax to vary the force exerted on the coelomic fluid and thus produce a variety of body movements.

Altogether the development of the coelom must be considered an important stepping stone in the evolution of larger and more complex forms. The three major phyla of coelomate protostomes are the molluscs, the annelids, and the arthropods. A number of smaller invertebrate phyla, the echinoderms, and the vertebrates are also coelomates. Ironically, despite the physiological advantages of a coelom, the molluscs do not seem to have exploited them. The coelom in molluscs is limited to a space around the heart and perhaps around the gonads. Nevertheless, the coelom of molluscs develops embryonically in a manner similar to that of the annelids and represents in early form an important body plan to be exploited more fully in other groups.

CHARACTERISTICS

1. Body bilaterally symmetrical (bilateral asymmetry in some); unsegmented; usually with definite head
2. Ventral body wall specialized as a muscular **foot,** variously modified but used chiefly for locomotion
3. Dorsal body wall forms pair of folds called the **mantle,** which encloses the **mantle cavity,** is modified into **gills** or **lungs,** and secretes the **shell** (shell absent in some)
4. Surface epithelium usually ciliated and bearing mucous glands and sensory nerve endings

5. **Coelom** limited mainly to area around heart and perhaps lumen of gonads
6. Complex digestive system; rasping organ (**radula**) usually present; anus usually emptying into mantle cavity
7. **Open circulatory system** (mostly closed in cephalopods) of heart (usually three chambered), blood vessels, and sinuses; respiratory pigments in blood
8. Gaseous exchange by **gills, lungs, mantle,** or **body surface**
9. One or two kidneys (**metanephridia**) opening into the pericardial cavity and usually emptying into the mantle cavity
10. Nervous system of paired cerebral, pleural, pedal, and visceral ganglia, with nerve cords and subepidermal plexus; ganglia centralized in nerve ring in gastropods and cephalopods
11. Sensory organs of touch, smell, taste, equilibrium, and vision (in some); eyes highly developed in cephalopods
12. Internal and external **ciliary tracts** often of great functional importance

CLASSIFICATION

Useful characteristics for distinction of classes of molluscs are the type of foot and the type of shell. Several other characteristics are important in particular classes.

Class Caudofoveata (kaw′do-fo-ve-at′a) (L., *cauda*, tail, + *fovea*, small pit). Wormlike; shell, head, and excretory organs absent; radula usually present; mantle with chitinous cuticle and calcareous scales; oral pedal shield near anterior mouth; mantle cavity at posterior end with pair of gills; sexes separate; formerly united with solenogasters in class Aplacophora. Examples: *Chaetoderma, Limifossor.*

Class Solenogastres (so-len′o-gas′trez) (Gr., *solen*, pipe, + *gaster*, stomach)—**solenogasters.** Wormlike; shell, head, and excretory organs absent; radula usually absent; mantle usually covered with scales or spicules; mantle cavity posterior, without true gills, but sometimes with secondary respiratory structures; foot represented by long, narrow, ventral pedal groove; hermaphroditic. Example: *Neomenia.*

Class Monoplacophora (mon′o-pla-kof′o-ra) (Gr., *monos*, one, + *plax*, plate, + *phora*, bearing). Body bilaterally symmetrical with a broad flat foot; a single limpetlike shell; mantle cavity with five or six pairs of gills; large coelomic cavities; radula present; six pairs of nephridia, two of which are gonoducts; separate sexes. Example: *Neopilina* (Fig. 13-6).

Class Polyplacophora (pol′y-pla-kof′o-ra) (Gr., *polys*, many, several, + *plax*, plate, + *phora*, bearing)—**chitons.** Elongated, dorsoventrally flattened body with reduced head; bilaterally symmetrical; radula present; shell of eight dorsal plates; foot broad and flat; gills multiple, along sides of body between foot and mantle edge; sexes usually separate, with a trochophore but no veliger larva. Examples: *Mopalia* (Fig. 13-7), *Tonicella* (Fig. 13-1, C).

Class Scaphopoda (ska-fop′o-da) (Gr., *skaphe*, trough, boat, + *pous, podos*, foot)—**tusk shells.** Body enclosed in a one-piece tubular shell open at both ends; conical foot; mouth with radula and tentacles; head absent; mantle for respiration; sexes separate; trochophore larva. Example: *Dentalium* (Fig. 13-9).

Class Gastropoda (gas-trop′o-da) (Gr., *gaster*, belly, + *pous, podos*, foot)—**snails** and others. Body asymmetrical and shows effects of torsion; body usually in a coiled shell (shell uncoiled or absent in some); head well developed, with radula; foot large and flat; one or two gills, or with mantle modified into secondary gills or a lung; most with single auricle and single nephridium; nervous system with cerebral, pleural, pedal, and visceral ganglia; dioecious or monoecious, some with trochophore, typically with veliger, some without pelagic larva. Examples: *Busycon, Polinices* (Fig. 13-13), *Physa, Helix, Aplysia* (Fig. 13-15).

Class Bivalvia (bi-val′ve-a) (L., *bi*, two, + *valva*, folding door, valve) (**Pelecypoda**)—**bivalves.** Body enclosed in a two-lobed mantle; shell of two lateral valves of variable size and form, with dorsal hinge; head greatly reduced, but mouth with labial palps; no radula; no cephalic eyes, a few with eyes on mantle margin; foot usually wedge shaped; gills platelike; sexes usually separate, typically with trochophore and veliger

larvae. Examples: *Anodonta, Venus, Tagelus* (Fig. 13-23), *Teredo* (Fig. 13-24).
Class Cephalopoda (sef′a-lop′o-da) (Gr., *kephalē*, head, + *pous, podos*, foot)—squids and octopuses. Shell often reduced or absent; head well developed with eyes and a radula; foot modified into arms or tentacles; siphon present; nervous system of well-developed ganglia, centralized to form a brain; sexes separate, with direct development. Examples: *Loligo* (Fig. 13-33), *Octopus* (Fig. 13-1, *D*), *Sepia* (Fig. 13-34).

___ Form and Function

The enormous variety, great beauty, and easy availability of the shells of molluscs have made shell collecting a popular pastime. However, many amateur shell collectors, even though able to name hundreds of the shells that grace our beaches, know very little about the living animals that created those shells and once lived in them. Reduced to its simplest dimensions, the mollusc body plan may be said to consist of a **head-foot** portion and a **visceral hump** portion. The head-foot is the more active area, containing the feeding, cephalic sensory, and locomotor organs. It depends primarily on muscular action for its function. The visceral hump is the portion containing digestive, circulatory, respiratory, and reproductive organs, and it depends primarily on ciliary tracts for its functioning. Two folds of skin, outgrowths of the dorsal body wall, make up a protective **mantle**, or **pallium**, which encloses a space between the mantle and body wall called the **mantle cavity** (**pallial cavity**). The mantle cavity houses the **gills** or lung, and in some molluscs the mantle secretes a protective **shell** over the visceral hump. Modifications of the structures comprising the head-foot and the visceral hump produce the great confusion of different patterns making up this major group of animals. Greater emphasis on either the head-foot portion or the visceral hump portion can be observed in the various classes of molluscs.

Head-foot

Most molluscs have well-developed heads, which bear the mouth and some specialized sensory organs. Photosensory receptors range from fairly simple up to the complex eyes of the cephalopods. Tentacles are often present. Within the mouth is a structure unique to molluscs, the radula, and usually posterior to the mouth is the chief locomotor organ, or foot.

Radula

The radula is a rasping, protrusible, tonguelike organ found in all molluscs except the bivalves and most solenogasters. It is a ribbonlike membrane on which are mounted rows of tiny teeth that point backward (Fig. 13-2). Complex muscles move the radula and its supporting cartilages (**odontophore**) in and out while the membrane is partly rotated over the tips of the cartilages. There may be a few or as many as 250,000 teeth, which, when protruded, can scrape, pierce, tear, or cut. The usual function of the radula is twofold: to rasp off fine particles of food material and to serve as a conveyor belt for carrying the particles in a continuous stream toward the digestive tract. As the radula wears away anteriorly, new rows of teeth are continuously replaced by secretion at its posterior end. The pattern and number of teeth in a row are specific for each species and are used in the classification of molluscs. Very interesting radular specializations, such as for boring through hard materials or for harpooning prey, are found in some forms.

Figure 13-2

A, Diagrammatic longitudinal section of gastropod head showing the radula and radula sac. The radula moves back and forth over the odontophore cartilage. As the animal grazes, the mouth opens, the odontophore is thrust forward, the radula gives a strong scrape backward bringing food into the pharynx, and the mouth closes. The sequence is repeated rhythmically. As the radula ribbon wears out anteriorly, it is continually replaced posteriorly. **B,** Radula of a snail (*Cittarium pica*) prepared for microscopic examination.

B, Photograph by K. Sandved.

Figure 13-3

A, Diagrammatic vertical section of shell and mantle of a bivalve. The outer mantle epithelium secretes the shell; the inner epithelium is usually ciliated. B, Formation of pearl between mantle and shell as a parasite or bit of sand under the mantle becomes covered with nacre.

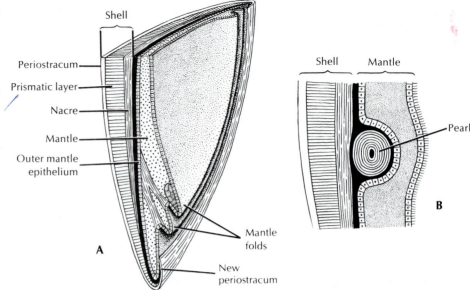

Foot

The molluscan foot may be adapted for locomotion, for attachment to a substratum, for food capture (in cephalopods), or for a combination of these functions. It is usually a ventral, solelike structure in which waves of muscular contraction effect a creeping locomotion (Fig. 13-14). However, there are many modifications, such as the attachment disc of the limpets, the laterally compressed "hatchet foot" of the bivalves, or the division of the foot into the suckered arms and tentacles of the squids and octopuses. Secreted mucus is often used as an aid to adhesion or as a slime track by small molluscs that glide on cilia.

The foot is manipulated by a combination of muscles and hydraulic mechanisms. Some molluscs glide by rhythmical waves of muscular action. In snails and bivalves the foot is extended from the body hydraulically, by engorgement with blood. Burrowing forms can extend the foot into the mud or sand, enlarge it with blood pressure, then use the engorged foot as an anchor to draw the body forward. In pelagic (free-swimming) forms the foot may be modified into winglike parapodia, or thin, mobile fins for swimming.

Visceral hump
Mantle and mantle cavity

The mantle is a sheath of skin extending from the visceral hump that hangs down on each side of the body, protecting the soft parts and creating between itself and the visceral mass the space called the mantle cavity. The outer surface of the mantle secretes the shell.

The mantle cavity plays an enormous role in the life of the mollusc. It usually houses the respiratory organs (gills or lung), which develop from the mantle, and the mantle's own exposed surface serves also for gaseous exchange. Into the mantle cavity are emptied products from the digestive, excretory, and reproductive systems. In aquatic molluscs a continuous current of water, kept moving by surface cilia or by muscular pumping, brings in oxygen and, in some forms, food; flushes out wastes; and carries reproductive products out to the environment. In aquatic forms the mantle is usually equipped with sensory receptors for sampling the environmental water. In cephalopods (squids and octopuses) the muscular mantle and its cavity create the jet propulsion used in locomotion. Many molluscs can withdraw the head or foot into the mantle cavity, which is surrounded by the shell, for protection.

Shell

The shell of the mollusc, when present, is secreted by the mantle and is lined by it. Typically there are three layers (Fig. 13-3). The **periostracum** is the outer horny layer, composed of an organic substance called conchiolin, which consists of quinone-tanned protein. It helps to protect the underlying calcareous layers from erosion by boring organisms. It is secreted by a fold of the mantle edge, and growth occurs only at the margin of the shell. On the older parts of the shell the periostracum often becomes worn away. The middle **prismatic layer** is composed of densely packed prisms of calcium carbonate laid down in a protein matrix. It is secreted by the glandular margin of the mantle, and increase in shell size occurs at the shell margin as the animal grows. The inner **nacreous layer** of the shell lies next to the mantle and is secreted continuously by the mantle surface, so that it increases in thickness during the life of the animal. The calcareous nacre is laid down in thin layers. Very thin and wavy layers produce the iridescent mother-of-pearl found in the abalones *(Haliotis),* the chambered nautilus *(Nautilus),* and many bivalves. Such shells may have 450 to 5000 fine parallel layers of crystalline calcium carbonate (aragonite) for each centimeter of thickness.

Freshwater molluscs usually have a thick periostracum that gives some protection against the acids produced in the water by the decay of leaf litter. In many marine molluscs the periostracum is relatively thin, and in some it is absent. There is a great variation in shell structure. Calcium for the shell comes from the environmental water or soil or from food. The first shell appears during the larval period and grows continuously throughout life.

Internal structure and function

In the molluscs, oxygen–carbon dioxide exchange occurs not only through the body surface, particularly that of the **mantle,** but in specialized respiratory organs such as gills or lungs, which are derivatives of the mantle. There is an **open circulatory system** with a pumping **heart,** blood vessels, and blood sinuses. Most cephalopods have a closed blood system with heart, vessels, and capillaries. The digestive tract is complex and highly specialized, according to the feeding habits of the various molluscs, and is usually provided with extensive ciliary tracts. Most molluscs have a pair of **kidneys (nephridia),** which connect with the coelom; the ducts of the kidneys in many forms serve also for the discharge of eggs and sperm. The **nervous system,** consisting of several pairs of ganglia with connecting nerve cords, is in general simpler than that of the annelids and arthropods. Neurosecretory cells have been identified in the nervous system that, at least in certain air-breathing snails, produce a growth hormone and function in osmoregulation. There are a number of types of highly specialized sense organs.

Reproduction and life history

Most molluscs are dioecious, although some are hermaphroditic. The free-swimming larva that emerges from the egg in primitive molluscs is the **trochophore,** which is also the primitive larval type of the annelids (Fig. 13-4). In most primitive molluscs the trochophore metamorphoses directly into a small juvenile, but in

Figure 13-4

Generalized trochophore larva. Molluscs and annelids with primitive embryonic development have trochophore larvae, as do several other phyla.

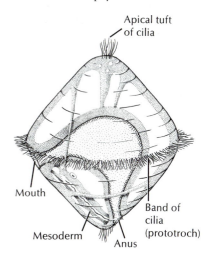

Apical tuft of cilia

Mouth

Mesoderm

Anus

Band of cilia (prototroch)

The trochophore larva (Fig. 13-4) is minute, translucent, and more or less pear shaped and has a prominent circlet of cilia (prototroch) and sometimes one or two accessory circlets. It is found in molluscs and annelids with primitive embryonic development and is considered one of the evidences for common phylogenetic origin of the two phyla. Some form of trochophore-like larva is also found in marine turbellarians, nemertines, brachiopods, phoronids, sipunculids, and echiurids, and it probably reflects some phylogenetic relationship among all these phyla.

Figure 13-5

Veliger of a snail, *Pedicularia*, swimming. The adults are parasitic on corals.
Photograph by K. Sandved.

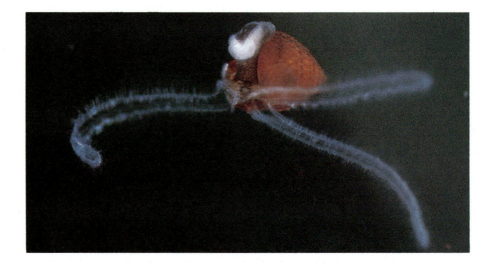

more advanced forms, another free-swimming larval stage, the **veliger**, intervenes (Fig. 13-5). The veliger has the beginnings of a foot, shell, and mantle. In many advanced molluscs the trochophore is passed in the egg, and a veliger hatches to become the only free-swimming stage. Cephalopods, freshwater and some marine snails, and some freshwater bivalves have no free-swimming larvae, and a juvenile hatches from the egg.

___ Classes of Molluscs

For more than 50 years five classes of living molluscs were recognized: Amphineura, Gastropoda, Scaphopoda, Bivalvia, and Cephalopoda. The discovery of *Neopilina* in the 1950s added another class (Monoplacophora), and Hyman (1967) contended that solenogasters and chitons comprise separate classes (Polyplacophora and Aplacophora), lapsing the name Amphineura. Recognition of important differences between organisms such as *Chaetoderma* and the other solenogasters has led to the separation of the Aplacophora into the Caudofoveata and the Solenogastres (Boss, 1982).

Class Caudofoveata

Members of the class Caudofoveata are wormlike, marine organisms ranging from 2 to 140 mm in length (Fig. 13-37). They are mostly burrowers and orient themselves vertically, with the terminal mantle cavity and gills at the entrance of the burrow. They feed on microorganisms and detritus. They have no shell, but their bodies are covered with calcareous scales. There are no spicules or scales on the oral pedal shield, an organ apparently associated with food selection and intake. A radula is present, although reduced in some, and the sexes are separate. Since this little group has fewer than 70 species, it does not represent a successful variation on the mollusc body plan. However, its features may be closer to the ancestral mollusc than any other living group.

Class Solenogastres

The solenogasters (Fig. 13-37) and the caudofoveates were formerly united in the class Aplacophora, and they are both wormlike, shell-less, with calcareous scales or spicules in their integument, with reduced head, and without nephridia. The

A

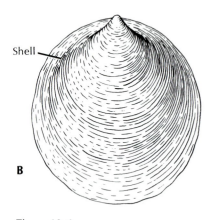

Shell

B

Figure 13-6

Neopilina, class Monoplacophora. Living specimens range from 3 mm to about 3 cm in length. **A**, Ventral view. **B**, Dorsal view.

solenogasters, however, usually have no radula and no gills (although secondary respiratory structures may be present). Their foot is represented by a midventral, narrow furrow, the pedal groove. They are hermaphroditic. Rather than burrowing, solenogasters live free on the bottom, and they often live and feed on cnidarians. The solenogasters are also a small group, numbering about 180 species.

Class Monoplacophora   Study

Until 1952 it was thought that the Monoplacophora were extinct; they were known only from Paleozoic shells. However, in that year living specimens of *Neopilina* (Gr., *neo,* new, + *pilos,* felt cap) were dredged up from the ocean bottom near the west coast of Costa Rica. Fewer than a dozen species of monoplacophorans are now known. These molluscs are small and have a low, rounded shell and a creeping foot (Fig. 13-6). They have a superficial resemblance to the limpets, but unlike most other molluscs, a number of organs are serially repeated. Such serial repetition occurs to a more limited extent in the chitons. *Neopilina* has five pairs of gills, two pairs of auricles, six pairs of nephridia, one or two pairs of gonads, and a ladderlike nervous system with 10 pairs of pedal nerves. The mouth bears the characteristic radula. Some authors (Lemche and Wingstrand; Hyman) have considered the monoplacophorans truly metameric and constituting evidence that the molluscs were descended from a metameric, annelid-like ancestor. Others (Clark; Vagvolgyi) believe that *Neopilina* shows only pseudometamerism, although the phylogenetic relationship of the annelids and molluscs, based on embryological evidence, is unquestioned.

Class Polyplacophora—chitons

The chitons (Gr., coat of mail, tunic) (Figs. 13-7 and 13-8) represent a somewhat more successful mollusc group. They are rather flattened dorsoventrally and have a convex dorsal surface that bears eight articulating limy plates, or valves, hence their name Polyplacophora ("bearing many plates"). The plates overlap posteriorly and are usually dull colored to match the rocks to which the chitons cling. Their head and cephalic sensory organs are reduced, but photosensitive structures (esthetes), which have the form of eyes in some chitons, pierce the plates.

Most chitons are small (2 to 5 cm); the largest, *Cryptochiton* (Gr., *crypto,* hidden, + *chiton,* coat of mail), rarely exceeds 30 cm. They prefer rocky surfaces in intertidal regions, although some live at great depths. Chitons are stay-at-home organisms, straying only very short distances for feeding. In feeding, the radula is projected from the mouth to scrape algae from the rocks. The radula is reinforced with the iron-containing mineral, magnetite. The chiton clings tenaciously to its rock with the broad, flat foot. If detached, it can roll up like an armadillo for protection.

The mantle forms a girdle around the margin of the plates, and in some species mantle folds cover part or all of the plates. Compared with the primitive condition, the mantle cavity has been extended along the sides of the foot, and the gills have been increased in number. Thus, the gills are suspended from the roof of the mantle cavity along each side of the broad ventral foot. With the foot and the mantle margin adhering tightly to the substrate, these grooves become closed chambers, open only at the ends. Water enters the grooves anteriorly, flows across the gills, and leaves posteriorly, bringing a continuous supply of oxygen to the

Figure 13-7

Mossy chiton, *Mopalia muscosa.* The upper surface of the mantle, or "girdle," is covered with hairs and bristles, an adaptation for defense.
Photograph by R. Harbo.

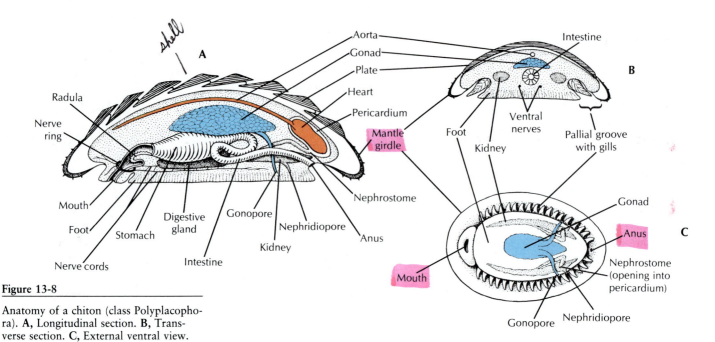

Figure 13-8

Anatomy of a chiton (class Polyplacophora). **A,** Longitudinal section. **B,** Transverse section. **C,** External ventral view.

Figure 13-9

Scaphopoda. **A,** *Dentalium* (class Scaphopoda), with its tubular shell, burrows into soft mud or sand and feeds by means of its prehensile tentacles. Water enters and leaves by way of the posterior aperture. **B,** Internal anatomy of *Dentalium.*

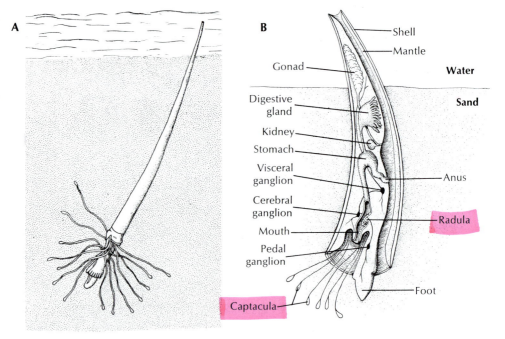

gills. At low tide the margins of the mantle can be tightly pressed to the substratum to diminish water loss. A pair of osphradia (sense organs for sampling water) are found in the mantle grooves near the anus of many chitons.

Blood pumped by the three-chambered heart reaches the gills by way of an aorta and sinuses. A pair of kidneys (metanephridia) carries waste from the pericardial cavity to the exterior. Two pairs of longitudinal nerve cords are connected in the buccal region.

Sexes are separate in most chitons, and the trochophore larva metamorphoses directly into a juvenile, without the intervention of a veliger.

Class Scaphopoda

The Scaphopoda, commonly called the tusk shells or tooth shells, are benthic marine molluscs found from the subtidal zone to over 6000 m in depth. They have a slender body covered with a mantle and a tubular shell open at both ends. In the scaphopods the molluscan body plan has taken a new direction, with the mantle wrapped around the viscera and fused to form a tube. Most scaphopods are 2.5 to 5 cm long, although they range from 4 mm to 25 cm long. *Dentalium* (L., *dentalis,* dental) is a common Atlantic genus.

The foot, which protrudes through the larger end of the shell, is used to burrow into mud or sand, always leaving the small end of the shell exposed to the water above (Fig. 13-9). Respiratory water is circulated through the mantle cavity both by movements of the foot and by ciliary action (Fig. 13-9). Gaseous exchange occurs in the mantle, for true gills are absent. Most of the food is detritus and protozoa from the substratum. It is caught on the cilia of the foot or on the mucus-covered, ciliated knobs of the long tentacles extending from the head, called captacula, and is conveyed to the nearby mouth. Eyes and tentacles are lacking. The radula carries the food to a crushing gizzard.

The sexes are separate, and the larva is a trochophore.

Class Gastropoda

Among the molluscs the class Gastropoda is by far the largest and most successful, containing about 35,000 living and 15,000 fossil species. It is made up of members of such diversity that there is no single general term in our language that can apply to them as a group. They include snails, limpets, slugs, whelks, conchs, periwinkles, sea slugs, sea hares, sea butterflies, and others. They range from some of the most primitive of marine molluscs to the highly evolved terrestrial air-breathing snails and slugs. These animals are basically bilaterally symmetrical, but because of **torsion,** a twisting process that occurs in the early larval stage, the visceral mass has become asymmetrical.

The shell, when present, is always of one piece (**univalve**) and may be coiled or uncoiled. Starting at the apex, which contains the oldest and smallest whorl, the whorls become successively larger and spiral about the central axis, or **columella** (Fig. 13-10). The shell may be right handed (**dextral**) or left handed (**sinistral**), depending on the direction of coiling. Dextral shells are far more common. The direction of coiling is genetically determined.

Gastropods range from microscopic forms to giant marine forms such as *Pleuroploca gigantea,* a snail with a shell up to 60 cm long, and the sea hare *Aplysia* (Fig. 13-15), some species of which reach 1 m in length. Most of them, however, are between 1 and 8 cm in length. Some fossil gastropods were as much as 2 m long.

The range of gastropod habitats is large. In the sea, gastropods are common both in the littoral zones and at great depths, and some are even pelagic. Some are adapted to brackish water and others to fresh water. On land they are restricted by such factors as the mineral content of the soil and extremes of temperature, dryness, and acidity. Even so, they are widespread, and some have been found at great altitudes and some even in polar regions. Snails occupy all kinds of habitats: in small pools or large bodies of water, in woodlands, in pastures, under rocks, in mosses, on cliffs, in trees, underground, and on the bodies of other animals. They have successfully undertaken every mode of life except aerial locomotion.

Figure 13-10

Shell of the whelk *Busycon.* **A** and **B,** *Busycon carica,* a dextral, or right-handed, shell. **C,** *B. contrarium,* a sinistral, or left-handed, shell.

Figure 13-11

Torsion in gastropods. **A,** Ancestral condition before torsion. **B,** Hypothetical intermediate condition. **C,** Early gastropod, torsion complete; direction of crawling now tends to carry waste products back into mantle cavity, resulting in fouling.

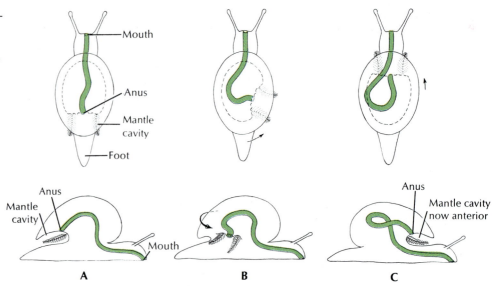

Gastropods are usually sluggish, sedentary animals because most of them have heavy shells and slow locomotor organs. Some are specialized for climbing, swimming, or burrowing. Shells are their chief defense, although they are also protected by coloration and by secretive habits. Many snails have an **operculum,** a horny plate that covers the shell aperture when the body is withdrawn into the shell. Others lack shells altogether. Some are distasteful to other animals, and a few such as *Strombus* can deal an active blow with the foot, which bears a sharp operculum. Nevertheless, they are eaten by birds, beetles, small mammals, fish, and other predators. Serving as intermediate hosts for many kinds of parasites, especially trematodes, snails are often harmed by the larval stages of parasites.

Torsion

Of all the molluscs, only gastropods undergo torsion. Torsion is a peculiar phenomenon that moves the mantle cavity, which was originally (primitively) posterior, to the front of the body, thus twisting the visceral organs as well through a 180-degree rotation to produce the typical gastropod asymmetry.

Torsion occurs very early in development (veliger stage), and in some species the entire action may take only a few moments. Before torsion occurs, the embryo is bilaterally symmetrical with an anterior mouth and a posterior anus and mantle cavity (Fig. 13-11). Torsion is brought about by an uneven growth of the right and left muscles that attach the shell to the head-foot.

After the organism undergoes torsion, the anus and mantle cavity open anteriorly above the mouth and head. Torsion also shifts the gill, kidney, and other organs, originally on the left side, to the right side and the organs originally on the right side to the left side, bends the digestive tract, and twists the nerve cords into a figure eight. Because of the space available in the mantle cavity, the sensitive head end of the animal can now be drawn into the protection of the shell, with the tougher foot forming a barrier to the outside.

There are varying degrees of torsion in the different groups of gastropods. In some gastropods, such as the sea hare, *Aplysia,* a reverse action, or **detorsion,** follows torsion, partially restoring the bilateral symmetry.

The curious arrangement that results from torsion poses a serious sanitation problem by creating the possibility of wastes being washed back over the gills

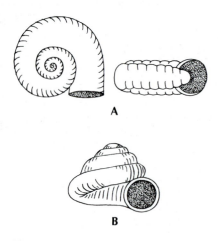

Figure 13-12

Coiling of the shell, which is independent of torsion. **A,** Two views of planospiral coiling, or coiling that occurs in a single plane. **B,** Conispiral coiling, which produces a cone-shaped shell.

(**fouling**) and causes us to wonder what strong evolutionary pressures selected for such a strange realignment of body structures. Several explanations have been proposed, but these have been little better than speculations. Certainly the consequences of torsion and the resulting need to avoid fouling have been very important in the subsequent evolution of gastropods. These consequences cannot be explored, however, until another unique aspect of gastropods—coiling—has been described.

Coiling

The coiling, or spiral winding, of the shell and visceral hump is not the same as torsion. Coiling may occur in the larval stage at the same time as torsion, but the fossil record shows that coiling was a separate evolutionary event and originated in gastropods earlier than torsion did. Nevertheless, all living gastropods have descended from coiled, torted ancestors, whether or not they now show these characteristics.

Early gastropods had a bilaterally symmetrical **planospiral** shell; that is, all the whorls lay in a single plane (Fig. 13-12, *A*). Such a shell was not very compact, since each whorl had to lie completely outside the preceding one. Curiously, a few modern species have secondarily returned to the planospiral form. The compactness problem of the planospiral shell was solved by the **conispiral** shape, in which each succeeding whorl was at the side of the preceding one (Fig. 13-12, *B*). However, this shape was clearly unbalanced, hanging as it was with much weight over to one side. Better weight distribution was achieved by shifting the shell upward and posteriorly, with the shell axis oblique to the longitudinal axis of the foot (Fig. 13-20). The weight and bulk of the main body whorl, the largest whorl of the shell, pressed on the right side of the mantle cavity, however, and apparently interfered with the organs on that side. Accordingly, the gill, auricle, and kidney of the right side have been lost in all except primitive living gastropods, leading to a condition of *bilateral asymmetry*.

Although the loss of the right gill was probably an adaptation to the mechanics of carrying the coiled shell, that condition made possible a way to avoid the problem of torsion—fouling—that is displayed in most modern prosobranchs. Water is brought into the left side of the mantle cavity and out the right side, carrying with it the wastes from the anus and nephridiopore, which lie near the right side. Ways in which fouling is avoided in other gastropods are mentioned later in the chapter.

Feeding habits

Feeding habits of gastropods are as varied as their shapes and habitats, but all include the use of some adaptation of the radula. The majority of gastropods are herbivorous, rasping off particles of algae. Some herbivores are grazers, some are browsers, and some are planktonic feeders. *Haliotis*, the abalone (Fig. 13-13, *A*), holds seaweed with the foot and breaks off pieces with the radula. Land snails forage at night for green vegetation.

Some snails, such as *Bullia* and *Buccinum*, are scavengers living on dead and decaying flesh; others are carnivores that tear their prey with the radular teeth. *Melongena* feeds on clams, especially *Tagelus*, the razor clam, thrusting its proboscis between the gaping shell valves. *Fasciolaria* and *Polinices* (Fig. 13-13, *B*) feed on a variety of molluscs, preferably bivalves. *Urosalpinx cinerea*, the oyster borer, or tingle, drills holes through the shell of the oyster. Its radula, bearing three

Figure 13-13

A, Red abalone, *Haliotus rufescens.* This huge, limpetlike snail is prized as food and extensively marketed. Abalones are strict vegetarians, feeding especially on sea lettuce and kelp. **B,** Moon snail, *Polinices lewisii.* A common inhabitant of West Coast sand flats, the moon snail is a predator of clams and mussels. It uses its radula to drill neat holes through its victim's shell, through which the proboscis is then extended to eat the bivalve's fleshy body.

Photographs by D.W. Gotshall.

A

B

Figure 13-14

Cone shell, *Conus californicus*. Water is drawn into the mantle cavity through the extended siphon.
Photograph by D.W. Behrens.

longitudinal rows of teeth, is used first to begin the drilling action, then the animal glides forward, everts an accessory boring organ through a pore in the anterior sole of its foot, and holds it against the shell, using a chemical agent to soften the shell. Short periods of rasping alternate with long periods of chemical activity until a neat round hole is completed. With its proboscis inserted through the hole, the snail may feed continuously for hours or days, using the radula to tear away the soft flesh. *Urosalpinx* is attracted to its prey at some distance by sensing some chemical, probably one released in the metabolic wastes of the prey.

Cyphoma gibbosum (p. 302) and related species live and feed on gorgonians (phylum Cnidaria, Chapter 10) on shallow, tropical coral reefs. This snail is commonly known as the flamingo tongue. During normal activity the brightly colored mantle entirely envelops the shell, but it can be quickly withdrawn into the shell aperture when the animal is disturbed.

Members of the genus *Conus* (Fig. 13-14) feed on worms, fish, and other gastropods. Their radula is highly modified for prey capture. A gland charges the radular teeth with a highly toxic venom. When *Conus* senses the presence of its prey, a single radular tooth is slid into position at the tip of the proboscis. When the proboscis strikes the prey, the tooth is expelled like a harpoon, and the poison quiets the prey at once. Some species of *Conus* can deliver very painful stings, and with several species the sting is lethal to humans. The venom is apparently a neurotoxin.

Some gastropods feed on organic deposits on the sand or mud. Others collect the same sort of organic debris but can digest only the microorganisms contained in it. Some of the sessile gastropods, such as the limpets, are ciliary feeders that use the gill cilia to draw in particulate matter that is rolled into a mucous ball and is carried to the mouth. Some of the sea butterflies secrete a mucous net to catch small planktonic forms; then they draw the web into the mouth.

After maceration by the radula or by some grinding device, such as the gizzard in the sea hare *Aplysia* (Fig. 13-15), digestion is usually extracellular in the lumen of the stomach or digestive glands. In ciliary feeders the stomachs are sorting regions, and most of the digestion is intracellular in the digestive glands.

Internal form and function

Respiration in most gastropods is carried out by a **gill** (two gills in primitive prosobranchs) located in the mantle cavity, although some aquatic forms, lacking gills, depend on the mantle and skin. The pulmonates have a highly vascular area in the mantle that serves as a **lung** (Fig. 13-16). Many aquatic pulmonates must surface to expel a bubble of gas from the lung. To take in air, they curl the edge of the mantle around the **pneumostome** (a pulmonary opening in the mantle cavity) to form a siphon.

Most gastropods have a single nephridium (kidney). The circulatory and nervous systems are well developed (Fig. 13-16). The latter includes three pairs of ganglia connected by nerves. Sense organs include eyes or simple photoreceptors, statocysts, tactile organs, and chemoreceptors. The simplest type of gastropod eye is simply a cuplike indentation in the skin lined with pigmented photoreceptor cells. In many gastropods the eyecup contains a lens and is covered with a cornea. A sensory area called the **osphradium,** located in the incurrent siphon of most gastropods, is known to be chemosensory in some forms, although its function may be mechanoreceptive in some and is still unknown in others.

A   **B**

Figure 13-15

A, The sea hare, *Aplysia dactylomela*, crawls and swims across a tropical sea-grass bed, assisted by large, winglike parapodia, here curled above the body. **B,** When attacked, the sea hare squirts a copious protective secretion from its "purple gland" in the mantle cavity.
Photographs by C.P. Hickman, Jr.

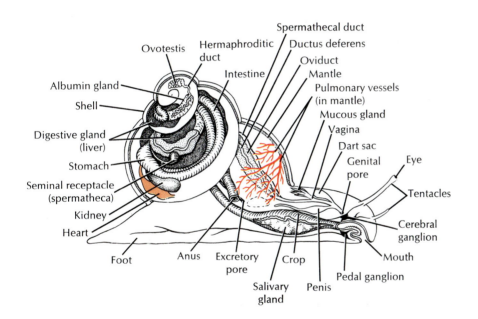

Figure 13-16

Anatomy of a pulmonate snail.

There are both dioecious and monoecious gastropods. Many gastropods perform courtship ceremonies. During copulation in monoecious species there is an exchange of spermatozoa or spermatophores (bundles of sperm). Many terrestrial pulmonates eject a dart from a dart sac (Fig. 13-16) into the partner's body to heighten excitement before copulation. After copulation each partner deposits its eggs in shallow burrows in the ground. The most primitive gastropods discharge ova and sperm into the seawater where fertilization occurs, and the embryo soon hatches as a free-swimming trochophore larva. In most gastropods fertilization is internal.

Fertilized eggs encased in transparent shells may be emitted singly to float among the plankton or may be laid in gelatinous layers attached to the substratum. In some marine forms, eggs are enclosed, either in small groups or in large numbers, in tough egg capsules, in a wide variety of egg cases (Fig. 13-17). The young generally emerge as veliger larvae (Fig. 13-5), or they may spend the veliger

A   B   C

Figure 13-17

Eggs of marine gastropods. **A,** The wrinkled whelk, *Thais lamelosa,* lays egg cases resembling grains of wheat; each contains hundreds of eggs. **B,** Urnlike egg case of the common Caribbean drupe snail *(Drupa).* **C,** The moon snail forms a collarlike egg case resembling a discarded rubber plunger. The case is covered with sand as it is extruded and cemented with mucus.

A and C, Photographs by R. Harbo; **B,** photograph by K. Sandved.

stage in the case or capsule and emerge as young snails. Some species, including many freshwater snails, are ovoviviparous, brooding their eggs and young in the pallial oviduct.

Major groups of gastropods

There are three subclasses of gastropods: the Prosobranchia, Opisthobranchia, and Pulmonata.

Prosobranchia

The mantle cavity is anterior as a result of torsion, with the gill or gills lying in front of the heart. Water enters the left side and exits from the right side, and the edge of the mantle is often extended into a long siphon to further separate exhalant from inhalant flow (Fig. 13-14). In the primitive prosobranchs with two gills (for example, the abalone *Haliotis* and the keyhole limpet *Diodora,* Figs. 13-13, *A,* and 13-18, *B*), fouling is avoided by having the exhalant water go up and out through one or more holes in the shell above the mantle cavity.

Prosobranchs have one pair of tentacles. The sexes are usually separate. An operculum is often present.

This group contains most of the marine snails and some of the freshwater and terrestrial gastropods. They range in size from the periwinkles and small limpets *(Patella* and *Diodora)* (Fig. 13-18, *B*) to the horse conch *(Pleuroploca),* the largest gastropod in America. Familiar examples of prosobranchs are the abalone *(Haliotis),* which has an ear-shaped shell; the whelk *(Busycon),* which lays its eggs in double-edged, disc-shaped capsules attached to a cord a meter long; the common periwinkle *(Littorina);* the moon snail *(Polinices,* Fig. 13-13, *B);* the oyster borer *(Urosalpinx),* which bores into oysters and sucks out their juices; the rock shell *(Murex),* a European species of which was used for making the royal purple of the ancient Romans; and the freshwater forms *(Goniobasis* and *Viviparus).*

Opisthobranchia

The opisthobranchs show partial or complete detorsion; thus, the anus and gill (if present) are displaced to the right side or rear of the body. Clearly, the fouling problem is obviated if the anus is moved to the posterior. Two pairs of tentacles

A

B

Figure 13-18

A, Cowry, *Jenneria pustulata,* crawls over zoanthid cnidarians. The brightly patterned and polished shells of cowries have been used as ornaments for thousands of years. **B,** Keyhole limpet, *Diodora aspera,* a prosobranch gastropod with a hole in the apex through which the water leaves the shell.

A, Photograph by K. Sandved; **B,** photograph by R. Harbo.

A

B

C

Figure 13-19

"Nudibranchs." **A,** Aeolid nudibranchs crawl across a hydroid colony. Their long, dorsal cerata contain nematocysts, which the animals obtain from their cnidarian diet. **B,** *Tridachia crispata* feeds on algae but does not destroy the chloroplasts in the algal cells it eats. The chloroplasts continue to function and contribute to the nutrition of the gastropod. **C,** The giant nudibranch, *Dendronotus irus,* may reach 30 cm in length.

A, Photograph by K. Sandved; **B,** photograph by L.S. Roberts; **C,** photograph by R. Harbo.

Figure 13-20

Pulmonate land snail. Note two pairs of tentacles; the second, larger pair bears the eyes.

Photograph by C.P. Hickman, Jr.

Figure 13-21

Bivalve molluscs. **A,** Mussels, *Mytilus edulis,* occur in northern oceans around the world; they form dense beds in the intertidal zone. A host of marine creatures lives protected beneath attached mussels. **B,** Scallops *(Chlamys opercularis)* swim to escape attack by starfish *(Asterias rubens).* When alarmed, these most agile of bivalves swim by clapping the two shell valves together.

A, Photograph by R. Harbo; B, photograph by D.P. Wilson.

are usually found, and the shell is typically reduced or absent. All are monoecious. The opisthobranchs are an odd assemblage of molluscs that include sea slugs, sea hares, sea butterflies, canoe shells, and others. They are nearly all marine; most of them are shallow-water forms, hiding under stones and seaweed; a few are pelagic. Currently nine or more orders of opisthobranchs are recognized, but for convenience they can be divided into two classical groups: tectibranchs, with gill and shell usually present, and nudibranchs, in which there is no shell or true gill, but in which secondary gills are present along the dorsal side or around the anus.

Among the tectibranchs are the large sea hare *Aplysia* (Fig. 13-15), which has large earlike anterior tentacles and a vestigial shell, and the pteropods, or sea butterflies (*Carolina* and *Clione*). In pteropods the foot is modified into fins for swimming; thus, they are pelagic and form a part of the plankton fauna.

The nudibranchs are represented by the sea slugs, which are often brightly colored and carnivorous. The plumed sea slug *Aeolis,* which lives on sea anemones and hydroids, often draws the color of its prey into the elongated papillae (cerata) that cover its back. It also salvages the nematocysts of the hydroids for its own use. The frilled sea slug *Tridachia* (Fig. 13-19, *B*) is a lovely little green or blue and white form common in Florida waters. *Hermissenda* is one of the common West Coast nudibranchs (Fig. 13-19, *A*).

Pulmonata

The pulmonates show torsion and include the land and freshwater snails and slugs (and a few brackish and saltwater forms). They have lost their ancestral gills, but the vascularized mantle wall has become a lung, which fills with air by contraction of the mantle floor (some aquatic species have developed secondary gills). The anus and nephridiopore open near the opening of the lung to the outside (pneumostome), and waste is expelled forcibly with air or water from the lung. They are monoecious. The aquatic species have one pair of nonretractile tentacles, at the base of which are the eyes; land forms have two pairs of tentacles, with the posterior pair bearing the eyes (Fig. 13-20). Among the thousands of land species, some of the most familiar American forms are *Helix, Polygyra, Succinea, Anguispira, Zonitoides, Limax,* and *Agriolimax.* Aquatic forms are represented by *Helisoma, Lymnaea,* and *Physa. Physa* is a left-handed (sinistral) snail.

A

B

Class Bivalvia (Pelecypoda)

The Bivalvia are also known as Pelecypoda (pel-e-sip'o-da), or "hatchet-footed" animals, as their name implies (Gr., *pelekys,* hatchet, + *pous, podos,* foot). They are the bivalved molluscs that include the mussels, clams, scallops, oysters, and shipworms (Figs. 13-21 to 13-24) and that range in size from tiny seed shells 1 to 2 mm in length to giant South Pacific clams *Tridacna,* which may reach more than 1 m in length and as much as 225 kg (500 pounds) in weight (Fig. 13-31). Most bivalves are sedentary **filter feeders** that depend on ciliary currents produced by the gills to bring in food materials. Unlike the gastropods, they have no head, no radula, and very little cephalization.

Most pelecypods are marine, but many live in brackish water and in streams, ponds, and lakes.

Form and function
Shell

Bivalves are laterally compressed, and their two shells (**valves**) are held together dorsally by a hinge ligament that causes the valves to gape ventrally. The valves are drawn together by adductor muscles that work in opposition to the hinge ligament (Fig. 13-23, *B* and *C*). The valves function largely for protection, but those of the shipworms *(Teredo)* have microscopic teeth for rasping wood, and the rock borers *(Pholas)* use spiny valves for boring into rock. The umbo is the oldest part of the shell, and growth occurs in concentric lines around it (Fig. 13-23, *A*).

Pearl production is the by-product of a protective device used by the animal when a foreign object (grain of sand, parasite, or other) becomes lodged between the shell and mantle. The mantle secretes many layers of nacre around the irritating object (Fig. 13-3). Pearls are cultured by inserting particles of nacre, usually taken from the shells of freshwater clams, between the shell and mantle of a certain species of oyster and by keeping the oysters in enclosures for several years. *Meleagrina* is an oyster used extensively by the Japanese for pearl culture.

One might get the impression that a "cultured" pearl is somehow artificial or imitation. However, a cultured pearl is just as real or genuine as a "natural" pearl; the difference is that humans have stimulated its production rather than gathering it from a "wild" oyster.

Figure 13-22

Representing groups that have evolved from burrowing ancestors, the surface-dwelling bivalves *Pecten* sp. (**A**) and *Lima scabra* (**B**) have developed sensory organs along their mantle edges. Tentacles are present in both, and the *Pecten* has a series of blue eyes.
A, Photograph by L.S. Roberts; **B**, photograph by K. Sandved.

A   **B**

Figure 13-23

Tagelus plebius, the stubby razor clam (class Bivalvia). **A,** External view of right valve. **B,** Inside of left shell showing scars where muscles were attached. The mantle was attached at the pallial line. **C** and **D,** Sections showing function of adductor muscles and hinge ligament. In **C** the adductor muscle is contracted, pulling the valves together. In **D** the adductor muscle is relaxed, allowing the hinge ligament to pull the valves apart.

Figure 13-24

A, Shipworms are bivalves that burrow in wood, causing great damage to unprotected wooden hulls and piers. **B,** The two small, anterior valves, seen at left, are used as rasping organs to extend the burrow.

Photographs by L.S. Roberts.

Body

The body is made up of the **visceral mass** suspended from the dorsal midline, a muscular **foot** attached to the visceral mass anteroventrally, and a pair of **gills** (ctenidia) on each side, each covered by a fold of the **mantle.** Some bivalves have a single gill rather than a double gill on each side.

Mantle

The mantle hangs down on each side of the visceral mass, adhering to the valves. The posterior edges of the mantle folds are modified to form dorsal **excurrent (exhalant)** and ventral **incurrent (inhalant) apertures** for regulating water flow (Fig. 13-25, *A*). In some marine bivalves the mantle is drawn out into long muscular siphons that allow the clam to burrow into the mud or sand and extend the siphons to the water above (Fig. 13-25, *B* to *D*). Cilia on the gills and inner surface of the mantle direct the flow of water over the gills.

Locomotion

Pelecypods move by extending a slender muscular foot between the valves (Fig. 13-25, *D*). Blood swells the end of the foot to anchor it in mud or sand, and then longitudinal muscles contract to shorten the foot and pull the animal forward. In most bivalves the foot is used for burrowing.

The scallops and file shells are able to swim jerkily by clapping their valves together to create a sort of jet propulsion, with water being expelled from the mantle cavity near the shell hinge (Figs. 13-21, *B*, and 13-22).

Gills

Gaseous exchange is carried on by both the mantle and the gills. In most bivalves each gill is formed of two walls (lamellae) joined together at their ventral margins. Each lamella is made up of many vertical gill filaments strengthened by chitinous rods. Water enters the gills through innumerable small pores in the walls and is propelled by ciliary action. Partitions between the walls divide the gill internally into many vertical **water tubes** that carry water upward (dorsally) into a common

Figure 13-25

Adaptations for inhalant and exhalant currents. **A,** In the northwest ugly clam, *Entodesma saxicola,* the inhalant and exhalant siphons are clearly visible. **B to D,** In many marine forms the mantle is drawn out into long siphons. In **A, B,** and **D** the inhalant current brings in both food and oxygen. In **C,** *Yoldia,* the siphons are respiratory; long ciliated palps feel about over the mud surface and convey food to the mouth.

A, Photograph by R. Harbo.

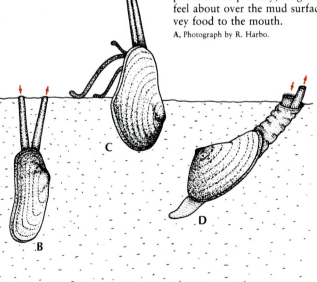

Figure 13-26

Section through heart region of a fresh-water clam to show relation of circulatory and respiratory systems. Respiratory water currents: water is drawn in by cilia, enters gill pores, and then passes up water tubes to suprabranchial chambers and out excurrent aperture. Blood in gills exchanges carbon dioxide for oxygen. Blood circulation: ventricle pumps blood forward to sinuses of foot and viscera, and posteriorly to mantle sinuses. Blood returns from mantle to auricles; it returns from viscera to the kidney, and then goes to the gills, and finally to the auricles.

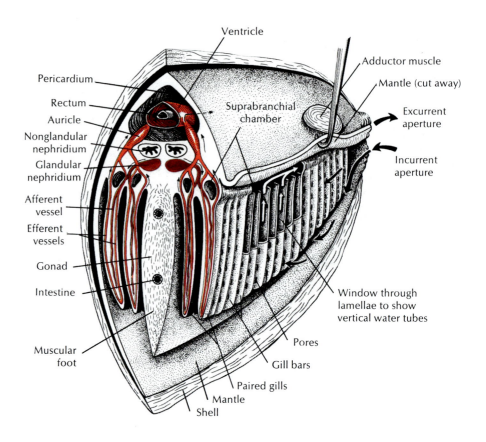

Figure 13-27

Feeding mechanism of freshwater clam. Left valve and mantle are removed. Water enters the mantle cavity posteriorly and is drawn forward by ciliary action to the gills and palps. As water enters the tiny openings of the gills, food particles are sieved out and caught up in strings of mucus that are carried by cilia to the palps and directed to the mouth. Sand and debris drop into the mantle cavity and are removed by cilia.

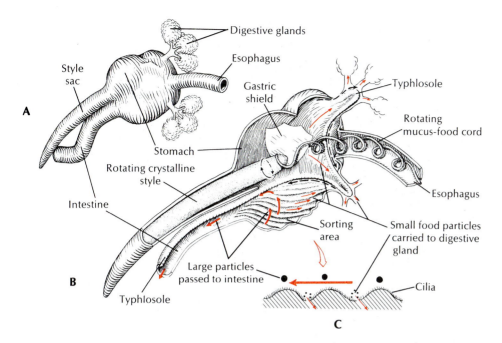

Figure 13-28

Stomach and crystalline style of ciliary-feeding clam. **A,** External view of stomach and style sac. **B,** Transverse section showing direction of food movements. Food particles in incoming water are caught in a cord of mucus that is kept rotating by the crystalline style. Ridged sorting areas direct large particles to the intestine and small food particles to digestive glands. **C,** Sorting action of cilia.
B, Modified from Morton, J.E. 1967. Mollusca, ed. 4. London, Hutchinson & Co.

suprabranchial chamber (Fig. 13-26) and through it to the excurrent aperture. Blood vessels or spaces in the interlamellar partitions are used for exchange of gases.

In most freshwater forms the water tubes in the female often double as brood pouches for eggs and larvae during the breeding season. The various orders of Bivalvia are classified on the basis of their gill type and hinge structure.

Feeding

Most bivalves are filter feeders. The respiratory currents bring both oxygen and organic materials to the gills where ciliary tracts direct them to the tiny pores of the gills. Gland cells on the gills and labial palps secrete copious amounts of mucus, which entangles particles too large to enter the gill pores. These mucous masses slide down the outside of the gills toward food grooves at the lower edge of the gills (Fig. 13-27). Heavier particles of sediment drop off the gills as a result of gravitational pull, but smaller particles travel along the food grooves toward the labial palps. The palps, being also grooved and ciliated, direct the mucous mass into the mouth.

Some bivalves, such as *Nucula* and *Yoldia,* are deposit feeders and have long proboscides attached to the labial palps (Fig. 13-25, C). These can be protruded onto the sand or mud to collect food particles, in addition to the particles attracted by the gill currents.

Septibranchs, another group of bivalves, draw small crustaceans or bits of organic debris into the mantle cavity by sudden inflow of water created by the pumping action of a muscular septum in the mantle cavity.

Internal structure and function

The floor of the stomach of filter-feeding bivalves is folded into ciliary tracts for sorting the continuous stream of particles. A cylindrical style sac opening into the stomach secretes a gelatinous rod called the crystalline style, which projects into the stomach and is kept whirling by means of cilia in the style sac (Fig. 13-28). Rotation of the style helps to dissolve its surface layers, freeing enzymes (such as

Figure 13-29

Life cycle of the oyster.

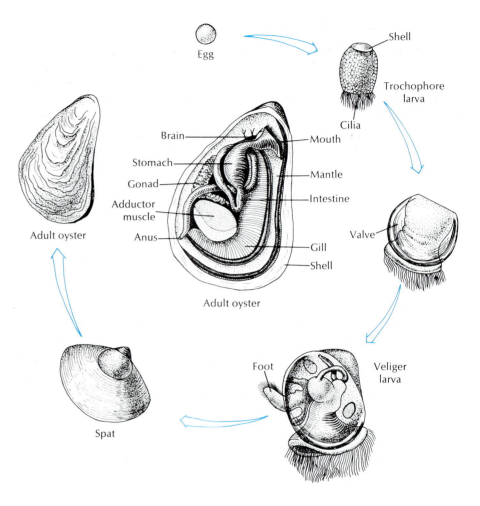

amylase) that it contains, and to roll the mucous food mass. Dislodged particles are sorted, and suitable ones are directed to the digestive gland or picked up by amebocytes. Further digestion is intracellular.

The stomach of the carnivorous septibranch is muscular and serves as a crushing gizzard. Digestible material, after being broken up, passes to the digestive diverticula and is phagocytized and digested intracellularly.

The three-chambered heart, which lies in the pericardial cavity (Fig. 13-26), is made up of two auricles and a ventricle and beats slowly, sometimes at the rate of about six times a minute. Part of the blood is oxygenated in the mantle and is returned to the ventricle through the auricles; the rest circulates through sinuses and passes in a vein to the kidneys, from there to the gills for oxygenation, and back to the auricles.

A pair of U-shaped kidneys (nephridial tubules) lies just below and behind the heart (Fig. 13-26). The glandular portion of each tubule opens into the pericardium; the bladder portion empties into the suprabranchial chamber.

The nervous system consists of three pairs of widely separated ganglia connected by commissures and a system of nerves. Sense organs are poorly developed. They include a pair of statocysts in the foot, a pair of osphradia of uncertain function in the mantle cavity, tactile cells, and sometimes simple pigment cells on the mantle. Scallops *(Pecten, Chlamys)* have a row of small blue eyes along each mantle edge (Figs. 13-21, *B*, and 13-22, *A*). Each is made up of cornea, lens, retina, and pigmented layer. Tentacles on the margin of the mantle of *Pecten* and *Lima* (Fig. 13-22) have tactile and chemoreceptor cells.

Reproduction and development

Sexes are usually separate. Gametes are discharged into the suprabranchial chamber to be carried out with the exhalant current. An oyster may produce 50 million eggs in a single season. In most bivalves fertilization is external. The embryo develops into trochophore, veliger, and spat stages (Fig. 13-29). Oyster larvae swim about for approximately 2 weeks before settling down for attachment to become spats. Oysters take about 4 years to grow to commercial size.

In most freshwater clams, fertilization is internal. Eggs drop into the water tubes of the gills where they are fertilized by sperm entering with the inhalant current. They develop there into a bivalved **glochidium larva** stage, which is a specialized veliger (Fig. 13-30). When discharged, the glochidia are carried by water currents, and if they come in contact with a passing fish, they attach to its gills or skin and live as parasites for several weeks. Then they sink to the bottom to begin independent lives. Larval "hitchhiking" helps distribute a form whose locomotion is very limited.

Boring

Many pelecypods can burrow into mud or sand, but some have evolved a mechanism for burrowing into much harder substances, such as wood or stone.

Teredo, Bankia, and some other genera are called shipworms. They can be very destructive to wooden ships and wharves. These strange little clams have a long, wormlike appearance, with a pair of slender siphons on the posterior end that keep water flowing over the gills, and a pair of small globular valves on the anterior end with which they burrow (Fig. 13-24). The valves have microscopic teeth so that they function as very effective wood rasps. The animals extend their burrows with an unceasing rasping motion of the valves. This sends a continuous flow of fine wood particles into the digestive tract where they are attacked intracellularly by the enzyme cellulase.

Fertilization is internal, with the zygotes sometimes becoming implanted in the gill tissue. The young *Teredo* are liberated as globular, ciliated larvae 0.5 μm in diameter that swim about looking for a likely spot to penetrate wood and metamorphose. Clinging to the new burrow with its foot and boring forward as it grows, the young *Teredo* may grow to a length of 100 to 125 mm and a diameter of 5 mm, always extending its siphons backward toward the opening to pump in the oxygen- and food-bearing water. One species of *Bankia* makes burrows up to 1 m long and 12 mm in diameter.

Some clams bore into rock. The piddock (*Pholas*) bores into limestone, shale, sandstone, and sometimes wood or peat. It has strong valves that bear spines by which it gradually cuts away the rock while anchoring itself by its foot. *Pholas* may grow to 15 cm long and make rock burrows up to 30 cm long.

Class Cephalopoda

The Cephalopoda are the most advanced of the molluscs; in some respects they are the most advanced of all the invertebrates. They include the squids, octopuses, nautiluses, devilfish, and cuttlefish. All are marine, and all are active predators.

Cephalopods are the "head-footed" molluscs (Gr., *kephalē*, head, + *pous, podos*, foot) in which the modified foot is concentrated in the head region. The edges of the foot are drawn out into arms and tentacles that bear sucking discs for seizing prey; also, part of the foot is modified to form a funnel for expelling water from the mantle cavity.

Figure 13-30

Glochidium, or larval form, of some freshwater clams. When the larva is released from brood pouch of mother, it may become attached to a fish's gill by clamping its valves closed. It remains as a parasite on the fish for several weeks. Its size is approximately 0.3 mm.

Figure 13-31

Clam *(Tridacna crocea)* lies buried in coral rock with only the richly colored fluted mantle edge visible. These bivalves bear enormous numbers of symbiotic single-celled plants (zooxanthellae) that provide much of the clam's nutriment.
Photograph by K. Sandved.

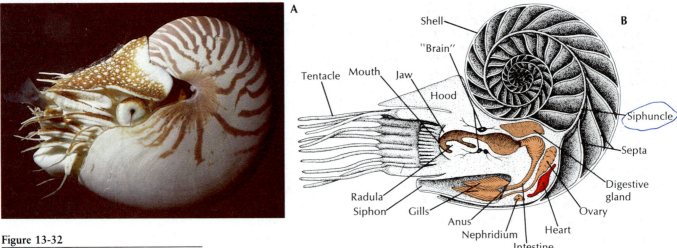

Figure 13-32

Nautilus, a cephalopod. **A,** Live *Nautilus,* feeding on a fish. **B,** Longitudinal section, showing gas-filled chambers of shell, and diagram of body structure.

A, Courtesy M. Butschler.

Cephalopods range upward in size from 2 or 3 cm. The squid *Loligo* is about 30 cm long. The giant squid *Architeuthis* is the largest invertebrate known.

Fossil records of cephalopods go back to Cambrian times. The earliest shells were straight cones; others were curved or coiled, culminating in the coiled shell similar to that of the modern *Nautilus,* the only remaining member of the once flourishing nautiloids (Fig. 13-32). Cephalopods without shells or with internal shells (such as octopuses and squids) are believed to have evolved from some early straight-shelled nautiloid.

The natural history of the cephalopods is known only in part. They are marine animals and appear sensitive to the degree of salinity. Few are found in the Baltic Sea, where the water has a low salt content. Cephalopods are found at various depths. The octopus is often seen in the intertidal zone, lurking among rocks and crevices, but occasionally is found at great depths. The more active squids are rarely found in shallow water, and some have been taken at depths of 5000 m. *Nautilus* is usually found near the bottom in water 50 to 560 m deep, near islands in the southwestern Pacific.

Major groups of cephalopods

There are three subclasses of cephalopods: the Nautiloidea, which have two pairs of gills; the entirely extinct Ammonoidea; and the Coleoidea, which have one pair of gills. The Nautiloidea populated the Paleozoic and Mesozoic seas, but there survives only one genus, *Nautilus* (Fig. 13-32), of which there are five or six species. The Ammonoidea were widely prevalent in the Mesozoic era but became extinct by the end of the Cretaceous period.

The subclass Coleoidea includes all living cephalopods except *Nautilus.* There are four orders of coleoids. Members of the order Sepioidea (cuttlefishes and their relatives) have a rounded or compressed, bulky body bearing fins (Fig. 13-34, *A*). They have eight arms and two tentacles. Both the arms and the tentacles have suckers, but the tentacles bear suckers only at their ends (Fig. 13-33). Members of the order Teuthoidea (squids, Fig. 13-33) have a more cylindrical body but also have eight arms and two tentacles. The order Vampyromorpha (vampire squid) contains only a single, deepwater species. It has eight arms with suckers; the arms are joined by an extensive membrane reminiscent of the membrane joining the digits of a bat's wing. Vampire squids also have a pair of tactile,

A, Squid *Loligo pealei* capturing a menhaden. **B,** Lateral view of squid anatomy, with the left half of the mantle removed.
A, Photograph by H.W. Pratt/BPS.

Figure 13-33

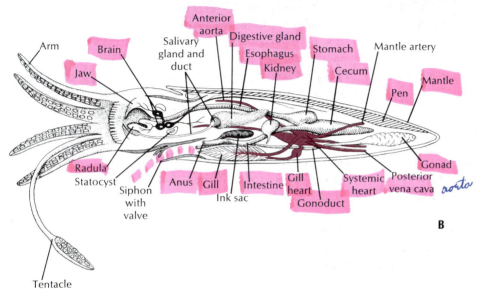

It was formerly believed that the gas in the chambers of *Nautilus* was the product of secretion by the siphuncle, but recent investigation has shown that the function of the siphuncle is *not* to secrete gas but to *bail fluid* out of the unoccupied chambers. The shell and septa are composed of calcium carbonate and protein, and as the animal grows, the mantle covering the visceral mass secretes more septa and creates additional chambers. Each new chamber is initially filled with a fluid similar in ionic composition to that of the *Nautilus*'s blood (and of seawater). The mechanism of fluid removal appears to involve the active secretion of ions into tiny intercellular spaces in the siphuncular epithelium, so that a very high local osmotic pressure is produced, and the water is drawn out of the chamber by osmosis. The gas in the chamber is only the respiratory gas from the siphuncle tissue that diffuses into the chamber as the fluid is removed. Thus, the gas pressure in the chamber is 1 atmosphere or less because it is in equilibrium with the gases dissolved in the seawater surrounding the *Nautilus,* which are in turn in equilibrium with air at the surface of the sea, despite the fact that the *Nautilus* may be swimming at 400 m beneath the surface. That the shell can withstand implosion by the surrounding 41 atmospheres (about 600 pounds per square inch), and that the siphuncle can remove water against this pressure are marvelous feats of natural engineering!

coiled filaments that are thought to be homologous to the tentacles of teuthoid squids; thus, vampire squids are intermediate between teuthoids and octopuses. Members of the order Octopoda have eight arms and no tentacles (Fig. 13-1, *D*). Their bodies are short and saclike, with no fins. The suckers in teuthoid squids are stalked (pedunculated), with horny rims bearing teeth; in octopuses the suckers are sessile and have no horny rims.

Form and function
Shell

Although early nautiloid and ammonoid shells were heavy, they were made buoyant by a series of **gas chambers,** as is that of *Nautilus* (Fig. 13-32), enabling the animal to swim while carrying its shell. The shell of *Nautilus,* although coiled, is quite different from that of a gastropod. The shell is divided by transverse septa into internal chambers (Fig. 13-32). The living animal inhabits only the last chamber. As it grows, it moves forward, secreting behind it a new septum. The chambers are connected by a cord of living tissue called the **siphuncle,** which extends from the visceral mass. Cuttlefishes also have a small, curved shell, but it is entirely enclosed by the mantle. In the squids most of the shell has disappeared, leaving only a thin, horny strip called a pen, which is enclosed by the mantle. In *Octopus* (Gr., *oktos,* eight, + *pous, podos,* foot) the shell has disappeared entirely.

Figure 13-34

A, *Sepia*, the cuttlefish. B, Octopus den with eggs. The female guards the eggs during incubation.

A, Photograph by D.P. Wilson; B, photograph by R. Harbo.

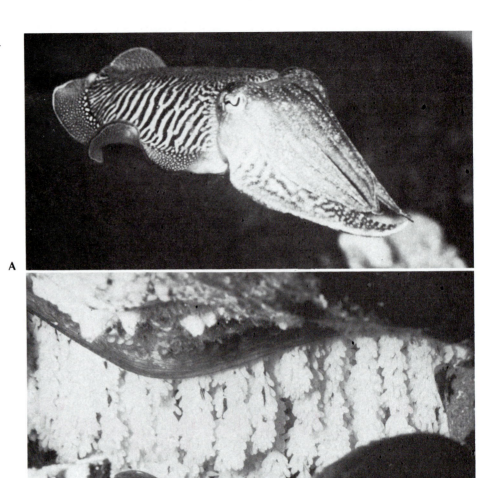

Locomotion

Most cephalopods swim by forcefully expelling water from the mantle cavity through a ventral **funnel**—a sort of jet propulsion method. The funnel is mobile and can be pointed forward or backward to control direction; speed is controlled by the force with which water is expelled.

Squids and cuttlefishes are excellent swimmers. The squid body is streamlined and built for speed (Fig. 13-33). Cuttlefishes swim more slowly. The lateral fins of squids and cuttlefishes serve as stabilizers, but they are held close to the body for rapid swimming.

Nautilus is active at night; its gas-filled chambers keep the shell upright. Although not as fast as the squid, it moves surprisingly well.

Octopus has a rather globular body and no fins (Fig. 13-1, *E*). The octopus can swim backward by spurting jets of water from its funnel, but it is better adapted to crawling about over the rocks and coral, using the suction discs on its arms to pull or to anchor itself. Some deep-water octopods have the arms webbed like an umbrella and swim in a sort of medusa fashion.

External features

During the embryonic development of the cephalopod, the head and foot become indistinguishable. The ring around the mouth, which bears the arms, or tentacles, is considered to be derived from the foot.

Selected references

Abbott, R.T. 1968. Seashells of North America, a guide to field identification. Racine, Wis., Golden Press. *Excellent illustrations, and only slightly less information than his more expensive* American seashells.

Abbott, R.T. 1974. American seashells, ed. 2. New York, Van Nostrand Reinhold Co.

Barnes, R.D. 1980. Invertebrate zoology, ed. 4. Philadelphia, Saunders College/Holt, Rinehart & Winston.

Boss, K.J. 1971. Critical estimate of the number of recent Mollusca. Occasional Papers on Mollusks, Mus. Comp. Zool., Harvard Univ. 3:81-135.

Boss, K.J. 1982. Mollusca. In S.P. Parker (ed.). Synopsis and classification of living organisms, vol. 1. New York, McGraw-Hill Book Co.

Clark, R.B. 1964. Dynamics in metazoan evolution: the origin of the coelom and segments. Oxford, Eng., Clarendon Press.

Cousteau, J., and P. Diolé. 1973. Octopus and squid, the soft intelligence. New York, Doubleday & Co. Inc. *Popular interest: beautiful color plates; illustrated glossary.*

Hyman, L.H. 1967. The invertebrates: Mollusca, vol. 6. New York, McGraw-Hill Book Co. *This volume covers four groups of the molluscs—Aplacophora, Polyplacophora, Monoplacophora, and Gastropoda—and upholds the fine tradition of the other volumes in this series.*

Kaestner, A. 1964. Invertebrate zoology, vol. 1. New York, John Wiley & Sons, Inc.

Keen, A.M., and J.H. McLean. 1971. Sea shells of tropical west America. Stanford, Calif., Stanford University Press.

Lemche, H. 1957. A new living deep-sea mollusk of the Cambro-Devonian class Monoplacophora. Nature 179:413. *An account of Neopilina.*

Lemche, H., and K.G. Wingstrand. 1959. The anatomy of *Neopilina galatheae*. Galathea Reports 3:9-71.

Light, S.F., R.I. Smith, F.A. Pitelka, D.P. Abbott, and F.M. Weesner. 1967. Intertidal invertebrates of the central California coast. Berkeley, University of California Press.

Linsley, R.M. 1978. Shell form and evolution of gastropods. Am. Sci. 66:432-441.

Morris, P.A. (W.J. Clench [ed.]) 1973. A field guide to shells of the Atlantic and Gulf coasts and the West Indies, ed. 3. Boston, Houghton Mifflin Co. *An excellent revision of a popular handbook.*

Moynihan, M.H., and A.F. Rodaniche. 1977. Communication, crypsis, and mimicry among cephalopods. In T.A. Sebeok (ed.). How animals communicate. Bloomington, Indiana University Press.

Nixon, M., and J.B. Messenger (eds.). 1977. The biology of cephalopods. Symposia of the Zoological Society of London, no. 38. London, Academic Press, Inc., Ltd. *A series of articles, including evolution, systematics, physiology, behavior, learning, and maturation of cephalopods.*

Pennak, R.W. 1978. Freshwater invertebrates of the United States, ed. 2. New York, John Wiley & Sons, Inc.

Purchon, R.D. 1968. The biology of the Mollusca. New York, Pergamon Press, Inc. *A readable book that reviews in eight essays the research of the past 40 to 50 years, stressing the fascinating adaptive radiation within the classes.*

Rice, T. 1971. Marine shells of the Pacific Northwest. Edmonds, Wash., Ellison Industries. *Handy field guide with color plates.*

Runham, N.W., and P.J. Hunter. 1970. Terrestrial slugs. London, Hutchinson University Library.

Russell-Hunter, W.D. 1979. A life of invertebrates. New York, Macmillan, Inc.

Solem, A. 1974. The shell makers: introducing mollusks. New York, John Wiley & Sons, Inc. *Good for the shell collector who wants to know more about the living molluscs.*

Stasek, C.R. 1972. The molluscan framework. In M. Florkin and B.T. Scheer (eds.). Chemical zoology, vol. 8. New York, Academic Press, Inc. *Discusses phylogeny of molluscs and derivation of the classes from functional viewpoint.*

Thompson, T.E. 1976. Biology of the Opisthobranch molluscs, vol. 1. London, The Ray Society. *Basically an identification guide; beautifully illustrated.*

Thompson, T.E. 1976. Nudibranchs. Neptune, N.J., T.F.H. Publications, Inc. *A slender handbook filled with superb color photographs.*

Vagvolgyi, J. 1967. On the origin of molluscs, the coelom, and coelomic segmentation. Syst. Zool. 16:153-168.

Yochelson, E.L. 1978. An alternative approach to the interpretation of the phylogeny of ancient mollusks. Malacologia 17:165-191. *Argues that there are several classes of extinct mollusks.*

Yonge, C.M., and T.E. Thompson. 1976. Living marine molluscs. London, William Collins Sons & Co., Ltd. *Interesting book about both the more common molluscs and those with particularly interesting adaptive features.*

Selected *Scientific American* articles

Boycott, B.B. 1965. Learning in the octopus. 212:42-50 (Mar.).

Feder, H.M. 1972. Escape responses in marine invertebrates. 227:92-100 (July).

Korringa, P. 1953. Oysters. 189:86-91 (Nov.). *Their life history is described.*

Lane, C.E. 1961. The teredo. 204:132-142 (Feb.). *Biology of the shipworm.*

Roper, C.R.E., and K.J. Boss. 1982. The giant squid. 246:96-105 (Apr.). *Many mysteries remain about the deep-sea squid, Architeuthis, because it has never been studied alive. It can reach a weight of 1000 pounds and a length of 18 m, and its eyes are as large as automobile headlights.*

Ward, P., L. Greenwald, and O.E. Greenwald. 1980. The buoyancy of the chambered nautilus. 243:190-203 (Oct.). *Reviews recent discoveries on how the nautilus removes the water from a chamber after secreting a new septum.*

Willows, H.O.D. 1971. Giant brain cells in mollusks. 224:68-75 (Feb.).

Yonge, C.M. 1975. Giant clams. 232:96-105 (Apr.).

CHAPTER 14

THE SEGMENTED WORMS

Phylum Annelida

Two beautiful Christmas-tree worms *(Spirobranchus giganteus)* extend their feathery
plumes from the mouths of their tubes to trap minute food particles on the
delicate radioles. They have built their tubes in a colony
of fire coral, *Millepora complanata.*

Photograph by L.S. Roberts

Position in Animal Kingdom

1. Annelids belong to the **protostome** branch of the animal kingdom and have spiral and determinate cleavage.
2. Annelids have a true **coelom** (body cavity).
3. Annelids as a group show a primitive metamerism with comparatively few differences between the different somites.
4. All organ systems are present and well developed.

Biological Contributions

1. The introduction of **metamerism** by the group represents the greatest advancement of this phylum and lays the groundwork for the more highly specialized metamerism of the arthropods.
2. A true coelomic cavity reaches a high stage of development in this group.
3. Specialization of the head region into differentiated organs, such as the tentacles, palps, and eyespots of the polychaetes, is carried further in some annelids than in other invertebrates so far considered.
4. The tendency toward **centralization of the nervous system** is more developed, with cerebral ganglia (brain), two closely fused ventral nerve cords with giant fibers running the length of the body, and various ganglia with their lateral branches.
5. The circulatory system is much more complex than any we have so far considered. It is a closed system with muscular blood vessels and aortic arches ("hearts") for propelling the blood.
6. The appearance of the fleshy **parapodia,** with their respiratory and locomotor functions, introduces a suggestion of the paired appendages and specialized gills found in the more highly organized arthropods.
7. The well-developed **nephridia** in most of the somites have reached a differentiation that involves removal of waste from the blood as well as from the coelom.
8. Annelids are the most highly organized animals capable of complete regeneration. However, this ability varies greatly within the group.

PHYLUM ANNELIDA

Annelida (an-nel′i-da) (L., *annellus*, little ring, + *ida*, pl. suffix) consists of the segmented worms. It is a large phylum, numbering approximately 9000 species, the most familiar of which are the earthworms and freshwater worms (oligochaetes) and the leeches (hirudineans). However, approximately two thirds of the phylum is comprised of the marine worms (polychaetes), which are less familiar to most people. Among the latter are many curious members; some are strange, even grotesque, whereas others are graceful and beautiful (see lead photograph). They include the clamworms, plumed worms, parchment worms, scaleworms, lugworms, and many others. The annelids are true coelomates and belong to the protostome branch, with spiral and determinate cleavage. They are a highly developed group in which the nervous system is more centralized and the circulatory system more complex than those of the phyla we have studied thus far.

The Annelida are worms whose bodies are divided into similar rings, or **segments,** arranged in linear series and externally marked by circular grooves called **annuli;** the name of the phylum is descriptive of this characteristic. Body segmentation, or **metamerism,** in the annelids is not merely an external feature but is also seen internally in the repetitive arrangement of organs and systems and in the partitioning off of segments (also called metameres or somites) by septa. Metamerism is not limited to annelids; it is shared by the arthropods (insects, crustaceans, and others), which are related to the annelids, and also by the vertebrates, in which it evolved independently.

Annelids are sometimes called "bristle worms" because, with the exception of the leeches, most annelids bear tiny chitinous bristles called **setae** (L., *seta,* hair or bristle). Short needlelike setae help anchor the somites during locomotion to prevent backward slipping; long, hairlike setae aid aquatic forms in swimming. Since many annelids either are burrowers or live in secreted tubes, the stiff setae also aid in preventing the worm from being pulled out or washed out of its home. Robins know from experience how effective the earthworms' setae are.

Annelids have a worldwide distribution and occur in marine and brackish waters, fresh water, and terrestrial soils. A few of the species may be called cosmopolitan.

Polychaetes are chiefly marine forms. Most are benthic, but some live free in the open sea. They are usually divided into two groups: the sedentary polychaetes, or Sedentaria, and the free-moving polychaetes, or Errantia. Sedentary polychaetes are mainly tubicolous; that is, they spend all or much of their time in tubes or permanent burrows. Many of them, especially those that live in tubes, have elaborate devices for feeding and respiration. In sabellids and serpulids the cirri or tentacles around the mouth give rise to great featherlike "branchial crowns" that are involved in both feeding and respiration (p. 338). By means of ciliary currents water passes between the tentacles and carries food entangled in mucus to the mouth. The errant, or free-moving, polychaetes have various habitats; some are strictly pelagic and others live in crevices or under rocks or shells, never straying far in open water.

Many polychaetes are euryhaline (can tolerate a wide range of environmental salinity) and occur in brackish water. Freshwater polychaete fauna is more diversified in warmer regions than in the temperate zones.

Clitellates (oligochaetes and leeches) occur predominantly in fresh water or terrestrial soils. Some freshwater species burrow in the bottom mud and sand and others among submerged vegetation. The swimming species usually have long setae, whereas the common earthworms, the most familiar example of the oligochaetes, have short setae.

Many of the leeches (class Hirudinea) are predators, and many are specialized for piercing their prey and feeding on blood or soft tissues. A few leeches are marine, but most of them live in fresh water or in damp regions. Suckers are typically found at both ends of the body for attachment to the substratum or to their prey. Some are adapted for forcing their pharynx or proboscis into soft tissues such as the gills of fish. The most specialized leeches, however, have sawlike chitinous jaws with which they can cut through tough skin. Many leeches live as carnivores on small invertebrates; some are temporary parasites; and some are permanent parasites, never leaving their host.

CHARACTERISTICS

1. Body **metamerically segmented**; symmetry bilateral
2. Body wall with outer circular and inner longitudinal muscle layers; outer transparent moist cuticle secreted by epithelium
3. **Chitinous setae,** often present on fleshy appendages called **parapodia;** setae absent in leeches
4. **Coelom** (schizocoel) well developed and divided by septa, except in leeches; coelomic fluid supplies turgidity and functions as hydrostatic skeleton
5. **Blood system closed** and segmentally arranged; respiratory pigments (hemoglobin, hemerythrin, or chlorocruorin) often present; amebocytes in blood plasma
6. Digestive system complete and not metamerically arranged
7. Respiratory gas exchange through skin, **gills,** or **parapodia**
8. Excretory system typically a **pair of nephridia for each metamere**

9. Nervous system with a double ventral nerve cord and a pair of ganglia with lateral nerves in each metamere; brain a pair of dorsal cerebral ganglia with connectives to cord
10. Sensory system of tactile organs, taste buds, statocysts (in some), photoreceptor cells, and eyes with lenses (in some)
11. Hermaphroditic or separate sexes; larvae, if present, are trochophore type; asexual reproduction by budding in some; spiral cleavage and mosaic development

CLASSIFICATION

The annelids are classified primarily on the basis of the presence or absence of parapodia, setae, metameres, and other morphological features. Because both the oligochaetes and the hirudineans (leeches) bear a saddlelike enlargement, called a **clitellum** (L., *clitellae*, packsaddle) (Fig. 14-2, *B*), that is involved in reproduction, these two groups are often placed under the heading Clitellata (cli-tel-la′ta) and members are called clitellates. On the other hand, because both the Oligochaeta and the Polychaeta possess setae, some authorities place them together in a group called Chaetopoda (ke-top′o-da) (N.L., *chaeta*, bristle, from Gr., *chaitē*, long hair, + *pous, podos*, foot).

Class Polychaeta (pol″e-ke′ta) (Gr., *polys*, many, + *chaitē*, long hair). Mostly marine; head distinct and bearing eyes and tentacles; most segments with parapodia (lateral appendages) bearing tufts of many setae; clitellum absent; sexes usually separate; gonads transitory; asexual budding in some; trochophore larva usually; mostly marine.

Subclass Errantia (er-ran′she-a) (L., *errare*, to wander, + *ia*, pl. suffix). Segments usually similar except in head and anal regions; parapodia alike and with acicula (long, stout setae); pharynx usually protrusible; head appendages usually present; free-living, tube-dwelling, and pelagic species. Examples: *Nereis, Aphrodita, Glycera*.

Subclass Sedentaria (sed-en-ta′re-a) (L., *sedere*, to sit, + *aria*, like or connected with). Body with unlike segments, parapodia, and regional differentiation; prostomium small or indistinct; head appendages modified or absent; pharynx without jaws and mostly nonprotrusible; parapodia reduced and without acicula; gills anterior or absent; tube-dwelling or in burrows. Examples: *Arenicola, Chaetopterus, Amphitrite*.

Class Oligochaeta (ol′i-go-ke′ta) (Gr., *oligos*, few, + *chaitē*, long hair). Body with conspicuous segmentation; number of segments variable; setae few per metamere; no parapodia; head absent; coelom spacious and usually divided by intersegmental septa; hermaphroditic; development direct, no larva; chiefly terrestrial and freshwater. Examples: *Lumbricus, Stylaria, Aeolosoma, Tubifex*.

Class Hirudinea (hir′u-din′e-a) (L., *hirudo*, leech, + *ea*, characterized by)—leeches. Body with fixed number of segments (34) with many annuli; body with anterior and posterior suckers usually; clitellum present; no parapodia; setae absent (except *Acanthobdella*); coelom closely packed with connective tissue and muscle; development direct; hermaphroditic; terrestrial, freshwater, and marine. Examples: *Hirudo, Placobdella, Macrobdella*.

The Branchiobdellida, a group of small annelids that are parasitic or commensal on crayfish and show similarities to both oligochaetes and leeches, are here placed with the oligochaetes, but they are considered by some authorities to be a separate class. They have 14 or 15 segments and bear a head sucker.

One genus of leech, *Acanthobdella*, is a primitive type with some characteristics of leeches and some of oligochaetes; it is sometimes separated from the other leeches into a special class, Acanthobdellida, that characteristically has 27 somites, setae on the first five segments, and no anterior sucker.

Body Plan

The annelid body typically has a head or prostomium, segmented body, and terminal portion bearing the anus. New segments form just in front of the terminal portion; thus, the oldest segments are at the anterior end and the youngest segments are at the posterior end. The prostomium and the terminal portion are not considered metameres.

The body wall is made up of strong circular and longitudinal muscles adapt-

Figure 14-1

Annelid body plan.

Figure 14-2

Earthworm anatomy. **A,** Internal structure of anterior portion of worm. **B,** External features, lateral view. **C,** Generalized transverse section through region posterior to clitellum. **D,** Portion of epidermis showing sensory, glandular, and epithelial cells.

ed for swimming, crawling, and burrowing and is covered with epidermis and a thin, outer layer of nonchitinous cuticle (Fig. 14-1).

In most annelids the coelom develops embryonically as a split in the mesoderm on each side of the gut (**schizocoel**), forming a pair of coelomic compartments in each segment. Each compartment is surrounded with **peritoneum** (a layer of mesodermal epithelium), which lines the body wall, forms dorsal and ventral **mesenteries,** and covers all the organs (Fig. 14-1). Where the peritonea of adjacent segments meet, the **septa** are formed. These are perforated by the gut and longitudinal blood vessels. Not only is the coelom metamerically arranged, but practically every body system is affected in some way by this segmental arrangement.

Except in the leeches, the coelom is filled with fluid and serves as a **hydrostatic skeleton.** Because the volume of the fluid is essentially constant, contraction of the longitudinal body wall muscles causes the body to shorten and become larger in diameter, whereas contraction of the circular muscles causes it to lengthen and become thinner. Separation of the hydrostatic skeleton into a metameric series of coelomic cavities increases its efficiency greatly because the force of local muscle contraction is not transferred throughout the length of the worm. Widening and elongation can occur in restricted areas. Crawling motions are effected by alternating waves of contraction of longitudinal and circular muscles (peristaltic contraction) passing down the body. Segments in which longitudinal muscles are contracted widen and anchor themselves against burrow walls or other substratum while other segments, in which circular muscles are contracted, elongate and stretch forward. Forces powerful enough for burrowing as well as locomotion can thus be generated. Swimming forms use undulatory rather than peristaltic movements in locomotion.

Class Oligochaeta

The more than 3000 species of oligochaetes are found in a great variety of sizes and habitats. They include the familiar earthworms and many species that live in fresh water. Most are terrestrial or freshwater forms, but some are parasitic, and a few live in marine or brackish water.

Oligochaetes, with few exceptions, bear setae, which may be long or short, straight or curved, blunt or needlelike, or arranged singly or in bundles. Whatever the type, they are less numerous in oligochaetes than in polychaetes, as is implied by the class name, which means "few long hairs." Aquatic forms usually have longer setae than do earthworms.

Earthworms

The most familiar of the oligochaetes are the earthworms ("night crawlers"), which burrow in moist, rich soil, emerging at night to explore their surroundings. In damp, rainy weather they stay near the surface, often with mouth or anus protruding from the burrow. In very dry weather they may burrow several feet underground, coil up in a slime chamber, and become dormant. *Lumbricus terrestris* (L., *lumbricum,* earthworm), the form commonly studied in school laboratories, is approximately 12 to 30 cm long (Fig. 14-2). Giant tropical earthworms may have from 150 to 250 or more segments and may grow to as much as 4 m in length. They usually live in branched and interconnected tunnels.

Aristotle called earthworms the "intestines of the soil." Some 22 centuries later Charles Darwin published his observations in his classic *The Formation of Vegetable Mould Through the Action of Worms.* He showed how worms enrich the soil by bringing subsoil to the surface and mixing it with the topsoil. An earthworm can ingest its own weight in soil every 24 hours, and Darwin estimated that from 10 to 18 tons of dry earth per acre pass through their intestines annually, thus bringing up potassium and phosphorus from the subsoil and also adding to the soil nitrogenous products from their own metabolism. They expose the mold to the air and sift it into small particles. They also drag leaves, twigs, and organic substances into their burrows closer to the roots of plants. Their activities are important in aerating the soil. Darwin's views were at odds with his contemporaries, who thought earthworms were harmful to plants. But recent research has amply confirmed Darwin's findings, and earthworm management is now practiced in many countries.

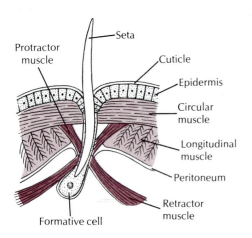

Figure 14-3

Seta with its muscle attachments showing relation to adjacent structures. Setae lost by wear and tear are replaced by new ones, which develop from formative cells.
Modified from Stephenson, J. 1972. The Oligochaeta. New York, Wheldon & Wesley Ltd., Stechert-Hafner Service Agency, Inc.; and others.

Form and function

In earthworms the mouth is overhung by a fleshy prostomium at the anterior end, and the anus is on the terminal end (Fig. 14-2, B). In most earthworms each segment bears four pairs of chitinous setae (Fig. 14-2, C), although in some oligochaetes each segment may have up to 100 or more. Each seta is a bristlelike rod set in a sac within the body wall and moved by tiny muscles (Fig. 14-3). The setae project through small pores in the cuticle to the outside. In locomotion and burrowing, setae anchor parts of the body to prevent slipping. Earthworms move by peristaltic movement. Contractions of circular muscles in the anterior end lengthen the body, pushing the anterior end forward where it is anchored by setae; contractions of longitudinal muscles then shorten the body, pulling the posterior end forward. As these waves of contraction pass along the entire body, it is gradually moved forward.

Nutrition

Most oligochaetes are scavengers. Earthworms feed mainly on decayed organic matter, bits of leaves and vegetation, refuse, and animal matter. After being moistened by secretions from the **mouth,** food is drawn in by the sucking action of the muscular **pharynx.** The liplike prostomium aids in manipulating the food into position. The calcium from the soil swallowed with the food tends to produce a high blood calcium level. **Calciferous glands** along the **esophagus** secrete calcium ions into the gut and so reduce the calcium ion concentration of the blood. Calciferous glands are really excretory, rather than digestive, organs. They also function in regulating the acid-base balance of the body fluids, maintaining the pH at a fairly stable value.

Leaving the **esophagus,** food is stored temporarily in the thin-walled **crop** before being passed on into the **gizzard,** which grinds the food into small pieces. Digestion and absorption take place in the **intestine.** Along the dorsal side, the wall of the intestine is infolded to form a **typhlosole,** which greatly increases the absorptive and digestive surface (Figs. 14-2, C, and 14-4, B). The digestive system secretes various enzymes to break down the food: pepsin, which acts on proteins; amylase, which acts on polysaccharides; cellulase, which acts on cellulose; and lipase, which acts on fats. The indigestible residue is discharged through the **anus.**

Surrounding the intestine and dorsal vessel and filling much of the typhlosole is a layer of yellowish **chlorogogue tissue** derived from the peritoneum. This tissue serves as a center for the synthesis of glycogen and fat, a function roughly equivalent to that of liver cells. The chlorogogue cells when ripe (full of fat) are released into the coelom where they float free as cells called **eleocytes** (Gr., *elaio,* oil, + *kytos,* hollow vessel [cell]), which transport materials to the body tissues. They apparently can pass from segment to segment and have been found to accumulate around wounds and regenerating areas, where they break down and release their contents into the coelom. Chlorogogue cells also function in excretion.

Circulation

Annelids have a double transport system: the coelomic fluid and the circulatory system. Food, wastes, and respiratory gases are carried by both coelomic fluid and blood in varying degrees. The blood is carried in a closed system of blood vessels, including capillary systems in the tissues. There are five main blood trunks, all running lengthwise through the body (Fig. 14-4).

Body wall

Esophagus

Anterior

Dorsal vessel (true heart)

Aortic arches

Lateral esophageal vessel

Typhlosolar vessel

Dorsointestinal vessel

Parietal vessel

Capillaries in body wall

Posterior

Region of nephridium

Ventral vessel

Nerve cord

Lateroneural vessel

Subneural vessel

Typhlosole

Ventrointestinal vessel

Segmental vessel

A

B

Figure 14-4

Scheme of circulation in the earthworm. **A,** Somites 9, 10, and 11, showing three of the five aortic arches that receive blood from the dorsal vessel and pass it down to the ventral vessel to be carried posteriorly and distributed to the body tissues. **B,** Any somite posterior to the esophagus, showing distribution of blood from ventral vessel to intestine, nerve cord, and body wall and return of blood to dorsal vessel by the parietal and intestinal vessels. The dorsal vessel is the chief pumping organ.

The **dorsal vessel** (single) runs above the alimentary canal from the pharynx to the anus. It is a pumping organ, provided with valves, and functions as the true heart. This vessel receives blood from vessels of the body wall and digestive tract and pumps it anteriorly into the five pairs of aortic arches. The function of the aortic arches is to maintain a steady pressure of blood into the ventral vessel.

The **ventral vessel** (single) serves as the aorta. It receives blood from the aortic arches and delivers it to the brain and rest of the body, giving off segmental vessels to the walls, nephridia, and digestive tract.

The direction of blood flow in the other longitudinal blood vessels is illustrated in Fig. 14-4. The blood contains colorless ameboid cells and a dissolved respiratory pigment, hemoglobin. The blood of the annelids may have respiratory pigments other than hemoglobin.

Excretion

The organs of excretion are the **nephridia,** a pair of which is found in each somite except the first three and the last one. Each one occupies parts of two successive somites (Fig. 14-5). A ciliated funnel, the **nephrostome,** lies just anterior to an intersegmental septum and leads by a small ciliated tubule through the septum into the somite behind, where it connects with the main part of the nephridium. This part of the nephridium is made up of several complex loops of increasing size, which finally terminate in a bladderlike structure leading to an aperture, the **nephridiopore;** this opens to the outside near the ventral row of setae. By means of cilia, wastes from the coelom are drawn into the nephrostome and tubule, where they are joined by organic wastes filtered from blood capillaries in the glandular part of the nephridium. All the waste is discharged to the outside through the nephridiopore.

Aquatic oligochaetes excrete ammonia; terrestrial oligochaetes excrete the much less toxic urea. *Lumbricus* produces both, the level of urea depending somewhat on environmental conditions. Both urea and ammonia are produced by chlorogogue cells, which may break off and enter the nephridia directly, or their products may be carried by the blood. Some nitrogenous waste is also eliminated through the body surface.

Oligochaetes are largely freshwater animals, and even such terrestrial forms

Figure 14-5

Nephridium of earthworm. Wastes are drawn into the ciliated nephrostome in one segment, then passed through the loops of the nephridium, and expelled through the nephridiopore of the next segment.

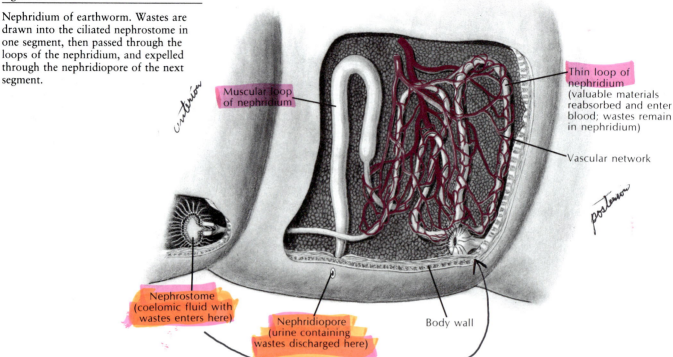

Muscular loop of nephridium

Thin loop of nephridium (valuable materials reabsorbed and enter blood; wastes remain in nephridium)

Vascular network

Nephrostome (coelomic fluid with wastes enters here)

Nephridiopore (urine containing wastes discharged here)

Body wall

Figure 14-6

Anterior portion of earthworm and its nervous system. Note concentration of sensory endings in this region.

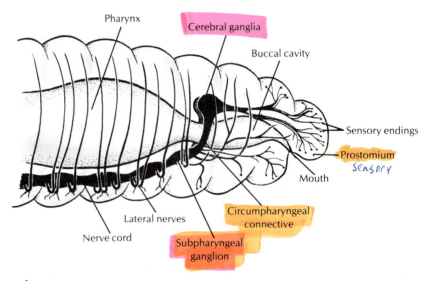

Pharynx

Cerebral ganglia

Buccal cavity

Sensory endings

Prostomium
sensory

Mouth

Circumpharyngeal connective

Subpharyngeal ganglion

Lateral nerves

Nerve cord

as earthworms must exist in a moist environment. Osmoregulation is a function of the body surface and the nephridia, as well as the gut and the dorsal pores. *Lumbricus* will gain weight when placed in tap water and lose it when returned to the soil. Salts as well as water can pass across the integument, apparently by active transport.

Respiration

The earthworm has no special respiratory organs, but gaseous exchange is made in the moist skin, where oxygen is picked up and carbon dioxide is given off. Blood capillaries are fairly numerous just below the cuticle, and the oxygen combines with the hemoglobin of the plasma and is carried to the various tissues.

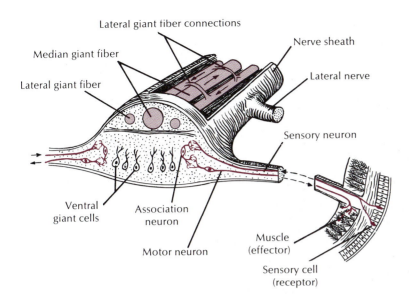

Figure 14-7

Portion of nerve cord of earthworm showing arrangement of simple reflex arc (*in foreground*) and the three dorsal giant fibers that are adapted for rapid reflexes and escape movements. Ordinary crawling involves a succession of reflex acts, the stretching of one somite stimulating the next to stretch, and so on. Impulses are transmitted much faster in giant fibers than in regular nerves so that all segments can contract simultaneously when quick withdrawal into a burrow is necessary.

Nervous system and sense organs

The nervous system in earthworms (Fig. 14-6) consists of a **central system** and **peripheral nerves**. The central system is made up of a pair of cerebral ganglia (the brain) above the pharynx and a pair of connectives passing around the pharynx connecting the brain with the first pair of ganglia in the nerve cord; a ventral nerve cord, really double, running along the floor of the coelom to the last somite; and a pair of fused ganglia on the nerve cord in each somite. Each pair of fused ganglia gives off nerves to the body structures, which contain both sensory and motor fibers.

Neurosecretory cells have been found in the brain and ganglia of annelids, both oligochaetes and polychaetes. They are endocrine in function and secrete neurohormones concerned with the regulation of reproduction, secondary sex characteristics, and regeneration.

For rapid escape movements most annelids are provided with from one to several very large axons commonly called **giant axons** (Fig. 14-7), or giant fibers, located in the ventral nerve cord. Their large diameter increases the rate of conduction and makes possible simultaneous contractions of muscles in many segments.

Simple **sense organs** are distributed all over the body. Earthworms have no eyes but do have many lens-shaped photoreceptors in the epidermis. Most oligochaetes are negatively phototactic to strong light but positively phototactic to weak light. Many single-celled sense organs are widely distributed in the epidermis. What are presumably chemoreceptors are most numerous on the prostomium. There are many free nerve endings in the integument, which are probably tactile.

In the dorsal median giant fiber of *Lumbricus*, which is 90 to 160 μm in diameter, the speed of conduction has been estimated at 20 to 45 m/second, several times faster than in ordinary neurons of this species. This is also much faster than in polychaete giant fibers, probably because in the earthworms the giant fibers are enclosed in myelinated sheaths. The speed of conduction may be altered by changes in temperature.

General behavior

Earthworms are among the most defenseless of creatures, yet their abundance and wide distribution indicate their ability to survive. Although they have no specialized sense organs, they are sensitive to many stimuli, such as **mechanical,** to which they react positively when it is moderate and negatively when it is a vibration (such as a footfall near them), which causes them to retire quickly into their

Figure 14-8

Two earthworms in copulation. Their anterior ends point in opposite direction as their ventral surfaces are held together by mucous bands secreted by the clitella. Mutual insemination occurs during copulation. After separation each worm secretes a cocoon to receive its eggs and sperm.

Courtesy Carolina Biological Supply Co., Burlington, N.C.

burrows; and **light,** which they avoid unless it is very weak. Chemical responses aid them in the choice of food.

Chemical as well as tactile responses are very important to the worm. It not only must be able to sample the organic content of the soil to find food, but also must sense its texture, acidity, and calcium content.

Experiments show that earthworms have some learning ability. They can be taught to avoid an electric shock, and thus an association reflex can be built up in them. Darwin credited earthworms with a great deal of intelligence in pulling leaves into their burrows, for they apparently seized the leaves by the narrow end, the easiest way for drawing a leaf-shaped object into a small hole. Darwin assumed that the seizure of the leaves by the worms did not result from random handling or from chance but was purposeful in its mechanism. However, investigations since Darwin's time have shown that the process is mainly one of trial and error, for they often seize a leaf several times before attaining the right position.

Reproduction and development

Earthworms are monoecious (hermaphroditic); that is, both male and female organs are found in the same animal (Fig. 14-2, *A*). In *Lumbricus* the reproductive systems are found in somites 9 to 15. Two pairs of small testes and two pairs of sperm funnels are surrounded by three pairs of large seminal vesicles. Immature sperm from the testes mature in the seminal vesicles, then pass into the sperm funnels and down sperm ducts to the male genital pores in somite 15, where they are expelled during copulation. Eggs are discharged by a pair of small ovaries into the coelomic cavity, where they are picked up by ciliated funnels and are carried by oviducts to the outside through female genital pores on somite 14. Two pairs of seminal receptacles in somites 9 and 10 receive and store sperm from the mate during copulation.

Reproduction in earthworms may occur at any season, but copulation usually occurs at night during warm, moist weather (Fig. 14-8). When mating, the worms extend their anterior ends from their burrows and bring their ventral surfaces together (Fig. 14-9). They are held together by mucus secreted by the **clitellum** and by special ventral setae, which penetrate each other's bodies in the regions of contact. Sperm are discharged and travel to the seminal receptacles of the other worm in its seminal grooves. After copulation each worm secretes, around its clitellum, first a mucous tube and then a tough, chitinlike band that forms a **cocoon.** As the cocoon passes forward, eggs from the oviducts, albumin from the skin glands, and sperm from the mate (stored in the seminal receptacles) are poured into it. Fertilization of the eggs then takes place within the cocoon. When the cocoon leaves the worm, its ends close, producing a lemon-shaped body. Embryonation occurs within the cocoon, and the form that hatches from the egg is a young worm similar to the adult. It does not develop a clitellum until it is sexually mature.

Freshwater oligochaetes

Freshwater oligochaetes usually are smaller and have more conspicuous setae than do the earthworms. They are more mobile than earthworms and tend to have better-developed sense organs. They are generally benthic forms that creep about on the bottom or burrow in the soft mud. Aquatic oligochaetes are an important food source for fishes. A few are ectoparasitic.

Some of the more common freshwater oligochaetes are *Aeolosoma* (Gr.,

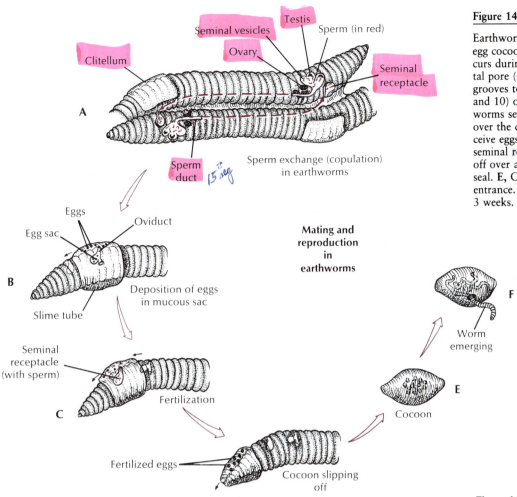

A, Sperm exchange (copulation) in earthworms

Clitellum

Seminal vesicles   Testis   Sperm (in red)

Ovary

Seminal receptacle

Sperm duct   15th seg

B, Eggs   Oviduct   Egg sac   Slime tube   Deposition of eggs in mucous sac

C, Seminal receptacle (with sperm)   Fertilization

D, Fertilized eggs   Cocoon slipping off

E, Cocoon

F, Worm emerging

Mating and reproduction in earthworms

Figure 14-9

Earthworm copulation and formation of egg cocoons. **A,** Mutual insemination occurs during copulation; sperm from genital pore (somite 15) pass along seminal grooves to seminal receptacles (somites 9 and 10) of each mate. **B** and **C,** After worms separate, a slime tube formed over the clitellum passes forward to receive eggs from oviducts and sperm from seminal receptacles. **D,** As cocoon slips off over anterior end, its ends close and seal. **E,** Cocoon is deposited near burrow entrance. **F,** Young worms emerge in 2 to 3 weeks.

aiolos, quick-moving, + *soma,* body) (Fig. 14-10) (1 mm long), which contains red or green pigments, has bundles of setae, and is often found in hay cultures; *Nais* (L., *nais,* water nymph) (2 to 4 mm long), which is brownish and has two or three bundles of setae on each segment; *Stylaria* (Gr., *stylos,* pillar) (10 to 25 mm long), which has two bunches of setae on each segment, with the prostomium extended into a long process, and black eyespots; *Dero* (Gr., *derē,* neck, throat) (5 to 10 mm long), which is reddish, lives in tubes, and has three tail gills; *Tubifex* (L., *tubus,* tube, + *faciens,* to make or do) (30 to 40 mm long), which is reddish and lives with its head in mud at the bottom of ponds and its tail waving in the water; *Chaetogaster* (N.L., *chaeta,* bristle, + *gastrula,* belly) (10 to 15 mm long), which has only ventral bundles of setae; and *Enchytraeus* (Gr., *enchytraeus,* living in an earthen pot), small whitish worms that live both in moist soil and in water. Some oligochaetes, such as *Aeolosoma,* may form chains of zooids asexually by transverse fission (Fig. 14-10, *B*).

Class Hirudinea—the Leeches

Leeches are found predominantly in freshwater habitats, but a few are marine, and some have even adapted to terrestrial life in warm, moist places. They are more abundant in tropical countries than in temperate zones. Some leeches attack human beings and are a nuisance.

Figure 14-10

Some freshwater oligochaetes. **A,** *Stylaria* has the prostomium drawn out into a long snout. **B,** *Aeolosoma* uses cilia around the mouth to sweep in food particles, and it buds off new individuals asexually. **C,** *Tubifex* lives head down in long tubes. **D,** *Aulophorus* is provided with ciliated anal gills.

Figure 14-11

The world's largest leech, *Haementeria ghilianii*, found in French Guiana, South America.

Photograph by T. Branning.

For centuries the "medicinal leech" *(Hirudo medicinalis)* was employed in medical practice for bloodletting because of the mistaken idea that bodily disorders and fevers were caused by a plethora of blood. Since the leech is 10 to 12 cm long and can extend to a much greater length when distended with blood, the amount of blood it can suck from a patient is considerable. Leech collecting and leech culture in ponds were practiced in Europe on a commercial scale during the nineteenth century. Wordsworth's interesting poem "The Leech-Gatherer" was based on this use of the leech.

Most leeches are between 2 and 6 cm in length, but some are smaller; some, including the "medicinal" leech, reach 20 cm, but the giant of all is the Amazonian *Haementeria* (Gr., *haimateros,* bloody) (Fig. 14-11), which reaches 30 cm.

Leeches are found in a variety of patterns and colors: black, brown, red, or olive green. They are usually flattened dorsoventrally.

Like the oligochaetes, leeches have a **clitellum** during the breeding season. The clitellum secretes a cocoon for the reception of eggs. Both groups are hermaphroditic, but leeches are more highly specialized. As fluid feeders and bloodsuckers, they have lost the setae used by the oligochaetes in locomotion and have developed **suckers** for attachment while sucking blood; their gut is specialized for storage of large quantities of blood.

Form and function

Unlike other annelids, leeches have a **fixed number of somites** (34), but they appear to have many more because each somite is marked by transverse grooves to form from two to 16 superficial rings (**annuli**) (Fig. 14-12).

The **coelom** represents another difference between leeches and other annelids; leeches lack distinct coelomic compartments. In all but one species the septa have disappeared, and the coelomic cavity is filled with connective tissue and a system of spaces called **sinuses**. The coelomic sinuses form a regular system of channels filled with coelomic fluid, which in some leeches serves as an auxiliary circulatory system.

Most leeches creep with looping movements of the body, by attaching first one sucker and then the other and pulling up the body. Aquatic leeches can also swim with a graceful undulatory movement.

Nutrition

Leeches are popularly considered parasitic, but it would be more accurate to call them predaceous. Even the true bloodsuckers rarely are host specific or remain on the host for a long period of time. Most freshwater leeches are active predators or scavengers equipped with a proboscis that can be extended to draw in small invertebrates or to take blood from cold-blooded vertebrates. Some freshwater leeches are true bloodsuckers, preying on cattle, horses, humans, and others. Some terrestrial leeches feed on insect larvae, earthworms, and slugs, which they hold by an anterior sucker while using a strong sucking pharynx to draw in the food. Other terrestrial forms climb brushes or trees to reach warm-blooded vertebrates such as birds or mammals.

Most leeches are fluid feeders. Many prefer to feed on tissue fluids and blood pumped from wounds already open. The true bloodsuckers, which include the so-called medicinal leech *Hirudo* (L., a leech), have cutting plates, or "jaws," for cutting through tissues. Some species are true parasites, living permanently on their hosts.

Respiration and excretion

Gas exchange occurs only through the skin except in some of the fish leeches, which have gills. There are 10 to 17 pairs of nephridia, in addition to coelomocytes and certain other specialized cells that may also be involved in excretory functions.

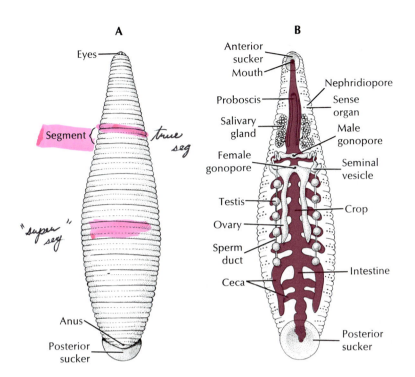

A

Eyes

Segment (*true seg*

"*super* seg"

Anus

Posterior sucker

B

Anterior sucker
Mouth

Proboscis

Salivary gland

Female gonopore

Testis

Ovary

Sperm duct

Ceca

Nephridiopore

Sense organ

Male gonopore

Seminal vesicle

Crop

Intestine

Posterior sucker

Figure 14-12

Structure of a leech, *Placobdella*. **A**, External appearance, dorsal view. **B**, Internal structure, ventral view.

Nervous and sensory systems

Leeches have two "brains," one in the head, composed of six pairs of fused ganglia forming a ring around the pharynx, and one in the tail, composed of seven pairs of fused ganglia. The additional 21 pairs of ganglia are segmentally arranged along the double nerve cord. In addition to free sensory nerve endings and photoreceptor cells in the epidermis, there is a row of sense organs, called sensillae, in the central annulus of each segment; there are also a number of pigment cup ocelli.

Reproduction

Leeches are hermaphroditic but practice cross-fertilization during copulation. Sperm are transferred by a penis or by hypodermic impregnation (a spermatophore is expelled from one worm and penetrates the integument of the other). After copulation the clitellum secretes a cocoon that receives the eggs and sperm. Cocoons are buried in bottom mud, attached to submerged objects, or, in terrestrial species, placed in damp soil. Development is similar to that of oligochaetes.

Circulation

In leeches the coelom has been reduced, by the invasion of connective tissue and in some by a proliferation of chlorogogue tissue, to a system of coelomic sinuses and channels. Some orders of leeches retain the typical oligochaete circulatory system, and in these the coelomic sinuses act as an auxiliary blood-vascular system. In other orders the traditional blood vessels have disappeared and the system of coelomic sinuses forms the only blood-vascular system. In those the blood (the equivalent of coelomic fluid) is propelled by contractions of certain longitudinal channels.

Figure 14-13

Polychaete tubeworms. **A,** *Protula* (family Serpulidae) builds a calcareous tube. **B,** *Spirographis spallanzani* (family Sabellidae) builds a noncalcareous tube.

Photographs by C.P. Hickman, Jr.

Class Polychaeta

The polychaetes are the largest and most primitive class of annelids, with more than 5300 species, most of them marine. Although the majority of them are 5 to 10 cm long, some are less than 1 mm, and others may be as long as 3 m. Some are brightly colored in reds and greens; others are dull or iridescent. Some are picturesque, such as the "featherduster" worms (Fig. 14-13).

Polychaetes live under rocks, in coral crevices, or in abandoned shells, or they burrow into mud or sand; some build their own tubes on submerged objects or in bottom material; some adopt the tubes or homes of other animals; some are pelagic, making up a part of the planktonic population. They are extremely abundant in some areas; for example, a square meter of mud flat may contain thousands of polychaetes. They play a significant part in marine food chains, since they are eaten by fish, crustaceans, hydroids, and many others.

Form and function

Polychaetes differ from other annelids in having a well-differentiated head with specialized sense organs; paired appendages, called parapodia, on most segments; and no clitellum (Fig. 14-14). As their name implies, they have many setae, usually arranged in bundles on the parapodia. They show a pronounced differentiation of some body somites and a specialization of sensory organs practically unknown among clitellates.

In contrast to clitellates, polychaetes have no permanent sex organs, possess no permanent ducts for their sex cells, and usually have separate sexes. Their development is indirect, for they undergo a form of metamorphosis that involves a trochophore larva.

Polychaetes are usually divided into two subclasses: Errantia and Sedentaria. These subclasses are convenient but probably artificial. The **Errantia,** or errant worms (L., *errare,* to wander), include the free-moving pelagic forms, active burrowers, crawlers, and the tube worms that leave their tubes for feeding or breeding. Most of these, like the clam worm *Nereis* (Gr., name of a sea nymph) (Fig. 14-14), are predatory forms equipped with jaws or teeth. They have a muscular eversible pharynx armed with teeth that can be thrust out with surprising speed and dexterity for capturing prey. The **Sedentaria** (L., *sedere,* to sit) are largely sedentary worms that rarely expose more than the head end from the tubes or burrows in which they live (p. 338 and Fig. 14-13).

Most sedentary tube and burrow dwellers are particle feeders, using ciliary or mucoid methods of obtaining food. The principal food source is plankton and detritus. Some, like *Amphitrite* (Gr., a sea nymph in mythology) (Fig. 14-15), with head peeping out of the mud, send out long extensible tentacles over the surface. Cilia and mucus on the tentacles entrap particles found on the sea bottom and move them toward the mouth.

The fanworms, or "featherduster" worms, are beautiful tubeworms, fascinating to watch as they emerge from their secreted tubes and unfurl their lovely tentacular crowns to feed. A slight disturbance, sometimes even a passing shadow, causes them to duck quickly into the safety of the homes they have built. Food attracted to the feathery arms, or **radioles,** by ciliary action is trapped in mucus and is carried down ciliated food grooves to the mouth (Fig. 14-16, *B* and *C*). Particles too large for the food grooves are carried along the margins and dropped off. Further sorting may occur near the mouth where only the small particles of

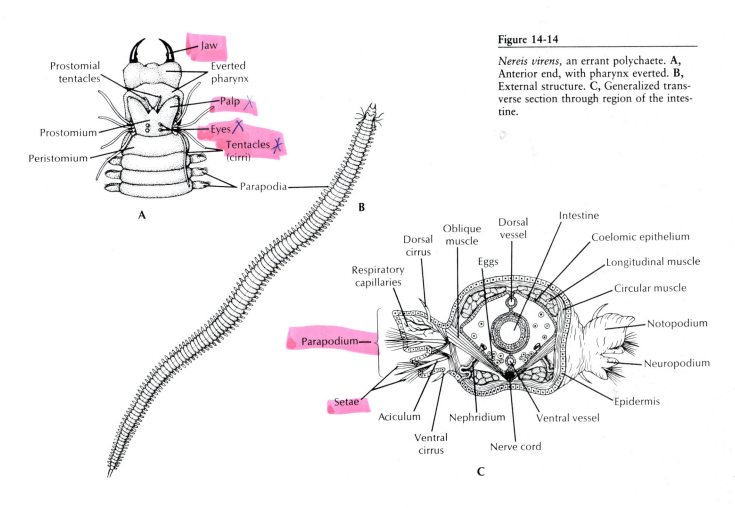

Figure 14-14

Nereis virens, an errant polychaete. **A,** Anterior end, with pharynx everted. **B,** External structure. **C,** Generalized transverse section through region of the intestine.

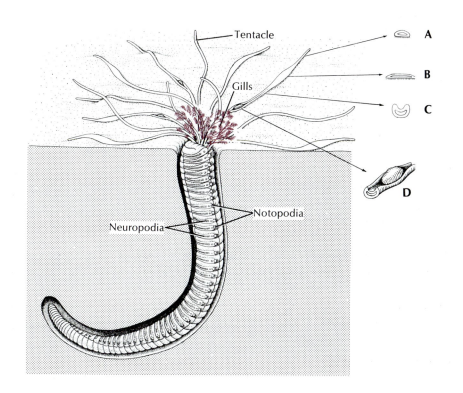

Figure 14-15

Amphitrite, which builds its tubes in mud or sand, extends long grooved tentacles out over the mud to pick up bits of organic matter. The smallest particles are moved along food grooves by cilia, larger particles by peristaltic movement. Its plumelike gills are blood red. **A,** Section through exploratory end of tentacle. **B,** Section through tentacle in area adhering to substratum. **C,** Section showing ciliary groove. **D,** Particle being carried toward mouth.

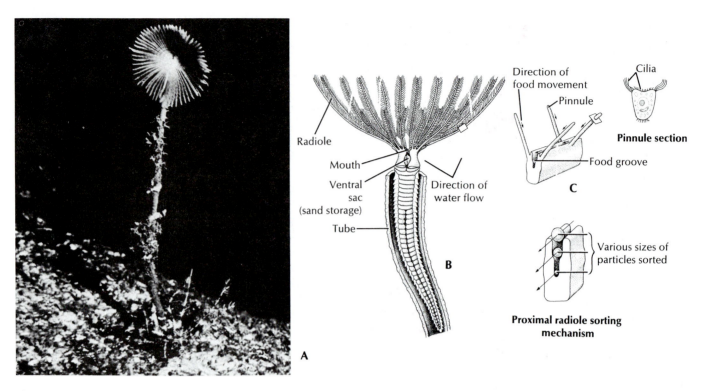

Figure 14-16

Sabella, a polychaete ciliary feeder. **A,** *Sabella pavonia* with its crown of feeding radioles extended from its leathery secreted tube, reinforced with sand and debris. **B,** Anterior view of the crown. Cilia direct small food particles along grooved radioles to mouth and discard larger particles. Sand grains are directed to storage sacs and later are used in tube building. **C,** Distal portion of radiole showing ciliary tracts of pinnules and food grooves.

A, Courtesy T. Lündalv.

food enter the mouth, and sand grains are stored in a sac to be used later in enlarging the tube.

Some worms, such as *Chaetopterus* (Gr., *chaitē,* long hair, + *pteron,* wing), secrete mucous filters through which they pump water to collect edible particles (Fig. 14-17). The lugworm *Arenicola* (L., *arena,* sand, + *colo,* inhabit) lives in an L-shaped burrow in which, by peristaltic movements, it keeps water filtering down through the sand and out the open end of the burrow. It ingests the food-laden sand brought by the water current (Fig. 14-18).

Tube dwellers secrete many types of tubes. Some are parchmentlike (Fig. 14-16); some are firm, calcareous tubes attached to rocks or other surfaces (Fig. 14-13, *A*); and some are simply grains of sand or bits of shell or seaweed cemented together with mucous secretions. Many burrowers in sand and mud flats simply line their burrows with mucus (Fig. 14-18).

The polychaete typically has a head, or **prostomium,** which may or may not be retractile and which often bears eyes, antennae, and sensory palps (Figs. 14-14 and 14-19). The first segment (**peristomium**) surrounds the mouth and may bear setae, palps, or, in predatory forms, chitinous jaws. Ciliary feeders may bear a tentacular crown that can be opened like a fan or withdrawn into the tube.

The trunk is segmented, and most segments bear appendages called **parapodia,** which may have lobes, cirri, setae, and other parts on them (Fig. 14-19). The parapodia are used in crawling, swimming, or anchoring in tubes. They usually serve as the chief respiratory organs, although some polychaetes may also have gills. *Amphitrite,* for example, has three pairs of branched gills and long extensible tentacles (Fig. 14-15). *Arenicola,* the lugworm (Fig. 14-18), which burrows through the sand leaving characteristic castings at the entrance to its burrow, has paired gills on certain somites.

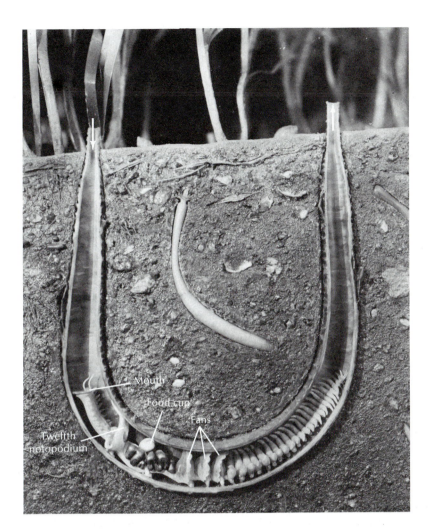

Figure 14-17

Chaetopterus, a sedentary polychaete (in U-tube) and *Phascolosoma,* a sipunculan worm (in center). *Chaetopterus* lives in a parchment tube through which it pumps water with its three pistonlike fans. The fans beat 60 times per minute to keep water currents moving. The winglike notopodia of the twelfth segment continuously secrete a mucous net that strains out food particles. As the net fills with food, the food cup rolls it into a ball and, when the ball is large enough (about 3 mm), the food cup bends forward and deposits the ball in a ciliated groove to be carried by cilia to the mouth and swallowed.

Courtesy The American Museum of Natural History, New York.

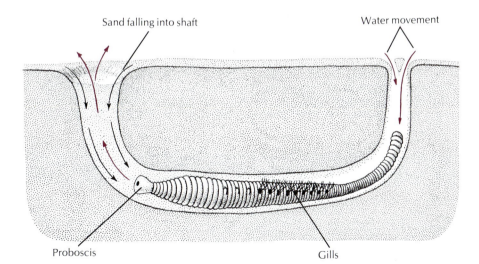

Figure 14-18

Arenicola, the lugworm, lives in an L-shaped burrow in intertidal mud flats. It burrows by successive eversions and retractions of its proboscis. By peristaltic movements it keeps water filtering down through the sand and out the open end of the burrow. The worm then ingests the food-laden sand.

Some polychaetes live most of the year as sexually unripe animals called atokes, but during the breeding season a portion of the body develops into a sexually ripe worm called an epitoke, which is swollen with gametes (Fig 14-20). One example is the palolo worm, which lives in burrows among the coral reefs of the South Seas. During the reproductive cycle, the posterior somites become swollen with gametes. During the swarming period, which occurs at the beginning of the last quarter of the October-November moon, these epitokes break off and swim to the surface. Just before sunrise, the sea is literally covered with them, and at sunrise they burst, freeing the eggs and sperm for fertilization. The anterior portions of the worms regenerate new posterior sections. A related form swarms in the Atlantic in the third quarter of the June-July moon. Swarming is of great adaptive value because the synchronous maturation of all the epitokes ensures the maximum number of fertilized eggs. However, it is very hazardous; many types of predators have a feast. In the meantime, the atoke remains safe in its burrow to produce another epitoke at the next cycle!

Sense organs are more highly developed in polychaetes than in oligochaetes and include eyes, nuchal organs, and statocysts. Eyes, when present, may range from simple eyespots to well-developed organs. They are most conspicuous in errant worms. Usually the eyes are retinal cups, with rodlike photoreceptor cells lining the cup wall and directed toward the lumen of the cup. The highest degree of development is found in the family Alciopidae, which has large, image-resolving eyes similar in structure to those of some cephalopod molluscs (Fig. 13-35), with cornea, lens, retina, and retinal pigment. The alciopid eye also has accessory retinas, a characteristic shared by deep-sea fishes and some deep-sea cephalopods. The accessory retinas are sensitive to different wavelengths of light, and their function may be to serve as a depth gauge for these pelagic animals because different wavelengths penetrate to different depths. Recent studies with electroencephalograms show that these eyes are especially well adapted to utilizing the dim light of the deep sea. Nuchal organs are ciliated sensory pits or slits that appear to be chemoreceptive, an important factor in food gathering. Some burrowing and tube-building polychaetes have statocysts that function in body orientation.

Reproductive systems are simple. Gonads appear as temporary swellings of the peritoneum and shed their gametes into the coelom. They are carried outside through gonoducts, through nephridia, or by rupture of the body wall. Fertilization is external, and the early larva is a trochophore.

Some interesting polychaetes
Clam worms—Nereis

The clam worms, or sand worms as they are sometimes called, are errant polychaetes that live in mucus-lined burrows in or near low tide (Fig. 14-19). Sometimes they are found in temporary hiding places such as under stones, where they stay, bodies covered and heads protruding. They are most active at night, when they wiggle out of their hiding places and swim about or crawl over the sand in search of food.

The body, containing about 200 somites, may grow to 30 or 40 cm in length. The head is made up of a prostomium and a peristomium. The prostomium bears

Figure 14-19

Nereis diversicolor, head and anterior segments. Note the well-defined segments, the lobed parapodia, and the prostomium with tentacles.
Photograph by D.P. Wilson.

a pair of stubby **palps,** sensitive to touch and taste; a pair of short sensory **tentacles;** and two pairs of small dorsal **eyes** that are light sensitive. The peristomium bears the ventral mouth, a pair of chitinous **jaws,** and four pairs of sensory tentacles (Fig. 14-14, *A*).

Each parapodium is formed of two lobes: a dorsal **notopodium** and a ventral **neuropodium** (Fig. 14-14, *C*). Each lobe is supported by one or more chitinous spines (acicula). The parapodia bear setae and are abundantly supplied with blood vessels. The parapodia are used for both creeping and swimming and are manipulated by oblique muscles that run from the midventral line to the parapodia in each somite. The worm swims by lateral undulatory wriggling of the body—unlike the peristaltic movement of the earthworms. It can dart through the water with considerable speed. These undulatory movements can also be used to suck water into or pump it out of the burrow. The worm will usually adapt some kind of burrow if it can find one. When a worm is placed near a glass tube, it will wriggle in without hesitation.

The clam worm feeds on small animals, other worms, larval forms, and the like. It seizes them with its chitinous jaws, which are protruded through the mouth when the pharynx is everted. When the pharynx is withdrawn, the food is swallowed. Movement of the food through the alimentary canal is by peristalsis.

Parchment worms—Chaetopterus

Chaetopterus lives in a U-shaped parchment tube buried, except for the tapered ends, in sand or mud along the shore (Fig. 14-17). The worm attaches to the side of the tube by ventral suckers. Fans (modified parapodia) on segments 14 to 16 pump water through the tube by rhythmical movements. A pair of enlarged parapodia in the twelfth segment secretes a long mucous bag that reaches back to a small food cup just in front of the fans. All the water passing through the tube is filtered through this mucous bag, the end of which is rolled up into a ball by cilia in the cup. When the ball is about the size of a BB shot, the fans stop beating and the ball of food and mucus is rolled forward by ciliary action to the mouth and is swallowed.

___ Significance of Metamerism

No truly satisfactory explanation has yet been given for the origins of metamerism and the coelom, although the subject has stimulated much speculation and debate over the years. All of the classical explanations of the origin of metamerism and the coelom have had important arguments leveled against them, and more than one may be correct, or none, as suggested by R.B. Clark (1964). The coelom and metamerism may have evolved independently in more than one group of animals, as, for example, in the chordates and in the protostome line. Clark stressed the functional and evolutionary significance of these features to the earliest animals that possessed them. He argued forcefully that the adaptive value of the coelom in the protostomes, at least, was as a **hydrostatic skeleton** in a burrowing animal. Thus, contraction of muscles in one part of the animal could act antagonistically on muscles in another part by transmission of the force of contraction through the enclosed constant volume of fluid in the coelom.

Although burrowing in the substrate may have selected for the coelom, certain other advantages accrued to its possessors. The coelomic fluid would have acted as a circulatory fluid for nutrients and wastes, making large numbers of

Figure 14-20

Eunice viridis, the Samoan palolo worm. The posterior segments make up the epitokal region, consisting of segments packed with gametes. Each segment has an eyespot on the ventral side. Once a year the worms swarm, and the epitokes detach, rise to the surface, and discharge their ripe gametes, leaving the water milky. By the next breeding season, the epitokes are regenerated.

After W.M. Woodworth, 1907; from Fauvel, P. 1959. Annélides polychétes. Reproduction. In P.P. Grassé (ed.). Traite de Zoologie, vol. 5, part 1. Paris, Masson et Cie.

Atoke

Epitoke

flame cells distributed throughout the tissues unnecessary. Gametes could be stored in the spacious coelom for release simultaneously with other individuals in the population, thus enhancing chances of fertilization, and this would have selected for greater nervous and endocrine control. Finally, separation of the coelom into a series of compartments by septa, resulting in metamerism, would have greatly increased the capacity for powerful burrowing. The force exerted by muscle contraction on the fluid in one coelomic compartment would not be transmitted to the fluid in other compartments, making possible independent and separate movements by the separate metameres. Independent movements of metameres in different parts of the body would have placed selective value on a more sophisticated nervous system for control of the movements and led to elaboration of the central nervous system.

Phylogeny and Adaptive Radiation
Phylogeny

There are so many similarities in the early development of the molluscs, annelids, and primitive arthropods that there seems little doubt about their close relationship. It is thought that the common ancestor of the three phyla was some type of flatworm. Many marine annelids and molluscs have an early embryogenesis typical of protostomes, in common with some marine flatworms, suggesting a real, if remote, relationship. Annelids share with the arthropods an outer secreted cuticle and have a similar nervous system, and the lateral appendages (parapodia) of many marine annelids are similar to the appendages of certain primitive arthropods. The most important resemblance, however, probably lies in the segmented plan of the annelid and the arthropod body structure.

Which of the annelids came first? This has been the subject of a long and continuing debate. It was long assumed that the archiannelids, a small group of minute polychaetes, were the most primitive of the annelids. This view is no longer widely held. Rather than primitive, they appear to be polychaetes that have become secondarily simplified as a result of their small size and their adaptation to a psammolittoral life—that is, living in the interstitial spaces between the grains of sand or on the mud bottom. R.B. Clark (1969) suggests that the origin of annelids needs to be viewed in terms of the origin of the metameric arrangement of worms. He emphasizes that the only consistent correlation between the structure and function of a segmented coelom is a mechanical one. The division of the coelom, a hydrostatic organ, into units is a mechanical device limiting the transfer of hydrostatic pressure from one part of the coelom to another. There is an advantage in such a locomotor device to macroscopic animals, but not to microscopic ones, so there is little reason to assume it evolved first in the microscopic archiannelids. Most hypotheses of annelid origin have assumed that the polychaetes were the earliest segmented worms and that metamerism arose in connection with the development of lateral appendages (parapodia). However, the oligochaete body is adapted to vagrant burrowing in the substratum with a peristaltic movement that is highly benefited by a metameric coelom. Polychaetes, on the other hand, are adapted to swimming and crawling in a medium too fluid for effective peristaltic locomotion. Although the parapodia do not prevent such locomotion, they do little to further it, and it seems unlikely that they evolved as an adaptation for swimming. Although the polychaetes are more primitive in some respects, such as in their reproductive system, some authorities have argued that the ancestral annelids were more similar to the oligochaetes in overall body plan and that these gave rise to the polychaetes and leeches. Others maintain that the oligochaetes developed from polychaete stock. The leeches are closely related to the oligochaetes and probably evolved from them in connection with a swimming existence and the abandonment of a burrowing mode of life.

Adaptive radiation

Annelids are an ancient group that has undergone extensive adaptive radiation. The basic body structure, particularly of the polychaetes, lends itself to almost endless modification. As marine worms, polychaetes have a wide range of habitats in an environment that is not physically or physiologically demanding. Unlike the earthworms, whose environment imposes strict physical and physiological selective pressure, the polychaetes have been free to experiment and thus have achieved a wide range of adaptive features.

A basic adaptive feature in the evolution of annelids is their septal arrangement, resulting in fluid-filled coelomic compartments. Fluid pressure in these compartments is used as a hydrostatic skeleton in precise movements such as burrowing and swimming. Powerful circular and longitudinal muscles have been adapted for flexing, shortening, and lengthening the body.

There is a wide variation in feeding adaptations, from the sucking pharynx of the oligochaetes and the chitinous jaws of carnivorous polychaetes to the specialized tentacles and cirri of the ciliary feeders.

In polychaetes the parapodia have been adapted in many ways and for many functions, chiefly locomotion and respiration.

In leeches many adaptations, such as suckers, cutting jaws, pumping pharynx, distensible gut, and the production of hirudin, are related to their predatory and bloodsucking habits.

_____ Summary

The phylum Annelida is a large group including the earthworms and freshwater oligochaetes, leeches, and marine polychaetes. They are metameric, having their bodies divided into a linear series of segments, each of which contains representatives of most body systems. Annelids, with the exception of leeches, bear chitinous bristles called setae. They are cosmopolitan. Many are burrowing, and there are many filter feeders and predators.

The body is comprised of many metameres. Because the coelom forms embryonically as a split in the mesoderm, it is lined with a mesodermal peritoneum, and the gut and other organs are suspended in mesenteries. The peritoneum between metameres forms septa. The fluid-filled coelomic cavities function as a hydrostatic skeleton except in the leeches.

The class Oligochaeta includes the earthworms and many freshwater forms; they have a small number of setae per segment (compared to the Polychaeta) and no parapodia. Most earthworms have four pairs of setae per segment, which function to keep the body from slipping in the burrow. The circulatory system is closed, and the dorsal blood vessel is the main pumping organ. There is a pair of nephridia in most somites, and the nephrostome of each nephridium lies in the intersegmental septum of the somite immediately preceding it. Earthworms have the typical annelid nervous system: dorsal cerebral ganglia connected to a double, ventral nerve cord with segmental ganglia, running the length of the worm. Giant axons with a high speed of conduction are present. Oligochaetes are hermaphroditic and practice cross-fertilization. The clitellum plays an important role in reproduction, including secretion of mucus to surround the worms during copulation and secretion of a cocoon to receive the eggs and sperm and in which embryonation occurs. A small, juvenile worm hatches from the cocoon.

Freshwater oligochaetes have longer setae than earthworms, and some have gills.

The leeches (class Hirudinea) are mostly freshwater, although a few are marine and a few are terrestrial. They feed mostly on fluids; many are predators, some are temporary parasites, and a few are permanent parasites. The hermaphroditic leeches reproduce in a fashion similar to oligochaetes, with cross-fertilization and cocoon formation by the clitellum.

Polychaetes are the largest class of annelids and are mostly marine. They have many setae on each somite, which are borne on paired parapodia. Parapodia show a wide variety of adaptations among polychaetes, including specialization for swimming, respiration, crawling, maintaining position in a burrow, pumping water through a burrow, and as accessory feeding organs. Errant polychaetes are mostly predaceous and have an eversible pharynx with jaws. Sedentary polychaetes rarely leave the burrows or tubes in which they live. Several styles of deposit and filter feeding are shown among the sedentary polychaetes. Polychaetes are dioecious, have a primitive reproductive system, have no clitellum, and practice external fertilization, and their larva is a trochophore.

It is probable that the coelom and metamerism evolved as a hydrostatic skeleton in adaptation for strong and sustained burrowing, but its origin had several important evolutionary implications, leading to more efficient nervous and endocrine control systems.

Embryological evidence supports a phylogenetic relationship of the annelids with the molluscs and arthropods. The question of whether the oligochaetes arose from polychaete stock or vice versa is unsettled. Leeches probably evolved from an oligochaete ancestor.

Adaptive radiation in the annelids shows exploitation of the hydrostatic skeleton, setae, parapodia, and other organs for locomotion, respiration, and feeding. Leeches have become specialized for predation and bloodsucking habits.

Selected references

Barnes, R.D. 1965. Tube-building and feeding in chaetopterid polychaetes. Biol. Bull. **129**:217-233.

Barnes, R.D. 1980. Invertebrate zoology, ed. 4. Philadelphia, Saunders College/Holt, Rinehart & Winston.

Brinkhurst, R.O., and B.G. Jamieson. 1972. Aquatic oligochaetes of the world. Toronto, Toronto University Press.

Brown, S.C. 1975. Biomechanics of water pumping by *Chaetopterus variopedatus* Renier: skeletomusculature and kinetics. Biol. Rev. **149**:136-156.

Clark, L.B., and W.N. Hess. 1940. Swarming of the Atlantic palolo worm, *Leodice fucata*. Tortugas Lab. Papers **332**:21-70. *The "clever" palolo worm lives to breed another day.*

Clark, R.B. 1964. Dynamics in metazoan evolution. The origin of the coelom and segments. Oxford, Eng., Clarendon Press. *An important treatise giving the author's hypotheses on the subject.*

Clark, R.B. 1969. Systematics and phylogeny: Annelida, Echiura, Sipuncula. In K. Florkin and B.T. Scheer (eds.). Chemical zoology, vol. 4. New York, Academic Press, Inc.

Dales, R.P. 1967. Annelids, ed. 2. London, The Hutchinson Publishing Group, Ltd. *A concise account of the annelids.*

Darwin, C.R. 1881. The formation of vegetable mould through the action of worms. *A classic account of the way in which earthworms improve and transform the surface of the soil.*

Edmondson, W.T. (ed.). 1959. Freshwater biology, ed. 2. New York, John Wiley & Sons, Inc. *Contains a guide to identification of freshwater annelids, with keys.*

Fauchald, K. 1977. The polychaete worms: definitions and keys to the orders, families, and genera. Natur. Hist. Mus. Los Angeles Co., Sci. Ser. **28**:1-190.

Gosner, K.L. 1971. Guide to identification of marine and estuarine invertebrates: Cape Hatteras to the Bay of Fundy. New York, Interscience.

Hartman, O., 1968. Atlas of the errantiate polychaetous annelids from California. Los Angeles, University of Southern California, Allan Hancock Foundation. *Extensive keys for identification.*

Light, S.F., R.I. Smith, F.A. Pitelka, D.P. Abbott, and F.M. Weesner. 1967. Intertidal invertebrates of the central California coast. Berkeley, University of California Press.

Mangum, C. 1970. Respiratory physiology in annelids. Am. Sci. **58**(6):641-647.

Mann, K.H. 1962. Leeches *(Hirudinea)*: their structure, physiology, ecology, and embryology. New York, Pergamon Press, Inc.

Mulloney, B. 1970. Structure of the giant fibers of earthworms. Science **168**:994-996.

Pennak, R.W. 1978. Freshwater invertebrates of the United States. ed. 2. New York, John Wiley & Sons, Inc. *A brief account with keys to families and genera of freshwater annelids.*

Pettibone, M.H. 1982. Annelida. In S.P. Parker (ed.). Synopsis and classification of living organisms, vol. 2. New York, McGraw-Hill Book Co.

Russell-Hunter, W.D. 1979. A life of invertebrates. New York, Macmillan, Inc.

Sawyer, R.T. 1972. North American freshwater leeches, exclusive of the Piscicolidae, with a key to all species. Ill. Biol. Monogr. No. 46. *Technical treatment of these parasitic leeches.*

Wald, G., and S. Rayport. 1977. Vision in annelid worms. Science **196**:1434-1439.

Selected *Scientific American* articles

Nicholls, J.C., and D. Van Essen. 1974. The nervous system of the leech. 230:38-48 (Jan.).

Wells, P. 1959. Worm autobiographies. 200:132-141 (June).

CHAPTER 15

THE ARTHROPODS

Phylum Arthropoda
Subphylum Trilobita
Subphylum Chelicerata

Galápagos shore crab *Grapsus grapsus* scurries across the rocks.

Photograph by C.P. Hickman, Jr.

Position in Animal Kingdom

1. Arthropods belong to the **protostome** branch, or schizocoelous coelomates, of the animal kingdom, and in primitive forms they have spiral cleavage and mosaic development.
2. Arthropods have the characteristic structure of higher forms: bilateral symmetry, three germ layers, coelomic cavity, and organ systems.
3. They share with the annelids the property of conspicuous segmentation, but in their somites they have greater variety and more grouping for specialized purposes, and to the somites have been added the jointed appendages, with pronounced division of labor, resulting in greater variety of action.

Biological Contributions

1. **Cephalization** makes additional advancements, with centralization of fused ganglia and sensory organs in the head.
2. The **somites** have gone beyond the sameness of the annelid type and are now **specialized** for a variety of purposes, forming functional groups of somites (**tagmosis**).
3. The presence of paired **jointed** appendages diversified for numerous uses produces greater adaptability.
4. Locomotion is by extrinsic limb muscles, in contrast to the body musculature of annelids. **Striated muscles** are emphasized, thus ensuring rapidity of movement.
5. Although **chitin** is found in a few other forms below arthropods, its use is better developed in the arthropods. The **cuticular exoskeleton**, containing chitin, is a great advance over that of the annelids, making possible a wide range of adaptations.
6. The gills, and especially the **tracheae**, represent a breathing mechanism more efficient than that of most invertebrates.
7. The alimentary canal shows greater specialization by having chitinous teeth, compartments, and gastric ossicles.
8. Behavior patterns have advanced far beyond those of most invertebrates, with a higher development of primitive intelligence and **social** organization.
9. **Metamorphosis** is common in development.
10. Many arthropods have well-developed protective coloration and protective resemblances.

PHYLUM ARTHROPODA

Phylum Arthropoda (ar-throp′o-da) (Gr., *arthron*, joint, + *pous, podos,* foot) is the most extensive phylum in the animal kingdom, comprised of more than three fourths of all known species. Approximately 900,000 species of arthropods have been recorded, and probably as many more remain to be classified. Arthropods include the spiders, scorpions, ticks, mites, crustaceans, millipedes, centipedes, insects, and some others. In addition, there is a rich fossil record extending to the very late Precambrian period.

Arthropods are eucoelomate protostomes with well-developed organ systems, and they share with the annelids the property of conspicuous segmentation.

Arthropods have an exoskeleton containing chitin, and their primitive pattern is that of a linear series of similar somites, each with a pair of jointed appendages. However, the pattern of somites and appendages varies greatly in the phylum. There is a tendency for the somites to be combined or fused into functional groups, called **tagmata** (sing., **tagma**), for specialized purposes; the appendages are frequently differentiated and specialized for pronounced division of labor.

Few arthropods exceed 60 cm in length, and most are far below this size. The largest is the Japanese crab *Macrocheira* (Gr., *makros,* large + *cheir,* hand), which has approximately a 3.7 m span; the smallest is the parasitic mite *Demodex* (Gr., *dēmos,* fat, + *dex,* a wood worm), which is less than 0.1 mm long.

Arthropods are usually active, energetic animals. Judging by their great diversity and their wide ecological distribution, as well as by the vast number of species, their success is surpassed by no other group of animals.

Although arthropods compete with humans for food and spread serious diseases, they are essential in pollination of many food plants, and they also serve as food, yield useful drugs and dyes, and produce useful products such as silk, honey, and beeswax.

The arthropods are more widely and more densely distributed throughout all regions of the earth than are members of any other phylum. They are found in all types of environment from low ocean depths to very high altitudes, and from the tropics far into both north and south polar regions. Different species are adapted for life in the air; on land; in fresh, brackish, and marine waters; and in or on the bodies of plants and other animals. Some species live in places where no other form could survive.

Although all types—carnivorous, omnivorous, and symbiotic—occur in this vast group, the majority are herbivorous. Most aquatic arthropods depend on algae for their nourishment, and the majority of land forms live chiefly on plants. In diversity of ecological distribution, the arthropods have no rivals.

CHARACTERISTICS

1. Bilateral symmetry; **metameric body** divided into **tagmata** consisting of head and trunk; head, thorax, and abdomen; or cephalothorax and abdomen
2. **Jointed appendages;** primitively, one pair to each somite, but number often reduced; appendages often modified for specialized functions
3. **Exoskeleton of cuticle** containing protein, lipid, chitin, and often calcium carbonate secreted by underlying epidermis and shed (molted) at intervals
4. **Complex muscular system,** with exoskeleton for attachment, **striated muscles** for rapid actions, smooth muscles for visceral organs; no cilia
5. **Reduced coelom** in adult; most of body cavity consisting of hemocoel (sinuses, or spaces, in the tissues) filled with blood
6. Complete digestive system; mouthparts modified from appendages and adapted for different methods of feeding
7. Open circulatory system, with dorsal **contractile heart,** arteries, and hemocoel (blood sinuses)
8. Respiration by **body surface, gills, tracheae** (air tubes), or **book lungs**
9. Paired excretory glands called coxal, antennal, or maxillary glands present in some, homologous to metameric nephridial system of annelids; some with other excretory organs, called malpighian tubules
10. Nervous system of annelid plan, with dorsal brain connected by a ring around the gullet to a double nerve chain of ventral ganglia; fusion of ganglia in some species; well-developed sensory organs
11. Sexes usually separate, with paired reproductive organs and ducts; usually internal fertilization; oviparous or ovoviviparous; often with **metamorphosis;** parthenogenesis in a few forms

CLASSIFICATION

Subphylum Trilobita (tri′lo-bi′ta) (Gr., *tri,* three, + *lobos,* lobe)—**trilobites.** All extinct forms; Cambrian to Carboniferous; body divided by two longitudinal furrows into three lobes; distinct head, thorax, and abdomen, biramous (two-branched) appendages.

Subphylum Chelicerata (ke-lis′-e-ra′ta) (Gr., *chēlē,* claw, + *keras,* horn, + *ata,* group suffix)—**eurypterids, horseshoe crabs, spiders, ticks.** First pair of appendages modified to form chelicerae; pair of pedipalps and four pairs of legs; no antennae, no mandibles; cephalothorax and abdomen usually unsegmented.

Class Merostomata (mer′o-sto′ma-ta) (Gr., *mēros*, thigh, + *stoma*, mouth, + *ata*, group suffix)—aquatic chelicerates. Cephalothorax and abdomen; compound lateral eyes; appendages with gills; sharp telson.

Subclass Eurypterida (yu-rip-ter′i-da) (Gr., *eurys*, broad, + *pteryx*, wing or fin, + *ida*, pl. suffix)—giant water scorpions. Extinct; cephalothorax covered by dorsal carapace; abdomen with 12 segments and postanal telson; pair of simple ocelli and pair of compound eyes. Example: *Eurypterus.*

Subclass Xiphosurida (zif-o-su′ri-da) (Gr., *xiphos*, sword, + *oura*, tail)—horseshoe crabs. Cephalothorax convex and horseshoe shaped; abdomen unsegmented and terminated by long spine; three-jointed chelicerae and six-jointed walking legs; pair of simple eyes and pair of compound eyes; book gills. Example: *Limulus.*

Class Pycnogonida (pik′no-gon′i-da) (Gr., *pyknos*, compact, + *gony*, knee, angle)—sea spiders. Small (3 to 4 mm), but some reach 500 mm; body chiefly cephalothorax; tiny abdomen; usually four pairs of long walking legs (some with five or six pairs); mouth on long proboscis; four simple eyes; no respiratory or excretory system. Example: *Pycnogonum.*

Class Arachnida (ar-ack′ni-da) (Gr., *arachnē*, spider)—scorpions, spiders, mites, ticks, harvestmen. Four pairs of legs; segmented or unsegmented abdomen with or without appendages and generally distinct from cephalothorax; respiration by gills, tracheae, or book lungs; excretion by malpighian tubules or coxal glands; dorsal bilobed brain connected to ventral ganglionic mass with nerves; simple eyes; sexes separate; chiefly oviparous; no true metamorphosis. Examples: *Argiope, Centruroides.*

Subphylum Mandibulata* (man-dib′u-la′ta) (L., *mandibula*, mandible, + *ata*, group suffix). Head appendages consisting of one or two pairs of antennae, one pair of mandibles, and one or two pairs of maxillae.

Class Crustacea (crus-ta′she-a) (L., *crusta*, shell, + *acea*, group suffix)—crustaceans. Mostly aquatic, with gills; hard exoskeleton; cephalothorax usually with dorsal carapace; biramous appendages, modified for various functions; two pairs of antennae; sexes usually separate; development primitively with nauplius stage (see résumé of subclasses, p. 395).

Class Diplopoda (di-plop′o-da) (Gr., *diploos*, double, + *pous, podos*, foot)—millipedes. Subcylindrical body; head with short antennae and simple eyes; body with variable number of somites; short legs, usually two pairs of legs to a somite; separate sexes; oviparous. Examples: *Julus, Spirobolus.*

Class Chilopoda (ki-lop′-o-da) (Gr., *cheilos*, lip, + *pous, podos*, foot)—centipedes. Dorsoventrally flattened body; variable number of somites, each with one pair of legs; one pair of long antennae; separate sexes; oviparous. Examples: *Cermatia, Lithobius, Geophilus.*

Class Pauropoda (pau-rop′o-da) (Gr., *pauros*, small + *pous, podos*, foot)—pauropods. Minute (1 to 1.5 mm); cylindrical body consisting of double segments and bearing nine or 10 pairs of legs; no eyes. Example: *Pauropus.*

Class Symphyla (sym′fy-la) (Gr., *syn*, together, + *phylon*, tribe)—garden centipedes. Slender (1 to 8 mm) with long, filiform antennae; body consisting of 15 to 22 segments with 10 to 12 pairs of legs; no eyes. Example: *Scutigerella.*

Class Insecta (in-sek′ta) (L., *insectus*, cut into)—insects. Body with distinct head, thorax, and abdomen; pair of antennae; mouthparts modified for different food habits; head of six fused somites; thorax of three somites; abdomen with variable number, usually 11 somites; thorax with two pairs of wings (sometimes one pair or none) and three pairs of jointed legs; separate sexes; usually oviparous; gradual or abrupt metamorphosis. (A brief description of insect orders is given on pp. 432 to 435.)

---

*The subphylum Mandibulata has traditionally included arthropods possessing mandibles and antennae: crustaceans, myriapods, and insects. However, some authorities now believe that crustacean mandibles and insect-myriapod mandibles have resulted from convergent evolution rather than a natural close relationship. They consider the Crustacea and Uniramia (insects and myriapods) to be subphyla. For the present we retain the traditional arrangement.

COMPARISON OF ARTHROPODA WITH ANNELIDA

Similarities between Arthropoda and Annelida are as follows:

1. External segmentation
2. Segmental arrangement of muscles
3. Metamerically arranged nervous system with dorsal cerebral ganglia

Arthropods differ from annelids in having the following:

1. Fixed number of segments
2. Usually a lack of intersegmental septa
3. Tagmatization
4. Coelomic cavity reduced; main body cavity a hemocoel
5. Open (lacunar) circulatory system
6. Special mechanisms (gills, tracheae, book lungs) for respiration
7. Exoskeleton containing chitin
8. Jointed appendages
9. Compound eyes (also present in a few annelids) and other well-developed sense organs
10. Absence of cilia
11. Metamorphosis in many cases

Why Have Arthropods Been So Successful?

The success of the arthropods is attested to by their diversity, number of species, wide distribution, variety of habitats and feeding habits, and power of adaptation to changing conditions. Some of the structural and physiological patterns that have been helpful to them are briefly summarized in the following discussion.

1. A versatile exoskeleton. The arthropods possess an exoskeleton that is highly protective without sacrificing mobility. This skeleton is the **cuticle,** an outer covering secreted by the underlying epidermis. The cuticle is made up of an inner and usually thicker **endocuticle** and an outer, relatively thin **epicuticle.** The endocuticle contains **chitin** bound with protein. Chitin is a tough, resistant, nitrogenous polysaccharide that is insoluble in water, alkalis, and weak acids. Thus the endocuticle not only is flexible and lightweight but also affords protection, particularly against dehydration. In some crustaceans the chitin may make up as much as 60% to 80% of the endocuticle, but in insects it is probably not more than 40%. In most crustaceans the endocuticle in some areas is also impregnated with **calcium salts,** which reduce its flexibility. In the hard shells of lobsters and crabs, for instance, this calcification is extreme. The outer epicuticle is composed of protein and lipid. The protein is stabilized and hardened by tanning, adding further protection. Both the endocuticle and epicuticle are laminated, that is, composed of several layers each (Fig. 28-1, p. 671).

The cuticle may be soft and permeable or may form a veritable coat of armor. Between body segments and between the segments of appendages it is thin and flexible, creating movable joints and permitting free movements. In crustaceans and insects the cuticle forms ingrowths (apodemes) that serve for muscle attachment. It may also line the foregut and hindgut, line and support the trachea, and be adapted for biting mouthparts, sensory organs, copulatory organs, and ornamental purposes. It is indeed a versatile material.

The nonexpansible cuticular exoskeleton does, however, impose important conditions on growth. To grow, an arthropod must shed its outer covering at intervals and grow a larger one—a process called **ecdysis,** or **molting.** Arthropods molt four to seven times before reaching adulthood, and some continue to molt after that. An exoskeleton is also relatively heavy and becomes proportionately heavier with increasing size. This tends to limit the ultimate body size.

2. Segmentation and appendages for more efficient locomotion. Typically each somite is provided with a pair of jointed appendages, but this arrangement is often modified, with both segments and appendages specialized for adaptive functions. The limb segments are essentially hollow levers that are moved by internal muscles, most of which are striated for rapid action. The jointed appendages are equipped with sensory hairs and have been modified and adapted for sensory functions, food handling, swift and efficient walking legs, and swimming appendages.

3. Air piped directly to cells. Most land arthropods have the highly efficient tracheal system of air tubes, which delivers oxygen directly to the tissues and cells and makes a high metabolic rate possible. Aquatic arthropods breathe mainly by some form of gill that is quite efficient.

4. Highly developed sensory organs. Sensory organs are found in great variety, from the compound (mosaic) eye to those simpler senses that have to do with touch, smell, hearing, balancing, chemical reception, and so on. Arthropods are keenly alert to what goes on in their environment.

5. Complex behavior patterns. Arthropods exceed most other invertebrates in the complexity and organization of their activities. Innate (unlearned) behavior unquestionably controls much of what they do, but learning also plays an important part in the lives of many of them.

6. Reduced competition through metamorphosis. Many arthropods pass through metamorphic changes, including a larval form quite different from the adult in structure. The larval form is often adapted for eating a different kind of food from that of the adult, resulting in less competition within a species.

Subphylum Trilobita

The trilobites probably had their beginnings before the Cambrian period, in which they flourished. They have been extinct some 200 million years, but were abundant during the Cambrian and Ordovician periods. Their name refers to the tri-lobed shape of the body, caused by a pair of longitudinal grooves. They were bottom dwellers, probably scavengers (Fig. 15-1, *A*). Most of them could roll up like pill bugs, and they ranged from 2 to 67 cm in length.

The exoskeleton contained chitin, strengthened in some areas by calcium carbonate. The body was comprised of three tagmata: head, thorax, and pygidium. The head was one piece but showed signs of former segmentation; the thorax had a variable number of somites; and the somites of the pygidium, at the posterior end, were fused into a plate. The head bore a pair of antennae, compound eyes, mouth, and four pairs of jointed appendages. Each body somite except the last also bore a pair of biramous (two-branched) appendages. One of the branches had a fringe of filaments that may have served as gills.

Subphylum Chelicerata

The chelicerate arthropods are an ancient group that includes the eurypterids (extinct), horseshoe crabs, spiders, ticks and mites, scorpions, and sea spiders. They are characterized by having six pairs of appendages that include a pair of chelicerae, a pair of pedipalps, and four pairs of walking legs. They have no mandibles and no antennae. Most chelicerates suck up liquid food from their prey.

A

B

Figure 15-1

Fossils of early arthropods. **A,** Trilobite, dorsal view; plaster-cast impression. These animals were abundant in mid-Cambrian period. **B,** Eurypterid fossil; eurypterids flourished in Europe and North America from Ordovician to Permian periods.

Photographs by F.M. Hickman.

Figure 15-2

Mating of horseshoe crabs, *Limulus*. At high tide the female digs a depression in the sand for her eggs, which the male fertilizes externally before the hole fills up with sand. The male *(right)* is following the female *(left)* as she selects the spot for her eggs. Sometimes she is followed by several males.

Photograph by L.L. Rue, III.

Class Merostomata

Class Merostomata is represented by the eurypterids, all now extinct, and the xiphosurids, or horseshoe crabs, an ancient group sometimes referred to as "living fossils."

Eurypterids—subclass Eurypterida

The eurypterids, or giant water scorpions (Fig. 15-1, *B*) were the largest of all fossil arthropods, some reaching a length of 3 m. Their fossils are found in rocks from the Ordovician to the Permian periods. They had many resemblances to the marine horseshoe crabs (Figs. 15-2 and 15-3) and also to the scorpions, their land counterparts. The head had six fused segments and bore both simple and compound eyes and six pairs of appendages. The abdomen had 12 segments and a spikelike tail.

Ideas regarding their early habitats differ. Some believe the eurypterids evolved mainly in fresh water; others hold that they arose in brackish lagoons.

Horseshoe crabs—subclass Xiphosurida

The xiphosurids are an ancient marine group that dates from the Cambrian period. Our common horseshoe crab *Limulus* (L., *limus*, sidelong, askew) (Fig. 15-2) goes back practically unchanged to the Triassic period. Only three genera (five species) survive today: *Limulus*, which lives in shallow water along the North American Atlantic coast; *Carcinoscorpius* (Gr., *karkinos*, a crab, + *skorpiōn*, scorpion), along the southern shore of Japan; and *Tachypleus*, in the East Indies and along the coast of southern Asia. They usually live in shallow water.

Xiphosurids have an unsegmented, horseshoe-shaped carapace (hard dorsal shield) and a broad abdomen, which has a long telson, or tailpiece. The cephalothorax bears five pairs of walking legs and a pair of chelicerae, whereas the abdomen has six pairs of broad, thin appendages that are fused in the median line (Fig. 15-3). On some of the abdominal appendages, book gills (flat, leaflike gills) are exposed. There are two compound and two simple eyes on the carapace. The horseshoe crab swims by means of its abdominal plates and can walk with its walking legs. It feeds at night on worms and small molluscs, which it seizes with its chelicerae.

During the mating season the horseshoe crabs come to shore at high tide to mate (Fig. 15-2). The female burrows into the sand where she lays her eggs, with one or more smaller males following her closely to add their sperm to the nest before she covers the eggs with sand. The eggs are warmed by the sun and protected from the waves until the young larvae hatch and return to the sea by another high tide. The larvae are segmented and are often called "trilobite larvae" because they resemble the trilobites, which are often considered to have been their ancestors.

Figure 15-3

Ventral view of horseshoe crab *Limulus* (class Merostomata). They grow to 0.5 m in length.

Photograph by F.M. Hickman.

Class Pycnogonida—sea spiders *don't study*

Some sea spiders are only a few millimeters long, but others are much larger. They have small, thin bodies and usually four pairs of long, thin walking legs. In addition, they have a feature unique among arthropods: somites are reduplicated in some groups, so that they possess five or six pairs of legs instead of the "normal" four pairs. The males of many species bear a subsidiary pair of legs (**ovigers**) (Fig. 15-4) on which they carry the developing eggs. The ovigers are often absent in females, and they are absent in males of at least one species. Many species also are equipped with chelicerae and palps.

The mouth is located at the tip of a long suctorial proboscis used to suck juices from cnidarians and soft-bodied animals. Most pycnogonids have four simple eyes. The circulatory system is limited to a simple dorsal heart, and excretory and respiratory systems are absent. The long, thin body and legs provide a large surface, in proportion to volume, that is evidently sufficient for diffusion of gases and wastes. Because of the small size of the body, the digestive system sends branches into the legs, and most of the gonads are also found there.

Sea spiders are found in all oceans, but they are most abundant in polar waters. *Pycnogonum* (Fig. 15-5) is a common intertidal genus found on both the Atlantic and Pacific coasts of the United States; it has relatively short, heavy legs. *Nymphon* (Fig. 15-4) is the largest genus of pycnogonids, with over 200 species, and it occurs from subtidal depths to 6800 m in all seas except the Black and Baltic seas.

Some authorities believe that the pycnogonids are more closely related to the crustaceans than to other arthropods (their larva is rather similar in appearance to the nauplius larva of crustaceans); others have placed them closer to the arachnids.

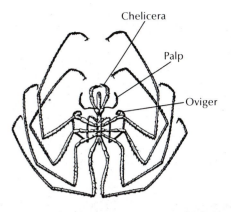

Figure 15-4

Pycnogonid, *Nymphon* sp. In this genus all the anterior appendages (chelicerae, palps, and ovigers) are present in both sexes, although ovigers are often not present in females of other genera.
From Hedgpeth, J.W. 1982. In S.P. Parker (ed.). Synopsis and classification of living organisms. New York, McGraw Hill Book Co.

Class Arachnida

The arachnids (Gr., *arachnē*, spider) are not as closely knit a group as the insects. In addition to spiders, the group includes scorpions, pseudoscorpions, whip scorpions, ticks, mites, daddy longlegs (harvestmen), and others. There are many differences among these with respect to form and appendages. They are mostly free living and are far more common in warm, dry regions than elsewhere.

The arachnid tagmata are a cephalothorax and abdomen, and the cephalothorax usually bears a pair of chelicerae, a pair of pedipalps, and four pairs of walking legs (Fig. 15-6). Antennae and mandibles are lacking. Most arachnids are predaceous and may be provided with claws, fangs, poison glands, or stingers. They usually have sucking mouthparts or a strong sucking pharynx with which they suck the fluids and soft tissues from the bodies of their prey. Among their interesting adaptations are the spinning glands of the spiders.

Arachnids have been extremely successful. More than 100,000 species have been described so far. They were the first of the arthropods to move into terrestrial habitats. Scorpions are found among Silurian fossils, and by the end of the Paleozoic period mites and spiders had appeared.

Most arachnids are harmless to humans and actually do much good by destroying injurious insects. A few, such as the black widow and brown recluse spiders, can give painful or even dangerous bites. The sting of the scorpion may be quite painful. Some ticks and mites are vectors of diseases as well as causes of

Figure 15-5

Pycnogonum, a pycnogonid with relatively short legs. Females of this genus have none of the anterior appendages, and only males have ovigers.
From Hedgpeth, J.W. 1982. In S.P. Parker (ed.). Synopsis and classification of living organisms. New York, McGraw-Hill Book Co.

Figure 15-6

Huntsman spider (family Lycosidae). They are also sometimes called wolf spiders.

Photograph by F.M. Hickman.

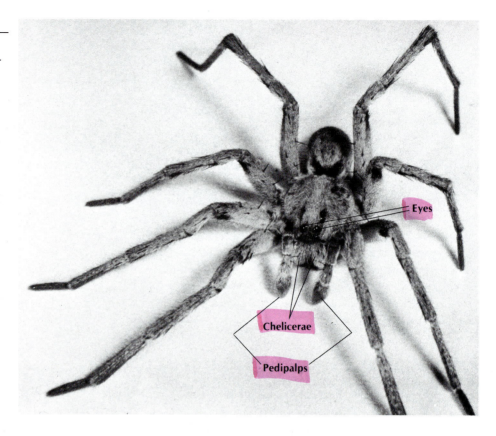

Figure 15-7

A, Crab spider, *Misumenoides aleatorius,* on a zinnia awaits its insect prey. Its coloration matches the petals among which it lies, deceiving insects that visit the flowers in search of pollen or nectar. **B,** A jumping spider, *Eris aurantius.* This species has excellent vision and stalks an insect until it is close enough to leap with unerring precision, fixing its chelicerae into its prey.

Photographs by J.H. Gerard.

annoyance and painful irritations. Certain mites damage a number of important food and ornamental plants by sucking their juices. Several smaller orders are not included in the following discussion.

Spiders—order Araneae

The spiders are a large group of 35,000 species, distributed all over the world. The spider body is compact: a **cephalothorax (prosoma)** and **abdomen (opisthosoma),** both unsegmented and joined by a slender pedicel.

The anterior appendages are a pair of **chelicerae** (Fig. 15-6), which have terminal **fangs** provided with ducts from poison glands, and a pair of **pedipalps**

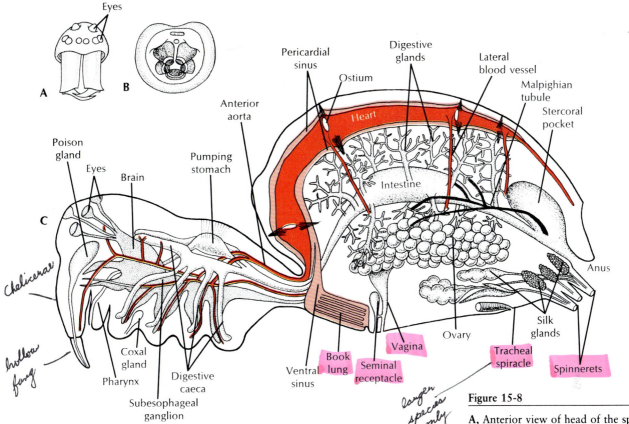

Figure 15-8

A, Anterior view of head of the spider, showing eyes and chelicerae with fangs. **B,** Ventral view of spinnerets. The type of chelicerae and the number, arrangement, and location of eyes, lung slits, tracheal spiracles, and spinnerets are all identifying characteristics used in classifying spiders. **C,** Internal structure.

having basal parts with which they chew (Fig. 15-6). Four pairs of **walking legs** terminate in claws.

All spiders are predaceous, feeding largely on insects (Fig. 15-7). They effectively dispatch their prey with their fangs and poison. Some spiders chase their prey, others ambush them, and many trap them in a net of silk. After the spider seizes its prey with its chelicerae and injects venom, it liquefies the tissues with a digestive fluid and sucks up the resulting broth into the stomach. Spiders with teeth at the bases of the chelicerae crush or chew up the prey, aiding digestion by enzymes from the mouth.

Spiders breathe by means of book lungs or tracheae or both. Book lungs, which are unique in spiders, consist of many parallel air pockets extending into a blood-filled chamber (Fig. 15-8). Air enters the chamber by a slit in the body wall. The tracheae make up a system of air tubes that carry air directly to the tissues from openings called spiracles. The tracheae are similar to those in insects (p. 416) but are much less extensive.

Spiders and insects have a unique **excretory system of malpighian tubules** (Fig. 15-8), which work in conjunction with specialized rectal glands. Potassium and other solutes and waste materials are secreted into the tubules, which drain the fluid, or "urine," into the intestine. The rectal glands reabsorb most of the potassium and water, leaving behind such wastes as uric acid. By this cycling of water and potassium, species living in dry environments may conserve body fluids, producing a nearly dry mixture of urine and feces. Many spiders also have **coxal glands,** which are modified nephridia that open at the coxa, or base, of the first and third walking legs.

Spiders usually have eight **simple eyes,** each provided with a lens, optic rods, and a retina (Figs. 15-8, *A,* and 15-9). They are used chiefly for perception of

Figure 15-9

Wolf spider, *Lycosa aspera*. Several of its eight eyes are visible as shiny black bulbs on its head.
Photograph by J.H. Gerard.

Figure 15-10

Grasshopper, snared and helpless in the web of a golden garden spider *(Miranda aurantia)*, is wrapped in silk while still alive. If the spider is not hungry, the prize will be saved for a later meal.
Photograph by J.H. Gerard.

Figure 15-11

Fisher spider, *Dolomedes triton,* feeds on a minnow. This handsome spider feeds mostly on aquatic and terrestrial insects but occasionally captures small fishes and tadpoles. It pulls its paralyzed victim from the water, pumps in digestive enzymes, then sucks out the predigested contents.
Photograph by J.H. Gerard.

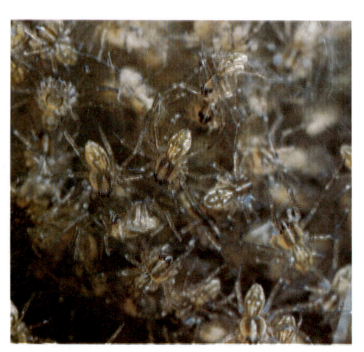

Figure 15-12

Newly hatched fisher spiders *(Dolomedes triton)*.
Photograph by J.H. Gerard.

moving objects, but some, such as those of the hunting and jumping spiders, may form images. Since a spider's vision is usually poor, its awareness of its environment depends a great deal on its hairlike **sensory setae**. Every seta on its surface, whether or not it is actually connected to receptor cells, is useful in communicating some information about the surroundings, air currents, or changing tensions in the spider's web. By sensing the vibrations of its web, the spider can judge the size and activity of its entangled prey or can receive the message tapped out by a prospective mate.

Web-spinning habits

The ability to spin silk is an important factor in the lives of spiders, as it is in some other arachnids. Two or three pairs of spinnerets containing hundreds of microscopic tubes run to special abdominal **silk glands** (Fig. 15-8, *B* and *C*). A scleroprotein secretion emitted as a liquid hardens on contact with air to form the silk thread. Spiders' silk threads are stronger than steel threads of the same diameter and are said to be second in strength only to fused quartz fibers. The threads will stretch one fifth of their length before breaking.

The spider web used for trapping insects is the use of silk familiar to most people. The kind of net varies with the species. Some are primitive and consist merely of a few strands of silk radiating out from a spider's burrow or place of retreat. Others spin the beautiful, geometrical orb webs. However, spiders use silk threads for many purposes besides web making. They use them to line their nests; form sperm webs or egg sacs; build draglines; make bridge lines, warning threads, molting threads, attachment discs, or nursery webs; or wrap up their prey securely (Fig. 15-10). Not all spiders spin webs for traps. Some, such as the wolf spiders (Figs. 15-6 and 15-9), jumping spiders (Fig. 15-7, *B*), and fisher spiders (Fig. 15-11), simply chase and catch their prey.

Reproduction

Before mating, the male spins a small web, deposits a drop of sperm on it, and then picks the sperm up and stores it in the special cavities of his pedipalps. When he mates, he inserts the pedipalps into the female genital opening to store the sperm in his mate's seminal receptacles. Before mating, there is usually a courtship ritual. The female lays her eggs in a silken net, which she may carry about or may attach to a web or plant. A cocoon may contain hundreds of eggs, which hatch in approximately 2 weeks. The young usually remain in the egg sac for a few weeks and molt once before leaving it (Fig. 15-12). Several molts occur before adulthood.

Are spiders really dangerous?

It is truly amazing that such small and helpless creatures as the spiders have generated so much unreasoning fear in the human heart. Spiders are timid creatures that, rather than being dangerous enemies to humans, are actually allies in the continuing battle with insects. The venom produced to kill the prey is usually harmless to humans. Even the most poisonous spiders bite only when threatened or when defending their eggs or young. The American tarantulas (Fig. 15-13), despite their fearsome size, are *not* dangerous. They rarely bite, and their bite is not considered serious.

There are, however, two species in the United States that can give severe or even fatal bites: the **black widow** and the **brown recluse**. The black widow, *Latrodectus mactans* (L., *latro*, robber, + *dēktes*, biter), is small and shiny black,

Figure 15-13

Tarantula, *Dugesiella lentzi*.
Photograph by J.H. Gerard.

Figure 15-14

A, Black widow spider, *Latrodectus mactans*, suspended on her web. Note the orange "hourglass" on the ventral side of her abdomen. B, Brown recluse spider, *Loxosceles reclusa*, is a small venomous spider. Note the small violin-shaped marking on its cephalothorax. The venom is hemolytic and dangerous.

Photographs by J.H. Gerard.

A

B

A

B

Figure 15-15

A, Striped scorpion, *Centruroides vittatus* (order Scorpionida). This species is not considered dangerous to humans. B, A harvestman, *Leiobunum* sp. (order Opiliones). Harvestmen run rapidly on their stiltlike legs. They are especially noticeable during the harvesting season, hence the common name.

A, Photograph by J.H. Gerard; B, photograph by C.P. Hickman, Jr.

with a bright orange or red "hourglass" on the underside of the abdomen (Fig. 15-14, *A*). The venom is neurotoxic; that is, it acts on the nervous system. Approximately four or five out of each 1000 bites reported have proved fatal.

The brown recluse, *Loxosceles reclusa* (Gr., *loxos*, crooked, + *skelos*, leg), is smaller than the black widow, is brown, and bears a violin-shaped dorsal stripe on its back (Fig. 15-14, *B*). Its venom is hemolytic rather than neurotoxic, producing death of the tissues surrounding the bite. Its bite is serious and occasionally fatal.

Scorpions—order Scorpionida

Although scorpions are more common in tropical and subtropical regions, some also occur in temperate zones. Scorpions are generally secretive, hiding in burrows or under objects by day and feeding at night. They feed largely on insects and spiders, which they seize with the pedipalps and tear up with the chelicerae.

Sand-dwelling scorpions apparently locate their prey by sensing surface waves generated by movements of insects on or in the sand. These waves are picked up by compound slit sensilla located on the basitarsal segments of the legs. The scorpion can locate a burrowing cockroach 50 cm away and reach it in three or four quick orientation movements.

The scorpion tagmata are a rather short **cephalothorax,** which bears the appendages, a pair of large median eyes, and two to five pairs of small lateral eyes; a **preabdomen** of seven segments; and a long slender **postabdomen,** or tail, of five segments, which ends in a stinging apparatus (Fig. 15-15). The chelicerae are small and three jointed; the pedipalps are large, chelate (pincerlike), and six jointed; and the four pairs of walking legs are eight jointed.

On the ventral side of the abdomen are curious comblike **pectines,** which are tactile organs used for exploring the ground and for sex recognition. The stinger on the last segment consists of a bulbous base and a curved barb that injects the venom. The venom of most species is not harmful to humans but may produce a painful swelling. However, the sting of certain species of *Androctonus* in Africa and *Centruroides* (Gr., *kenteō*, to prick, + *oura*, tail, + *oides*, form) in Mexico can be fatal unless antivenom is available.

Scorpions perform a complex mating dance, the male holding the female's chelae and stepping back and forth. He taps her genital area with his forelegs and stings her pedipalp. Finally, he deposits a spermatophore and pulls the female over it until the sperm mass is taken up in the female orifice. Scorpions are either ovoviviparous or truly viviparous; that is, the females brood their young within the female reproductive tract. After several months or a year of development, anywhere from six to 90 young are produced, depending on the species. The young, only a few millimeters long, crawl up on the mother's back until after the first molt. They mature in about a year.

Harvestmen—order Opiliones

Harvestmen, often known as "daddy longlegs," are common in the United States and other parts of the world (Fig. 15-15, B). These curious creatures are easily distinguished from spiders by the fact that their abdomen and cephalothorax are broadly joined, without the constriction of the pedicel, and their abdomen shows external segmentation. They have four pairs of usually long, spindly legs, and without apparent ill effect, they can cast off one or more of these if they are grasped by a predator (or human hand). The ends of their chelicerae are pincerlike, and they feed much more as scavengers than do arachnids.

Ticks and mites—order Acari

Members of the order Acari are without doubt the most medically and economically important group of arachnids. They far exceed the other orders in number of individuals and species. Although about 30,000 species have been described, some authorities estimate that from 500,000 to 1 million species exist. Hundreds of individuals of several species of mites may be found in a small portion of leaf mold in forests. They are found throughout the world in both terrestrial and aquatic habitats, even extending into such inhospitable regions as deserts, polar areas, and hot springs. Many acarines are parasitic during one or more stages of their life cycle.

Most mites are 1 mm or less in length. Ticks, which comprise only one suborder of the Acari, range from a few millimeters to occasionally 3 cm. A tick may become enormously distended with blood after feeding on its host.

Acarines differ from all other arachnids in having complete fusion of the cephalothorax and abdomen, with no sign of external division or segmentation (Fig. 15-16). Their mouthparts are carried on a little anterior projection, the **capitulum.** The capitulum is mainly made up of the feeding appendages surrounding the mouth. On each side of the mouth is a **chelicera,** which functions in piercing, tearing, or gripping food. The form of the chelicerae varies greatly in different families. Lateral to the chelicerae is a pair of segmental **pedipalps,** which also vary greatly in form and function related to feeding. Ventrally the bases of the pedipalps are fused to form a **hypostome,** whereas a **rostrum,** or **tectum,** extends dorsally over the mouth. Adult mites and ticks usually have four pairs of legs, although there may be only one to three in some specialized forms.

Sperm are transferred directly by most acarines, but many species transfer sperm indirectly by means of a spermatophore. A larva with six legs hatches from the egg, and this is followed by one or more eight-legged nymphal stages before the adult stage is reached.

Many species of mites are entirely free living. Beetle mites (oribatid mites) (Fig. 15-17) have a very convex dorsal surface and are abundant in humus and moss. There are some marine mites, but most aquatic species are found in fresh water. They have long, hairlike setae on their legs for swimming, and their larvae may be parasitic on aquatic invertebrates. Such abundant organisms must be important ecologically, but many acarines have more direct effects on our food

American dog tick

A

B

Figure 15-16 *chigger*

A, Wood tick, *Dermacentor variabilis* (order Acari). Larvae, nymphs, and adults are all parasitic but drop off their hosts to molt to the next stage. B, Red velvet (harvest) mite, *Trombidium* sp. As with the chigger (*Trombicula*), only the larvae of *Trombidium* are parasitic. Nymphs and adults are free living and feed on insect eggs and small soil invertebrates.

Photographs by J.H. Gerard.

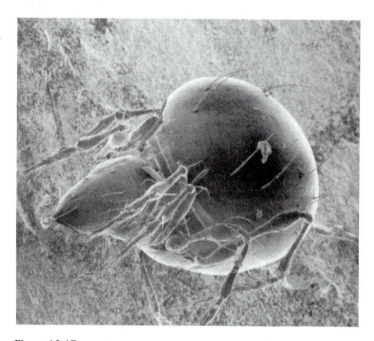

Figure 15-17

Scanning electron micrograph of *Oppia coloradensis*, a beetle mite.
Courtesy T. Woolley.

Figure 15-18

Demodex folliculorum, the human follicle mite.
From Desch, C., and W.B. Nutting. 1972. J. Parasitol. **58:**169-178.

Figure 15-19

Sarcoptes scabiei, the itch mite.
Courtesy J. Georgi.

Figure 15-20

Boophilus annulatus, a tick that carries Texas cattle fever.
Courtesy J. Georgi.

supply and health. The spider mites (family Tetranychidae) are serious agricultural pests on fruit trees, cotton, clover, and many other plants. They suck out the contents of plant cells, causing a mottled appearance to the leaves, and construct a protective web from silk glands opening near the base of the chelicerae. The larvae of the genus *Trombicula* are called chiggers or redbugs. They feed on the dermal tissues of terrestrial vertebrates, including humans, and may cause an irritating dermatitis; some species of chiggers transmit a disease called Asiatic scrub typhus. The hair follicle mite, *Demodex* (Fig. 15-18), is apparently nonpathogenic in humans; it infects most of us although we are unaware of it. Other species of *Demodex* and other genera of mites cause mange in domestic animals. The human itch mite, *Sarcoptes scabiei* (Fig. 15-19), causes intense itching as it burrows beneath the skin. Many species of ticks transmit diseases of humans and domestic animals. Species of *Dermacentor* (Fig. 15-16, *A*) and other ticks transmit Rocky Mountain spotted fever, a poorly named disease because most cases occur in the eastern United States. *Dermacentor* also transmits tularemia and the agents of several other diseases. Texas cattle fever, also called red-water fever, is caused by a protozoan parasite transmitted by the cattle tick *Boophilus annulatus* (Fig. 15-20). Many more examples could be cited.

___ Phylogeny and Adaptive Radiation
Phylogeny

The similarities between the annelids and the arthropods give strong support to the hypothesis that both phyla originated from a line of coelomate segmented protostomes, which in time diverged to form a protoannelid line with laterally located parapodia and one or more protoarthropod lines with more ventrally located parapodia. The protoannelid line gave rise eventually to the polychaetes. The protoarthropod lines apparently diverged into three branches: (1) the trilobites and the chelicerates (spiders and horseshoe crabs), (2) the crustaceans, and (3) the insects, millipedes, and centipedes. The phylum Onychophora also may have come from a part of a protoarthropod line.

Some biologists consider the arthropods to be three separate phyla, each organized at the arthropod level. This is in accord with the three-stem origin of the arthropods, since a phylum is supposed to be monophyletic.

The morphological diversity of the Acari has suggested to acarologists that this order arose from at least two separate arachnid ancestors.

Adaptive radiation

Annelids show relatively little specialization or fusion of somites and little differentiation of appendages. However, in arthropods the adaptive trend has been toward tagmatization of the body by differentiation or fusion of somites, giving rise in more advanced groups to such tagma as head and trunk; head, thorax, and abdomen; or cephalothorax (fused head and thorax) and abdomen. Primitive arthropods tend to have similar appendages, whereas the more advanced forms have appendages specialized for specific functions, or some appendages may be lost entirely.

Much of the amazing diversity in arthropods seems to have developed because of modification and specialization of their cuticular exoskeleton and their jointed appendages, resulting in a wide variety of locomotor and feeding adaptations.

W.S. Bristowe (1971) estimated that at certain seasons a Sussex field that had been undisturbed for several years had a population of 2 million spiders to the acre. He concluded that so many could not successfully compete except for the many specialized adaptations they had evolved. These include adaptations to cold and heat, wet and dry conditions, and light and darkness.

Some spiders capture large insects, some only small ones; web-builders snare mostly flying insects, whereas hunters seek those that live on the ground. Some lay eggs in the spring, others in the late summer. Some feed by day, others by night, and some have developed flavors that are distasteful to birds or to certain predatory insects. As it is with the spiders, so has it been with other arthropods; their adaptations are many and diverse and contribute in no small way to their long success.

___ Summary

The Arthropoda is the largest, most successful phylum in the world. They are metameric, coelomate protostomes with well-developed organ systems. Most show marked tagmatization. They are extremely diverse and occur in all habitats capable of supporting life. Perhaps more than any other single factor, the success of the arthropods is accounted for by adaptations made possible by their cuticular exoskeleton. Other important elements in their success are jointed appendages, tracheal respiration, efficient sensory organs, complex behavior, and metamorphosis.

The trilobites were a dominant Paleozoic subphylum, now extinct. Members of the subphylum Chelicerata have no antennae, and their main feeding appendages are chelicerae. In addition, they have a pair of pedipalps (which may be similar to the walking legs) and four pairs of walking legs. The class Merostomata includes the extinct eurypterids and the ancient, although still extant, horseshoe crabs. The class Pycnogonida contains the sea spiders, which are odd little animals with a large suctorial proboscis and vestigial abdomen. The great majority of living chelicerates are in the class Arachnida: spiders (order Araneae), scorpions (order Scorpionida), harvestmen (order Opiliones), ticks and mites (order Acari), and others.

The tagmata of spiders (cephalothorax and abdomen) show no external segmentation and are joined by a waistlike pedicel. Spiders are predaceous, and their chelicerae are provided with poison glands for paralyzing or killing their prey. They breathe by book lungs, tracheae, or both. Spiders can spin silk, which they use for a variety of purposes, including webs for trapping prey in some cases.

Scorpions are distinguished by their large, clawlike pedipalps and their clearly segmented abdomen, which bears a terminal stinging apparatus. Harvestmen have small, ovoid bodies with very long, slender legs. Their abdomen is segmented and broadly joined to the cephalothorax.

The cephalothorax and abdomen of ticks and mites are completely fused, and the mouthparts are borne on the anterior capitulum. They are most numerous of any arachnids; some are important carriers of disease, and others are serious plant pests.

This spider, *Microthena schreibersci,* from Panama is thought to resemble the thorny terminal buds of tropical trees.
Courtesy D.K. Hoffmaster.

Selected references

Barnes, R.D. 1980. Invertebrate zoology, ed. 4. Philadelphia, Saunders College/Holt, Rinehart & Winston.

Bristowe, W.S. 1971. The world of spiders. London, William Collins Sons & Co., Ltd. *The author is a supreme spider-watcher and tells of spider activities in a style that should convince any reader that spiders can be fun. Well-illustrated.*

Brownell, P.H. 1977. Compressional and surface waves in sand: used by desert scorpions to locate prey. Science **197**:477-479.

Carthy, J.D. 1965. The behavior of arthropods. Edinburgh, Oliver & Boyd. *A slim book and not too difficult.*

Carthy, J.D. 1968. The pectines of scorpions. In J.D. Carthy and G.E. Newell (eds.). Invertebrate receptors. Symposium of the Zoological Society of London, no. 23. New York, Academic Press, Inc., pp. 251-261.

Clarke, K.U. 1973. The biology of the Arthropoda. New York, American Elsevier Publishers, Inc. *Gives a basis of facts and some theoretical material suitable for first- and second-year students.*

Cloudsley-Thompson, J.L. 1968. Spiders, scorpions, centipedes and mites. New York, Pergamon Press, Inc. *Deals with seven orders, emphasizing their general behavior, feeding habits, and mating behavior.*

Foelix, R.F. 1982. Biology of spiders. Cambridge, Mass., Harvard University Press. *Attractive, comprehensive book with extensive references; of interest to both amateurs and professionals.*

Harwood, R.F., and M.T. James. 1979. Entomology in human and animal health, ed. 7. New York, Macmillan, Inc. *Authoritative and readable account of medical entomology with chapters on ticks and mites.*

Headstrom, R. 1973. Spiders of the United States. Cranbury, N.J., A.S. Barnes & Co., Inc. *Both for information and for identification of the spiders (omitting the tarantulas and trap-door spiders).*

Kaestner, A. 1968. Invertebrate zoology, vol. 2. Arthropod relatives, Chelicerata, Myriapoda. New York, Interscience.

Kaston, B.J. 1972. How to know the spiders, ed. 2. Dubuque, William C. Brown Co., Publishers. *Spiral-bound identification manual.*

King, P.E. 1973. Pycnogonids. New York, St. Martin's Press, Inc.

Krantz, G.W. 1978. A manual of acarology, ed. 2. Corvallis, Oregon State University Press.

Levi, H.W., and L.R. Levi (H.S. Zim, ed.). 1968. A guide to spiders and their kin. Golden Nature Guide. Racine, Wis., Western Publishing Co., Inc. *A useful field guide.*

Manton, S.M. 1977. The Arthropoda: habits, functional morphology, and evolution. Oxford, Eng., Clarendon Press. *A full and technical exposition of the author's hypothesis regarding the polyphyletic origins of the Arthropoda.*

McDaniel, B. 1979. How to know the ticks and mites. Dubuque, Iowa, William C. Brown Co., Publishers. *Useful, well-illustrated keys to genera and higher categories of ticks and mites in the United States.*

Moore, R.C., C.G. Lalicker, and A.G. Fisher. 1952. Invertebrate fossils. New York, McGraw-Hill Book Co. *Has two chapters dealing with trilobites and chelicerates.*

Naegle, J.A. (ed.). 1963. Advances in acarology, vol. 1. Ithaca, N.Y., Cornell University Press. *For the specialist.*

Sankey, J.H.P., and T.H. Savory. 1974. The British harvestmen, Linnean Society's Synopsis, 2nd Series. Synopses Br. Fauna, N. S. No. 4:1-76.

Savory, T.H. 1977. Arachnida, ed. 2. New York, Academic Press, Inc. *Fairly advanced account, covering morphology, physiology, embryology, ethology, and more about the group. Devotes a chapter to each of the orders.*

Schmidt, G.D., and L.S. Roberts. 1981. Foundations of parasitology, ed. 2. St. Louis, The C.V. Mosby Co. *Has chapters on general form and function of arthropods and on Acari.*

Snow, K.R. 1970. The Arachnida: an introduction. New York, Columbia University Press. *A short account of the class. Emphasis is on mites, ticks, and spiders; other orders given more briefly; includes* Limulus.

Tuttle, D.M., and E.W. Baker. 1968. Spider mites of the southwestern United States and a revision of the Tetranychidae. Tucson, University of Arizona Press.

Selected *Scientific American* articles

Burgess, J.W. 1976. Social spiders. **234**:100-107 (Mar.). *Gregarious spiders are rare but some form communal webs for catching prey.*

Llano, G.A. 1962. The terrestrial life of the Antarctic. **207**:213-230 (Sept.).

Savory, T.H. 1962. Daddy longlegs. **207**:119-128 (Oct.).

Savory, T.H. 1966. False scorpions. **214**:95-100 (Mar.).

Savory, T.H. 1968. Hidden lives. **219**:108-114 (July). *Almost half of the cryptozoic species are arachnids.*

CHAPTER 16

THE AQUATIC MANDIBULATES

Phylum Arthropoda

Class Crustacea

The thoracic legs of barnacles have become modified into long cirri, which they sweep through the water to filter out food particles.

Photograph by K. Sandved.

Mandibulates are those arthropods that possess mandibles (jawlike appendages). They include the crustaceans, insects, and myriapods (centipedes, millipedes, pauropods, and symphylans). As noted in the previous chapter, some investigators contend that the mandibles of the crustaceans and those of the insects-myriapods are not homologous but the result of convergent evolution. There is not yet sufficient agreement on this point for us to give up the concept of a subphylum Mandibulata; therefore we are retaining the traditional arrangement. Nonetheless, all of these forms have, at least, a pair of **antennae**, a pair of **mandibles**, and a pair of **maxillae** on the head. These appendages perform sensory, mastigatory, and food-handling functions, respectively. The body may consist of a head and trunk, but in the more advanced forms, a high degree of tagmosis (p. 363) has occurred so that there is a well-defined head, thorax, and abdomen. In most Crustacea one or more thoracic segments have become fused with the head to form a **cephalothorax**. The thoracic and abdominal appendages are mainly for walking or swimming, but in some groups they are highly specialized in function. Among the mandibulates, the Crustacea are mainly marine; however, there are many freshwater and a few terrestrial species, whereas the insects and myriapods are mainly terrestrial. There are numerous species of insects in freshwater habitats, and a few in marine. The myriapods and insects are discussed in Chapter 17.

CLASS CRUSTACEA

The class Crustacea (L., *crusta*, shell) gets its name from the hard shells most of them bear. The 30,000 or more species in this class include lobsters, crayfish, shrimp, crabs, water fleas, copepods, barnacles, and some others. It is the only arthropod class that is primarily aquatic. The majority are free living and free moving, but many are sessile, commensal, or parasitic. Although crustaceans differ from other arthropods in a variety of ways, the only truly distinguishing characteristic is that crustaceans are the only arthropods with **two pairs of antennae.**

General Nature of a Crustacean

In addition to the two pairs of antennae and a pair of mandibles, crustaceans have two pairs of maxillae on the head, followed by a pair of appendages on each body segment (in some crustaceans not all somites bear appendages). All appendages, except perhaps the first antennae, are primitively **biramous** (two main branches), and at least some of the appendages of present-day adults show that condition. Organs specialized for respiration, if present, are in the form of **gills.**

Most crustaceans have between 16 and 20 segments, but some primitive forms have 60 segments or more. The more advanced crustaceans tend to have fewer segments and increased tagmatization. The major tagmata are the head, thorax, and abdomen, but these are not homologous throughout the class (or even within some subclasses) because of varying degrees of fusion of segments (somites), for example, as in the cephalothorax.

The most advanced and by far the largest group of crustaceans is the subclass Malacostraca, which includes the lobsters, crabs, shrimps, beach fleas, sow bugs, and many others. These show a surprisingly constant arrangement of body segments and tagmata that is often referred to as the **caridoid facies*** and is con-

---

*"Caridoid" derives from the scientific name of a group of crustaceans; "facies" means face or general appearance.

Figure 16-1

Archetypical plan of the Malacostraca. The maxillae and maxillipeds have been separated diagrammatically to illustrate the general plan. Typically in the living animal only the third maxilliped is visible externally.

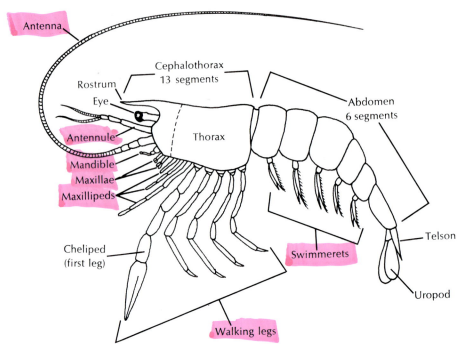

sidered the ancestral plan of the group (Fig. 16-1). This typical body plan has a head of five (six embryonically) fused somites, a thorax of eight somites, and an abdomen of six somites (seven in a few species). At the anterior end is the nonsegmented **rostrum** and at the posterior end is the nonsegmented **telson,** which with the last abdominal somite and its **uropods** forms the tail fan in many forms.

In many crustaceans the dorsal cuticle of the head may extend posteriorly and around the sides of the animal to cover or be fused with some or all of the thoracic and abdominal somites. This covering is called the **carapace.** In some groups the carapace forms clamshell-like valves that cover most or all of the body. In the decapods (including lobsters, shrimp, crabs, and others), the carapace covers the entire cephalothorax but not the abdomen.

___ Form and Function

Because of their size and easy availability, large crustaceans such as crayfish have been studied more than other groups. They are also commonly studied in introductory laboratories. Therefore many of the comments that follow apply specifically to crayfishes and their relatives.

External features

The bodies of crustaceans are covered with a secreted cuticle composed of chitin, protein, and limy, calcareous material. The harder, heavy plates of the larger crustaceans are particularly high in calcareous deposits. The hard protective covering is soft and thin at the joints between the somites, allowing flexibility of movement. The carapace, if present, covers much or all of the cephalothorax; in decapods such as crayfish, all of the head and thoracic segments are enclosed dorsally by the carapace. Each somite not enclosed by the carapace is covered by a dorsal cuticular plate, or **tergum** (Fig. 16-2), and a ventral transverse bar, the **sternum,** lies between the segmental appendages (Fig. 16-3). The abdomen termi-

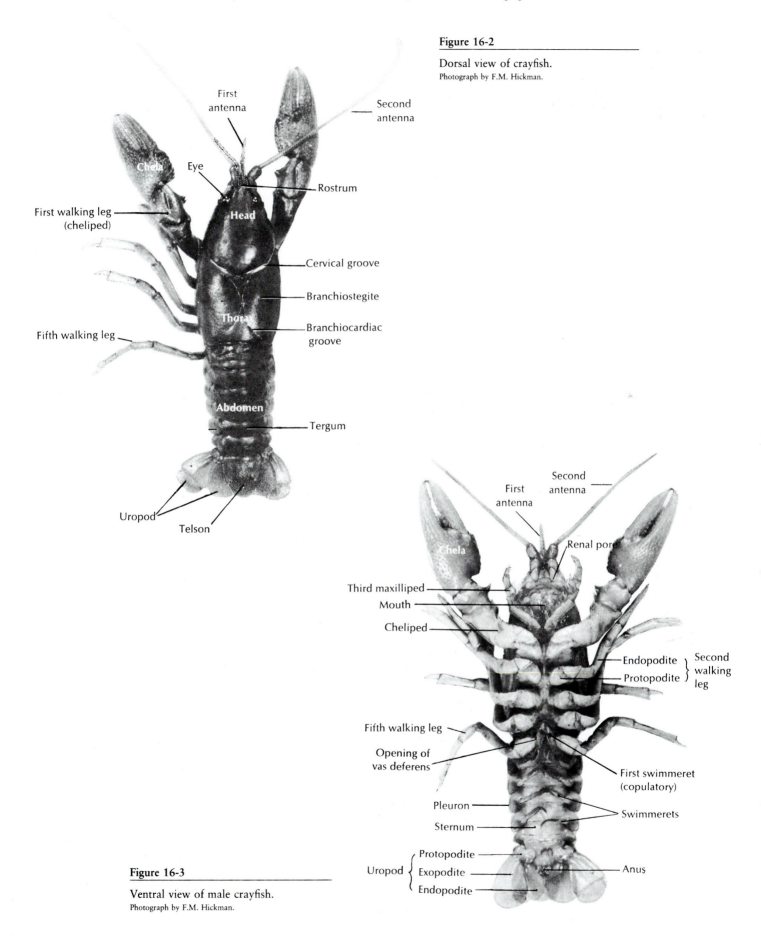

Figure 16-2

Dorsal view of crayfish.
Photograph by F.M. Hickman.

First antenna

Second antenna

Eye

Chela

Rostrum

First walking leg (cheliped)

Head

Cervical groove

Branchiostegite

Thorax

Branchiocardiac groove

Fifth walking leg

Abdomen

Tergum

Uropod

Telson

Second antenna

First antenna

Renal pore

Chela

Third maxilliped

Mouth

Cheliped

Endopodite

Protopodite

Second walking leg

Fifth walking leg

Opening of vas deferens

First swimmeret (copulatory)

Pleuron

Swimmerets

Sternum

Protopodite

Uropod { Exopodite

Endopodite

Anus

Figure 16-3

Ventral view of male crayfish.
Photograph by F.M. Hickman.

Table 16-1 Crayfish appendages

Appendage	Protopod	Endopod	Exopod	Function
First antenna	3 segments, statocyst in base	Many-jointed feeler	Many-jointed feeler	Touch, taste, equilibrium
Second antenna	2 segments, excretory pore in base	Long, many-jointed feeler	Thin, pointed blade	Touch, taste
Mandible	2 segments, heavy jaw and base of palp	2 distal segments of palp	Absent	Crushing food
First maxilla	2 thin medial lamellae	Small unjointed lamella	Absent	Food handling
Second maxilla	2 bilateral lamellae, extra plate, epipod	1 small pointed segment	Dorsal plate, the scaphognathite (bailer)	Drawing currents of water into gills
First maxilliped	2 medial plates and epipod	2 small segments	1 basal segment, plus many-jointed filament	Touch, taste, food handling
Second maxilliped	2 segments plus gill	5 short segments	2 slender segments	Touch, taste, food handling
Third maxilliped	2 segments plus gill	5 larger segments	2 slender segments	Touch, taste, food handling
First walking leg (cheliped)	2 segments plus gill	5 segments with heavy pincer	Absent	Offense and defense
Second walking leg	2 segments plus gill	5 segments plus small pincer	Absent	Walking and prehension
Third walking leg	2 segments plus gill; genital pore in female	5 segments plus small pincer	Absent	Walking and prehension
Fourth walking leg	2 segments plus gill	5 segments, no pincer	Absent	Walking
Fifth walking leg	2 segments; genital pore in male; no gill	5 segments, no pincer	Absent	Walking
First swimmeret	In female reduced or absent; in male fused with endopod to form tube			In male, transferring sperm to female
Second swimmeret Male	Structure modified for transfer of sperm to female			
Female	2 segments	Jointed filament	Jointed filament	Creating water currents; carrying eggs and young
Third, fourth, and fifth swimmerets	2 short segments	Jointed filament	Jointed filament	Creating current of water; in female carrying eggs and young
Uropod	1 short, broad segment	Flat, oval plate	Flat, oval plate; divided into 2 parts with hinge	Swimming; egg protection in female

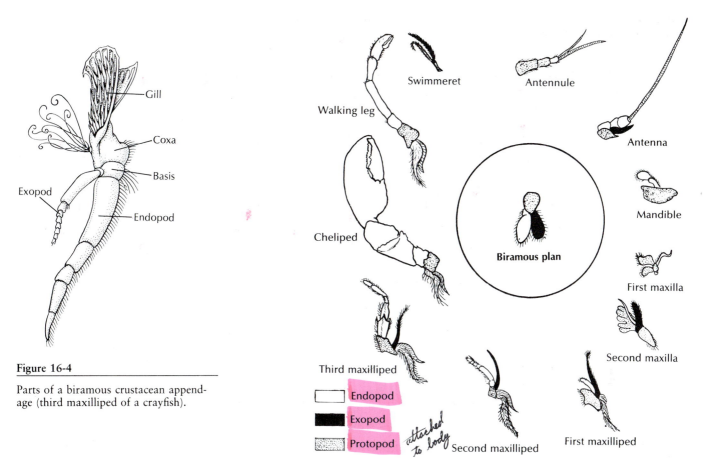

Figure 16-4

Parts of a biramous crustacean appendage (third maxilliped of a crayfish).

Figure 16-5

Appendages of the crayfish showing how they have become modified from the basic biramous plan, as found in a swimmeret.

nates in a **telson,** which is not considered a somite and bears the anus. In several subclasses the telson bears a pair of processes, forming the **caudal furca.**

The position of the **gonopores** varies according to sex and group of crustaceans. They may be on or at the base of a pair of appendages, at the terminal end of the body, or on somites without legs. In crayfish the openings of the vasa deferentia are on the median side at the base of the fifth pair of walking legs, and those of the oviducts are at the base of the third pair. In the female the opening to the seminal receptacle is located in the midventral line between the fourth and fifth pairs of walking legs.

Appendages

Members of the subclass Malacostraca (including crayfishes) and the primitive subclasses typically have a pair of jointed appendages on each somite (Fig. 16-3), although the abdominal somites in most other subclasses do not bear appendages. Considerable specialization is evident in the appendages of the advanced crustaceans such as the crayfishes. All, however, are variations of the basic, biramous plan, illustrated by a crayfish appendage such as a maxilliped (Figs. 16-4 and 16-5). The basal portion, the **protopod,** bears a lateral **exopod** and a medial **endopod.** The **protopod** is made up of two joints (**basis** and **coxa**), whereas the exopod and endopod have from one to several segments each. Some appendages, such as the walking legs of crayfishes, have become secondarily uniramous. Medial or lateral processes may be found on crustacean limbs, called **endites** and **exites,** respectively, and an exite on the protopod is called an **epipod.** Epipods are often modified as gills. Table 16-1 shows how the various appendages have become modified from the biramous plan to fit specific functions.

The terminology applied by various workers to crustacean appendages has not been blessed with uniformity. At least two systems are in wide use. Alternative terms to those we have used, for example, are protopodite, exopodite, endopodite, basipodite, coxopodite, and epipodite. The first and second pairs of antennae may be referred to as the antennules and antennae, and the first and second maxillae are often called maxillules and maxillae. A rose by any other name . . .

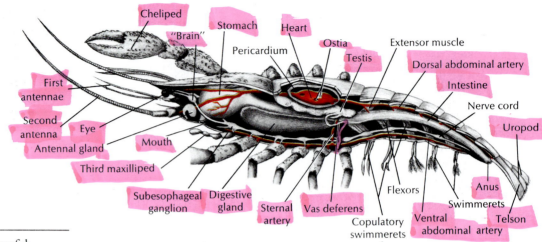

Figure 16-6

Internal structure of male crayfish.

Structures that have a similar basic plan and have descended from a common form are said to be **homologous,** whether they have the same function or not. Since the specialized walking legs, mouthparts, chelipeds, and swimmerets have all developed from a common biramous type but have become modified to perform different functions, they are all homologous to each other (serially homologous). In primitive forms they were all very similar to one another. During the evolution of this structural modification, some branches have been reduced, some lost, some greatly altered, and some new parts added. The crayfish and their allies possess the best examples of **serial homology** in the animal kingdom.

Internal features

The muscular and nervous systems and segmentation in the thorax and abdomen clearly show the metamerism inherited from the annelid ancestors, but there are marked modifications in other systems. Most of the changes involve concentration of parts in a particular region or else reduction or complete loss of parts, such as the intersepta.

Hemocoel

The major body space in the arthropods is not a true coelom but a blood-filled **hemocoel.** The hemocoel is a *primary* body cavity that is actually a persistent blastocoel. A true coelom, on the other hand, is a *secondary* body cavity that forms within the mesoderm. The only remaining coelomic compartments in the crustaceans are the end sacs of the excretory organs and the space around the gonads.

Muscular system

Striated muscles make up a considerable part of the body of most Crustacea. The muscles are usually arranged in antagonistic groups: **flexors,** which draw a part toward the body, and **extensors,** which straighten it out. The abdomen of a crayfish has powerful flexors (Fig. 16-6), which are used when the animal swims backward—its best means of escape. Strong muscles on either side of the stomach control the mandibles.

Figure 16-7

Diagrammatic cross section through heart region of crayfish showing direction of blood flow in this "open" blood system. Blood is pumped from heart to body tissues through arteries, which empty into tissue sinuses. Returning blood enters sternal sinus, is carried to gills for gas exchange, and then is carried back to pericardial sinus by branchiocardiac canals. Note absence of veins.

Respiratory system

Respiratory gas exchange in the smaller crustaceans takes place over thinner areas of the cuticle (for example, in the legs) or over the entire body, and specialized structures may be absent. The larger crustaceans have gills, which are delicate, featherlike projections with very thin cuticle. In the decapods the sides of the carapace enclose the gill cavity, which is open anteriorly and ventrally (Fig. 16-7). Gills may project from the pleural wall into the gill cavity, from the articulation of the thoracic legs with the body, or from the thoracic coxopodites. The latter two types are typical of crayfish. The "bailer," a part of the second maxilla, draws water over the gill filaments, into the gill cavity at the bases of the legs, and out of the gill cavity at the anterior.

Circulatory system

Crustaceans and other arthropods have an "open" or lacunar type of circulatory system. This means that there are no veins, but that the hemolymph (blood) leaves the heart by way of arteries, circulates through the hemocoel, and returns to venous sinuses, or spaces, instead of veins before it reenters the heart. The annelids have a closed system, as do the vertebrates.

A dorsal heart is the chief propulsive organ. It is a single-chambered sac of striated muscle. Hemolymph enters the heart from the surrounding pericardial sinus through paired ostia, with valves that prevent backflow into the sinus (Fig. 16-6). From the heart the hemolymph enters one or more arteries. Valves in the arteries prevent a backflow of hemolymph. Small arteries empty into the tissue sinuses, which in turn often discharge into the large sternal sinus (Fig. 16-7).

From there, afferent sinus channels carry hemolymph to the gills, if any, where oxygen and carbon dioxide are exchanged. The hemolymph is then returned to the pericardial sinus by efferent channels (Fig. 16-6).

Hemolymph in arthropods is largely colorless. It includes ameboid cells of at least two types. Hemocyanin, a copper-containing respiratory pigment, or hemo-

Figure 16-8

Scheme of antennal gland (green gland) of crayfish. (In natural position organ is much folded.) Most selective resorption takes place in the labyrinth, a complicated spongy mass. Some crustaceans lack a labyrinth, and the excretory tubule (nephridial canal) is a much-coiled tube.

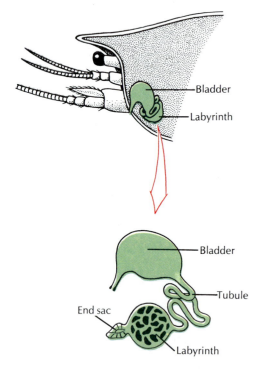

globin, an iron-containing pigment, may be carried in solution. Hemolymph has the property of clotting, which prevents its loss in minor injuries. Some ameboid cells release a thrombinlike coagulant that precipitates the clotting.

Excretory system

The excretory organs of adult crustaceans are a pair of tubular structures located in the ventral part of the head anterior to the esophagus (Fig. 16-6). They are called **antennal glands** or **maxillary glands,** depending on whether they open at the base of the antennae or of the second maxillae. A few adult crustaceans have both. The excretory organs of the decapods are antennal glands, also called **green glands** in this group. Crustaceans do not have malpighian tubules.

The **end sac** of the antennal gland, which is derived from an embryonic coelomic compartment, consists of a small vesicle (**saccule**) and a spongy mass called a **labyrinth.** The labyrinth is connected by an **excretory tubule** to a dorsal **bladder,** which opens to the exterior by a pore on the ventral surface of the basal antennal segment (Fig. 16-8). Hydrostatic pressure within the hemocoel provides the force for filtration of fluid into the end sac, and as the filtrate passes through the excretory tubule, it is modified by resorption of salts, amino acids, glucose, and some water and is finally excreted as urine.

Excretion of nitrogenous wastes (mostly ammonia) takes place by diffusion across thin areas of cuticle, especially the gills, and the so-called excretory organs function principally to regulate the ionic and osmotic composition of the body fluids. Freshwater crustaceans, such as the crayfish, are constantly threatened with overdilution of the blood by water, which diffuses across the gills and other water-permeable surfaces. The green glands, by forming a dilute, low-salt urine, act as an effective "flood-control" device. In marine crustaceans such as lobsters and crabs the kidney functions to adjust the salt composition of the hemolymph by selective modification of the salt content of the tubular urine. In these forms the urine remains isosmotic to the blood.

Nervous system

The nervous systems of crustaceans and annelids have much in common, although those of crustaceans have more fusion of ganglia (Fig. 16-6). The **brain** is a pair of **supraesophageal ganglia** that supply nerves to the eyes and the two pairs of antennae. It is joined by connectives to the **subesophageal ganglion,** a fusion of at least five pairs of ganglia that supply nerves to the mouth, appendages, esophagus, and antennal glands. The double ventral nerve cord has a pair of ganglia for each somite and gives off nerves to the appendages, muscles, and other parts (Fig. 16-9, *B*). In addition to this central system, there may be a sympathetic nervous system associated with the digestive tract.

In primitive crustaceans such as branchiopods the ventral nerve cord has the ladder arrangement characteristic of flatworms and annelids, for the two parts of the cord are separate and are connected by transverse commissures (Fig. 16-9, *A*).

Sensory system

Crustaceans have better-developed sense organs than do the annelids. The largest sense organs of the crayfish are the eyes and the statocysts. Tactile organs are widely distributed over the body in the form of **tactile hairs,** delicate projections of the cuticle that are especially abundant on the chelae, mouthparts, and telson. The chemical senses of **taste** and **smell** are found in hairs on the antennae, mouthparts, and other places.

A saclike **statocyst,** opening to the surface by a dorsal pore, is found on the basal segment of each first antenna of crayfishes. The statocyst contains a ridge that bears sensory hairs formed from the chitinous lining and grains of sand that serve as **statoliths.** Whenever the animal changes its position, corresponding changes in the position of the grains on the sensory hairs are relayed as stimuli to the brain, and the animal can adjust itself accordingly. The cuticular lining of the statocyst is shed at each molting (ecdysis), and with it the sand grains are also lost. New grains are picked up through the dorsal pore after ecdysis.

The eyes in many crustaceans are **compound,** since they are made up of many photoreceptor units called **ommatidia** (Fig. 16-10). Covering the rounded surface of each eye is a transparent area of the cuticle, the **cornea,** which is divided into many small squares known as facets. These are the outer ends of the ommatidia. Each ommatidium behaves like a tiny eye and is comprised of several kinds of cells arranged in a columnar fashion (Fig. 16-10). Black pigment cells are found between adjacent ommatidia.

The movement of pigment in the arthropod compound eye permits it to adjust for different amounts of light. In each ommatidium are three sets of pigment cells: distal retinal, proximal retinal, and reflecting; these are so arranged that they can form a more or less complete collar or sleeve around each ommatidium. For strong light or day adaptation the distal retinal pigment moves inward and meets the outward-moving proximal retinal pigment so that a complete pigment sleeve is formed around the ommatidium (Fig. 16-10). In this condition only rays that strike the cornea directly will reach the photoreceptor (retinular) cells, for each ommatidium is shielded from the others. Thus, each ommatidium will see only a limited area of the field of vision (a mosaic, or apposition, image). In dim light the distal and proximal pigments separate so that the light rays, with the aid of the reflecting pigment cells, have a chance to spread to adjacent ommatidia and to form a continuous, or superposition, image. This second type of vision is less precise but takes maximum advantage of the limited amount of light received.

Figure 16-9

Types of crustacean nervous systems. **A,** *Branchinecta,* a fairy shrimp. **B,** *Astacus,* a crayfish. **C,** *Argulus,* a branchiuran. Note tendency toward concentration and fusion of ganglia. Ladderlike arrangement in **A** may be considered a primitive condition, whereas that in **B** is similar to nervous system of annelid type.

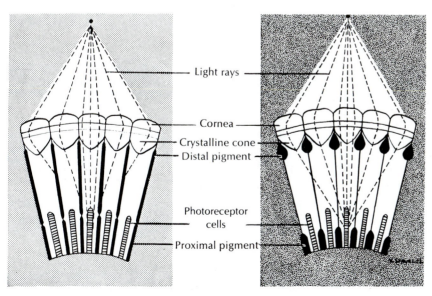

Day-adapted   **Night-adapted**

Light rays · Cornea · Crystalline cone · Distal pigment · Photoreceptor cells · Proximal pigment

Figure 16-10

Portion of compound eye of arthropod showing migration of pigment in ommatidia for day and night vision. Five ommatidia represented in each diagram. In daytime each ommatidium is surrounded by a dark pigment collar so that each ommatidium is stimulated only by light rays that enter its own cornea (mosaic vision); in nighttime, pigment forms incomplete collars and light rays can spread to adjacent ommatidia (continuous, or superposition, image).
Redrawn from Moment, G.B. 1967. General zoology. Boston, Houghton Mifflin Co.

Figure 16-11

Life cycle and distribution *(in red)* of the Gulf shrimp *Pennaeus*. Pennaeids spawn at depths of 20 to 50 fathoms. The young larval forms make up part of the plankton fauna. Older shrimp spend their days hidden in the loose deposits on the bottom, coming up at night to feed. Development is considered slightly metamorphic.

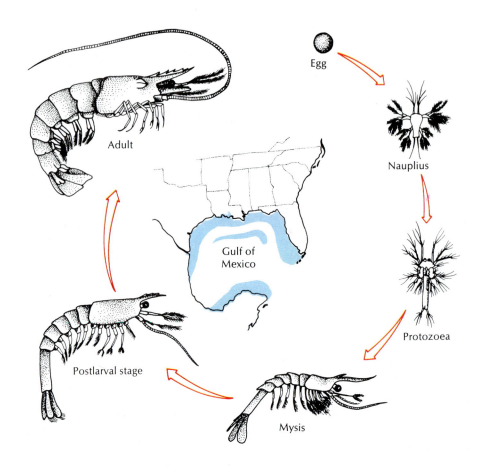

Egg

Nauplius

Protozoea

Gulf of Mexico

Adult

Postlarval stage

Mysis

Reproduction, life cycles, and endocrine function

Most crustaceans have separate sexes, and there are a variety of specializations for copulation among the different groups. The barnacles are monoecious but generally practice cross-fertilization. In some of the ostracods males are scarce, and reproduction is usually parthenogenetic. Most crustaceans brood their eggs in some manner: branchiopods and barnacles have special brood chambers, the copepods have egg sacs attached to the sides of the abdomen (Fig. 16-15), and the malacostracans usually carry eggs and young attached to their appendages.

From the egg of a crayfish hatches a tiny juvenile with the same form as the adult and a complete set of appendages and somites. This type of development is described as **epimorphic**: the juvenile that hatches from the egg resembles a miniature adult, and there is no larval form. In the majority of crustaceans, however, a larva quite unlike the adult in structure and appearance hatches from the egg (p. 394). The primitive and most widely occurring larva in the Crustacea is the **nauplius** (Figs. 16-11 and 16-15). The nauplius bears only three pairs of appendages: uniramous first antennae, biramous second antennae, and biramous mandibles. They all function as swimming appendages at this stage. Through a series of molts, the organism grows and adds somites and appendages, slowly becoming more like the adult. Such development is described as **anamorphic.** In many crustaceans the development is neither epimorphic nor anamorphic, but **metamorphic,** in which assumption of the adult form involves radical changes. For example, the metamorphosis of a barnacle proceeds from a free-swimming nauplius to a larva with a bivalve carapace called a cyprid and finally to the sessile adult with calcareous plates.

Figure 16-12

Cuticle secretion and resorption in preecdysis. **A,** Interecdysis condition. **B,** Old endocuticle separates from epidermis, which secretes new epicuticle. **C,** As new endocuticle is secreted, molting fluid dissolves old endocuticle, and the solution products are resorbed. **D,** At ecdysis, little more than the old epicuticle is left to discard. In postecdysis, new cuticle is stretched and unfolded, and more endocuticle is secreted.

Modified from Schmidt, G.D., and L.S. Roberts. 1981. Foundations of parasitology, ed. 2. St. Louis, The C.V. Mosby Co.

Ecdysis

Ecdysis (ek′duh-sis) (Gr., *ekdyein,* to strip off), or molting, is necessary for the body to increase in size because the exoskeleton is nonliving and does not grow as the animal grows. Much of the crustacean's functioning, including its reproduction, behavior, and many metabolic processes, is directly affected by the physiology of the molting cycle.

The **cuticle,** which is secreted by an underlying cell layer, the epidermis, is composed of several layers. The outermost is the **epicuticle,** a very thin layer of lipid-impregnated protein. The bulk of the cuticle is made up of the several layers of the **endocuticle:** (1) the **pigmented layer,** which is just beneath the epicuticle and contains protein, calcium salts, and chitin; (2) the **calcified layer,** which contains more chitin and less protein and is heavily mineralized with calcium salts; and (3) the **uncalcified layer,** which is a relatively thin layer of chitin and protein.

Some time before the actual ecdysis, the epidermis separates from the uncalcified layer and secretes a new epicuticle (Fig. 16-12). Enzymes are released through canals to the area above the new epicuticle. The enzymes begin to dissolve the old endocuticle, and the soluble products are resorbed and stored within the body of the crustacean. Some of the calcium salts are stored as gastroliths (mineral accretions) in the walls of the stomach. Finally, little more than the epicuticle is left. The animal swallows water, which it absorbs through its gut, and its blood volume increases greatly. The internal pressure causes the cuticle to split, and the animal pulls itself out of its old exoskeleton (Fig. 16-13). Then follow a stretching of the still soft cuticle, redeposition of the salvaged inorganic salts and other constituents, hardening of the new cuticle, and deposition of more endocuticular material. During the period of molting, the animal is defenseless and remains hidden away.

When the crustacean is young, ecdysis must occur frequently to allow growth, and the molting cycle is relatively short. As the animal approaches maturity, intermolt periods become progressively longer, and in some species molting ceases altogether. During intermolt periods, increase in tissue mass occurs as water is replaced by living tissue.

Hormonal control of the ecdysis cycle

Although ecdysis is hormonally controlled, the cycle is often initiated by an environmental stimulus perceived by the central nervous system. Such stimuli may include temperature, day length, and humidity (in the case of land crabs). The action of the signal from the central nervous system is to decrease the production of a **molt-inhibiting hormone** by the **X-organ.** The X-organ is a group of neurosecretory cells in the medulla terminalis of the brain. In the crayfish and other decapods, the medulla terminalis is found in the eyestalk. The hormone is carried in the axons of the X-organ to the **sinus gland** (which is probably not glandular in function), also in the eyestalk, where it is released into the hemolymph.

Figure 16-13

Molting sequence in the lobster *Homarus americanus*. **A,** Membrane between carapace and abdomen ruptures, and carapace begins slow elevation. This step may take up to 2 hours. **B to E,** Head, thorax, and finally abdomen are withdrawn. This process usually takes no more than 15 minutes. **F,** Immediately after ecdysis, chelipeds are desiccated and body is very soft. Lobster continues rapid absorption of water so that within 12 hours body increases about 20% in length and 50% in weight. Tissue water will be replaced by protein in succeeding weeks.

Drawn from photographs by D.E. Aiken.

When the level of molt-inhibiting hormone drops, release of a **molting hormone** from the **Y-organs** is promoted. The Y-organs are located beneath the adductor muscles of the mandibles and are homologus to the prothoracic glands of insects, which produce the hormone ecdysone. The action of the molting hormone is to initiate the processes leading to ecdysis (proecdysis). Once initiated, the cycle proceeds automatically without further action of hormones from either the X- or Y-organs.

Other endocrine functions

Not only does removal of eyestalks accelerate molting, it was also found over 100 years ago that crustaceans whose eyestalks have been removed can no longer

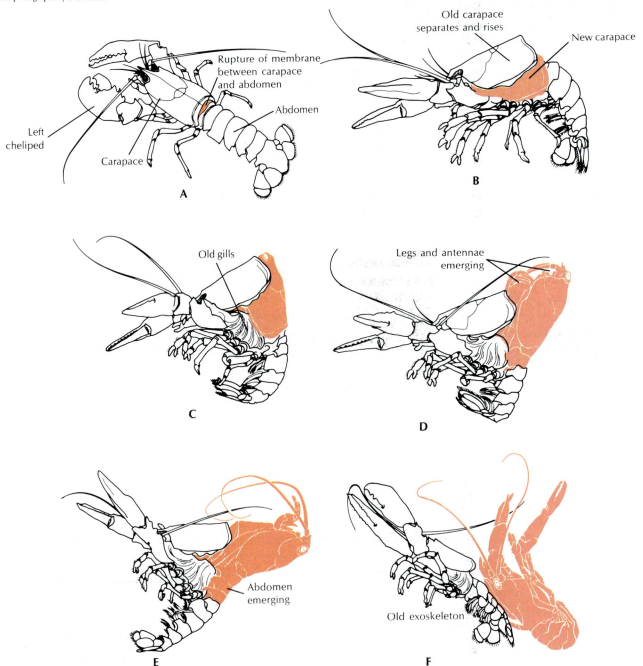

adjust body coloration to background conditions. About 50 years later it was discovered that the defect was not caused by loss of vision but by loss of hormones in the eyestalks. Body color of crustaceans is largely a result of pigments in special branched cells (chromatophores) in the epidermis. Color change is achieved by concentration of the pigment granules in the center of the cells, which causes a lightening effect, or by dispersal of the pigment throughout the cells, which causes a darkening effect. The pigment behavior is controlled by hormones from neurosecretory cells in the eyestalk, as is migration of retinal pigment for light and dark adaptation in the eyes (Fig. 16-10).

Release of neurosecretory material from the pericardial organs in the wall of the pericardium causes an increase in the rate and amplitude of the heartbeat.

Androgenic glands, which were first found in an amphipod (*Orchestia,* the common beach flea), probably occur in all male malacostracans. These are not neurosecretory organs. Their secretion stimulates the expression of male sexual characteristics. Young malacostracans have rudimentary androgenic glands, but in females these glands fail to develop. If they are artificially implanted in a female, her ovaries transform to testes and begin to produce sperm, and her appendages begin to take on male characteristics at the next molt. In isopods the androgenic glands are found in the testes; in all other malacostracans they are between the muscles of the coxopodites of the last thoracic legs and partly attached near the ends of the vasa deferentia. Although females do not possess organs similar to androgenic glands, their ovaries produce one or two hormones that influence secondary sexual characteristics.

Hormones that influence other body processes in Crustacea may be present, and evidence suggests that a neurosecretory substance produced in the eyestalk regulates blood sugar level.

Feeding habits

Feeding habits and adaptations for feeding vary greatly among crustaceans. Many forms can shift from one type of feeding to another depending on environment and food availability, but fundamentally the same set of mouthparts is used by all. The mandibles and maxillae are involved in the actual ingestion; maxillipeds hold and crush food. In predators the walking legs, particularly the chelipeds, serve in food capture.

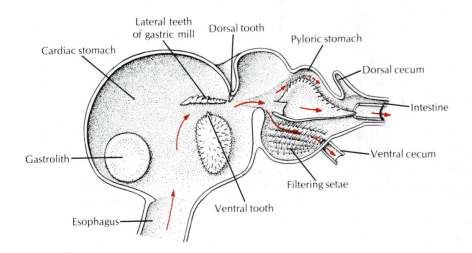

Figure 16-14

Malacostracan stomach showing gastric "mill" and directions of food movements. Mill is provided with chitinous ridges, or teeth, for mastication, and setae for straining the food before it passes into the pyloric stomach.

Figure 16-15

Group of smaller crustaceans. A nauplius hatches from the egg in most cases, except in the Branchiura, in which the nauplius is passed embryonically and a post-larva hatches. Not drawn to same scale.

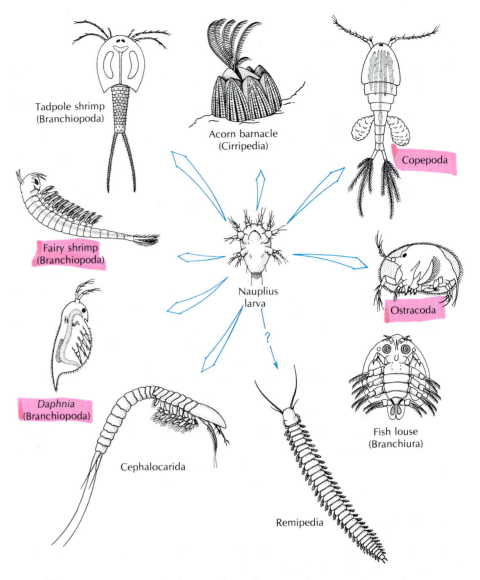

Tadpole shrimp (Branchiopoda)

Acorn barnacle (Cirripedia)

Copepoda

Fairy shrimp (Branchiopoda)

Nauplius larva

Ostracoda

Daphnia (Branchiopoda)

Fish louse (Branchiura)

Cephalocarida

Remipedia

Figure 16-16

Water flea, *Daphnia* (order Cladocera), photographed with polarized light. These microscopic forms occur in great numbers in northern lakes and are an important component of the food chain leading to fishes.

Courtesy Carolina Biological Supply Co., Burlington, N.C.

Many crustaceans, both large and small, are predatory, and some have interesting adaptations for killing their prey. One shrimplike form, *Lygiosquilla*, has on one of its walking legs a specialized digit that can be drawn into a groove and released suddenly to pierce a passing prey. The pistol shrimp *Alpheus* has one enormously enlarged chela that can be cocked like the hammer of a gun and snapped with a force that stuns its prey.

The food of crustaceans ranges from plankton, detritus, and bacteria, used by the **filter feeders,** to larvae, worms, crustaceans, snails, and fishes, used by **predators,** and dead animal and plant matter, used by **scavengers.** Filter feeders, such as the fairy shrimps, water fleas, and barnacles, use their legs, which bear a thick fringe of setae, to create water currents that sweep food particles through the setae. The mud shrimp *Upogebia* uses long setae on its first two pairs of thoracic appendages to strain food material from water circulated through its burrow by movements of its swimmerets.

Crayfishes have a two-part stomach (Fig. 16-14). The first part contains a **gastric mill** in which food, already torn up by the mandibles, can be further ground up by three calcareous teeth into particles fine enough to pass through a setose filter in the second part; the food particles then pass into the intestine for chemical digestion.

___ Brief Résumé of the Crustaceans

The crustaceans are an extensive group with many subdivisions. They have many patterns of structure, habitat, and mode of living. Some are much larger than the crayfish; others are smaller, even microscopic. Some are highly developed and specialized; others have simpler organization.

The reader should realize that the following summary of crustacean groups is misleadingly brief. Although all subclasses are mentioned, a complete presentation would require coverage of a surprisingly large number of taxa in the hierarchy below the subclass level. Among the Malacostraca, for example, some very unusual taxa such as "series" and "section" are used.

Subclass Cephalocarida

Cephalocarida (sef'a-lo-kar'i-da) (Gr., *kephalē*, head, + *karis*, shrimp, + *ida*, pl. suffix) (Fig. 16-15) is a small group, with only four species described so far, that is found along both coasts of the United States, in the West Indies, and in Japan. They are 2 to 3 mm long and have been found in bottom sediments from the intertidal zone to a depth of 300 m. They are even more primitive than the oldest known fossil crustacean, dating from the Devonian period. The thoracic limbs are very similar to each other, and the second maxillae are similar to the thoracic limbs. The serial similarity of the body somites and the musculature is primitive. The second maxillae and the first seven thoracic legs may be considered triramous, bearing a pseudepipod in addition to the exopod and endopod. The eighth legs lack the endopod. Cephalocarids do not have eyes, a carapace, or abdominal appendages. True hermaphrodites, they are unique among the Arthropoda in discharging both eggs and sperm through a common duct.

Subclass Remipedia

Remipedia (ri-mi-pee'dee-a) (L., *remipedes,* oar-footed) (Fig. 16-15) is another very small group, described even more recently than the Cephalocarida. The single species was found in a marine cave in the Bahamas, and like the cephalocarids, it is very primitive. It has 31 to 32 trunk segments (thorax and abdomen), all bearing paired, biramous, swimming appendages that are all essentially alike. It has biramous antennules. Both pairs of maxillae and a pair of maxillipeds, however, are prehensile and apparently adapted for feeding. The shape of the swimming appendages is similar to that found in the Copepoda, but unlike copepods and cephalocarids, the swimming legs are directed laterally rather than ventrally.

Subclass Branchiopoda

Branchiopoda (bran'kee-op'o-da) (Gr., *branchia*, gills, + *pous, podos*, foot) also represents a primitive crustacean type. Four orders are recognized: **Anostraca** (fairy shrimp and brine shrimp, Fig. 16-15), which lack a carapace; **Notostraca** (tadpole shrimp such as *Triops*, Fig. 16-15), whose carapace forms a large dorsal shield covering most of the trunk somites; **Conchostraca** (clam shrimp such as *Lynceus*), whose carapace is bivalve and usually encloses the entire body; and **Cladocera** (water fleas such as *Daphnia*, Figs. 16-15 and 16-16), with a carapace typically covering the entire body but not the head. Branchiopods have reduced first antennae and second maxillae. Their legs are flattened and leaflike (**phyllo-**

Yager (1981) described the Remipedia as a new *class* of Crustacea; however, because we are considering the groups of equivalent rank as subclass (Levi, 1982), we must regard Remipedia as a subclass. In the most recent classification of the Crustacea, Bowman and Abele (1982) suggest that readers may choose for themselves whether to consider Crustacea a phylum, a subphylum, or a superclass, and they regard the subclasses in this chapter as classes. Nonetheless, their choice is, for us, no choice. If we call the Crustacea a phylum, subphylum, or super-class, we must then relegate the other major groups of arthropods to the proper taxa, a reclassification for which Bowman and Abele themselves admit there is insufficient evidence.

podia) and are the chief respiratory organs (hence the name branchiopods). The legs also are used in filter feeding in most branchiopods, and in groups other than the cladocerans, they are used for locomotion as well.

Most branchiopods are freshwater forms. The most important and successful order is the Cladocera, which often forms a large segment of the freshwater zooplankton. Their reproduction is very interesting and is reminiscent of that occurring in some rotifers (Chapter 12). During the summer they often produce only females, by parthenogenesis, rapidly increasing the population. With the onset of unfavorable conditions, some males are produced, and eggs that must be fertilized are produced by normal meiosis. The fertilized eggs are highly resistant to cold and desiccation, and they are very important for survival of the species over the winter and for passive transfer to new habitats. Cladocera are mostly epimorphic, whereas other branchiopods are mainly anamorphic.

Subclass Ostracoda

Members of Ostracoda (os-trak′o-da) (Gr., *ostrakodes,* testaceous, that is, having a shell) are, like the conchostracans, enclosed in a bivalve carapace and resemble tiny clams, 0.25 to 8 mm long (Fig. 16-15). Ostracods show considerable fusion of trunk somites, and numbers of thoracic appendages are reduced to two or none. Feeding and locomotion are principally by use of the head appendages. Most ostracods live on the bottom or climb on plants, but some are planktonic, burrowing, or parasitic. Feeding habits are diverse; there are particle, plant, and carrion feeders and predators. They are widespread in both marine and freshwater habitats. Development is anamorphic.

Subclass Mystacocarida

The Mystacocarida (mis-tak′o-kar′i-da) (Gr., *mystax,* mustache, + *karis,* shrimp, + *ida,* pl. suffix) is a subclass of tiny crustaceans (less than 0.5 mm long) that live in the interstitial water between sand grains of marine beaches (psammolittoral habitat). Only 10 species have been described, but mystacocarids are widely distributed through many parts of the world. They are primitive in several characteristics and are believed to be related to the Copepoda.

Subclass Copepoda

The Copepoda (ko-pep′o-da) (Gr., *kōpē,* oar, + *pous, podos,* foot) is an important subclass of Crustacea, second only to the Malacostraca in numbers of species. The copepods are small (usually a few millimeters or less in length) and rather elongate, tapering toward the posterior. They lack a carapace and retain the simple, median, nauplius eye in the adult (Fig. 16-15). They have a single pair of uniramous maxillipeds and four pairs of rather flattened, biramous, thoracic swimming appendages. The fifth pair of legs is reduced. The posterior part of the body is usually separated from the anterior, appendage-bearing portion by a major articulation. The first antennae are often longer than the other appendages. The Copepoda have been very successful and evolutionarily enterprising, with large numbers of symbiotic as well as free-living species. Many of the parasites are highly modified, and the adults may be so highly modified (and may depart so far from the description just given) that they can hardly be recognized as arthropods.

Ecologically, the free-living copepods are of extreme importance, often dominating the primary consumer level (p. 1026) in aquatic communities. In many marine localities the copepod *Calanus* is the most numerous organism in the zooplankton and has the greatest proportion of the total biomass (p. 1028). In other localities it may be surpassed in the biomass only by euphausids (p. 400). *Calanus* forms a major portion of the diet of such economically and ecologically important fish as herring, menhaden, sardines, and the larvae of larger fish and (along with euphausids) is an important food item for whales and sharks. Other genera commonly occur in the marine zooplankton, and some forms such as *Cyclops* and *Diaptomus* may form an important segment of the freshwater plankton. Many species of copepods are parasites of a wide variety of other marine invertebrates and marine and freshwater fish, and some of the latter are of economic importance. Some species of free-living copepods serve as intermediate hosts of parasites of humans, such as *Diphyllobothrium* (a tapeworm) and *Dracunculus* (a nematode), and of other animals.

Development in the free-living species is commonly anamorphic or slightly metamorphic, but in some of the highly modified parasites, it is strongly metamorphic.

Subclass Branchiura

Branchiura (brank-i-ur'a) (Gr., *branchia*, gills, + *ura*, tail) is a small group of primarily fish parasites, which, despite its name, has no gills (Fig. 16-15). Members of this group are usually between 5 and 10 mm long and may be found on marine or freshwater fish. They typically have a broad, shieldlike carapace, compound eyes, four biramous thoracic appendages for swimming, and a short, unsegmented abdomen. The second maxillae have become modified as suction cups, enabling the parasites to move about on their fish host or even from fish to fish. Development is almost epimorphic: there is no nauplius, and the young resemble the adults except in size and degree of development of the appendages.

Subclass Cirripedia

The Cirripedia (sir-ri-ped'i-a) (L., *cirrus*, curl of hair, + *pes, pedis*, foot) includes the barnacles (order Thoracica), which are usually enclosed in a shell of calcareous plates, as well as three smaller orders of burrowing or parasitic forms. Barnacles are sessile as adults and may be attached to the substrate by a stalk (goose barnacles) (Fig. 16-17, *B*) or directly (acorn barnacles) (Figs. 16-15 and 16-17, *A*). Typically the carapace (mantle) surrounds the body and secretes a shell of calcareous plates. The head is reduced, the abdomen is absent, and the thoracic legs are long, many-jointed cirri with hairlike setae. The cirri are extended through an opening between the calcareous plates to filter from the water the small particles on which the animal feeds (Fig. 16-17). Although all barnacles are marine, they are often found in the intertidal zone and are therefore exposed to drying and sometimes fresh water for some periods of time. During these periods the aperture between the plates can be closed to a very narrow slit.

Barnacles are hermaphroditic and undergo a striking metamorphosis during development. Most hatch as nauplii, which soon become cyprid larvae, so called because of their resemblance to the ostracod genus *Cypris*. They have a bivalve carapace and compound eyes. The cyprid attaches to the substrate by means of its

A
B

Figure 16-17

A, Giant barnacles, *Balanus nubilis* (subclass Cirripedia), of the Pacific coast may be 7.5 cm (3 inches) high and are the largest barnacles in the world. **B,** Common gooseneck barnacles, *Lepas anatifera*. Note the feeding legs, or cirri, on both *Lepas* and *Balanus*. Barnacles attach themselves to a variety of firm substrates, including rocks, pilings, and boat bottoms. A boat's speed may be decreased by as much as 35% because of increased friction caused by barnacles.

A, Photograph by R. Harbo; B, photograph by K. Sandved.

Figure 16-18

Life cycle of *Sacculina*, a rhizocephalan (subclass Cirripedia) parasite of crabs (*Carcinus*).

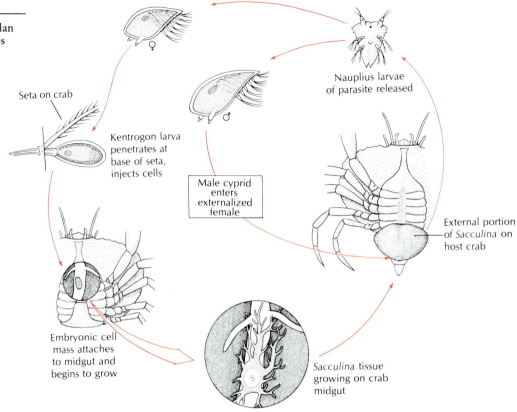

Seta on crab

Kentrogon larva penetrates at base of seta, injects cells

Male cyprid enters externalized female

Nauplius larvae of parasite released

External portion of *Sacculina* on host crab

Embryonic cell mass attaches to midgut and begins to grow

Sacculina tissue growing on crab midgut

The exact position at which the reproductive structures become externalized from the crab's body is of great adaptive value for the rhizocephalan parasite. Because the crab's egg mass (if it had one) would be borne in this position, the crab treats the parasite as if it were a mass of eggs. It protects, ventilates, and grooms the parasite and actually assists in the parasite reproduction by performing spawning behavior at the appropriate time. It has been shown experimentally that the crab's grooming is necessary to the continued good health of the parasite. But what if the rhizocephalan's larva is so unlucky as to infect a male crab? No problem. During the parasite's internal growth in the male crab, the crab is castrated, and it becomes structurally and behaviorally like a female!

first antennae, which have adhesive glands associated with them, and begins its metamorphosis. This involves several dramatic changes, including secretion of the calcareous plates, loss of the eyes, and transformation of the swimming appendages to cirri.

Barnacles frequently foul ship bottoms by settling and growing there. So great may be their number that the speed of the ship may be reduced 30% to 40%, necessitating drydocking the ship to clean them off.

Members of the cirripede order Rhizocephala, such as *Sacculina*, are highly modified parasites of crabs. They start life as cyprid larvae, just as other cirripedes, but when they find a host, most species metamorphose into a **kentrogon,** which injects cells of the parasite into the hemocoel of the crab (Fig. 16-18). Eventually, rootlike absorptive processes grow throughout the crab's body, and the parasite's reproductive structures become externalized between the cephalothorax and the reflexed abdomen of the crab.

Subclass Malacostraca

The Malacostraca (mal-a-kos′tra-ka) (Gr., *malakos*, soft, + *ostrakon*, shell) is the largest subclass of Crustacea and shows great diversity. The diversity is indicated by the higher classification of the group, which includes two series, four superorders, 12 or 13 orders, 16 suborders, and numerous sections, subsections, and superfamilies. We confine our coverage to mentioning a few of the most important orders. The characteristic caridoid facies of the malacostracans is described on p. 381.

A

B

Figure 16-19

A, Four pill bugs, *Armadillidium vulgare* (order Isopoda), common terrestrial forms. **B,** Freshwater sow bug, *Asellus* sp., an aquatic isopod.

A, Photograph by C.P. Hickman, Jr.; B, photograph by J.H. Gerard.

Figure 16-20

Some crustaceans of the subclass Malacostraca.

Meganyctiphanes
(order Euphausiacea)
"northern krill"

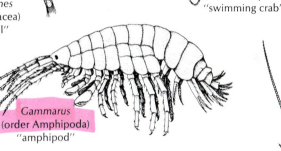

Callinectes
(order Decapoda)
"swimming crab"

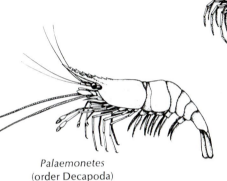

Palaemonetes
(order Decapoda)
"prawn"

Gammarus
(order Amphipoda)
"amphipod"

Asellus
(order Isopoda)
"aquatic isopod"

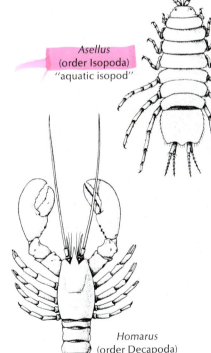

Homarus
(order Decapoda)
"lobster"

Order Isopoda

The Isopoda (i-sop'o-da) (Gr., *isos*, equal, + *pous, podos,* foot) is one of the few crustacean groups to have successfully invaded terrestrial habitats in addition to freshwater and seawater habitats.

Isopods are commonly dorsoventrally flattened, lack a carapace, and have sessile compound eyes; their first pair of thoracic limbs are maxillipeds. The remaining thoracic limbs lack exopods and are similar, while the abdominal appendages bear the gills and, except the uropods, also are similar to each other (hence the name isopods).

Common land forms are the sow bugs, or pill bugs *(Porcellio* and *Armadillidium,* Fig. 16-19, *A),* which live under stones and in damp places. Although they are terrestrial, they do not have the efficient cuticular covering and other adaptations possessed by insects to conserve water; therefore, they must live in moist conditions. *Asellus* (Figs. 16-19, *B,* and 16-20) is a common freshwater form found under rocks and among aquatic plants. *Ligia* is a common marine form that scurries about on the beach or rocky shore. Some isopods are parasites of fish or crustaceans and may be highly modified.

Development is essentially epimorphic but may be highly metamorphic in the specialized parasites.

Order Amphipoda

Amphipoda (am-fip'o-da) (Gr., *amphis*, on both sides, + *pous, podos,* foot) resembles isopods in that the members lack a carapace and have sessile compound eyes and one pair of maxillipeds (Fig. 16-21). However, they are usually com-

A   B   C

Figure 16-21

Marine amphipods. **A,** Free-swimming amphipod, *Anisogammarus* sp. **B,** Skeleton shrimp, *Caprella* sp., shown on a bryozoan colony, resemble praying mantids. **C,** *Phronima*, a marine pelagic amphipod, takes over the tunic of a salp (subphylum Urochordata, Chapter 22). Swimming by means of its abdominal swimmerets, which protrude from the opening of the barrel-shaped tunic, the amphipod maneuvers to catch its prey.
A, Photograph by R. Harbo; *B* and *C*, photographs by K. Sandved.

pressed laterally, and their gills are in the typical thoracic position. Furthermore, their thoracic and abdominal limbs are each arranged in two or more groups that differ in form and function. For example, one group of abdominal legs may be for swimming and another for jumping. There are many marine amphipods, including some beach-dwelling forms (for example, the beach flea, *Orchestia*), numerous freshwater species (*Hyalella* and *Gammarus,* Fig. 16-20), and a few parasites. Development is epimorphic.

Order Euphausiacea

The Euphausiacea (u-faws-i-a′si-a) (Gr., *eu,* well, + *phausi,* shining bright, + L., *acea,* suffix, pertaining to) is a group of only about 90 species, but they are important as the oceanic plankton known as "krill." They are about 3 to 6 cm long, have a carapace that is fused with all the thoracic segments but does not entirely enclose the gills, have no maxillipeds, and have all thoracic limbs with exopods (Fig. 16-20). Most are bioluminescent, with a light-producing substance in an organ called a **photophore.** Some species may occur in enormous swarms, up to 45 m^2 and extending 100 to 500 m in one direction. They form a major portion of the diet of baleen whales and many fishes. Eggs hatch as nauplii, and development is anamorphic.

Order Decapoda

Decapoda (de-cap′o-da) (Gr., *deka,* ten, + *pous, podos,* foot) have three pairs of maxillipeds and five pairs of walking legs, of which the first is modified to form pincers (chelae). They range in size from a few millimeters to the largest of all arthropods, the Japanese spider crab, whose chelae span 4 m. The crayfishes, lobsters, crabs, and "true" shrimp belong in this group (Figs. 16-20 and 16-22 to 16-24). There are over 8500 species of decapods, and the order is extremely diverse. They are very important ecologically and economically, and numerous species are items of food for humans.

The crabs, especially, exist in a great variety of forms. Although resembling the pattern of crayfish, they differ from the latter in having a broader cephalothorax and a reduced abdomen. Familiar examples along the seashore are the hermit crabs (Fig. 16-22, *B*), which live in snail shells because their abdomens are not protected by the same heavy exoskeleton as the anterior parts are; the fiddler crabs, *Uca* (Fig. 16-22, *C*), which burrow in the sand just below the high-tide level

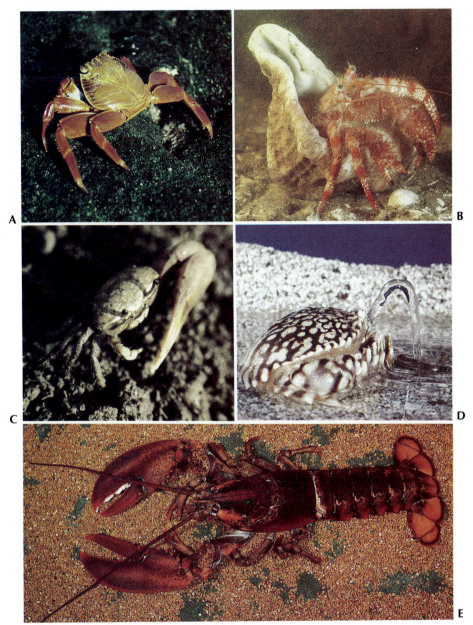

Figure 16-22

Decapod crustaceans. **A,** The bright orange tropical rock crab, *Grapsus grapsus,* is a conspicuous exception to the rule that most crabs bear cryptic coloration. **B,** The hermit crab, *Dardanus venosus,* which has a soft abdominal exoskeleton, lives in a snail shell that it carries about and into which it can withdraw for protection. **C,** The male fiddler crab, *Uca* sp., uses its enlarged cheliped to wave territorial displays and in threat and combat. **D,** The massive chelipeds of box crabs, *Calappa ocellata,* are well adapted for crushing the shells of their snail prey. Here the crab is "exhaling" water from its branchial chamber. **E,** Northern lobster *Homarus americanus.*

A and C, Photographs by C.P. Hickman, Jr.; B and D, photographs by K. Sandved; E, photograph by J.H. Gerard.

and come out to run about over the sand while the tide is out; and the spider crabs such as *Libinia* and the interesting decorator crabs *Oregonia* and others, which cover their carapaces with sponges and sea anemones for protective camouflage (Fig. 16-23).

___ Phylogeny and Adaptive Radiation

The relationship of the crustaceans to other arthropods has long been a puzzle. According to a widely held hypothesis, the trilobites are the ancestors of the crustaceans, but some zoologists have proposed that both these groups evolved independently from different nonarthropod ancestors.

Some light was shed on the problem when the primitive crustacean *Hutch-*

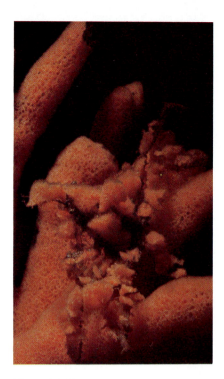

Figure 16-23

Decorator crab, *Oregonia gracilis*, covered with orange sponge. This species is one of several spider crab species that deliberately mask themselves with material from their immediate environment. This crab is so thoroughly masked with pieces of the sponge on which it sits that little of its carapace is visible.

Photograph by R. Harbo.

insoniella macracantha was discovered in 1954 in Long Island Sound. This form was assigned to a new subclass of its own (Cephalocarida) because of its several very primitive characteristics. These include thoracic appendages that are similar to each other and second maxillae that are similar to the thoracic appendages. Except for the eighth thoracic legs, which lack the innermost branch, they are all essentially three branched, or **triramous.** Many authorities see similarities between these appendages and those of the trilobites, and the many specialized limbs of other crustaceans are derivable from the triramous cephalocarid appendages. The characteristics of this little form (about 4 mm long) support the idea that crustaceans were derived from primitive trilobites or that the two groups were derived from a common ancestor. The position of the newly discovered Remipedia awaits determination by investigators of crustacean phylogeny. The differentiation of both pairs of maxillae and a pair of maxillipeds for food handling is a more advanced character than is shown by cephalocarids. Remipedians show several similarities to fossil crustaceans from the Devonian and the Pennsylvanian periods.

A

B

Figure 16-24

A, River crayfish, *Orconectes virilis.* **B,** Painted shrimp, *Hymenocera picta. Hymenocera* is known to feed on sea stars (phylum Echinodermata, p. 469).

A, Photograph by J.H. Gerard; **B,** photograph by K. Sandved.

The adaptive radiation demonstrated by the crustaceans is great, with all manner of aquatic niches exploited. They are unquestionably the dominant arthropod group in the marine environment, and they share dominance of freshwater habitats with insects. Invasion of terrestrial environments has been much more limited, with isopods being the only notable success. There are a few other terrestrial examples, such as land crabs. The most important subclass, in both numbers and diversity, is the Malacostraca, followed by the Copepoda. Both groups include planktonic filter feeders and numerous scavengers. Copepods have been particularly successful as parasites of both vertebrates and invertebrates, and it is clear that the present parasitic copepods are the products of numerous invasions of such niches.

_____ Summary

In addition to a pair of mandibles, mandibulate arthropods (subphylum Mandibulata) have a pair of antennae, a pair of maxillae, and often other head appendages. Their tagmata are a head and trunk or a head, thorax, and abdomen.

The Crustacea is a large, primarily aquatic class of mandibulates. Crustaceans have two pairs of antennae, their appendages are primitively biramous, and many have a carapace.

The two branches of the crustacean leg are the exopod and the endopod, which are both attached to the basal protopod. Appendages are variously specialized, such as chelipeds, maxillipeds, swimmerets, and uropods.

All arthropods must periodically cast off their cuticle (ecdysis) and grow in dimensional size before the newly secreted cuticle hardens. Premolt and postmolt periods are hormonally controlled, as are several other processes, such as change in body color and expression of sexual characteristics.

Feeding habits vary greatly in Crustacea, and there are many predators, scavengers, filter feeders, and parasites. Respiration is through the body surface or by gills, and excretory organs take the form of maxillary or antennal glands. Circulation, as in other arthropods, is through an open system of sinuses (hemocoel), and a dorsal, tubular heart is the chief pumping organ. Most crustaceans have compound eyes composed of units called ommatidia. Sexes are usually separate.

The crustacean subclass Branchiopoda is characterized by the possession of phyllopodia and contains, among others, the order Cladocera, which is ecologically important as zooplankton. Members of the subclass Copepoda lack a carapace and abdominal appendages. They are abundant and are among the most important of the primary consumers in many freshwater and marine ecosystems. Most members of the subclass Cirripedia (barnacles) are sessile as adults, secrete a shell of calcareous plates, and filter feed by means of their thoracic appendages.

The Malacostraca are the largest crustacean subclass, and the most important orders are the Isopoda, Amphipoda, Euphausiacea, and Decapoda. All have both abdominal and thoracic appendages. Isopods lack a carapace and are usually dorsoventrally flattened. Amphipods also lack a carapace but are usually laterally flattened. Euphausiaceans are important oceanic plankton called krill. Decapods include crabs, shrimp, lobster, crayfish, and others; they have five pairs of walking legs (including the chelipeds) on their thorax.

Selected references

Adiyodi, K.G., and R.G. Adiyodi. 1970. Endocrine control of reproduction in decapod Crustacea. Biol. Rev. 45:121-165.

Barnes, R.D. 1980. Invertebrate zoology, ed. 4. Philadelphia, Saunders College/Holt, Rinehart & Winston.

Barrington, E.J.W. 1979. Invertebrate structure and function, ed. 2. New York, John Wiley & Sons, Inc.

Bliss, D.E. (ed. in chief). 1982. The biology of Crustacea, vols. 1-5. New York, Academic Press, Inc. *Five volumes in this series, planned as a 10-volume comprehensive publication, have been published. The series is likely to become a standard reference for all aspects of crustacean biology.*

Bowman, T.E., and L.G. Abele. 1982. Classification of the recent Crustacea. In L.G. Abele (ed.). The biology of Crustacea, vol. 1. Systematics, the fossil record, and biogeography. New York, Academic Press, Inc. *This classification is likely to be the one followed by many authors in the near future. It recognizes the following classes: Cephalocarida, Branchiopoda, Remipedia, Maxillopoda (containing subclasses Mystacocarida, Cirripedia, Copepoda, and Branchiura), Ostracoda, and Malacostraca.*

Clarke, K.U. 1973. The biology of the Arthropoda. New York, American Elsevier Publishers, Inc.

Gosner, K.L. 1971. Guide to identification of marine and estuarine invertebrates. New York, Interscience.

Kabata, Z. 1970. Diseases of fishes, book I. Crustacea as enemies of fishes. In S.F. Snieszko and H.R. Axelrod (eds.). Jersey City, N.J., T.F.H. Publications, Inc. *An excellent account of the crustacean parasites of fishes, from the little modified to the bizarre; includes pathology and treatment of affected hosts.*

Kabata, Z. 1982. Parasitic Copepoda of British fishes. Ray Society Publication No. 152. London, British Museum (Natural History). *There is much in this book that is applicable to the study of copepods in general.*

Kaestner, A. 1970. Invertebrate zoology, vol. 3. New York, Interscience. *The best and fullest account of the class in one volume in English; a must for serious students of Crustacea.*

Levi, H.W. 1982. Crustacea. In S.P. Parker (ed.). Synopsis and classification of living organisms, vol. 2. New York, McGraw-Hill Book Co.

Marshall, S.M. 1973. Respiration and feeding in copepods. In F.S. Russell and M. Yonge (eds.). Advances in marine biology, vol. 11. New York, Academic Press, Inc., pp. 57-120.

Marshall, S.M., and A.P. Orr. 1955. The biology of a marine copepod *Calanus finmarchicus* (Gunnerus). Edinburgh, Oliver & Boyd.

Mauchline, J., and L.R. Fisher. 1969. The biology of euphausiids. In F.S. Russell and M. Yonge (eds.). Advances in marine biology, vol. 7. New York, Academic Press, Inc.

Newell, R.C. 1970. Biology of intertidal animals. London, Logos Press, Ltd.

Pennak, R.W. 1978. Freshwater invertebrates of the United States, ed. 2. New York, John Wiley & Sons, Inc. *Unusually clear taxonomic keys and illustrative drawings.*

Ritchie, L.E., and J.T. Høeg. 1981. The life history of *Lernaeodiscus porcellanae* (Cirripedia: Rhizocephala) and co-evolution with its porcellanid host. J. Crust. Biol. 1:334-347. *The life history and description of the maternal care given the parasite by its host. A fascinating story.*

Russell-Hunter, W.D. 1979. A life of invertebrates. New York, Macmillan, Inc.

Sanders, H.L. 1957. The Cephalocarida and crustacean phylogeny. Syst. Zool. 6:112-128.

Schmidt, G.D., and L.S. Roberts. 1981. Foundations of parasitology, ed. 2. St. Louis, The C.V. Mosby Co. *Includes treatment of parasitic Crustacea.*

Schmitt, W.L. 1965. Crustaceans. Ann Arbor, The University of Michigan Press. *A good little book by one of the most eminent students of the group; very interesting reading and easy to understand.*

Tombes, A.S. 1970. An introduction to invertebrate endocrinology. New York, Academic Press, Inc.

Yager, J. 1981. Remipedia, a new class of Crustacea from a marine cave in the Bahamas. J. Crust. Biol. 1:328-333.

Selected *Scientific American* articles

Benson, A.A., and R.F. Lee. 1975. The role of wax in oceanic food chains. 232:77-86 (Mar.).

Brown, F.A., Jr. 1954. Biological clocks and the fiddler crab. 190:34-37 (Apr.).

Caldwell, R.L., and H. Dingle. 1976. Stomatopods. 234:81-89 (Jan.).

Murphy, R.C. 1962. The oceanic life of the Antarctic. 207:187-210 (Sept.).

Palmer, J.D. 1975. Biological clocks of the tidal zone. 232:70-79 (Feb.).

Wicksten, M.D. 1980. Decorator crabs. 242:146-154 (Feb.). *Many species of spider crabs camouflage themselves with materials from their environment, which they attach with specialized, hooked setae on their carapace and legs.*

CHAPTER   17

THE TERRESTRIAL
MANDIBULATES

The Myriapods and Insects

Phylum Arthropoda

Classes Chilopoda, Diplopoda, Pauropoda, Symphyla, and Insecta

Luna moth *Actias luna* is one of the largest, most beautiful moths found in North America.
Its larva feeds on walnut, sweet-gum, hickory, and other trees.

Photograph by C.P. Hickman, Jr.

Figure 17-1

Centipede *Scolopendra* (class Chilopoda). Most segments have one pair of appendages each. First segment bears a pair of poison claws, which in some species can inflict serious wounds. Centipedes are carnivorous.

Photograph by F.M. Hickman.

Along with the arachnids, the insects and myriapods are primarily terrestrial arthropods. Only a few of them have returned to aquatic life, usually in fresh water.

The term "myriapod," meaning "many footed," is commonly used for a group of several classes of mandibulate arthropods that have evolved a pattern of two tagmata—head and trunk—with paired appendages on all trunk somites except the last. The myriapods include the Chilopoda (centipedes), Diplopoda (millipedes), Pauropoda (pauropods), and Symphyla (symphylans).

The insects have evolved a pattern of three tagmata—head, thorax, and abdomen—with appendages on the head and thorax but greatly reduced on or absent from the abdomen. Insects may have arisen from an early myriapod or protomyriapod form.

The terrestrial mandibulates have no antennules, and their appendages are unlike those of the crustaceans in being always uniramous, never biramous. Although some insect young are aquatic and have gills, the gills are not homologous to those of the crustaceans.

The insects and myriapods share with the onychophorans and some of the arachnids the use of tracheae for carrying the respiratory gases directly to and from all body cells.

Excretion is usually by malpighian tubules.

CLASS CHILOPODA

The Chilopoda (ki-lop′o-da) (Gr., *cheilos*, margin, lip, + *pous, podos,* foot), or centipedes, are land forms with somewhat flattened bodies that may contain from a few to 177 somites (Fig. 17-1). Each somite, except the one behind the head and the last two in the body, bears a pair of jointed appendages. The appendages of the first body segment are modified to form poison claws.

The head appendages are similar to those of an insect. There are a pair of antennae, a pair of mandibles, and one or two pairs of maxillae. A pair of eyes on the dorsal side of the head consists of groups of ocelli.

The digestive system is a straight tube into which salivary glands empty at the anterior end. Two pairs of malpighian tubules empty into the hind part of the intestine. There is an elongated heart with a pair of arteries to each somite. Res-

Figure 17-2

Seven-inch-long millipedes from Ecuador, mating. Note the typical doubling of appendages on most segments.

Photograph by K. Sandved.

406

piration is by means of a tracheal system of branched air tubes that come from a pair of spiracles in each somite. The nervous system is typically arthropod, and there is also a visceral nervous system.

Sexes are separate, with unpaired gonads and paired ducts. Some centipedes lay eggs and others are viviparous. The young are similar to the adults.

Centipedes prefer moist places such as under logs, bark, and stones. They are very agile and are carnivorous in their eating habits, living on earthworms, cockroaches, and other insects. They kill their prey with their poison claws and then chew it with their mandibles. The common house centipede, *Scutigera* (L., *scutum*, shield, + *gera*, bearing), which has 15 pairs of legs, is often seen scurrying around bathrooms and damp cellars, where it catches insects. Most species are harmless to humans. Some of the tropical centipedes may reach a length of 30 cm.

CLASS DIPLOPODA

The Diplopoda (Gr., *diplos*, double, two + *pous*, *podos*, foot) are commonly called millipedes, which literally means "thousand feet" (Fig. 17-2). Even though they do not have that many legs, they do have a large number of appendages, since each abdominal somite has two pairs of appendages, a condition that may have arisen from the fusion of pairs of somites. Their cylindrical bodies are made up of 25 to 100 somites. The short thorax consists of four somites, each bearing one pair of legs.

The head bears two clumps of simple eyes and a pair each of antennae, mandibles, and maxillae. The general body structures are similar to those of centipedes, with a few variations here and there. Two pairs of spiracles on each abdominal somite open into air chambers that give off the tracheal air tubes. Two genital apertures are found toward the anterior end.

In most millipedes the appendages of the seventh somite are specialized for copulatory organs. After copulation the eggs are laid in a nest and are carefully guarded by the mother. The larval forms have only one pair of legs to each somite.

Millipedes are not so active as centipedes. They walk with a slow, graceful motion, not wriggling as the centipedes do. They prefer dark, moist places under logs or stones. They are herbivorous, feeding on decayed plant or animal matter, although sometimes they eat living plants. When disturbed, they often roll up into a coil. Common examples of this class are *Spirobolus* and *Julus*, both of which have wide distribution.

CLASS PAUROPODA

The Pauropoda (Gr., *pauros*, small, + *pous*, *podos*, foot) are a group of minute (2 mm or less), soft-bodied myriapods, numbering almost 500 species. They have a small head with branched antennae and no eyes, but they have a pair of sense organs that have the appearance of eyes (Fig. 17-3, *A*). Their 12 trunk segments usually bear nine pairs of legs (none on the first or the last two segments). They have only one tergal plate covering each two segments.

Tracheae, spiracles, and circulatory system are lacking. Pauropods are probably most closely related to the diplopods but are considered to be more primitive.

Figure 17-3

A, Pauropod. Pauropods are minute, whitish myriapods with three-branched antennae and nine pairs of legs. They live in leaf litter and under stones. They are eyeless but have sense organs that resemble eyes. **B**, *Scutigerella*, a symphylan, is a minute whitish myriapod that is sometimes a greenhouse pest.

B, Modified from Snodgrass, R.E. 1952. A textbook of arthropod anatomy. Ithaca, N.Y., Cornell University Press.

Although widely distributed, the pauropods are the least well known of the myriapods. They live in moist soil, leaf litter, or decaying vegetation and under bark and debris. Representative genera are *Pauropus* and *Allopauropus*.

CLASS SYMPHYLA dont study

The Symphyla (Gr., *sym*, together, + *phylon*, tribe) are small (2 to 10 mm) and have centipede-like bodies (Fig. 17-3, *B*). They live in humus, leaf mold, and debris. *Scutigerella* (L., dim. of *Scutigera*) are often pests on vegetables and flowers, particularly in greenhouses. They are soft bodied, with 14 segments, 12 of which bear legs and one a pair of spinnerets. The antennae are long and unbranched. Only 160 species have been described.

Symphylans are eyeless but have sensory pits at the bases of the antennae. The tracheal system is limited to a pair of spiracles on the head and tracheal tubes to the anterior segments only.

CLASS INSECTA

The Insecta (L., *insectus*, cut into) are the most successful biologically of all the groups of arthropods. There are more species of insects than species in all the other classes of animals combined. The recorded number of insect species has been estimated to be close to 800,000, but this figure represents only about half the species that exist. There is also striking evidence that evolution is continuing among insects at the present time, even though the group as a whole is considered to be stable, according to the fossil record.

It is difficult to appreciate fully the significance of this extensive group and its role in the biological pattern of animal life. The study of insects (**entomology**) occupies the time and resources of skilled men and women all over the world. The struggle between humans and their insect competitors seems to be endless, yet paradoxically insects have so interwoven themselves into the economy of nature in so many useful roles that we would have a difficult time without them.

Insects differ from other arthropods in having **three pairs of legs** and usually **two pairs of wings** on the thoracic region of the body, although some have one pair of wings or none. In size insects range from less than 1 mm to 20 cm in length, the majority being less than 2.5 cm long. Generally, the largest insects live in tropical areas.

Distribution

Insects are among the most abundant and widespread of all land animals. They have spread into practically all habitats that will support life except the deeper waters of the sea. Relatively few are marine. The marine water striders *(Halobates),* which live on the surface of the ocean, are the only marine invertebrates that live on the sea-air interface. Insects are common in brackish water, in salt marshes, and on sandy beaches. They are abundant in fresh water, in soils, in forests, and in plants, and they are found even in deserts and wastelands, on mountaintops, and as parasites in and on the bodies of plants and animals.

Their wide distribution is made possible by their powers of flight and their highly adaptable nature. In most cases they can easily surmount barriers that are

The mating behavior of *Scutigerella* is unusual. The male places a spermatophore at the end of a stalk. When the female finds it, she takes it into her mouth, storing the sperm in special buccal pouches. Then she removes the eggs from her gonopore with her mouth and attaches them to moss or lichen, or to the walls of crevices, smearing them during the handling with some of the semen and so fertilizing them. The young at first have only six or seven pairs of legs.

well nigh impassable to many other animals. Their small size allows them to be carried by currents of both wind and water to far regions. Their well-protected eggs can withstand rigorous conditions and can be carried long distances by birds and animals. Their agility and aggressiveness enable them to fight for every possible niche in a habitat. No single pattern of biological adaptation can be applied to them.

___ Adaptability

Insects, during their evolution, have shown an amazing adaptability, as evidenced by their wide distribution and enormous diversity of species. Most of their structural modifications have taken place in the wings, legs, antennae, mouthparts, and alimentary canal. Such wide diversity enables this vigorous group to take advantage of all available resources of food and shelter. Some are parasitic, some suck the sap of plants, some chew up the foliage of plants, some are predaceous, and some live on the blood of various animals. Within these different groups, specialization occurs, so that a particular kind of insect will eat, for instance, the leaves of only one kind of plant. This specificity of eating habits lessens competition and to a great extent accounts for their biological success.

Insects are well adapted to dry and desert regions. The hard and protective exoskeleton helps prevent evaporation, but some insects also extract the utmost in fluid from food and fecal material, as well as moisture from the water by-product of bodily metabolism.

As in other arthropods, the exoskeleton is made up of a complex system of plates known as **sclerites,** connected to one another by concealed, flexible hinge joints. The muscles between the sclerites enable the insect to make precise movement. The rigidity of its exoskeleton is attributable to the unique scleroproteins and not to its chitin component, and its lightness makes flying possible. By contrast, the cuticle of crustaceans is stiffened mostly by mineral matter.

___ External Form and Function

Insects show a remarkable variety of morphological characters. Some are fairly generalized in body structure, some are highly specialized. The grasshopper, or locust, is a generalized type that is usually used in laboratories to demonstrate the general features of insects (Fig. 17-4).

Figure 17-4

A, External features of a female grasshopper. The terminal segment of a male with external genitalia is shown in inset. **B,** Spur-throated grasshopper, *Melanoplus* sp. (order Orthoptera). This large genus contains many agricultural pest species.

B, Photograph by C.P. Hickman, Jr.

A

B

Figure 17-5

A few of the various types of insect antennae. *Left to right:* mosquito (plumose); May beetle (laminate); click beetle (serrate); tenebrionid beetle (moniliform); and water scavenger beetle (clavate). Photomicrograph by F.M. Hickman.

The insect tagmata are the head, thorax, and abdomen. The cuticle of each body segment is typically composed of four plates (sclerites), a dorsal notum (tergum), a ventral sternum, and a pair of lateral pleura. The pleura of abdominal segments is membranous rather than sclerotized.

The head usually bears a pair of relatively large compound eyes, a pair of antennae, and usually three ocelli. The antennae, which vary greatly in size and form (Fig. 17-5), act as tactile organs, organs of smell, and in some cases organs of hearing. Mouthparts, formed from specially hardened cuticle, typically consist of a labrum, a pair each of mandibles and maxillae, a labium, and a tonguelike hypopharynx. The type of mouthparts an insect possesses determines how it feeds. Some of these modifications will be discussed later.

The thorax is composed of the prothorax, mesothorax, and metathorax, each bearing a pair of legs (Fig. 17-4, *A*). In most insects the mesothorax and metathorax each bear a pair of wings. The wings are cuticular extensions formed by the epidermis. They consist of a double membrane containing veins of thicker cuticle that serve to strengthen the wing. Although these veins vary in their patterns among the different species, they are constant within a species and serve as one means of classification and identification.

Legs of insects are often modified for special purposes. Terrestrial forms have walking legs with terminal pads and claws as in beetles. These pads may be sticky for walking upside down, as in houseflies. The hindlegs of the grasshoppers and crickets are adapted for jumping (Fig. 17-6). The mole cricket has the first pair of legs modified for burrowing in the ground. Water bugs and many beetles have paddle-shaped appendages for swimming. For grasping its prey, the forelegs of the praying mantis are long and strong (Fig. 17-7).

The legs of the honeybee are good examples of how an insect's appendages can be developed for special purposes (Fig. 17-8). The first pair of legs in this insect is suited to collecting pollen by having a feathery **pollen brush** on the metatarsus and a fringe of hairs on the medial edge of the tibia for cleaning the head and the compound eye. A semicircular indentation lined with teeth is found in the metatarsus, and this is covered over with a spine, the **velum**, from the tibia. As the antenna is pulled through this notch, it is cleaned of pollen; hence this structure is called the **antennae cleaner**. The middle leg also has a **pollen brush** on the metatarsus and a **spur** on the tibia for removing wax from the wax glands on the abdomen. The hindlimb is the most specialized of all, for it bears the **pollen basket**, the **pollen packer**, and **pollen brushes**. The pollen basket is a concavity on the tibia, with hairs along both edges that are kept moist with secretions from the mouth. The pollen packer consists of a row of stout bristles on the tibia and the auricle, a smooth plate on the metatarsus. The pecten removes the pollen from the pollen brush of the opposite leg onto the auricle. When the leg is flexed, the auricle presses against the end of the tibia, compressing the pollen. The inner surface of the metatarsus bears pollen brushes (combs) consisting of rows of stout spines.

The abdomen of insects is composed of nine to 11 segments; the eleventh, when present, is reduced to a pair of cerci (appendages at the posterior end). Larval or nymphal forms have a variety of abdominal appendages, but these are lacking in the adults. The end of the abdomen bears the external genitalia (Fig. 17-4).

There are innumerable variations in body form among the insects. Beetles are usually thick and plump (Fig. 17-9, *A*); damselflies, crane flies, and walking sticks are long and slender (Fig. 17-9, *B*); aquatic beetles are streamlined; and cockroaches are flat, adapted to living in crevices. The ovipositor of the female

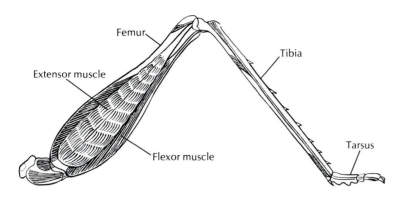

Figure 17-6

Hindleg of grasshopper. Muscles that operate the leg are found within a hollow cylinder of exoskeleton. Here they are attached to the internal wall, from which they manipulate segments of limb on the principle of a lever. Note pivot joint and attachment of tendons of extensor and flexor muscles, which act reciprocally to extend and flex the limb.

Figure 17-7

A, Praying mantis *Tenodera sinensis* (order Orthoptera), feeding on an insect. **B,** Praying mantis laying eggs.

Photographs by J.H. Gerard.

A

B

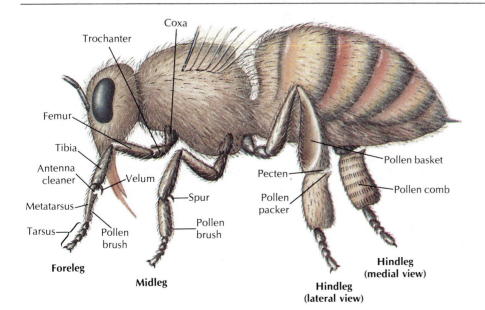

Foreleg

Midleg

Hindleg (lateral view)

Hindleg (medial view)

Figure 17-8

Adaptive legs of worker honeybee. In the foreleg, toothed indentation covered with velum is used to comb out antennae. Spur on the middle leg removes wax from wax glands on the abdomen. Pollen picked up on body hairs is combed off by pollen brushes on the front and middle legs and deposited on pollen brushes of the hindlegs. Long hairs of pecten on the hindleg remove pollen from the brush of the opposite leg; then the auricle is used to press it into a pollen basket when the leg joint is flexed back. A bee carries her load in both baskets to the hive and pushes pollen into a cell, to be cared for by other workers.

ichneumon wasp is extremely long (Fig. 17-10). The cerci form horny forceps in the earwigs and are long and many jointed in stoneflies and mayflies. Antennae are long in cockroaches and katydids, short in dragonflies and most beetles, knobbed in butterflies, and plumed in most moths. Dobsonflies have greatly enlarged mandibles, which in males resemble long, thin forceps (Fig. 17-11).

Locomotion
Walking

Most insects, when walking, use a triangle of legs involving the first and last leg of one side together with the middle leg of the opposite side. In this way, insects keep three of their six legs on the ground, a tripod arrangement for stability. A slow-moving insect alternates its movement first on one side and then on the other. When it goes faster, the two phases tend to overlap and one side may begin before the other side has finished.

Some insects, such as the water strider *Gerris* (L., *gero*, to carry), are able to walk on the surface of water. The water strider has on its footpads nonwetting hairs that do not break the surface film of water but merely indent it. As it skates along, *Gerris* uses only the two posterior pairs of legs and steers with the anterior pair (Fig. 17-12). The body of the marine water strider *Halobates* (Gr., *halos*, the sea, + *bātes*, one that treads), an excellent surfer on rough ocean waves, is further protected by a water-repellent coat of close-set hairs shaped like thick hooks.

Power of flight

Insects share the power of flight with birds and flying mammals. However, their wings have evolved in a different manner from that of the limb buds of birds and mammals and are not homologous to them. Insect wings are formed by outgrowths from the body wall of the mesothoracic and metathoracic segments and are composed of cuticle.

Most insects have two pairs of wings, but the Diptera (true flies) have only one pair, the hindwings being represented by a pair of tiny **halteres** (balancers) that vibrate and are responsible for equilibrium during flight. Males of order Strepsiptera have only the hind pair of wings and an anterior pair of halteres. The males of the scale insects also have one pair of wings but no halteres. Some insects are wingless. Ants and termites, for example, have wings only on males, and on females during certain periods; workers are always wingless. Lice and fleas are always wingless.

Wings may be thin and membranous, as in flies and many others (Fig. 17-10); thick and horny, such as the front wings of beetles (Fig. 17-9, *A*); parchmentlike, such as the front wings of grasshoppers; covered with fine scales, as in butterflies and moths; or covered with hairs, as in caddis flies.

Wing movements are controlled by a complex of muscles in the thorax. These include some of the largest and strongest of all insect muscles. Dragonflies, orthopterans, moths, butterflies, and some other insects have **direct flight muscles** that insert directly on the base of the wings and control usually the tilting, or "feathering," of the wing. However, in the horizontal wings of the dragonflies they also provide the up and down movements (Fig. 17-13, *A*). Most of the more highly specialized insects have the more powerful **indirect flight muscles**. These include both longitudinal muscles and dorsoventral muscles, which attach to the walls of the thorax instead of directly on the wings. These raise or lower the wings by changing the shape of the thoracic walls (Fig. 17-13, *B*). Contraction of the

A

B

Figure 17-9

A, A giant horned beetle *Diloboderus abderus* (order Coleoptera) from Uruguay. Though the ferocious-looking processes from the head and thorax might appear to be for pinching or stabbing an opponent, they actually are used to lift or pry up a rival of the same species away from resources. **B,** Walking sticks *Diapheromera femorata* (order Orthoptera), mating. This species is common in much of North America. It is wingless, and despite its camouflage as a twig, it is fed upon by numerous predators.
Photographs by K. Sandved.

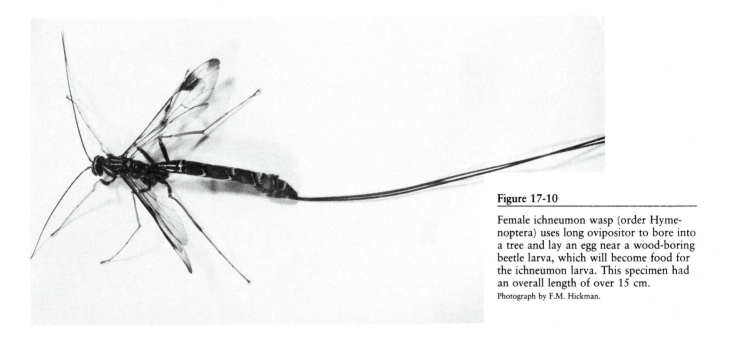

Figure 17-10

Female ichneumon wasp (order Hymenoptera) uses long ovipositor to bore into a tree and lay an egg near a wood-boring beetle larva, which will become food for the ichneumon larva. This specimen had an overall length of over 15 cm.
Photograph by F.M. Hickman.

Figure 17-11

Dobsonfly (order Neuroptera) has aquatic naiad, the hellgrammite, often used by fishermen as bait.
Photograph by C.P. Hickman, Jr.

Figure 17-12

Water strider, *Gerris* sp. (order Hemiptera). The animal is supported on its long, slender legs by the water's surface tension.
Photograph by J.H. Gerard.

longitudinal muscles causes the notum to bulge upward and thus lowers the wings. Contraction of the dorsoventral muscles depresses the notum and forces the wings upward. The wing behaves as a lever, pivoting on the pleural process, and the base of the wing, which projects inward from the pivot, moves as the notum moves but in the opposite direction.

Obviously flying entails more than a simple flapping of the wings; a forward thrust is necessary. As the indirect flight muscles alternate rhythmically to raise and lower the wings, the direct flight muscles alter the angle of the wings so that they act as lifting airfoils during both the upstroke and the downstroke, twisting the leading edge of the wings downward during the downstroke and upward during the upstroke. This produces a figure-eight movement that aids in spilling air from the trailing edges of the wings. The quality of the forward thrust depends, of course, on several factors, such as variations in wing venation, how much the wings are tilted, and how they are feathered.

Flight speeds vary. The fastest flyers usually have narrow, fast-moving wings with a strong tilt and a strong figure-eight component. Sphinx moths and horse-

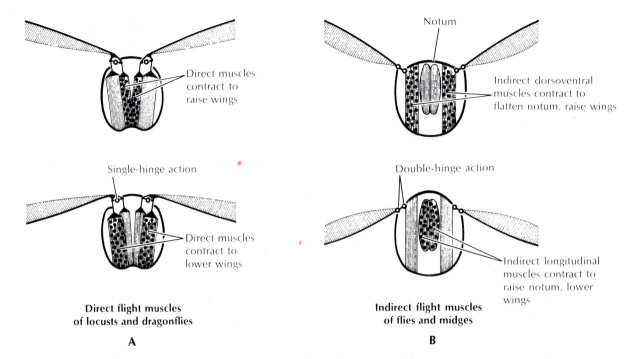

Direct muscles
contract to
raise wings

Single-hinge action

Direct muscles
contract to
lower wings

**Direct flight muscles
of locusts and dragonflies**

A

Notum

Indirect dorsoventral
muscles contract to
flatten notum, raise wings

Double-hinge action

Indirect longitudinal
muscles contract to
raise notum, lower
wings

**Indirect flight muscles
of flies and midges**

B

Figure 17-13

Insect flight muscles. **A,** Direct muscles are attached to the base of the wings at their articulation and raise, lower, or tilt the wings by direct action. **B,** Indirect muscles are attached to the thoracic walls and exert a lever action on the wings by changing the shape of the thorax.

flies are said to achieve approximately 48 km (30 miles) per hour and dragonflies approximately 40 km (25 miles) per hour. Some insects are capable of long continuous flights. The migrating monarch butterfly *Danaus plexippus* (Gr., after Danaus, mythical king of Arabia) (Fig. 17-21) travels south for hundreds of miles in the fall, flying at a speed of approximately 10 km (6 miles) per hour.

The frequency of wing beat also varies. Light insects with large wings, such as butterflies, may beat as few as four times per second. The small wings of heavy insects, such as flies and bees, may vibrate at 100 beats per second or more. The fruit fly *Drosophila* (Gr., *drosos*, dew, + *philos*, loving) can fly at 300 beats per second, and midges have been clocked at more than 1000 beats per second.

_____ Internal Form and Function
Nutrition

The digestive system (Fig. 17-14) consists of a foregut (mouth with salivary glands, esophagus, crop for storage, and gizzard for grinding); a midgut (stomach and gastric ceca); and a hindgut (intestine, rectum, and anus). Since the foregut and hindgut are lined with cuticle, absorption of food takes place largely in the midgut, although some absorption may take place in all sections. The majority of insects feed on plant juices and plant tissues. Such a food habit is called **phytophagous.** Some insects feed on specific plants; others, such as grasshoppers, will eat almost any plant. The caterpillars of many moths and butterflies eat the foliage of only certain plants. Certain species of ants and termites cultivate fungous gardens as a source of food.

Many beetles and the larvae of many insects live on dead animals (**saprophagous**). A number of insects are **predaceous,** catching and eating other insects as well as other types of animals (Fig. 17-7). The so-called predaceous diving beetle *Cybister fimbriolatus* (Gr., *kybistētēr,* diver), however, has been found not to be as predaceous as supposed but is largely a scavenger.

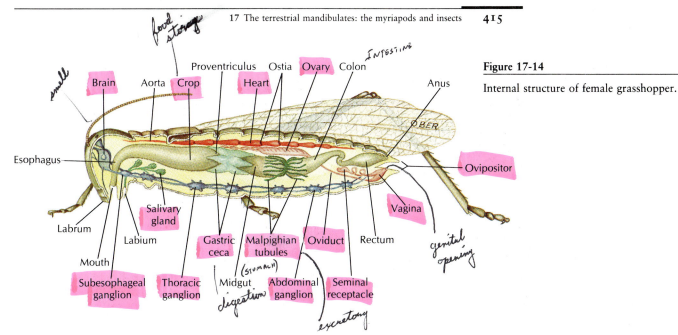

food storge

smell

INTESTINE

ØBER

(STOMACH)

digestion

excretory

genital opening

Figure 17-14

Internal structure of female grasshopper.

Many insects, adults as well as larvae, are **parasitic.** Fleas, for instance, live on the blood of mammals, and the larvae of many varieties of wasps live on spiders and caterpillars (Fig. 17-15). In turn, many are parasitized by other insects. Some of the latter are beneficial to humans by controlling the numbers of injurious insects. Parasitism of parasitic insects by other insects, a condition known as **hyperparasitism,** often becomes quite involved.

For each type of feeding, the mouthparts are adapted in a specialized way. The **sucking mouthparts** are usually arranged in the form of a tube and can pierce the tissues of plants or animals. This arrangement is well shown in the water scorpion (*Ranatra fusca),* a member of the order Hemiptera. This elongated, stick-like insect with a slender caudal respiratory tube has a beak in which there are four piercing, needlelike stylets made up of two mandibles and two maxillae. These parts are fitted together to form two tubes, a salivary tube for injecting saliva into the prey and a food tube for drawing out the body fluid of the prey. The mosquito also combines piercing with needlelike stylets and sucking through a food channel (Fig. 17-16, *B*). In honeybees the labium forms a flexible and contractile "tongue" covered with many hairs. When the bee plunges its proboscis into nectar, the tip of the tongue bends upward and moves back and forth rapidly. Liquid enters the tube by capillarity and is drawn up continuously by a pumping pharynx. In butterflies and moths, mandibles are usually absent, and the maxillae are modified into a long sucking proboscis (Fig. 17-16, *C*) for drawing nectar from flowers. At rest the proboscis is coiled up into a flat spiral. In feeding it is extended, and fluid is pumped up by pharyngeal muscles.

Houseflies, blowflies, and fruit flies have **sponging and lapping mouthparts** (Fig. 17-16, *D*). At the apex of the labium is a pair of large, soft lobes with grooves on the lower surface that serve as food channels. These flies lap up liquid food or liquefy food first with salivary secretions. Horseflies are fitted not only to sponge up surface liquids but to bite into the skin with slender, tapering mandibles and then sponge up blood.

Biting mouthparts such as those of the grasshopper and many other herbivorous insects are adapted for seizing and crushing food (Fig. 17-16, *A*); those of most carnivorous insects are sharp and pointed for piercing their prey. The mandibles of chewing insects are strong, toothed plates whose edges can bite or tear while the maxillae hold the food and pass it toward the mouth. Enzymes secreted by the salivary glands add chemical action to the chewing process.

A

B

Figure 17-15

A, Hornworm, larval stage of a sphinx moth (order Lepidoptera). The more than 100 species of North American sphinx moths are strong fliers and mostly nocturnal feeders. Their larvae, called hornworms because of the large, fleshy posterior spine, are often pests of tomatoes, tobacco, and other plants. **B,** Hornworm parasitized by a tiny wasp *Apanteles,* which laid its egg inside the caterpillar. The wasp larvae have emerged, and their pupae are on the caterpillar's skin. Young wasps emerge in 5 to 10 days, but the caterpillar usually dies.

A, Photograph by C.P. Hickman, Jr.: B, photograph by J.H. Gerard.

The kind of mouthparts an insect has may determine the type of insecticide used in destroying it. For those that bite and chew their food the poison can be applied directly to the food; those that suck may be smothered with gaseous mixtures that interfere with their respiration.

Circulation

A tubular heart in the pericardial cavity (Fig. 17-14) moves hemolymph (blood) forward through the only blood vessel, a dorsal aorta. The heartbeat is a peristaltic wave. Accessory pulsatory organs help move the hemolymph into the wings and legs, and flow is also facilitated by various body movements. The hemolymph consists of plasma and amebocytes and apparently has little to do with oxygen transport.

Gas exchange

Terrestrial animals require efficient respiratory systems that permit rapid oxygen–carbon dioxide exchange but at the same time restrict water loss. In insects this is the function of the **tracheal system,** an extensive network of thin-walled tubes that branch into every part of the body (Fig. 17-17). The tracheal trunks open to the outside by paired **spiracles,** usually two on the thorax and seven or eight on the abdomen. A spiracle may be merely a hole in the integument, as in primary wingless insects, but it is usually provided with a valve or some sort of closing mechanism that cuts down water loss. The evolution of such a device must have been very important in enabling insects to move into drier habitats. The spiracle may also possess a filtering device such as a sieve plate or a set of interlocking bristles that may prevent entrance of water, parasites, or dust into the tracheae. The **tracheae** are composed of a single layer of cells and are lined with cuticle that is shed, along with the outer cuticle, during the molt. They are supported by spiral thickenings of the cuticle (called taenidia) that prevent their collapse. The tracheae branch out into smaller tubes, ending in very fine, fluid-filled tubules called **tracheoles** (not lined with cuticle), which branch into a fine network over the cells. In large insects the largest tracheae may be several millimeters in diameter but taper down to 1 to 2 μm. The tracheoles then taper to 0.5 to 0.1 μm in diameter. In one of the stages of the silkworm larva, it is estimated that there are 1.5 million tracheoles! Scarcely any living cell is located more than a few micrometers away from a tracheole. In fact, the ends of some tracheoles actually indent the membranes of the cells they supply, so that they terminate close to the mitochondria.

**Chewing
(grasshopper)**

**Piercing and sucking
(mosquito)**

Figure 17-16

Four types of insect mouthparts. (See text for description of types and examples.)

**Siphoning tube
(butterfly)**

**Sponging
(housefly)**

The tracheal system affords an efficient system of transport without the use of oxygen-carrying pigments in the hemolymph.

The tracheal system may also include **air sacs,** which appear to be dilated tracheae without taenidia (Fig. 17-18, A). They are thin walled and flexible and are located largely in the body cavity but also in appendages. In some insects the sacs may have functions other than respiratory. For example, they may allow internal organs to change in volume during instar stages without changing the shape of the larvae; they reduce the weight of large insects; or they may act as sound resonators or heat insulators.

In some very small insects, gas transport occurs entirely by diffusion along a concentration gradient. As oxygen is used, a partial vacuum develops in the tracheae and air is sucked in through the spiracles. Larger or more active insects employ some ventilation device for moving air in and out of the tubes. Usually muscular movements in the abdomen perform the pumping action that draws air in or expels it. In some insects—locusts, for example—additional pumping is provided by telescoping the abdomen, pumping with the prothorax, or thrusting the head forward and backward.

The tracheal system is primarily adapted for air breathing, but many insects (nymphs, larvae, and adults) live in water. In small, soft-bodied aquatic nymphs, the gaseous exchange may occur by diffusion through the body wall, usually into and out of a tracheal network just under the integument. The aquatic nymphs of stoneflies and mayflies are equipped with **tracheal gills,** which are thin extensions of the body wall containing a rich tracheal supply. The gills of dragonfly nymphs are ridges in the rectum (rectal gills) where gas exchange occurs as water moves in and out.

Although the diving beetle *Dytiscus* (Gr., *dytikos,* able to swim) can fly, it spends most of its life in the water as an excellent swimmer. It uses an "artificial gill" in the form of a bubble of air held under its wing covers. The bubble is kept stable by a layer of hairs on top of the abdomen and is in contact with the spiracles on the abdomen. Oxygen from the bubble diffuses into the tracheae and is replaced by diffusion of oxygen from the water. Thus, the bubble can last for several hours before the beetle must surface to replace it. Mosquito larvae are not good swimmers but live just below the surface, putting out short breathing tubes like snorkels to the surface for air (Fig. 17-19). Spreading oil on the water, a favorite method of mosquito control, clogs the tracheae with oil and so suffocates the larvae. "Rattailed maggots" of the syrphid flies have an extensible tail that can stretch as much as 15 cm to the water surface.

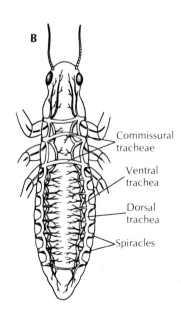

Figure 17-17

A, Relationship of spiracle, tracheae, taenidia (chitinous bands that strengthen the tracheae), and tracheoles (diagrammatic). **B,** Generalized arrangement of insect tracheal system (diagrammatic). Air sacs and tracheoles not shown.

Figure 17-18

Malpighian tubules of insect. **A,** Malpighian tubules are located at the juncture of the midgut and hindgut (rectum) as shown in the cutaway view of a wasp. **B,** Function of malpighian tubules. Solutes, especially potassium, are actively secreted into the tubules. Water and wastes follow. This fluid moves into the rectum where solutes and water are actively resorbed, leaving wastes to be excreted.

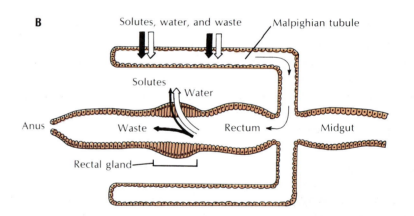

Excretion and water balance

Insects and spiders have a unique excretory system consisting of **malpighian tubules** that operate in conjunction with specialized glands in the wall of the rectum. The malpighian tubules, variable in number, are thin, elastic, blind tubules attached to the juncture between the midgut and hindgut (Figs. 17-14 and 17-18, *A*). The free ends of the tubules lie free in the hemocoel and are bathed in hemolymph.

Since the malpighian tubules are closed and lack an arterial supply, urine formation cannot be initiated by hemolymph ultrafiltration as in the crustaceans and vertebrates. Instead potassium is actively secreted into the tubules (Fig. 17-18, *B*). This primary secretion of ions pulls water along with it by osmosis to produce a potassium-rich fluid. Other solutes and waste materials also are secreted or diffuse into the tubule. The fluid, or "urine," then drains from the tubules into the intestine. In the rectum, specialized rectal glands actively resorb potassium and water as needed, leaving behind wastes such as uric acid.

Since water requirements vary among different types of insects, this ability to cycle water and salts is very important. Insects living in dry environments may resorb nearly all water from the rectum, producing a nearly dry mixture of urine

A B

Figure 17-19

A, Mosquito *Culex* (order Diptera) lays her eggs in small packets or rafts on the surface of standing or slowly moving water. **B,** Mosquito larvae are the familiar wrigglers of ponds and ditches. To breathe, they hang head down, with respiratory tubes projecting through the surface film of water. Motion of vibratile tufts of fine hairs on the head brings a constant supply of food.

From *Mosquito,* an Encyclopaedia Britannica film.

and feces. Leaf-feeding insects take in and excrete quantities of fluid. Freshwater larvae need to excrete water and conserve salts. Insects that feed on dry grains need to conserve water and excrete salt.

Nervous system

The nervous system in general resembles that of the larger crustaceans, with a similar tendency toward fusion of ganglia (Fig. 17-14). A giant fiber system has been demonstrated in a number of insects. There is also a stomodeal nervous system that corresponds in function to the autonomic nervous system of vertebrates. Neurosecretory cells located in various parts of the brain have an endocrine function, but, except for their role in molting and metamorphosis, little is known of their activity.

Sense organs

Along with neuromuscular coordination, insects have unusually keen sensory perception. Their sense organs are mostly microscopic and are located chiefly in the body wall. Each type usually responds to a specific stimulus. The various organs are receptive to mechanical, auditory, chemical, visual, and other stimuli.

Mechanoreception

Mechanical stimuli, or those dealing with touch, pressure, vibration, and the like, are picked up by sensilla. A sensillum may be simply a seta, or hair, connected with a nerve cell process, a nerve ending just under the cuticle and lacking a seta, or a more complex organ (scolopophorous organ) consisting of sensory cells with their endings attached to the body wall. Such organs are widely distributed over the antennae, legs, and body.

Auditory reception

Airborne sounds may be detected by very sensitive hairs (hair sensilla) or by tympanal organs. In tympanal organs a number of sensory cells (ranging from a few to hundreds) extend to a very thin tympanic membrane that encloses an air space in which vibrations can be detected. Tympanal organs are found in certain Orthoptera (Fig. 17-4), Homoptera, and Lepidoptera. Some insects are fairly insensitive to airborne sounds but can detect vibrations reaching them through the substrate. Vibrations of the substrate are detected by organs usually on the legs.

A

B

Figure 17-20

Copulation in insects (see also Fig. 17-9, *B*). **A,** Bluet damselflies *Enallagma* sp. (order Odonata) are common throughout North America. **B,** *Omura congrua* (order Orthoptera) are a kind of grasshopper found in Brazil.

Photographs by K. Sandved.

Chemoreception

Chemoreceptors (for taste or smell) are usually bundles of sensory cell processes that are often located in sensory pits. These are usually on mouthparts, but in ants, bees, and wasps they are also found on the antennae, and butterflies, moths, and flies also have them on the legs. The chemical sense is generally keen, and some insects can detect certain odors for several kilometers. Many of the patterns of insect behavior such as feeding, mating, habitat selection, and host-parasite relations are mediated through the chemical senses. These senses are also involved in the responses of insects to man-made repellents and attractants.

Visual reception

Insect eyes are of two types, simple and compound. Simple eyes are found in some nymphs and larvae and in many adults. Most insects have three ocelli on the head. Recent experiments indicate that the honeybee uses them to monitor light intensity but not to form images.

Compound eyes are found in most adults and may cover most of the head. They consist of thousands of ommatidia—6300 in the eye of a honeybee, for example. The structure of the compound eye is similar to that of crustaceans (Fig. 16-10). An insect such as a honeybee can see simultaneously in almost all directions around its body, but it is more myopic than the human, and images, even of nearby objects, are fuzzy. However, most flying insects rate much higher than humans in flicker-fusion tests. Flickers of light become fused in the human eye at a frequency of 45 to 55 per second, but bees and blowflies can distinguish as many as 200 to 300 separate flashes of light per second. This should be an advantage in analyzing a fast-changing landscape during flight.

A bee can distinguish colors, but its sensitivity begins in the ultraviolet range, which the human eye cannot see, and extends into the orange; the honeybee cannot distinguish shades of red from shades of gray.

Other senses

Insects also have well-developed senses for temperature, especially on the antennae and legs, and for humidity, proprioception, gravity, and others.

Neuromuscular coordination

Insects are active creatures with excellent neuromuscular coordination. Arthropod muscles are typically cross-striated, just as vertebrate skeletal muscles are. A flea can leap a distance of 100 times its own length, and an ant can carry in its jaws a load greater than its own weight. This sounds as though insect muscle were stronger than that of other animals. Actually, however, the force a particular muscle can exert is related directly to its cross-sectional area, not its length. Based on maximum load moved per square centimeter of cross section, the strength of insect muscle is relatively the same as that of vertebrate muscle.

Reproduction

Sexes are separate in insects, and fertilization is usually internal. Insects have various means of attracting mates. The female moth gives off a powerful pheromone that can be detected for a great distance by the male. Fireflies use flashes of light; some insects find each other by means of sounds or color signals and by various kinds of courtship behavior.

A

B

C

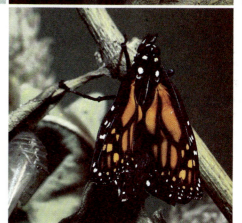

D

Sperm are usually deposited in the vagina of the female at the time of copulation (Fig. 17-20). In some orders the sperm are encased in spermatophores that may be transferred at copulation or deposited on the substratum to be picked up by the female. The silverfish deposits a spermatophore on the ground, then spins signal threads to guide the female to it. During evolutionary transition from aquatic to terrestrial life, spermatophores were widely used, with copulation evolving much later.

Usually the sperm are stored in the spermatheca of the female in numbers sufficient to fertilize more than one batch of eggs. Many insects mate only once during their lifetime, and none mates more than a few times.

Insects usually lay a great many eggs. The queen honeybee, for example, may lay more than 1 million eggs during her lifetime. On the other hand, some flies are viviparous and bring forth only a single offspring at a time. Insect forms that make no provision for the care of their young may lay many more eggs than do insects that provide for their young or those that have a very short life cycle.

Most species normally lay their eggs in a particular type of place to which they are guided by visual, chemical, or other clues. Butterflies and moths lay their eggs on the specific kind of plant on which the caterpillar must feed (p. 405). The tiger moth may look for a pigweed, the sphinx moth for a tomato or tobacco plant, and the monarch butterfly for a milkweed plant (Fig. 17-21). Insects whose immature stages are aquatic lay their eggs in water (Fig. 17-19, *A*). A tiny braconid wasp lays her eggs on the caterpillar of the sphinx moth where they will feed and pupate in tiny white cocoons (Fig. 17-15). The ichneumon wasp, with unerring accuracy, seeks out a certain kind of larva in which her young will live as internal parasites. Her long ovipositors may have to penetrate 1 to 2 cm of wood to find the larva of a wood wasp or a wood-boring beetle in which she will deposit her eggs (Fig. 17-22).

Figure 17-21

Complete metamorphosis. **A,** Monarch butterfly, *Danaus plexippus* (order Lepidoptera), lays eggs on a milkweed plant. **B,** Hatched larva feeds on milkweed leaves. **C,** When mature, the larva hangs on the milkweed plant and transforms into a chrysalis, or pupa, an inactive stage that does not feed and is covered by a cocoon or protective covering. **D,** Adult has emerged. The wings quickly expand and harden, pigmentation develops, and the butterfly goes on its way.

A, Photograph by C.P. Hickman, Jr.; **B** to D, photographs by J.H. Gerard.

Figure 17-22

An ichneumon wasp with the end of the abdomen raised to thrust her long ovipositor into wood to find a tunnel made by the larva of a wood wasp or wood-boring beetle. She can bore 13 mm or more into the wood to lay her eggs in the larva of the wood-boring beetle, which will become host for her own larvae. Other ichneumon species attack spiders, moths, flies, crickets, caterpillars, and others. (See also Fig. 17-10.)

Photograph by L.L. Rue, III.

Metamorphosis and Growth

Early development occurs within the egg, and the hatching young escape from the egg in various ways. During the postembryonic development most insects change in form; that is, they undergo **metamorphosis** (Fig. 17-21). During this period they must undergo a number of molts in order to grow, and each stage of the insect between molts is called an **instar.**

Although metamorphosis is not limited to insects, insects illustrate it more dramatically than any other group. The transformation, for instance, of the hickory horned devil caterpillar into the beautiful royal walnut moth represents an astonishing morphological change in development. In insects metamorphosis is associated with the evolution of wings, which are restricted to the reproductive stage where they can be of the most benefit. Not all insects undergo metamorphosis, but most of them do in some form or other.

Complete metamorphosis

Approximately 88% of insects undergo a complete metamorphosis, which separates the physiological processes of growth (**larva**) from those of differentiation (**pupa**) and reproduction (**adult**) (Fig. 17-21). Each stage functions efficiently without competition with the other stages, for the larvae often live in entirely different surroundings and eat different foods from the adults. The wormlike larvae, which usually have chewing mouthparts, are known as caterpillars, maggots, bagworms, fuzzy worms, grubs, and so on. After a series of instar stages during which the wings are developing internally, the larva forms a case or cocoon about itself and becomes a pupa, or chrysalis, a nonfeeding stage in which many insects pass the winter. When the final molt occurs over winter, the full-grown adult emerges, pale and with wings wrinkled. In a short time the wings expand and harden, and the insect is on its way. The stages, then, are egg, larva (several instars), pupa, and adult. The adult undergoes no further molting. Insects that undergo complete metamorphosis are said to be **holometabolous** (Gr., *holo*, complete + *metabolē*, change).

Gradual metamorphosis

Some insects undergo a type of gradual, or incomplete, metamorphosis. These include the grasshoppers, cicadas, and mantids, which have terrestrial young, and mayflies, stoneflies, and dragonflies, which lay their eggs in water. The young are

Figure 17-23

A, Ecdysis in the dog-day cicada, *Tibicen pruinosa* (order Homoptera). The old cuticle splits along a dorsal midline as a result of increased blood pressure and of air forced into the thorax by muscle contraction. The emerging insect is pale, and its new cuticle is soft. The wings will be expanded by blood pumped into veins, and the insect enlarges by taking in air. **B,** Seventeen-year cicada, *Magicicada septendecim.*

A, Photograph by J.H. Gerard; **B,** photograph by L.L. Rue, III.

A   B

called **nymphs** (or **naiads** if aquatic), and their wings develop externally as budlike outgrowths in the early instars and increase in size as the animal grows by successive molts and becomes a winged adult (Fig. 17-23). The aquatic naiads have tracheal gills or other modifications for aquatic life (Fig. 17-24). The stages are egg, nymph (several instars), and adult. Insects that undergo gradual metamorphosis are called **hemimetabolous** (Gr., *hemi*, half, + *metabolē*, change).

Epimorphosis

A few insects, such as silverfish and springtails, undergo epimorphosis (p. 390). The young, or juveniles, are similar to the adults except in size. The stages are egg, juvenile, and adult. Such insects include the wingless insects (apterygote orders).

Physiology of metamorphosis

Metamorphosis in insects is controlled and regulated by hormones. Three major endocrine organs are involved in development through the larval stages to the pupa and eventually to the emergence of the adult. These organs are the **brain,** the **prothoracic (ecdysial) glands,** and the **corpora allata** (Fig. 33-5, p. 796).

The intercerebral part of the brain and the ganglia of the nerve cord contain several groups of neurosecretory cells that produce an endocrine substance called the **brain hormone (prothoracicotropic hormone).** These neurosecretory cells may send their axons to paired organs behind the brain, the **corpora allata,** which serve as a storage place for the brain hormone. The brain hormone is carried in the hemolymph to the prothoracic gland, a glandular organ in the head or the prothorax that is stimulated to produce the **molting hormone,** or ecdysone (ek'duh-sone). This hormone sets in motion certain processes that lead to the casting off of the old skin (ecdysis) by proliferation of the epidermal cells.

If the larval form is retained at the end of this process, it is called simple molting; if the insect undergoes changes into pupa or adult, it may be referred to as metamorphosis. Simple molting persists as long as a certain **juvenile hormone** (neotenine) is present in sufficient amounts, along with the molting hormone in the hemolymph, and each molting simple produces a larger larva. The juvenile hormone is produced by the corpora allata (Fig. 33-5).

Even the kind of cuticle produced depends on the amount of juvenile hormone present. If only a small amount of this hormone is present, a pupal cuticle is the result. When the corpora allata cease to produce the juvenile hormone, the molting hormone alone is secreted into the hemolymph and the adult emerges (metamorphosis). Thus, the molting hormone is necessary for each molt but is modified by the juvenile hormone, whose action is to maintain larval characters in the young insect.

Experimental evidence shows that when the corpora allata (and thus the juvenile hormone) are removed surgically from the larva, the following molt will result in metamorphosis into the adult. Conversely, if the corpora allata from a young larva are transplanted into an old larva, the latter can be converted into a giant larva, because metamorphosis to the pupa or adult stage cannot occur. Many other experimental modifications on this theme have been performed. Progress has also been made in determining the chemical nature of the hormones (p. 796).

The mechanism of molting and metamorphosis just described is that found

A

B

C

Figure 17-24

A, Stonefly, *Perla* sp. (order Plecoptera). B, Ten-spot dragonfly, *Libellula pulchella* (order Odonata). C, Naiad of dragonfly. Both stoneflies and dragonflies have aquatic larvae, called naiads, which undergo gradual metamorphosis.

A, Photograph by C.P. Hickman, Jr.; B, photograph by J.H. Gerard; C, courtesy Carolina Biological Supply Co., Burlington, N.C.

A   B

Figure 17-25

Mimicry in butterflies. **A,** Monarch butterfly is distasteful to, and avoided by, birds because as a caterpillar it fed on the acrid milkweed. **B,** It is mimicked by the smaller viceroy butterfly, *Limenitis archippus,* which feeds on willows and is presumably tasteful to birds, but is not eaten because it so closely resembles the monarch in color and markings. This kind of mimicry is called "Batesian" mimicry.
Photographs by J.H. Gerard.

in holometabolous insects, but the same factors also apply in general to the molting nymphal stages of hemimetabolous insects, in which there are no pupal stages. A recent method of insect control involves the use of compounds that mimic the juvenile hormones. These prevent insects from becoming sexually competent when treated just before they become adults.

What factors initiate the sequence of secretion and the role of these three different hormones? How are they correlated with cyclical events in the life histories of insects? Experimentally it has been shown that in some insects low temperature activates the neurosecretory cells of the intercerebral gland of the brain, which then sets in motion the sequence of events already related. The chilling of the brain seems to be all important in the initiation of metamorphosis. Adults do not molt and grow, since the ecdysial glands degenerate after the last ecdysis. Many aspects of the control mechanism of these interesting processes have not yet been worked out.

___ Diapause

Many animals, including many types of insects, undergo a period of dormancy in their annual life cycle. In temperate zones there may be a period of winter dormancy, called hibernation, or a period of summer dormancy, called estivation, or both. It is well known that there are periods in the life cycle of many insects when eggs, larvae, pupae, or even adults remain dormant for a long time because external conditions of climate, moisture, and the like are too harsh or unfavorable for survival in states of normal activity. Thus, the life cycle is synchronized with periods of suitable environmental conditions and abundance of food. Most insects enter such a state when some factor of the environment, such as temperature, becomes unfavorable, and the state continues until conditions again become favorable.

Some species, however, become dormant at a certain time *before* conditions become unsuitable and remain so for a definite period, even if conditions do not change. This type of dormancy is called **diapause** (di'a-poz) (Gr., *dia,* through, dividing into two parts, + *pausis,* a stopping). Diapause, or the capacity to anticipate periods of stressful conditions, is genetically determined in each species but is set off by some certain signal. The most constant and reliable indicator of extensive temperature changes to come is the lengthening or shortening of the days. It is not surprising, then, that photoperiod, or day length, is often the signal that initiates diapause. The arrival of a critical length of day starts the physiological machinery for establishing diapause, which continues until the proper day length or other signal is received. In the American silkworm *Hyalophora* the pupa goes into diapause. Activity is resumed *only* if the pupa is chilled for approximately 10 weeks at 3° to 5° C, after which the final metamorphosis occurs. In this instance chilling seems to be the necessary stimulus for the resumption of neurosecretory action and ecdysone production; no juvenile hormone is produced at the end of diapause.

Sometimes in insects a distinction is made between this obligatory type of dormancy, known as **primary** or **obligatory diapause,** and the dormancy that is initiated directly by stressful environmental conditions, which is then called **facultative diapause.**

Diapause always occurs at the end of an active growth stage of the molting cycle so that, when the diapause period is over, the insect is ready for another molt. One species of the ant *Myrmica* reaches the third instar stage in late summer. Many of the larvae do not develop beyond this point until the following spring, even if temperatures are mild or if the larvae are kept in a warm laboratory.

Protection

Insects as a group display many colors. This is especially true of butterflies, moths, and beetles. Even in the same species the color pattern may vary in a seasonal way, and there also may be color differences between males and females. Some of the color patterns in insects are probably highly adaptive, such as those for **protective coloration, warning coloration,** and **mimicry** (Figs. 17-25 and 17-26).

Besides color, insects have other methods of protecting themselves. The cuticular exoskeleton affords good protection for many of them; some, such as stinkbugs, have repulsive odors and tastes; others protect themselves by a good offense, for many are very aggressive and can put up a good fight (for example, bees and ants); and still others are swift in running for cover when danger threatens.

Monarch butterflies (Fig. 17-25, *A*) are known to be poisonous to birds because their caterpillars assimilate cardiac glycosides from certain species of milkweed (Asclepiadaceae). This substance confers unpalatability on the butterflies after metamorphosis and induces vomiting in their predators. Certain leaf beetles that are toxic or unpalatable to their predators produce defensive secretions containing cardiac glycosides, which are not sequestered from their foods but are synthesized by the beetles themselves. Bats detect their insect prey by echolocation, but certain moths have evolved special ultrasonic ears (tympanic membranes) by which they can pick up the bat chirps and thus evade capture (Fig. 32-22, p. 781).

Many insects practice chemical warfare in a variety of ingenious ways. Some use chemical exudates that repel an assault because of their bad taste, odor, or poisonous properties or that mechanically prevent a predator from attacking. When certain aphids are touched by a parasitic wasp, they secrete a waxy substance that hardens in air and may fatally entangle the wasp. A social wasp of the American tropics hangs its comb from the end of a very thin stalk, then secretes onto the stalk a repellent from its abdominal gland. Its comb is then safe from marauding ants, which will not walk down the treated stalk.

Some repellents are injected directly into the enemy. The stings of bees,

A

B

C

Figure 17-26

Camouflage in insects. **A,** *Estigena pardalis* (order Lepidoptera) in Java resembles a dead leaf. **B,** Bizarre processes from the thorax of a treehopper from Mexico, *Sphongophorus* sp. (order Homoptera), masquerade as parts of the twig where it feeds. **C,** Broken outlines and color of a katydid (*Dysonia* sp., order Orthoptera) in Costa Rica give it the appearance of the leaves on which it has been feeding.

Photographs by K. Sandved.

wasps, and ants are good examples. The bombardier beetle, on the other hand, produces an irritating spray that it aims accurately at attacking ants or other enemies.

Migration

Some insect species practice seasonal mass movements somewhat similar to the migrations of birds, except that the migrating individuals do not usually make the return flight; this is made by members of the next generation. The monarch butterfly *Danaus plexippus* is among the best known of the migratory insects. In late summer they start the southern flight from all over the United States and Canada. The farther they go, the more numerous they become, with huge swarms of them congregating in some places. They winter in the southern United States and Mexico and reproduce there or on the spring flight north. Most of the adult monarchs that drift southward in the fall have developed during the preceding summer. In the spring they spread northward, following the emergence of milkweed, the only food the caterpillars can eat. Several generations are produced during the summer. Each new hatch flies farther north, mates, and lays its eggs. The caterpillars hatch, grow fat on milkweed, and pupate. Butterflies from the last hatch to emerge in the fall do not mate but instead use their energy to migrate south. By tagging the wings of thousands of monarchs, it has been determined that some of them make flights of close to 3200 km (about 2000 miles).

In California the ladybug beetles, which have been of great help in conquering the scale insect, migrate from the valleys to the mountains for a part of their life cycle. Some insects breed in the south, then migrate north in the spring and summer. Some breed in the north but do not winter there. Among such migrating insects are certain leafhoppers and noctuid moths. Mass migrations of grasshoppers have been known since biblical times. They used to occur in the United States but have been uncommon in the past century. Such mass migrations have involved billions of individuals and covered thousands of square miles, with the grasshoppers eating everything in sight wherever they landed.

Behavior and Communication

The keen sensory perceptions of insects make them extremely responsive to many stimuli. The stimuli may be internal (physiological) or external (environmental), and the responses are governed by both the physiological state of the animal and the pattern of nerve pathways traveled by the impulses. Many of the responses are simple, such as orientation toward or away from the stimulus, for example, attraction of a moth to light, avoidance of light by a cockroach, or attraction of carrion flies to the odor of dead flesh.

Much of the behavior of insects, however, is not a simple matter of orientation but involves a complex series of responses. A pair of tumble bugs, or dung beetles, chews off a bit of dung, rolls it into a ball, and rolls the ball laboriously to where they intend to bury it, after laying their eggs in it (Fig. 17-27). The cicada slits the bark of a twig and then lays an egg in each of the slits. The female potter wasp *Eumenes* scoops up clay into pellets, carries them one by one to her building site, and fashions them into dainty little narrow-necked clay pots, into each of which she lays an egg. Then she hunts and paralyzes a number of caterpillars, pokes them into the opening of a pot, and closes up the opening with clay. Each egg, in its own protective pot, hatches to find a well-stocked larder of food.

Figure 17-27

Tumble bugs, or dung beetles, *Canthon pilularis* (order Coleoptera), chew off a bit of dung, roll it into a ball, and then roll it to where they will bury it in soil. One beetle pushes while the other pulls. Eggs are laid in the ball, and the larvae feed on the dung. Tumble bugs are black, an inch or less in length, and common in pasture fields.

Photograph by J.H. Gerard.

Much of such behavior is "innate"; that is, entire sequences of actions apparently have been genetically programmed. However, a great deal more learning is involved than was once believed. The potter wasp, for example, must learn where she has left her pots if she is to return to fill them with caterpillars one at a time. Social insects, which have been studied extensively, have been found capable of most of the basic forms of learning used by mammals. The exception is insight learning. Apparently insects, when faced with a new problem, cannot reorganize their memories to construct a new response.

Insects communicate with other members of their species by means of chemical, visual, auditory, and tactile signals. **Chemical signals** take the form of **pheromones,** which are substances secreted by one individual that affect the behavior or physiological processes of another individual. Pheromones include sex attractants, releasers of certain behavior patterns, trail markers, alarm signals, territorial markers, and the like. Like hormones, pheromones are effective in minute quantities. Social insects, such as bees, ants, wasps, and termites, can recognize a nestmate—or an alien in the nest—by means of identification pheromones. An intruder from another species is violently attacked at once. If the intruder is from the same species but another colony, there may be a variety of responses. It may be attacked and killed; it may be investigated but finally accepted; or it may be accepted but given less food than the others until it has had time to acquire the colony odor. Caste determination in termites, and to some extent in ants and bees, is determined by pheromones. In fact, pheromones are probably a primary integrating force in populations of social insects. Many insect pheromones have been extracted and chemically identified.

Sound production and **reception** (phonoproduction and phonoreception) in insects have been studied extensively, and it is evident that, although a sense of hearing is not present in all insects, this means of communication is meaningful to insects that use it. Sounds serve as warning devices, advertisement of territorial claims, or courtship songs. The sounds of crickets and grasshoppers seem to be concerned with courtship and aggression. Grasshoppers rub the femur of the third pair of legs over the ridges of the forewings. Male crickets scrape the rough edges of the forewings together to produce their characteristic chirping. The hum of mosquitoes is caused by the rapid vibration of their wings. The long, drawn-out sound of the male cicada, a recruitment call, is produced by the vibrating membranes in a pair of organs on the ventral side of the basal abdominal segment.

Certain kinds of flies, springtails, and beetles manufacture their own **visual signals** in the form of **bioluminescence.** The best known of the luminescent beetles are the fireflies, or lightning bugs (which are neither flies nor bugs, but beetles), in which the flash of light is a means of locating a prospective mate. Each species has its own characteristic flashing rhythm produced on the ventral side of the last abdominal segments. The male flashes his species-specific pattern while flying. If a female flashes the proper answer after the appropriate interval, he flies toward her, giving his signal again. The dialogue usually culminates in copulation. An interesting instance of aggressive mimicry has been observed in females of several species of *Photuris,* which prey on male fireflies of other species by mimicking the female mating signals of the prey species and then capturing and devouring the luckless males that court them (Fig. 17-28).

There are many forms of **tactile communication,** such as tapping, stroking, grasping, and antennae touching, which evoke responses varying from recognition to recruitment and alarm. The food-begging behavior of the larvae of the ant *Formica* is to tap the mandibles of the worker with their own mouthparts, trig-

Some insects can memorize and perform in sequence tasks involving multiple signals in various sensory areas. Worker honeybees have been trained to walk through mazes that involved five turns in sequence, using such clues as the color of a marker, the distance between two spots, or the angle of a turn. The same is true of ants. Workers of one species of *Formica* learned a six-point maze at a rate only two or three times slower than that of laboratory rats. The foraging trips of ants and bees often wind and loop about in a circuitous route, but once the forager has found food, the return trip is relatively direct. One investigator suggests that the continuous series of calculations necessary to figure the angles, directions, distance, and speed of the trip and to convert it into a direct return could involve a stopwatch, a compass, and integral vector calculus. How the insect does it is unknown.

Figure 17-28

Firefly femme fatale, *Photuris versicolor,* eating a male *Photinus tanytoxus,* which she has attracted with false mating signals.
Photograph by J.E. Lloyd.

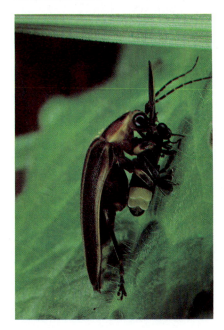

gering the regurgitation of liquid food by the worker. When an adult *Formica* worker taps another worker with its antennae, the signal is to stop moving about.

Social behavior

Insects rank very high in the animal kingdom in their organization of social groups, and cooperation within the more complex groups depends heavily on chemical and tactile communication. Social communities are not all complex, however. Some community groups are temporary and uncoordinated, as are the hibernating associations of carpenter bees or the feeding gatherings of aphids. Some are coordinated for only brief periods, such as the mating swarms of mosquitoes or mayflies. Others cooperate more fully, such as the tent caterpillars *Malacosoma,* which not only gather in sleeping and feeding communities but join in building a home web and a feeding net. However, even these are still open communities, and their social behavior is limited to the larval stage of the life cycle.

In the true societies of some orders, such as the Hymenoptera (honeybees and ants) and Isoptera (termites), a complex social life is necessary for the perpetuation of the species. Such societies are closed. In them all stages of the life cycle are involved, the communities are usually permanent, all activities are collective, and there is reciprocal communication. There is a high degree of efficiency in the division of labor. Such a society is essentially a family group in which the mother or perhaps both parents remain with the young, sharing the duties of the group in a cooperative manner. The society is usually characterized by polymorphism, or **caste** differentiation, along with differences in behavior that are associated with the division of labor.

The honeybees have one of the most complex organizations in the insect world. Instead of lasting one season, their organization continues for a more or less indefinite period. As many as 60,000 to 70,000 honeybees may be found in a single hive. Of these, there are three castes: a single sexually mature female, or **queen;** a few hundred **drones,** which are sexually mature males; and the **workers,** which are sexually inactive genetic females (Fig. 17-29).

The workers take care of the young, secrete wax with which they build the six-sided cells of the honeycomb, gather the nectar from flowers, manufacture honey, collect pollen, and ventilate and guard the hive. Each worker appears to be responsible for a specific task, depending on its age, but during its lifetime of a few weeks it performs all of the various tasks.

One drone, sometimes more, fertilizes the queen during the mating flight, at which time enough sperm is stored in her spermatheca to last her a lifetime. Drones have no stings and are usually driven out or killed by the workers at the end of the summer. A queen may live as long as five seasons, laying thousands of eggs in that time. She is responsible for keeping the hive going through the winter, and only one reigning queen is tolerated in a hive at one time.

Castes are determined partly by fertilization and partly by what is fed to the larvae. Drones develop from unfertilized eggs (and consequently are haploid); queens and workers develop from fertilized eggs (and thus are diploid). Female larvae that are destined to become queens are fed royal jelly, a secretion from the salivary glands of the nurse workers. Royal jelly differs from the "worker jelly" fed to ordinary larvae, but the components in it that are essential for queen determination have not yet been identified. Honey and pollen are added to the worker

Figure 17-29

Queen bee surrounded by her court. The queen is the only egg layer in the colony. The attendants, attracted by her pheromones, constantly lick her body. As food is transferred from these bees to others, the queen's presence is communicated throughout the colony.

Photograph by K. Lorenzen © 1979. Educational Images, Lyons Falls, N.Y.

Figure 17-30

A, Termite workers, *Reticulitermes flavipes* (order Isoptera), eating yellow pine. Workers are wingless sterile adults that tend the nest, care for the young, and so forth. **B,** Termite queen (*Macrotermes bellicosus* from Ghana) becomes a distended egg-laying machine. The queen and several workers and soldiers are shown here.
A, Photograph by J.H. Gerard; **B,** photograph by K. Sandved.

diet about the third day of larval life. Female workers are prevented from maturing sexually by pheromones in the "queen substance," which is produced by the queen's mandibular glands. Royal jelly is produced by the workers only when the level of "queen substance" pheromone in the colony drops. This occurs when the queen becomes too old, dies, or is removed. Then the workers' ovaries develop, and they start enlarging a larval cell and feeding the larva the royal jelly that produces a new queen.

Honeybees have evolved an efficient system of communication by which, through certain body movements, their scouts inform the workers of the location and quantity of food sources (Fig. 34-18, p. 828).

Termite colonies contain several castes, consisting of fertile individuals, both males and females, and sterile individuals (Fig. 17-30). Some of the fertile individuals may have wings and may leave the colony, mate, lose their wings, and as **king** and **queen** start a new colony. Wingless fertile individuals may under certain conditions substitute for the king or queen. Sterile members are wingless and become **workers** and **soldiers.** Soldiers have large heads and mandibles and serve for the defense of the colony. As in bees and ants, caste differentiation is caused by extrinsic factors. Reproductive individuals and soldiers secrete inhibiting pheromones that are passed throughout the colony to the nymphs through a mutual feeding process, called **trophallaxis,** so that they become sterile workers. Workers also produce pheromones, and if the level of "worker substance" or "soldier substance" falls, as might happen after an attack by marauding predators, for example, compensating proportions of the appropriate caste are produced in the next generation.

The phenomenon of trophallaxis, or exchange of nutrients, appears to be common among all social insects because it integrates the colony by passage of pheromones. The process involves feeding of the young by the queen and workers, which in turn may receive a drop of saliva from the young. It may also involve mutual licking, grooming, and the like.

Ants also have highly organized societies. Superficially, they resemble termites, but they are quite different (belong to a different order) and can be distin-

Figure 17-31

Ants attending treehopper nymphs on a
jackfruit in Brazil.
Photograph by K. Sandved.

guished easily. In contrast to termites, ants are usually dark in color, are hard
bodied, and have a constriction between the thorax and abdomen.

In ant colonies the males die soon after mating and the queen either starts
her own new colony or joins some established colony and does the egg laying. The
sterile females are wingless workers and soldiers that do the work of the colony:
gather food, care for the young, and protect the colony. In many larger colonies
there may be two or three types of individuals within each caste.

Ants have a varied diet. In some the larvae are the real food digesters for the
colony, since they can digest solid food and the adults feed on liquid foods. Nutrients are distributed among the members by means of trophallaxis.

Ants have evolved some striking patterns of "economic" behavior, such as
making slaves, farming fungi, herding "ant cows" (aphids or other homopterans)
(Fig. 17-31), sewing their nests together with silk, and using tools.

Insects and Human Welfare

Beneficial insects

Although most of us think of insects primarily as pests, humanity would have
great difficulty in surviving if all insects were suddenly to disappear. Some of them
produce useful materials: honey and beeswax from bees, silk from silkworms, and
shellac from a wax secreted by the lac insects. More important, however, insects
are necessary for the cross-fertilization of many fruits and other crops.

Very early in their evolution, insects and higher plants formed a relationship
of mutual adaptations that have been to each other's advantage. Insects exploit
flowers for food, and flowers exploit insects for pollination. Each floral development of petal and sepal arrangement is correlated with the sensory adjustment of
certain pollinating insects. Among these mutual adaptations are amazing devices
of allurements, traps, specialized structures, and precise timing.

Many predaceous insects, such as tiger beetles, aphid lions, ant lions, praying mantids, and lady bird beetles, destroy harmful insects. Some insects control
harmful ones by parasitizing them or by laying their eggs where their young, when

Figure 17-32

Fly maggots (order Diptera) feeding on a
deer carcass.
Photograph by L.L. Rue, III.

hatched, may devour the host. Dead animals are quickly consumed by maggots hatched from eggs laid in carcasses (Fig. 17-32).

Insects and their larvae serve as an important source of food for many birds, fish, and other animals.

Harmful insects

Harmful insects include those that eat and destroy plants and fruits, such as grasshoppers, chinch bugs, corn borers, boll weevils, grain weevils, San Jose scale, and scores of others (Fig. 17-33). Practically every cultivated crop has some insect pest. Lice, bloodsucking flies, warble flies, botflies, and many others attack humans or domestic animals or both. Malaria, carried by the *Anopheles* mosquito, is still one of the world's killers; yellow fever and filariasis are also transmitted by mosquitoes. Fleas carry plague, which at many times in history has almost wiped out whole human populations. The housefly is the vector for typhoid, as is the louse for typhus fever; the tsetse fly carries African sleeping sickness; and a bloodsucking bug, *Rhodnius,* is a carrier of Chagas' disease. In addition there is tremendous destruction of food, clothing, and property by weevils, cockroaches, ants, clothes moths, termites, and carpet beetles. Not the least of the insect pests is the bedbug, *Cimex,* a bloodsucking hemipterous insect that humans may have contracted, probably early in their evolution, from bats that shared their caves.

Control of insects

Because all insects are an integral part of the ecological communities to which they belong, their total destruction would probably do more harm than good. Food chains would be disturbed, some of our most loved birds would disappear, and the biological cycles by which dead animal and plant matter disintegrates and returns to enrich the soil would be seriously impeded. The beneficial role of insects in our environment has often been overlooked, and in our zeal to control the pests we have indiscriminately sprayed the landscape with extremely effective "broad-spectrum" insecticides that eradicate the good, as well as the harmful, insects. We have also found, to our chagrin, that many of the chemicals we have used persist in the environment and accumulate as residues in the bodies of animals higher up in the food chains. Also, many strains of insects have developed a resistance to the insecticides in common use.

In recent years an effort has been made to use pesticides that are specific in their targets. In addition to chemical control, other methods of control have been under intense investigation and experimentation.

The development of **insect-resistant crops** is one area of investigation. So many factors, such as yield and quality, are involved in developing resistant crops that the teamwork of specialists from many related fields is required. Some progress, however, has been made.

Several types of biological controls have been developed and are under investigation. All of these areas present problems but also show great possibilities. One is the use of bacterial and viral pathogens. A bacterium, *Bacillus thuringiensis,* has been used to control several lepidopteran pests (cabbage looper, imported cabbage worm, tomato worm), and several other bacteria show some potential. Many viruses that seem to have potential as insecticides have been isolated. However, specific viruses are difficult to rear and could be expensive to put into commercial production.

A

B

C

Figure 17-33

Insect pests. **A,** Japanese beetles, *Popillia japonica* (order Coleoptera), are serious pests of fruit trees and ornamental shrubs. They were introduced into the United States from Japan in 1917. **B,** Walnut caterpillars, *Datana ministra* (order Lepidoptera), defoliating a hickory tree. **C,** Corn ear worms, *Heliothis zea* (order Lepidoptera). An even more serious pest of corn is the infamous corn borer, an import from Europe in 1908 or 1909.

A, Photograph by L.L. Rue, III; B and C, photographs by J.H. Gerard.

Introduction of natural predators or parasites of the insect pests has met with some success. In the United States the vedalia beetle was brought from Australia to counteract the work of the cottony-cushion scale on citrus plants, and numerous instances of control by use of insect parasites have been recorded.

Another approach to biological control is to interfere with the reproduction or behavior of insect pests with sterile males or with naturally occurring organic compounds that act as hormones or pheromones. Such research, although very promising, is slow because of our limited understanding of insect behavior and the problems of isolating and identifying complex compounds that are produced in such minute amounts. Nevertheless, pheromones will probably play an important role in biological pest control in the future.

The sterile male approach has been used effectively in eradicating screwworm flies, a livestock pest. Large numbers of male insects, sterilized by irradiation, are introduced into the natural population; females that mate with the sterile flies lay infertile eggs.

CLASSIFICATION

Insects are divided into orders on the basis of wing structure, mouthparts, metamorphosis, and so on. Entomologists do not all agree on the names of the orders or on the limits of each order. Some choose to combine and others to divide the groups. However, the following synopsis of the orders is one that is rather widely accepted.

[handwritten: WINGLESS NO STUDY]

Subclass Apterygota (ap-ter-y-go′ta) (Gr., *a*, not + *pterygōtos*, winged) (**Ametabola**). Primitive **wingless** insects, anamorphic or epimorphic.

   Order Protura (pro-tu′ra) (Gr., *protos*, first + *oura*, tail). Minute (1 to 1.5 mm); no eyes or antennae; appendages on abdomen as well as thorax; live in soil and dark, humid places; anamorphic.

   Order Diplura (dip-lu′ra) (Gr., *diploos*, double, + *oura*, tail)—**japygids**. Usually less than 10 mm; pale, eyeless; a pair of long terminal filaments or pair of caudal forceps; live in damp humus or rotting logs; epimorphic.

   Order Collembola (col-lem′bo-la) (Gr., *kolla*, glue, + *embolon*, peg, wedge)—**springtails and snow fleas**. Small (5 mm or less); no eyes; respiration by trachea or body surface; a springing organ folded under the abdomen for leaping (Fig. 17-34, *B* to *D*); abundant in soil; sometimes swarm on pond surface film or on snowbanks in spring; epimorphic.

   Order Thysanura (thy-sa-nu′ra) (Gr., *thysanos*, tassel, + *oura*, tail)—**silverfish and bristletails** (Fig. 17-34, *A*). Small to medium size; large eyes; long antennae; three long terminal cerci; live under stones and leaves and around human habitations; epimorphic.

Subclass Pterygota (ter-y-go′ta) (Gr., *pterygōtos*, winged) (**Metabola**). **Winged** insects (some secondarily wingless) **with metamorphosis**; includes 97% of all insects.

   Superorder Exopterygota (ek-sop-ter-i-go′ta) (Gr., *exo*, outside + *pterygōtos*, winged) (**Hemimetabola**). **Metamorphosis gradual; wings develop externally** on larvae; compound eyes present on larvae; larvae called **nymphs** (or **naiads** if aquatic).

[handwritten: division 1, incomplete metamorphosis]

   Order Ephemeroptera (e-fem-er-op′ter-a) (Gr., *ephēmeros*, lasting but a day, + *pteron*, wing)—**mayflies** (Fig. 17-35). Wings membranous; forewings larger than hindwings; adult mouthparts vestigial; nymphs aquatic, with lateral tracheal gills.

Figure 17-34

A, Silverfish *Lepisma* (order Thysanura) is often found in homes. **B to D**, Springtails (order Collembola). **B**, *Anurida*. **C** and **D**, *Orchesetta* in resting and leaping positions.

A

B

C   D

Order Odonata (o-do-na′ta) (Gr., *odontos*, tooth, + *ata,* characterized by)—**dragonflies, damselflies** (Figs. 17-20, *A,* and 17-24, *B*). Large; membranous wings are long, narrow, net veined, and similar in size; long and slender body; aquatic nymphs with aquatic gills and prehensile labium for capture of prey.

Order Orthoptera (or-thop′ter-a) (Gr., *orthos,* straight, + *pteron,* wing)—**grasshoppers** (Fig. 17-4), **locusts, crickets, cockroaches, walking sticks** (Fig. 17-9, *B*), **praying mantids** (Fig. 17-7). Wings, when present, with forewings thickened and hindwings folded like a fan under forewings; chewing mouthparts.

Order Dermaptera (der-map′ter-a) (Gr., *derma,* skin, + *pteron,* wing)—earwigs (Fig. 17-36). Very short forewings; large and membranous hindwings folded under forewings when at rest; biting mouthparts; forcepslike cerci.

Order Plecoptera (ple-kop′ter-a) (Gr., *plekein,* to twist, + *pteron,* wing)—stoneflies (Fig. 17-24, *A*). Membranous wings; larger and fanlike hindwings; aquatic nymph with tufts of tracheal gills.

Order Isoptera (i-sop′ter-a) (Gr., *isos,* equal, + *pteron,* wing)—**termites** (Fig. 17-30). Small; membranous, narrow wings similar in size with few veins; wings shed at maturity; erroneously called "white ants"; distinguishable from true ants by broad union of thorax and abdomen; complex social organization.

Order Embioptera (em-bi-op′ter-a) (Gr., *embios,* lively, + *pteron,* wing)—**webspinners.** Small; male wings membranous, narrow, and similar in size; wingless females; chewing mouthparts; colonial; make silk-lined channels in tropical soil.

Order Psocoptera (so-cop′ter-a) (Gr., *psoco,* rub small, + *pteron,* wing) (**Corrodentia**)—psocids, "book lice," "bark lice." Body usually small, may be as large as 10 mm; membranous, narrow wings with few veins, usually held rooflike over abdomen when at rest; some wingless species; found in books, bark, bird nests, on foliage.

Order Zoraptera (zo-rap′ter-a) (Gr., *zōros,* pure, + *apterygos,* wingless)—zorapterans. As large as 2.5 mm; membranous, narrow wings usually shed at maturity; colonial and termitelike.

Order Mallophaga (mal-lof′a-ga) (Gr., *mallos,* wool, + *phagein,* to eat)—**biting lice.** As large as 6 mm; wingless; chewing mouthparts; legs adapted for clinging to host; live on birds and mammals.

Order Anoplura (an-o-plu′ra) (Gr., *anoplos,* unarmed, + *oura,* tail)—**sucking lice.** Depressed body; as large as 6 mm; wingless; mouthparts for piercing and sucking; adapted for clinging to warm-blooded host; includes the head louse, body louse, crab louse, others.

Order Thysanoptera (thy-sa-nop′ter-a) (Gr., *thysanos,* tassel, + *pteron,* wing)—**thrips.** Length 0.5 to 5 mm (a few longer); wings, if present, long, very narrow, with few veins, and fringed with long hairs; sucking mouthparts; destructive plant-eaters, but some feed on insects.

Order Hemiptera (he-mip′ter-a) (Gr., *hemi,* half, + *pteron,* wing) (**Heteroptera**)—**true bugs.** Size 2 to 100 mm; wings present or absent; forewings with basal portion leathery, apical portion membranous; hindwings membranous; at rest, wings held flat over abdomen; piercing-sucking mouthparts; many with odorous scent glands; include water scorpions, water striders (Fig. 17-12), bedbugs, **squash bugs,** assassin bugs, **chinch bugs, stinkbugs,** plant bugs, lace bugs, others.

Order Homoptera (ho-mop′ter-a) (Gr., *homos,* same, + *pteron,* wing)—**cicadas** (Fig. 17-23), **aphids, scale insects, leafhoppers,** treehoppers (Fig. 17-26, *B*). (Often included as suborder under Hemiptera.) If winged, either membranous or thickened front wings and membranous hindwings; wings held rooflike over body; piercing-sucking mouthparts; all plant-eaters; some destructive; a few serving as source of shellac, dyes, and so on; some with complex life histories.

Superorder Endopterygota (en-dop-ter-y-go′ta) (Gr., *endon,* inside, + *pterygotos,* winged) (**Holometabola**). Metamorphosis complete; wings develop internally; larvae without compound eyes.

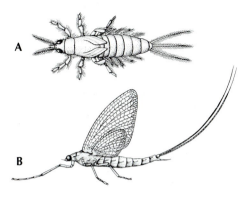

Figure 17-35

A and **B,** Mayfly (order Ephemeroptera) naiad and adult.

Figure 17-36

Earwig (order Dermaptera). Forcepslike cerci at posterior end are usually better developed in male and are used as organs for defense and offense. (Stained preparation, greatly enlarged.) Photograph by F.M. Hickman.

Figure 17-37

A, *Papilio krishna* (order Lepidoptera) is a beautiful swallowtail butterfly from India. Members of the Papilionidae grace many areas of the world, both tropical and temperate, including North America. Compare the knobbed antennae with the plumed antennae in **B,** *Rothschildia jacobaea,* a saturniid moth from Brazil. *Hyalophora cecropia* is a common saturniid in North America. C, Paper wasp (order Hymenoptera) attending her pupae. **D,** *Curculio proboscideus,* the chestnut weevil, is a member of the largest family (Curculionidae) of the largest insect order (Coleoptera). This family includes many serious agricultural pests.

Photographs by K. Sandved.

A

B

C

Order Neuroptera (neu-rop′ter-a) (Gr., *neuron,* nerve, + *pteron,* wing)—**dobsonflies, ant lions, lacewings.** Medium to large size; similar, membranous wings with many cross veins; chewing mouthparts; dobsonflies with greatly enlarged mandibles in males, and with aquatic larvae (doodlebugs) make craters in sand to trap ants.

Order Coleoptera (ko-le-op′ter-a) (Gr., *koleos,* sheath, + *pteron,* wing)—**beetles** (Figs. 17-9, *A,* 17-27, and 17-33, *A*), **fireflies** (Fig. 17-28), **weevils** (Fig. 17-37, *D*). The largest order of animals in the world; front wings (elytra) thick, hard, opaque; membranous hindwings folded under front wings at rest; mouthparts for biting and chewing; includes ground beetles, carrion beetles, whirligig beetles, darkling beetles, stag beetles, dung beetles (Fig. 17-27), diving beetles, boll weevils, others.

Order Strepsiptera (strep-sip′ter-a) (Gr., *strepsis,* a turning, + *pteron,* wing)—**stylops.** Females with no wings, eyes, or antennae; males with vestigial forewings and fan-shaped hindwings; females and larvae parasitic in bees, wasps, and other insects.

Order Mecoptera (me-kop′ter-a) (Gr., *mekos,* length, + *pteron,* wing)—**scorpionflies** (Fig. 17-38, *A* and *B*). Small to medium size; wings long, slender, with many veins; at rest, wings held rooflike over back; scorpion-like male clasping organ at end of abdomen; carnivorous; live in moist woodlands.

Order Lepidoptera (lep-i-dop′ter-a) (Gr., *lepidos,* scale, + *pteron,* wing)—**butterflies and moths.** Membranous wings covered with overlapping scales, wings coupled at base; mouthparts a sucking tube, coiled when not in use; larvae (caterpillars) with chewing mandibles for plant eating, stubby prolegs on the abdomen, and silk glands for spinning cocoons; antennae knobbed in butterflies and usually plumed in moths (Fig. 17-37, *A* and *B*).

Order Diptera (dip′ter-a) (Gr., *dis,* two, + *pteron,* wing)—**true flies.** Single pair of wings, membranous and narrow; hindwings reduced to inconspicuous balancers (halteres); sucking mouthparts or adapted for sponging, lapping, or piercing; legless larvae called maggots or, when aquatic, wrigglers (Fig. 17-19); includes crane flies, mosquitoes, moth flies, midges, fruit flies, flesh flies, houseflies, horseflies, botflies, blowflies, and many others.

Order Trichoptera (tri-kop′ter-a) (Gr., *trichos,* hair, + *pteron,* wing)—**caddis flies** (Fig. 17-38, *C* and *D*). Small, soft bodied; wings well veined and hairy,

D

folded rooflike over hairy body; chewing mouthparts; aquatic larvae construct cases of leaves, sand, gravel, bits of shell, or plant matter, bound together with secreted silk or cement; some make silk feeding nets attached to rocks in stream.

Order Siphonaptera (si-fon-ap′ter-a) (Gr., *siphon*, a siphon, + *apteros*, wingless)—**fleas.** Small; wingless; bodies laterally compressed; legs adapted for leaping; no eyes; ectoparasitic on birds and mammals; larvae legless and scavengers.

Order Hymenoptera (hi-men-op′ter-a) (Gr., *hymen*, membrane, + *pteron*, wing)—**ants, bees, wasps** (Fig. 17-37, C). Very small to large; membranous, narrow wings coupled distally; subordinate hindwings; mouthparts for biting and lapping up liquids; ovipositor sometimes modified into stinger, piercer, or saw (Fig. 17-22); both social and solitary species, most larvae legless, blind, and maggotlike.

_____ Phylogeny and Adaptive Radiation

Insect fossils, although not abundant, have been found in numbers sufficient to give a general idea of the evolutionary history of insects. Although several groups of marine arthropods, such as trilobites, crustaceans, and xiphosurans, were present in the Cambrian period, the first terrestrial arthropods—the scorpions and millipedes—did not appear until the Silurian period. The first insects, which were wingless, date from the Devonian period. By the Carboniferous period, several orders of winged insects, most of which are now extinct, had appeared.

Not all zoologists have put the same interpretation on the comparative data that are available, but certain general relationships are evident. It is believed that the insects arose from a myriapod ancestor that had paired leglike appendages. Both myriapods and insects have clearly defined heads with antennae and mandibles. However, the evolution of insects involved specialization of the next three segments to become the locomotor segments (thorax) and a loss or reduction of appendages on the rest of the body (abdomen). The primitively wingless apterygotes are undoubtedly the most primitive of the insects, and traits similar to those of the myriapods are found in them. Probably some ancestral form similar to the Protura or Thysanura gave rise to two major lines of winged insects, which differed in their ability to flex their wings. One of these led to the Odonata and Ephemeroptera, which have outspread wings that cannot be folded back over the abdomen. The other line branched into three groups, all of which were present by the Permian period. One group with gradual metamorphosis, chewing mouthparts, and cerci includes the Orthoptera, Dermaptera, Isoptera, and Embioptera; another with gradual metamorphosis and a tendency toward sucking mouthparts includes the Thysanoptera, Hemiptera, and Homoptera and perhaps also the Psocoptera, Zoraptera, Mallophaga, and Anoplura, although there is some disagreement among authorities about the last group. Insects with complete metamorphosis are the most specialized, and the Neuroptera, which were probably the earliest of these, may have given rise to the other endopterygote orders, with the social insects being the most advanced.

The adaptive nature of the insects has been stressed throughout this chapter. The direction and range of their adaptive radiation, both structurally and physiologically, have been amazingly varied. Whether it be in the area of habitat, feeding adaptations, means of locomotion, reproduction, or general mode of living, the adaptive achievements of the insects are truly remarkable.

Figure 17-38

A, Male scorpionfly *Panorpa* (order Mecoptera) has recurved abdomen with scorpion-like claspers. **B,** Scorpionfly larva. **C,** Caddis fly (order Trichoptera). **D,** Several types of larval cases built by aquatic caddis fly larvae, often on the underside of stones.

A

B

C

D

Larva with case

___ Summary

The terrestrial mandibulates include several small classes of myriapods and the largest class of animals, the Insecta. All have only one pair of antennae and have uniramous appendages.

The tagmata of the myriapods are head and trunk, and the most important groups are the centipedes (class Chilopoda) and millipedes (class Diplopoda). Centipedes are predators and bear one pair of legs on most somites. Millipedes are mostly scavengers and have two pairs of legs on most somites. All myriapods are terrestrial.

The Insecta are easily recognized by the combination of their tagmata (head, thorax, and abdomen) and the possession of three pairs of thoracic legs.

The evolutionary success of insects is largely explained by several features allowing them to exploit terrestrial habitats, such as waterproofing their cuticle and other mechanisms to minimize water loss and the ability to enter dormancy during adverse conditions.

Many insects bear two pairs of wings on their thorax, although some have one pair and some are wingless. Wing movements in some insects are controlled by direct flight muscles, which insert directly on the base of the wings in the thorax, whereas others have indirect flight muscles, which move the wings by changing the shape of the thorax.

Feeding habits vary greatly among insects and can be described as phytophagous, saprophagous, predaceous, and parasitic. Within the general categories of biting, chewing, sucking, and piercing, there is an enormous variety of specialization reflecting the particular feeding habits of a given insect. Insects breathe by means of a tracheal system, which is a system of tubes that open by spiracles on the thorax and abdomen and conduct respiratory gases to and from internal tissues. Aquatic forms often have tracheal gills. Excretory organs are malpighian tubules. Insects possess efficient sense organs that can respond to mechanical, auditory, chemical, visual, and other stimuli.

Sexes are separate in insects, and fertilization is usually internal. Almost all insects undergo metamorphosis during development. In hemimetabolous (gradual) metamorphosis, the juvenile instars (nymphs) have externally developing wing buds (hence, exopterygote). The adult emerges at the last nymphal molt. In holometabolous (complete) metamorphosis, the juvenile instars (larvae) have internally developing wings (hence, endopterygote), and the last larval molt gives rise to a nonfeeding stage (pupa). A winged adult emerges at the final, pupal, molt. Hormonal control of metamorphosis is the same for both types: the activation hormone produced in the brain stimulates ecdysone production from the prothoracic glands, which initiates the processes of the premolt stage. The amount of juvenile hormone secreted by the corpora allata determines the degree of maturation at each molt. The ability to undergo a state of dormancy (facultative or obligatory diapause) at some stage is of great value in surviving harsh conditions.

Insects can communicate with one another and affect one another's behavior or physiological state by various means, the most important of which is chemical signals (pheromones). Pheromones and some other stimuli coordinate the functioning of very complex insect societies, such as those of bees, ants, and termites. In each of these, functions in the society are divided among three or more castes.

Insects are important to human welfare, particularly because they pollinate food crop plants, control populations of other, harmful insects by predation and parasitism, and serve as food for other animals. Many insects are harmful to human interests because they feed on food and other crop plants, and many are carriers of important diseases of humans and domestic animals. There are grave difficulties with control of harmful insects by chemical insecticides, but these may be overcome by the development and more widespread use of natural and biological control methods.

Modern insects and myriapods show certain basic similarities, and insects are probably descended from one or more myriapod-like ancestors. The apterygote orders of insects are the most primitive, and the holometabolous orders are the most advanced.

Adaptive radiation and the evolutionary success of the arthropods have been enormous.

Selected references

Andersen, S.O. 1976. Cuticular enzymes and sclerotization in insects. In H.R. Hepburn (ed.). The insect integument. Amsterdam, Elsevier Scientific Publishing Co., pp. 121-144.

Askew, R.R. 1971. Parasitic insects. New York, American Elsevier Publishers, Inc.

Birch, M.C. (ed.). 1974. Pheromones. New York, American Elsevier Publishers, Inc.

Borror, D.J., D.M. Delong, and C.A. Triplehorn. 1976. An introduction to the study of insects, ed. 4. New York, Holt, Rinehart & Winston.

Boudreaux, H.B. 1979. Arthropod phylogeny with special reference to insects. New York, John Wiley & Sons, Inc.

Butler, C.G. 1975. The world of the honeybee, rev. ed. Collins, London. *Updated to add queen substances, pheromones, communication, and so on.*

Chu, H.F. 1949. How to know the immature insects. Dubuque, Iowa, William C. Brown Co., Publishers. *An identification guide.*

Corning, W.C., J.A. Dyal, and A.O.D. Willows. 1973. Invertebrate learning, vol. 2. New York, Plenum Publishing Corp.

Debach, P. 1974. Biological control by natural enemies. New York, Cambridge University Press.

Dethier, V.G. 1976. The hungry fly. Cambridge, Mass., Harvard University Press.

Gillot, C. 1980. Entomology. New York, Plenum Publishing Corp. *Comprehensive textbook.*

Harwood, R.F., and M.T. James. 1979. Entomology in human and animal health, ed. 7. New York, Macmillan, Inc. *Up to date, and one of the best texts available in medical entomology.*

Hölldobler, B. 1976. Tournaments and slavery in a desert ant. Science 192:912-914.

Hölldobler, B., and C.P. Haskins. 1977. Sexual calling behavior in primitive ants. Science **195**:793-794.

Jacobson, M. 1972. Insect sex pheromones. New York, Academic Press, Inc.

Jaques, H.E. 1947. How to know the insects, ed. 2. Dubuque, Iowa, William C. Brown Co., Publishers. *A good key to the families of insects.*

Jaques, H.E. 1951. How to know the beetles. Dubuque, Iowa, William C. Brown Co., Publishers. *A useful and compact manual for the coleopterist.*

Matthews, R.W., and J.R. Matthews. 1978. Insect behavior. New York, John Wiley & Sons, Inc.

McCafferty, W.P. 1981. Aquatic entomology: the fisherman's and ecologist's illustrated guide to insects and their relatives. Boston, Science Books International. *Unsurpassed for identification of aquatic insects. Fine illustrations.*

Milne, L., and M. Milne. 1980. The Audubon Society field guide to North American insects and spiders. New York, Alfred A. Knopf, Inc.

Richards, O.W., and R.G. Davies. 1978. Imms' outlines of entomology, ed. 6. London, Chapman & Hall, Ltd.

Riddiford, L.M., and J.W. Truman. 1978. Biochemistry of insect hormones and insect growth regulators. In R. Rockstein (ed.). Biochemistry of insects. New York, Academic Press, Inc., pp. 307-357.

Rockstein, M. 1973, 1974. The physiology of Insecta, vols. 1 to 6, ed. 2. New York, Academic Press, Inc. *An extensive review of this large group.*

Scheller, U. 1982. Pauropoda. In S.P. Parker (ed.). Synopsis and classification of living organisms, vol. 2. New York, McGraw-Hill Book Co., pp. 724-726.

Schmidt, G.D., and L.S. Roberts. 1981. Foundations of parasitology, ed. 2. St. Louis, The C.V. Mosby Co. *Contains chapters on parasitic and medically important insects.*

Spoczynski, J.O.I. 1975. The world of the wasp. New York, Crane, Russak & Co., Inc. *An interesting little book.*

Swan, L.A., and C.S. Papp. 1972. The common insects of North America. New York, Harper & Row, Publishers, Inc.

von Frisch, K. 1974. Decoding the language of the bee. Science **185**:663-668. *A Nobel lecture.*

Wigglesworth, V.B. 1972. Principles of insect physiology, ed. 7. New York, John Wiley & Sons, Inc. *A comprehensive account.*

Wigglesworth, V.B. 1974. Insect physiology, ed. 7. New York, John Wiley & Sons, Inc. *A brief and easily understandable summary.*

Wilson, E.O. 1971. The insect societies. Cambridge, Mass., Harvard University Press.

Selected *Scientific American* articles

Batra, S.W.T., and L.R. Batra. 1967. The fungus gardens of insects. 217:112-120 (Nov.).

Bentley, D., and R.R. Hoy. 1974. The neurobiology of cricket song. 231:34-44 (Aug.). *The songs give clues linking genetic information, development, the nervous system, and behavior.*

Buck, J., and E. Buck. 1976. Synchronous fireflies. 234:74-85 (May). *Discusses the evolutionary role of some fireflies flashing in unison and some being unsynchronized.*

Camhi, J.M. 1980. The escape system of the cockroach. 243:158-172 (Dec.). *With tiny, hairlike receptors, the insect detects air movement generated by an approaching object.*

Eberhard, W.G. 1980. Horned beetles. 242:166-182 (Mar.).

Edwards, C.A. 1969. Soil pollutants and soil animals. 220:88-90 (Apr.). *The effect of pesticides on soil invertebrates, the majority of which are arthropods.*

Heinrich, B. 1973. The energetics of the bumblebee. 228:96-102 (Apr.).

Heinrich, B., and G.A. Bartholomew. 1972. Temperature control in flying moths. 226:71-77 (June). *Muscles of insects cannot contract fast enough for flight unless they reach a certain temperature; therefore it may be necessary for them to warm up by a process similar to shivering.*

Heinrich, B., and G.A. Bartholomew. 1979. The ecology of the African dung beetle. 241:146-156 (Nov.). *Dung beetles play a vital role in dispersal of feces left by herds of mammals.*

Hölldobler, B. 1971. Communication between ants and their guests. 224:86-93 (Mar.).

Hölldobler, B.K., and E.O. Wilson. 1977. Weaver ants. 237:146-154 (Dec.). *Weaver ants use their larvae as shuttles to weave nests in the tropical rain forest.*

Horridge, G.A. 1977. The compound eye of insects. 237:108-120 (July).

Jacobson, M., and M. Beroza. 1964. Insect attractants. 211:20-27 (Aug.).

Jones, J.C. 1978. The feeding behavior of mosquitoes. 238:138-148 (June). *The mouthparts of the female mosquito are complex structures, exquisitely adapted for piercing skin and sucking blood.*

Manzel, R., and J. Erber. 1978. Learning and memory in bees. 239:102-110 (July). *Bees can learn the color and odor of flowers that yield nectar and pollen.*

Milne, L.J., and M. Milne. 1976. The social behavior of burying beetles. 235:84-89 (Aug.).

Milne, L.J., and M. Milne. 1978. Insects of the water surface. 238:134-142 (Apr.). *The surface tension of a calm body of water creates an unusual environment, and the same four types of insects are associated with it all over the world: water striders (Hemiptera), backswimmers (Hemiptera), whirligig beetles (Coleoptera), and springtails (Collembola).*

Rothschild, M. 1965. Fleas. 213:44-53 (Dec.). *The reproduction of the rabbit flea is remarkably controlled by that of its host.*

Rothschild, M., Y. Schlein, K. Parker, C. Neville, and S. Sternberg. 1973. The flying leap of the flea. 222:92-101 (Nov.).

Schneider, D. 1974. The sex-attractant receptor of moths. 231:28-35 (July).

Seeley, T.D. 1982. How honeybees find a home. 247:158-168 (Oct.). *To survive winters in temperate climates, the swarm must occupy a nest site that meets rigorous requirements. Finding a suitable site is the job of the "scout" bees, which must then reach agreement among themselves on the site and guide the swarm to its new home.*

von Frisch, K. 1962. Dialects in the language of the bees. 207:78-86 (Aug.).

Waterhouse, D.F. 1974. The biological control of dung. 230:100-109 (Apr.).

Weis-Fogh, T. 1975. Unusual mechanisms for the generation of lift in flying. 233:80-87 (Nov.).

Wenner, A.M. 1964. Sound communication in honeybees. 210:116-124 (Apr.).

Williams, C.M. 1967. Third-generation pesticides. 217:13-17 (July).

Wilson, D.M. 1968. The flight-control system of the locust. 218:83-90 (May).

Wilson, E.O. 1972. Animal communication. 227:52-71 (Sept.).

Wright, R.H. 1975. Why mosquito repellents repel. 233:104-111 (July).

CHAPTER 18

THE LESSER PROTOSTOMES

Phylum Sipuncula

Phylum Echiura

Phylum Pogonophora

Phylum Priapulida

Phylum Pentastomida

Phylum Onychophora

Phylum Tardigrada

This little creature, which resembles some prehistoric monster but is only 300 to 500 μm long, is *Echiniscus spiniger,* one of the "water bears" of phylum Tardigrada. Unable to swim, it clings to moss or water plants with its claws. If the environment dries up, it goes into a state of suspended animation and "sleeps away" the drought.

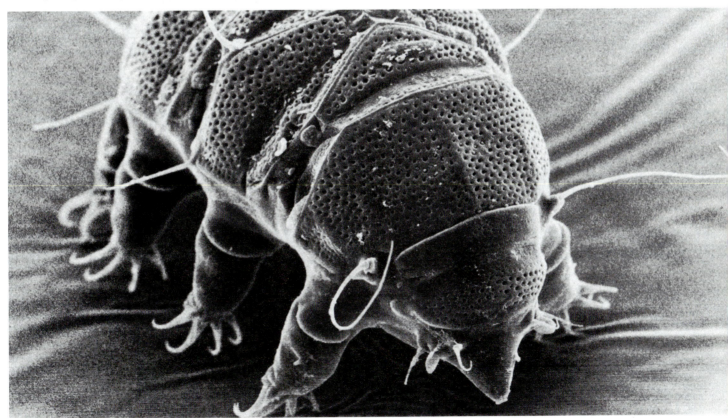

Scanning electron micrograph by D.R. Nelson.

Position in Animal Kingdom
The phyla discussed in this chapter are all coelomate protostomes, although some also have some deuterostome characteristics in their embryological development. Their relationship to each other and to the major protostome phyla is often puzzling, but they all probably digressed at different times from the annelid-arthropod stem line. Possible phylogenetic relationships will be mentioned in the discussion of each group.

THE LESSER PROTOSTOMES

This chapter includes a brief discussion of seven phyla whose positions in the phylogenetic lines of the animal kingdom are somewhat problematical, as are their relationships to each other. The great evolutionary flow that began with the appearance of the coelom and led to the three major phyla—Mollusca, Annelida, and Arthropoda—also produced a number of other lines. Some are now extinct, whereas others, although small in number of species and marked by very little evolutionary divergence within each phylum, have survived. The seven phyla grouped here probably stemmed from the annelid-arthropod line, all following different adaptive trends.

Four of the phyla, Sipuncula, Echiura, Priapulida, and Pogonophora, are benthic (bottom-dwelling) marine worms that seem to have some affinity with the annelids. The first three have a variety of proboscis devices used in burrowing and food gathering. The pogonophores live in tubes, mostly in deep-sea mud, have long anterior tentacles, and lack a digestive tract. The Pentastomida, Onychophora, and Tardigrada have sometimes been grouped together and called the pararthropods because they have unjointed limbs with claws (at some stage) and a cuticle that undergoes molting and thus show a relationship with arthropods. The Pentastomida are entirely parasitic; the Onychophora are terrestrial but are limited to damp areas; the Tardigrada are found in marine, freshwater, and terrestrial habitats.

Phylum Sipuncula

The phylum Sipuncula (sigh-pun'kyu-la) (L., *sipunculus*, little siphon, + *ida*, pl. suffix) consists of benthic marine worms, predominantly littoral or sublittoral. They live sedentary lives in burrows in mud or sand (Fig. 14-17, p. 355), occupy borrowed snail shells, or live in coral crevices or among vegetation. Some species construct their own rock burrows by chemical and perhaps mechanical means. More than half the species are restricted to tropical zones. Some are tiny, slender worms, but the majority range from 15 to 30 cm in length. Some of them are commonly known as "peanut worms" because, when disturbed, they can contract to a peanut shape (Fig. 18-1).

Sipunculans have no segmentation or setae. They are most easily recognized by a slender retractile introvert, or proboscis, that is continually and rapidly being run in and out of the anterior end. The walls of the trunk are muscular. When the introvert is everted, the mouth can be seen at its tip surrounded by a crown of ciliated tentacles. Undisturbed sipunculans usually extend the anterior end from the burrow or hiding place and stretch out the tentacles to explore and feed. They are largely deposit feeders living on organic matter collected in mucus on the tentacles and moved to the mouth by ciliary action. The introvert is extended by hydrostatic pressure produced by contraction of the body wall muscles against the

Figure 18-1

Dendrostomum, a sipunculan.

coelomic fluid. It is retracted by special retractor muscles. Its surface is often rough because of surface spines, hooks, or papillae.

There is a large, fluid-filled coelom traversed by muscle and connective tissue fibers. The digestive tract is a long tube that doubles back on itself to end in the anus near the base of the introvert (Fig. 18-2). A pair of large nephridia open to the outside to expel waste-filled coelomic amebocytes; they also serve as gonoducts. Circulatory and respiratory systems are lacking, but the coelomic fluid contains red corpuscles that bear a respiratory pigment, hemerythrin, used in the transportation of oxygen. The nervous system has a bilobed cerebral ganglion just behind the tentacles and a ventral nerve cord extending the length of the body. The sexes are separate. Permanent gonads are lacking, and ovaries or testes develop seasonally in the connective tissue covering the origins of one or more of the retractor muscles. Sex cells are released through the nephridia. Asexual reproduction also occurs by transverse fission, the posterior one fifth of the parent constricting off to become the new individual. The larval form is usually a trochophore.

There are approximately 330 species and 16 genera, which are placed by some authorities into four families. The best-known genera are probably *Sipunculus*, *Phascolosoma* (Gr., *phaskōlos*, leather bag, pouch, + *sōma*, body), *Aspidosiphon* (Gr., *aspidos*, shield, + *siphōn*, siphon), and *Golfingia*.

The early embryological development of sipunculans, echiurans, and annelids is almost identical, showing a very close relationship among the three. It is also similar to the molluscan development. The four phyla are grouped together by some authors into a supraphyletic assemblage called the "Trochozoa" because of the common possession of a trochophore larva. There are other similarities, too, that point to the close relationship of the sipunculans to the echiurans and annelids. The sipunculans and echiurans are simpler animals than the annelids and probably represent collateral evolutionary lines that have retained more primitive features than the annelids have.

___ Phylum Echiura

The phylum Echiura (ek-ee-yur′a) (Gr., *echis*, adder, + *oura*, tail, + *ida*, pl. suffix) consists of marine worms that burrow into mud or sand or live in empty snail shells or sand dollar tests, rocky crevices, and so on. They are found in all oceans—most commonly in littoral zones of warm waters—but some have been found in polar waters and some have been dredged from depths of 2000 m. They vary in length from a few millimeters to 40 or 50 cm.

The echiurans have only one third as many species (about 100) as the sipunculans, but they are much more diverse and are found in greater densities. There are two classes: Echiurida and Sactosomatida. Echiurida is much larger and includes two orders and five families.

The body of the echiuran is cylindrical and somewhat sausage shaped (Fig. 18-3). Anterior to the mouth is a flattened, extensible proboscis (introvert), which, unlike that of the sipunculids, cannot be retracted into the trunk. Echiurids are often called "spoonworms" because of the shape of the contracted proboscis in some worms. The proboscis, which contains the brain, is actually a cephalic lobe, probably homologous to the annelid prostomium. The proboscis has a ciliated groove leading to the mouth. While the animal lies buried, the proboscis can extend out over the mud for exploration and deposit feeding (Fig. 18-4). *Bonellia viridis* picks up very small particles and moves them along the proboscis by cilia;

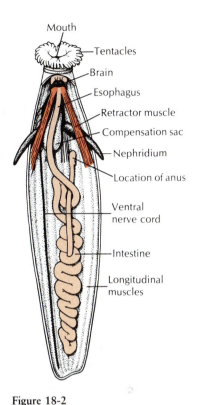

Figure 18-2

Internal structure of *Sipunculus*.

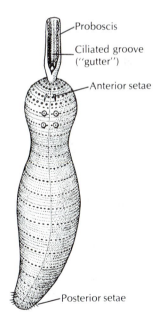

Figure 18-3

Echiurus, an echiurid common on both Atlantic and Pacific coasts. The shape of the proboscis lends them the common name of "spoon worms."

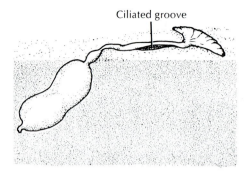

Ciliated groove

Figure 18-4

Tatjanellia (phylum Echiurida) is a detritus feeder. Lying buried in the sand, it explores the surface with its long proboscis, which picks up organic particles and carries them along a ciliated groove to the mouth.

After Zenkevitch; modified from Dawydoff, C. 1959. Classe des Echiuriens. In P. Grassé (ed.). Traité de Zoologie, vol. 5. Paris, Masson et Cie.

In some species sexual dimorphism is pronounced, with the female being much the larger of the two. *Bonellia* has an extreme sexual dimorphism, and sex is determined in a very interesting way. At first the free-swimming larvae are sexually undifferentiated. Those that come into contact with the proboscis of a female become tiny males (1 to 3 mm long) that migrate to the female uterus. About 20 males are usually found in a single female. Larvae that do not contact a female proboscis metamorphose into females. It is not known whether the stimulus for male development is a chemical from the female proboscis, a matter of the chemical content of the environmental water, or a dimorphism in the eggs.

larger particles are moved by a combination of cilia and muscular action or by muscular action alone. Unwanted particles can be rejected along the route to the mouth. The proboscis is short in some forms and long in others. *Bonellia*, which is only 8 cm long, can extend its proboscis to a meter in length.

One common form, *Urechis* (Gr., *oura*, tail, + *echis*, viper, serpent), lives in a U-shaped burrow in which it secretes a funnel-shaped mucous net. It pumps water through the net, capturing bacteria and fine particulate material in it. When loaded with food, the net is swallowed. *Lissomyena* (Gr., *lissos*, smooth, + *mys*, muscle) lives in empty gastropod shells in which it constructs galleries irrigated by rhythmical pumping of water and feeds on sand and mud drawn in by the irrigation process.

The muscular body wall is covered with cuticle and epithelium, which may be smooth or ornamented with papillae. There may be a pair of anterior setae or a row of bristles around the posterior end. The coelom is large. The digestive tract is long and coiled and terminates at the posterior end. A pair of anal vesicles may have an excretory and osmoregulatory function. Most echiurans have a closed circulatory system with colorless blood but contain hemoglobin in coelomic corpuscles and certain body cells. Two or three pairs of nephridia serve mainly as gonoducts. A nerve ring runs around the pharynx and forward into the proboscis, and there is a ventral nerve cord. There are no specialized sense organs.

The sexes are separate, with a single gonad in each sex. The mature sex cells break loose from the gonads and leave the body cavity by way of the nephridia, and fertilization is usually external.

Early cleavage and trochophore stages are very similar to those of annelids and sipunculans. The trochophore stage, which may last from a few days to 3 months, according to the species, is followed by gradual metamorphosis to the wormlike adult.

The relationship of the echiurans to annelids and sipunculans has already been mentioned. Echiurans show a transitory metamerism during their embryogenesis and so may have descended from a metameric ancestor. Sipunculans, however, show no trace of metamerism.

Phylum Pogonophora

The phylum Pogonophora (po'-go-nof'e-ra) (Gr., *pōgōn*, beard, + *phora*, bearing), or beardworms, was entirely unknown before the twentieth century. The first specimens to be described were collected from deep-sea dredgings off the coast of Indonesia in 1900. They have since been discovered in several seas, including the western Atlantic off the U.S. eastern coast. Some 80 species have been described so far; they have been divided into two orders: Athecanephria and Thecanephria.

These elongated tube-dwelling forms have left no known fossil record. Their closest affinity seems to be to the annelids.

Most pogonophores live in the bottom ooze on the ocean floor, always below the intertidal zone and usually at depths of more than 200 m. This accounts for their delayed discovery, for they are obtained only by dredging. Their usual length is from 5 to 85 cm, with a diameter usually of a fraction of a millimeter. They are sessile animals that secrete very long chitinous tubes in which they live, probably extending the anterior end only for feeding. The tubes are generally oriented upright in the bottom ooze. The tube is usually about the same length as the animal, which can move up or down inside the tube but cannot turn around.

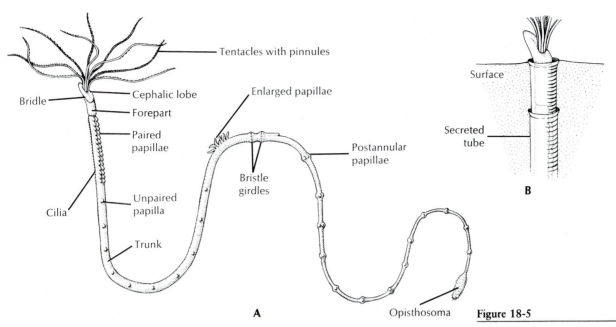

Figure 18-5

Diagram of a typical pogonophoran. **A,** External features. The body, in life, is much more elongated than shown in this diagram. **B,** Position in tube.

Form and function
External features

The beardworm has a long, cylindrical body covered with cuticle. The body is divided into a short anterior forepart; a long, very slender trunk; and a small, segmented opisthosoma (Fig. 18-5). It is difficult to determine which is the ventral and which is the dorsal side of the animal because the pogonophore lives in a vertical position, and if removed, simply curls up and never crawls. Therefore, rather than using the terms "dorsal" and "ventral," the side of the body containing the main nerve trunk is called the adneural side, and the other side the antineural. The **forepart** is made up of the anterior cephalic lobe, which contains the central nervous ganglion and a short muscular region following the lobe. On the antineural side the **cephalic lobe** bears some long **tentacles** (the "beard" that gives the phylum its name). There may be from one to 260 or more tentacles depending on the species. They are hollow extensions of the coelom and bear minute pinnules. For a part or all of their length the tentacles lie parallel with each other, enclosing a cylindrical intertentacular space into which the pinnules project (Fig. 18-6). Each tentacle contains an afferent and an efferent blood vessel. The forepart also bears a pair of slanting ridges consisting of thickened cuticle and called the **bridle,** which may help the animal cling to the inner surface of the tube as it moves up and down or which may be the means of distributing the glandular exudate that forms the tube.

The long **trunk** bears **papillae** and, about midway back, two rings of short toothed setae called **girdles,** or **belts,** which are used to grip the wall of the tube, allowing the two halves of the body to contract or extend independently in the tube. Anterior to the girdles is the preannular region of the trunk, which usually bears longitudinal bands of cilia on the neural side and papillae on the opposite side. The postannular part of the trunk is very thin and is easily broken when the animals are collected. In fact, the segmented tail end of the animal, or **opisthosoma,** was not found and described until after 1963! It is thicker than the trunk, is divided into five to 23 short segments that bear setae, and ends in a small depression.

The mucus-coated **cuticle** that covers the body is made up of crisscross layers

Figure 18-6

Cross section of tentacular crown of pogonophore *Lamellisabella*. Tentacles arise from ventral side of forepart at base of cephalic lobe. Tentacles (which vary in number in different species) enclose a cylindrical space, with the pinnules forming a kind of food-catching network. Food may be digested in this pinnular meshwork and absorbed into the blood supply of tentacles and pinnules.

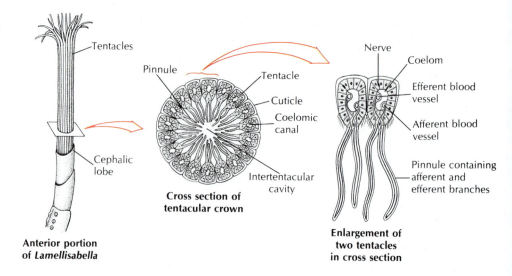

Anterior portion
of *Lamellisabella*

Cross section of
tentacular crown

Enlargement of
two tentacles
in cross section

Among the most amazing animals found in the deep-water, Pacific rift communities (Chapter 41, p. 1025) are the giant pogonophorans, *Riftia pachyptila*. Much larger than any pogonophorans reported before this discovery, they measure up to 3 m in length and 2 to 3 cm in diameter. Like other members of their phylum, they have no mouth or digestive tract. Their blood-red plume of tentacles provides a large surface area for absorption of nutrients from the seawater; the tentacles are partially fused into lamellae, with about 340 tentacles per lamella and 335 lamellae on each side, for a total of approximately 2.28×10^5 tentacles in the plume. Even so, it seems unlikely that sufficient dissolved nutrients would be present in seawater to support such a large animal. Evidence suggests that the bodies of the worms contain large numbers of symbiotic, chemoautotrophic bacteria in a highly vascularized organ in the trunk called the trophosome. The discovery of enzymes of sulfur metabolism in the trophosome indicates that the bacteria can oxidize the sulfide from the vent water and make use of the ATP and reducing power generated by sulfur oxidation to reduce and fix carbon dioxide. Thus, *Riftia* fixes enough carbon in the trophosome to nourish the rest of the worm.

of fibers with microvilli protruding through the mesh. Its structure is similar to that of the cuticle of annelids and sipunculans. The pogonophoran cuticle has characteristic thickenings that seem to help the animal grip the tube wall. The **setae** are chitinous and are structurally and chemically similar to annelid setae.

Internal features

The body wall is composed of cuticle, epidermis, and circular and longitudinal muscles.

There is a compartment in each of the body divisions, and septa between the segments of the opisthosoma also divide it into compartments. These compartments have not been shown to be lined by peritoneum; therefore they may not be true coeloms.

Pogonophores are remarkable in having **no mouth or digestive tract,** making their mode of nutrition a rather puzzling matter. Evidence suggests that they absorb nutrients dissolved in the seawater, such as glucose, amino acids, and fatty acids, through the pinnules and microvilli of their tentacles. This absorption is against a concentration gradient and is therefore an active transport process. Absorption of dissolved substances may be supplemented by phagocytosis and pinocytosis in some species. Pogonophorans are the *only nonparasitic metazoans* that lack any trace of a digestive system.

Gas exchange probably also occurs principally in the tentacles. There is a well-developed **closed blood-vascular system.**

Sexes are separate in pogonophores, with a pair of gonads and a pair of gonoducts in the trunk compartment. They often live in dense populations, facilitating cross-fertilization. As a male *Siboglinum* ejects spermatophores from the genital openings, it reaches into the tube with its tentacles, picks up the spermatophores, and draws them toward the top of the tube. As more spermatophores are drawn forward, they push the earlier ones out. Presumably the waterborne spermatophores are captured by the tentacles of nearby females or are caught in their tubes. Fertilization occurs in the female's tube, and the zygotes accumulate in the top part of the tube.

The cleavage is unequal but atypical. It seems to be closer to radial than to spiral. Gastrulation is by epiboly; there is no blastocoel or blastopore. The development of the apparent coelom is schizocoelic, not enterocoelic as was originally described. The worm-shaped embryo is ciliated but a poor swimmer. It is probably swept along by water currents until it settles.

Phylogeny and adaptive radiation

Because the first specimens of Pogonophora that were dredged up lacked the segmented opisthosoma, Ivanov and other early workers, who believed they were working with whole specimens, described the coelom as trimeric (composed of three parts), like that of the hemichordates, and assumed that the organisms were deuterostomes. Ivanov also described the larval coelom as being trimeric. The later discovery of the segmented posterior end brought about some revision of the hypothesis. The adult coelom has proved to be polymeric, not trimeric. That fact and the schizocoelic development of the larva point toward an affinity with protostomes rather than deuterostomes. The pogonophore tubes were originally thought to resemble those of the hemichordate pterobranchs, but analysis of their amino acid and chitin content shows no relationship to the pterobranchs. Pogonophores have photoreceptor cells very similar to those of annelids (oligochaetes and leeches), and the structure of the cuticle, the makeup of the setae, and the segmentation of the opisthosoma all strongly suggest a relationship with the annelids. However, the phylogenetic position of the Pogonophora must be considered still unsettled until the embryology of more species of more than one family is studied.

Adaptive radiation has not been extensive. The chief areas of diversity are in the structure of the tentacular crown and the tube.

—— Phylum Priapulida

The Priapulida (pri'a-pyu'li-da) (Gr., *priapos,* phallus, + *ida,* pl. suffix) are a small group (only nine species) of marine worms found chiefly in the colder waters of both hemispheres. They have been reported along the Atlantic coast from Massachusetts to Greenland and along the Pacific coast from California to Alaska. They live in the mud and sand of the sea floor and range from intertidal zones to depths of several thousand meters.

Their cylindrical bodies are rarely more than 12 to 15 cm long. Most of them are burrowing predaceous animals that usually orient themselves upright in the mud with the mouth at the surface. They are adapted for burrowing by body contractions. *Tubiluchus* (L., *tubulus,* dim. of *tubus,* waterpipe) is a minute detritus feeder adapted to interstitial life in warm coralline sediments. *Maccabeus* (named for a Judean patriot who died in 160 BC) is a tiny tube-dweller discovered in muddy Mediterranean bottoms.

Form and function
External features

The body includes a proboscis, trunk, and usually one or two caudal appendages (Fig. 18-7). The eversible proboscis is ornamented with papillae and ends with rows of curved spines that surround the mouth. When the proboscis is everted, the spines point forward; when it is invaginated, they are directed posteriorly (Fig. 18-8). The proboscis is used in sampling the surroundings as well as for the capture of small, soft-bodied prey. One genus, *Maccabeus,* has a crown of branchial tentacles around the mouth.

Figure 18-7

Priapulus caudatus (phylum Priapulida) with proboscis *(top)* partially invaginated. The warty trunk is annulated but not truly segmented. The caudal appendages are probably respiratory and chemoreceptive organs.
Courtesy W.L. Shapeero.

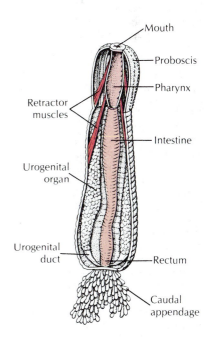

Figure 18-8

Major internal structures of *Priapulus.*

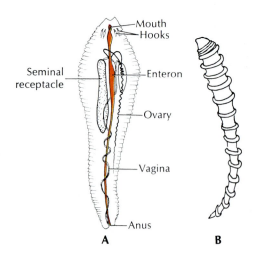

Figure 18-9

Two pentastomids. **A,** *Pentastomum,* found in lungs of snakes and other vertebrates. Female is shown with some internal structures. **B,** Female *Armillifer,* a pentastomid with pronounced body rings. In parts of Africa and Asia, humans are parasitized by immature stages; adults (10 cm long or more) live in lungs of snakes. Human infection may occur from eating snakes or from contaminated food or water.

The trunk is not truly segmented but is superficially divided into 30 to 100 rings and is covered with tubercles and spines. The tubercles are probably sensory in function. The anus and urogenital pores are located at the posterior end of the trunk. The caudal appendages (one in *Priapulus caudatus* and two in *Priapulopsis bicaudatus* [Gr., *priapos,* phallus, + *opsis,* aspect, appearance]) are hollow stems bearing many hollow vesicles that communicate with the coelom. They are believed to be respiratory and probably chemoreceptive in function. *Tubiluchus* bears a long terminal tail instead of caudal appendages. The body is covered with a chitinous cuticle that is molted periodically throughout life.

Internal features

The muscular body wall contains a single layer of epithelium beneath the cuticle, layers of circular and longitudinal muscles, and a thin peritoneum.

The digestive system consists of the proboscis, a muscular pharynx, and a straight intestine and rectum. There are a nerve ring around the pharynx and a midventral nerve cord. The coelom contains amebocytes and, at least in *Priapulus caudatus,* corpuscles bearing hemerythrin.

Sexes are separate. The paired urogenital organs are each made up of a gonad and clusters of solenocytes, both connected to a protonephridial tubule that carries both gametes and urinary products to the outside. Fertilization is external. Spawning has been observed in *Priapulus caudatus,* in which the male usually spawns first, the female's spawning apparently being stimulated by that of the male. Sexual dimorphism is absent in priapulids except for *Tubiluchus,* in which the abdomen of the male is covered with setae.

The embryology of the Priapulida is poorly known. In *Priapulus* and *Halicryptus* (Gr., *hals,* the sea, + *kryptos,* secret, hidden), the egg undergoes radial cleavage and develops into a stereogastrula. The larvae develop a strong cuticle, forming a lorica, much like that of rotifers, into which the animal can wholly withdraw. The larvae of *Priapulus* dig into the mud and become detritus feeders. The cuticle is molted between successive stages, and development may take as long as 2 years. Metamorphosis occurs at the last molt.

Phylogeny and adaptive radiation

Priapulids were formerly placed with the pseudocoelomates by some authorities, but a peritoneum has been identified, placing them among the true coelomates. However, their relationship to other coelomates is obscure. Some authors believe them to be remnants of an ancient group because they have retained several primitive features. They bear a fairly close resemblance to the Kinorhyncha. A better knowledge of their embryogeny is needed to understand their phylogeny.

The small number of species indicates either that the priapulids have undergone little adaptive radiation or that only remnants remain of groups that were once more widely distributed. Their stable ecological niche has given them little opportunity or necessity for wide evolutionary diversification within the group.

___ Phylum Pentastomida

The Pentastomida (pen-ta-stom'i-da) (Gr., *pente,* five, + *stoma,* mouth), or tongue worms, are a phylum of about 60 to 70 species of wormlike parasites of the respiratory system of vertebrates. The adults live mostly in the lungs of reptiles, such as snakes, lizards, and crocodiles, but one species, *Reighardia sternae,* lives in

Figure 18-10

Anterior end of a pentastome. Note both the mouth *(arrow)* between the middle hooks and the apical sensory papillae.

Courtesy J. Ubelaker. From Schmidt, G.D., and L.S. Roberts. 1981. Foundations of parasitology, ed. 2. St. Louis, The C.V. Mosby Co.

the air sacs of terns and gulls, and another, *Linguatula serrata* (Gr., *lingua,* tongue), lives in the nasopharynx of canines and felines (and occasionally humans). Although more common in tropical areas, they are also found in North America, Europe, and Australia.

Form and function
Morphology

The adults range from 1 to 13 cm in length. Transverse rings give their bodies a segmented appearance (Fig. 18-9). The body is covered with a chitinous cuticle that is molted periodically during larval stages. The anterior end may bear five short protuberances (hence the name Pentastomida). Four of these bear claws. The fifth bears the mouth and two pairs of sclerotized hooks for attachment to the host tissues (Fig. 18-10). There is a simple straight digestive system, adapted for sucking. The nervous system, similar to that of annelids and arthropods, has paired ganglia along the ventral nerve cord. The only sense organs appear to be papillae. There are no circulatory, excretory, or respiratory organs.

Reproduction and life cycles

Sexes are separate, and the females are usually larger than the males. Fertilization is internal. A female may produce several million eggs, which pass up the trachea of the host, are swallowed, and pass out with the feces. The larvae hatch out as oval, tailed creatures with four stumpy legs, each with one or two retractile claws and a penetration apparatus at the anterior end of the body.

Most pentastomid life cycles require an intermediate vertebrate host such as a fish, a reptile, or, rarely, a mammal, which is eaten by the definitive vertebrate host. After ingestion by the intermediate host, the larva penetrates the intestine, migrates randomly in the body, and finally metamorphoses into a nymph, which lacks the legs and penetration apparatus. After several molts the nymph develops mouth hooks and a segmented appearance and grows in size. It finally becomes encapsulated and dormant. When eaten by the final host, the nymph finds its way to the lung, feeds on blood and tissue, and matures. Females of *Linguatula serrata* live 2 years or more in the nasopharyngeal mucosa. Their eggs leave the host via nasal secretions or feces.

Several species have been found encysted in humans, the most common being *Armillifer armillatus* (L., *armilla,* ring, bracelet, + *fero,* to bear), but usually they cause few symptoms. *Linguatula serrata* is a cause of nasopharyngeal pentastomiasis, or "halzoun," a disease of humans in the Middle East and India.

Phylogeny

The phylogenetic affinities of the Pentastomida are uncertain. They have some similarities to the Annelida, and some workers have believed that they are offshoots from the polychaetes. Their larval appendages and molting cuticle, however, are arthropod characters. Their larvae resemble tardigrade larvae. Most modern taxonomists align them with the arthropods, but there is little agreement as to where they fit in that phylum. Some authors suggest that they are related to the myriapods; others see an affinity with the Acarina because the larvae resemble mite larvae. Wingstrand (1972) says pentastomid spermatozoa are identical to those of the crustacean subclass Branchiura and suggests that they should be classed with the Branchiura. Because their modifications for parasitic life make it difficult to do more than guess at the free-living forms from which they arose, it seems best to keep them in a separate phylum.

Phylum Onychophora

Members of the phylum Onychophora (on-y-kof′o-ra) (Gr., *onyx,* claw, + *pherein,* to bear) are commonly called the "velvet worms," or "walking worms." They comprise approximately 70 species of caterpillar-like animals, ranging from 1.4 to 15 cm in length. They live in rain forests and other moist, leafy habitats in tropical and subtropical regions and in some temperate regions of the Southern Hemisphere.

The fossil record of the onychophorans shows that they have changed little in their 500 million year history. A fossil form, *Aysheaia,* discovered in the Burgess shale deposit of British Columbia and dating back to mid-Cambrian times, is very much like the modern onychophorans. Onychophorans have been of unusual interest to zoologists because they share so many characteristics with both the annelids and the arthropods. They have been called, a bit too hopefully perhaps, the "missing link" between the two phyla. According to the fossil record, onychophorans were originally marine animals and were probably far more common at one time than they are now. Today they are terrestrial and extremely retiring, coming out only at night or when the air is nearly saturated with moisture.

These curious animals have been dubbed velvet worms because they are covered with a velvety skin, and walking worms because they have from 14 to 43 pairs of stumpy, unjointed legs (Fig. 18-11), each ending with a flexible pad and a pair of claws. It was for this characteristic that the first onychophorans, discovered in 1825, were given the generic name *Peripatus,* from the Greek *peripatos,* meaning "a walking about."

Form and function
External features

The onychophoran body is more or less cylindrical and shows no external segmentation except for the paired appendages. The skin is soft and velvety and is covered with a thin, flexible cuticle that contains protein and chitin. In structure

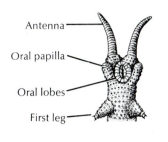

Antenna

Oral papilla

Oral lobes

First leg

**Ventral view
of head**

In natural habitat

Figure 18-11

Peripatus, a caterpillar-like onychophoran that has both annelid and arthropod characteristics.

and chemical composition it resembles arthropod cuticle; however, it never hardens like arthropod cuticle, and it is molted in patches rather than all at one time. The body is studded with tiny **tubercles,** some of which bear sensory bristles. The color may be green, blue, orange, dark gray, or black, and minute scales on the tubercles give the body an iridescent and velvety appearance. The head bears a pair of large **antennae,** each with an annelid-like **eye** at the base (Fig. 18-11). The ventral mouth has a pair of clawlike **mandibles** and is flanked by a pair of **oral papillae** from which a defensive secretion can be expelled.

The **unjointed legs** are short, stubby, and clawed. Locomotion is achieved by waves of contraction passing from anterior to posterior. When a segment is extended, the legs are lifted up and moved forward. The legs are more ventrally located than are the parapodia of annelids.

Internal features

The body wall is muscular like that of the annelids. The body cavity is a **hemocoel,** imperfectly divided into compartments, or sinuses, much like those of the arthropods. **Slime glands** on each side of the body cavity open on the oral papillae. When disturbed by a predator, the animal can eject from the slime glands two streams of a sticky substance that rapidly hardens.

The mouth, surrounded by lobes of skin, contains a dorsal tooth and a pair of lateral mandibles used for grasping and cutting prey. There is a muscular pharynx and a straight digestive tract. Most velvet worms are predaceous, feeding on caterpillars, insects, snails, worms, and the like. Some onychophorans live in termite nests and feed on termites. Prey discovered by the tentacles is held by the lips and sucking pharynx while the mandibles slit open the body wall. A pair of **salivary glands** secretes salivary enzymes into the wound, and the digested tissues are sucked into the mouth.

Each segment contains a pair of **nephridia,** each nephridium with a vesicle, ciliated funnel and duct, and nephridiopore opening at the base of a leg. There is some evidence that the chief excretory product is uric acid, a water-salvaging device used by birds, lizards, land snails, and most insects. Absorptive cells in the midgut excrete crystalline uric acid, and certain pericardial cells function as nephrocytes, storing excretory products taken from the blood.

For respiration there is a **tracheal system** that ramifies to all parts of the body and communicates with the outside by many openings, or **spiracles,** scattered all over the body. The spiracles cannot be closed to prevent water loss, so although the tracheae are efficient, the animals are restricted to moist habitats. The tracheal system is somewhat different from that of arthropods and probably has evolved independently.

The open circulatory system has, in the pericardial sinus, a dorsal, tubular heart with a pair of ostia in each segment.

There are a pair of cerebral ganglia with connectives and a pair of widely separated nerve cords with connecting commissures. The brain gives off nerves to the antennae and head region, and the cords send nerves to the legs and body wall. Sense organs include the pigment cup ocelli, taste spines around the mouth, tactile papillae on the integument, and hygroscopic receptors that orient the animal toward water vapor.

Onychophorans are dioecious, with paired reproductive organs. The males usually deposit their sperm in spermatophores in the female seminal receptacle. The South African *Peripatopsis* (Gr., *peripatos,* a walking about, + *opsis,* aspect, appearance) has no seminal receptacles. The male deposits the spermatophores on the female's back, which may accumulate a number of them. White blood cells dissolve the skin beneath the spermatophores. The sperm can then enter the body cavity and migrate in the blood to the ovaries to fertilize the eggs. Onychophorans may be oviparous, ovoviparous, or viviparous. Only the Australian genera *Ooperipatus* (Gr., *ōon,* an egg, + *peripatos,* a walking about) and *Symperipatus* (Gr., *sym,* together, + *peripatos,* a walking about) are oviparous, laying shell-covered eggs in moist places. In all other onychophorans the eggs develop in the uterus, and living young are produced. Female *Peripatus acacioi,* raised in the laboratory (Lavallard and Campiglia, 1975), could give birth by 15 months of age. They usually had an annual brood of one to eight young. Parturition took about half an hour, with the young freeing themselves gradually, head first. In some species there is a placental attachment between mother and young (viviparous); in others the young develop in the uterus without attachment (ovoviviparous).

Phylogeny

Onychophorans resemble the annelids with their soft body, nonjointed appendages, segmentally arranged nephridia, muscular body wall, pigment cup ocelli, and ciliated reproductive ducts. Arthropod characteristics are the cuticle, the tubular heart and open circulatory system, the presence of tracheae, a hemocoel for a body cavity, and the large size of the brain. They differ from either phylum in their scanty metamerism, structure of the mandibles, and the separate arrangement of the nerve cords. They are more primitive than insects and are somewhat like the centipedes in the arrangement of internal metamerism.

Some authors believe the onychophorans should be included with the arthropods, but that would involve redefining the phylum Arthropoda. Manton (1977) recommends placing the Onychophora, myriapods, and insects in a phylum called Uniramia. Despite the onychophorans' obvious relationship to the myriapods and insects, however, most authors believe that the differences seem to warrant keeping them in a separate phylum.

___ Phylum Tardigrada

Tardigrada (tar-di-gray′da) (L., *tardus,* slow, + *gradus,* step), or "water bears," are minute forms usually less than a millimeter in length. Most of the 300 to 400 species are terrestrial forms that live in the water film surrounding mosses and lichens. Some live in freshwater algae or mosses or in the bottom debris, and a few are marine, inhabiting the interstitial spaces between sand grains, in both deep and shallow seawater. They share many characteristics with the arthropods.

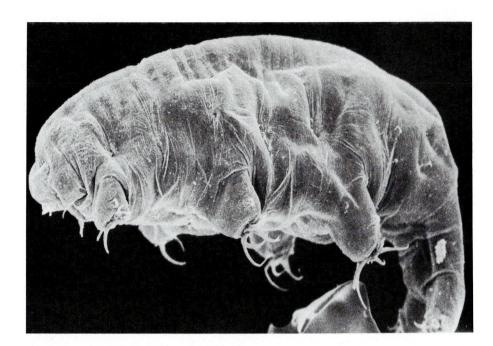

Figure 18-12

Scanning electron micrograph of an aquatic tardigrade, *Pseudobiotus*.
Photograph by D.R. Nelson.

Form and function
External features

The body is elongated, cylindrical, or a long oval and is unsegmented. The head is merely the anterior part of the trunk. The trunk bears four pairs of short, stubby, unjointed legs, each armed with four to eight claws, which may be unequal in size and are used for clinging to the substrate (Fig. 18-12 and p. 439). The last pair of appendages lies at the posterior end of the body. The body is covered by a non-chitinous cuticle, secreted by the epidermis, that is molted along with the claws and buccal apparatus four or more times in its life history. Cilia are absent. Common American species are *Macrobiotus* (Gr., *makros*, large, + *biotos*, life), *Echiniscus* (Gr., *echinos*, hedgehog, + *iskos*, dim. suffix), and *Hypsibius* (Gr., *hypsos*, high height, + *bios*, life).

Internal features

The mouth is at the anterior end and opens into a buccal tube that empties into a muscular pharynx that is adapted for sucking. Two needlelike stylets flanking the buccal tube can be protruded through the mouth. The stylets are used for piercing the cellulose walls of plant cells, and the liquid contents are sucked in by the pharynx. Some tardigrades suck the body juices of nematodes, rotifers (Fig. 18-13), and other small animals. Glands empty into both the pharynx and the digestive tract. Some tardigrades, such as *Echiniscus*, expel feces when molting, leaving the feces in the discarded cuticle.

At the junction of the stomach and rectum, three glands, often called malpighian tubules, empty into the digestive system. They are thought to be excretory in function.

Most of the body cavity is a hemocoel, with the true coelom restricted to the gonadal cavity. There are no circulatory or respiratory systems; fluids freely circulate through the body spaces, and gaseous exchange can occur through the body surface.

The muscular system consists of a number of long muscle bands, each com-

Figure 18-13

Scanning electron micrograph of tardigrade *(Milnesium tardigradum)* feeding on a bdelloid rotifer.
Photograph by D.R. Nelson.

posed of a single smooth muscle cell. Most have their origins and insertions on the body wall. Circular muscles are absent, but the hydrostatic pressure of the body fluid may act as a type of skeleton. Being unable to swim, the water bear creeps about awkwardly, clinging to the substrate with its claws.

The brain is large and covers most of the dorsal surface of the pharynx. It connects by way of circumpharyngeal connectives to the subpharyngeal ganglion, from which the double ventral nerve cord extends posteriorly as a chain of four ganglia. Sense organs usually consist of a pair of pigmented eyespots (in most species) and various sensory spines and bristles.

Sexes are separate in tardigrades. In some freshwater and moss-dwelling species, males are unknown and parthenogenesis seems to be the rule. In marine species, however, males and females occur with approximately equal frequency. The gonad is single, and the gonoduct may end at a gonopore or may join the rectum. Year-round reproduction is typical of marine species. Eggs of some species are highly ornate (Fig. 18-14). Egg laying, like defecation, apparently occurs only at molting, when the volume of coelomic fluid is reduced. Females of some species deposit the eggs in the molted cuticle (Fig. 18-15). Males gather around the old cuticle and shed sperm into it. Other species are fertilized internally but only at the time of molting.

Cleavage is holoblastic but atypical, and a stereogastrula is formed. Six pairs of coelomic pouches arise from the gut, but all except the last pair disaggregate to form the buccal apparatus, pharynx, and body musculature. The last pair fuses to form the gonad. Thus, the gonocoel (which is enterocoelic) is the only true coelom left in the adult. Development is direct, and the young juveniles use stylets and claws to open the eggs. Further growth and development occur through periodic molting. The life span of marine tardigrades is thought to be about 3 to 4 months.

Figure 18-14

Scanning electron micrograph of the highly ornate egg of the tardigrade, *Macrobiotus hufelandii*.
Photograph by D.R. Nelson.

Figure 18-15

Molted cuticle of a tardigrade, containing a number of fertilized eggs.
From Sayre, R.M. 1969. Trans. Am. Microsc. Soc. 88:266-274.

Cryptobiosis

One of the most intriguing features of terrestrial tardigrades is their capacity to enter a state of suspended animation, called cryptobiosis (formerly called anabiosis), during which metabolism is virtually imperceptible; the organism can withstand harsh environmental conditions. Under gradual drying conditions, the water content of the body is reduced from 85% to only 3%, movement ceases, and the body becomes barrel shaped. In a cryptobiotic state tardigrades can resist temperature extremes, ionizing radiation, oxygen deficiency, and other adverse conditions and may survive for years. Activity resumes when moisture is again available.

Phylogeny

The affinities of tardigrades are among the most puzzling of all animal groups. They have some similarities to the rotifers, particularly in their reproduction and their cryptobiotic tendencies, and some authors call them pseudocoelomates. Their embryology, however, would seem to put them among the coelomates. The nervous system indicates a relationship to the annelids and arthropods. Some authors place them close to the arthropods, particularly the mites. Their enterocoelic origin of the mesoderm is a deuterostome characteristic. For the present, at least, their status is quite uncertain.

___ Summary

The seven small phyla covered in this chapter are grouped together here for convenience. The Sipuncula, Echiura, and probably the Pogonophora are related to the annelids; the Pentastomida, Onychophora, and Tardigrada seem closer to the arthropods. The relationship of the Priapulida to other coelomates is obscure.

Sipunculans are small, burrowing marine worms with an eversible introvert at their anterior end. The introvert bears tentacles with which they deposit feed. They are not metameric.

Echiurans are more diverse than sipunculans, but fewer in number of species. They are also burrowing marine worms, and most deposit feed with a proboscis anterior to their mouth. They show a transitory metamerism during their embryogenesis.

Pogonophorans live in tubes on the deep ocean floor, and they are metameric. They have no mouth or digestive tract but apparently absorb nutrient by the crown of tentacles at their anterior end.

The Priapulida are a tiny group of burrowing, marine worms with an eversible proboscis. They are mostly predaceous, and in most species the mouth is surrounded by recurved spines for capturing prey. They are not metameric but show superficial segmentation.

The Pentastomida are wormlike parasites in the lungs and nasal passages of carnivorous vertebrates. They are clearly related to the arthropods, possibly closest to the branchiuran Crustacea.

The Onychophora are caterpillar-like animals found in humid, mostly tropical habitats. They are metameric and crawl by means of a series of unjointed, clawed appendages. They show both annelid and arthropod characteristics.

Tardigrades are minute animals, mostly terrestrial, living in the water film that surrounds mosses and lichens. They have eight unjointed legs and a nonchitinous cuticle. Their chief body cavity is a hemocoel, as in arthropods. They can undergo cryptobiosis, withstanding adverse conditions for long periods.

Batillipes bullacaudatus, a marine tardigrade.
Courtesy R.P. Higgins.

Selected references

Barnes, R.D. 1980. Invertebrate zoology, ed. 4. Philadelphia, Saunders College/Holt, Rinehart & Winston.

Clark, R.B. 1972. Systematics and phylogeny: Annelida, Echiura, Sipuncula. In M. Florkin and B.T. Scheer (eds.). Chemical zoology, vol. 4. New York, Academic Press, Inc.

Cutler, E.B. 1982. Pogonophora. In S.P. Parker (ed.). Synopsis and classification of living organisms, vol. 2. New York, McGraw-Hill Book Co.

Gosner, K.L. 1971. Guide to identification of marine and estuarine invertebrates: Cape Hatteras to the Bay of Fundy. New York, Interscience.

Gould-Somero, M. 1974. Echiura. In A.C. Giese and J.S. Pearse (eds.). Reproduction of marine invertebrates, vol. 3. New York, Academic Press, Inc.

Hackman, R.H., and M. Goldberg. 1975. Peripatus: its affinities and its cuticle. Science **190**:582-583.

Hyman, L.H. 1959. The invertebrates, vol. 5. New York, McGraw-Hill Book Co.

Ivanov, A.V. 1963. Pogonophora. New York, Consultants Bureau.

Jaccarini, V., and P.J. Schembri. 1977. Feeding and particle selection in the echiurian worm *Bonellia viridis* Rolando (Echiura: Bonellidae). J. Exp. Mar. Biol. Ecol. **28**(2):163-182.

Jones, M.L. 1981. *Riftia pachyptila* Jones: observations on the vestimentiferan worm from the Galapagos Rift. Science **213**:333-336. *This article concerns primarily the structure of the giant pogonophoran. Following it in the same issue of Science are five more papers on the worm's nutrition, blood, and bacterial symbionts.*

Kaestner, A. 1967, 1968. Invertebrate zoology, vols. 1 and 2. New York, Interscience.

Lavallard, R., and S. Campiglia. 1975. Contribution to the biology of *Peripatus acacioi* Marcus and Marcus (Onychophora). V. Studies of the breeding in a laboratory culture. Zool. Anz. **195**(5/6):338-350. *In French with French and English summaries.*

Light, S.F., R.I. Smith, F.A. Pitelka, D.P. Abbott, and F.M. Weesner. 1967. Intertidal invertebrates of the central California coast. Berkeley, University of California Press.

Manton, S.M. 1977. The Arthropoda: habits, functional morphology, and evolution. Oxford, Eng., Clarendon Press. *The Onychophora is considered part of the phylum Uniramia, along with the Myriapoda, and Hexapoda (Insecta) as subphyla.*

Nelson, D.R. 1975. The hundred-year hibernation of the water bear. Nat. Hist. **84**(7):62-65.

Peck, S.B. 1975. A review of the New World Onychophora with the description of a new cavernicolous genus and species from Jamaica. Psyche **82**(3/4):341-358. *A key to the two families and eight genera of New World onychophorans.*

Pennak, R.W. 1978. Freshwater invertebrates of the United States, ed. 2. New York, John Wiley & Sons, Inc.

Pollock, L.W. 1975. Tardigrada. In A.C. Giese and J.S. Pearse (eds.). Reproduction of marine invertebrates, vol. 2. New York, Academic Press, Inc., pp. 43-54.

Rice, M.E. 1975. Sipuncula. In A.C. Giese and J.S. Pearse (eds.). Reproduction of marine invertebrates, vol. 2. New York, Academic Press, Inc., pp. 67-128.

Schmidt, G.D., and L.S. Roberts. 1981. Foundations of parasitology, ed. 2. St. Louis, The C.V. Mosby Co. *A chapter is devoted to the Pentastomida.*

Shapeero, W. 1961. Phylogeny of Priapulida. Science **133**:879-880.

Southward, E.C. 1975. Fine structure and phylogeny of the Pogonophora. In E.J.W. Barrington and R.P.S. Jefferies (eds.). Protochordates. London, Zoological Society of London, no. 36.

Southward, E.C. 1975. Pogonophora. In A.C. Giese and J.S. Pearse (eds.). Reproduction of marine invertebrates, vol. 2. New York, Academic Press, Inc., pp. 129-156.

Stephen, A.C., and S.J. Edmonds. 1972. The phyla Sipuncula and Echiura. London, British Museum (Natural History).

van der Land, J. 1975. Priapulida. In A.C. Giese and J.S. Pearse (eds.). Reproduction of marine invertebrates, vol. 2. New York, Academic Press, Inc., pp. 55-66.

Wingstrand, K.G. 1972. Comparative spermatology of a pentastomid, *Raillietiella hemidactyli,* and a branchiuran crustacean, *Argulus foliaceus,* with a discussion of pentastomid relationships. Kongelige Danske Videnskabernes Selskab Biol. Skrifter **19**(4):1-72.

Selected *Scientific American* article

Crowe, J.H., and A.F. Cooper, Jr. 1971. Cryptobiosis. **225**(6):30-36 (Dec.).

CHAPTER 19

THE LOPHOPHORATE ANIMALS

Phylum Phoronida

Phylum Ectoprocta (Bryozoa)

Phylum Brachiopoda

The lophophorate animals are distinguished by a crown of delicate ciliated tentacles surrounding the mouth and used for particle feeding. Colonies of individuals are commonly encrusting or branching and bushy, like this *Bugula neritina*.

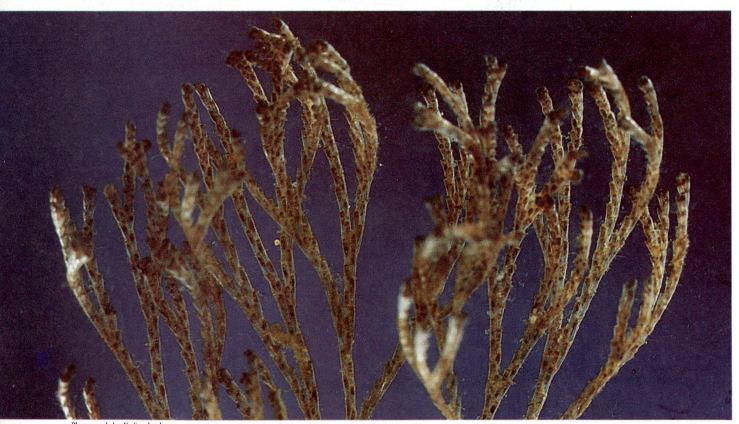

Photograph by K. Sandved.

Position in Animal Kingdom

1. The lophophorate phyla possess a **true coelom,** that is, a body cavity lined with a layer of mesodermal epithelium called the peritoneum.
2. They belong to the **protostome** branch of the **bilateral** animals, but they have some of the characteristics of the deuterostomes.
3. The three phyla are usually grouped together because they all possess the crown of tentacles called a **lophophore,** which is specialized for sedentary filter feeding. The lophophore **surrounds the mouth but not the anus,** thus differing from the tentacular crown of Entoprocta.

Biological Contributions

1. The lophophore, a unique ridge that bears hollow, ciliated tentacles, is an efficient specialized filter-feeding device, forming a ciliated route, or trough, for trapping and directing food particles to the mouth.
2. The brachiopods and phoronids possess vascular systems for circulation of food nutrients and other materials.
3. The blood in phoronids possesses red blood corpuscles that contain hemoglobin for carrying oxygen.

THE LOPHOPHORATES

The Phoronida are wormlike marine forms that live in secreted tubes in sand or mud or attached to rocks or shells. The Ectoprocta are minute forms, mostly colonial, whose protective cases often form encrusting masses on rocks, shells, or plants. The Brachiopoda are bottom-dwelling marine forms that superficially resemble molluscs because of their bivalved shells.

One might wonder why these three apparently different types of animals are lumped together in a group called Lophophorata. Actually they have more in common than first appears. They are all coelomate; all have some protostome characteristics; all are sessile; and none has a distinct head. But these characteristics are also shared by other phyla. What really sets them apart from other phyla is the common possession of a **ciliary feeding device** called a **lophophore** (Gr., *lophos,* crest or tuft, + *phorein,* to bear).

A lophophore is a unique arrangement of ciliated tentacles borne on a ridge (a fold of the body wall), which surrounds the mouth but not the anus. The lophophore with its crown of tentacles contains within it an extension of the coelom, and the thin, ciliated walls of the tentacles are not only an efficient feeding device but also serve as a respiratory surface for exchange of gases between the environmental water and the coelomic fluid. The lophophore can usually be extended for feeding or withdrawn for protection.

In addition, all three phyla have a **U-shaped alimentary canal,** with the anus placed near the mouth but **outside the lophophore.** All have a **free-swimming larval stage** but are **sessile as adults.**

Phylum Phoronida

The phylum Phoronida (fo-ron'i-da) (L., surname of Io, in mythology) is comprised of approximately 10 species of small, wormlike animals that live on the bottom of shallow coastal waters, especially in temperate seas. They range from a few millimeters to 30 cm in length. Each worm secretes a leathery or chitinous tube in which it lies free but which it never leaves. The tubes may be anchored singly or in a tangled mass on rocks, shells, or pilings or buried in the sand. The

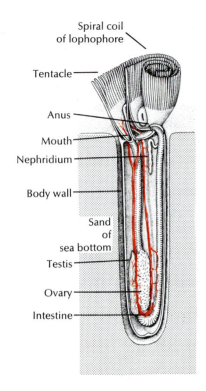

Spiral coil of lophophore

Tentacle

Anus

Mouth

Nephridium

Body wall

Sand of sea bottom

Testis

Ovary

Intestine

Figure 19-1

Internal structure of *Phoronis* (phylum Phoronida), in diagrammatic vertical section, showing one half of lophophore.

tentacles on the lophophore are thrust out for feeding, but if the animal is disturbed, it can withdraw completely into its tube.

The lophophore is made up of two parallel ridges curved in a horseshoe shape, the bend located ventrally and the mouth lying between the two ridges (Fig. 19-1). The horns of the ridges are often coiled into twin spirals. Each ridge carries hollow ciliated tentacles, which, like the ridges themselves, are extensions of the body wall.

The cilia on the tentacles direct a water current toward a groove between the two ridges, which leads toward the mouth. Plankton and detritus caught in this current become entangled in mucus and are carried by the cilia to the mouth. The anus lies dorsal to the mouth, outside the lophophore, flanked on each side by a nephridiopore (Fig. 19-1). Water leaving the lophophore passes over the anus and nephridiopores, carrying away the wastes. Cilia in the stomach area of the U-shaped gut aid in food movement.

The body wall is made of cuticle, epidermis, and both longitudinal and circular muscles. The coelomic cavity is subdivided by mesenteric partitions into compartments similar to those of the deuterostomes. The phoronids have a closed system of contractile blood vessels but no heart; the red blood contains hemoglobin. There is a pair of metanephridia. A nerve ring sends nerves to the tentacles and body wall; a single giant motor fiber lies in the epidermis; and an epidermal nerve plexus supplies the body wall and epidermis.

There are both monoecious (the majority) and dioecious species of Phoronida, and at least one species reproduces asexually. Cleavage seems to be related to both the spiral and the radial types. The free-swimming, ciliated larva, called an actinotroch, metamorphoses into the adult, which sinks to the bottom, secretes a tube, and becomes sessile.

Phoronopsis californica is a large, orange form about 30 cm long found along the west coast of the United States. *Phoronis architecta* is a smaller (approximately 12 cm long) Atlantic coast species that has a very wide distribution.

___ Phylum Ectoprocta (Bryozoa)

The Ectoprocta (ek-to-prok'ta) (Gr., *ektos*, outside, + *proktos*, anus) have long been called bryozoans, or moss animals (Gr., *bryon*, moss, + *zōon*, animal), a term that originally included the Entoprocta also. However, because the entoprocts are pseudocoelomates and have the anus located within the tentacular crown, they are no longer classed with the ectoprocts, which, like the other lophophorates, are eucoelomate and have the anus outside the circle of tentacles. Some authors continue to use the name "Bryozoa" but now exclude the entoprocts from the group.

Of the 4000 or so species of ectoprocts, few are more than 0.5 mm long. All are aquatic, both freshwater and marine, but are found largely in shallow waters. With very few exceptions they are colony builders. Ectoprocts have been very successful. They have left a rich fossil record since the Ordovician period. Marine forms today exploit all kinds of firm surfaces, such as shells, rocks, large brown algae, mangrove roots, and ship bottoms.

Each member of a colony lives in a tiny chamber, called a **zoecium**, which is secreted by its epidermis (Fig. 19-2). Each individual, or **zooid**, consists of a feeding polypide and a case-forming cystid. The **polypide** includes the lophophore, digestive tract, muscles, and nerve centers. The **cystid** is the body wall of the animal, together with its secreted exoskeleton. The exoskeleton, or zoecium, may,

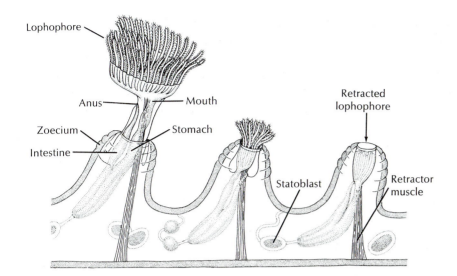

Figure 19-2

Small portion of freshwater colony of *Plumatella* (phylum Ectoprocta), which grows on the underside of rocks. These tiny individuals disappear into their chitinous zoecia when disturbed.

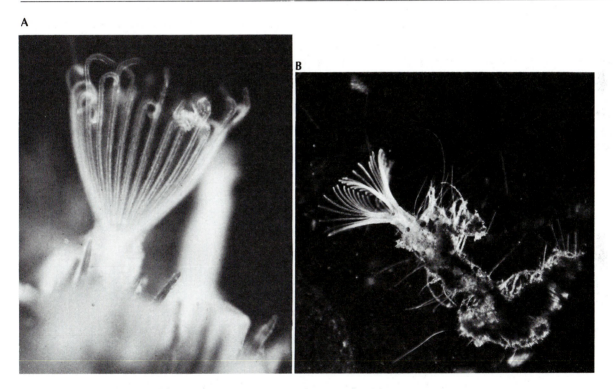

according to the species, be gelatinous, chitinous, or stiffened with calcium and possibly also impregnated with sand. The shape may be boxlike, vaselike, oval, or tubular.

Some colonies form limy encrustations on seaweed, shells, and rocks; others form fuzzy or shrubby growths on erect, branching colonies that look like seaweed. Some ectoprocts might easily be mistaken for hydroids but can be distinguished under a microscope by the fact that their tentacles are ciliated (Fig. 19-3). In some freshwater forms the individuals are borne on finely branching stolons that form delicate tracings on the underside of rocks or plants. Other freshwater ectoprocts are embedded in large masses of gelatinous material. Although the zooids are minute, the colonies may be several centimeters in diameter, some encrusting colonies may be a meter or more in width (Fig. 19-4), and erect forms

Figure 19-3

A, Ciliated lophophore of *Flustrella,* a marine ectoproct. **B,** *Plumatella repens,* a freshwater bryozoan (phylum Ectoprocta). It grows in branching, threadlike colonies on the underside of rocks and vegetation in lakes, ponds, and streams.

Figure 19-4

Skeletal remains of a colony of *Membranipora,* a marine encrusting form of Ectoprocta. Each little oblong zoecium is the calcareous former home of a tiny ectoproct.

Photograph by B. Tallmark.

may reach 30 cm or more in height. Freshwater ectoprocts may form mosslike colonies on the stems of plants or on rocks, usually in shallow ponds or pools. They may be able to slide along slowly on the object that supports them.

The polypide lives a type of jack-in-the-box existence, popping up to feed and then quickly withdrawing into its little chamber, which often has a tiny trapdoor (operculum) that shuts to conceal its inhabitant. To extend the tentacular crown, certain muscles contract, which increases the hydraulic pressure within the body cavity and pushes the lophophore out. Other muscles can contract to withdraw the crown to safety with great speed.

The lophophore ridge tends to be circular in marine ectoprocts (Fig. 19-3, *A*) and U-shaped in freshwater species (Fig. 19-3, *B*). When feeding, the animal extends the lophophore and spreads the tentacles out into a funnel. Cilia on the tentacles draw water into the funnel and out between the tentacles. Food particles trapped in mucus in the funnel are drawn into the mouth, both by the pumping action of the muscular pharynx and by the action of cilia in the pharynx. Undesirable particles can be rejected by reversing the ciliary action, by drawing the tentacles close together, or by retracting the whole lophophore into the zoecium. Digestion in the ciliated, U-shaped digestive tract appears to be extracellular for protein and starches and intracellular for fats.

Respiratory, vascular, and excretory organs are absent. Gaseous exchange is through the body surface, and since the ectoprocts are small, coelomic fluid is adequate for internal transport. Coelomocytes engulf and store waste materials. There are a ganglionic mass and a nerve ring around the pharynx, but no sense organs are present. The coelom is divided by a septum into an anterior portion in the lophophore and a larger posterior portion. Pores in the walls between adjoining zooids permit exchange of materials by way of the coelomic fluid.

Most colonies are made up of feeding individuals, but polymorphism also occurs. One type of modified zooid resembles a bird beak that snaps at small invading organisms that might foul a colony. Another type has a long bristle that sweeps away foreign particles.

Most ectoprocts are hermaphroditic. Some species shed eggs into the seawater, but most brood their eggs, some within the coelom and some externally in a special ovicell, which is a modified zoecium in which the embryo develops. Marine species have radial cleavage but a highly modified trochophore larva with a vibratile plume of sensory cilia, an adhesive sac, and a piriform organ. After swimming about for a time, the larva uses the vibratile plume to select a suitable site for settling, then attaches temporarily with a sticky acid mucopolysaccharide secreted from the piriform organ. Later, the adhesive sac produces acid mucopolysaccharide and protein secretions that effect a permanent attachment.

Freshwater species reproduce both sexually and asexually. Asexual reproduction is by budding or by means of **statoblasts**, hard, resistant capsules containing a mass of germinative cells that are formed during the summer and fall (Fig. 19-2). When the colony dies in late autumn, the statoblasts are released, and in spring they can give rise to new polypides and eventually to new colonies.

Brooding is often accompanied by degeneration of the lophophore and gut of the adults, the remains of which contract into minute dark balls, or **brown bodies**. Later, new internal organs may be regenerated in the old chambers. The brown bodies may remain passive or may be taken up and eliminated by the new digestive tract—an unusual kind of storage excretion.

_____ Phylum Brachiopoda

The Brachiopoda (brak-i-op′o-da) (Gr., _brachiōn,_ arm, + _pous, podos,_ foot), or lamp shells, are an ancient group. Although fewer than 300 species are now living, some 30,000 fossil species, which once flourished in the Paleozoic and Mesozoic seas, have been described. Modern forms have changed little from the early ones. _Lingula_ (L., tongue) (Fig. 19-5, _A_) is probably the most ancient of these "living fossils," having existed virtually unchanged since Ordovician times. Most modern brachiopod shells range between 5 to 80 mm in length, but some fossil forms reached 30 cm.

Brachiopods are attached, bottom-dwelling, marine forms that mostly prefer shallow water. Their name, which means "arm-footed," refers to the arms of the **lophophore**. Externally brachiopods resemble the bivalved molluscs in having two calcareous shell valves secreted by the mantle. They were, in fact, classed with the molluscs until the middle of the nineteenth century. Brachiopods, however, have **dorsal** and **ventral valves** instead of right and left lateral valves as do the bivalve molluscs and, unlike the bivalves, most of them are attached to a substrate either directly or by means of a fleshy stalk called a **pedicel** (or pedicle). Some, such as _Lingula,_ live in vertical burrows in sand or mud. Muscles open and close the valves and provide movement for the stalk and tentacles.

In most brachiopods the ventral (pedicel) valve is slightly larger than the dorsal (brachial) valve, and one end projects in the form of a short pointed beak that is perforated where the fleshy stalk passes through (Fig. 19-5, _B_). In many the shape of the pedicel valve is that of the classic oil lamp of ancient Greece and Rome, so that the brachiopods came to be known as the "lamp shells."

There are two classes of brachiopods, based on shell structure. The shell valves of Articulata are connected by a hinge with an interlocking tooth-and-socket arrangement, as in _Terebratella_ (L., _terebratus,_ a boring, + _ella,_ dim. suffix); those of Inarticulata lack the hinge and are held together by muscles only, as in _Lingula_ and _Glottidia_ (Gr., _glōttidos,_ mouth of windpipe).

The body occupies only the posterior part of the space between the valves (Fig. 19-6), and extensions of the body wall form mantle lobes that line and secrete the shell. The large horseshoe-shaped lophophore in the anterior mantle cavity bears long, ciliated tentacles used in respiration and feeding. Ciliary water currents carry food particles between the gaping valves and over the lophophore. Food is caught in mucus on the tentacles and carried in a ciliated food groove along the arm of the lophophore to the mouth. Unwanted particles are carried

Figure 19-5

Brachiopods. **A,** _Lingula,_ an inarticulate brachiopod that normally occupies a burrow. The contractile pedicel can withdraw the body into the burrow. **B,** An articulate brachiopod, _Terebratella._ The valves have a tooth-and-socket articulation, and a short pedicel projects through the pedicel valve to attach to the substratum.

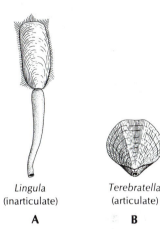

Lingula
(inarticulate)

A

Terebratella
(articulate)

B

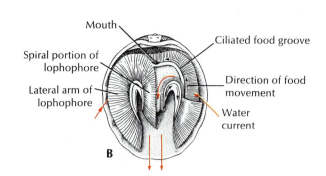

Figure 19-6

Phylum Brachiopoda. **A,** An articulate brachiopod (longitudinal section). **B,** Feeding and respiratory currents. Large arrows show water flow over lophophore; small arrows indicate food movement toward mouth in ciliated food groove.

B, Modified from Russell-Hunter, W.D. 1969. A biology of higher invertebrates. New York, Macmillan, Inc.

down rejection tracts to the mantle lobe and carried out in ciliary currents. Organic detritus and some algae are apparently primary food sources. The brachiopod lophophore not only can create food currents, as do other lophophorates, but also seems to be able to absorb dissolved nutrients directly from the environmental seawater.

The coelom, like that of other lophophorates, has an anterior mesocoel and a posterior metacoel. One or two pairs of nephridia open into the coelom and empty into the mantle cavity. Coelomocytes, which ingest particulate wastes, are carried out by the nephridia. There is an open circulatory system with a contractile heart. The lophophore and mantle are probably the chief sites of gaseous exchange. There is a nerve ring with a small dorsal and a larger ventral ganglion.

Sexes are separate, and paired gonads discharge gametes through the nephridia. Most fertilization is external, but a few species brood their eggs and young.

The development of brachiopods is similar in some ways to that of the deuterostomes, with radial, mostly equal, holoblastic cleavage and the coelom forming enterocoelically in the articulates. The free-swimming larva resembles the trochophore. In the articulates, metamorphosis occurs after the larva has attached by a pedicel. In inarticulates the juvenile resembles a minute brachiopod with a coiled pedicel in the mantle cavity. There is no metamorphosis. As the larva settles, the pedicel attaches to the substratum, and adult existence begins.

Phylogeny and Adaptive Radiation

The possession of a lophophore by all three phyla is considered evidence of their close relationship, but each phylum has specialized along its own lines and developed its own life-style. As a group they seem to occupy a phylogenetic position somewhere between the protostomes and the deuterostomes. The coelom is divided into three regions as in deuterostomes, although the anterior portion, or protocoel, is repressed, since there is no head. The lack of a head in lophophorates may be correlated with their ciliary method of feeding. In their embryology they display both protostome and deuterostome characteristics, with radial cleavage and, in the brachiopods, enterocoelic development of the coelom. All have a trochophore type of larva. Some authorities consider them the most primitive of the deuterostomes or at least ancestral to the other deuterostomes.

All lophophorates are **filter feeders,** and most of their evolutionary diversification has been guided by this function. The tubes of phoronids vary according to their habitats. Various ectoprocts tend to build their protective exoskeletons of chitin or gelatin, which may or may not be impregnated with calcium and sand. Brachiopod variations occur largely in their shells and lophophores.

___ Summary

The Phoronida, Ectoprocta, and Brachiopoda all bear a lophophore, which is a crown of ciliated tentacles surrounding the mouth but not the anus and containing an extension of the coelomic cavity. They are also sessile as adults, have a U-shaped digestive tract, and have free-swimming larvae. The lophophore functions as both a respiratory and a feeding structure, its cilia creating water currents from which food particles are filtered.

Phoronida are the least successful of the lophophorates, living in tubes mostly in shallow coastal waters. The lophophore is thrust out of the tube for feeding.

Ectoprocts are abundant in marine habitats, living on a variety of submerged substrata, and a number of species are common in fresh water. Ectoprocts are colonial, and although each individual is quite small, the colonies are commonly several centimeters or more in width or height. Each individual lives in a chamber (zoecium), which is a secreted exoskeleton of chitinous, calcium carbonate, or gelatinous material.

Brachiopods were a very successful phylum in the Paleozoic era but have been declining since the early Mesozoic era. Their bodies and lophophores are covered by a mantle, which secretes a dorsal and a ventral valve (shell). They are usually attached to the substrate directly or by means of a pedicel.

The lophophorates have coelomic compartments that apparently correspond to two of the three compartments (mesocoel and metacoel) found in many deuterostomes. Their embryogenesis shows both protostome and deuterostome characteristics.

Selected references

American Society of Zoology. 1977. Biology of lophophorates. Am. Zool. **17**(1):3-150. *A collection of 13 papers.*

Barnes, R.D. 1980. Invertebrate zoology, ed. 4. Philadelphia, Saunders College/Holt, Rinehart & Winston.

Emig, C.C. 1977. The lophophore: significant structures in Lophophorata (Brachiopoda, Bryozoa, Phoronida). Zool. Ser. **5**(3/4):133-138.

Emig, C.C. 1977. Embryology of Phoronida. Am. Zool. **17**:21-37.

Gosner, K.L. 1971. Guide to identification of marine and estuarine invertebrates: Cape Hatteras to the Bay of Fundy. New York, Interscience.

Hyman, L.H. 1959. The invertebrates, vol. 5. Smaller coelomate groups. New York, McGraw-Hill Book Co. *Phoronida, Ectoprocta, Brachiopoda, and Sipuncula are covered in this volume.*

Light, S.F., R.I. Smith, F.A. Pitelka, D.P. Abbott, and F.M. Weesner. 1967. Intertidal invertebrates of the central California coast. Berkeley, University of California Press.

McCammon, H.M. 1969. The food of articulate brachiopods. J. Paleontol. **43**(4):976-985.

Nielson, C. 1977. The relationships of Entoprocta, Ectoprocta and Phoronida. Am. Zool. **17**:149-150.

Pennak, R.W. 1978. Freshwater invertebrates of the United States, ed. 2. New York, John Wiley & Sons, Inc. *Accounts of the freshwater ectoprocts and the tardigrades, with keys to the common species.*

Rudwick, M.J.S. 1970. Living and fossil brachiopods. London, Hutchinson Educational.

Ryland, J.S. 1970. Bryozoans. London, Hutchinson Educational.

Steele-Petrovic, H.M. 1976. Brachiopod food and feeding processes. Palaeontology **19**(3):417-436.

Woollacott, R.M., and R.C. Zimmer (eds.). 1977. Biology of bryozoans. New York, Academic Press, Inc. *Contains 15 articles on ectoprocts. Advanced.*

CHAPTER 20

THE ECHINODERMS

Phylum Echinodermata

Beautiful brittle star, *Ophiothrix suensonii,* clinging to its host sponge. Suenson's brittle stars are always associated with sponges or horny corals.

Photograph by W.C. Ober.

Position in Animal Kingdom

Phylum Echinodermata (e-ki'no-der'ma-ta) (Gr., *echinos,* sea urchin, hedgehog, + *derma,* skin, + *ata,* characterized by) belongs to the **Deuterostomia** branch of the animal kingdom, the members of which are enterocoelous coelomates. The other phyla of this group are Chaetognatha, Hemichordata, and Chordata. Primitively, deuterostomes have the following embryological features in common: anus developing from or near the blastopore, and mouth developing elsewhere; coelom budded off from the archenteron (enterocoel); radial and indeterminate cleavage; and endomesoderm (mesoderm derived from or with the endoderm) from enterocoelic pouches. Although only distantly related, the Echinodermata is the only major invertebrate group showing affinities with the vertebrates. The typical deuterostome embryogenesis is shown only by some of the lower vertebrates, but the similarity probably has real evolutionary meaning. Thus, the echinoderms, the chordates, and the lesser deuterostome phyla presumably have been derived from a common ancestor. Nevertheless, their evolutionary history has taken the echinoderms to the point where they are very much unlike any other animal group.

Biological Contributions

There is one word that best describes the echinoderms: strange. They are a major group, but they occupy the end of a side branch of the phylogenetic tree, so none of their characteristics can be said to presage those of any more advanced group. They have a unique constellation of characteristics that are found in no other phylum. Although an enormous amount of research has been devoted to the echinoderms, we are still far from a satisfactory understanding of many aspects of their biology. As Libbie Hyman (1955) wrote, echinoderms are a "noble group especially designed to puzzle the zoologist."

Among the more striking of the features shown by the echinoderms are the system of coelomic channels comprising the **water-vascular system,** the calcareous **dermal endoskeleton,** the **hemal system,** and the **metamorphosis** from bilateral larva to radial adult.

——THE ECHINODERMS

The echinoderms are marine forms and include the sea stars, brittle stars, sea urchins, sea cucumbers, and sea lilies. They represent a bizarre group sharply distinguished from all other members of the animal kingdom. Their name is derived from their external spines or protuberances. A calcareous endoskeleton is found in all members of the phylum, either in the form of plates or represented by scattered tiny ossicles.

The most noticeable characteristics of the echinoderms are (1) the spiny endoskeleton of plates, (2) the water-vascular system, (3) the pedicellariae, (4) the dermal branchiae, and (5) radial or biradial symmetry. Radial symmetry is not limited to echinoderms, but no other group with such complex organ systems has radial symmetry.

Echinoderms are an ancient group of animals extending back to the Cambrian period. Despite the excellent fossil record, the origin and early evolution of the echinoderms are still obscure. It seems clear that they descended from bilateral ancestors because their larvae are bilateral but become radially symmetrical later in their development. Many zoologists believe that early echinoderms were sessile and evolved radiality as an adaptation to the sessile existence. Bilaterality is of adaptive value to animals that travel through their environment, while radiality is of value to animals whose environment meets them on all sides equally. Hence, the body plan of present-day echinoderms seems to have been derived from one that was attached to the bottom by a stalk, had radial symmetry and radiating grooves (ambulacra) for food gathering, and had an upward-facing oral side. Attached forms were once plentiful, but only about 80 species, all in the class Crinoidea, still

Figure 20-1

Some sea stars (subclass Asteroidea) from the Pacific coast of North America. **A,** Cushion star *Pteraster tessellatus* can secrete incredible quantities of mucus when disturbed, presumably as a defense reaction. **B,** Leather star *Dermasterias imbricata* lacks spines and feeds on sea anemones. **C,** *Mediaster aequalis* has a brilliant red color. **D,** *Crossaster papposus,* one of the sun stars, feeds on other sea stars. **E,** *Pisaster ochraceus* is the most abundant sea star on the Pacific coast of the United States, sometimes occurring in great numbers. This and many other species of sea stars show a diversity of individual coloration (see also p. 251).

A, B, D, and E, Photographs by R. Harbo; C, photograph by D.W. Gotshall.

A

B

C

D

survive. Oddly, conditions have favored the survival of their free-moving descendants, although they are still quite radial, and among them are some of the most abundant marine animals. Nevertheless, in the exception that proves the rule, at least three groups of echinoderms (two groups of echinoids and the holothuroids) seem to be evolving back toward bilaterality.

Echinoderms have no ability to osmoregulate and thus are rarely found in brackish waters. They are found in all oceans of the world and at all depths, from the intertidal to the abyssal regions. Often the most common animals in the deep ocean are echinoderms. The most abundant species found in the Philippine Trench (10,540 m) was a holothurian. Echinoderms are virtually all bottom dwellers, although there are a few pelagic species.

No parasitic echinoderms are known, but a few are commensals. On the other hand, a wide variety of other animals make their homes in or on echinoderms, including parasitic or commensal algae, protozoa, ctenophores, turbellarians, cirripedes, copepods, decapods, snails, clams, polychaetes, fish, and other echinoderms.

The asteroids, or sea stars (Fig. 20-1), are commonly found in various types of bottom habitats, often on hard, rocky surfaces, but numerous species are at home on sandy or soft bottoms. Some species are particle feeders, but many are predators, feeding particularly on sedentary or sessile prey, since the sea stars themselves are relatively slow moving.

Ophiuroids—brittle stars, or serpent stars (Fig. 20-10)—are by far the most active echinoderms, moving by their arms rather than by tube feet. A few species are reported to have swimming ability, and some burrow. They may be scavengers, browsers, or deposit or filter feeders. Some are commensal in large sponges, in whose water canals they may live in great numbers.

Holothurians, or sea cucumbers (Fig. 20-20), are widely prevalent in all seas.

E

Many are found on sandy or mucky bottoms, where they lie concealed. Compared with other echinoderms, holothurians are greatly extended in the oral-aboral axis. They are oriented with that axis more or less parallel to the substrate and lying on one side. Most are suspension or deposit feeders.

Echinoids, or sea urchins (Fig. 20-15), are adapted for living on the ocean bottom and always keep their oral surface in contact with the substratum. The "regular" sea urchins prefer hard bottoms, but the sand dollars and heart urchins ("irregular" urchins) are usually found on sand. The regular urchins, which are radially symmetrical, feed chiefly on algae or detritus, while the irregulars, which are secondarily bilateral, feed on small particles.

Crinoids (Fig. 20-25) stretch their arms out and up like a flower's petals and feed on plankton and suspended particles. Most living species become detached from their stems as adults, but they nevertheless spend most of their time on the substrate, holding on by means of aboral appendages called cirri.

The zoologist who admires the fascinating structure and function of echinoderms can share with the layperson an admiration of the beauty of their symmetry, often enhanced by bright colors. Many species are rather drab, but others may be orange, red, purple, blue, and often bicolor.

Because of the spiny nature of their structure, echinoderms are not often the prey of other animals—except other echinoderms (sea stars). Some fish have strong teeth and other adaptations that enable them to feed on echinoderms. In scattered parts of the world, humans relish sea urchin gonads, either raw or roasted on the half shell. Trepang, the cured body wall of certain large holothurians, is considered a delicacy, particularly in some Oriental countries. It is highly nutritious, since more than 50% is easily digestible protein, and it is said to impart a delicate flavor to soups.

Sea stars feed on a variety of molluscs, crustaceans, and other invertebrates, but their chief economic impact is on clams and oysters. A single star may eat as many as a dozen oysters or clams in a day. To rid shellfish beds of these pests, large rope "mops" in which the sea stars become entangled are sometimes dragged over oyster beds, and the collected sea stars are destroyed in hot water vats. A more effective method is to distribute lime over areas where they abound. Lime damages the delicate epidermal membrane, destroying the dermal branchiae and ultimately the animal itself. Meanwhile, the oysters remain with their shells tightly closed until the lime dissipates.

Echinoderms have been widely used in experimental embryology, for their gametes are usually abundant and easy to collect and handle in the laboratory. The investigator can follow the embryonic developmental stages with great accuracy. We know more about the molecular biology of sea urchin development than that of almost any other embryonic system. Artificial parthenogenesis was first discovered in sea urchin eggs, when it was found that, by treating the eggs with hypertonic seawater or subjecting them to a variety of other stimuli, development would take place without the presence of sperm.

CHARACTERISTICS

1. Body unsegmented (nonmetameric) with **radial, pentamerous symmetry**; body rounded, cylindrical, or star shaped, with five or more radiating areas, or ambulacra, alternating with interambulacral areas
2. **No head or brain;** few specialized sensory organs; sensory system of tactile and chemoreceptors, podia, terminal tentacles, photoreceptors, and statocysts
3. Nervous system with circumoral ring and radial nerves; usually two or three systems of networks located at different levels in the body, varying in degree of development according to group

4. **Endoskeleton** of **dermal calcareous ossicles** with **spines** or of calcareous **spicules** in dermis; covered by an epidermis (ciliated in most); **pedicellariae** (in some)

5. A unique **water-vascular system** of coelomic origin that extends from the body surface as a series of tentacle-like projections (**podia**, or **tube feet**) that are protracted by increase of fluid pressure within them; an opening to the exterior (**madreporite** or **hydropore**) usually present

6. Locomotion by tube feet, which project from the ambulacral areas, by movement of spines, or by movement of arms, which project from central disc of body

7. Digestive system usually complete; axial or coiled; anus absent in ophiuroids

8. Coelom extensive, forming the perivisceral cavity and the cavity of the water-vascular system; coelom of enterocoelous type; coelomic fluid with amebocytes

9. Blood-vascular system (**hemal system**) much reduced, playing little if any role in circulation, and surrounded by extensions of coelom (**perihemal sinuses**); main circulation of body fluids (coelomic fluids) by peritoneal cilia

10. Respiration by **dermal branchiae**, by tube feet, by **respiratory tree** (holothuroids), and by **bursae** (ophiuroids) *[margin note: variable]*

11. **Excretory organs absent**

12. Sexes separate (except a few hermaphroditic) with large gonads, single in holothuroids but multiple in most; simple ducts, with no elaborate copulatory apparatus or secondary sexual structures; fertilization usually external; eggs brooded in some

13. Development through **free-swimming, bilateral, larval stages** (some with direct development); metamorphosis to radial adult or subadult form

14. Autotomy and regeneration of lost parts conspicuous

CLASSIFICATION

There are about 6000 living and 20,000 extinct or fossil species of Echinodermata. The traditional classification of the echinoderms placed all the free-moving forms that were oriented with oral side down in the subphylum Eleutherozoa, containing most of the living species. The other subphylum, Pelmatozoa, contained mostly forms with stems and oral side up; most of the extinct classes and the living Crinoidea belong to this group. There has been growing recognition that these subphyla were each polyphyletic, and most students of echinoderms have adopted the following classification (proposed by Fell and used in Moore, 1966, 1967). Characteristics for strictly fossil classes are omitted here.

Subphylum Homalozoa (ho-mal'o-zo'a) (Gr., *homalos,* level, even, + *zōon,* animal). Ancient fossil echinoderms called carpoids, which were not radially symmetrical; fossil classes Homostelea, Homoiostelea, Stylophora (Fig. 22-3, p. 504), and Ctenocystoidea.

Subphylum Crinozoa (krin'o-zo'a) (Gr., *krinon,* lily, + *zōon,* animal). Radially symmetrical, with rounded or cup-shaped theca and brachioles or arms. Attached by stem during part or all of life. Oral surface directed upward. Fossil classes: Eocrinoidea, Paracrinoidea, Cystoidea, and Blastoidea.

    Class Crinoidea (krin-oi'de-a) (Gr., *krinon,* lily, + *eidos,* form, + *ea,* characterized by)—sea lilies and feather stars. Aboral attachment stalk of dermal ossicles; mouth and anus on oral surface; five arms branching at base and bearing pinnules; ciliated ambulacral grooves on oral surface with tentacle-like tube feet for food gathering; spines, madreporite, and pedicellariae absent. Examples: *Antedon, Nemaster* (Fig. 20-25).

Subphylum Asterozoa (as'ter-o-zo'a) (Gr., *aster,* star, + *zōon,* animal). Radially symmetrical, star-shaped echinoderms, unattached as adults.

    Class Stelleroidea (stel'ler-oi'de-a) (L., *stella,* star, + Gr., *eidos,* form). With characteristics of subphylum, body a central disc with radially arranged rays or arms.

        Subclass Somasteroidea (som'ast-er-oi'de-a) (Gr., *soma,* body, + *aster,* star, + *eidos,* form). Mostly extinct sea stars with primitive skeletal structure; single

Figure 20-2

Asterias forbesi is a heavy predator on oysters and other molluscs along the Atlantic coast of the United States. Also note the green sea urchins *Strongylocentrotus droebachiensis* and a human artifact. Trash such as the latter all too commonly detracts from the underwater scenery.
Photograph by L.S. Roberts.

living species, *Platasterias latiradiata,* from deep water off western coast of Mexico.

Subclass Asteroidea (as′ter-oi′de-a) (Gr., *aster,* star, + *eidos,* form, + *ea,* characterized by)—**sea stars.** Star-shaped echinoderms, with the arms not sharply marked off from the central disc; ambulacral grooves open, with tube feet on oral side; tube feet often with suckers; anus and madreporite aboral; pedicellariae present. Example: *Asterias* (Fig. 20-2).

Subclass Ophiuroidea (o′fe-u-roi′de-a) (Gr., *ophis,* snake, + *oura,* tail, + *eidos,* form)—**brittle stars and basket stars.** Star shaped, with the arms sharply marked off from the central disc; ambulacral grooves closed, covered by ossicles; tube feet without suckers and not used for locomotion; pedicellariae absent. Examples: *Ophiura* (Fig. 20-10, *A*), *Gorgonocephalus* (Fig. 20-13, *B*).

Subphylum Echinozoa (ek′in-o-zo′a) (Gr., *echinos,* sea urchin, hedgehog, + *zōon,* animal). Unattached, globoid, discoid, or more or less cylindrical echinoderms without arms. Fossil classes: Helicoplacoidea, Edriosteroidea, Ophiocistioidea.

Class Echinoidea (ek′i-noi′de-a) (Gr., *echinos,* sea urchin, hedgehog, + *eidos,* form)—**sea urchins, sea biscuits, and sand dollars.** More or less globular or disc-shaped echinoderms with no arms; compact skeleton or test with closely fitting plates; movable spines; ambulacral grooves covered by ossicles, closed; tube feet with suckers; pedicellariae present. Examples: *Arbacia, Strongylocentrotus* (Fig. 20-15, *D*), *Lytechinus, Mellita.*

Class Holothuroidea (hol′o-thu-roi′de-a) (Gr., *holothourion,* sea cucumber + *eidos,* form)—**sea cucumbers.** Cucumber-shaped echinoderms with no arms; spines absent; microscopic ossicles embedded in thick muscular wall; anus present; ambulacral grooves closed; tube feet with suckers; circumoral tentacles (modified tube feet); pedicellariae absent; madreporite plate internal. Examples: *Sclerodactyla, Parastichopus, Cucumaria* (Fig. 20-20, *C*).

Class Stelleroidea
Sea stars—subclass Asteroidea

Sea stars are familiar along the shoreline where large numbers of them may aggregate on the rocks. Sometimes they cling so tenaciously that they are difficult to dislodge without tearing off some of their tube feet. They also live in muddy or sandy bottoms and among coral reefs. They are often brightly colored and range in size from a centimeter in greatest diameter to about a meter across. *Asterias* (Gr., *asteros,* a star) (Fig. 20-2) is one of the common genera of the east coast of the United States and is commonly studied in zoology laboratories. *Pisaster* (Gr., *pisos,* a pea, + *asteros,* a star) (Fig. 20-1, *E*) is common on the California coast, as is *Dermasterias* (Gr., *dermatos,* skin, leather, + *asteros,* a star), the leather star (Fig. 20-1, *B*).

Figure 20-3

Asterias. **A,** Aboral view. **B,** Oral view.
Photographs by F.M. Hickman.

A

B

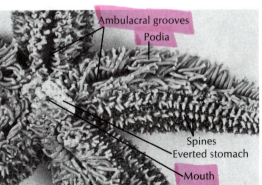

Form and function
External features

Sea stars are composed of a central disc that merges gradually with the tapering arms (rays). They tend to be pentamerous and typically have five arms, but they may have more (Fig. 20-1, *D*). The body is flattened, flexible, and covered with a ciliated pigmented epidermis. The mouth is centered on the under, or oral, side, surrounded by a soft peristomial membrane. An **ambulacral groove** along the oral side of each arm is bordered by movable **spines** that protect the rows of **tube feet**

Figure 20-4

A, Sea star dissection, aboral view; at right, portions of two arms with digestive glands lifted aside to expose gonads and ampullae. At lower left, two undissected arms show madreporite and spines. **B,** Water-vascular system. Podia penetrate between ossicles. (Polian vesicles are not present in *Asterias*.) **C,** Cross section of arm at level of gonads, illustrating open ambulacral grooves.

A, Photograph by F.M. Hickman.

(podia) projecting from the groove (Fig. 20-3). Viewed from the oral side, the large **radial nerve** can be seen in the center of each ambulacral groove (Fig. 20-4, C), between the rows of tube feet. The nerve is very superficially located, covered only by thin epidermis. Under the nerve is an extension of the coelom and the radial canal of the water-vascular system, all of which are external to the under-lying ossicles (Fig. 20-4, C). In all other classes of living echinoderms except the crinoids, these structures are covered over by ossicles or other dermal tissue; thus, the ambulacral grooves in asteroids and crinoids are said to be **open,** and those of the other groups are **closed.**

The aboral surface is usually rough and spiny, although the spines of many species are flattened, so that the surface appears smooth (Fig. 20-1, C). Around the bases of the spine are groups of minute, pincerlike **pedicellariae,** bearing tiny jaws manipulated by muscles (Fig. 20-5). These help keep the body surface free of debris, protect the papulae, and sometimes aid in food capture. The **papulae (dermal branchiae** or **skin gills)** are soft delicate projections of the coelomic cavity, covered only with epidermis and lined internally with peritoneum; they extend out through spaces between the ossicles and are concerned with respiration (Figs. 20-4, C, and 20-5, F). Also on the aboral side are the inconspicuous **anus** and the circular **madreporite** (Fig. 20-3, A), a calcareous sieve leading to the water-vascular system.

Endoskeleton

Beneath the epidermis of the sea star is a mesodermal endoskeleton of small calcareous plates, or **ossicles,** bound together with connective tissue. From these ossicles project the spines and tubercles that are responsible for the spiny surface. Muscles in the body wall move the rays and can partially close the ambulacral grooves by drawing their margins together.

Coelom, excretion, and respiration

The coelomic compartments of the larval echinoderm give rise to several structures in the adult, one of which is a spacious body **coelom** filled with fluid. The fluid contains amebocytes (**coelomocytes**), bathes the internal organs, and projects

Figure 20-5

Pedicellariae of sea stars and sea urchins. **A,** Forceps-type pedicellaria of *Asterias.* **B** and **C,** Scissors-type pedicellariae of *Asterias;* size relative to spine is shown in **B. D,** Tridactyl pedicellaria of *Strongylocentrotus,* cutaway showing muscle. **E,** Globiferous pedicellaria of *Strongylocentrotus.* **F,** Close-up view of the aboral surface of the sea star *Pycnopodia helianthoides.* Note the large pedicellariae, as well as the groups of small pedicellariae around the spines. Many thin-walled papulae can be seen.

A to **E,** Drawings by T. Doyle; **F,** photograph by R. Harbo.

into the papulae. The coelomic fluid is circulated around the body cavity and into the papulae by the ciliated peritoneal lining. Exchange of respiratory gases and excretion of nitrogenous waste, principally ammonia, take place by diffusion through the thin walls of the papulae and tube feet. Some wastes may be picked up by the coelomocytes, which migrate through the epithelium of the papulae or tube feet to the exterior, or the tips of papulae containing the waste-laden coelomocytes may be pinched off.

Water-vascular system

The water-vascular system is another coelomic compartment and is unique to the echinoderms. Showing exploitation of hydraulic mechanisms to a greater degree than in any other animal group, it is a system of canals and specialized tube feet that, together with the dermal ossicles, has determined the evolutionary potential and limitations of this phylum. In sea stars the primary functions of the water-vascular system are locomotion and food gathering, in addition to respiration and excretion.

Structurally, the water-vascular system opens to the outside through small pores in the **madreporite.** The madreporite of asteroids is on the aboral surface (Fig. 20-3, *A*) and leads into the **stone canal,** which descends toward the **ring canal** around the mouth (Fig. 20-4, *B*). **Radial canals** diverge from the ring canal, one into the ambulacral groove of each ray. Also attached to the ring canal are four or five pairs of folded, pouchlike **Tiedemann's bodies** and from one to five **polian vesicles** (polian vesicles are absent in some sea stars, such as *Asterias*). The Tiedemann's bodies are thought to produce coelomocytes, and the polian vesicles are apparently for fluid storage.

A series of small **lateral canals,** each with a one-way valve, connects the radial canal to the cylindrical **podia,** or **tube feet,** along the sides of the ambulacral groove in each ray. Each podium is a hollow, muscular tube, the inner end of which is a muscular sac, the **ampulla,** that lies within the body coelom (Fig. 20-4, *A* and *C*), and the outer end of which usually bears a **sucker.** Some species lack the suckers. The podia pass to the outside between the ossicles in the ambulacral groove.

The function of the madreporite is still obscure. One suggestion is that it allows rapid adjustment of hydrostatic pressure within the water-vascular system in response to changes in external hydrostatic pressure resulting from depth changes, as in tidal fluctuations and wave surges.

Figure 20-6

A, *Orthasterias koehleri* eating a clam. **B,** This *Pycnopodia helianthoides* has been overturned while eating a large sea urchin *Strongylocentrotus franciscanus.* This sea star has 20 to 24 arms and can range up to 1 m in diameter (arm tip to arm tip).

A, Photograph by R. Harbo; **B,** photograph by D.W. Gotshall.

A

B

The water-vascular system operates hydraulically and is an effective locomotor mechanism. The valves in the lateral canals prevent backflow of fluid into the radial canals. The tube foot has in its walls connective tissue that maintains the cylinder at a relatively constant diameter. On contraction of muscles in the ampulla, fluid is forced into the podium, extending it. Conversely, contraction of the longitudinal muscles in the tube foot retracts the podium, forcing fluid back into the ampulla. Contraction of muscles in one side of the podium bends the organ toward that side. Small muscles at the end of the tube foot can raise the middle of the disclike end, creating a suction-cup effect when the end is applied to the substrate. It has been estimated that by combining mucous adhesion with suction, a single podium can exert a pull equal to 25 to 30 g. Coordinated action of all or many of the tube feet is sufficient to draw the animal up a vertical surface or over rocks.

On a soft surface, such as muck or sand, the suckers are ineffective (numerous sand-dwelling species have no suckers), so the tube feet are employed as legs. Locomotion becomes mainly a stepping process. Most sea stars can move only a few centimeters per minute, but some very active ones can move 75 to 100 cm per minute; for example, *Pycnopodia* (Gr., *pyknos*, compact, dense, + *pous, podos*, foot) (Fig. 20-6, *A*). When inverted, the sea star bends its rays until some of the tubes reach the substratum and attach as an anchor; then the sea star slowly rolls over.

Tube feet are innervated by the central nervous system rather than through the diffuse subepidermal plexus. Nervous coordination enables the tube feet to move in a single direction, although not in unison, so that the sea star may progress. If the radial nerve in an arm is cut, the podia in that arm lose coordination, although they can still function. If the circumoral nerve ring is cut, the podia in all arms become uncoordinated, and movement ceases.

Feeding and digestive system

The **mouth** on the oral side leads through a short **esophagus** to a large **stomach** in the central disc. The lower (**cardiac**) part of the stomach can be everted through the mouth during feeding (Fig. 20-3, *B*), and excessive eversion is prevented by gastric ligaments. The upper (**pyloric**) part is smaller and connects by ducts to a pair of large **pyloric ceca** (**digestive glands**) in each arm (Fig. 20-4, *A*). Digestion is mostly extracellular, although some intracellular digestion may occur in the ceca.

Figure 20-7

A, Crown-of-thorns star *Acanthaster planci* feeding on coral. **B**, Close-up view of arm of *A. planci*. Puncture wounds from these spines are painful; the spines are equipped with poison glands.
Photographs by J.L. Rotman.

A   B

A short **intestine** leads aborally from the pyloric stomach, and there are usually a few small, saclike **intestinal ceca** (Fig. 20-4, *A*). The **anus** is inconspicuous, and some sea stars lack an intestine and anus.

Many sea stars are carnivorous and feed on molluscs, crustaceans, polychaetes, echinoderms, other invertebrates, and sometimes small fish. Sea stars consume a wide range of food items, but many show particular preferences (Fig. 20-7). Some select brittle stars, sea urchins, or sand dollars, swallowing them whole and later regurgitating undigestible ossicles and spines (Fig. 20-6, *A*). Some attack other sea stars, and if they are small compared to their prey, they may attack and begin eating at the end of one arm.

Asteroids feed heavily on molluscs (Fig. 20-6, *B*), and *Asterias* is a significant predator on commercially important clams and oysters. When feeding on a bivalve, a sea star will hump over its prey, attaching its podia to the valves, and then exert a steady pull, using its feet in relays. A force of some 1300 g can thus be exerted. In half an hour or so the adductor muscles of the bivalve fatigue and relax. With a very small gap available, the star inserts its soft everted stomach into the space between the valves and wraps it around the soft parts of the shellfish. After feeding, the sea star draws in its stomach by contraction of the stomach muscles and relaxation of body wall muscles.

Some sea stars feed on small particles, either entirely or in addition to carnivorous feeding. Plankton and other organic particles coming in contact with the animal's surface are carried by the epidermal cilia to the ambulacral grooves and then to the mouth.

Hemal system

The so-called hemal system is not very well developed in asteroids, and its function in all echinoderms is unclear. The hemal system has little or nothing to do with circulation of body fluids. It is a system of tissue strands enclosing unlined sinuses and is itself enclosed in another coelomic compartment, the **perihemal channels.** The main channel is the **axial sinus,** which extends up through a spongy mass of tissue (the **axial gland**) lying along the stone canal. At its oral end it connects to a **periesophageal hemal ring,** which in turn gives rise to **radial hemal lacunae** that run out into each arm between the radial nerve and the radial water canal. The axial gland also connects to a **gastric hemal ring,** with branches to each pyloric cecum, and to an **aboral hemal ring,** with branches to the gonads. Coelomocytes are present in the hemal fluid, and they may be produced in the hemal system. The hemal system may be useful in distributing digested products, but its specific functions are not really known.

Nervous system

The nervous system consists of three units at different levels in the disc and arm. The chief of these systems is the **oral (ectoneural)** system composed of a **nerve ring** around the mouth and a main **radial nerve** into each arm. It appears to coordinate the tube feet. A **deep (hyponeural)** system lies aboral to the oral system, and an **aboral** system consists of a ring around the anus and radial nerves along the roof of the rays. An **epidermal nerve plexus** or nerve net freely connects these systems with the body wall and related structures. The epidermal plexus has been shown to coordinate the responses of the dermal branchiae to tactile stimulation—the only instance known in echinoderms in which coordination occurs through a nerve net.

The sense organs are not well developed. Tactile organs and other sensory

Since 1963 there have been numerous reports of increasing numbers of the crown-of-thorns sea star (*Acanthaster planci* [Gr., *akantha*, thorn, + *asteros*, star]) (Fig. 20-7) that were damaging large areas of coral reef in the Pacific Ocean. The crown-of-thorns star feeds on coral polyps, and it sometimes occurs in large aggregations, or "herds." Among the suggested reasons for its increase were human destruction of the giant triton, a gastropod that feeds on sea stars, or that dredging, blasting, and other activities had destroyed the creatures that feed on the sea star larvae. Various attempts have been made to correct the problem. Indications at present are that the crown-of-thorns epidemic is tapering off and that recovery of the damaged reefs may be more rapid than was formerly believed.

cells are scattered over the surface, and an ocellus is at the tip of each arm. Their reactions are mainly to touch, temperature, chemicals, and differences in light intensity. Sea stars are usually more active at night.

Reproductive system, regeneration, and autotomy

Most sea stars have separate sexes. A pair of gonads lies in each interradial space (Fig. 20-4, *A*). Fertilization is external and occurs in early summer when the eggs and sperm are shed into the water. The maturation and shedding of sea star eggs are stimulated by a secretion from neurosecretory cells located on the radial nerves.

Echinoderms can regenerate lost parts. Sea star arms can regenerate readily, even if all are lost. Stars also have the power of autotomy and can cast off an injured arm near the base. It may take months to regenerate a new arm.

If an arm is broken off or removed, and it contains a part (about one fifth) of the central disc, the arm can regenerate a complete new sea star (Fig. 20-8)! In former times fishermen used to dispatch sea stars they collected from their oyster beds by chopping them in half with a hatchet—a worse than futile activity. Some sea stars reproduce asexually under normal conditions by cleaving the central disc, each part regenerating the rest of the disc and missing arms.

Development

In some species the liberated eggs are brooded, either under the oral side of the animal or in specialized aboral structures, and development is direct, but in most species the embryonating eggs are free in the water and hatch to free-swimming larvae.

Early embryogenesis shows the typical primitive deuterostome pattern. Gastrulation is by invagination, and the anterior end of the archenteron pinches off to become the coelomic cavity, which expands in a U shape to fill the blastocoel. Each of the legs of the U, at the posterior, constricts to become a separate vesicle, and these eventually give rise to the main coelomic compartments of the body (**somatocoels**). The anterior portion of the U gives rise to the water-vascular system and the perihemal channels. The free-swimming larva has cilia arranged in bands and is called a **bipinnaria** (Fig. 20-9, *A*). The ciliated tracts become extended into larval arms. Soon the larva grows three adhesive arms and a sucker at its

Figure 20-8

"Comet" form of the sea star *Linckia* in which one arm is regenerating the rest of the animal. Although asteroids characteristically can regenerate new arms as necessary if a part of the central disc is present, species of *Linckia* can accomplish this feat from an arm only.
Photograph by K. Sandved.

The mesocoel and metacoel compartments of the coelom, as found in the lophophorates, are present in echinoderms. Echinoderms also have a more anterior compartment, the protocoel, although the protocoel often is not completely separated from the mesocoel. In echinoderms the metacoel, mesocoel, and protocoel are referred to as somatocoel, hydrocoel, and axocoel.

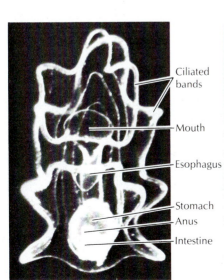

Ciliated bands

Mouth

Esophagus

Stomach
Anus
Intestine

A

B

Figure 20-9

Bilaterally symmetrical larvae of asteroids and echinoids. **A,** Bipinnaria of *Asterias rubens.* **B,** Echinopluteus of *Psammechinus miliaris;* as in the ophiopluteus, the ciliated bands extend onto the long, graceful arms.
Photographs by D.P. Wilson.

Figure 20-10

A, Brittle star *Ophiura lutkeni* (subclass Ophiuroidea). Brittle stars do not use their tube feet for locomotion but can move rapidly (for an echinoderm) by means of their arms. **B,** Basket star *Astrophyton muricatum* (subclass Ophiuroidea). Basket stars extend their many-branched arms to filter feed, usually at night.

A, Photograph by R. Harbo; **B,** photograph by D.W. Gotshall.

anterior end and is then called a **brachiolaria.** At that time it attaches to the substratum, forms a temporary attachment stalk, and undergoes metamorphosis.

Metamorphosis involves a dramatic reorganization of a bilateral larva into a radial juvenile. The anteroposterior axis of the larva is lost, and *what was the left side becomes the oral surface, and the larval right side becomes the aboral surface.* Correspondingly, the larval mouth and anus disappear, and a new mouth and anus form on what was originally the left and right sides, respectively. The portion of the anterior coelomic compartment from the left side expands to form the ring canal of the water-vascular system around the mouth, and then it grows branches to form the radial canals. As the short, stubby arms and the first podia appear, the animal detaches from its stalk and begins life as a young sea star.

Brittle stars—subclass Ophiuroidea

The brittle stars are the largest of the major groups of echinoderms in numbers of species, and they are probably the most abundant also. They abound in all types of benthic marine habitats, even carpeting the abyssal sea bottom in many areas.

Form and function

Apart from the typical possession of five arms, the brittle stars are surprisingly different from the asteroids. The arms of brittle stars are slender and sharply set off from the central disc (Fig. 20-10). They have no pedicellariae or papulae, and their ambulacral grooves are closed and covered with arm ossicles. The tube feet are without suckers; they aid in feeding but are of limited use in locomotion. In contrast to that in the asteroids, the madreporite of the ophiuroids is located on the oral surface, on one of the oral shield ossicles (Fig. 20-11). Ampullae on the podia are absent, and force for protrusion of the podium is generated by a proximal muscular portion of the podium.

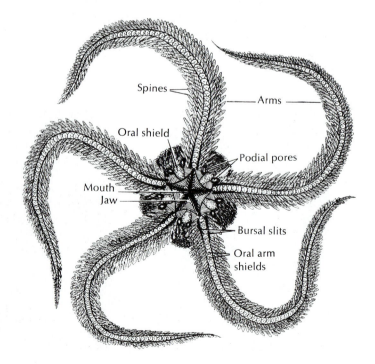

Figure 20-11

Oral view of spiny brittle star *Ophiothrix.*

Each of the jointed arms consists of a column of articulated ossicles (the so-called **vertebrae**), connected by muscles and covered by plates. Locomotion is by arm movement. The arms are moved forward in pairs and are placed against the substratum, while one (any one) is extended forward or trailed behind, and the animal is pulled or pushed along in a jerky fashion.

The mouth is surrounded by five movable plates that serve as **jaws** (Fig. 20-11). There is no anus. The skin is leathery, with dermal plates and spines arranged in characteristic patterns. Surface cilia are mostly lacking.

The visceral organs are confined to the central disc, since the rays are too slender to contain them (Fig. 20-12). The **stomach** is saclike, and there is no intestine. Indigestible material is cast out of the mouth.

Five pairs of **bursae** (peculiar to ophiuroids) open toward the oral surface by **genital slits** at the bases of the arms. Water circulates in and out of these sacs for exchange of gases. On the coelomic wall of each bursa are small **gonads** that discharge into the bursa their ripe sex cells, which pass through the genital slits into the water for fertilization (Fig. 20-13, *A*). Sexes are usually separate; a few ophiuroids are hermaphroditic. Some brood their young in the bursae; the young escape through the genital slits or by rupturing the aboral disc. The larva is called the **ophiopluteus,** and its ciliated bands extend onto delicate, beautiful larval arms, like those of the echinopluteus of the echinoids (Fig. 20-9, *B*). During the metamorphosis to the juvenile, there is no temporarily attached phase, as there is in asteroids.

Water-vascular, nervous, and hemal systems are similar to those of the sea stars. Each arm contains a small coelom, a radial nerve, and a radial canal of the water-vascular system.

Biology

Brittle stars tend to be secretive, living on hard bottoms where light penetrates. They are generally negatively phototropic and insinuate themselves into small crevices between rocks, becoming more active at night. They are commonly fully exposed on the bottom in the permanent darkness of the deep sea. Ophiuroids feed on a variety of small particles, either browsing food from the bottom or filter feeding. Podia are important in transferring food to the mouth. Some brittle stars extend arms into the water and catch suspended particles in mucous strands between the arm spines.

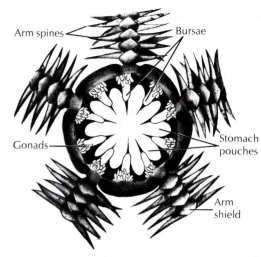

Figure 20-12

Ophiuroid with aboral disc wall cut away to show principal internal structures. The bursae are fluid-filled sacs in which water constantly circulates for respiration. They also serve as brood chambers. Only bases of arms are shown.

Figure 20-13

A, This brittle star *Ophiopholis aculeata* has its bursae swollen with eggs, which it is ready to expel. The arms have been broken and are regenerating. **B,** Oral view of a basket star *Gorgonocephalus eucnemis,* showing pentaradial symmetry. Photographs by R. Harbo.

A

B

Figure 20-14

Diadema antillarum (class Echinoidea) is a common species in the West Indies and Florida and its spines are a hazard to swimmers.

Photograph by A. Kerstitch.

Figure 20-15

Diversity among regular sea urchins (class Echinoidea). **A,** Pencil urchin *Eucidaris tribuloides*. Members of this order are the most primitive living sea urchins, surviving since the Paleozoic era, and may be ancestral to all other extant echinoids. **B,** Slate-pencil urchin *Heterocentrotus mammilatus*. The large, triangular spines of this urchin were formerly used for writing on slates. **C,** Aboral spines of the intertidal urchin *Colobocentrotus atratus* are flattened and mushroom shaped, while the marginal spines are wedge shaped, giving the animal a streamlined form to withstand pounding surf. **D,** Purple sea urchin *Strongylocentrotus purpuratus* is common along the Pacific coast of North America where there is heavy wave action. **E,** *Astropyga magnifica* is one of the most spectacularly colored sea urchins, with bright-blue spots along its interambulacral areas.

A, Photograph by A. Kerstitch; **B to D,** photographs by R. Harbo; **E,** photograph by K. Sandved.

A

B

Figure 20-16

Two sand dollar species. **A,** *Encope grandis* as they are normally found burrowing near the surface on a sandy bottom. **B,** Removed from the sand. The short spines and petaloids on the aboral surface of this *Encope micropora* are easily seen.

Photographs by A. Kerstitch.

Regeneration and autotomy are even more pronounced in brittle stars than in sea stars. Many seem very fragile, releasing an arm or even part of the disc at the slightest provocation. Some can reproduce asexually by cleaving the disc; each progeny then regenerates the missing parts.

Some common ophiuroids along the coast of the United States are *Amphipholis* (Gr., *amphi,* both sides of, + *pholis,* horny scale) (viviparous and hermaphroditic), *Ophioderma* (Gr., *ophis,* snake, + *dermatos,* skin), *Ophiothrix* (Gr., *ophis,* snake, + *thrix,* hair), and *Ophiura* (Gr., *ophis,* snake, + *oura,* tail) (Fig. 20-10, *A*). The basket stars *Gorgonocephalus* (Gr., *Gorgo,* name of a female monster of terrible aspect, + *kephalē,* a head) (Fig. 20-13, *B*) and *Astrophyton* (Gr., *asteros,* star, + *phyton,* creature, animal) (Fig. 20-10, *B*) have arms that branch repeatedly. Most ophiuroids are drab, but some are attractive, with variegated color patterns (p. 486).

____ Class Echinoidea
Sea urchins, sand dollars, and heart urchins

The echinoids have a compact body enclosed in an endoskeletal **test,** or shell. The dermal ossicles, which have become closely fitting plates, make up the test. Echinoids lack arms, but their tests reflect the typical pentamerous plan of the echinoderms in their five ambulacral areas. The most notable modification of the ancestral body plan is that the oral surface has expanded over the sides and top, so that the ambulacral areas extend up to the area around the anus (**periproct**). The majority of living species of sea urchins are referred to as "regular"; they have a hemispherical shape, radial symmetry, and medium to long spines (Figs. 20-14 and 20-15). Sand dollars (Fig. 20-16) and heart urchins (Fig. 20-17) are "irregular" because the orders to which they belong have become secondarily bilateral; their spines are usually very short. Regular urchins move by means of their tube feet, with some assistance from their spines, and irregular urchins move chiefly by their spines (Fig. 20-16). Some echinoids are quite colorful.

Echinoids have a wide distribution in all seas, from the intertidal regions to the deep oceans. Regular urchins often prefer rocky or hard bottoms, whereas sand dollars and heart urchins like to burrow into a sandy substrate. Distributed along one or both coasts of North America are common genera of regular urchins

A

B

Figure 20-17

An irregular echinoid *Meoma,* one of the largest heart urchins (test up to 18 cm). *Meoma* occurs in the West Indies and from the Gulf of California to the Galápagos Islands. **A,** Aboral view. Anterior ambulacral area is not modified as a petaloid in the heart urchins, although it is in sand dollars. **B,** Oral view. Note curved mouth at anterior end and periproct at posterior end.

Photographs by L.S. Roberts.

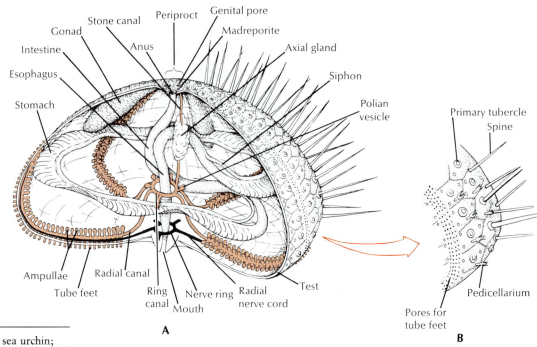

Figure 20-18

A, Internal structure of the sea urchin; water-vascular system in red. **B,** Detail of portion of endoskeleton.

Figure 20-19

Aristotle's lantern, the complex mechanism used by the sea urchin for masticating its food. Five pairs of retractor muscles draw the lantern and teeth up into the test; five pairs of protractors push the lantern down and expose the teeth. Other muscles produce a variety of movements. Only major skeletal parts and muscles are shown in the diagram.

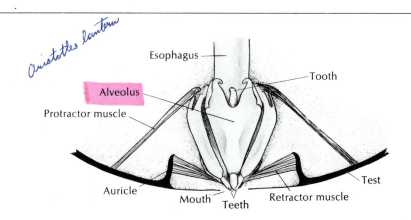

(*Arbacia* [Gr., Arbakēs, first king of Media], *Strongylocentrotus* [Gr., *strongylos*, round, compact, + *kentron*, point, spine] [Figs. 20-2 and 20-15, *D*], and *Lytechinus* [Gr., *lytos*, dissolvable, broken, + *echinos*, sea urchin]) and sand dollars (*Dendraster* [Gr., *dendron*, tree, stick, + *asteros*, star] and *Echinarachnius* [Gr., *echinos*, sea urchin, + *arachnē*, spider]). The West Indies–Florida region is rich in echinoderms, including echinoids, of which *Diadema* (Gr., *diadeō*, to bind around), with its long, needle-sharp spines, is a prominent example (Fig. 20-14).

Form and function

The echinoid **test** is a compact skeleton of 10 double rows of plates that bear movable, stiff spines (Fig. 20-18). The plates are firmly sutured. The five pairs of ambulacral rows are homologous to the five arms of the sea star and have pores (Fig. 20-18, *B*) through which the long tube feet extend. The plates bear small

A

B

C

Figure 20-20

Sea cucumbers (class Holothuroidea). **A,** Common along the Pacific coast of North America, *Parastichopus californicus* grows to 50 cm in length. Its tube feet on the dorsal side are reduced to papillae and warts. **B,** In sharp contrast to most sea cucumbers, the surface ossicles of *Psolus chitonoides* are developed into a platelike armor. The ventral surface is a flat, soft, creeping sole, and the mouth (surrounded by tentacles) and anus are turned dorsally. **C,** Tube feet are found in all ambulacral areas of *Cucumaria miniata* but are better developed on its ventral side, shown here.
Photographs by R. Harbo.

tubercles on which the round ends of the spines articulate as ball-and-socket joints. The spines are moved by small muscles around the bases.

There are several kinds of **pedicellariae,** the most common of which are three jawed and are mounted on long stalks (Fig. 20-5). Pedicellariae help keep the body clean and capture small organisms. The pedicellariae of many species bear poison glands, and the toxin paralyzes small prey.

The mouth of regular urchins is surrounded by five converging teeth. In some sea urchins branched **gills** (modified podia) encircle the peristome. The **anus, genital openings,** and **madreporite** are located aborally in the periproct region (Fig. 20-18). The sand dollars also have teeth, and the mouth is located at about the center of the oral side, but the anus has shifted to the posterior margin or even the oral side of the disc, so that an anteroposterior axis and bilateral symmetry can be recognized. Bilateral symmetry is even more accentuated in the heart urchins, with the anus near the posterior on the oral side and the mouth moved away from the oral pole toward the anterior (Fig. 20-17).

Inside the test (Fig. 20-18) are the coiled digestive system and a complex chewing mechanism (in the regular urchins and in sand dollars), called **Aristotle's lantern** (Fig. 20-19), to which the teeth are attached. A ciliated siphon connects the esophagus to the intestine and enables the water to bypass the stomach to concentrate the food for digestion in the intestine. Sea urchins eat algae and other organic material, which they graze with their teeth. Sand dollars have short club-shaped spines that move the sand and its organic contents over the aboral surface and down the sides. Fine food particles drop between the spines and are carried by ciliated tracts on the oral side to the mouth.

The hemal and nervous systems are basically similar to those of the asteroids. The ambulacral grooves are closed, and the radial canals of the water-vascular system run just beneath the test, one in each of the ambulacral radii (Fig. 20-18). The podia are supplied with ampullae within the test, each of which usually communicates with its podium by *two* canals through pores in the ambulacral plate; consequently, such pores in the plates are in pairs. The peristomial gills, where present, are of little or no importance in respiratory gas exchange, this function being carried out principally by the other podia. In the irregular urchins the respiratory podia are thin walled, flattened, or lobulate and are arranged in ambulacral fields called **petaloids** on the aboral surface. The irregular urchins also

Figure 20-21

Anatomy of the sea cucumber *Sclerodactyla*. **A,** Internal. **B,** External. *Red,* Hemal system.

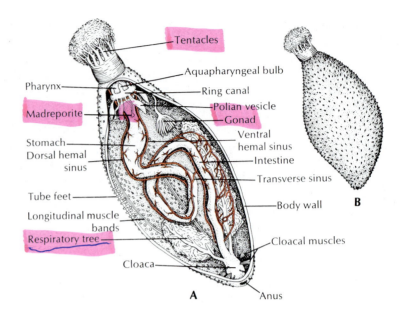

have short, suckered, single-pored podia in the ambulacral and sometimes interambulacral areas; these function in food handling.

Sexes are separate, and both eggs and sperm are shed into the sea for external fertilization. Some, such as certain of the pencil urchins, brood their young in depressions between the spines. The **echinopluteus larvae** (Fig. 20-9, *B*) of nonbrooding echinoids may live a planktonic existence for several months and then metamorphose quickly into young urchins.

⎯ Class Holothuroidea

Sea cucumbers

In a phylum characterized by odd animals, class Holothuroidea contains members that both structurally and physiologically are among the strangest. These animals have a remarkable resemblance to the vegetable after which they are named (Fig. 20-20). Compared with the other echinoderms, the holothurians are greatly elongated in the oral-aboral axis, and the ossicles are much reduced in most, so that the animals are soft bodied. Some species characteristically crawl on the surface of the sea bottom, others are found beneath rocks, and some are burrowers.

Common species along the east coast of North America are *Cucumaria frondosa* (L., *cucumis,* cucumber), *Sclerodactyla briareus* (Gr., *skleros,* hard, + *daktylos,* finger) (Fig. 20-21), and the translucent, burrowing *Leptosynapta* (Gr., *leptos,* slender, + *synapsis,* joining together). Along the Pacific coast there are several species of *Cucumaria* (Fig. 20-20, C) and the striking reddish brown *Parastichopus* (Gr., *para,* beside, + *stichos,* line or row, + *pous, podos,* foot) (Fig. 20-20, A), with very large papillae.

Form and function

The body wall is usually leathery, with tiny ossicles embedded in it (Fig. 20-22), although a few species have large ossicles forming a dermal armor (Fig. 20-20, *B*). Because of the elongate body form of the sea cucumbers, they characteristically lie on one side. In some species the locomotor tube feet are equally distributed to the five ambulacral areas (Fig. 20-20, C) or all over the body, but most have tube feet

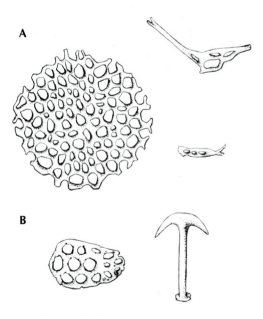

Figure 20-22

Ossicles of sea cucumbers are usually tiny and buried in the leathery dermis. They can be extracted from the tissue with caustic solutions and are important taxonomic characteristics. **A,** *Sclerodactyla.* **B,** *Leptosynapta.*

Drawings by T. Doyle.

well developed only in the ambulacra normally applied to the substratum (Fig. 20-20, *A* and *B*). Thus, a secondary bilaterality is present, albeit of quite different origin from that of the irregular urchins. The side applied to the substratum has three ambulacra and is called the **sole;** the tube feet in the dorsal ambulacral areas, if present, are usually without suckers and may be modified as sensory papillae. All tube feet, except oral tentacles, may be absent in burrowing forms.

The **oral tentacles** are 10 to 30 retractile, modified tube feet around the mouth. The body wall contains circular and longitudinal muscles along the ambulacra.

The **coelomic cavity** is spacious and fluid filled and has many coelomocytes. The digestive system empties posteriorly into a muscular **cloaca** (Fig. 20-21). A **respiratory tree** composed of two long, many-branched tubes also empties into the cloaca, which pumps seawater into it. The respiratory tree serves for both respiration and excretion and is not found in any other group of living echinoderms. Gas exchange also occurs through the skin and tube feet.

The hemal system is more well developed in holothurians than in other echinoderms. The **water-vascular system** is peculiar in that the madreporite lies free in the coelom.

The sexes are separate, but some holothurians are hermaphroditic. Among the echinoderms, only the sea cucumbers have a single gonad, and this is considered a primitive character. The gonad is usually in the form of one or two clusters of tubules that join at the gonoduct. Fertilization is external, and the free-swimming larva is called an **auricularia.** Some species brood the young either inside the body or somewhere on the body surface.

Biology

Sea cucumbers are sluggish, moving partly by means of their ventral tube feet and partly by waves of contraction in the muscular body wall. The more sedentary species trap suspended food particles in the mucus of their outstretched oral tentacles or pick up particles from the surrounding bottom. They then stuff the tentacles into their pharynx, one by one, sucking off the food material (Fig. 20-23, *A*). Others crawl along, grazing the bottom with their tentacles (Fig. 20-23, *B*).

Sea cucumbers have a peculiar power of what appears to be self-mutilation but is really a mode of defense. Some, when irritated, may cast out a part of their viscera by a strong muscular contraction that may either rupture the body wall or evert its contents through the anus. The lost parts are soon regenerated.

There is an interesting commensal relationship between some sea cucumbers and a small fish, *Carapus,* that uses the cloaca and respiratory tree of the sea cucumber as shelter.

Class Crinoidea
Sea lilies and feather stars

The crinoids are the most primitive of the living echinoderms. As fossil records reveal, crinoids were once far more numerous than now. They differ from other echinoderms by being attached during a substantial part of their lives. Sea lilies have a flower-shaped body that is placed at the tip of an attached stalk (Fig. 20-24). The feather stars have long, many-branched arms, and the adults are free moving, though they may remain in the same spot for long periods (Fig. 20-25). During metamorphosis feather stars become sessile and stalked, but after several

A

B

Figure 20-23

A, *Eupentacta quinquesemita* extends its tentacles to collect particulate matter in the water, then puts them one by one into its mouth and cleans the food from them. **B,** Moplike tentacles of *Parastichopus californicus* are used for deposit feeding on the bottom.
Photographs by R. Harbo.

Figure 20-24

Crinoid structure. **A,** Feather star (stalked crinoid) with portion of stalk. Modern crinoid stalks rarely exceed 60 cm, but fossil forms were as much as 20 m long. **B,** Oral view of calyx of the crinoid *Antedon,* showing direction of ciliary food currents. Ambulacral grooves with podia extend from mouth along arms and branching pinnules. Food particles touching podia are tossed into ambulacral grooves and carried, tangled in mucus, by strong ciliary currents toward mouth. Particles falling on interambulacral areas are carried by cilia first toward mouth and then outward and finally dropped off the edge, thus keeping the oral disc clean.

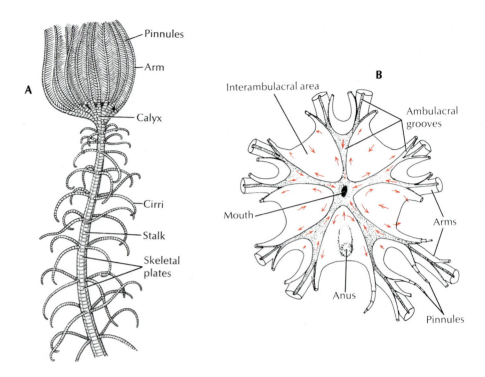

months they detach and become free moving. Many crinoids are deep-water forms, but feather stars may inhabit shallow waters, especially in the Indo-Pacific and West Indian–Caribbean regions, where the largest numbers of species are found.

Form and function

The body disc, or **calyx,** is covered with a leathery skin (**tegmen**) containing calcareous plates. The epidermis is poorly developed. Five flexible arms branch to form many more arms, each with many lateral **pinnules** arranged like barbs on a feather (Fig. 20-24). The calyx and arms together are called the **crown.** Sessile forms have a long, jointed **stalk** attached to the aboral side of the body. This stalk is made up of plates, appears jointed, and may bear **cirri.** Madreporite, spines, and pedicellariae are absent.

The upper (oral) surface bears the mouth, which opens into a short esophagus, from which the long **intestine** with diverticula proceeds aborally for a distance and than makes a complete turn to the **anus,** which may be on a raised cone (Fig. 20-24, *B*). With the aid of tube feet and mucous nets, crinoids feed on small organisms that are caught in the ambulacral grooves. The **ambulacral grooves** are open and ciliated and serve to carry food to the mouth (Fig. 20-24, *B*). Tube feet in the form of tentacles are also found in the grooves.

The **water-vascular system** has the echinoderm plan. The nervous system is made up of an **oral ring** and a **radial nerve** that runs to each arm. The aboral or entoneural system is more highly developed in crinoids than in most other echinoderms. Sense organs are scanty and primitive.

The sexes are separate. The gonads are simply masses of cells in the genital cavity of the arms and pinnules. The gametes escape without ducts through a rupture in the pinnule wall. Brooding is known in some forms. The **doliolaria** larvae are free swimming for a time before they become attached and metamorphose. Most living crinoids are from 15 to 30 cm long, but some fossil species had stalks 25 m in length.

____ Phylogeny and Adaptive Radiation
Phylogeny

Based on the embryological evidence of the bilateral larvae of echinoderms, there can be little doubt that their ancestors were bilateral and that their radial symmetry is secondary. Some recent investigators believe that the radial symmetry arose in a free-moving echinoderm ancestor and that sessile groups were derived several times independently from the free-moving ancestors. However, this view does not account for the adaptive significance of the radial symmetry, that is, as an adaptation for the sessile existence. The more traditional view is that the first echinoderms were sessile, became radial as an adaptation to that existence, and then gave rise to the free-moving groups. Certainly, the most primitive living echinoderms are the crinoids, and the existence of a transitory stalked phase in the asteroids, which also have some primitive characteristics such as open ambulacra, supports the traditional sequence. It is also believed that the endoskeleton was an adaptation for a sessile existence and that the original function of the water-vascular system was in feeding.

The nature of the hypothetical preechinoderm has also been subject to debate. Some have held that it was a **dipleurula** ancestor, which was a creeping, soft-bodied animal with three, paired coelomic compartments. Hyman and others have suggested that it was a **pentacula** ancestor, more like a lophophorate animal, with tentacles around the mouth. According to the latter hypothesis, the water-vascular system was derived from the five tentacles around one side, which contained extensions of the middle coelomic compartment of the ancestor.

Adaptive radiation

The radiation of the echinoderms has been determined by the limitations and potentials of their most important characteristics: radial symmetry, the water-vascular system, and their dermal endoskeleton. If their ancestors had a brain and specialized sense organs, these were lost in the adoption of radial symmetry. Thus, it is unsurprising that there are large numbers of creeping, benthic forms with filter-feeding, deposit-feeding, scavenging, and herbivorous habits, comparatively few predators, and very rare pelagic forms. In this light the relative success of the asteroids as predators is impressive and probably attributable to the extent to which they have exploited the hydraulic mechanism of the tube feet.

The basic body plan of echinoderms has severely limited their evolutionary opportunities to become parasites. Indeed, the most mobile of the echinoderms, the ophiuroids, which are also the ones most able to insert their bodies into small spaces, are the only group with significant numbers of commensal species.

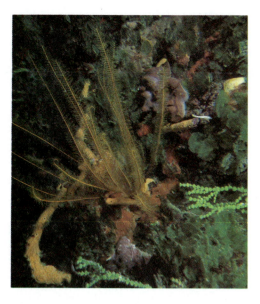

Figure 20-25

Nemaster spp. are crinoids found on Caribbean coral reefs. They extend their arms into the water to catch food particles while maintaining their body in a crevice.
Photograph by D.W. Gotshall.

____ Summary

The phylum Echinodermata shows the characteristics of the Deuterostomia division of the animal kingdom. The echinoderms are an important marine group sharply distinguished from other phyla of animals. They have a radial symmetry but were derived from bilateral ancestors. They fill a variety of benthic niches, including particle feeders, browsers, scavengers, and predators.

The sea stars (class Stelleroidea, subclass Asteroidea) can be used to illustrate the echinoderms. They usually have five arms, which merge gradually with a

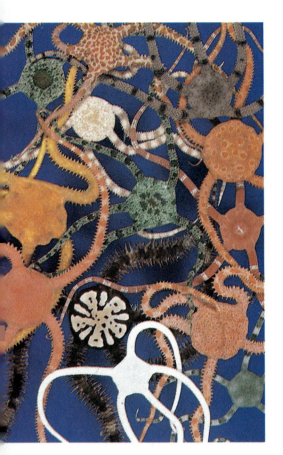

Brittle stars (subclass Ophiuroidea) are usually dull gray or brown, but some are quite showy, like these specimens from Puerto Rico.
Photograph by K. Sandved.

central disc. In common with other echinoderms they have no head and few specialized sensory organs. The mouth is central on the under (oral) side of the body. They have an endoskeleton of dermal ossicles. Open ambulacral areas occupy the grooves of the oral sides of the arms. Many sea stars have tiny, pincerlike pedicellariae around the bases of the spines on the aboral surface. Papulae (dermal branchiae) project between ossicles and are concerned with respiration. Like other echinoderms, sea stars have a water-vascular system, an elaborate hydraulic system derived from one of the coelomic cavities. It opens to the outside through the madreporite on the aboral surface. The madreporite is connected to the ring canal around the esophagus by way of the stone canal, and radial canals extend from the ring canal along each ambulacral area. Along the radial canals, branches lead to the many tube feet, structures that are important in locomotion, food gathering, respiration, and excretion. The tube feet often end in suckers. Many sea stars are predators, whereas others feed on small particles. Like other echinoderms, sea stars have a hemal system, enclosed by another coelomic compartment, which is of uncertain function. Sexes are separate, and reproductive systems are very simple. The bilateral, free-swimming larva becomes attached, transforms to a radial juvenile, then detaches and becomes a motile sea star.

Brittle stars (subclass Ophiuroidea) differ from asteroids in that their arms are slender and sharply set off from the central disc, they have no pedicellariae or ampullae, and their ambulacral grooves are closed. Their tube feet have no suckers, and their madreporite is on the oral side. They crawl by means of their arms, and they can move around more rapidly than other echinoderms. As in other echinoderms, their bilateral larva metamorphoses to a radial juvenile, but in common with sea urchins and sea cucumbers, there is no attached phase.

In sea urchins (class Echinoidea), the dermal ossicles have become closely fitting plates, the body is compact, and there are no arms. Their ambulacral areas are closed and extend up around their bodies. They move by means of tube feet or by their spines. Some urchins (sand dollars and heart urchins) are evolving a return to bilateral symmetry.

The dermal ossicles in sea cucumbers (class Holothuroidea) are very small; therefore the body wall is soft. Holothuroids are greatly elongated in the oral-aboral axis and lie on their side. Because certain of the ambulacral areas are characteristically against the substratum, sea cucumbers have also undergone some return to bilateral symmetry. The tube feet around the mouth are modified into tentacles, with which they feed. They have an internal respiratory tree connected to the cloaca, and the madreporite hangs free in the coelom.

Sea lilies and feather stars (class Crinoidea) are the only group of living echinoderms, other then the asteroids, with open ambulacral areas. They are mucociliary particle feeders and lie with their oral side up. They become attached to the substratum by a stem during metamorphosis, although the feather stars later detach from the stem.

Although it is clear that the ancestor of the echinoderms was bilaterally symmetrical, a point still debated is whether radiality arose in a free-moving ancestor, which then gave rise to sessile groups, or whether a sessile ancestor evolved radiality and then gave rise to the free-moving forms. A hypothetical preechinoderm called the pentacula would relate the echinoderms to the lophophorates.

The basic body plan of echinoderms (including radial symmetry, water-vascular system, and dermal endoskeleton) has limited their radiation but has produced surprising evolutionary success.

Selected references

Barnes, R.D. 1980. Invertebrate zoology, ed. 4. Philadelphia, Saunders College/Holt, Rinehart & Winston.

Barrington, E.J.W. 1979. Invertebrate structure and function, ed. 2. New York, John Wiley & Sons, Inc. *Excellent account of function in echinoderms and hemichordates.*

Binyon, J. 1972. Physiology of echinoderms. Elmsford, N.Y., Pergamon Press, Inc.

Boolootian, R.A. (ed.). 1966. Physiology of Echinodermata. New York, Interscience. *A valuable account of the physiology of this group.*

Brown, T., and K. Willey. 1972. Crown of thorns: the death of the Great Barrier Reef? Sydney, Angus & Robertson, Publishers.

Burnett, A.L. 1960. The mechanism employed by the starfish *Asterias forbesi* to gain access to the interior of the bivalve *Venus mercenaria*. Ecology **41**:583-584. *This investigator and others have shown that the starfish uses no narcotic agent to produce a small gap between the clam's valves through which the starfish can squeeze its stomach.*

Collins, A.R.S. 1975. Biochemical investigation of two responses involved in the feeding behaviour of *Acanthaster planci* (L.). III. Food preferences. J. Exp. Mar. Biol. **17**:87-94.

Corning, W.C., J.A. Dyal, and A.O.D. Willows (eds.). 1975. Invertebrate learning, vol. 3. New York, Plenum Publishing Corp.

Davidson, E.H., B.R. Hough-Evans, and R.J. Britten. 1982. Molecular biology of the sea urchin embryo. Science **217**:17-26. *Many fundamental insights into the process of embryogenesis have been revealed through studies of sea urchins.*

Dungan, M.L., T.E. Miller, and D.A. Thomson. 1982. Catastrophic decline of a top carnivore in the Gulf of California rocky intertidal zone. Science **216**:989-991. *A devastating disease led to a population crash of the predatory sea star,* Heliaster kubiniji. *Significant change in the intertidal community can be expected.*

Fell, H.B. 1972. Phylum Echinodermata. In A.J. Marshall and W.D. Williams (eds.). Textbook of zoology: invertebrates. New York, American Elsevier Publishers, Inc.

Fell, H.B. 1982. Echinodermata. In S.P. Parker (ed.). Synopsis and classification of living organisms, vol. 2. New York, McGraw-Hill Book Co.

Fontaine, A.R. 1965. Feeding mechanisms of the ophiuroid *Ophiocomina nigra*. J. Mar. Biol. Assoc. U.K. **45**:373.

Goodbody, I. 1960. The feeding mechanism in the sand dollar *Mellita sexiesperforata*. Biol. Bull. **119**(1):80-86.

Gosner, K.L. 1971. Guide to identification of marine and estuarine invertebrates. New York, Interscience. *A comprehensive identification aid for invertebrates of the east coast of North America, especially from Cape Hatteras to the Bay of Fundy.*

Haugh, B.N., and B.M. Bell. 1980. Fossilized viscera in primitive echinoderms. Science **209**:653-657. *Anatomical reconstructions of fossilized viscera suggest division of the Echinodermata into three subphyla, designated by these authors as I (to include crinoids and some extinct classes), II (all extinct), and III (including the other extant classes).*

Hyman, L.H. 1955. The invertebrates, vol. 4. Echinodermata. New York, McGraw-Hill Book Co. *The most comprehensive work yet published on the echinoderms; an invaluable reference.*

Moore, R.C. (ed.). 1966, 1967. Treatise on invertebrate paleontology: Echinodermata, Parts U and S. Lawrence, Kan., Geological Society of America and University of Kansas Press.

Nichols, D. 1966. Echinoderms. London, Hutchinson & Co., Ltd.

Ormond, R.F.G., A.C. Campbell, S.H. Head, R.J. Moore, P.R. Rainbow, and A.P. Saunders. 1973. Formation and breakdown of aggregations of the crown-of-thorns starfish, *Acanthaster planci* (L.). Nature **246**:167-169.

Ricketts, E.F., and J. Calvin. 1968. Between Pacific tides, ed. 4 (revised by J.W. Hedgpeth). Stanford, Calif., Stanford University Press. *In many ways this is a unique book of seashore life. It stresses the habits and habitats of the Pacific coast invertebrates (including echinoderms), and the illustrations are revealing. It includes an excellent systematic index and annotated bibliography.*

Russell-Hunter, W.D. 1979. A life of invertebrates. New York, Macmillan, Inc.

Smith, R.I., F.A. Pitelka, D.P. Abbott, and F.M. Weesner (eds.). 1957. Intertidal invertebrates of the central California coast. Berkeley, University of California Press. *This is a revision of S.F. Light's* Laboratory and Field Text in Invertebrate Zoology. *Consists mainly of taxonomic keys to the forms found in the intertidal zone.*

Selected *Scientific American* articles

Benson, A.A., and R.F. Lee. 1975. The role of wax in oceanic food chains. **232**:77-86 (Mar.). *The possession of enzymes to digest the wax in corals may account for the ability of* Acanthaster planci, *a sea star, to feed on coral polyps.*

Feder, H.M. 1972. Escape responses in marine invertebrates. **227**:93-100 (July). *Slow-moving molluscs and other echinoderms can undergo some remarkable antics in efforts to escape predatory sea stars.*

CHAPTER 21

THE LESSER DEUTEROSTOMES

Phylum Chaetognatha

Phylum Hemichordata

These acorn worms, *Saccoglossus pusillus,* have been removed from their burrows. Their body regions (proboscis, collar, trunk) can be distinguished easily.

Courtesy J.W. Evans.

The deuterostomes include, along with the Echinodermata, three other phyla: Chaetognatha, Hemichordata, and Chordata. Two of the chordate subphyla—Urochordata and Cephalochordata—are also invertebrate groups.

The term "lesser (or minor) deuterostomes" is usually used in reference to the hemichordates and chaetognaths, but only in the sense that they have a relatively small number of species. However, they are widespread and include some commonly found invertebrate forms. Often smaller groups deserve much more attention than is usually given them, for they contribute much to our understanding of evolutionary diversity and relationships.

These phyla have enterocoelous development of the coelom and some form of radial cleavage. The hemichordates were formerly included as a subphylum of the Chordata, but they are probably more closely related to the Echinodermata. The Chaetognatha apparently are not closely related to any other group.

▬ PHYLUM CHAETOGNATHA

A common name for the chaetognaths is arrowworms. They are all marine animals and are considered by some to be related to the nematodes and by others to be related to the annelids. However, they actually seem to be aberrant and show no distinct relationship to any other group. Only their embryology indicates their position as deuterostomes.

The name Chaetognatha (ke-tog'na-tha) (Gr., *chaitē*, long flowing hair, + *gnathos*, jaw) refers to the sickle-shaped bristles on each side of the mouth. This is not a large group, for only some 65 species are known. Their small, straight bodies resemble miniature torpedoes, or darts, ranging from 2.5 to 10 cm in length.

The arrowworms are all adapted for a planktonic existence, except for *Spadella* (Gr., *spadix*, palm frond, + *ella*, dim. suffix), a benthic genus. They usually swim to the surface at night and descend during the day. Much of the time they drift passively, but they can dart forward in swift spurts, using the caudal fin and longitudinal muscles—a fact that no doubt contributes to their success as planktonic predators. Horizontal fins bordering the trunk are used in flotation rather than in active swimming.

▬ Form and Function

The body of the arrowworm is unsegmented and is made up of head, trunk, and postanal tail (Fig. 21-1). On the underside of the head is a large vestibule leading to the mouth. The vestibule contains teeth and is flanked on both sides by curved chitinous spines used in seizing the prey. A pair of eyes is on the dorsal side. A peculiar hood formed from a fold of the neck can be drawn forward over the head and spines. When the animal captures prey, the hood is retracted, and the teeth and raptorial spines spread apart and then snap shut with startling speed. Arrowworms are voracious feeders, living on planktonic forms, especially copepods, and even small fish.

The body is covered with a thin cuticle and with epidermis that is single layered except along the sides of the body, where it is stratified in a thick layer. These are the only invertebrates with a many-layered epidermis.

Arrowworms are fairly advanced worms in that they have a complete digestive system, a well-developed coelom, and a nervous system with a nerve ring containing large dorsal and ventral ganglia and a number of lateral ganglia. Sense

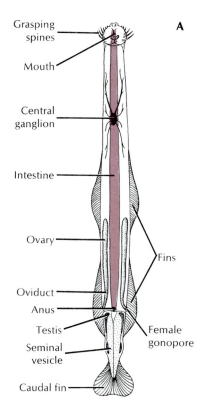

Figure 21-1

Arrowworm *Sagitta*. **A,** Internal structure. **B,** Head *(top)* is largely covered with hood formed from epidermis. When worm is engaged in catching its prey, hood is retracted to neck region. (Preserved specimen.)

B, Photograph by L.S. Roberts.

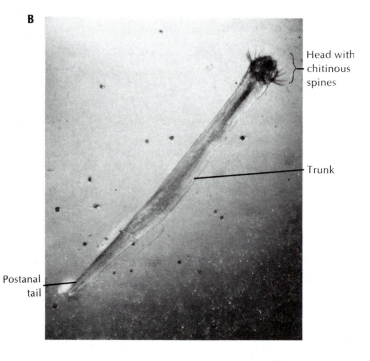

organs include the eyes, sensory bristles, and a U-shaped ciliary loop that extends over the neck from the back of the head and may detect water currents or may be chemosensory. Vascular, respiratory, and excretory systems, however, are entirely lacking.

Arrowworms are hermaphroditic with either cross- or self-fertilization. The eggs of *Sagitta* (L., arrow) are coated with jelly and are planktonic. Eggs of other arrowworms may be attached to the body and carried about for a time. The juveniles develop directly without metamorphosis. Chaetognath embryogenesis differs from that of other deuterostomes in that the coelom is formed by a backward extension from the archenteron rather than by pinched-off coelomic sacs. There is no true peritoneum lining the coelom. Cleavage is radial, complete, and equal.

The best-known species is *Sagitta*, the common arrowworm (Fig. 21-1).

PHYLUM HEMICHORDATA

Position in Animal Kingdom
1. Hemichordates belong to the deuterostome branch of the animal kingdom and are enterocoelous coelomates with radial cleavage.
2. Hemichordates show some of both echinoderm and chordate characteristics.
3. A chordate plan of structure is suggested by gill slits and a restricted dorsal tubular nerve cord.
4. Similarity to the echinoderms is shown in larval characteristics.

Biological Contributions
1. A **tubular dorsal nerve cord** in the collar zone may represent an early stage of the condition in chordates; a diffused net of nerve cells is similar to the uncentralized, subepithelial plexus of echinoderms.
2. The **gill slits** in the pharynx, which are also characteristic of chordates, are used primarily for filter feeding and only secondarily for breathing and are thus comparable to those in the protochordates.

The Hemichordata (hem'i-kor-da'ta) (Gr., *hemi,* half, + *chorda,* string, cord) are marine animals that were formerly considered a subphylum of the chordates, based on their possession of gill slits and a rudimentary notochord. However, it is now generally agreed that the so-called hemichordate notochord is really a stomochord and not homologous with the chordate notochord, so the hemichordates are given the rank of a separate phylum.

Hemichordates are vermiform bottom dwellers, living usually in shallow waters. Some are colonial and live in secreted tubes. Most are sedentary or sessile. Their distribution is fairly worldwide, but their secretive habits and fragile bodies make collecting them difficult.

Members of class Enteropneusta (Gr., *enteron,* intestine, + *pneustikos,* of, or for, breathing) (acorn worms) range from 20 mm to 2.5 m in length and 3 to 200 mm in breadth. Members of class Pterobranchia (Gr., *pteron,* wing, + *branchia,* gills) are smaller, usually 5 to 14 mm, not including the stalk. About 70 species of enteropneusts and three small genera of pterobranchs are recognized.

Hemichordates have the typical tricoelomate structure of deuterostomes.

CHARACTERISTICS
1. Soft bodied; wormlike or short and compact with stalk for attachment
2. Body divided into proboscis, collar, and trunk; coelomic pouch single in proboscis, but paired in other two; buccal diverticulum in posterior part of proboscis
3. Enteropneusta free moving and of burrowing habits; pterobranchs sessile, mostly colonial, living in secreted tubes
4. Circulatory system of dorsal and ventral vessels and dorsal heart
5. Respiratory system of gill slits (few or none in pterobranchs) connecting the pharynx with outside as in chordates
6. No nephridia; a single glomerulus connected to blood vessels may have excretory function
7. A subepidermal nerve plexus thickened to form dorsal and ventral nerve cords, with a ring connective in the collar; dorsal nerve cord of collar hollow in some
8. Sexes separate in Enteropneusta, with gonads projecting into body cavity; in pterobranchs reproduction may be sexual or asexual (in some) by budding; tornaria larva in some Enteropneusta

____ Class Enteropneusta

The enteropneusts, or acorn worms, are sluggish, wormlike animals that live in burrows or under stones, usually in mud or sand flats of intertidal zones. *Balanoglossus* (Gr., *balanos,* acorn, + *glōssa,* tongue) and *Saccoglossus* (Gr., *sakkos,* sac, strainer, + *glōssa,* tongue) (Fig. 21-2) are common genera.

Form and function

The mucus-covered body is divided into a tonguelike **proboscis,** a short **collar,** and a long **trunk** (protosome, mesosome, and metasome).

Proboscis

The proboscis is the active part of the animal. It probes about in the mud, examining its surroundings and collecting food in mucous strands on its surface. These are carried by cilia to the groove at the edge of the collar, are directed to the mouth on the underside, and are swallowed. Large particles can be rejected by covering the mouth with the edge of the collar (Fig. 21-3).

Figure 21-2

Acorn worm *Saccoglossus* (Hemichordata, class Enteropneusta). **A,** External lateral view. **B,** Longitudinal section through anterior end.

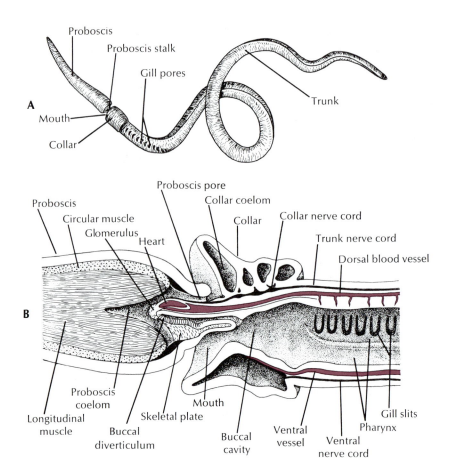

Burrow dwellers use the proboscis to excavate, thrusting it into the mud or sand and allowing cilia and mucus to move the sand backward. Or they may eat the sand and mud as they go, extracting its organic contents. They build U-shaped mucus-lined burrows, usually with two openings 10 to 30 cm apart and with the base of the U 50 to 75 cm below the surface. They can thrust the proboscis out the front opening for feeding. Defecation at the back opening builds characteristic spiral fecal mounds that leave a telltale clue to the location of the burrows.

In the posterior end of the proboscis is a small coelomic sac (protocoel) into which extends the **buccal diverticulum,** a slender, blindly ending pouch of the gut that reaches forward into the buccal region and was formerly believed to be a notochord. A slender canal connects the protocoel with a **proboscis pore** to the outside (Fig. 21-2, *B*). The paired coelomic cavities in the collar also open by pores. By taking in water through the pores into the coelomic sacs, the proboscis and collar can be stiffened to aid in burrowing. Contraction of the body musculature then forces the excess water out through the gill slits, reducing the hydrostatic pressure and allowing the animal to move forward.

Branchial system

A row of **gill pores** is located dorsolaterally on each side of the trunk just behind the collar (Fig. 21-3, *A*). These open from a series of gill chambers that in turn connect with a series of **gill slits** in the sides of the pharynx. No gills are attached to the gill slits, but some respiratory gaseous exchange occurs in the vascular branchial epithelium, as well as in the body surface. Ciliary currents keep a fresh supply of water moving from the mouth through the pharynx and out the gill slits and branchial chambers to the outside.

Feeding and the digestive system

Hemichordates are largely ciliary-mucus feeders. Behind the buccal cavity lies the large pharynx containing in its dorsal part the U-shaped gill slits (Fig. 21-2, *B*). Since there are no gills, the primary function of the branchial mechanism of the pharynx is presumably food gathering. Food particles caught in mucus and brought to the mouth by ciliary action on the proboscis and collar are strained out of the branchial water that leaves through the gill slits and are directed along the ventral part of the pharynx and esophagus to the intestine, where digestion and absorption occur (Fig. 21-3).

Circulatory and excretory systems

A middorsal vessel carries blood forward above the gut. In the collar the vessel expands into a sinus and a heart vesicle above the buccal diverticulum. Blood is then driven into a network of blood sinuses called the **glomerulus,** which partially surrounds these structures. The glomerulus is assumed to have an excretory function (Fig. 21-2, *B*). Blood travels posteriorly through a ventral vessel below the gut, passing through extensive sinuses to the gut and body wall. The blood is colorless.

Nervous and sensory systems

The nervous system consists mostly of a subepithelial network, or plexus, of nerve cells and fibers to which processes of epithelial cells are attached. Thickenings of this net form dorsal and ventral nerve cords that are united posterior to the collar by a ring connective. The dorsal cord continues into the collar and furnishes many fibers to the plexus of the proboscis. The collar cord is hollow in some species and contains giant nerve cells with processes running to the nerve trunks. This primitive nerve plexus system is highly reminiscent of that of the cnidarians and echinoderms.

Sensory receptors include neurosensory cells throughout the epidermis (especially in the proboscis, a preoral ciliary organ that may be chemoreceptive) and photoreceptor cells.

Reproductive system and development

Sexes are separate in enteropneusts. Gonads are arranged in a dorsolateral row on each side of the anterior part of the trunk. Fertilization is external, and in some species a ciliated **tornaria** larva develops that at certain stages is so similar to the echinoderm bipinnaria that it was once believed to be an echinoderm larva. The familiar *Saccoglossus* of American waters has direct development without a tornaria stage.

____ Class Pterobranchia

The basic plan of the class Pterobranchia is similar to that of the Enteropneusta, but certain structural differences are correlated with the sedentary mode of life of pterobranchs. The first pterobranch ever reported was obtained by the famed *Challenger* expedition of 1872 to 1876. Although first placed among the Polyzoa (Entoprocta and Ectoprocta), its affinities to the hemichordates were later recognized. Only two genera (*Cephalodiscus* and *Rhabdopleura*) are known in any detail.

Pterobranchs are small animals, usually within the range of 1 to 7 mm in length, although the stalk may be longer. Many individuals of *Cephalodiscus* (Gr.,

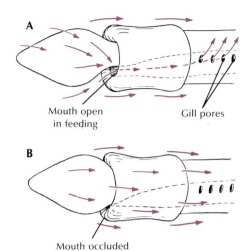

Figure 21-3

Food currents of enteropneust hemichordate. **A,** Side view of acorn worm with mouth open, showing direction of currents created by cilia on proboscis and collar. Food particles are directed toward mouth and digestive tract. Rejected particles move toward outside of collar. Water leaves through gill pores. **B,** When mouth is occluded, all particles are rejected and passed onto the collar. Nonburrowing and some burrowing hemichordates use this feeding method.
Modified from Russell-Hunter, W.D. 1969. A biology of the higher invertebrates. New York, Macmillan, Inc.

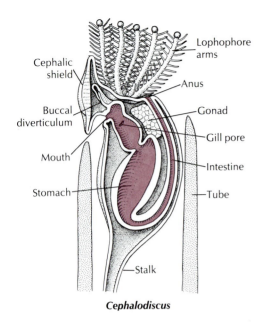

Cephalodiscus

Figure 21-4

Cephalodiscus, a pterobranch hemichordate. These tiny (5 to 7 mm) forms live in coenecium tubes in which they can move about. Ciliated tentacles and arms direct currents of food and water toward mouth. These deep-sea animals may be close to the ancestral stock of echinoderms and chordates.

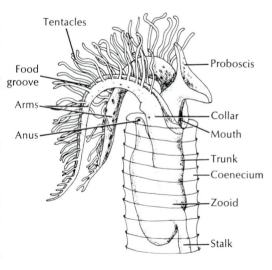

Figure 21-5

Rhabdopleura, a pterobranch hemichordate in its tube. Individuals live in branching tubes, connected by stolons, and protrude the tentacled lophophore for feeding.

kephalē, head, + *diskos,* disc) (Fig. 21-4) live together in gelatinous tubes, which often form an anastomosing system. The zooids are not connected, however, and live independently in the tubes. Through apertures in these tubes, they extend their crown of tentacles. They are attached to the walls of the tubes by extensible stalks that can jerk the owners back into the tubes when necessary.

The body of *Cephalodiscus* is divided into the three regions—proboscis, collar, and trunk—characteristic of the hemichordates. There is only one pair of gill slits, and the alimentary canal is U shaped, with the anus near the mouth. The proboscis is shield shaped. At the base of the proboscis are five to nine pairs of branching arms with tentacles containing an extension of the coelomic compartment of the mesosome, as in a lophophore. Ciliated grooves on the tentacles and arms collect food. Some species are dioecious, and others are monoecious. Asexual reproduction by budding may also occur.

In *Rhabdopleura* (Gr., *rhabdos,* rod, + *pleura,* a rib, the side), which is smaller than *Cephalodiscus,* the members remain together to form a colony of zooids connected by a stolon and enclosed in coenecium tubes (Fig. 21-5). The collar in these forms bears two branching arms or lophophores. No gill clefts or glomeruli are present. New individuals are reproduced by budding from a creeping basal stolon, which branches on a substratum. None of the pterobranchs has a tubular nerve cord in the collar, but otherwise their nervous system is similar to that of the Enteropneusta.

Atubaria (Gr., *a,* prefix meaning absence of, + L., *tubus,* tube), a little-known genus, has no tube but attaches its stalk to colonial hydroids.

The fossil graptolites of the middle Paleozoic era are often placed as an extinct class under Hemichordata. Their tubular chitinous skeleton and colonial habits indicate an affinity with *Rhabdopleura.* They are considered important index fossils of the Ordovician and Silurian geological strata.

Phylogeny and Adaptive Radiation
Phylogeny

Hemichordate phylogeny has long been puzzling. Hemichordates share characteristics with both the echinoderms and the chordates. They share with the chordates the gill slits, which are used primarily for filter feeding and secondarily for breathing as in some of the protochordates. A short dorsal, somewhat hollow nerve cord in the collar zone foreshadows the nerve cord of the chordates. The buccal diverticulum in the hemichordate mouth cavity, which was long believed to be a rudimentary notochord homologous with the notochord of chordates, is now considered of no phylogenetic importance. The relationship to the echinoderms is striking. The early embryogenesis is remarkably like that of echinoderms, and the early tornaria larva is almost identical to the bipinnaria larva of asteroids. The similarity between the hydraulic action of the coelomic pouches and that of the water-vascular system in echinoderms and the similarity in plan of the subepithelial nerve plexus of the two groups are further evidence of their relationship.

Within the phylum the class Pterobranchia is considered more primitive than the class Enteropneusta and shows affinities with the Ectoprocta, Brachiopoda, and others because of its lophophore and sessile habits. Some believe that the pterobranchs may be similar to the common ancestors of both the hemichordates and the echinoderms.

Adaptive radiation

The pterobranchs, because of their sessile lives and habitat in secreted tubes in ocean bottoms, where conditions are fairly stable, have undergone little adaptive divergence. They have retained a tentacular type of ciliary feeding. The enteropneusts, on the other hand, although sluggish, are more active than the pterobranchs. Having lost the tentaculated arms, they use a proboscis to trap small organisms in mucus, or they eat sand as they burrow and digest organic sediments from the sand. Their evolutionary divergence, although greater than that of the pterobranchs, is still modest.

_____ Summary

The arrowworms (phylum Chaetognatha) are a small group but are important as a component of marine plankton. They have a well-developed coelom and are effective predators, catching other planktonic organisms with the teeth and chitinous spines around their mouth.

Members of the phylum Hemichordata are marine worms that were formerly considered chordates because their buccal diverticulum was believed to be a notochord. However, in common with the chordates, some of them do have gill slits and a hollow, dorsal nerve cord. The divisions of their body (proboscis, collar, trunk) contain the typical deuterostome coelomic compartments (protocoel, mesocoel, metacoel). The hemichordate class Enteropneusta contains burrowing worms that feed on particles strained out of the water by their gill slits. Members of the class Pterobranchia are tube dwellers, filter feeding with tentacles. The hemichordates are important phylogenetically because they show affinities with the chordates, echinoderms, and lophophorates.

Selected references

Alvarino, A. 1965. Chaetognaths. Oceanogr. Mar. Biol. Ann. Rev. 3:115-194.

Barrington, E.J.W. 1965. The biology of Hemichordata and Protochordata. San Francisco, W.H. Freeman & Co. Publishers. *Concise account of behavior, physiology, and reproduction of hemichordates, urochordates, and cephalochordates.*

Barrington, E.J.W. 1979. Invertebrate structure and function, ed. 2. New York, John Wiley & Sons, Inc. *Contains accounts of the feeding, nervous system, and behavior of hemichordates.*

Benito, J. 1982. Hemichordata. In S.P. Parker (ed.). Synopsis and classification of living organisms, vol. 2. New York, McGraw-Hill Book Co.

Bieri, R. 1959. The distribution of planktonic Chaetognatha in the Pacific and their relationship to the water masses. Limnol. Oceanogr. 4:1-28.

Dilly, P.N. 1975. The pterobranch *Rhabdopleura compacta*: its nervous system and phylogenetic position. Symp. Zool. Soc. Lond. 36:1-16.

Ghirardelli, E. 1968. Some aspects of the biology of the chaetognaths. Adv. Mar. Biol. 6:271-375.

Gosner, K.L. 1971. Guide to the identification of marine and estuarine invertebrates. New York, Interscience.

Hyman, L.H. 1959. The invertebrates, vol. 5. Smaller coelomate groups. New York, McGraw-Hill Book Co. *The best appraisal in English of this strange group.*

Michel, H.B. 1982. Chaetognatha. In S.P. Parker (ed.). Synopsis and classification of living organisms, vol. 2. New York, McGraw-Hill Book Co.

Newell, G.E. 1951. The stomochord of Enteropneusta. Proc. Zool. Soc. 121:741. *An appraisal of the status of the stomochord in comparison with a true notochord.*

Parry, D.A. 1944. Structure and function of the gut in *Spadella* and *Sagitta*. J. Marine Biol. Assoc. U.K. 26:16-36.

Russell-Hunter, W.D. 1979. A life of invertebrates. New York, Macmillan, Inc.

Stebbing, A.R.D., and P.N. Dilly. 1972. Some observations on living *Rhabdopleura compacta* (Hemichordata). J. Mar. Biol. Assoc. U.K. 52:443-449.

CHAPTER 22

THE CHORDATES

Ancestry and Evolution, General Characteristics, Protochordates

Sea squirts *(Clavelina sp.)*, sessile marine protochordates of the subphylum Urochordata.
Although adult sea squirts (ascidians) are highly specialized chordates,
their free-swimming "tadpole" larvae bear the chordate hallmarks—
notochord, gill slits, dorsal nerve cord, and postanal
tail—and occupy an important position in hypotheses
of chordate ancestry.

Photograph by S.K. Webster, Monterey Bay Aquarium/BPS.

___ THE CHORDATES

The animals most familiar to most people belong to the great phylum Chordata (kor-da′ta) (L., *chorda*, cord). Humans themselves are members and share one of the common characteristics from which the phylum derives its name—the **notochord** (Gr., *nōton*, back, + L., *chorda*, cord) (Fig. 22-1). This structure is possessed by all members of the phylum, in either the larval or the embryonic stages or throughout life. The notochord is a rodlike, semirigid body of vacuolated cells, which extends, in most cases, the length of the body between the enteric canal and the central nervous system. Its primary purpose is to support and stiffen the body, that is, to act as a skeletal axis.

The structural plan of chordates retains many of the features of nonchordate invertebrates, such as bilateral symmetry, anteroposterior axis, coelom tube-within-a-tube arrangement, metamerism, and cephalization. Yet, although the kinship of chordates and nonchordates is obvious, it has not been possible to establish the exact relationship with certainty.

Two possible lines of descent have been proposed. Earlier speculations that focused on the arthropod-annelid-mollusc group (Protostomia branch) of the invertebrates have fallen from favor. It is now believed that only the echinoderm group (Deuterostomia branch) deserves serious consideration as a chordate ancestor. The echinoderms and chordates share several important characteristics: **radial cleavage** (p. 129), **type of mesoderm and coelom formation,** and **anus derivation from the first embryonic opening (blastopore)** with mouth derivation from an opening of secondary origin. These common characteristics indicate a natural, if remote, kinship between the two groups.

As a whole, there is more fundamental unity of plan throughout all the organs and systems of this phylum than there is in many of the invertebrate phyla. Ecologically the chordates are among the most adaptable of organic forms and are able to occupy most kinds of habitat. From a purely biological viewpoint, chordates are of primary interest because they illustrate so well the broad biological principles of evolution, development, and relationship. They represent as a group the background of the human species.

CHARACTERISTICS
1. Bilateral symmetry; segmented body; three germ layers; well-developed coelom
2. **Notochord** (a skeletal rod) present at some stage in life cycle
3. **Single, dorsal, tubular nerve cord;** anterior end of cord usually enlarged to form brain
4. **Pharyngeal gill slits** present at some stage in life cycle and may or may not be functional
5. **Postanal tail,** usually projecting beyond the anus at some stage but may or may not persist
6. **Ventral heart,** with dorsal and ventral blood vessels; closed blood system
7. Complete digestive system
8. Exoskeleton often present; well developed in some vertebrates
9. A cartilage or bony **endoskeleton** present in the majority of members (vertebrates)

___ Four Chordate Hallmarks

The four distinctive characteristics that set chordates apart from all other phyla are the **notochord, dorsal tubular nerve cord, pharyngeal gill slits,** and **postanal tail.** These characteristics are always found at some embryonic stage, although

Notochord

Fibrous sheath

Elastic sheath

A

Notochord

B

Figure 22-1

A, Structure of notochord and its surrounding sheaths. Cells of notochord proper are thick walled, pressed together closely, and filled with semifluid. Stiffness is caused mainly by turgidity of fluid-filled cells and surrounding connective tissue sheaths. This primitive type of endoskeleton is characteristic of all chordates at some stage of the life cycle. The notochord provides longitudinal stiffening of the main body axis, a base for myomeric muscles, and an axis around which the vertebral column develops. **B,** In hagfishes and lampreys it persists throughout life, but in higher vertebrates it is largely replaced by the vertebrae. In humans slight remnants are found in nuclei pulposi of intervertebral discs. Its method of formation is different in the various groups of animals. In amphioxus it originates from the endoderm; in birds and mammals it arises as an anterior outgrowth of the embryonic primitive streak.

they may be altered or may disappear in later stages of the life cycle. These four features are so important that each merits an introduction of its own.

Notochord

The notochord is a flexible, rodlike structure, extending the length of the body; it is the first part of the endoskeleton to appear in the embryo. The notochord is an axis for muscle attachment, and because it can bend without shortening, it permits undulatory movements of the body. In most of the protochordates and in primitive vertebrates, the notochord persists throughout life (Fig. 22-1). In all vertebrates a series of cartilaginous or bony vertebrae is formed from the connective tissue sheath around the notochord and replaces the notochord as the chief mechanical axis of the body.

Dorsal, tubular nerve cord

In most invertebrate phyla that have a nerve cord, it is ventral to the alimentary canal and is solid, but in the chordates the single cord is dorsal to the alimentary canal and is a tube (although the hollow center may be nearly obliterated during growth). The anterior end becomes enlarged to form the brain. The hollow cord is produced in the embryo by the infolding of ectodermal cells on the dorsal side of the body above the notochord. Among the vertebrates, the nerve cord lies in the neural arches of the vertebrae, and the anterior brain is surrounded by a bony or cartilaginous cranium.

Pharyngeal gill slits

Pharyngeal gill slits are perforated slitlike openings that lead from the pharyngeal cavity to the outside. They are formed by the invagination of the outside ectoderm and the evagination of the endodermal lining of the pharynx. The two pockets break through when they meet, forming the slit. In higher vertebrates these pockets may not break through and only grooves are formed instead of slits; all traces of them usually disappear. In forms that use the slits for breathing, gills with blood vessels develop at the margins of the slits; here gaseous exchange (oxygen and carbon dioxide) proceeds between the blood and the water that flows over the gills. The slits have in their walls supporting frameworks of gill bars. Primitive forms such as amphioxus have a large number of slits, but only six or seven are the rule in the fishes. The transitory appearance of the slits in the embryos of land vertebrates is evidence for their evolutionary ancestry.

Postanal tail

The postanal tail, together with somatic musculature and the stiffening notochord, provides the motility that larval tunicates and amphioxus need for their free-swimming existence. As a structure added to the body behind the end of the digestive tract, it clearly has evolved specifically for propulsion in water. Its efficiency is later increased in fishes with the addition of fins.

____ Adaptations That Have Guided Chordate Evolution

From gilled filter-feeding ancestors to the highest vertebrates, the evolution of chordates has been guided by the specialized basic adaptations of the living endoskeleton, paired limbs, efficient respiration, and an advanced nervous system.

Living endoskeleton

The endoskeleton of chordates, as in the echinoderms, is an internal supportive structure and framework for the body. This is a departure in animal architecture, since invertebrate skeletons generally enfold the body. As compared with the dead, noncellular exoskeleton of arthropods, the living endoskeleton of chordates possesses a powerful and overriding advantage: it permits continuous growth without the necessity of shedding. For this reason vertebrate animals can attain great size; some of them are the most massive in the animal kingdom. Endoskeletons provide ample surface for muscle attachment, and size differences between animals result mainly from the amount of muscle tissue they possess. More muscle tissue necessitates greater development of body systems, such as circulatory, digestive, respiratory, and excretory. Thus, the endoskeleton is a chief factor in the development and specialization of the higher animals.

We should note that the chordates did not wholly discard the exoskeleton, which after all does provide excellent defensive armor for its owner. Most fishes have dermal scales, and many higher vertebrates developed epidermal scales, beaks, claws, and feathers from the protein keratin (p. 672). The endoskeleton also plays a protective role—for example, the cranium that encloses the brain and the thoracic rib cage that surrounds important visceral structures.

The endoskeleton was probably composed initially of cartilage that later gave way to bone. Cartilage forms a perfectly suitable endoskeleton, especially for an aquatic existence, and still is the first skeleton to appear in all larval and embryonic vertebrates. In the agnathans (hagfish and lampreys), the sharks and their kin, and even some primitive bony fishes such as sturgeons, the adult endoskeleton is composed strictly of cartilage. Bone appears in the endoskeleton of more advanced vertebrates, perhaps because it offers two clear advantages to cartilage. First, it serves as a reservoir for phosphate, an indispensable component of compounds with high-energy bonds, of membranes, and of DNA. Second, only bone could provide the structural strength required for life on land, where mechanical stresses on the endoskeleton are far greater than they are in water.

Paired limbs

Pectoral and pelvic appendages are present in most vertebrates in the form of paired fins or legs. They originated as swimming stabilizers and later became prominently developed into legs for travel on land.

Pharynx and efficient respiration

The perforated pharynx (gill slits), present in all chordates at some stage in their life cycle, evolved as a filter-feeding apparatus. In primitive chordates (such as amphioxus), water with suspended food particles is drawn through the mouth by ciliary action and flows out through the gill slits where the food is trapped in mucus. A later improvement was the replacement of cilia with a muscular feeding apparatus that pumps water through the pharynx by expanding and contracting the pharyngeal cavity. This adaptation led to the development of **internal gills.** Many invertebrate groups have gills, but they are typically feathery projections from the body surface, and all lack the pharyngeal suction pump that makes the vertebrate gill an exceedingly effective device. Some fish gills can remove 85% of the oxygen from water in its single pass across the gill surface. No invertebrate aquatic respiratory device can approach this efficiency. The tracheal system of arthropods is a highly efficient aerial respiratory device but is effective only in small animals. The chordate paired gill clefts and the internal gills that evolve from them are one of the most distinctive chordate features.

Advanced nervous system

No single system in the body is more strongly associated with functional and structural advancement than is the nervous system. Longitudinal nerve cords appear in various invertebrate groups but are typically paired and ventrally situated and contain nerve fibers mixed with clusters of nerve cells (ganglia). Only the chordates have a single, hollow, dorsal nerve cord, with clear separation of the **brain,** wherein are concentrated nerve cells, and the **spinal cord,** which contains principally nerve fibers. Such a system permits the greatest possible utilization of space for well-integrated nervous patterns. Sense organs are developed well beyond those of any invertebrate group: paired eyes with lens and inverted retinas; pressure receptors, such as paired ears designed for equilibrium and later redesigned to include sound reception; and chemical receptors, including taste receptors and the exquisitely sensitive olfactory organs of many vertebrates.

CLASSIFICATION

There are three subphyla under phylum Chordata. Two of these subphyla are small groups of few genera, their members lack a vertebral column, and they are of interest primarily as borderline or first chordates (protochordates). The third subphylum, Vertebrata, is subdivided into eight classes.

> **Phylum Chordata**
> > **Group Protochordata (Acrania)**
> > > **Subphylum Urochordata** (u′ro-kor-da′ta) (Gr., *oura,* tail + L., *chorda,* cord, + *ata,* characterized by) (**Tunicata**)—**tunicates.** Notochord and nerve cord in free-swimming larva only; sessile adults encased in tunic.
> > > **Subphylum Cephalochordata** (sef′a-lo-kor-da′ta) (Gr., *kephalē,* head, + L., *chorda,* cord)—**lancelets (amphioxus).** Notochord and nerve cord found along entire length of body and persist throughout life; fishlike in form.
> > **Group Craniata**
> > > **Subphylum Vertebrata** (ver′te-bra′ta) (L., *vertebratus,* backboned). Bony or cartilaginous vertebrae surrounding spinal cord; notochord in all embryonic stages, persisting in some of the fish; also may be divided into two groups (superclasses) according to presence of jaws.
> > > > **Superclass Agnatha** (ag′na-tha) (Gr., *a,* without, + *gnathos,* jaw) (**Cyclostomata**)—**hagfishes, lampreys.** Without true jaws or appendages.

Table 22-1 Divisions of the Phylum Chordata

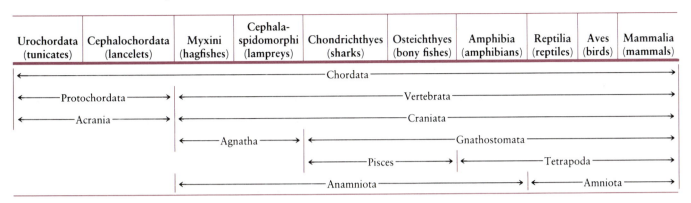

Urochordata (tunicates)	Cephalochordata (lancelets)	Myxini (hagfishes)	Cephala-spidomorphi (lampreys)	Chondrichthyes (sharks)	Osteichthyes (bony fishes)	Amphibia (amphibians)	Reptilia (reptiles)	Aves (birds)	Mammalia (mammals)

Class **Myxini** (mik-sy′ny) (Gr., *myxa*, slime)—**hagfishes.** Terminal mouth with four pairs of tentacles; buccal funnel absent; nasal sac with duct to pharynx; five to 15 pairs of gill pouches; partially hermaphroditic.

Class **Cephalaspidomorphi** (sef-a-lass′pe-do-morf′e) (Gr., *kephalē*, head, + *aspidos*, shield, + *morphē*, form)—**lampreys.** Suctorial mouth with horny teeth; nasal sac not connected to mouth; seven pairs of gill pouches.

Superclass **Gnathostomata** (na′tho-sto′ma-ta) (Gr., *gnathos*, jaw, + *stoma*, mouth)—**jawed fishes, all tetrapods.** With jaws and (usually) paired appendages.

Class **Chondrichthyes** (kon-drik′thee-eez) (Gr., *chondros*, cartilage, + *ichthys*, a fish)—**sharks, skates, rays, chimaeras.** Streamlined body with heterocercal tail; cartilaginous skeleton; five to seven gills with separate openings, no operculum, no swim bladder.

Class **Osteichthyes** (os′te-ik′thee-eez) (Gr., *osteon*, bone, + *ichthys*, a fish) (Teleostomi)—**bony fishes.** Primitively fusiform body but variously modified; mostly ossified skeleton; single gill opening on each side covered with operculum; usually swim bladder or lung.

Class **Amphibia** (am-fib′e-a) (Gr., *amphi*, both or double, + *bios*, life)—**amphibians.** Ectothermic tetrapods; respiration by lungs, gills, or skin; development through larval stage; skin moist, containing mucous glands, and lacking scales.

Class **Reptilia** (rep-til′e-a) (L., *repere*, to creep)—**reptiles.** Ectothermic (some endothermic) tetrapods possessing lungs; embryo develops within shelled egg; no larval stage; skin dry, lacking mucous glands, and covered by epidermal scales.

Class **Aves** (ay′veez) (L., pl. of *avis*, bird)—**birds.** Endothermic vertebrates with front limbs modified for flight; body covered with feathers; scales on feet.

Class **Mammalia** (ma-may′lee-a) (L., *mamma*, breast)—**mammals.** Endothermic vertebrates possessing mammary glands; body more or less covered with hair; well-developed brain.

The basic taxonomic division of the phylum Chordata is only one of several systems used to characterize different groups within the phylum. These are summarized in Table 22-1. A fundamental separation is the Protochordata from the Vertebrata. Since the former lack a well-developed head, they are also called Acrania. All vertebrates have a well-developed skull case enclosing the brain and are called Craniata.

Two basic branches of the vertebrates are the Agnatha, forms lacking jaws (lampreys and hagfishes), and Gnathostomata, forms having jaws (all other vertebrates). These two groups represent early separations within the Vertebrata. The

Gnathostomata in turn can be subdivided into Pisces, jawed aquatic vertebrates with limbs, if any, in the shape of fins, and the Tetrapods, jawed vertebrates with two pairs of limbs. Another fundamental separation among the vertebrates is based on embryological patterns. The embryos of reptiles, birds, and mammals develop within a fluid-filled membranous sac, the amnion. These are called the Amniota. Fishes and amphibians, the Anamniota, lack this important adaptation.

___ Ancestry and Evolution

Since the mid–nineteenth century when the theory of organic evolution became the focal point for ferreting out relationships between groups of living organisms, zoologists have debated the question of vertebrate origins. It has been very difficult to reconstruct lines of descent because the earliest protochordates were in all probability soft-bodied creatures that stood little chance of being preserved as fossils even under the most ideal conditions. Consequently, such reconstructions largely come from the study of living organisms, especially from an analysis of early developmental stages that tend to be more insulated from evolutionary changes than the differentiated adult forms that they become.

The earliest speculations understandably focused on the most successful and in many respects most advanced of invertebrate groups, the Arthropoda. It was quickly recognized that, if an arthropod (a cockroach, for example) with its segmented body, ventral nerve cord, and dorsal heart were turned on its back, the basic plan of a vertebrate would result. Later, the ancestral award was transferred to the Annelida, because this group shares a basic body plan with the arthropods and in addition has an excretory system that strikingly resembles that of primitive vertebrates.

Although the annelid-vertebrate theory continued to receive support as late as 1922, it contained unresolvable difficulties. An inverted annelid has its brain and mouth in the wrong relative positions. The annelid's nerve cord is ventral but connects to a dorsal brain by way of circumpharyngeal connectives through which the digestive tube passes (Fig. 14-2, A, p. 342). When an annelid is inverted, as was required for the annelid-vertebrate theory, the mouth ends up on top of the head and the brain below. Despite efforts to explain this discrepancy, the annelid theory was eventually discarded like the arthropod theory before it.

Early in this century when further theorizing became rooted in developmental patterns of animals, it immediately became apparent that only the echinoderms deserved serious consideration as the vertebrates' ancestor. Echinoderms and chordates belong to the deuterostome branch of the animal kingdom, in which the anus forms from the blastopore or at the end of the gastrula, and the mouth is formed as a secondary opening, usually on the opposite end. The coelom of both phyla is primitively enterocoelous: it is budded off from the archenteron of the embryo. Both echinoderm and chordate embryos show indeterminate cleavage; that is, each of the early blastomeres has equivalent potentiality for supporting full development of a complete embryo. These characteristics are shared by brachiopods and pterobranchs (a hemichordate group), as well as by echinoderms, protochordates, amphioxus, and vertebrates. This is probably a natural grouping and almost certainly indicates interrelationships, although remote (Fig. 22-2).

More recently, another piece of evidence linking chordates with the starfishes and their allies has come from the detailed study of a curious group of fossil echinoderms, the Stylophora. These small, nonsymmetrical forms have a head resembling a long-toed medieval boot, a series of branchial slits covered with flaps

Most of the early efforts to prove invertebrate and chordate kinship are now recognized as based on similarities related to analogy rather than homology. As discussed in Chapter 6 (p. 143), analogous structures are those that perform similar functions but have altogether different origins (such as wings of birds and butterflies). Homologous structures, on the other hand, share a common origin but may look quite different (at least superficially) and perform quite different functions. For example, all vertebrate forelimbs are homologous because they are derived from a pentadactyl limb, even though they may be modified as differently as the human arm and a bird's wing. Homologous structures share a genetic heritage; analogous structures do not. Obviously, only homologous similarities have any bearing in ancestral connections.

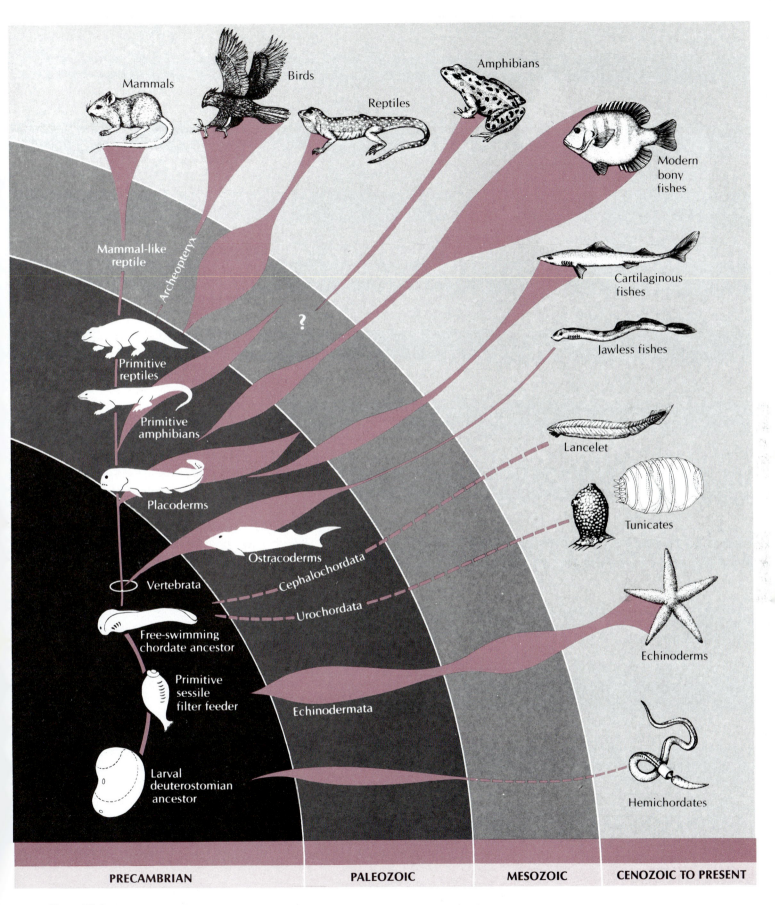

Figure 22-2

Family tree of the chordates, suggesting probable origin and relationships. Other schemes have been suggested and are possible. *White,* Extinct stem groups. *Black,* Living groups. *Red,* Lines of descent. The relative success in numbers of species of each group through geological time, as indicated by the fossil record, is suggested by the bulging and thinning of that group's line of descent. Dashed lines indicate a poor or nonexistent fossil record.

Gill slits   Mouth

Anus   Tail

Figure 22-3

Fossil of a primitive echinoderm, *Cothurnocystis*, that lived during the Ordovician period (450 million years BP). It shows affinities with both echinoderms and chordates and may belong to a group that was ancestral to the chordates.

Courtesy R.P.S. Jeffries, The British Museum.

The once exalted position of amphioxus in zoological circles was put to rhyme by Philip Pope. Sung to the tune of "Tipperary," the poem ends:

My notochord shall grow into
   a chain of vertebrae;
As fins my metapleural folds
   shall agitate the sea;
This tiny dorsal nervous tube
   shall form a mighty brain,
And the vertebrates shall
   dominate the animal domain.
Chorus
It's a long way from
   Amphioxus
It's a long way to us.
It's a long way from
   Amphioxus
To the meanest human cuss.
It's good-bye fins and gill slits,
Welcome skin and hair.
It's a long way from
   Amphioxus
But we came from there.

much like the gill openings of sharks, a postanal tail with a central rod resembling a notochord, and muscle blocks and a dorsal nerve cord (Fig. 22-3). These creatures were apparently adapted to use their gill slits for filter feeding, as do the primitive chordates today. Are they the long-sought chordate ancestors? Unfortunately we are not yet, and perhaps will never be, in a position to know.

Unable to narrow further the search for a prechordate-chordate connecting link, zoologists are now focusing on groups within the chordate phylum itself, which share enough anatomical and developmental features to make unraveling the evolutionary past a more profitable effort.

Candidates for vertebrate ancestral stock

The three subphyla that bear the four chordate hallmarks are the Cephalochordata (of which the lancelet, amphioxus, is the best-known representative), the Urochordata (tunicates or sea squirts), and the Vertebrata. Since the vertebrates comprise by far the greatest number of the chordates, the terms "vertebrate" and "chordate" are frequently used (somewhat incorrectly) as synonyms. The backboneless members of the phylum—cephalochordates and urochordates—are usually referred to as protochordates or prevertebrates and have long been considered good candidates for the vertebrate ancestral stock.

The Hemichordata, described in the preceding chapter, previously were also assigned to the phylum Chordata, since they possess a perforated pharynx (gill slits) and a middorsal thickening of nervous tissue, which may be a forerunner of the vertebrate tubular nerve cord. However, the stomochord of the hemichordates cannot be homologized to the notochord as was once believed. Furthermore, the gill slits and dorsal nerve center may represent a convergent resemblance to similar chordate structures rather than a true homology. Consequently, the hemichordates have been excluded from chordate membership, but most biologists agree that a real, although remote, relationship exists.

Position of amphioxus

The problems of sorting out lines of descent within the phylum Chordata are enormous because most of the prechordates and protochordates are highly specialized remnants of once successful and well-represented groups. The first approach was to place the chordate and prechordate groups in order of increasing morphological complexity leading to the vertebrates.

By this analysis, amphioxus becomes the logical structural ancestor of the vertebrates because it possesses as an adult all four chordate characteristics previously mentioned plus several vertebrate hallmarks: segmented musculature, the beginning of optic and olfactory sense organs, a liver diverticulum, beginnings of a ventral heart, and separation of dorsal and ventral spinal roots in the vertebrate style (Fig. 22-13). Little wonder that amphioxus once attained a pinnacle position among zoologists searching for their vertebrate ancestor.

On closer scrutiny, however, amphioxus fails to meet the qualifications for a generalized ancestral type. Its notochord is overdeveloped into a forward extension for its specialized burrowing mode of life, and this prevents the development of a proper brain. Its kidney is a solenocyte type that bears little resemblance to the vertebrate glomerular-tubular nephron. Its unique atrium has no vertebrate counterpart, and there is a nonvertebrate-like proliferation of gill slits. Amphioxus today is usually regarded as a highly specialized member of the chordate family: it lies in an offshoot, rather than in the main line, of chordate descent.

Urochordata and the theory of recapitulation

After amphioxus, attention became focused on the alternative protochordate group, the Urochordata (tunicates). The urochordates are divided into three groups of which the ascidians (sea squirts) are the simplest and most common.

At first glance, more unlikely candidates for vertebrate ancestors could hardly be imagined. As adults, ascidians are virtually immobile forms surrounded by a tough, cellulose-containing tunic of variable color. Their adult life is spent in one spot attached to some submarine surface, filtering vast amounts of seawater from which they extract their planktonic food. As adults they lack a notochord, tubular nerve cord, postanal tail, sense organs, and segmented musculature. Superficially they resemble sponges far more than they resemble any known vertebrate (Fig. 22-8). Yet the chordate nature of ascidians is abundantly evident in their larvae, which, because of their superficial resemblance to larval amphibians, are referred to as "tadpole larvae." These tiny, active, site-seeking forms have all the right qualifications for membership in the prevertebrate club: notochord, hollow dorsal nerve cord, gill slits, postanal tail, brain, and sense organs (an otolith balance organ and an eye complete with a lens).

The discovery of this form in 1869 not only placed the urochordates squarely in the vertebrate camp but greatly influenced the great German zoologist Ernst Haeckel in formulating his concept of recapitulation (biogenetic law, see Principle 7, p. 12). According to this theory, adult stages of ancestors are repeated during the development of their descendants; in other words, the development of a living organism is an accurate record of past evolutionary history.

We recognize now that this record is very slurred and telescoped and must be interpreted with caution. But at the time that the nature of the ascidian tadpole larva was first understood, it was considered to be a relic of an ancient free-swimming chordate ancestor of the ascidians. Adult ascidians then came to be regarded as degenerate, sessile descendants of the ancient chordate form.

Garstang's hypothesis of chordate larval evolution

In 1928 W. Garstang in England introduced totally fresh thinking to the vertebrate ancestor debates. In effect, Garstang turned the sequence around: rather than the ancestral tadpole larva giving rise to a degenerative sessile ascidian adult, he suggested that sessile ascidian adults *were* the ancestral stock from which the tadpole larvae were evolved to seek out new habitats. Thus, the planktonic tadpole larva was visualized as an ascidian creation, evolved within the group to spread it far and wide. Garstang next suggested that at some point the tadpole larva became neotenous, becoming capable of maturing gonads and reproducing in the larval stage. With continued larval evolution, a new group of free-swimming animals would appear (Fig. 22-4).

The best evidence for this hypothesis is found in the living tunicates today, especially among the two planktonic groups, the thaliaceans and the larvaceans (p. 510). In the latter group the basic larval form is retained throughout life; they are in effect neotenous tunicates, although extremely specialized.

Garstang departed from previous thinking by suggesting that evolution may occur in the larval stages of animals. Zoologists accepted this idea slowly because they were accustomed to thinking of developmental stages as being largely insulated from change, as embodied in the "biogenetic law."

The ascidian tadpole larva with its propulsive tail, stiffening notochord, and dorsal nerve cord, which integrates sensory information and motor activity, clear-

Neoteny is well known among living amphibians. The larvae of the American axolotl, for example, may become sexually mature and reproduce without ever undergoing metamorphosis. In some lakes, generation after generation reproduce in the neotenous larval state, and true adults never occur. In other lakes having different environmental conditions, the axolotls metamorphose to reproducing adults. Other examples of neoteny are known; indeed, many believe the human species is neotenous! Certainly, neoteny *could* have occurred among the early chordates, and if it did, the sessile adult stage would be dropped, leaving a new free-swimming chordate.

Figure 22-4

Garstang's hypothesis of vertebrate origins. Adult ascidians live on the sea floor but reproduce through a free-swimming tadpole larva. More than 500 million years ago, some larvae began to reproduce in the swimming stage. These evolved into the ostracoderms, the first known vertebrates.

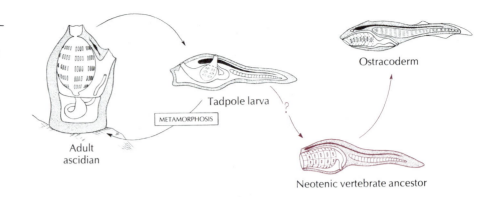

Ostracoderm

Tadpole larva

METAMORPHOSIS

Adult ascidian

Neotenic vertebrate ancestor

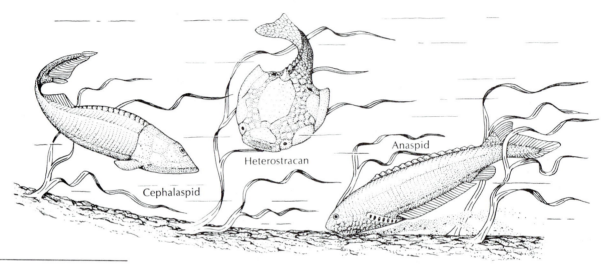

Anaspid

Heterostracan

Cephalaspid

Figure 22-5

Three ostracoderms, jawless fishes of Silurian and Devonian times. Representatives of three of the best-known ostracoderm groups are illustrated as they might have appeared while searching for food on the floor of a Devonian sea or lake. All were filter feeders, drawing water and organic debris into the mouth, straining out the organic matter, and expelling the water through the gill openings and between the ventral head plates.

ly suggests and foreshadows the vertebrate line. The resemblance of an early vertebrate ostracoderm to this hypothetical ancestor is suggested in Fig. 22-4.

Jawless ostracoderms—earliest vertebrates

The earliest vertebrate fossils are fragments of bony armor discovered in Ordovician rock in Russia and the United States. They were small, jawless creatures collectively called **ostracoderms** (os-trak′o-derm) (Gr., *ostrakon*, shell, + *derma*, skin), which belong to the Agnatha division of the vertebrates. These earliest ostracoderms, called **heterostracans** (Fig. 22-5), lacked paired lateral fins that subsequent fishes found so important for stability. Their swimming movements must have been inefficient and clumsy, although sufficient to propel them from one mud bed to another where they practiced their mud-grubbing search for nutrients in the form of organic debris on the sea bottom. Later in the Silurian period and especially in the Devonian period, the heterostracan ostracoderms underwent a major radiation, resulting in the appearance of several peculiar-looking forms varying in shape and length of the snout, dorsal spines, and dermal plates. Most continued their mud-loving existence, although at least one species became a surface feeder. Without ever evolving paired fins or jaws, the heterostracans dominated the early Devonian period until eclipsed by another ostracoderm group, the **cephalaspids.**

The cephalaspids improved the efficiency of a benthic life by evolving paired fins. These fins, located just behind the head shield, provided control over pitch and yaw that ensured well-directed forward movement. The best-known genus in this group is *Cephalaspis* (Gr., *kephalē*, head, + *aspis*, shield) (Fig. 22-5), the subject of a brilliant and classical series of studies by the Swedish paleozoologist E.A. Stensiö. *Cephalaspis* was a small animal, seldom exceeding 30 cm in length, and was covered by a well-developed armor, the head by a solid shield (rounded anteriorly) and the body by bony plates. It had no axial skeleton or vertebrae. Its mouth was ventral and anterior, and it was jawless and toothless. Its paired eyes were located close to the middorsal line. A pineal eye was also present, in front of which was a single nasal opening. At the lateroposterior corners of the head shield were flaplike fins. The trunk and tail were apparently adapted for active swimming. Between the margin of the head shield and the ventral plates there were 10 gill openings on each side. They also had a lateral line system. They were adapted for filter feeding, which may explain the large, expanded size of the head, made up as it was of a large pharyngeal gill-slit filtering apparatus.

A third major group of ostracoderms, the **anaspids,** were clearly related to the cephalaspids although they looked very different (Fig. 22-5). The most significant of the anaspids (although not the earliest to appear) was the genus *Jamoytius* (named in honor of J.A. Moy-Thomas, a British paleontologist). *Jamoytius* was jawless like other ostracoderms and had simple myotomes like amphioxus. It had paired fins, but these were peculiar, elongate, posterior stabilizers that formed a part of the caudal (tail) fin. The anaspids were much more streamlined than other ostracoderms and are believed to have had an active mode of life. Some paleontologists believe that one of the two groups of living agnathans, the lampreys, may have evolved from the anaspids (Fig. 23-1, pp. 522 and 523).

As a group, the ostracoderms were basically fitted for a simple, bottom-feeding life. Yet despite their anatomical limitations, they enjoyed a respectable radiation in the Silurian and Devonian periods. Their overall contribution was enormous, for they provided a blueprint for subsequent vertebrate evolution. But they could not survive the competition of the more advanced jawed fishes that began to dominate the Devonian period, and in the end they disappeared.

Early jawed vertebrates

All jawed vertebrates, whether extinct or living, are collectively called gnathostomes ("jaw mouth"), in contrast to jawless vertebrates, the agnathans ("without jaw"). The latter are also often referred to as cyclostomes ("circle mouth").

Erik Stensiö was the first paleozoologist to approach fossil anatomy with the same painstaking attention to minute detail that morphologists have long applied to the anatomical study of living fishes. He developed novel and exacting methods for gradually grinding away a fossil, a few micrometers at a time, to reveal internal features. He was able to reconstruct not only bony anatomy, but nerves, blood vessels, and muscles in numerous groups of Paleozoic and early Mesozoic fishes. His innovative methods are now widely used by paleozoologists.

Figure 22-6

Early jawed fishes of the Devonian period, 400 million years ago. The placoderm *(left)* and a related acanthodian *(right)* were highly mobile and voracious forms. Although more successful than the less maneuverable ostracoderms, they eventually failed in competition with their successors, the bony and cartilaginous fishes.

Devonian placoderm

Acanthodian

Gill bar   Gill slit

Jawless, filter-feeding ancestor

Spiracle

Early jaw formation

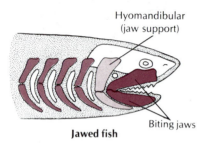

Hyomandibular
(jaw support)

Biting jaws

Jawed fish

Figure 22-7

How the vertebrates got their jaw. The mud-loving Silurian fish converted the first gill opening into a spiracle that opened on the upper head, allowing water to be drawn in without fouling the gills. The first gill bars, no longer required for gill support, became enlarged and armed with teeth. Relics of this transformation are seen during the development of sharks.

The first jawed vertebrates to appear in the fossil record were the **placoderms** (plak′o-derm) (Gr., *plax*, plate, + *derma*, skin) (Fig. 22-6). The advantages of jaws are obvious, since they allowed predation on large and active forms of food. The possessors of jaws would enjoy a tremendous advantage over jawless vertebrates, which were restricted to a wormlike existence of sifting out organic debris and small organisms in the bottom mud. Jaws arose through modifications of the first two of the serially repeated cartilaginous gill arches. The beginnings of this trend can be seen in some of the jawless ostracoderms where the mouth became bordered by strong dermal plates that could be manipulated somewhat as jaws with the gill arch musculature. The more anterior arches continued a gradual modification to permit more efficient seizing, and the skin surrounding the mouth was modified into teeth. Eventually the anterior gill arches became bent into the characteristic position of vertebrate jaws, as seen in the placoderms (Fig. 22-7).

The early jawed fishes had well-developed lateral fins. These may have arisen as lateral folds in the body wall, which broke up into a series of fins, such as is found in the **acanthodians,** a primitive group contemporary with the placoderms (Fig. 22-6). In these, however, the anterior and posterior pairs were larger than the others and eventually became the pectoral and pelvic fins; the intermediate ones disappeared. Some paleontologists believe that these numerous paired fins may have arisen independently as separate structures. Their internal skeleton so far as is known was composed of bone.

Placoderms evolved into a great variety of forms, some large and grotesque in appearance. They were armored fishes, covered with diamond-shaped scales or with large plates of bone. All became extinct by the end of the Paleozoic era.

Evolution of modern fishes and tetrapods

Reconstruction of the origins of the vast and varied assemblage of modern living vertebrates is, as we have seen, based largely on fossil evidence. Unfortunately, the fossil evidence for the earliest vertebrates is often incomplete and tells us much less than we would like to know about subsequent trends in evolution. Affinities become much easier to establish as the fossil record improves. For instance, the descent of birds and mammals from reptilian ancestors has been worked out in a highly convincing manner from the relatively abundant fossil record available. By contrast, the ancestry of modern fishes is shrouded in uncertainty.

The Swedish paleontologist E. Jarvik has emphasized that the main vertebrate stem groups (such as cyclostomes, lungfishes, sharks, bony fishes, and stem tetrapods) became anatomically specialized some 400 to 500 million years ago and have changed relatively little since then. Thus, main evolutionary lines, as seen in the fossil record, run back almost in parallel; if extended backward to their illogical extreme, they would hardly ever meet. Obviously they must meet at some point in the distant past, but this exercise reveals that the crucial separations in vertebrate evolution occurred in the Cambrian period, perhaps even the Precambrian period, long before the fossil record became established for the convenience of paleozoologists (Jarvik, 1967).

Despite the difficulty of establishing early lines of descent for the vertebrates, they are clearly a natural, monophyletic group, distinguished by a great number of common characters. They have almost certainly descended from a common ancestor, the nature of which we have already discussed. Very early in their evolution, the vertebrates divided into two important stems, the agnathans and the gnathostomes. These two groups differ from each other in many fundamental ways, in addition to the obvious lack of jaws in the former group and their presence in the latter. Thus, both groups are very old and of approximately the same age. On this basis we cannot say that agnathans are more "primitive" than gnathostomes, even though the latter have continued a marvelous evolutionary advance that produced most of the modern fishes, all of the tetrapods, and the reader of this book. Although the agnathans are represented today only by the hagfishes and the lampreys, these creatures too are successful in their own way.

___ Subphylum Urochordata (Tunicata)

The tunicates (Fig. 22-8) are widely distributed in all seas from near the shoreline to great depths. Most of them are sessile, at least as adults, although some are free living. The name "tunicate" is suggested by the nonliving tunic (test) that surrounds them and contains cellulose. A common name for them is sea squirt because some of them discharge water through the excurrent siphon when irritated. They vary in size from microscopic forms to several centimeters in length. As a group they may be considered degenerative or specialized chordates, for the adults lack many of the common characteristics of chordates.

Urochordata is divided into three classes: **Ascidiacea** (Gr., *askiolion*, little bag, + *acea,* suffix), **Larvacea** (L., *larva,* ghost, + *acea,* suffix), and **Thaliacea** (Gr., *thalia,* luxuriance, + *acea,* suffix). Of these, the members of **Ascidiacea,** commonly known as the ascidians, or sea squirts, are by far the most common and are the best known. Ascidians may be solitary, colonial, or compound. Each of the solitary and colonial forms has its own test, but among the compound forms many individuals may share the same test (Fig. 22-9). In some of these compound ascidians each member has its own incurrent siphon, but the excurrent opening is common to the group.

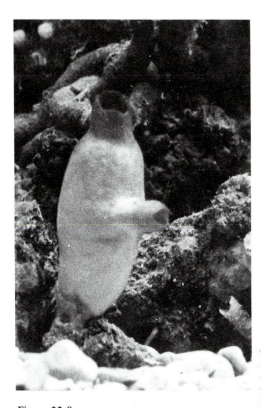

Figure 22-8

Typical solitary ascidian, the sea peach *Halocynthia pyriformis* of the northwestern Atlantic.
Photograph by C.P. Hickman, Jr.

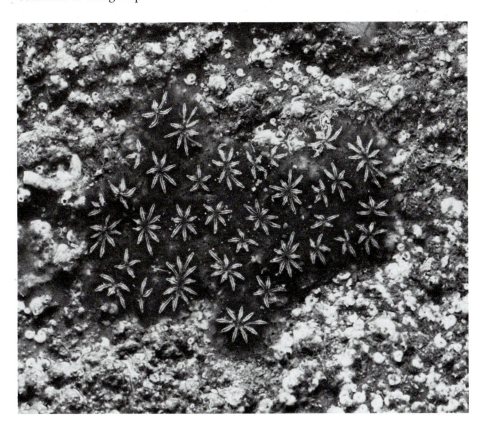

Figure 22-9

Compound sea squirt *Botryllus schlosseri,* common in shallow coastal waters and rock tide pools. Each of the star-shaped patterns represents a colonial arrangement in which the arms of the star are individuals, each with its own incurrent siphon at the end of the arm. All are united centrally where they share a common test, forming a compound ascidian. (Approximately ×2.)
Photograph by D.P. Wilson.

The **Larvacea** and **Thaliacea** are pelagic (open-sea) forms and are not often found in the intertidal zones where ascidians are common. The members of Larvacea are small, tadpolelike forms less than 5 mm in length and resemble ascidian tadpoles (Fig. 22-10, *B*). They perhaps represent persistent larval forms that have become neotenic. They secrete around themselves cellulose tunics and are filter feeders. *Oikopleura* is a larvacean form often collected in tow-net samplings of ocean plankton.

The class Thaliacea is made up of members that may reach a length of 8 to 10 cm. Their transparent body is spindle shaped or cylindrical and is surrounded by bands of circular muscle, with their incurrent and excurrent siphons at opposite ends (Fig. 22-10, *A*). They are mostly carried along by currents, although by contracting their circular muscle bands they can force water out of their excurrent siphons and can move by jet propulsion. Many are provided with luminous organs and give a brilliant light at night. Most of the body is hollow, with the viscera forming a compact mass on the ventral side. They appear to have come from attached ancestors as did the ascidians. Some of them have complex life histories. In forms such as *Doliolum* there is alternation of generations between sexual and asexual forms. After hatching from the egg, the larval tadpole changes into a barrel-shaped nurse or asexual stage, which produces small buds on a ventral stolon. These buds break free, become attached to another part of the parent, and develop into three kinds of individuals; one kind breaks free to become the sexual stage. *Salpa* also has alternation of generations and is a common form along the Atlantic coast.

Adult ascidian—Molgula

Molgula is globose in form and is attached by its base to piles and stones. Lining the test or tunic is a membrane or **mantle**. On the outside are two projections: the **incurrent** and **excurrent siphons** (Fig. 22-11). Water enters the incurrent siphon and passes into the pharynx (branchial sac) through the mouth. On the midventral side of the pharynx is a groove, the **endostyle,** which is ciliated and secretes mucus. Food material in the water is entangled by the mucus in this endostyle and carried into the esophagus and stomach. The intestine leads to the anus near the excurrent siphon. The water passes through the pharyngeal slits in the walls of the pharynx into the atrial cavity. As the water passes through the slits, respiration occurs.

Figure 22-10

A, Thaliacean *Doliolum nationalis*—a member of the class Thaliacea. (Approximately ×25.) **B,** Larvacean *Oikopleura dioca*—a typical tadpolelike member of the class Larvacea. (Approximately ×55.)
Photographs by D.P. Wilson.

A   B

The circulatory system contains a ventral **heart** near the stomach and two large vessels, one connected to each end of the heart. The action of the heart is peculiar in that it drives the blood first in one direction and then in the other. This reversal of blood flow is found in no other chordate. The excretory system is a type of nephridium near the intestine. The nervous system is restricted to a nerve ganglion and a few nerves that lie on the dorsal side of the pharynx. A notochord is lacking. The animals are hermaphroditic, for both ovaries and testes are found in the same animal. Ducts lead from the gonads close to the intestines and empty near the anus. The germ cells are carried out the excurrent siphon into the surrounding water, where cross-fertilization occurs.

Of the four chief characteristics of chordates, adult tunicates have only one: the pharyngeal gill slits. However, the larval form gives away the secret of their true relationship. The tadpole larva (Fig. 22-11) is an elongate, transparent form with all four chordate characteristics: a notochord, a hollow dorsal nerve cord, a propulsive postanal tail, and a large pharynx with endostyle and gill slits. The larva does not feed but swims about for some hours before fastening itself vertically by its adhesive papillae to some solid object. It then undergoes a retrograde metamorphosis to become the sessile adult (Fig. 22-11).

Subphylum Cephalochordata

Amphioxus

Subphylum Cephalochordata is the most interesting of all the protochordates, for one of its members is the lancelet *Branchiostoma* (formerly *Amphioxus*) (Fig. 22-12), one of the classical animals in zoology. Cephalochordates are found mainly on the sandy marine beaches of southern waters, where they burrow in the sand, with the anterior end projecting out. One American species, *Branchiostoma virginiae* (Gr., *branchia*, gills, + *stoma*, mouth) is found from Florida to the Chesapeake Bay. Altogether there are 28 species, of which four are North American, scattered over the world. They can swim in open water by swift lateral movements of the body.

Amphioxus (Gr., *amphi*, both sides [ends], + *oxys*, sharp) is especially interesting, for it has the four distinctive characteristics of chordates in simple form, and in other ways it may be considered a blueprint of the phylum. It has a slender,

Figure 22-11

Metamorphosis of a solitary ascidian from a free-swimming tadpole larva stage.

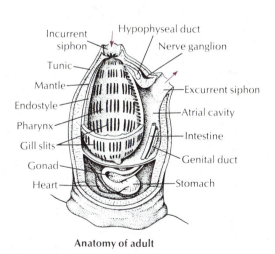

Anatomy of adult

Figure 22-12

Amphioxus. This interesting bottom-dwelling cephalochordate possesses the four distinctive chordate characteristics (notochord, dorsal nerve cord, pharyngeal gill slits, and postanal tail) that once made it the prime candidate for our vertebrate ancestor. However, because it also bears many specialized and degenerate features, zoologists now consider it a divergent offshoot from the main line of chordate evolution.
Photograph by B. Tallmark.

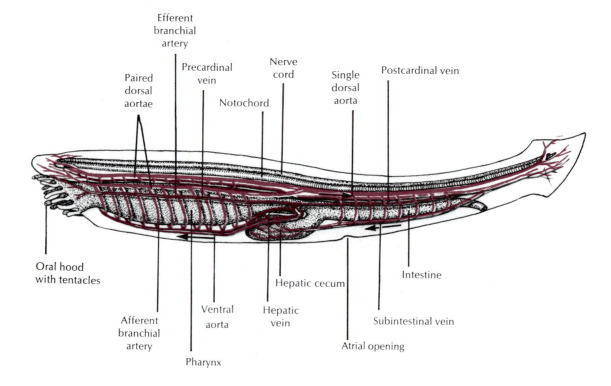

Figure 22-13

Structure of amphioxus showing scheme of the circulation.

laterally compressed, transparent body, 5 to 7 cm long (Fig. 22-12). It is a filter feeder. Water enters the mouth, driven by cilia in the buccal cavity, then passes through the numerous gill slits in both sides of the compressed pharynx into an atrium. It leaves by an atrial opening. A groove in the floor of the pharynx, known as the endostyle, secretes mucus, which is moved by cilia along the gill slits. Food particles in the water passing through the slits are trapped in the mucus, which is then moved to the intestine. Here the food particles are separated from the mucus and passed into a cecum where they are digested. Although amphioxus lacks a liver and pancreas, these organs of higher vertebrates develop as pouches that grow out of the gut in the position of the cecum of amphioxus.

The closed circulatory system is complex for so simple a chordate (Fig. 22-13). The flow pattern is similar to that of the fishes, although there is no heart. Blood flows posteriorly in a dorsal aorta, is distributed to the body tissues by a microcirculation, and is then collected into veins. These empty into a ventral aorta that pumps the blood forward by peristaltic-like contractions of the vessel wall.

The blood passes into branchial vessels in the gill bars where it is oxygenated and then passed into the dorsal aorta.

Excretion in amphioxus is by numerous nephridia called solenocytes, which resemble modified flame cells. Each solenocyte is a blind-ended tube containing a beating flagellum that excretes a fluid, presumably urine, into the atrium.

The nervous system is centered around a hollow dorsal nerve cord lying above the notochord. The nerve cord is enclosed in a collagenous sheath that provides protection much as vertebrae protect the spinal cord of fishes. There is no brain. The nerve cord gives off a pair of spinal nerve roots at each body segment, or myotome. Although this arrangement resembles the vertebrate spinal cord, the ventral root actually does not contain nerves but rather the drawn-out extensions of myotomic muscle fibers. Ciliated cells with sensory functions are found in various parts of the body.

Sexes are separate, and each sex has about 25 pairs of gonads located on the wall of the atrium. The sex cells are set free in the atrial cavity and pass through the atriopore to the outside, where fertilization occurs. Cleavage is total (holoblastic), and a gastrula is formed by invagination. The larva hatches soon after deposition and gradually assumes the shape of the adult.

No other chordate shows the basic diagnostic chordate characteristics as clearly as the amphioxus. Not only are the four chief characters of chordates—dorsal nerve cord, notochord, pharyngeal gill slits, and postanal tail—well represented but so are secondary characteristics, such as liver diverticulum, hepatic portal system, and the beginning of a ventral heart. Indicative also of the condition in vertebrates is the much thicker dorsal portion of the muscular layer. This is in contrast to the invertebrate phyla in which the muscular layer is about the same thickness around the body cavity. The metameric arrangement of the muscles is suggestive of a similar plan in the embryos of vertebrates.

Just where amphioxus belongs in the evolutionary blueprint of the chordates and the vertebrates is a controversial point. Many authorities place it near the primitive fishes, ostracoderms, but whether it comes before or after these fishes in the evolutionary line is not settled. Because many regard the amphioxus as a highly specialized or degenerate member of the early chordates, it is often assigned to a divergent side branch of some stage intermediate between the early filter-feeding prevertebrates and the vertebrates (Fig. 22-2).

____ Subphylum Vertebrata

The third subphylum of the chordates is the large and eminently successful Vertebrata, the subject of the next five chapters of this book. The subphylum Vertebrata shares the basic chordate characteristics with the other two subphyla, but in addition it has a number of features that the others do not share. The characteristics that give the members of this group the name "Vertebrata" or "Craniata" are a spinal column of vertebrae, which forms the chief skeletal axis of the body, and a braincase, or cranium.

CHARACTERISTICS
1. Chief diagnostic features of chordates—**notochord, dorsal nerve cord, pharyngeal gill slits,** and **postanal tail**—all present at some stage of the life cycle
2. **Integument** basically of two divisions, an outer **epidermis** of stratified epithelium from the ectoderm and an inner **dermis** of connective tissue derived from the mesoderm; many modifications of skin among the various classes, such as glands, scales, feathers, claws, horns, and hair

3. Notochord more or less replaced by the spinal column of vertebrae composed of cartilage or bone or both; distinctive **endoskeleton** consisting of vertebral column with the cranium, visceral arches, limb girdles, and two pairs of jointed appendages

4. **Many muscles** attached to the skeleton to provide for movement

5. Complete digestive system ventral to the spinal column and provided with large digestive glands, liver, and pancreas

6. Circulatory system consisting of the **ventral heart** of two to four chambers; a closed blood vessel system of arteries, veins, and capillaries; blood fluid containing red blood corpuscles with hemoglobin and white corpuscles; paired aortic arches connecting the ventral and dorsal aortas and giving off branches to the gills among the aquatic vertebrates; in the terrestrial types modification of the aortic arch plan into pulmonary and systemic systems

7. Well-developed **coelom** largely filled with the visceral systems

8. Excretory system consisting of **paired kidneys** (mesonephric or metanephric types in adults) provided with ducts to drain the waste to cloaca or anal region

9. Brain typically divided into five vesicles

10. Ten or 12 pairs of **cranial nerves** with both motor and sensory functions usually; a pair of spinal nerves for each primitive myotome; an **autonomic nervous system** in control of involuntary functions of internal organs

11. **Endocrine system** of ductless glands scattered through the body

12. Nearly always separate sexes; each sex containing paired gonads with ducts that discharge their products either into the cloaca or into special openings near the anus

13. **Body plan** consisting typically of **head, trunk,** and **postanal tail; neck** present in some, especially terrestrial forms; two pairs of appendages usually, although entirely absent in some; coelom divided into a pericardial space and a general body cavity; mammals with a thoracic cavity

___ Ammocoete Larva of the Lamprey as a Chordate Archetype

The lampreys (jawless fishes of the class Petromyzontes, discussed in the next chapter) have a freshwater larval stage known as the ammocoete stage. In body form, appearance, life habit, and most anatomical details, the ammocoete larva resembles amphioxus. In fact, the lamprey larva was given the genus name *Ammocoetes* (Gr., *ammos,* sand, + *koite,* bed, referring to the preferred larval habitat) in the nineteenth century when it was erroneously thought to be an adult cephalochordate, closely allied to amphioxus. The ammocoete larva is so different from the adult lamprey that the mistake is understandable; not until it was shown to metamorphose into the adult lamprey was the exact relationship explained. This eel-like larva spends several years buried in the sand and mud of shallow streams,

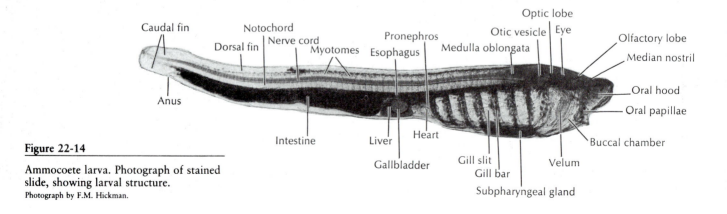

Figure 22-14

Ammocoete larva. Photograph of stained slide, showing larval structure.
Photograph by F.M. Hickman.

until it finally emerges as an adult that may continue to live in fresh water (freshwater lampreys) or else may migrate to the sea (marine lampreys).

The lamprey larva has a long, slender body with an oral hood surrounding the mouth much like amphioxus (Fig. 22-14). The ammocoete feeds like amphioxus, drawing water by ciliary action into the pharynx and pumping it out through gill slits. In the floor of the pharynx is an endostyle, as in amphioxus, that produces a food-ensnaring mucus that is passed directly to the intestine. The arrangement of body muscle into myotomes, the presence of a notochord serving as the chief skeletal axis, and the plan of the circulatory system all closely resemble these features in amphioxus.

The ammocoete does have several characteristics lacking in amiphioxus that foreshadow the vertebrate body plan. These include a two-chambered heart (atrium and ventricle), two median eyes each consisting of a simple lens and receptor cells, a three-part brain (forebrain, midbrain, hindbrain), a thyroid gland, and a pituitary gland. The kidney is pronephric (p. 730) and conforms to the basic vertebrate plan, whereas the solenocyte flame-cell kidney of amphioxus is altogether different. Instead of the numerous gill slits of amphioxus, there are only seven pairs of gill pouches and slits in ammocoetes (there are six pairs in shark embryos). The ammocoete also has a true liver replacing the hepatic cecum of amphioxus, a gallbladder, and pancreatic tissue (but no distinct pancreas gland).

Thus, the ammocoete larva clearly bears many vertebrate hallmarks and approaches the supposed blueprint of the ancestral chordate. Yet the ammocoete and amphioxus have much in common and share many true homologies, strengthening the conclusion that the protochordates and vertebrates share a common ancestry.

____ Summary

The vertebrates, backboned members of the animal kingdom, are characterized as a group by their comparatively large size, high degree of motility, and distinctive body plan, which embodies several distinguishing features that have led to the eminent evolutionary success of the group. Most important of these are the living endoskeleton that allows continuous growth and provides a sturdy framework for efficient muscle attachment and action; paired limbs; a pharynx perforated with gill slits (lost or greatly modified in higher vertebrates) with vastly increased respiratory efficiency; and advanced nervous and sensory systems with clear separation of the brain, which is enclosed within a protective, bony cranium, and the spinal cord, which is enclosed within a flexible vertebral column.

The vertebrates comprise one subphylum of the phylum Chordata, named for the rodlike notochord that appears at some stage in the life cycle of every chordate. Two other chordate subphyla lack a vertebral column and well-developed head. They are the Urochordata (tunicates), most of which are sessile as adults, but all of which have a free-swimming larval stage; and the Cephalochordata (lancelets), fishlike forms that include among their members the famous amphioxus. Amphioxus was once believed to be an ancestor of the vertebrates but it is now considered a specialized side branch of chordate evolution. All the chordates share four distinctive hallmarks that set them apart from all other phyla: a notochord, a dorsal tubular nerve cord, pharyngeal gill slits, and a postanal tail.

Sea squirts (ascidians) in an intertidal community.
Photograph by C.P. Hickman, Jr.

The chordates are believed to have descended from echinoderm-like ancestors, probably in the Precambrian era, but the true origin of the chordates is not yet, and may never be, known with certainty. Taken as a whole, the chordates have a greater fundamental unity of organ systems and body plan than have many of the invertebrate phyla.

Selected references

Barrington, E.J.W. 1965. The biology of Hemichordata and Protochordata. San Francisco, W.H. Freeman & Co. Publishers. *A synthesis of recent work on these deuterostomes most closely related to vertebrates. Discusses the possible homologies between the endostyle and the vertebrate thyroid gland.*

Barrington, E.J.W., and R.P.S. Jeffries (eds.). 1975. Protochordates. Symp. Zool. Soc. London, No. 36. New York, Academic Press, Inc. *Contributed chapters on aspects of amphioxus biology and on chordate evolution.*

Berrill, N.J. 1955. The origin of vertebrates. New York, Oxford University Press. *The author stresses the tunicates as the basic stock from which other protochordates and vertebrates arose. He believes that such a sessile filter feeder was really the most primitive animal and was not a mere degenerate side branch of chordate evolution.*

Cloney, R.A. 1982. Ascidian larvae and the events of metamorphosis. Amer. Zool. 22:817-826.

Garstang, W. 1928. The morphology of the Tunicata, and its bearings on the phylogeny of the Chordata. Quar. J. Micr. Sci. 72:51.

Halstead, L.B. 1968. The pattern of vertebrate evolution. San Francisco, W.H. Freeman & Co. Publishers. *In this thoughtful interpretation of fossil evidence, the author considers physiological and ecological aspects of evolution.*

Halstead, L.B. 1973. The heterostracan fishes. Biol. Rev. 48:279-332. *Thorough review of the earliest known vertebrates.*

Jarvik, E. 1967. Aspects of vertebrate phylogeny. In T. Ørvig (ed.). Nobel Symposium 4. Stockholm, Almqvist & Wiksell.

Jarvik, E. 1980. Basic structure and evolution of vertebrates, 2 vols. New York, Academic Press, Inc. *Advanced reference work worth perusing if only to see the superb illustrations and scholarly paleontological work that has emerged from the "Stockholm school" founded 60 years ago by E. Stensiö.*

Jeffries, R.P.S. 1975. Fossil evidence concerning the origin of the chordates. Symp. Zool. Soc. Lond. 36:253-318. *Closely argued view that the chordates are derived from a peculiar group of echinoderms, which the author places in a new subphylum, the Calcichordata, allied to the Chordata.*

Løvtrup, S. 1977. The phylogeny of vertebrata. New York, John Wiley & Sons, Inc. *Controversial and personal view of vertebrate evolution, but a rich source of information.*

Romer, A.S. 1966. Vertebrate paleontology, ed. 3. Chicago, University of Chicago Press. *An authoritative work by a distinguished paleontologist.*

Romer, A.S., and T.S. Parsons. 1977. The vertebrate body, ed. 5. Philadelphia, W.B. Saunders Co. *Early chapters of this popular comparative anatomy text deal with vertebrate adaptations, ancestry, and body plan.*

Stahl, B.J. 1974. Vertebrate history: problems in evolution. New York, McGraw-Hill Book Co. *Vertebrate evolution and paleontology.*

Wessells, N.K. 1974. Vertebrate structures and functions: readings from *Scientific American*. San Francisco, W.H. Freeman & Co. Publishers. *An anthology of* Scientific American *articles with excellent introductions by N.K. Wessells.*

Young, J.Z. 1981. The life of vertebrates, ed. 3. New York, Oxford University Press. *A classic.*

C H A P T E R   2 3

T H E   F I S H E S

Phylum Chordata

Classes Myxini, Cephalaspidomorphi, Chondrichthyes,

and Osteichthyes

Anterior end of a flounder, *Scophthalmus aquosus*, known commonly as the "windowpane." Flounders
begin life as conventional symmetrical and upright larvae (Fig. 36-1, p. 864), but during
a remarkable transformation early in life, one eye migrates across the head to join the
other eye. From then on they lie and swim on the blind side, which usually becomes
colorless. These changes, together with the loss of the swim bladder
and the presence of cryptic coloration on the eyed side, fit them
for their life role as effective, well-camouflaged,
bottom-dwelling predators.

Fishes are the undisputed masters of the aquatic environment. Because they live in a habitat that is basically alien to humans, we have not always found it easy to appreciate the incredible success of these vertebrates. Plato considered fishes "senseless beings . . . which have received the most remote habitations as a punishment for their extreme ignorance." And average North Americans today are probably unaware of and uninformed about fishes unless they happen to be fishermen or tropical fish enthusiasts.

Nevertheless, the world's fishes have enjoyed an adaptive radiation easily as spectacular as that of all the land vertebrates, with the possible exception of the mammals (the latter having succeeded in the air and in the sea as well as on land). Their numerous structural adaptations have produced a great variety of forms ranging from gracefully streamlined trout to grotesque creatures that dwell in the blackness of the ocean's abyssal depths. Considered either in numbers of species (more than 21,000 valid named species) or in numbers of individuals (countless billions), they easily outnumber the four terrestrial vertebrate classes combined.

Although fishes are the oldest vertebrate group, there is not the slightest evidence that, like their amphibian and reptile successors, they are declining from a period of earlier glory; certain groups of ancient fishes have become extinct but have been replaced by successful modern fishes. There are indeed more bony fishes today than ever before, and no other group threatens their domination of the seas.

Their success can be attributed to perfect adaptation to their dense medium. A trout or pike can hang motionless in the water at any depth, varying its neutral buoyancy by adding or removing gas from the swim bladder, or it can dart forward or at angles, using its fins as brakes and tilting rudders. Fish have excellent olfactory and visual senses and a unique lateral line system, which with its exquisite sensitivity to water currents and vibrations provides a "distance touch" in water. Their gills are the most effective respiratory devices in the animal kingdom for extracting oxygen from water. With highly developed organs of salt and water exchange, bony fishes are excellent osmotic regulators, capable of fine-tuning their body fluid composition in their chosen freshwater or seawater environment. Fishes have evolved complex behavioral mechanisms for dealing with emergencies, and many have evolved elaborate reproductive behavior concerned with courtship, nest building, and care of the young. These are only a few examples of many such adaptations evident in this varied phylogenetic assemblage, which includes four of the eight vertebrate classes.

ANCESTRY AND RELATIONSHIPS OF MAJOR GROUPS OF FISHES

Theories of chordate and vertebrate origins were described in the preceding chapter. The fishes, like all other vertebrates, take their origin from an unknown common ancestor that may have arisen from a free-swimming larval form of an ancient ascidian or ascidian-like stock. During the Cambrian period, or perhaps even in the Precambrian, the earliest fishlike vertebrates branched into the jawless agnathans and the jawed gnathostomes (Fig. 23-1). All subsequent vertebrates descended from one or the other of these two important stems.

The agnathans include such extinct groups as the heterostracans, cephalaspids, and anaspids (commonly and collectively referred to as ostracoderms [Fig. 23-1]), and the living hagfishes (Myxini) and lampreys (Cephalaspidomorphi).

The evidence points to an affinity between the anaspids and the living lampreys, but the heritage of the hagfishes is unknown. It has long been recognized that hagfishes and lampreys only superficially resemble each other. There are numerous anatomical and physiological contrasts, as well as important differences in their mode of life and life cycles. This suggests that the hagfishes and lampreys have been phylogenetically independent for a very long time and should be considered as belonging to entirely separate lineages, as ichthyologists now regard them. Lampreys appear to be more closely related to the fossil ostracoderms than are the hagfishes.

All the rest of the fishes are gnathostomes that have descended from one or more early jawed ancestors. The placoderms have often been suggested as the early ancestors, but the fossil evidence is so fragmentary that it is impossible to pick out ancestral groups with certainty. Whatever the early lines of descent, ichthyologists now recognize several natural groups of living jawed fishes, which are depicted in Fig. 23-1.

The sharks, skates, and rays comprise one natural, compact group, the subclass Elasmobranchii of the class Chondrichthyes. These animals lost the heavy armor of the early placoderms and adopted cartilage instead of bone for the skeleton (thought to be a secondary degeneration), an active and predatory habit, and a sharklike body form that has undergone only minor changes over the ages. The elasmobranchs flourished during the Devonian and Carboniferous periods but declined dangerously close to extinction in the Permian period. They staged a recovery in the early Mesozoic era and radiated into the modest but thoroughly successful assemblage of modern sharks.

Sharing a remote relationship to the elasmobranchs are the bizarre chimaeras of the subclass Holocephali. They appeared in the Jurassic period of the Mesozoic, apparently as an offshoot of some now extinct elasmobranch stock. These peculiar yet strangely appealing fishes have many internal elasmobranch structures and consequently have been included with the latter in the class Chondrichthyes (cartilaginous fishes).

The bony fishes (class Osteichthyes) are the dominant fishes today. This diverse assemblage offers perplexing classification problems. We can recognize three great stems of descent: first are the actinopterygians, or **ray-finned fishes,** which radiated into the modern bony fishes; second are the crossopterygians, the **lobe-finned fishes,** from which the amphibians are descended; and third are the dipneusts, or **lungfishes.** Ichthyologists formerly classified the last two of these three groups together as Choanichthyes ("funnel-fish") in the belief that they shared internal nostrils, that is, funnel-shaped nostrils that open into the mouth cavity in the style of higher vertebrates. But more thorough studies of fossil forms revealed that the internal nostril of the lungfish has a completely different origin; this and other differences in the skeleton have now set the lungfishes apart from the mainline of vertebrate descent.

The distinction of being ancestors of the tetrapods (vertebrates with four legs, that is, all higher vertebrates) probably rests with the crossopterygians, which are represented today by a single living species, the coelacanth *Latimeria chalumnae.* Both the crossopterygians, with one species, and the dipneusts, with six, are relic groups. These seven survivors are meager evidence of stocks that flourished in the Devonian period. Having remained mostly unchanged over the subsequent 400 million years to the present, they are in a sense "living fossils." The lobe-finned fishes and lungfishes are now grouped with the ray-finned fishes under the class Osteichthyes (Teleostomi in some classifications), to produce a highly unbal-

Recently some ichthyologists have argued that the lungfishes should not be placed out of the running as our ancestral forebears. The weight of opinion, however, still favors the crossopterygians as the tetrapod ancestors. Such disagreements are an expected outcome of a sketchy fossil record that readily lends itself to different interpretations, and they illustrate the kind of controversy that has always surrounded fish evolution.

anced living representation: one lobe-fin (the coelacanth), six species (three genera) of lungfishes, and some 20,000 species of ray-finned fishes. The last are divided into three superorders as shown in Fig. 23-1. The evolution of these groups is discussed later in this chapter.

One further point of evolutionary importance must be mentioned. The great weight of paleontological opinion now favors a marine origin for the vertebrates. But at some later time, probably in the Silurian or Lower Devonian period, most of the major groups of fishes penetrated into estuaries and then into freshwater rivers. This invasion was of momentous importance to subsequent vertebrate evolution. It compelled the development of physiological mechanisms to maintain osmotic and ionic balance in the highly dilute freshwater environment. These Devonian invaders established a body fluid concentration (about one-third that of seawater) and ionic composition that fixed the body fluid pattern for all vertebrates to evolve later, whether aquatic, terrestrial, or aerial. Thus it was that when the early bony fishes (Osteichthyes) and elasmobranchs *returned* to the sea in the Triassic period, they encountered a new osmotic challenge: they were now much more dilute than their surroundings. Rather than sliding back into osmotic equilibrium with seawater, they became osmotic and ionic regulators. In bony fishes and sharks this physiological problem is solved in different ways that are described later. Our interest at this point is that both the marine elasmobranchs and marine bony fishes are descendants of freshwater stocks: they have come full circle by returning to their ancestral home in the sea.

The fishes seem to have been uncertain about where they preferred to live. It is probable that the move back and forth between the sea and freshwater environments took place several times; several marine families independently have given rise to freshwater families, and the reverse has also occurred.

CLASSIFICATION

The following broad classification mostly follows that of Nelson (1984). No one scheme is accepted by even a majority of ichthyologists. When we contemplate the incredible difficulty of ferreting out relationships among some 21,000 living species and a vast number of fossils of varying ages, we can appreciate why fish classification has undergone, and will continue to undergo, continuous change.

Subphylum Vertebrata
Superclass Agnatha (ag′na-tha) (Gr., *a*, not, + *gnathos*, jaw) (Cyclostomata). No jaws; cartilaginous skeleton; ventral fins absent; one or two semicircular canals; notochord persistent.
    Class Myxini (mik-sy′ny) (Gr., *myxa*, slime)—**hagfishes.** Mouth terminal with four pairs of tentacles; buccal funnel absent; nasal sac with duct to pharynx; gill pouches, five to 15 pairs; partially hermaphroditic. Examples: *Myxine, Bdellostoma.*
    Class Cephalaspidomorphi (sef-a-lass′pe-do-morf′e) (Gr., *kephalē*, head, + *aspidos*, shield, + *morphē* form)—**lampreys.** Mouth suctorial with horny teeth; nasal sac not connected to mouth; gill pouches, seven pairs. Examples: *Petromyzon, Lampetra.*
Superclass Gnathostomata (na′tho-sto′ma-ta) (Gr., *gnathos*, jaw, + *stoma*, mouth). Jaws present; usually paired limbs; three pairs of semicircular canals; notochord persistent or replaced by vertebral centra.
    Class Chondrichthyes (kon-drik′thee-eez) (Gr., *chondros*, cartilage, + *ichthys*, fish)—**cartilaginous fishes.** Cartilaginous skeleton; teeth not fused to jaws; no swim bladder; intestine with spiral valve.
        Subclass Elasmobranchii (e-laz′mo-bran′kee-i) (Gr., *elasmos*, metal plate, + *branchia*, gills)—**sharks, skates, rays.** Placoid scales or no scales; five to seven gill arches and gills in separate clefts along pharynx. Examples: *Squalus, Raja.*
        Subclass Holocephali (hol′o-sef′a-li) (Gr., *holos*, entire, + *kephalē*, head)—**chimaeras, or ghostfish.** Gill slits covered with operculum; jaws with tooth

plates; single nasal opening; without scales; accessory clasping organs in male; lateral line an open groove. Examples: *Chimaera, Hydrolagus*.

Class Osteichthyes (os′te-ik′thee-eez) (Gr., *osteon*, bone, + *ichthys*, a fish) (Teleostomi)—**bony fishes.** Body primitively fusiform but variously modified; skeleton mostly ossified; single gill opening on each side covered with operculum; usually swim bladder or lung.

Subclass Crossopterygii (cros-sop-te-rij′ee-i) (Gr., *krossoi*, fringe or tassels, + *pteryx*, fin, wing)—**lobe-finned fishes.** Heavy bodied; paired fins lobed with internal skeleton of basic tetrapod type; premaxillae, maxillae present; scales large with tubercles and heavily overlapped; three-lobed diphycercal tail; skeleton with much cartilage; bony spines hollow; air bladder vestigial; gills hard with teeth; intestine with spiral valve; spiracle present. Example: *Latimeria*.

Subclass Dipneusti (dip-nyu′sti) (Gr., *di*, two, + *pneustikos*, of breathing)—**lungfishes.** All median fins fused to form diphycercal tail; fins lobed or of filaments; scales of cycloid bony type; teeth of grinding plates; no premaxillae or maxillae; air bladder of single or paired lobes and specialized for breathing; intestine with spiral valve; spiracle absent. Examples: *Neoceratodus, Protopterus, Lepidosiren*.

Subclass Actinopterygii (ak′ti-nop-te-rij′ee-i) (Gr., *aktis*, ray, + *pteryx*, fin, wing)—**ray-finned fishes.** Paired fins supported by dermal rays and without basal lobed portions; nasal sacs open only to outside. Examples: *Salmo, Perca*.

JAWLESS FISHES—SUPERCLASS AGNATHA

The living members of the Agnatha are represented by some 60 species almost equally divided between two classes: Myxini (hagfishes) and Cephalaspidomorphi (lampreys) (Fig. 23-2). Members of both groups lack jaws, internal ossification, scales, and paired fins, and both share porelike gill openings and an eel-like body form. At the same time there are so many important differences, some of which are indicated in the following list, that they have been assigned to separate vertebrate classes.

CHARACTERISTICS
1. Body slender, eel-like, rounded, with soft skin containing mucous glands but no scales
2. Median fins with cartilaginous fin rays, but no paired appendages
3. Fibrous and cartilaginous skeleton; notochord persistent
4. Suckerlike oral disc with well-developed teeth in lampreys; mouth with two rows of eversible teeth in hagfishes
5. Heart with one auricle and one ventricle; aortic arches in gill region; blood with erythrocytes and leukocytes
6. Seven pairs of gills in lampreys; five to 15 pairs of gills in hagfishes
7. Mesonephric kidney in lampreys; pronephric kidney anteriorly and mesonephric kidney posteriorly in hagfishes
8. Dorsal nerve cord with differentiated brain; eight to 10 pairs of cranial nerves
9. Digestive system without stomach; intestine with spiral fold in lampreys; spiral fold absent in hagfishes
10. Sense organs of taste, smell, hearing; eyes moderately developed in lampreys but highly degenerate in hagfishes; one pair of semicircular canals (hagfishes) or two pairs (lampreys)
11. External fertilization; gonad single without duct; sexes separate and long larval stage (ammocoete) in lampreys; hermaphroditic and direct development with no larval stage in hagfishes

Figure 23-1

Family tree of the fishes, showing their evolution through geological time. Widened areas in the lines of descent indicate periods of adaptive radiation and the relative success of each group. The lungfishes, for example, flourished in the Devonian period, but declined and are today represented by only three surviving genera. The sharks and rays radiated during the Carboniferous period and at that time were rulers of the sea (their successful contemporaries, the early chondrosteans, were freshwater fishes). The sharks came dangerously close to extinction during the Permian period but staged a recovery in the Mesozoic era and are a secure group today. Johnny-come-latelies in fish evolution are the spectacularly successful modern bony fishes, or teleosts, which make up 90% of all living fishes.

Early amphibians

Crossopterygii

Dipneusti

Actinopterygii

Osteichthyes

Placoderms

Chondrichthyes

Gnathostomata

Ostracoderms

Common chordate ancestor

Vertebrata

Agnatha

Cambrian   Ordovician   Silurian   Devonian   Carboniferous

PALEOZOIC

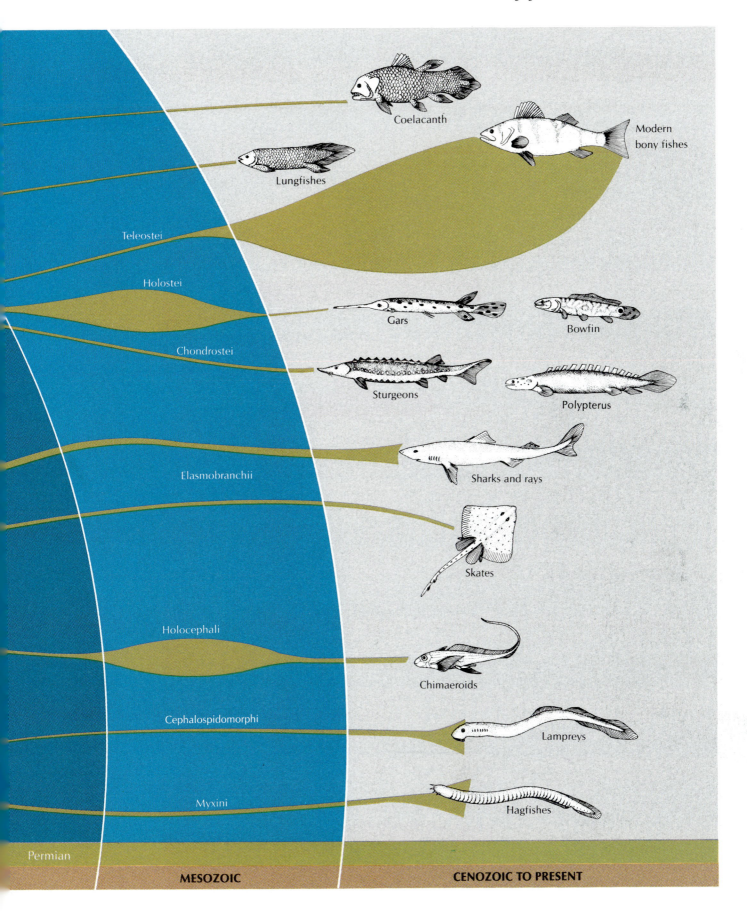

Coelacanth

Modern bony fishes

Lungfishes

Teleostei

Holostei

Gars

Bowfin

Chondrostei

Sturgeons

Polypterus

Elasmobranchii

Sharks and rays

Skates

Holocephali

Chimaeroids

Cephalospidomorphi

Lampreys

Myxini

Hagfishes

Permian

MESOZOIC

CENOZOIC TO PRESENT

Figure 23-2

Comparison of hagfish (class Myxini) and lamprey (class Cephalaspidomorphi), representatives of the superclass Agnatha.

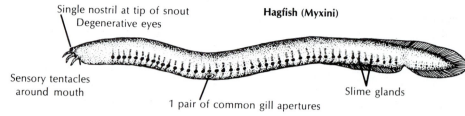

Single nostril at tip of snout
Degenerative eyes
Hagfish (Myxini)
Sensory tentacles around mouth
1 pair of common gill apertures
Slime glands

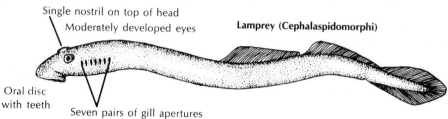

Single nostril on top of head
Moderately developed eyes
Lamprey (Cephalaspidomorphi)
Oral disc with teeth
Seven pairs of gill apertures

Hagfishes—Class Myxini

The hagfishes are an entirely marine group that feeds on dead or dying fishes, annelids, molluscs, and crustaceans. Thus, they are neither parasitic like lampreys nor predaceous, but are scavengers. There are only 32 described species of hagfishes, of which the best known in North America are the Atlantic hagfish *Myxine glutinosa* (Gr., *myxa,* slime) (Fig. 23-2) and the Pacific hagfish *Bdellostoma stouti* (Gr., *bdella,* leech, + *stoma,* mouth).

Hagfishes have long been of interest to comparative physiologists. Unlike any other vertebrate, they are isosmotic to seawater like marine invertebrates. They are the only vertebrates to have both pronephric and mesonephric kidneys in the adult, although only the latter forms urine. They have no fewer than four sets of hearts positioned at different places in the body to boost blood flow through their low-pressure circulatory system.

Despite other unique anatomical and physiological features of interest to biologists, hagfishes probably have fewer human admirers than any other group of fishes. The sports fisherman who catches one discovers that the hook is so deeply swallowed that retrieval is impossible. To cap the sportsman's misfortune, the animal secretes enormous quantities of slimy mucus from large and small mucous glands located all over the body and from special slime glands positioned along its sides (Fig. 23-2). A single hagfish is said to be capable of converting a bucket of water into a mass of whitish jelly in minutes. Their habit of biting into and entering the bodies of gill-netted fish has not endeared them to commercial fishermen either. Entering through the anus or gills, hagfishes set about eating out the contents of the body, leaving behind a loose sack of skin and bones. But as fishing methods have passed from the use of drift nets and set lines to large and efficient otter trawls, hagfishes have ceased to be an important pest.

The yolk-filled egg of the hagfish may be 14 to 25 mm in diameter and is enclosed in a horny shell. There is no larval stage, and growth is direct. They are hermaphroditic but can produce only one kind of gamete at a time; a single individual may produce sperm in one season and eggs the next.

Lampreys—Class Cephalaspidomorphi

All the lampreys of the Northern Hemisphere belong to the family Petromyzontidae (Gr., *petros,* stone, + *myzon,* sucking). The group name refers to the lamprey's habit of grasping a stone with its mouth to hold position in a current. The destructive marine lamprey *Petromyzon marinus* is found on both sides of the Atlantic Ocean (in America and Europe) and may attain a length of 1 m. *Lampetra* (L., *lambo,* to lick or lap up) also has a wide distribution in North America and Eurasia and ranges from 15 to 60 cm long. There are 19 species of lampreys in North America. About half of these belong to the nonparasitic brook type; the others are parasitic. The nonparasitic species have probably descended from the parasitic forms by degeneration of the teeth, alimentary canal, and so on. The genus *Ichthyomyzon* (Gr., *ichthyos,* fish, + *myzon,* sucking), which includes three parasitic and three nonparasitic species, is restricted to eastern North America. On the west coast of North America the chief marine form is *Lampetra tridentatus.*

Figure 23-3

Brook lampreys *Lampetra lamottei* clearing pebbles for a spawning nest in a small creek.
Courtesy J.W. Jordan, Jr.

All lampreys ascend freshwater rivers or streams to breed. The marine forms are anadromous (Gr., *ana,* up, + *dramein,* to run); that is, they leave the sea where they spend their adult lives to run up rivers and streams to spawn. In North America all lampreys spawn in the spring, but some European lampreys are autumn breeders. The males begin nest building and are joined later by females. Using their oral discs to lift stones and pebbles and vigorous body vibrations to sweep away light debris, they form an oval depression (Fig. 23-3). At spawning, with the female attached to a rock to maintain her position over the nest, the male attaches to the dorsal side of her head. He curls the posterior part of his body tightly about that of the female so that their cloacal openings are together. As the eggs are shed into the nest, they are fertilized by the male. Only small numbers of eggs are shed at each mating, and the process may be repeated numerous times over a period of 1 to 2 days. The sticky eggs adhere to pebbles in the nest and quickly become covered with sand. The adults die a short time after spawning.

The eggs hatch in about 2 weeks, releasing small larvae (ammocoete), which are so unlike their parents that early biologists were deceived into giving them distinct scientific names (such as *Ammocoetes branchioles*). The larva bears a remarkable resemblance to amphioxus and possesses the basic chordate characters in such simplified and easily visualized form that it has been considered a chordate archetype (p. 514). After absorbing the remainder of its yolk supply, the young ammocoete, now about 7 mm long, leaves the nest gravel and drifts downstream to burrow in some suitable sandy, low-current area. Here it remains for an extraordinarily long time, 3 to 7 years, feeding on minute organisms and debris in the mud. During this time the ammocoete grows and then in the fall rapidly metamorphoses into an adult. This change involves the development of larger eyes, the replacement of the hood by the oral disc with teeth, a shifting of the nostril to the top of the head, and the development of a rounder but shorter body.

Parasitic lampreys either migrate to the sea, if marine, or remain in fresh water, where they attach themselves by their suckerlike mouth to fish and, with their sharp horny teeth, rasp away the flesh and suck out the blood (Fig. 23-4). In order to promote the flow of blood, the lamprey injects an anticoagulant into the wound. When the lamprey is gorged, it releases its hold but leaves the fish with a large, gaping wound that may prove fatal. The parasitic freshwater adults live a year or more before spawning and then die; the anadromous forms live longer.

The nonparasitic lampreys do not feed after emerging as adults, for their alimentary canal degenerates to a nonfunctional strand of tissue. Within a few months they also spawn and die.

Figure 23-4

A, Sea lamprey *Petromyzon marinus* attached to the head of a sucker, on which it is feeding. **B,** Head of sea lamprey attached to the glass side of an aquarium, showing the horny teeth surrounding the rasping tongue in the center.

Courtesy L.L. Marking, National Fishery Research Laboratory, La Crosse, Wis.

A

B

The invasion of the Great Lakes by the landlocked sea lamprey *Petromyzon marinus* in this century has had a devastating effect on the fisheries there. No lampreys were present in the Great Lakes west of Niagara Falls until the Welland Ship Canal was built in 1829. Even then nearly 100 years elapsed before sea lampreys were first seen in Lake Erie. After that the spread was rapid, and the sea lamprey was causing extraordinary damage in all the Great Lakes by the late 1940s. No fish species was immune from attack, but the lampreys preferred lake trout, and this multimillion dollar fishing industry was brought to total collapse in the early 1950s. Lampreys then turned to rainbow trout, whitefish, turbot, yellow perch, and lake herring, all important commercial species. These stocks were decimated in turn. The lampreys then began attacking chubs and suckers. Coincident with the decline in attacked species, the sea lampreys themselves began to decline after reaching a peak abundance in 1951 in Lakes Huron and Michigan and in 1961 in Lake Superior. The fall has been attributed both to depletion of food and to the effectiveness of control measures (mainly chemical larvicides in selected spawning streams). Lake trout, aided by a restocking program begun in 1967, are now recovering. Wounding rates are low in Lake Michigan but still high in Lake Huron. Fishery organizations are experimenting with the introduction into the Great Lakes of species that appear to be more resistant to lamprey attack, such as kokanee salmon (landlocked Pacific sockeye salmon).

CARTILAGINOUS FISHES—CLASS CHONDRICHTHYES

There are more than 625 living species in the class Chondrichthyes, an ancient, compact, and highly developed group. Although a much smaller and less diverse assemblage than the bony fishes, their impressive combination of well-developed sense organs, powerful jaws and swimming musculature, and predaceous habits ensures them a secure and lasting niche in the aquatic community. One of their distinctive features is their cartilaginous skeleton. Although there is some calcification here and there, bone is entirely absent throughout the class—a curious evolutionary feature, since the Chondrichthyes are derived from ancestors having well-developed bone.

With the exception of whales, sharks are the largest living vertebrates. The larger sharks may reach 15 m in length. The dogfish sharks so widely studied in zoological laboratories rarely exceed 1 m.

Sharks, Skates, and Rays—Subclass Elasmobranchii

The elasmobranchs are carnivores that track their prey using their lateral line system and large olfactory organs. Their vision is not well developed.

Fertilization is internal (a curiously "modern" feature in an ancient group), and many sharks have evolved elaborate reproductive modes; some are live-bearers with gestation periods up to 2 years—the longest of any vertebrate.

According to Nelson (1984), there are five living orders of elasmobranchs. All of the more notorious sharks belong to the order Lamniformes, including the requiem sharks, hammerhead sharks (Fig. 23-5, *A*), whale sharks, mackerel sharks, nurse sharks, and sand sharks (Fig. 23-5, *B*). The order Squaliformes includes the dogfish shark, familiar to generations of comparative anatomy students. The skates and several groups of rays (sawfish rays, electric rays, stingrays, eagle rays, manta rays, and devil rays) belong to the order Rajiformes.

Much has been written about the propensities of sharks to eat humans, both by those exaggerating their ferocious nature and by those seeking to write them off as harmless. It is true, as the latter group of writers argues, that sharks are by nature timid and cautious. But it also is a fact that certain of them are dangerous to humans and deserve respect. There are numerous authenticated cases of shark attacks by *Carcharodon* (Gr., *karcharos*, sharp, + *odous*, tooth), the great white shark (commonly reaching 6 m and often larger); the mako shark *Isurus* (Gr., *is*, equal, + *ouros*, tail); the tiger shark *Galeocerdo* (Gr., *galeos*, shark, + *kerdō*, fox); and the hammerhead shark *Sphyrna* (Gr., *sphyra*, hammer). More shark casualties have been reported from the tropical and temperate waters of the Australian region than from any other. During World War II there were several reports of mass shark attacks on the victims of ship sinkings in tropical waters.

Outside of North America, sharks and skates are commonly used for food. They make up about 1% of the present market for fish. There is a small market for shark leather, which has greater tensile strength and lasting qualities than mammalian leather.

CHARACTERISTICS
1. **Body fusiform,** with a **heterocercal** caudal fin (Fig. 23-16); paired pectoral and pelvic fins, two dorsal median fins; pelvic fins in male modified for "claspers"; fin rays present
2. **Mouth ventral; two olfactory sacs that do not open into the mouth cavity;** jaws present
3. Skin with **placoid** scales (Fig. 23-8) and **mucous glands;** modified placoid scales for teeth
4. **Endoskeleton entirely cartilaginous;** notochord persistent; vertebrae complete and separate; appendicular, girdle, and visceral skeletons present
5. Digestive system with a J-shaped stomach and intestine with a spiral valve; liver, gallbladder, and pancreas present
6. Circulatory system of several pairs of aortic arches; dorsal and ventral aorta, capillary and venous systems, hepatic portal and renal portal systems; two-chambered heart
7. Respiration by means of five to seven pairs of gills with separate and exposed gill slits; **no operculum** except in chimaeras
8. No swim bladder
9. Brain of two olfactory lobes, two cerebral hemispheres, two optic lobes, a cerebellum, and a medulla oblongata; 10 pairs of cranial nerves; three pairs of semicircular canals
10. Sexes separate; gonads paired; reproductive ducts open into cloaca; oviparous, ovoviviparous, or viviparous; direct development; fertilization internal
11. Kidneys of mesonephros (opisthonephros) type

A

B

Figure 23-5

Sharks of the order Lamniformes (subclass Elasmobranchii). **A,** Hammerhead shark *Sphyrna tudes* may reach a length of 4.5 m. **B,** Sand tiger shark *Carcharias* sp. Large individuals of both species are considered highly dangerous.
Photographs by K. Sandved.

Figure 23-6

Dogfish shark *Squalus acanthias* (subclass Elasmobranchii).

Figure 23-7

Head of sand tiger shark *Carcharias* sp. Note the series of successional teeth; each tooth generation grows toward the jaw margin and is eventually shed.
Photograph by J.L. Rotman.

Figure 23-8

Skin of a shark showing the toothlike tubercles of placoid scales.
Photograph by J.L. Rotman.

Form and function

Although to most people sharks have a sinister appearance and fearsome reputation, they are at the same time among the most gracefully streamlined of all fishes. The body of a shark such as a dogfish shark (Fig. 23-6) is fusiform (spindle shaped). In front of the ventral mouth is a pointed **rostrum;** at the posterior end the vertebral column turns up to form the **heterocercal** tail. The fins consist of the paired **pectoral** and **pelvic** fins supported by appendicular skeletons, two median **dorsal** fins (each with a spine in *Squalus* [L., a kind of sea fish]), and a median **caudal** fin. A median **anal** fin is present in the smooth dogfish (*Mustelus* [L., *mustela,* weasel]). In the male the medial part of the pelvic fin is modified to form a **clasper,** which is used in copulation. The paired **nostrils** (blind pouches) are ventral and anterior to the mouth (Fig. 23-7). The lateral eyes are lidless, and behind each eye is a spiracle (remnant of the first gill slit). Five gill slits are found anterior to each pectoral fin. The tough, leathery skin is covered with **placoid scales** (Figs. 23-8 and 23-17), which are modified anteriorly to form replaceable rows of teeth in both jaws (Fig. 23-7). Placoid scales consist of dentin enclosed by an enamel-like substance, and they very much resemble the teeth of other vertebrates.

Figure 23-9

Internal anatomy of dogfish shark *Squalus acanthias.*

Sharks are well equipped for their predatory life. Their vision is less acute than that of most bony fishes, but this is more than compensated for by a keen sense of smell used to guide them to food. A well-developed **lateral line system** serves as a "distance touch" in water for detecting and locating objects and moving animals (predators, prey, and social partners). It is composed of a canal system extending along the side of the body and over the head. The canal opens at intervals to the surface. Inside are special receptor organs (**neuromasts**) that are extremely sensitive to vibrations and currents in the water. Sharks also can detect and aim attacks at prey buried in the sand by sensing the bioelectric fields that surround all animals.

Internally the cartilaginous skeleton is made up of a **chondrocranium,** which houses the brain and auditory organs and partially surrounds the eyes and olfactory organs; a vertebral column; a visceral skeleton; and an appendicular skeleton. The jaws are suspended from the chondrocranium by ligaments and cartilages. Both the upper and the lower jaws are provided with many sharp, triangular teeth that, when lost, are replaced by other rows of teeth. Teeth serve to grasp the prey, which is usually swallowed whole. The muscles are segmentally arranged and are especially useful in the undulations of swimming.

The mouth cavity opens into the large **pharynx,** which contains openings to the separate gill slits and spiracles. A short, wide esophagus runs to the J-shaped stomach. A **liver** and **pancreas** open into the short, straight **intestine,** which contains the unique **spiral valve** that delays the passage of food and increases the absorptive surface (Fig. 23-9). Attached to the short rectum is the **rectal gland,** which secretes a colorless fluid containing a high concentration of sodium chloride. It assists the kidney in regulating the salt concentration of the blood. The chambers of the **heart** are arranged in tandem formation (Fig. 23-9), and the circulatory system is basically the same as that of the embryonic vertebrate and of the ammocoete.

The **mesonephric kidneys** are two long, slender organs above the coelom;

Figure 23-10

Egg case of a skate ("mermaid's purse"). The horny case protects the developing young. Skate egg cases have coiling tendrils on the corners that entangle seaweeds.

Photograph by R. Harbo.

they are drained by the **wolffian ducts,** which open into a single urogenital sinus at the **cloaca.** The wolffian ducts also carry the sperm from the testes of the male, which uses a clasper to deposit the sperm in the female oviduct. The müllerian duct, or oviduct (paired), carries the eggs from the **ovary** and coelom and is modified into a **uterus** in which a primitive placenta may attach the embryo shark until it is born. Such a relationship is actually **viviparous reproduction;** other species simply retain the developing egg in the uterus without attachment to the mother's wall (**ovoviviparous reproduction**). Still others lay large, yolky eggs immediately after fertilization (**oviparous reproduction**). Some sharks and rays deposit their fertilized eggs in a horny capsule called the "mermaid's purse," which often is attached by tendrils to seaweed (Fig. 23-10). Later the young shark emerges from this "cradle."

The embryonic brain is the basic tripartite vertebrate brain: forebrain, midbrain, and hindbrain. These three parts develop into five subdivisions or regions—telencephalon, diencephalon, mesencephalon, metencephalon, and myelencephalon—each with certain functions. There are 10 pairs of cranial nerves that are distributed largely to the head regions. Surrounding the spinal cord are the neural arches of the vertebrae. Along the spinal cord a pair of spinal nerves, with united dorsal and ventral roots, is distributed to each body segment.

Elasmobranchs have developed an interesting solution to the physiological problem of living in a hyperosmotic medium. Like the ancestors of the bony fishes, those of sharks and their kin lived in fresh water, only returning to the sea in the Triassic period (about 230 million years ago) after becoming thoroughly adapted to freshwater existence. Their body fluid salt concentration was then much lower than the surrounding seawater; to prevent water from being drawn out of the body osmotically, the elasmobranchs have retained nitrogenous wastes, especially urea and trimethylamine oxide, in the blood. These solutes, combined with the blood salts, raised the blood solute concentration to slightly exceed that of seawater, eliminating an osmotic inequality between their bodies and the surrounding seawater.

Figure 23-11

Yellow stingray *Urolophus jamaicensis* (subclass Elasmobranchii) of the Caribbean.

Photograph by L.S. Roberts.

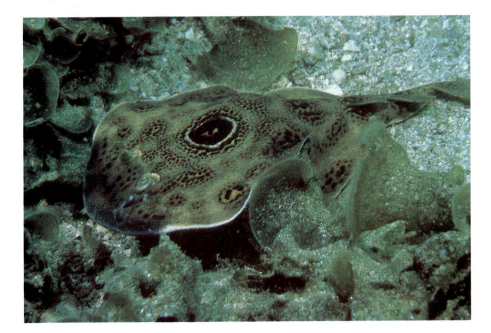

Figure 23-12

Bullseye electric ray *Diplobatis ommata* (subclass Elasmobranchii). The two electric organs of muscular origin lie anteriorly on either side of the body. Electric rays are sluggish swimmers.
Photograph by D.W. Gotshall.

The skates and rays (Fig. 23-11) are specialized for bottom dwelling. In these the pectoral fins are greatly enlarged and are used like wings in swimming. The gill openings are on the underside of the head, but the large spiracles are on top. Water for breathing is taken in through these spiracles to prevent clogging the gills, for the mouth is often buried in sand. Their teeth are adapted for crushing their prey: molluscs, crustaceans, and an occasional small fish. Two members of this group—the stingrays and the electric rays—are of special interest. In the stingrays the caudal and dorsal fins have disappeared and the tail is slender and whiplike. The tail is armed with one or more saw-edged spines, which can inflict dangerous wounds. Such wounds may heal slowly and leave complications. Electric rays (Fig. 23-12) have smooth, naked skins and have certain dorsal muscles modified into powerful electric organs, which can give severe shocks and stun their prey. Stingrays also have electric organs in the tail.

Chimaeras—Subclass Holocephali

The members of the small subclass Holocephali, distinguished by such suggestive names as ratfish (Fig. 23-13), rabbitfish, spookfish, and ghostfish, are remnants of an aberrant line that diverged from the elasmobranchs at least 300 million years ago (Carboniferous or Devonian period). Fossil chimaeras (ky-meer′uz) first occurred in the Jurassic period, reached their zenith in the Cretaceous and early Tertiary periods (120 million to 50 million years ago), and have declined ever since.

Today there are only about 25 species extant. Anatomically they present an odd mixture of sharklike and bony fish–like features. Instead of a toothed mouth, their jaws bear large flat plates. The upper jaw is completely fused to the cranium, a most unusual development in fishes. Their food is seaweed, molluscs, echinoderms, crustaceans, and fishes—a surprisingly mixed diet for such a specialized grinding dentition. Chimaeras are not commercial species and are seldom caught. Despite their grotesque shape, they are beautifully colored with a pearly iridescence.

Figure 23-13

Ratfish *Hydrolagus colliei*, a chimaera of the Pacific coast of North America (subclass Holocephali).
Photograph by R. Harbo.

s *Catastomus occidentalis*
...formes, superorder Teleostei). These freshwater fishes are aptly named for their habit of grubbing along the bottom, drawing in food through their protrusible jaws with thick, fleshy lips.
Photograph by D.W. Gotshall.

BONY FISHES—CLASS OSTEICHTHYES (TELEOSTOMI)

In no other major animal group do we see better examples of adaptive radiation than among the bony fishes. Their adaptations have fitted them for every aquatic habitat except the most completely inhospitable. Body form alone is indicative of this diversity. Some have fusiform, streamlined bodies and other adaptations for reducing friction. Predaceous, pelagic fish have trim, elongate bodies, powerful tail fins, and other mechanical advantages for swift pursuit. Sluggish bottom-feeding forms have flattened bodies for movement and concealment on the ocean floor. The elongate body of the eel is an adaptation for wriggling through mud and reeds and into holes and crevices. Some, such as pipefishes, are so whiplike that they are easily mistaken for filaments of marine algae waving in the current. Many other grotesque body forms are obviously cryptic or mimetic adaptations for concealment from predators or as predators. Such few examples cannot begin to express the amazing array of physiological and anatomical specializations for defense and offense, food gathering, navigation, and reproduction in the diverse aquatic habitats to which bony fishes have adapted themselves. More of these adaptations are described in the following pages.

CHARACTERISTICS

1. **Skeleton more or less bony**, representing the primitive skeleton; vertebrae numerous; notochord may persist in part; **tail usually homocercal**
2. Skin with mucous glands and with embedded dermal scales of three types: **ganoid, cycloid, or ctenoid**; some without scales; no placoid scales
3. Fins both median and paired, with **fin rays of cartilage or bone**
4. **Mouth terminal** with many teeth (some toothless); jaws present; olfactory sacs paired and may or may not open into mouth
5. Respiration by gills supported by bony gill arches and covered by a **common operculum**
6. **Swim bladder** often present with or without duct connected to pharynx
7. Circulation consisting of a two-chambered heart, arterial and venous systems, and characteristically four pairs of aortic arches; blood containing nucleated red cells

8. Nervous system of a brain with small olfactory lobes and cerebrum; large optic lobes and cerebellum; 10 pairs of cranial nerves; three pairs of semicircular canals
9. Sexes separate (sex reversal in some), gonads paired; fertilization usually external; larval forms may differ greatly from adults

Bony fishes vary greatly in size. Some species are less than 2 cm long; other forms may exceed 3 m in length. The swordfish is one of the largest and may attain a length of 4 m. Most fishes, however, fall between 2 and 30 cm in length.

Figure 23-15

Yellow bullhead *Ictalurus natalis* (family Siluriformes, superorder Teleostei). The characteristic barbels are used to detect food.

Photograph by J.H. Gerard.

CLASSIFICATION

Class Osteichthyes—bony fishes. Three subclasses, 69 orders.

Subclass Crossopterygii—lobe-finned fishes. Three extinct orders, one living order (Coelacanthimorpha) containing one species, *Latimeria chalumnae*.

Subclass Dipneusti—lungfishes. Six extinct orders, two living orders containing three genera: *Neoceratodus*, *Lepidosiren*, and *Protopterus*.

Subclass Actinopterygii—ray-finned fishes. Three superorders and 59 orders.

Superorder Chondrostei (kon-dros′tee-i) (Gr., *chondros*, cartilage, + *osteon*, bone)—**primitive ray-finned fishes.** Ten extinct orders; two living orders containing the bichir (*Polypterus*), sturgeons, and paddlefish.

Superorder Holostei (ho-los′tee-i) (Gr., *holos*, entire, + *osteon*, bone)—**intermediate ray-finned fishes.** Four extinct orders; two living orders containing the bowfin (*Amia*) and gars (*Lepidosteus*).

Superorder Teleostei (tel′e-os′tee-i) (Gr., *teleos*, perfect, + *osteon*, bone)—**climax bony fishes.** Body covered with thin scales without bony layer (cycloid or ctenoid) or scaleless; dermal and chondral parts of skull closely united; caudal fin mostly homocercal; mouth terminal; notochord a mere vestige; swim bladder mainly a hydrostatic organ and usually not opened to the esophagus; endoskeleton mostly bony. According to Nelson (1984), there are 10 extinct orders and 31 living orders. The latter are comprised of 415 families, and approximately 20,000 living species, representing 96% of all living fishes. Seven of the larger orders are as follows:

Anguilliformes—21 families; freshwater eels, moray eels, conger eels, snipe eels.

Salmoniformes—23 families; pikes, whitefish, salmon, trout, smelts, deep-sea luminescent fishes.

Cypriniformes—25 families; suckers (Fig. 23-14), minnows, carp, electric eels.

Siluriformes—30 families; catfish (Fig. 23-15).

Atheriniformes—15 families; flying fish, medakas, killifish, live-bearers.

Scorpaeniformes—20 families; rockfish, searobins, greenlings, sculpins, poachers, scorpionfish (Fig. 23-31).

Perciformes—146 families; barracudas, mullets, perch, darters, sunfishes, grunters, croakers, Moorish idols, damsel fish, viviparous perch, wrasses, parrot fish, trumpeters, sand perch, stargazers, blennies, wolffish, eel pouts, mackerels, tunas, swordfish, and others.

___ Origin, Evolution, and Diversity

The Osteichthyes are divided into three distinct groups: Crossopterygii (lobe-finned fishes), Dipneusti (lungfishes), and Actinopterygii (ray-finned fishes). What are their origins? As pointed out previously, it seems safest to steer a middle course through current paleontological debate and assign equal rank to all three groups in the class Osteichthyes. In other words, it is impossible to decide which one of these three groups, if any, might have served as ancestral stock for the other two. It is apparent from fossil evidence that all three groups were distinct in the Devonian period, some 400 million years ago. They are believed to have descended from an acanthodian of the Silurian period (Fig. 22-6, p. 507).

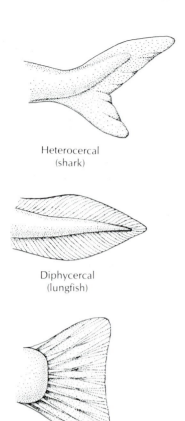

Figure 23-16

Types of caudal fins among fishes.

__Lobe-Finned Fishes—Subclass Crossopterygii

Crossopterygii has had the least spectacular evolutionary radiation of all the Osteichthyes. It is by far the most important in an evolutionary sense because the tetrapods arose from one or more of its ancient members. The crossopterygians had nostrils (choanae) that opened into the mouth, lungs as well as gills, and paired **lobed fins.** They first appeared in Devonian times, a capricious period of alternating droughts and floods when their lungs would have been a decided asset, if not absolutely essential, for their survival. They used their strong lobed fins as four legs to scuttle from one disappearing swamp to another that offered more promise for a continuing aquatic existence.

The crossopterygians are divided broadly into two groups. The **rhipidistians** appeared in the Devonian period, flourished in the late Paleozoic era, and then disappeared. This is the stock from which the amphibians have descended (Fig. 23-1). Among the primitive characteristics of the rhipidistians were the fusiform shape, two dorsal fins, and a **heterocercal** tail (Fig. 23-16). The paired fins bore sharp resemblances to a tetrapod limb, for they consisted of a basal arrangement of median or axial bones, with other bones radiating from these median ones. Some of the proximal bones seem to correspond to the three chief bones of the tetrapod limb. The scales of these primitive fish were of the **cosmoid** type, a thick complex scale of dentinlike cosmine, enamel, and vascular pulp cavities. This type of scale is not found in modern fishes but has been replaced by the bony **cycloid** type (Fig. 23-17).

The other group of crossopterygians was the **coelacanths.** These also arose in the Devonian period, radiated somewhat, and reached their evolutionary peak in the Mesozoic era. At the end of the Mesozoic era they nearly disappeared but left one remarkable surviving species, the living coelacanth *Latimeria chalumnae* (named for M. Courtenay-Latimer, South African museum director) (Fig. 23-18). Since the last coelacanths were believed to have become extinct 70 million years ago, the astonishment of the scientific world can be imagined when the remains of

Figure 23-17

Types of fish scales. Placoid scales are small, conical toothlike structures characteristic of the Chondrichthyes. Diamond-shaped ganoid scales, present in primitive bony fishes such as the gar, are composed of layers of silvery enamel (ganoin) on the upper surface and bone on the lower. Advanced bony fishes have either cycloid or ctenoid scales. These are thin and flexible and are arranged in overlapping rows.

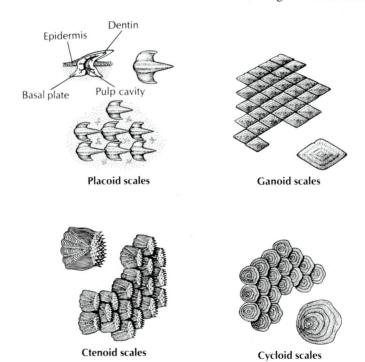

a coelacanth were found on a dredge off the coast of South Africa in 1938. An intensive search was begun in the Comoro Islands area near Madagascar where, it was learned, native Comoran fishermen occasionally caught them with hand lines at great depths. Numerous specimens have now been caught, many in excellent condition, although none has been kept alive beyond a few hours after capture.

The "modern" marine coelacanth is a descendant of the Devonian freshwater stock. The tail is of the **diphycercal** type (Fig. 23-16) but possesses a small lobe between the upper and lower caudal lobes, producing a three-pronged structure (Fig. 23-18). Coelacanths also show some degenerative features, such as more cartilaginous parts and a swim bladder that was either calcified or else persisted as a mere vestige. They also lack the internal nostril so characteristic of crossopterygians, but this is probably a secondary loss after the adoption of a deep-sea existence; obviously neither nostrils nor functional lungs have any relevance for such a life habit.

Lungfishes—Subclass Dipneusti

The lungfishes are another relic group of fishes, represented today by only three genera (Fig. 23-19). These resemble the lobe-finned fishes in having lobe-shaped paired fins and lungs. However, all lungfishes, extinct or living, differ from the crossopterygians in several significant skeletal features, including the totally different origin of the internal nostrils.

Of the three surviving genera of lungfishes, the least specialized is *Neoceratodus* (Gr., *neos,* new, + *keratos,* horn, + *odes,* form), the living Australian lungfish, which may attain a length of 1.5 m. This lungfish is able to survive in stagnant, oxygen-poor water by coming to the surface and gulping air into its single lung, but it cannot live out of water. The South American lungfish *Lepidosiren* (L., *lepidus,* pretty, + *siren,* mythical mermaid) and the African lungfish *Protopterus* (Gr., *prōtos,* first, + *pteron,* wing) are evolutionary side branches of the Dipneusti, and they can live out of water for long periods of time. *Protopterus* lives in African streams and rivers that run completely dry during the dry season, with their mud beds baked hard by the hot tropical sun. The fish burrows down at the approach of the dry season and secretes a copious slime that is mixed with mud to form a hard cocoon in which it estivates until the rains return.

Ray-Finned Fishes—Subclass Actinopterygii

The huge subclass Actinopterygii contains all the familiar bony fishes. The fossil record reveals that the group had its beginnings in Devonian freshwater lakes and streams. The earliest actinopterygians were small fishes with large eyes and extended mouths. Their tails were **heterocercal** (Fig. 23-16). They had a single dorsal fin and a single anal fin; paired fins were represented by the anterior pectoral fins and the posterior pelvic fins. Their skeletons were largely bone. Their trunks and tails were encased in an armor of heavy, rhombic **ganoid scales** (Fig. 23-17). Most of these early fishes had functional lungs, as did all the Devonian fishes, but they lacked internal nostrils. All had gills (five pairs or fewer) and spiracles.

These early actinopterygians belonged to the order Palaeonisciformes (pay'lee-o-nis-sif-for'meez). One common genus in the fossil record was *Cheirolepis* (Gr., *cheir,* hand, + *lepis,* scale), a generalized type that had some resem-

Figure 23-18

Coelacanth *Latimeria chalumnae*. This surviving marine relic of the crossopterygians that flourished some 350 million years ago has fleshy-based ("lobed") fins with which its ancestors used to pull themselves across land from pond to pond.
Courtesy Vancouver Public Aquarium, British Columbia.

Neoceratodus (Australia)
Direct descendant of ancient lungfish
Cannot withstand complete drying up of water

Protopterus (Africa)
Side branch of lungfish evolution
Can burrow in mud when water dries up

Lepidosiren (South America)
Side branch of lungfish evoluton
Can burrow in mud when water dries up

Figure 23-19

The three surviving lungfishes of the subclass Dipneusti. The approximate range of each genus is shown on map insets.

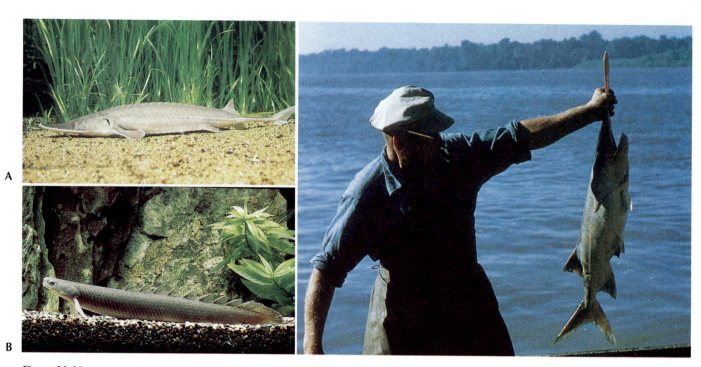

A

B

C

Figure 23-20

Chondrostean fishes. **A,** Shovelnose sturgeon *Scaphirhynchus platorhyncus* of the Mississippi basin. **B,** Bichir *Polypterus bichir* of the African Congo. It is a nocturnal predator. **C,** Paddlefish *Polyodon spatula* of the Mississippi River reaches a length of 2 m and a weight of 90 kg. It is sought by commercial fishermen, but catches are now very low because of river pollution.

A and B, Courtesy John G. Shedd Aquarium/Patrice Ceisel; C, photograph by J.H. Gerard.

blance to certain acanthodians (Fig. 22-6, p. 507). The palaeoniscids were distinctly different from their freshwater contemporaries, the crossopterygians and the lungfishes, with which they shared the Devonian swamps and rivers. The palaeoniscids were rare in the Devonian period, became a more secure group in the Carboniferous and Permian periods, but nearly disappeared in the Triassic period when their descendants returned to the sea.

In their evolution the actinopterygians have passed through three stages. The most primitive group includes the Chondrostei, represented today by the freshwater and marine sturgeons, paddlefishes, and the bichir *Polypterus* (Gr., *poly,* many, + *pteros,* winged) of African rivers (Fig. 23-20). *Polypterus* is an interesting relic with a lunglike swim bladder and many other primitive characteristics; it resembles an ancient palaeoniscid more than any other living descendant. There is no satisfactory explanation for the survival to the present of certain fishes such as this one and the coelacanth *Latimeria* when all of their kin perished millions of years ago.

A second, less primitive group of ray-finned fishes is the Holostei. There were several lines of descent within this group, which flourished during the Triassic and Jurassic periods. They declined toward the end of the Mesozoic era as their successors, the teleosts, crowded them out. There are only two surviving genera, the bowfin *Amia* (Gr., name of perchlike fish) of shallow, weedy waters of the Great Lakes and Mississippi Valley, and the gars *Lepisosteus* (Gr., *lepidos,* scale, + *osteon,* bone) of eastern North America (Fig. 23-21). The Holostei is now considered an artificial grouping because the gars appear to be more closely related to the teleosts (described below) than to the bowfin.

The third group is the Teleostei, the modern bony fishes (Fig. 23-22). Diversity appeared early in teleost evolution, foreshadowing the truly incredible variety of body forms among teleosts today. The skeleton of primitive fishes was largely ossified, but this condition regressed to a partly cartilaginous state among many of the Chondrostei and Holostei. Teleosts, however, have an internal skeleton almost completely ossified like the primitive members. The dermal investing bones

A

B

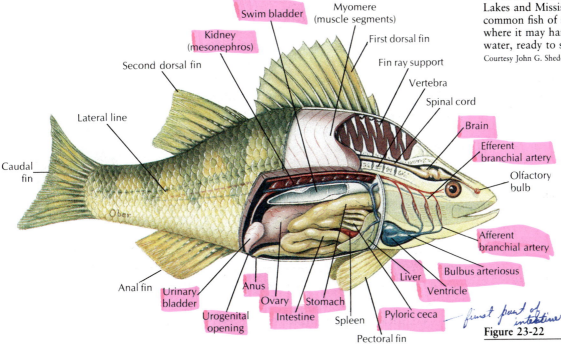

Figure 23-21

Holostean fishes. **A,** Bowfin *Amia calva*.
B, Longnose gar *Lepisosteus osseus*. Both
the bowfin and the gars live in the Great
Lakes and Mississippi basin. The gar is a
common fish of slow-moving streams,
where it may hang motionless in the
water, ready to snatch a passing fish.
Courtesy John G. Shedd Aquarium/Patrice Ceisel.

Swim bladder
Kidney (mesonephros)
Myomere (muscle segments)
First dorsal fin
Second dorsal fin
Fin ray support
Vertebra
Lateral line
Spinal cord
Brain
Efferent branchial artery
Caudal fin
Olfactory bulb
Ober
Afferent branchial artery
Liver
Bulbus arteriosus
Anal fin
Urinary bladder
Anus
Ventricle
Ovary
Stomach
Urogenital opening
Intestine
Spleen
Pyloric ceca
Pectoral fin

first part of intestine

Figure 23-22

Internal anatomy of the yellow perch
Perca flavescens (superorder Teleostei), a
freshwater teleost.

of the skull (dermatocranium) and the neurocranium around the brain and sense
organs form a closer union among the teleosts than they did in the primitive bony
fishes. Other evolutionary changes among the teleosts were the shifting of the
pelvic fins forward to the head and thoracic region, the transformation of the
lungs of primitive forms into swim bladders (Fig. 23-22) with hydrostatic functions and without ducts, the changing of the heterocercal tail of primitive fishes
and of the intermediate superorders into a homocercal form (Fig. 23-16), and the
development of the thin **cycloid** and **ctenoid scales** (Fig. 23-17) from the thick
ganoid type of early fishes. Among other changes were the loss of the spiracles and
the development of stout spines in the fins, especially in the pectoral, dorsal, and
anal fins.

Figure 23-23

Trunk musculature of a teleost fish. Segmental myotomes are arranged as bands, each shaped like a **W** lying on its side. The musculature has been dissected away in two places to show internal anterior and posterior deflection of myotomes.

STRUCTURAL AND FUNCTIONAL ADAPTATIONS OF FISHES
Locomotion in Water

To the human eye, some fishes appear capable of swimming at extremely high speeds. But our judgment is unconsciously tempered by our own experience that water is a highly resistant medium to move through. Most fishes, such as a trout or a minnow, can swim maximally about 10 body lengths per second, obviously an impressive performance by human standards. Yet when these speeds are translated into kilometers per hour it means that a 30 cm (1 foot) trout can swim only about 10.4 km (6.5 miles) per hour. The larger the fish, the faster it can swim. A 60 cm salmon can sprint 22.5 km (14 miles) per hour, and a 1.2 m barracuda, the fastest fish measured, is capable of 43 km (27 miles) per hour. Swordfish and marlin are thought to be capable of incredible bursts of speed approaching, or even exceeding, 110 km per hour (68 mph). No fish can swim at such record speeds for more than brief moments; cruising speeds are much lower.

The propulsive mechanism of a fish is its trunk and tail musculature. The axial, locomotory musculature is composed of zigzag muscle bands (myotomes) that on the surface take the shape of a **W** lying on its side (Fig. 23-23). Internally the muscle bands are deflected forward and backward in a complex fashion that apparently promotes efficiency of movement. The muscles are bound to broad sheets of tough connective tissue, which in turn tie to the highly flexible vertebral column.

Understanding how fishes swim can be approached by studying the motion of a very flexible fish such as an eel (Fig. 23-24). The movement is serpentine, not unlike that of a snake, with waves of contraction moving backward along the body by alternate contraction of the myotomes on either side. The anterior end of the body bends less than the posterior end, so that each undulation increases in amplitude as it travels along the body. While undulations move backward, the bending of the body pushes laterally against the water, producing a **reactive force** that is directed forward, but at an angle. It can be analyzed as having two components: **thrust,** which is used to overcome drag and propels the fish forward, and **lateral force,** which tends to make the fish's head "yaw," or deviate from the course in the same direction as the tail. This side-to-side head movement is very obvious in a swimming eel or shark, but many fishes have a large, rigid head with enough surface resistance to minimize yaw.

The movement of an eel is reasonably efficient at low speed, but its body shape generates too much frictional drag for rapid swimming. Fishes that swim rapidly, such as trout, are less flexible and limit the body undulations mostly to the caudal region (Fig. 23-24). Muscle force generated in the large anterior muscle mass is transferred through tendons to the relatively nonmuscular caudal peduncle and tail where thrust is generated. This form of swimming reaches its highest development in the tunas, whose bodies do not flex at all. Virtually all the thrust is derived from powerful beats of the tail fin. Many fast oceanic fishes such as marlin, swordfish, amberjacks, and wahoo have swept-back tail fins shaped much like a sickle. Such fins are the aquatic counterpart of the high–aspect ratio wings of the swiftest birds (p. 619).

Swimming is possible only because the density and noncompressibility of water offer great purchase for forward thrust. As a medium for locomotion, water offers another advantage: since the density of water is only slightly less than that of living tissue, most aquatic animals are almost perfectly supported and need expend little energy overcoming the force of gravity. Consequently, swimming is actually the most economical form of animal locomotion. For example, the energy cost per kilogram of body weight of traveling 1 km is 0.39 kcal for a salmon (swimming), 1.45 for a gull (flying), and 5.43 for a ground squirrel (walking). However, the low energy cost of swimming by fish is by no means fully understood. Relatively simple calculations show that a fish moves through water with only about one-tenth the drag of a rigid model of the fish's body.

Aquatic mammals and fishes create virtually no turbulence, a feat that humans with twentieth-century ingenuity are a long way from matching. The secret lies in the way aquatic animals bend their bodies and fins (or flukes) to swim and in the textural properties of the body surface. For example, the slimy surface of a fish reduces water friction by at least 66% as compared with the same surface from which the slime has been removed. Understanding the energetics of swimming remains part of the unfinished business of biology.

Neutral Buoyancy and the Swim Bladder

All fishes are slightly heavier than water because their skeletons and other tissues contain heavy elements that are present only in trace amounts in natural waters. To keep from sinking, sharks must always keep moving forward in the water. The asymmetrical (heterocercal) tail of a shark provides the necessary tail lift as it sweeps to and fro in the water, and the broad head and flat pectoral fins (Fig. 23-6) act as angled planes to provide head lift. Sharks are also aided in buoyancy by having very large livers containing a special fatty hydrocarbon called **squalene** that has a density of only 0.86. The liver thus acts like a large sack of buoyant oil that helps to compensate for the shark's heavy body.

By far the most efficient flotation device is a gas-filled space. The **swim bladder** serves this purpose in the bony fishes. It arose from the paired lungs of the primitive Devonian bony fishes. Lungs were probably a ubiquitous feature of the Devonian freshwater bony fishes when, as we have seen, the alternating wet and dry climate would have made such an accessory respiratory structure essential for life. The primitive lung may have been similar to the lungs found in the existing *Polypterus* (Fig. 23-20, *B*), the chondrostean fish of tropical Africa that so resembles the palaeoniscid ancestors of modern body fishes (Fig. 23-25). Swim bladders are present in most pelagic bony fishes but are absent in tunas, most abyssal fishes, and most bottom dwellers, such as flounders and sculpins.

By adjusting the volume of gas in the swim bladder, a fish can achieve neutral buoyancy and remain suspended indefinitely at any depth with no mus-

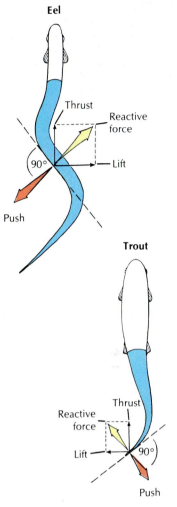

Figure 23-24

Movements of swimming fishes, showing the forces developed by an eel-shaped and a spindle-shaped fish.

From McFarland, W.N., and others. 1979. Vertebrate life. New York, Macmillan, Inc.

Figure 23-25

Evolution of lung and swim bladder. Most primitive fishes were provided with lungs, adaptations for the oxygen-depleted environments that existed during the evolution of the Osteichthyes. The lung originated as a diverticulum of the foregut. From this early, generalized lung two lines of evolution occurred. One led to the swim bladder of the modern teleost fish. Various transitional stages show that the swim bladder shifted to a dorsal position above the esophagus, becoming a buoyancy organ. The duct has been lost in most teleosts, and the swim bladder, with specialized gas secretion and reabsorption areas, is served by an independent blood supply. The second line of evolution has led to the tetrapod lung found in land forms. There has been extensive internal folding but no radical change in lung position.

cular effort. There are severe technical problems, however. If the fish descends to a greater depth, the swim bladder gas is compressed so that the fish becomes heavier and tends to sink. Gas must be added to the bladder to establish a new equilibrium buoyancy. If the fish swims up, the gas in the bladder expands, making the fish lighter. Unless gas is removed, the fish will rise with ever-increasing speed while the bladder continues to expand, until the fish pops helplessly out of the water. (This is a very real hazard for divers in helmeted diving suits, who must carefully adjust the air pressure to prevent overinflation or underinflation of their suits.)

Fishes adjust gas volume in the swim bladder in two ways. The less specialized fishes (trout, for example) have a **pneumatic duct** that connects the swim bladder to the esophagus (Fig. 23-25); these forms must come to the surface and gulp air to charge the bladder and obviously are restricted to relatively shallow depths. More specialized teleosts have lost the pneumatic duct (upper diagram in Fig. 23-25). In these fishes, the gas must originate in the blood and be secreted into the swim bladder. Gas exchange depends on two highly specialized areas: a **gas gland** that secretes gas into the bladder and a **resorptive area,** or "oval," that can remove gas from the bladder. The gas gland contains a remarkable network of blood capillaries, called the **rete mirabile** ("marvelous net") that acts to transfer gas, especially oxygen, from the blood to the swim bladder.

The amazing effectiveness of this device is exemplified by a fish living at a depth of 2400 m (8000 feet). To keep the bladder inflated at that depth, the gas inside (mostly oxygen, but also variable amounts of nitrogen, carbon dioxide, carbon monoxide, and argon) must have a pressure exceeding 240 atmospheres, much greater than the pressure in a fully charged steel gas cylinder. Yet the oxygen pressure in the fish's blood cannot exceed 0.2 atmosphere—equal to the oxygen pressure at the sea surface.

Physiologists who were at first baffled by the secretion mechanism now understand how it operates. In brief, the gas gland secretes lactic acid, which

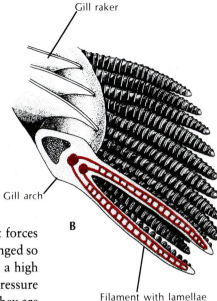

enters the blood, causing a localized high acidity in the rete mirabile that forces hemoglobin to release its load of oxygen. The capillaries in the rete are arranged so that the released oxygen accumulates in the rete, eventually reaching such a high pressure that the oxygen diffuses into the swim bladder. The final gas pressure attained in the swim bladder depends on the length of the rete capillaries; they are relatively short in fishes living near the surface but extremely long in deep-sea fishes.

___ Respiration

Fish gills are composed of thin filaments covered with a thin epidermal membrane that is folded repeatedly into platelike **lamellae** (Fig. 23-26). These are richly supplied with blood vessels. The gills are located inside the pharyngeal cavity and are covered with a movable flap, the **operculum.** This arrangement provides excellent protection to the delicate gill filaments, streamlines the body, and makes possible a pumping system for moving water through the mouth, across the gills, and out the operculum. Instead of opercular flaps as in bony fishes, the elasmobranchs have a series of **gill slits** out of which the water flows. In both elasmobranchs and bony fishes the branchial mechanism is arranged to pump water continuously and smoothly over the gills, even though to an observer it appears that fish breathing is pulsatile. The flow of water is opposite to the direction of blood flow (countercurrent flow), the best arrangement for extracting the greatest possible amount of oxygen from the water. Some bony fishes can remove as much as 85% of the oxygen from the water passing over their gills. Very active fishes, such as herring and mackerel, can obtain sufficient water for their high oxygen demands only by continuously swimming forward to force water into the open mouth and across the gills. This is called ram ventilation. Such fish will be asphyxiated if placed in an aquarium that restricts free swimming movements, even though the water is saturated with oxygen.

A surprising number of fishes can live out of water for varying lengths of time by breathing air. Several devices are employed by different fishes. We have already described the lungs of the lungfishes, *Polypterus,* and the extinct crossopterygians. Freshwater eels often make overland excursions during rainy weather, using the skin as a major respiratory surface. The bowfin, *Amia* (Fig. 23-21, *A*), has both gills and a lunglike swim bladder. At low temperatures it uses only its gills, but as the temperature and the fish's activity increase, it breathes mostly air with its swim bladder. The electric eel has degenerate gills and must supplement gill respiration by gulping air through its vascular mouth cavity. One of the best

Figure 23-26

Gills of fish. Bony, protective flap covering the gills (operculum) has been removed, **A,** to reveal branchial chamber containing the gills. Four gill arches are on each side, each bearing numerous filaments. A portion of gill arch, **B,** shows gill rakers that project forward to strain out food and debris and gill filaments that project to the rear. A single gill filament, **C,** is dissected to show the blood capillaries within the platelike lamellae. Direction of water flow (*large arrows*) is opposite the direction of blood flow (*small arrows*).

air breathers of all is the Indian climbing perch, which spends most of its time on land near the water's edge, breathing air through special air chambers above the much-reduced gills.

___ Osmotic Regulation

Fresh water is an extremely dilute medium with a salt concentration (0.001 to 0.005 gram moles per liter [M]) much below that of the blood of freshwater fishes (0.2 to 0.3 M). Water therefore tends to enter their bodies osmotically, and salt is lost by diffusion outward. Although the scaled and mucus-covered body surface is almost totally impermeable to water, water gain and salt loss do occur across the thin membranes of the gills. Freshwater fishes are **hyperosmotic regulators** that have several defenses against these problems (Fig. 23-27). First, the excess water is pumped out by the **mesonephric** kidney (p. 730), which is capable of forming a very dilute urine. Second, special **salt-absorbing cells** located in the gill epithelium actively move salt ions, principally sodium and chloride, from the water to the blood. This, together with salt present in the fish's food, replaces diffusive salt loss. These mechanisms are so efficient that a freshwater fish devotes only a small part of its total energy expenditure to keeping itself in osmotic balance.

Marine bony fishes are **hypoosmotic regulators** that encounter a completely different set of problems. Having a much lower blood salt concentration (0.3 to 0.4 M) than the seawater around them (about 1 M), they tend to lose water and gain salt. The marine teleost fish quite literally risks drying out, much like a desert mammal deprived of water. Again, marine bony fishes, like their freshwater counterparts, have evolved an appropriate set of defenses (Fig. 23-27). To compensate for water loss, the marine teleost drinks seawater. Although this behavior obviously brings needed water into the body, it is unfortunately accompanied by a great deal of unneeded salt. Unwanted salt is disposed of in two ways: (1) the major sea salt ions (sodium, chloride, and potassium) are carried by the blood to the gills where they are secreted outward by special **salt-secretory cells;** and (2) the remaining ions, mostly the divalent ions (magnesium, sulfate, and calcium), are left in the intestine and voided with the feces. However, a small but significant fraction of these residual divalent salts in the intestine, some 10% to 40% of the total, penetrates the intestinal mucosa and enters the bloodstream. These ions are excreted by the kidney. Unlike the freshwater fish kidney, which forms its urine by the usual filtration-resorption sequence typical of most vertebrate kidneys (pp. 732 to 734), the marine fish's kidney excretes divalent ions by tubular secretion. Since very little if any filtrate is formed, the glomeruli have lost their importance and disappeared altogether in some marine teleosts. The pipefishes and the goosefish, shown in Fig. 23-35, are examples of "aglomerular" marine fishes.

Most bony fishes are restricted to either a freshwater or a seawater habitat. However, some 10% of all teleosts can pass back and forth with ease between both habitats. Examples of these **euryhaline fishes** (Gr., *eurys*, broad, + *hals*, salt), which must have highly adaptable osmoregulatory mechanisms, are salmon, steelhead trout, many flounders and sculpins, killifish, sticklebacks, and eels. Fishes that can tolerate only very narrow ranges of salt concentration—most freshwater and marine fishes—are said to be **stenohaline** (Gr., *stenos*, narrow, + *hals*, salt). Fishes that migrate from the sea to spawn in fresh water—such as salmon, shad, and marine lampreys—are **anadromous** (Gr., *ana*, up, + *dramein*, to run). Freshwater forms that swim to the sea to spawn—such as the freshwater eel *Anguilla*—are **catadromous** (Gr., *kata*, down, + *dramein*, to run).

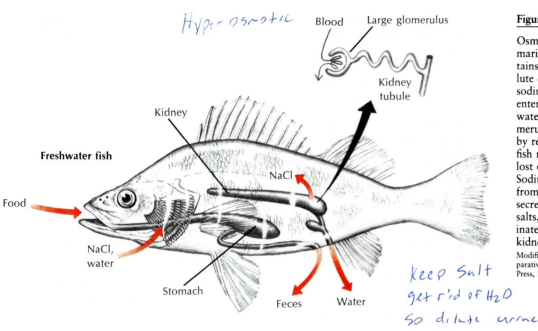

Hyper-osmotic (handwritten)

Blood   Large glomerulus

Kidney tubule

Kidney

Freshwater fish

Food

NaCl

NaCl, water

Stomach

Feces   Water

Keep salt (handwritten)
get rid of H₂O (handwritten)
so dilute urine (handwritten)

Figure 23-27

Osmotic regulation in freshwater and marine bony fishes. Freshwater fish maintains osmotic and ionic balance in its dilute environment by actively absorbing sodium chloride across gills (some salt enters with food). To flush out excess water that constantly enters body, glomerular kidney produces a dilute urine by reabsorbing sodium chloride. Marine fish must drink seawater to replace water lost osmotically to its salty environment. Sodium chloride and water are absorbed from stomach. Excess sodium chloride is secreted outward by gills. Divalent sea salts, mostly magnesium sulfate, are eliminated with feces and secreted by tubular kidney.

Modified from Webster, D., and M. Webster. 1974. Comparative vertebrate morphology. New York, Academic Press, Inc.

Glomerulus reduced or absent

Blood

Hyposmotic (handwritten)

Kidney tubule

Kidney

Marine fish

Food, seawater

NaCl, water

MgSO₄

NaCl, water

Stomach

MgSO₄, water, feces   MgSO₄, urea, little water

get rid of salt (handwritten)
keep H₂O (handwritten)

____ Feeding Behavior

For any fish, feeding is one of the main concerns of day-to-day living. Although many a luckless angler would swear otherwise, the fact is that a fish devotes more time and energy to eating, or searching for food to eat, than to anything else. Throughout the long evolution of fishes, there has been unrelenting selective pressure for those adaptations that enable a fish to come out on the better end of the eat-or-be-eaten contest. Certainly the most far-reaching single event was the evolution of jaws. Their possessors were freed from a mud-grubbing or parasitic existence and could adopt a predatory mode of life. Improved means of capturing larger prey demanded stronger muscles, more agile movement, better balance, and improved special senses. More than any other aspect of its life habit, feeding behavior shapes the fish.

Figure 23-28

Wolf eel, *Anarrhichthys ocellatus,* feeding on a sea cucumber (*Parastichopus* sp.) it has captured and pulled to the opening of its den.
Photograph by D.W. Gotshall.

Most fishes are **carnivores** that prey on a myriad of animal foods from zooplankton and insect larvae to large vertebrates. Some deep-sea fishes are capable of eating victims nearly twice their own size—an adaptation for life in a world where meals are necessarily infrequent. Most advanced ray-finned fishes cannot masticate their food as we can because doing so would block the current of water across the gills. Some, however, such as the wolf eel (Fig. 23-28), have molarlike teeth in the jaws for crushing their prey, which may include hard-bodied crustaceans. Others that do grind their food use powerful pharyngeal teeth in the throat. Most carnivores almost invariably swallow their prey whole, using sharp-pointed teeth in the jaws and on the roof of the mouth to seize their prey. The incompressibility of water makes the task even easier for many large-mouthed predators. When the mouth is opened, a negative pressure is created that sweeps the victim inside.

A second group of fishes are **herbivores** that eat flowering plants, algae, and grasses. Although the plant eaters are relatively few in number, they are crucial intermediates in the food chain, especially in freshwater rivers, lakes, and ponds that contain very little plankton.

Figure 23-29

School of plankton-feeding glassy sweepers, *Pempheris* sp.
Photograph by J.L. Rotman.

The **filter feeders** that crop the abundant microorganisms of the sea form a third and diverse group of fishes ranging from fish larvae to basking sharks. However, the most characteristic group of plankton feeders are the herringlike fishes (menhaden, herring, anchovies, capelin, pilchards, and others) that are for the most part **pelagic** (open-sea dwellers) and travel in large schools (Fig. 23-29). Both phytoplankton and the smaller zooplankton are strained from the water with a sievelike device, the gill rakers (Fig. 23-26). Because plankton feeders are the most abundant of all fishes, they are important food for numerous larger but less abundant carnivores. Many freshwater fishes, especially members of the large cichlid family, also depend on plankton for food.

A fourth group of fishes are **omnivores** that feed on both plant and animal food. Finally there are the **scavengers** that feed on organic debris (detritus) and the **parasites** that suck the body fluids of other fishes.

Digestion in most fishes follows the vertebrate plan. Except in several fishes

Figure 23-30

Fishes of a Red Sea coral reef, illustrating the great variety of species that inhabit the shallow waters of the tropical reef. Photograph by J. and C. Church.

that lack stomachs altogether, the food proceeds from stomach to tubular intestine, which tends to be short in carnivores but may be extremely long and coiled in herbivorous forms. In the carp, for example, the intestine may be nine times the body length, an adaptation for the lengthy digestion required for plant carbohydrates. In carnivores, some protein digestion may be initiated in the acid medium of the stomach, but the principal function of the stomach is to store the often large and infrequent meals while awaiting their reception by the intestine.

Digestion and absorption proceed simultaneously in the intestine. A curious feature of ray-finned fishes, especially the teleosts, is the presence of numerous **pyloric ceca** (Fig. 23-22) found in no other vertebrate group. Their primary function appears to be fat absorption, although all classes of enzymes (protein-, carbohydrate-, and fat-splitting) are secreted there. They number from two or three to several hundred in some advanced teleost species.

Coloration and Concealment

Tropical coral reef fishes bear some of the most resplendent hues and strikingly brilliant color patterns in the animal kingdom (Fig. 23-30). Viewed against the coral reef background of invertebrate and plant life that creates a riot of color, the vivid markings and coloration of reef fishes attract relatively little attention. Their coloration is not always for concealment, however, since tropical bony fishes tend toward vivid coloration even in areas of dull and somber backgrounds. Although

Figure 23-31

Spotted scorpionfish *Scorpaena plumieri*. Its color match with the background is almost perfect.
Photograph by L.S. Roberts.

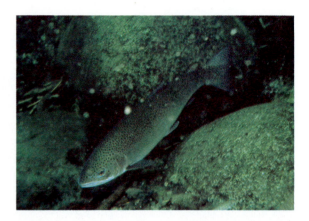

Figure 23-32

Camouflage in the rainbow trout *Salmo gairdnerii*. Note the countershading of dark, disruptive coloration above changing to lighter coloration of underparts.
Photograph by D.W. Gotshall.

A   **B**

Figure 23-33

Camouflage in flatfishes. Many flatfishes match not only the color but also the pattern of their surroundings. **A,** Rock sole *Lepidopsetta bilineata*. **B,** Sand sole *Psettichthys melanostictus*.
Photographs by R. Harbo.

conspicuous in these circumstances, they are protected by alertness and agility or by their poisonous flesh. In this instance the coloration is an advertisement, warning would-be predators to seek their meal elsewhere.

Outside of coral reefs and other shallow-water habitats of the tropical seas, fishes, like most other animals, characteristically bear colors and patterns that serve to conceal them from enemies (Fig. 23-31). Freshwater fishes wear subdued shades of green, brown, or blue above, grading to silver and yellow-white below. This is **obliterative shading.** Seen from above against its normal background of water and stream bottom, the fish becomes almost invisible (Fig. 23-32). Seen from beneath as it might be viewed by an aquatic predator, the pale belly of the fish blends with the water surface and sky above. The obliterative coloration is frequently enhanced by blotches, spots, and bars—conflicting patterns that, like the camouflaged ships of World War II, tend to break up the outline of the body. Some fishes, such as many flatfish species, can change their color to harmonize with the patterns of their background (Fig. 23-33).

Fish colors are chiefly the result of pigment within **chromatophores** in the

Figure 23-34

Seahorse is almost indistinguishable from the surrounding dead staghorn coral encrusted with algae and other marine life. Photograph by J. and C. Church.

Figure 23-35

Goosefish *Lophius piscatorius* awaits its meal. Above its head swings a modified dorsal fin spine ending in a fleshy tentacle that contracts and expands in a convincing wormlike manner. When a fish approaches the alluring bait, the huge mouth opens suddenly, creating a strong current that sweeps the prey inside. In a split second all is over.
Photograph by J.L. Rotman.

dermal layer of the skin. The pigments are red, orange, yellow, and black and can be blended to produce other shades. Pigment dispersion within the branched chromatophores is controlled by the autonomic nervous system. Fish also bear **guanine** in their skin, a purine compound that gives many fishes their silvery appearance.

Another form of concealment is protective resemblance, or **mimicry.** Pipefishes, for example, are of the shape and color of the seaweeds among which they live. Pipefishes even sway slowly like seaweeds in a gentle current. There are many other examples of protective body form that appear to turn their owners into fragmented seaweed, or a leaf, or floating debris, or a weed-covered rock on the bottom (Fig. 23-34). The goosefish, or angler, with its obliterative coloration and numerous fringes and branched appendages of skin, not only becomes nearly invisible when bedded down on the ocean floor but sways a tempting bait above its huge mouth to attract prey (Fig. 23-35).

Electric Fishes

The ability to produce strong electric shocks is confined to two groups of vertebrates: elasmobranchs (for example, electric ray) and teleosts (for example, electric eel, electric catfish). The best known and most studied is the famous electric eel, *Electrophorus* (Gr., *ēlektron,* amber, something bright, + *pherō,* to bear), of the Amazon and Orinoco river systems of South America (Fig. 23-36). This large, sluggish creature contains powerful electric organs that in 1 to 2.5 m adults can

Figure 23-36

Electric eel *Electrophorus electricus.* This animal, the most electrically powerful of freshwater electric fishes, produces brief bursts of pulses that may exceed 500 volts.
Courtesy John G. Shedd Aquarium/Patrice Ceisel.

Figure 23-37

Electric ray *Torpedo* with electric organs uncovered from above. Organs are built up of disclike, multinucleated cells called electrocytes, which are embedded in a jel-lylike substance. Each vertical column in an electric ray is made up of a stack of electrocytes piled on top of each other. Nerve fibers run to electrocytes, and blood capillaries course through the jelly layer. In addition to defensive and offensive purposes, electric organs may be used for recognition among members of a species when other methods of communication are absent.

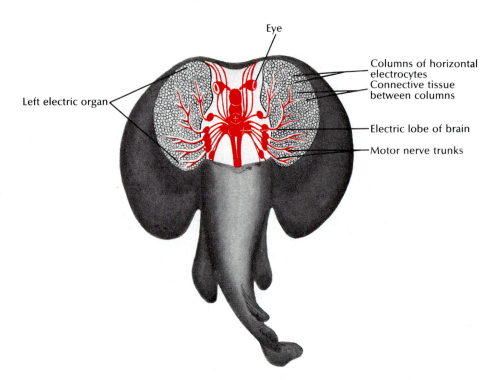

Eye

Columns of horizontal electrocytes
Connective tissue between columns

Left electric organ

Electric lobe of brain

Motor nerve trunks

Not all electric fishes are able to generate powerful shocks. There are hundreds of weakly electric fish species that generate oscillating electrical fields around their bodies for navigation and detection of prey. Many have weakly developed eyes and live in muddy, turbid tropical rivers and streams where vision would be of marginal usefulness. Any nearby object creates a disturbance in the electrical dipolar field, which is detected by numerous special sense organs (mormyromasts) embedded in the skin.

produce paralyzing discharges exceeding 600 volts, quite ample to stun or kill its prey or to discourage potential enemies, including large mammals. People who have accidentally met the electric eel under the latter's own terms report that it is about as pleasant as coming in contact with an uninsulated high-voltage wire. It is not necessary for the eel to actually touch its victims, since the shocks stretch out in an electric field for several meters around the fish. Even small eels less than 30 cm long can discharge pulses exceeding 200 volts.

The source of this impressive performance is the pair of electric organs lying on either side of the vertebral column and extending almost the entire length of the fish. Together they make up about 40% of the body weight. Each organ is composed of longitudinal columns of 6000 to 10,000 thin, waferlike plates (electrocytes) stacked one on another like a long cylinder of coins. There are about 60 such columns in each organ. Each plate, or electrocyte, is a modified muscle cell innervated by a nerve fiber and has very special electric properties. One side of the plate is a nervous layer that will depolarize when stimulated; the opposite side is a nutritive layer that remains inactive. All the nervous sides of the plates face the tail of the animal. When the eel chooses to discharge its organ, motor impulses are sent out to the electric organs from a special neural center in the brain. These impulses travel to the numerous plates in a highly synchronized way so that all of the thousands of plates discharge simultaneously. Each plate develops a potential charge of about 150 millivolts. Because the plates are arranged in series, the individual voltages summate like batteries arranged in series. Thus a high-voltage current flows from the tail to the head of the eel and completes the circuit in the water surrounding the eel. Electric eels must develop high voltages to overcome the high resistance of the fresh water in which they live.

Electric fishes living in the sea, such as the electric ray *Torpedo* (L., benumbing) (Fig. 23-37), live in a low-resistance medium where high voltages are not required. They generate high amperages instead. In *Torpedo* each electric organ contains some 2000 columns made up of about 1000 electrocytes arranged in vertical stacks. With fewer plates per column, the voltage produced is relatively

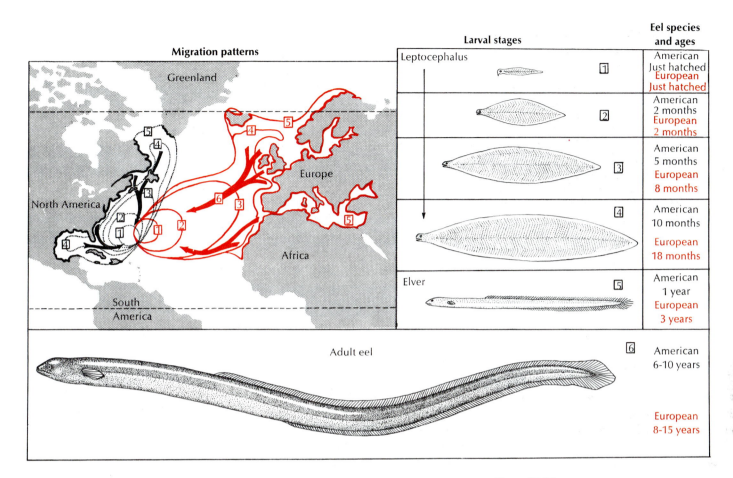

Figure 23-38

Life histories of the European eel *(Anguilla anguilla)* and American eel *(A. rostrata)*. *Red,* Migration patterns of European species. *Black,* Migration patterns of American species. Boxed numbers refer to stages of development. Note that the American eel completes its larval metamorphosis and sea journey in 1 year. It requires nearly 3 years for the European eel to complete its much longer journey.

low (about 50 volts), but the power output may be as much as 6 kilowatts! It is easy to understand why, when seasoned commercial fishermen happen to pick up one of these animals in their trawl, they leave it strictly alone until it is dead and safe to handle.

___ Migration

Eel

For centuries naturalists had been puzzled about the life history of the freshwater eel *Anguilla* (an-gwil'la) (L., eel), a common and commercially important species of coastal streams of the North Atlantic. Each fall, large numbers of eels were seen swimming down the rivers toward the sea, but no adults ever returned. And each spring countless numbers of young eels, called "elvers" (Fig. 23-38), each about the size of a wooden matchstick, appeared in the coastal rivers and began swimming upstream. Beyond the assumption that eels must spawn somewhere at sea, the location of their breeding grounds was totally unknown.

The first clue was provided by two Italian scientists, Grassi and Calandruccio, who in 1896 reported that elvers were not larval eels but rather were relatively advanced juveniles. The true larval eels, the Italians discovered, were tiny, leaf-shaped, completely transparent creatures that bore absolutely no resemblance to an eel. They had been called **leptocephali** (Gr., *leptos,* slender, + *kephalē,* head) by early naturalists, who never suspected their true identity. In 1905 Johann Schmidt, supported by the Danish government, began a systematic study of eel biology that

Figure 23-39

Migrating Pacific sockeye salmon.
Photographs by M. Trim.

he continued until his death in 1933. With the cooperation of captains of commercial vessels plying the Atlantic, thousands of the leptocephali were caught in different areas of the Atlantic with the plankton nets Schmidt supplied them. By noting where in the ocean larvae in different stages of development were captured, Schmidt and his colleagues eventually reconstructed the spawning migrations.

When the adult eels leave the coastal rivers of Europe and North America, they swim steadily and apparently at great depth for 1 to 2 months until they reach the Sargasso Sea, a vast area of warm oceanic water southeast of Bermuda (Fig. 23-38). Here, at depths of 300 m or more, the eels spawn and die. The minute larvae then begin an incredible journey back to the coastal rivers of Europe. Drifting with the Gulf Stream and preyed on constantly by numerous predators, they reach the middle of the Atlantic after 2 years. By the end of the third year they reach the coastal waters of Europe where the leptocephali metamorphose into elvers, with an unmistakable eel-like body form (Fig. 23-38). Here the males and females part company; the males remain in the brackish waters of coastal rivers and estuaries while the females continue up the rivers, often traveling hundreds of miles upstream. After 8 to 15 years of growth, the females, now 1 m or more long, return to the sea to join the smaller males; both return to the ancestral breeding grounds thousands of miles away to complete the life cycle.

Schmidt found that the American eel *(Anguilla rostrata)* could be distinguished from the European eel *(A. vulgaris)* because it had fewer vertebrae—an average of 107 in the American eel as compared with an average 114 in the European species. Since the American eel is much closer to the North American coastline, it requires only about 8 months to make the journey.

Homing salmon

The life history of salmon is nearly as remarkable as that of the eel and certainly has received far more popular attention. Salmon are **anadromous**; that is, they spend their adult lives at sea but return to fresh water to spawn. The Atlantic salmon *(Salmo salar)* and the Pacific salmon (six species of the genus *Oncorhynchus* [on-ko-rink′us]) have this practice, but there are important differences among the seven species. The Atlantic salmon (as well as the closely related steelhead trout) make upstream spawning runs year after year. The six Pacific salmon species (king, sockeye, silver, humpback, chum, and Japanese masu) each make a single spawning run (Fig. 23-39), after which they die.

The virtually infallible homing instinct of the Pacific species is legend: after migrating downstream as a smolt, a sockeye salmon ranges many hundreds of miles over the Pacific for nearly 4 years, grows to 2 to 5 kg in weight, and then returns almost unerringly to spawn in the headwaters of its parent stream. Some straying does occur and is an important means of increasing gene flow and populating new streams.

Many years ago Canadian biologists marked and released nearly a half million young sockeyes born in a tributary of British Columbia's Fraser River. Eleven thousand of these were recovered 4 years later in the same parent stream; not one was discovered to have strayed into any of the dozens of other Fraser River tributaries.

Experiments have shown that homing salmon are guided upstream by the characteristic odor of their parent stream. The salmon are apparently imprinted with the stream's odor while they are still unhatched embryos, since if the eggs are flown from the parent stream to another stream miles away, the adults still return to the parent stream after their residence at sea. The odor compound is a volatile organic substance, but its exact chemical nature remains unidentified; the embryonic salmon are probably conditioned to a mosaic of compounds released by the characteristic vegetation and soil in the watershed of the parent stream.

How do salmon find their way to the mouth of the river from the trackless miles of the open ocean? We know that they are incapable of distinguishing the parent stream odor while still hundreds of miles at sea. Recent experiments suggest that some migrating fish, like birds, are guided by celestial cues (stars or azimuth position of the sun). To do this, the salmon would require time-keeping abilities, certainly not an unreasonable possibility in view of the widespread presence of "biological clocks" in many organisms from the simplest to the most advanced.

___ Reproduction and Growth

In a group as diverse as the fishes, it is no surprise to find extraordinary variations on the basic theme of sexual reproduction. Fortunately, most fishes favor a simple theme, and it is with these that we begin our discussion.

The vast majority of fishes are **dioecious,** with **external fertilization** and **external development** of the eggs and embryos (**oviparous**). The **testes** of the male are elongate, whitish organs divided into lobules that contain cysts of maturing sperm cells in the same stage of development (Fig. 35-2, p. 847). This contrasts with the familiar pattern of higher vertebrates in which the seminiferous tubules at any point contain germ cells in all stages of development. The lobules open into a spermatic duct that runs into a urogenital sinus. The **ovaries** may run the length of the abdominal cavity and are made up of many ovarian follicles supported by connective tissue. The eggs develop within individual follicles. When the eggs are mature, they are shed either directly into the body cavity or into oviducts. In some teleosts, particularly salmon and trout, the oviducts are reduced or absent.

Most fishes spawn at certain times or seasons within a restricted range of temperature. Temperature is critical both for successful spawning and for the survival of the sensitive eggs and young. Many, perhaps most, fish spawn in the spring or early summer when the water temperature is rising. Others, such as cod, many flatfishes, salmon, and certain trout species, spawn in fall or winter, often when water temperatures are at their lowest. In polar water, fishes may live out their existence at temperatures between 0° and −2° C.

Many marine fishes have what appear to be extraordinarily wasteful modes of reproduction. Males and females come together in great schools and, without mating, release vast numbers of germ cells into the water to drift with the current. Large female cod may release 4 to 6 million eggs at a single spawning. Less than one in a million will survive the numerous perils of the ocean to reach reproductive maturity.

Unlike the minute, buoyant, transparent eggs of pelagic marine teleosts, those of near-shore species are larger, typically yolky, nonbuoyant, and adhesive. On the whole, fishes living in coastal waters where wave action and along-shore currents are prevalent dispose of their eggs in a more conservative manner. Some bury their eggs, many attach them to vegetation, some deposit them in nests, and some even incubate them in their mouths (Fig. 23-40). Many coastal species guard their eggs (Fig. 23-41). Intruders expecting an easy meal of eggs may be met with a vivid and often belligerent display by the guard, which is almost always the male.

Figure 23-40

Male banded jawfish *Opistognathus macrognathus* orally brooding its eggs. The male retrieves the female's spawn and incubates the eggs until they hatch. During brief periods when the jawfish is feeding, the eggs are left in the burrow.
Photograph by F. McConnaughey.

Figure 23-41

Lingcod *Ophiodon elongatus* guarding eggs.
Photograph by R. Harbo.

Figure 23-42

Spawning of Pacific salmon and development of the egg and young. **A,** Courting chum salmon. Male is nosing female's vent, possibly checking for spawning readiness. **B,** Male chum attacking uncooperative female during spawning. **C,** Female chum digging nest. **D,** Two coho salmon fertilizing eggs from female spawning between them. **E,** Fertilization. Sperm are guided to the opening in the egg (micropyle) by chemical attractant. **F,** "Eyed" stage. **G,** Developing embryo. **H,** Hatching larva. **I,** Emergent larva (alevin stage). **J,** Developing alevin. When the yolk is absorbed, the salmon emerges from the gravel as a fry and begins feeding.

Courtesy Joey Morgan/Hoot Productions, Ltd. From Childerhose, R.J., and M. Trim. 1979. Pacific salmon. Seattle, University of Washington Press.

Freshwater fishes almost invariably produce nonbuoyant eggs. Those, such as perch, that provide no parental care simply scatter their myriads of eggs among weeds or along the bottom. Freshwater fishes that do provide some form of egg care produce fewer, larger eggs that enjoy a better chance for survival.

Elaborate preliminaries to mating are the rule for freshwater fishes. The female Pacific salmon, for example, performs a ritualized mating "dance" with her breeding partner after arriving at the spawning bed in a fast-flowing, gravel-bottomed stream (Fig. 23-42, *A*). She then turns on her side and scoops out a nest with her tail (Fig. 23-42, *C*). As the eggs are laid by the female, they are fertilized by the male (Fig. 23-42, *D*). After the female covers the eggs with gravel, the exhausted fish die and drift downstream.

There are two other principal modes of reproduction in fishes: **internal fertilization with external development** and **internal fertilization with internal development.** The second of these two modes is practiced by the **live-bearers.** Several unrelated groups have live-bearing members; for example, the ever-popular guppies and mollies, the economically valuable redfish, the mosquito fish *Gambusia,* and all members of the surfperch family Embiotocidae (Fig. 23-43). In one surfperch, *Cymatogaster aggregatus,* male fishes may be retained in the ovary until they are sexually mature! The guppy, however, is a more typical example. The eggs are fertilized within the ovarian follicles where they develop for a period. The follicles then rupture, releasing the embryos into the cavity of the ovary, where they complete their gestation, nourished by their own yolk and possibly by secretions from the follicles.

Live-bearers actually comprise two groups: **ovoviviparous** forms (all of the examples given so far), in which the eggs are retained and nourished by egg yolk

Figure 23-43

Surfperch *Hypsurus caryi* giving birth at the time it was captured. All of the West Coast surfperches (family Embiotocidae) are viviparous. Brood size ranges from 3 to 80 young depending on the size of the mother.
Photograph by D.W. Gotshall.

within the mother, and **viviparous** forms, in which the young develop some type of placental attachment with the follicle, ovarian wall, or specialized uterus. True viviparity is known only in certain sharks, such as hammerhead and blue sharks, and a few teleost species, such as the dwarf top-minnow *Heterandria* and the four-eyed fishes of the genus *Anableps*. Many authorities consider the distinction between ovoviviparity and viviparity to be a rather artificial one because one can find examples among fishes in which the degree of placental development ranges from almost none to complete. Furthermore, in some live-bearing sharks the placenta develops only after several months of an ovoviviparous existence.

Soon after the eggs of oviparous species are fertilized and laid, they take up water and harden. Cleavage follows, and the blastoderm is formed, sitting astride a relatively enormous yolk mass. Soon the yolk mass is enclosed by the developing blastoderm, which then begins to assume a fishlike shape. The fish hatches as a larva that may be very different in appearance from the adult. The eyes and segmented muscles (myotomes) are well formed, but most conspicuous is the semi-transparent, globular mass of yolk, so large that larval movement is nearly impossible (Fig. 23-42, *1*). Not until the yolk is totally absorbed and the mouth and digestive tract are formed does the larva begin searching for its own food. After a period of growth the larva undergoes a **metamorphosis,** especially dramatic in many marine species such as the freshwater eel described previously (Fig. 23-38). Body shape is refashioned, fin and color patterns change, and the animal becomes a juvenile bearing the unmistakable definitive body form of its species.

Growth is temperature dependent. Consequently, fish living in temperate regions grow rapidly in summer when temperatures are high and food is abundant but nearly stop growing in winter. Seasonal growth is reflected as annual rings in the scales (Fig. 23-44), a distinctive record of convenience to fishery biologists who wish to determine a fish's age. Unlike birds and mammals, which reach a definitive adult size, most fishes after attaining reproductive maturity continue to grow for as long as they live. This is possible because their dense medium is so buoyant that it offsets the pull of gravity. It also is probably a selective advantage for the species, since the larger the fish, the more germ cells it produces and the greater its contribution to future generations.

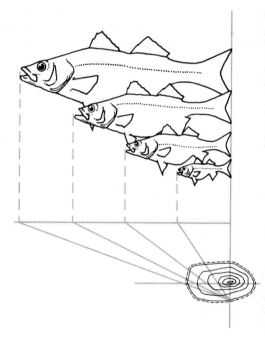

Figure 23-44

Scale growth. Fish scales disclose seasonal changes in growth rate. Growth is interrupted during winter, producing year marks (annuli). Each year's increment in scale growth is a ratio to the annual increase in body length. Otoliths (ear stones) and certain bones can also be used in some species to determine age and growth rate.

____ Summary

Fishes are poikilothermic, gill-breathing aquatic vertebrates with fins. They are the oldest vertebrates, having originated from an unknown chordate ancestor in the Cambrian period or possibly earlier. Four classes of fishes are recognized. Most primitive are the jawless hagfishes (class Myxini) and lampreys (class Cephalaspidomorphi), remnant groups having an eel-like body form without paired fins; a cartilaginous skeleton (although their ancestors, the ostracoderms, had bony skeletons); a notochord that persists throughout life; and a disclike mouth adapted for sucking or biting. All other vertebrates have jaws, a major development in vertebrate evolution. Members of the class Chondrichthyes (sharks, rays, skates, and chimaeras) are a successful group having a cartilaginous skeleton (a degenerative feature), paired fins, excellent sensory equipment, and an active, characteristically predaceous habit. The fourth class of fishes is the bony fishes (class Osteichthyes), which may be subdivided into three stems of descent. Two stems are relic groups, the lobe-finned fishes (subclass Crossopterygii, represented by one living species, the coelacanth) and the lungfishes (subclass Dipneusti). The third stem is the ray-finned fishes (subclass Actinopterygii), a huge and diverse modern assemblage containing nearly all of the familiar freshwater and marine fishes.

The modern bony fishes (teleost fishes) have radiated into nearly 20,000 species that reveal an enormous diversity of adaptations, body form, behavior, and habitat preference. Fishes swim by undulatory contractions of the body muscles, which generate thrust (propulsive force) and lift (lateral force). Flexible fishes oscillate the whole body, but in more rapid swimmers the undulations are limited to the caudal region or tail fin alone.

Most pelagic bony fishes achieve neutral buoyancy in water using a gas-filled swim bladder, the most effective gas-secreting device known in the animal kingdom. The gills of fishes, having efficient countercurrent flow between water and blood, facilitate high rates of oxygen exchange. All fishes but the hagfishes show well-developed osmotic and ionic regulation, achieved principally by the kidneys and the gills.

With the exception of the jawless agnathans, all fishes have jaws that are variously modified for carnivorous, herbivorous, planktivorous, and omnivorous feeding modes. Some fishes have specialized muscle tissue capable of generating and discharging high voltages in fresh water or high amperage in salt water for offensive and defensive behavior.

Most fishes are migratory to some extent, and some, such as freshwater eels and anadromous salmon, make remarkable migrations of great length and precision. Fishes reveal an extraordinary range of sexual reproductive strategies. Most fishes are oviparous, but ovoviviparous and viviparous fishes are not uncommon. The reproductive investment may be in large numbers of germ cells with low survival (many marine fishes) or in fewer germ cells with greater parental care for better survival (freshwater fishes).

Selected references

Bond, C.E. 1979. Biology of fishes. Philadelphia, W.B. Saunders Co. *Excellent textbook of ichthyology with a functional emphasis.*

Curtis, B. 1949. The life story of the fish, ed. 2. New York, Harcourt Brace Jovanovich, Inc. *Nontechnical account.*

Greenwood, P.H., and J.R. Norman. 1976. A history of fishes, ed. 3. New York, Halsted Press. *This classic provides a wealth of information on fish biology.*

Harden Jones, F.R. 1968. Fish migrations. London, Edward Arnold, Ltd. *Scholarly review of fish migration and orientation.*

Hardisty, M.W. 1979. Biology of the cyclostomes. London, Chapman & Hall, Ltd. *Comprehensive monograph by one who has spent a lifetime studying the hagfishes and lampreys.*

Hasler, A.D., A.T. Scholz, and R.M. Horrall. 1978. Olfactory imprinting and homing in salmon. Am. Sci. **66:**347-355. *Review of evidence supporting the olfactory hypothesis for salmon homing.*

Hoar, W.S., and D.J. Randall (eds.). 1969-1979. Fish physiology, 8 vols. New York, Academic Press, Inc. *This series represents the most complete and authoritative treatise on the functional biology of fishes published. Technical and detailed.*

Hobson, E.S. 1975. Feeding patterns among tropical reef fishes. Am. Sci. **63:**382-392. *Excellent description of day-night feeding activities over a reef.*

Lagler, K.F., J.E. Bardach, R.R. Miller, and D.R.M. Passino. 1977. Ichthyology, ed. 2. New York, John Wiley & Sons, Inc.

Lineaweaver, T.H., III, and R.H. Backus. 1970. The natural history of sharks. Philadelphia, J.B. Lippincott Co. *One of the best of many books dealing with these intriguing animals.*

Marshall, N.B. 1970. The life of fishes. New York, Universe Books. *Excellent general biology of fishes.*

Miller, D.J., and R.N. Lea. 1972. Guide to the coastal marine fishes of California. State of California, Dept. of Fish and Game Fish Bull. 157. *Comprehensive identification guidebook.*

Moriarty, C. 1978. Eels: a natural and unnatural history. New York, Universe Books. *Semipopular treatment.*

Moyle, P.B., and J.J. Cech. 1982. Fishes: an introduction to ichthyology. Englewood Cliffs, N.J., Prentice-Hall, Inc. *Clearly written, comprehensive textbook.*

Nelson, J.S. 1984. Fishes of the world, ed. 2. New York, John Wiley & Sons, Inc. *A modern classification of all major groups of fishes.*

Netboy, A. 1974. The salmon: their fight for survival. Boston, Houghton Mifflin Co. *Thorough and readable treatise of the biology of the magnificent but embattled salmon.*

Popper, A.N., and S. Coombs. 1980. Auditory mechanisms in teleost fishes. Am. Sci. **68:**429-440.

Schultz, L.P., and E.M. Stern. 1948. The ways of fishes. New York, D. Van Nostrand Co. *Despite its age, this is still an excellent account of fish biology at the semipopular level. Recommended for the beginning student.*

Shaw, E. 1978. Schooling fishes. Am. Sci. **66:**166-175. *How they are organized and what the benefits are.*

Tesch, F.-W. 1977. The eel: biology and management of anguillid eels. (English-language edition edited by P.H. Greenwood.) New York, John Wiley & Sons, Inc. *Comprehensive and authoritative standard reference on eels.*

Ursin, M.J. 1977. A guide to fishes of the temperate Atlantic Coast. New York, E.P. Dutton. *Guidebook with illustrations, descriptions, and distribution maps.*

Selected *Scientific American* articles

Brett, J.R. 1965. The swimming energetics of salmon. **213:**80-85 (Aug.). *Describes studies on the remarkable efficiency of swimming by fish.*

Carey, F.G. 1973. Fishes with warm bodies. **228:**36-44 (Feb.). *Some tuna and mackerel shark species employ a circulatory heat exchanger to conserve body heat and increase swimming power.*

Gilbert, P.W. 1962. The behavior of sharks. **207:**60-68 (July).

Gray, J. 1957. How fishes swim. **197:**48-54 (Aug.). *This British biologist's calculations of the seemingly impossible swimming efficiency of fishes have been referred to as "Gray's paradox."*

Grundfest, H. 1960. Electric fishes. **203:**115-124 (Oct.).

Jensen, D. 1966. The hagfish. **214:**82-90 (Feb.).

Johansen, K. 1968. Air-breathing fishes. **219:**102-111 (Oct.). *Not all fishes are water breathers. Many remarkable alternatives for air breathing evolved in fishes; several are described in this article.*

Leggett. W.C. 1973. The migrations of the shad. **228:**92-98 (Mar.).

Levine, J.S., and E.F. MacNichol, Jr. 1982. Color vision in fishes. **246:**140-149 (Feb.). *How color sensitivity is matched to visual habitat.*

Lissmann, H.W. 1963. Electric location by fishes. **208:**50-59 (Mar.). *Certain fishes generate weak electric fields to sense their environment and locate prey.*

Lühling, K.H. 1963. The archer fish. **209:**100-108 (July). *This small fish of Southeast Asia spouts a stream of water to down insects it sights on plants above the water.*

Millot, J. 1955. The coelacanth. **193:**34-39 (Dec.). *Its biology and evolutionary relationships are discussed.*

Partridge, B.L. 1982. The structure and function of fish schools. **246:**114-123 (June).

Ruud, J.T. 1965. The ice fish. **213:**108-114 (Nov.). *A family of transparent Antarctic fishes possesses neither red blood cells nor hemoglobin. The physiological consequences are described.*

Scholander, P.F. 1957. The wonderful net. **196:**96-107 (Apr.). *Describes the arrangement of blood vessels that form a countercurrent exchange system in the swim bladder of fishes.*

T H E   A M P H I B I A N S

Phylum Chordata
Class Amphibia

Green tree frog *Litoria caerulea* solemnly sits awaiting evening when it will become active
to feed. This vivid green Australian species is commonly seen in outdoor toilets,
which provide both shelter and insect food. As the name implies, tree frogs
are well adapted for an arboreal life, possessing suction discs on their toes.
Nevertheless, many tree frogs prefer brushy thickets, swampy woodlands,
or even the ground to high places in trees.

Photograph by C.P. Hickman, Jr.

The chorus of frogs beside a pond on a spring evening heralds one of nature's dramatic events. Masses of frog eggs soon hatch into limbless, gill-breathing, fishlike tadpole larvae. Warmed by the late spring sun, they feed and grow. Then, almost imperceptibly, a remarkable transformation takes place. Hindlegs appear and gradually lengthen. The tail shortens. The larval teeth are lost, and the gills are replaced by lungs. The eyelids develop. The forelegs emerge. In a matter of weeks the aquatic tadpole has completed its metamorphosis to an adult frog.

The early members of the class Amphibia (am-fib'e-a) (Gr., *amphi,* both or double, + *bios,* life), of which our chorusing frogs are among the more vociferous modern descendants, originated not in weeks but over millions of years by a lengthy series of almost imperceptible alterations that gradually fitted the vertebrate body plan for life on land. The origin of land vertebrates is no less a remarkable feat for this fact—a feat that incidentally would have a poor chance of succeeding today because well-established competitors make it impossible for a poorly adapted transitional form to gain a foothold.

Even now after some 350 million years of evolution, the amphibians are not completely land adapted; they are quasiterrestrial, hovering between aquatic and land environments. This double life is expressed in their name. Structurally they are between fishes and reptiles. Although adapted for a terrestrial existence, few can stray far from moist conditions. Many, however, have developed devices for keeping their eggs out of open water where the larvae would be exposed to enemies.

The more than 2500 species of amphibians are grouped into three living orders: the newts and salamanders (order Urodela), which are the least specialized and most aquatic of all amphibians; the frogs and toads (order Salientia), which are the largest and most successful group of amphibians and the closest to the stock from which the higher tetrapods (animals with four legs) descended; and the highly specialized, secretive, earthwormlike tropical caecilians (order Gymnophiona).

___MOVEMENT ONTO LAND

The movement from water to land is perhaps the most dramatic event in animal evolution, since it involves the invasion of a habitat that in many respects is more hazardous for life. Life was conceived in water, animals are mostly water in composition, and all cellular activities occur in water. Nevertheless, organisms eventually invaded the land, carrying their watery composition with them. To survive and maintain this fluid matrix, it was necessary that various structural, functional, and behavioral changes evolve. Considering that almost every system in the body required some modification, it is remarkable that all vertebrates are basically alike in fundamental structural and functional pattern: whether aquatic or terrestrial, vertebrates are obviously descendants of the same evolutionary branch.

Amphibians were not the first living things to move onto land. Insects made the transition earlier and plants much earlier still. The pulmonate snails were experimenting with land as a suitable place to live about the same time the early amphibians were. Yet of all these, the amphibian story is of particular interest because their descendants became the most successful and advanced animals on earth.

___ Physical Contrast between Aquatic and Land Habitats

Beyond the obvious difference in water content of aquatic and terrestrial habitats, there are several sharp differences between the two environments of significance to animals attempting to move from water to land.

Greater oxygen content of air

Air contains at least 20 times more oxygen than water. Air has approximately 210 ml of oxygen per liter; water contains 3 to 9 ml per liter, depending on temperature, presence of other solutes, and degree of saturation. Furthermore, the diffusion rate of oxygen is low in water. Consequently, aquatic animals must expend far more effort extracting oxygen from water than land animals expend removing oxygen from air.

Greater density of water

Water is approximately 1000 times denser than air and approximately 50 times more viscous. Although water is a much more resistant medium to move through, its high density, only a little less than that of animal protoplasm, buoys up the body. One of the major problems encountered by land animals was the need to develop strong limbs and remodel the skeleton to support their bodies in air.

Constancy of temperature in water

Natural bodies of water, containing a medium with tremendous thermal capacity, have little fluctuation in temperature. The temperature of the oceans remains almost constant day after day. In contrast, both the range and fluctuation in temperature are acute on land. Its harsh cycles of freezing, thawing, drying, and flooding, often in unpredictable sequence, presented severe thermal problems to terrestrial animals, which had to evolve behavioral and physiological strategies to protect themselves from thermal extremes. The most successful strategy, homeothermy (regulated constant body temperature), appeared in the birds and mammals.

Variety of land habitats

The variety of cover and shelter on land was a great inducement for its colonization. The rich offerings of terrestrial habitats include coniferous, temperate, and tropical forests, grasslands, deserts, mountains, oceanic islands, and polar regions. Even so, earth's hydrosphere (oceans, seas, lakes, rivers, and ice sheets), although offering a less diverse range of habitats, contains the greatest number and variety of living things on earth.

Opportunities for breeding on land

The provision of safe shelter for the protection of vulnerable eggs and young is much more readily accomplished on land than in water habitats.

ORIGIN AND RELATIONSHIPS OF AMPHIBIANS

The movement onto land required structural modifications of the fish body plan. Unlike a fish, which is supported and wetted by its medium and supplied with dissolved oxygen, a terrestrial animal must support its own weight, resist drying and rapid temperature change, and extract oxygen from air.

Appearance of Lungs

The Devonian period, beginning some 400 million years ago, was a time of mild temperatures and alternating droughts and floods. During dry periods, pools and streams began to dry up, water became foul, and the dissolved oxygen disappeared. Only those fishes able to use the abundance of atmospheric oxygen could survive such conditions. Gills were unsuitable because in air the filaments collapsed into clumps that soon dried out.

Virtually all freshwater fish surviving this period, including the lobe-finned fishes and the lungfishes, had a kind of lung developed as an outgrowth of the pharynx. It was relatively simple to enhance the efficiency of the air-filled cavity by improving its vascularity with a rich capillary network and by supplying it with arterial blood from the last (sixth) pair of aortic arches. Oxygenated blood was returned directly to the heart by a pulmonary vein to form a complete pulmonary circuit. Thus, the double circulation characteristic of all tetrapods originated: a systemic circulation, serving the body, and a pulmonary circulation, supplying the lungs.

Development of Limbs for Travel on Land

The evolution of limbs was also a product of difficult times during the Devonian period. When pools dried up, fishes were forced to move to another pool that still contained water. Only the lobe-finned fishes (crossopterygians) were preadapted for the task. They had strong lobed fins, used originally as swimming stabilizers, that could be adapted as paddles to lever their way across land in search of water. The pectoral fins were especially well developed, containing a series of skeletal elements in the fins and pectoral girdle that clearly foreshadowed the pentadactyl limb of tetrapods. We should note that the development first of strong fins and later of limbs did not happen so that fish could colonize land but rather as an adaptation to find water and continue living like fish. Land travel was simply and paradoxically a means for survival in water. But lungs and limbs were fortunate developments and essential specializations that preadapted vertebrates for life on land.

Earliest Amphibians

All evidence points to the lobe-finned fishes (crossopterygians) as ancestors of the modern amphibians. The lobe-fins, abundant and successful in the Devonian period, possessed lungs and strong, mobile fins. Their skull and tooth structure was similar to that of the earliest known amphibians, the Labyrinthodontia, a distinct salamander-like group of the late Devonian period.

Figure 24-1

Figure 24-1

Reconstruction of the skeleton and body of the very early amphibian *Ichthyostega*. Modified from Jarvik, E. 1955. Sci. Monthly 80:141-154.

A representative of this group was a 350 million year old fossil called *Ichthyostega* (Gr., *ichthyos,* fish, + *stegos,* covering) (Fig. 24-1). *Ichthyostega* possessed several new adaptations that equipped it for life on land. It had jointed, pentadactyl limbs for crawling on land, a more advanced ear structure for picking up airborne sounds, a foreshortening of the skull, and a lengthening of the snout that announced improved olfactory powers for detecting dilute airborne odors. Yet *Ichthyostega* was still fishlike in retaining a fish tail complete with fin rays and in having opercular (gill) bones.

The capricious Devonian period was followed by the Carboniferous period, characterized by a warm, wet climate during which mosses and large ferns grew in profusion on a swampy landscape. Conditions were ideal for the amphibians. They radiated quickly into a great variety of species, feeding on the abundance of insects, insect larvae, and aquatic invertebrates available: this was the age of amphibians.

With water everywhere, however, there was little selective pressure to encourage movement onto land and many amphibians actually improved their adaptations for living in water. Their bodies become flatter for moving about in shallow water. Many of the urodeles (newts and salamanders), which may have descended from the lepospondyls (Fig. 24-2), developed weak limbs. The tail became better developed as a swimming organ. Even the anurans (frogs and toads), which are the most terrestrial of all amphibians, developed specialized hindlimbs with webbed feet better suited for swimming than for movement on land. All groups of amphibians use their porous skin as an accessory breathing organ. This specialization was encouraged by the swampy surroundings of the Carboniferous period but presented serious desiccation problems for life on land.

Amphibians' Contribution to Vertebrate Evolution

Amphibians have met the problems of independent life on land only halfway. To be sure, they made several important contributions to the transition that required the evolution of their descendants, the reptiles, to complete. Of crucial importance were the change from gill to lung breathing and the development of limbs for locomotion on land. Amphibians also show strengthening changes in the skeleton so that the body can be supported on land. A start was also made toward shifting special sense priorities from the lateral line system of fish to the senses of smell and hearing. For this, both the olfactory epithelium and the ear required redesigning to improve sensitivities to airborne odors and sounds.

Despite these modifications, the amphibians are basically aquatic animals. They are ectothermic; that is, their body temperature is determined by and varies with the environmental temperature. Their skin is thin, moist, and unprotected from desiccation in air. An intact frog loses water nearly as rapidly as a skinless

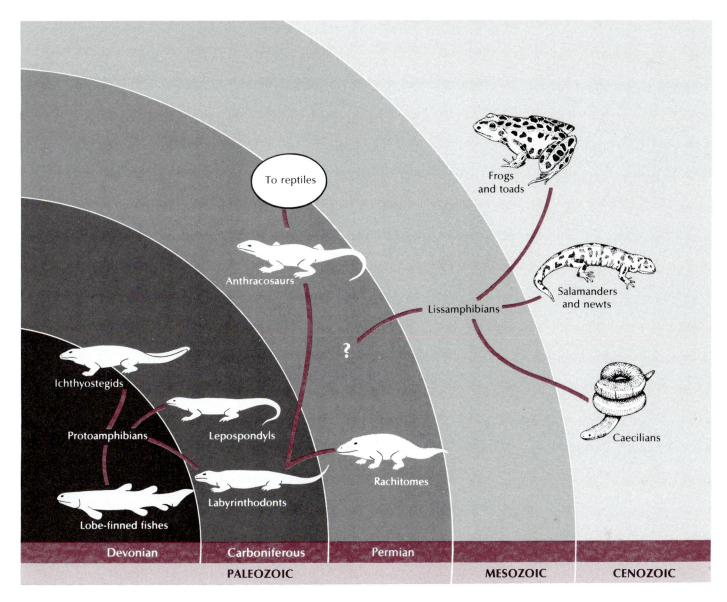

Labels in figure:
To reptiles
Frogs and toads
Anthracosaurs
Lissamphibians
Salamanders and newts
Ichthyostegids
?
Protoamphibians
Lepospondyls
Caecilians
Labyrinthodonts
Rachitomes
Lobe-finned fishes
Devonian — Carboniferous — Permian
PALEOZOIC — MESOZOIC — CENOZOIC

frog. Most important, the amphibians remain chained to the aquatic environment by their mode of reproduction. Eggs are shed directly into the water or laid in moist surroundings and are externally fertilized (with very few exceptions). The larvae that hatch typically pass through an aquatic tadpole stage.

Many amphibians have developed ingenious devices for laying their eggs elsewhere to give their young protection and a better chance for life. They may lay eggs under logs or rocks, in the moist forest floor, in flooded tree holes, in pockets on the mother's back (Fig. 24-3), or in folds of the body wall. One species of Australian frog even broods its young in its stomach.

However, it remained for the reptiles to complete the conquest of land with the development of a shelled (amniotic) egg, which finally freed the vertebrates from a reproductive attachment to the aquatic environment. With the appearance of reptiles at the end of the Paleozoic era, the halcyon era for the amphibians began to fade. The reptiles captured rule of both water and land and replaced most amphibians in both environments. From the survivors have descended the three modern orders of amphibians.

Figure 24-2

Evolution of the amphibians. The early amphibians arose from the lobe-finned fishes and radiated successfully during the Carboniferous period (the age of amphibians). Modern amphibians have radiated from the Lissamphibians of the Mesozoic era, a group of uncertain connection to the Paleozoic amphibians.

Figure 24-3

The female Surinam toad, carrying young on her back. As eggs are laid, the male assists in positioning them on the rough back skin of female. The skin swells, enclosing eggs. The approximately 60 young pass through the tadpole stage beneath the skin and emerge as small frogs. The Surinam "toad," actually a frog, is found mainly in Amazon and Orinoco river systems of equatorial South America.

Courtesy American Museum of Natural History.

CHARACTERISTICS

1. Skeleton mostly bony, with varying number of vertebrae; ribs present in some, absent in others; notochord does not persist; **exoskeleton absent**
2. Body forms vary greatly from an elongated trunk with distinct head, neck, and tail to a compact, depressed body with fused head and trunk and no intervening neck
3. **Limbs, usually four (tetrapod),** although some are legless; forelimbs of some much smaller than hindlimbs, in others all limbs small and inadequate; **webbed feet often present;** no true nails or claws
4. **Skin smooth and moist with many glands,** some of which may be poison glands; pigment cells (chromatophores) common, of considerable variety, and in a few capable of undergoing color and pattern changes in accordance with different backgrounds; **no scales,** except concealed dermal ones in some
5. Mouth usually large with small teeth in upper or both jaws; **two nostrils open into anterior part of mouth cavity**
6. Respiration by gills, lungs, skin, and pharyngeal region either separately or in combination; external gills in the larval form and may persist throughout life in some
7. **Circulation with three-chambered heart,** two atria and one ventricle, and a double circulation through the heart; skin abundantly supplied with blood vessels
8. Ectothermal
9. Excretory system of paired mesonephric kidneys; urea main nitrogenous waste
10. Ten pairs of cranial nerves
11. Separate sexes; fertilization mostly internal in salamanders and caecilians, mostly external in frogs and toads; predominantly oviparous, rarely ovoviviparous; metamorphosis usually present; **mesolecithal eggs with jellylike membrane coverings**

CLASSIFICATION

Order Gymnophiona (jim'no-fy'o-na) (Gr., *gymnos,* naked, + *ophineos,* of a snake) **(Apoda)**—caecilians. Body wormlike; limbs and limb girdle absent; mesodermal scales may be present in skin; tail short or absent; tropical; one family, 17 genera, approximately 160 species.

Order Urodela (yu'ro-dee'la) (Gr., *oura,* tail, + *dēlos,* visible) **(Caudata)**—salamanders, **newts.** Body with head, trunk, and tail; no scales; usually two pairs of equal limbs; eight families, 51 genera, approximately 300 species.

Order Salientia (say'lee-ench'e-a) (L., *saliens,* leaping, + *ia,* pl. suffix) **(Anura)**—frogs, **toads.** Head and trunk fused; no tail; no scales; two pairs of limbs; large mouth; lungs; 10 vertebrae, including urostyle; 13 families, 100 genera, approximately 2000 species.

___STRUCTURE AND NATURAL HISTORY
___ Caecilians—Order Gymnophiona (Apoda)

The little-known order Gymnophiona (Gr., *gymnos,* naked, + *ophiona,* snake) contains some 160 species of burrowing, wormlike creatures commonly called **caecilians** (L., *caecilia,* kind of lizard, from *caecus,* blind) (Fig. 24-2). They are distributed in tropical forests of South America (their principal home), Africa, and Southeast Asia. They are characterized by their long, slender body, small scales in the skin, many vertebrae, long ribs, no limbs, and terminal anus. The eyes are small, and most species are totally blind as adults (Fig. 24-4). Replacing eyes, which would be useless for a subterranean existence, are special sensory tentacles on the snout. Because they are almost all burrowing forms, they are seldom seen by humans. Their food is mostly worms and small invertebrates, which they find underground. Fertilization is internal, and the male is provided with a protrusible cloaca by which he copulates with the female. The eggs are usually deposited in moist ground near the water. The larvae may be aquatic, or the complete larval development may occur in the egg. In some species the eggs are carefully guarded in folds of the body during their development. Viviparity also is common among caecilians, with the embryos obtaining nourishment probably by eating the wall of the oviduct.

___ Salamanders and Newts—Order Urodela (Caudata)

As its name suggests, the order Urodela (Gr., *oura*, tail, + *dēlos*, visible) consists of tailed amphibians: the salamanders and newts. This compact, natural group is the least specialized of all the amphibians. Although urodeles are found in almost all temperate and tropical regions of the world, most species occur in North America. Urodeles are typically small; most of the common North American salamanders are less than 15 cm long. Some aquatic forms are considerably longer, and the carnivorous Japanese giant salamander may exceed 1.5 m in length.

Urodeles have primitive limbs set at right angles to the body, with forelimbs and hindlimbs of approximately equal size. In some the limbs are rudimentary. One group, the sirens, with minute forelimbs and no hindlimbs at all, is so different from other urodeles that some authorities place them in a completely separate order, Trachystomata.

Salamanders and newts are carnivorous, preying on worms, small arthropods, and small molluscs. Most eat only things that are moving. Since their food is rich in proteins, they do not usually store in their bodies great quantities of fat or glycogen. Like all amphibians, they are ectotherms and have a low metabolic rate.

Breeding behavior

Some urodeles are wholly aquatic throughout their life cycle, but most are terrestrial, living in moist places under stones and rotten logs, usually not far from water. They do not show as great a diversity of breeding habits as do frogs and toads. The eggs of most salamanders are fertilized internally, usually after the female picks up a packet of sperm (**spermatophore**) that previously has been deposited by the male on a leaf or stick (Fig. 24-5). Aquatic species lay their eggs in clusters or stringy masses in the water. Terrestrial species deposit eggs in small,

Figure 24-4

Head and anterior region of caecilian (order Gymnophiona [Apoda]). These legless and wormlike amphibians may reach lengths of 55 cm and diameters of 2 cm. Their body folds give them the appearance of a segmented worm. They have many sharply pointed teeth, a pair of tiny eyes mostly hidden beneath the skin, and a small tentacle between the eye and nostril; some forms have embedded mesodermal scales.

Courtesy General Biological Supply House, Inc., Chicago.

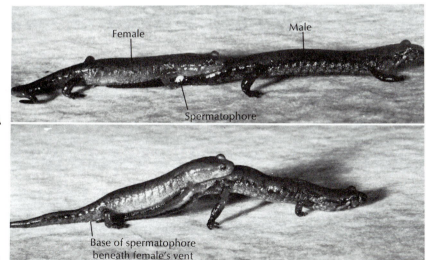

A

Female   Male

Spermatophore

B   Base of spermatophore beneath female's vent

Figure 24-5

Courtship and sperm transfer in the pigmy salamander *Desmognathus wrighti.* After judging the female's receptivity by the presence of her chin on his tail base, the male deposits a spermatophore on the ground, then moves forward a few paces. **A,** The white mass of the sperm atop a gelatinous base is visible at the level of the female's forelimb. The male moves ahead, the female following until the spermatophore is at the level of her vent. **B,** The female has recovered the sperm mass in her vent, while the male arches his tail, tilting the female upward and presumably facilitating recovery of the sperm mass.

Courtesy L. Houck.

Figure 24-6

Red-backed salamander *Plethodon cinereus* encircles her hatching brood in their nest of forest humus. Females of many species of the large North American family Plethodontidae remain with their eggs during incubation and may even return to the same nest site year after year.
Drawn from a photograph by P.A. Zahl.

grapelike clusters under logs or in excavations in soft earth, and many species remain to guard the eggs (Fig. 24-6). Unlike frogs and toads, which hatch into fishlike tadpole larvae, the embryos of urodeles hatch from their eggs resembling their parents. The larvae undergo metamorphosis in the course of development, but it is not nearly as revolutionary a change as is the metamorphosis of frog and toad tadpoles to the adult body form.

Respiration

All urodeles hatch with gills, but during development these are lost in all except the aquatic forms or in those that fail to undergo a complete metamorphosis. Gills would be useless for terrestrial salamanders, since the filaments would collapse and dry out to become functionless. Lungs, the characteristic respiratory organ of terrestrial vertebrates, replace the larval gills in most adult amphibians.

Yet many salamanders have dispensed with lungs altogether and thus bear the distinction of being the only vertebrates to have neither lungs nor gills. Members of the large family Plethodontidae, a group containing most of the familiar North American salamanders (Fig. 24-6), are completely lungless, and some members of other urodele families exhibit reductions in lung development. In all amphibians the skin contains extensive vascular nets that serve in varying degrees for the respiratory exchange of oxygen and carbon dioxide. In lungless salamanders the efficiency of cutaneous respiration is increased by the penetration of a capillary network into the epidermis or by the thinning of the epidermis over superficial dermal capillaries. Cutaneous respiration is supplemented by the pumping of air in and out of the mouth where the respiratory gases are exchanged across the vascularized membranes of the buccal (mouth) cavity (buccopharyngeal breathing). Lungless plethodontid salamanders are believed to have originated in swift streams of the Appalachian mountains, where lungs would have been a disadvantage by providing too much buoyancy, and the water is so cool and well oxygenated that cutaneous respiration alone was sufficient for life.

Figure 24-7

Red-spotted newt *Diemictylus viridescens*. Most newts have a land stage interposed between the aquatic larva and aquatic adult stages. This specimen is an adult female posing uncharacteristically out of water. The coral-colored land stage is popularly called the red eft.
Photograph by C.P. Hickman, Jr.

Figure 24-8

Mud puppy *Necturus maculosus*, an example of a paedomorphic species. Gills are retained in the breeding adult.

From The biology of the Amphibia by G.K. Nobel. Copyright © 1931, McGraw-Hill Book Co. Used with permission of McGraw-Hill Book Co.

Paedomorphosis

Whereas most urodeles complete their development to the definitive adult body form by metamorphosis, there are some species that retain their gills and other larval characteristics even after becoming sexually mature. This condition is called **paedomorphosis** (Gr., *pais*, child, + *morphē*, form). Some are **permanent larvae,** a genetically fixed condition in which the developing tissues fail to respond to the thyroid hormone that, in other amphibians, stimulates metamorphosis (Fig. 24-7). This condition is called obligatory paedomorphosis.

Examples of permanent larvae are mud puppies of the genus *Necturus* (Gr., *nekton*, swimming, + *oura*, tail) (Fig. 24-8), which live on bottoms of ponds and lakes and keep their external gills throughout life, and the amphiuma (*Amphiuma means* [Gr., *amphi*, double, + *pneuma*, breath]) of the southeastern United States, which with its nearly useless, rudimentary legs superficially resembles an eel more than an amphibian.

There are other species of salamanders that become sexually mature and breed in the larval state, but unlike the permanent larvae, they may metamorphose to adults if environmental conditions change. This is called **neoteny** (Gr., *neos*, young, + *teinen*, to extend).

Examples are species of the genus *Ambystoma* (Gr., *ambyx*, cup, + *stoma*, mouth) and of the genus *Triturus* (N.L., *Triton*, a sea god, + *oura*, tail). The American axolotl, *Ambystoma tigrinum*, widely distributed over Mexico and the southwestern United States, remains in the aquatic, gill-breathing, and fully reproductive larval form unless the water begins to dry up; then it metamorphoses to an adult, loses its gills, develops lungs, and assumes the appearance of an ordinary salamander.

Axolotls can be made to metamorphose by treating them with the thyroid hormone, thyroxine. Thyroxine is essential for normal metamorphosis in all amphibians. Recent research suggests that the pituitary gland fails to become fully active in neotenous forms and does not release thyrotropin, a pituitary hormone that is required to stimulate the production of thyroxine by the thyroid gland.

Although the British zoologist Walter Garstang is best remembered for his ideas on the origin of chordates and vertebrates, he also wrote numerous clever, unorthodox poems about larval forms and their development. Some of his verses were so complex as to require reference books to unravel, but the following charming poem about the axolotl can be enjoyed by all.

> *Ambystoma's* a giant newt who
>   rears in swampy waters,
> As other newts are wont to do,
>   a lot of fishy daughters:
> These axolotls, having gills,
>   pursue a life aquatic,
> But, when they should
>   transform to newts, are
>   naughty and erratic.
> They change upon compulsion,
>   if the water grows too foul,
> For then they have to use their
>   lungs, and go ashore to
>   prowl;
> But when a lake's attractive,
>   nicely aired, and full of food,
> They cling to youth perpetual,
>   and rear a tadpole brood.

Frogs and Toads—Order Salientia (Anura)

The more than 2000 species of frogs and toads that make up the order Salientia are the most familiar and most successful of amphibians. Frogs and toads are highly specialized for a jumping mode of locomotion, as suggested by the preferred name of the order, Salientia, meaning leaping. The alternate order name, Anura (Gr., *an*, without, + *oura*, tail), refers to another obvious group characteristic, the absence of tails in adults (although all pass through a tailed larval stage during development).

In addition to their importance in biomedical research and education, frogs have long served the epicurean market. In 1979, for example, nearly 6 million pounds of frog legs, worth more than 9 million dollars, were consumed by Americans alone. Most were imported from overseas because the domestic supply has been hard hit by the draining and pollution of wetlands. Most vulnerable is the bullfrog, mainstay of the frog leg market. Attempts to raise them in farms have not been successful, mainly because bullfrogs are voracious eating machines that prefer insects, crayfish, and other frogs and normally will accept only moving prey.

The Salientia are further distinguished from the Urodela by their larvae and a dramatic metamorphosis during development. The eggs of most frogs hatch into a tadpole ("polliwog") stage, with a long, finned tail, both internal and external gills, no legs, specialized mouthparts for herbivorous feeding (salamander larvae, in distinction, are carnivorous), and a highly specialized internal anatomy. They look and act altogether differently from adult frogs. The metamorphosis of the frog tadpole to the adult frog is thus a striking transformation. Neoteny and paedomorphosis are never exhibited in frogs and toads as they are among salamanders.

The Salientia are an old group—fossil frogs are known from the Jurassic period, 150 million years ago—and today they are a secure and successful group. Frogs and toads occupy a great variety of habitats, despite their aquatic mode of reproduction and water-permeable skin, which prevent them from wandering too far afield from sources of water, and their ectothermy, which bars them from polar and subarctic habitats.

Notwithstanding their success as a distinct group, the frogs and toads are really a specialized side branch of amphibian evolution, and despite their popularity for education purposes—approximately 20 million are used each year in the United States alone—they are not good representatives of the vertebrate body plan. They lack a visible neck, the caudal vertebrae are fused into a urostyle, ribs

Figure 24-9

Two common North American frogs. **A,** Bullfrog *Rana catesbeiana*, largest American frog (family Ranidae). **B,** Spring peeper *Hyla crucifer* (family Hylidae). Note adhesive pads on the feet of this singing male.

A, Photograph by L.L. Rue, III; **B,** photograph by C.P. Hickman, Jr.

A   **B**

Figure 24-10

American toad *Bufo americanus* (family Bufonidae). This principally nocturnal yet familiar amphibian feeds on large numbers of insect pests as well as snails and earthworms. The warty skin contains numerous poison glands that produce a surprisingly poisonous milky fluid, providing the toad with excellent protection from a variety of potential predators.

Photograph by L.L. Rue, III.

Figure 24-11

Gigantorana goliath (family Ranidae) of West Africa, the world's largest frog. This specimen weighed 3.3 kg (approximately 7½ pounds).
Courtesy American Museum of Natural History.

are absent in most species, and the hindlegs are much enlarged for leaping locomotion. The primitive and unspecialized salamander would be a much superior choice for the zoology laboratory were not frogs so readily available.

Frogs and toads are divided into 12 families. The best-known frog families in North America are Ranidae, containing most of our familiar frogs, and Hylidae, the tree frogs (Fig. 24-9). True toads, belonging to the family Bufonidae (L., *bufo*, toad, + *idae,* suffix), have short legs, stout bodies, and thick skins usually with prominent warts (Fig. 24-10). However, the term "toad" is used rather loosely to refer to more or less terrestrial members of several other families.

The largest anuran is the West African *Gigantorana goliath* (Gr., *gigantos,* giant, + *rana,* frog), which is more than 30 cm long from tip of nose to anus (Fig. 24-11). This giant eats animals as big as rats and ducks. The smallest frog recorded is *Phyllobates limbatus* (Gr., *phyllon,* leaf, + *batēs,* climber), which is only approximately 1 cm long. This tiny frog, which can be more than covered by a dime, is found in Cuba. The largest American frog is the bullfrog, *Rana catesbeiana* (Fig. 24-9, *A*), which reaches a head and body length of 20 cm.

Habitats and distribution

Probably the most abundant and successful of frogs are the 200 to 300 species of the genus *Rana* (Gr., frog), found all over the temperate and tropical regions of the world except in New Zealand, the oceanic islands, and southern South America. They are usually found near water, although some, such as the wood frog *R. sylvatica,* spend most of their time on damp forest floors, often some distance from the nearest water. The wood frog probably returns to pools only for breeding in early spring. The larger bullfrogs *R. catesbeiana* and green frogs *R. clamitans* are nearly always found in or near permanent water or swampy regions. The leopard frog *R. pipiens* has a wider variety of habitats and, with all its subspecies and forms, is the most widespread of all the North American frogs. This is the species most commonly used in biology laboratories and for classical electrophysiological research. It has been found in some form in nearly every state, although sparingly represented along the extreme western part of the Pacific coast. It also extends far into northern Canada and as far south as Panama.

Within the range of any species of frogs, they are often restricted to certain habitats (for instance, to certain streams or pools) and may be absent or scarce in similar habitats of the range. The pickerel frog *(R. palustris)* is especially noteworthy in this respect because it is known to be abundant only in certain localized regions.

Most of the larger frogs are solitary in their habits except during the breeding season. During the breeding period most of them, especially the males, are very noisy. Each male usually takes possession of a particular perch, where he may remain for hours or even days, trying to attract a female to that spot. At times frogs are mainly silent, and their presence is not detected until they are disturbed. When they enter the water, they dart about swiftly and reach the bottom of the pool, where they kick up a cloud of muddy water. In swimming, they hold the

While native American amphibians continue to disappear as wetlands are drained, an exotic frog introduced into southern California has found the climate quite to its liking. The African clawed frog *Xenopus laevis* (Fig. 24-12) is a voracious, aggressive, primarily aquatic frog that is rapidly displacing native frogs and fish from several waterways and is spreading rapidly. The species was introduced into North America in the 1940s when they were used extensively in human pregnancy tests. When more efficient tests appeared in the 1960s, some hospitals simply dumped surplus frogs into nearby streams, where the prolific breeders have become almost indestructible pests. As is so often the case with alien wildlife introductions, benign intentions frequently lead to serious problems.

Figure 24-12

African clawed frog *Xenopus laevis* (family Pipidae). The claws, an unusual feature in frogs, are visible on the hindfeet. This species also lacks a tongue. Clawed frogs are wholly aquatic.

Photograph by T. Branning.

forelimbs near the body and kick backward with the webbed hindlimbs, which propel them forward. When they come to the surface to breathe, only the head and foreparts are exposed, and, since they usually take advantage of any protective vegetation, they are difficult to see.

During the winter months most frogs hibernate in the soft mud of the bottom of pools and streams. Naturally their life processes are at a very low ebb during their hibernation period, and such energy as they need is derived from the glycogen and fat stored in their bodies during the spring and summer months. The more terrestrial frogs, such as tree frogs, bed down for the winter in the humus of the forest floor. They are tolerant of low temperatures, and many actually survive prolonged freezing of all the extracellular fluid, representing 35% of the body water. Such frost-tolerant frogs prepare for winter by accumulating glycerol in body fluids, which protects tissues from the normally damaging effects of ice crystal formation.

Adult frogs have numerous enemies, such as snakes, aquatic birds, turtles, raccoons, and humans; only a few tadpoles survive to maturity. Although usually defenseless, in the tropics and subtropics many frogs and toads are aggressive, jumping and biting at predators. Some defend themselves by feigning death. Most anurans can blow up their lungs so that they are difficult to swallow. When disturbed along the margin of a pond or brook, a frog often remains quite still; when it thinks it is detected, it jumps, not always into the water where enemies may be lurking but into grassy cover on the bank. When held in the hand, a frog may cease its struggles for an instant to put its captor off guard and then leap violently, at the same time voiding its urine. Their best protection is their ability to leap and their use of poison glands. Bullfrogs in captivity do not hesitate to snap at tormenters and are capable of inflicting painful bites.

Integument and coloration

The skin of the frog is thin and moist and is attached loosely to the body only at certain points. Histologically the skin is made up of two layers: an outer stratified **epidermis** and an inner spongy **dermis** (Fig. 24-13). The outer layer of epidermal cells (which are shed periodically when a frog or toad "molts") contains deposits of **keratin,** a tough, fibrous protein that provides a certain measure of protection against abrasion and loss of water from the skin. The more terrestrial amphibians such as toads have especially heavy deposits of keratin. But amphibian keratin is soft, unlike the hard keratin that forms scales, claws, feathers, horns, and hair of the higher vertebrates.

The inner layer of the epidermis gives rise to two types of integumentary glands that grow down into the loose dermal tissues below. Small **mucous** glands secrete a protective mucous waterproofing onto the skin surface, and large **serous** glands produce a whitish, watery poison that is highly irritating to would-be predators. All amphibians produce a skin poison, but its effectiveness varies from species to species and with different predators. The poison of *Dendrobates,* a small South American frog, is used by Indian tribes to poison the points of their arrows. This and the poisons of other dendrobatid frogs are the most lethal animal secretions known, drop for drop more poisonous even than the venoms of sea snakes or any of the most poisonous arachnids.

Skin color in the frog is produced by pigment granules scattered through the epidermis and by special pigment cells, **chromatophores,** located in the dermis

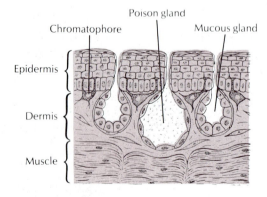

Chromatophore   Poison gland   Mucous gland

Epidermis

Dermis

Muscle

Figure 24-13

Section through frog skin.

A   B

Figure 24-14

Pigment cells (chromatophores). **A,** Pigment dispersed. **B,** Pigment concentrated. The pigment cell does not contract or expand; color effects are produced by streaming of cytoplasm, carrying pigment granules into cell branches for maximum color effect or to the center of the cell for minimum effect. Control over dispersal or concentration of pigment is mostly through light stimuli to eye. The melanophore-stimulating hormone is known to influence the activity of chromatophore (see text).

(Figs. 24-13 and 24-14). The chromatophores of amphibians, like those of many fishes and reptiles, are branched cells containing pigment that may be concentrated in a small area or dispersed throughout the branching processes to control skin coloration. Three types of chromatophores are recognized in amphibians: **xanthophores** just under the epidermis, containing red or yellow pigment; **iridiophores,** containing a silvery, crystalline pigment; and deeper-lying **melanophores,** containing black or brown melanin. Of the three types of chromatophores, the melanophores have especially long processes and are the most important for adjusting coloration to blend with the background. Some frogs and toads possess excellent powers of camouflage (Fig. 24-15).

The ability of many frogs to harmonize their skin with the surroundings is controlled by the amount of light reflected from the background onto the upper surface of the retina. This in turn controls the release of melanophore-stimulating hormone (MSH) from the intermediate lobe of the pituitary. When the frog is on a dark, light-absorbing background, little light is reflected onto the dorsal retina. Under these conditions, MSH is released from the pituitary, inducing pigment dispersion in the melanophores and darkening of the skin. On a light background the increased reflection of light onto the retina reflexly inhibits MSH release. The pigment remains concentrated in the centers of the melanophores, and the frog becomes pale in color. Other factors such as temperature, humidity, and diet also affect skin coloration.

Skeletal and muscular systems

In amphibians, as in their fish ancestors, the well-developed **endoskeleton** of bone and cartilage provides a framework for the muscles in movement and protection for the viscera and nervous systems. But movement onto land and the necessity of transforming paddlelike fins into tetrapod legs capable of supporting the body's weight introduced a new set of stress and leverage problems. The changes are most noticeable in the anurans, whose entire musculoskeletal system is specialized for jumping and swimming by simultaneous extensor thrusts of the hindlimbs.

Skeleton

In amphibians the vertebral column assumes a new role as a support from which the abdomen is slung and to which the limbs are attached. Since amphibians move with limbs instead of swimming with serial contractions of myotomic trunk musculature, the vertebral column has lost much of the original flexibility character-

Figure 24-15

Cryptic coloration of the tree frog (*Hyla*). Instead of the excellent protective markings borne by this harmless North America species, several of the dangerously poisonous South American tree frogs display vivid coloration that warns predators to keep away. All tree frogs have suction pads at ends of fingers and toes, enabling them to grip vertical surfaces.
Photograph by L.L. Rue, III.

istic of fishes. Rather it has become a rigid frame for transmitting force from the hindlimbs to the body. The anurans are further specialized by an extreme shortening of the body. Typical frogs have only nine trunk vertebrae and a rodlike **urostyle,** which represents several fused caudal vertebrae. The primitive, limbless caecilians, which obviously have not shared these specializations for tetrapod locomotion, may have as many as 200 vertebrae.

The frog skull is also vastly altered as compared with its crossopterygian ancestors; it is much lighter in weight and more flattened in profile and has fewer bones and less ossification. The front part of the skull, wherein are located the nose, eyes, and brain, is better developed, whereas the back of the skull, which contained the gill apparatus of fishes, is much reduced. Lightening of the skull was essential to mobility on land, and the other changes fitted the frog for its improved special senses and means for feeding and breathing.

The pattern of bones and muscles in the limbs is the typical tetrapod type. There are three main joints in each limb (hip, knee, and ankle; or shoulder, elbow, and wrist). The hand or foot is basically a five-rayed (pentadactyl) form with several joints in each of the digits. It is a repetitive system that can be plausibly derived from the bone structure of the crossopterygian fin, which is distinctly suggestive of the amphibian limb; it is not difficult to imagine how selective pressures through millions of years remodeled the former into the latter.

Musculature

The muscles of the limbs are presumably derived from the radial muscles that moved the fins of fishes up and down, but the muscular arrangement has become so complex in the tetrapod limb that it is no longer possible to see parallels between this and fin musculature. Despite its complexity, we can recognize two great groups of muscles on any limb: an anterior and ventral group that pulls the limb forward and toward the midline (protraction and adduction), and a second set of posterior and dorsal muscles that serves to draw the limb back and away from the body (retraction and abduction).

The trunk musculature, which in fishes is segmentally organized into powerful muscular bands (myotomes) for locomotion by lateral flexion, was much modified during amphibian evolution. The dorsal (epaxial) muscles are arranged to support the head and brace the vertebral column. The ventral (hypaxial) muscles of the belly are more developed in amphibians than in fishes, since they must support the viscera in air without the buoying assistance of water.

Respiration and vocalization

Amphibians use three respiratory surfaces for gas exchange: the skin (cutaneous breathing), the mouth (buccal breathing), and the lungs. These surfaces are used to varying degrees by different groups and under different environmental conditions. Frogs and toads show a much greater dependence on lung breathing than do salamanders, since cutaneous breathing, simple and direct as it obviously is, suffers from two disadvantages: (1) the skin must be kept thin and moist for gas exchange and consequently is too delicate for a wholly aerial life, and (2) the amount of gas exchange across the skin is mostly constant and cannot be varied to match changing demands of the body for more or less oxygen. Nevertheless, the skin continues to serve as an important supplementary avenue for gas exchange in anurans, especially during hibernation in winter. Even under normal conditions when lung breathing predominates, most of the carbon dioxide is lost across the skin while most of the oxygen is taken up across the lungs.

The lungs are supplied by pulmonary arteries (derived from the sixth aortic arches) and blood is returned directly to the left atrium by the pulmonary veins. Frog lungs are ovoid, elastic sacs with their inner surfaces divided into a network of septa that are in turn subdivided into small terminal air chambers called **alveoli.** The alveoli of the frog lung are much larger than those of more advanced vertebrates, and consequently the frog lung has a smaller relative surface available for gas exchange: the respiratory surface of the common *Rana pipiens* is about 20 cm^2 per cubic centimeter of air contained, compared with 300 cm^2 for humans. The problem in lung evolution was not the development of a good internal vascular surface, but rather the problem of moving air. A frog is a positive-pressure breather that fills its lungs by forcing air into them; this contrasts with the negative-pressure system of all the higher vertebrates. The sequence and explanation of breathing in a frog are shown in Fig. 24-16. One can easily follow this sequence in a living frog at rest: rhythmical throat movements of mouth breathing may continue some time before flank movements indicate that the lungs are being emptied.

Both male and female frogs have **vocal cords,** but those of the male are much better developed. They are located in the **larynx,** or voice box. Sound is produced by passing air back and forth over the vocal cords between the lungs and a large pair of sacs (vocal pouches) in the floor of the mouth. The latter also serve as effective resonators in the male. The chief function of the voice is to attract mates. Most species utter characteristic sounds that identify them. Nearly everyone is familiar with the welcome springtime calls of the spring peeper, which produces a high-pitched sound surprisingly strident for such a tiny frog. Another sound familiar to residents of the more southern United States is the resonant "jug-o-rum" call of the bullfrog. The bass notes of the green frog are banjolike, and those of the leopard frog are long and guttural. Many frog sounds are now available on phonograph records.

Circulation

As in fishes, circulation in amphibians is a closed system of arteries and veins serving a vast peripheral network of capillaries through which blood is forced by the action of a single pressure pump, the heart.

The principal changes in circuitry involve the shift from gill to lung breathing. With the elimination of gills, a major obstacle to blood flow was removed from the arterial circuit. But two new problems arose. The first was to provide a blood circuit to the lungs. As we have seen, this was solved by converting the sixth aortic arch into pulmonary arteries to serve the lungs and by developing new pulmonary veins for returning oxygenated blood to the heart. The second and evidently more difficult evolutionary problem was to separate the new pulmonary circulation from the rest of the body's circulation in such a way that oxygenated blood from the lungs would be selectively sent to the body and deoxygenated venous return from the body would be selectively sent to the lungs. In effect this meant creating a double circulation consisting of separate pulmonary and systemic circuits. This was eventually solved by the development of a partition down the center of the heart, creating a double pump, one for each circuit. Amphibians and reptiles have made the separation to variable degrees, but the task was completed

Figure 24-16

Breathing in frog. The frog, a positive-pressure breather, fills its lungs by forcing air into them. **A,** Floor of mouth is lowered, drawing air in through nostrils. **B,** With nostrils closed and glottis open, the frog forces air into its lungs by elevating floor of mouth. **C,** Mouth cavity rhythmically ventilates for a period. **D,** Lungs are emptied by contraction of body wall musculature and by elastic recoil of lungs.

Modified from Gordon, M.S., and others. 1968. Animal function: principles and adaptations. New York, Macmillan, Inc.

Figure 24-17

Structure of the frog heart. *Red arrows,* Oxygenated blood. *Black arrows,* Deoxygenated blood.

by the birds and mammals, which have a completely divided heart of two atria and two ventricles.

The frog heart (Fig. 24-17) has two separate atria and a single undivided ventricle. Blood from the body (systemic circuit) first enters a large receiving chamber, the **sinus venosus,** which forces it into the **right atrium.** The **left atrium** receives freshly oxygenated blood from the lungs. Up to this point the deoxygenated blood from the body and oxygenated blood from the lungs are separated. But now both atria contract almost simultaneously, driving both right and left atrial blood into the single undivided **ventricle.** We should expect that complete admixture of the two circuits would happen here. In fact there is evidence that in at least some amphibians they remain mostly separated, so that when the ventricle contracts, oxygenated pulmonary blood is sent to the systemic circuit and deoxygenated systemic blood is sent to the pulmonary circuit. The **spiral valve** in the **conus arteriosus** (Fig. 24-17) may play an important role in maintaining selective distribution. The matter is controversial and has defied complete analysis despite the application of advanced techniques using radiopaque media and high-speed cineradiography.

Feeding and digestion

Frogs are carnivorous like most other adult amphibians and feed on insects, spiders, worms, slugs, snails, millipedes, or nearly anything else that moves and is small enough to swallow whole. They snap at moving prey with their protrusible tongue, which is attached to the front of the mouth and is free behind. The free end of the tongue is highly glandular and produces a sticky secretion, which adheres to the prey. The teeth on the premaxillae, maxillae, and vomers are used to prevent escape of prey, not for biting or chewing. The digestive tract is relatively short in adult amphibians, a characteristic of most carnivores, and it produces a variety of enzymes for breaking down proteins, carbohydrates, and fats.

The larval stages of anurans (tadpoles) are usually herbivorous, feeding on pond algae and other vegetable matter; they have a relatively long digestive tract, since their bulky food must be submitted to time-consuming fermentation before useful products can be absorbed.

Nervous system and special senses

The frog nervous system is of the basic vertebrate plan that was established in the early jawless fishes. It is commonly divided into (1) the **central nervous system,** consisting of the brain and spinal cord; (2) the **peripheral nervous system,** consisting of the cranial and spinal nerves; and (3) the **autonomic nervous system,** composed of a chain of special ganglia on each side of the spinal column.

The three fundamental parts of the brain—forebrain (telencephalon), concerned with the sense of smell; midbrain (mesencephalon), concerned with vision; and hindbrain (rhombencephalon), concerned with hearing and balance—have undergone dramatic developmental trends as the vertebrates moved onto land and improved their environmental awareness. In general there is increasing cephalization with emphasis on information processing by the brain and a corresponding loss of independence of the spinal ganglia, which are capable of only stereotyped reflexive behavior. Nonetheless, a headless frog preserves an amazing degree of purposive and highly coordinated behavior. With only the spinal cord intact, it maintains normal body posture and can with purposive accuracy raise its leg to wipe from its skin a piece of filter paper soaked in dilute acid. It will even use the opposite leg if the closer leg is held.

The forebrain is divided into the **telencephalon** and the **diencephalon** (Fig. 24-18). The telencephalon contains the olfactory center, which has assumed greatly increased importance for the detection of dilute airborne odors on land. The sense of smell is in fact one of the dominant special senses in frogs. The remainder of the telencephalon is the cerebrum, which is of little importance in amphibians and provides no hint of the magnificent development it is destined to attain in the higher mammals. The diencephalon consists of **thalamus, hypothalamus,** and **posterior pituitary,** which are important relay channels and regulative centers. The thalamus and hypothalamus are primitive integrative areas concerned with thirst, hunger, sexual drive, pleasure, and pain.

The most complex integrative activities of the frog brain are centered in the midbrain. The **optic lobe** (tectum) is a dorsal enlargement that integrates sensory information from the eyes as well as from other senses.

The hindbrain is divided into an anterior **metencephalon,** or cerebellum, and a posterior **myelencephalon,** or medulla. The cerebellum is concerned with equilibrium and movement coordination and is not well developed in amphibians, which stay close to the ground and are not noted for dexterity of movement. The cerebellum becomes vastly developed in the fast-moving birds and mammals. The medulla is really the enlarged anterior end of the spinal cord through which pass all sensory neurons except those of vision and smell. Here are located centers for auditory reflexes, respiration, swallowing, and vasomotor control.

The evolution of a semiterrestrial life for the amphibians has necessitated a reordering of sensory receptor priorities on land. The pressure-sensitive lateral line (acousticolateral) system of fishes remains only in the aquatic larvae of amphibians and in a few strictly aquatic adult amphibian species. This system of course can serve no useful purpose on land, since it was designed to detect and localize objects in water by reflected pressure waves. Instead the task of detecting airborne sounds devolved on the ear.

The **ear** of a frog is by higher vertebrate standards a primitive structure: a middle ear closed externally by a large **tympanic membrane** (eardrum) and containing a **stapes** (columella) that transmits vibrations to the inner ear. The latter

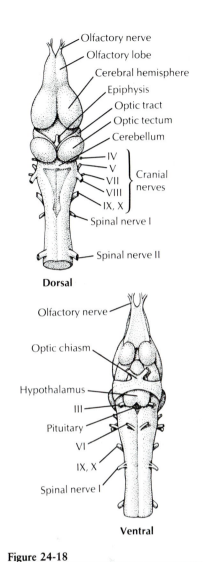

Figure 24-18

Brain of the frog, dorsal and ventral views.

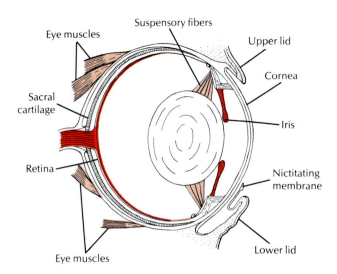

Keeping a sharp image on the retina for approaching or receding objects requires accommodation, and this is accomplished in different ways by different vertebrates. The eye of the bony fishes and lampreys is adjusted for near vision; to focus on distant objects, the lens must be moved backward. In amphibians, sharks, and snakes, the relaxed eye is focused on distant objects and the lens is moved *forward* to focus on nearby objects. In birds, mammals, and all reptiles except snakes, the lens accommodates by changing its *curvature* rather than by being moved forward or backward. The resting eye in these forms is adjusted for distant vision, and to focus on nearby objects the lens curvature is increased; that is, the lens is squeezed (or allowed to relax) into a rounder shape.

contains the **utricle**, from which arise the semicircular canals, and a **saccule** bearing a diverticulum, the **lagena**. The lagena is partly covered with a **tectorial membrane** that in its fine structure is not unlike that of the much more advanced mammalian cochlea. In most frogs this structure is sensitive to low-frequency sound energy not greater than 4000 Hz (cycles per second); in the bullfrog the main frequency response is in the 100 to 200 Hz range, which matches the energy of the male frog's low-pitched call.

Vision is the dominant special sense in most amphibians (the mostly blind caecilians are obvious exceptions). Several modifications were required to adapt the fish eye for use on dry land. Lachrymal glands and eyelids evolved to keep the eye moist, wiped free of dust, and shielded from injury. Since the cornea is exposed to air, it is an important refractive surface, removing much of the burden from the lens of bending light rays and focusing the image on the retina. As in the fishes, accommodation (adjusting focus for near and distant objects) is accomplished by moving the lens. But unlike the eyes of most fishes, the amphibian eye at rest is adjusted for distant objects and is moved forward to focus on nearby objects.

The **retina** contains both **rods** and **cones**, providing frogs with color vision. The **iris** contains well-developed circular and radial muscles and can rapidly expand or contract the aperture (pupil) to adjust to changing illumination. The upper lid of the eye is fixed, but the lower is folded into a transparent **nictitating membrane** capable of moving across the eye surface (Fig. 24-19). In all, frogs and toads possess good vision, a fact of crucial importance to animals that rely on quick escape to avoid their numerous predators.

Other sensory receptors include tactile and chemical receptors in the skin, taste buds on the tongue and palate, and a well-developed olfactory epithelium lining the nasal cavity.

Reproduction

Because frogs and toads are ectothermic, they breed, feed, and grow only during the warmer seasons of the year. One of the first drives after the dormant period is breeding. In the spring males croak and call vociferously to attract females. When their eggs are mature, the females enter the water and are clasped by the males in a process called **amplexus** (L., *amplexus,* embrace). As the female lays the eggs, the male discharges seminal fluid containing sperm over the eggs to fertilize them.

Figure 24-20

Eggs of American toad. Toads lay eggs in strings; frogs lay eggs in clusters.
Photograph by L.L. Rue, III.

Tadpole begins feeding on algae at 7 days; skin fold (operculum) grows over external gill, leaving pore or spiracle on left side for exit of water (11 days)

Eye
Spiracle

Olfactory organ
External gills

Hatches at 6 days as tadpole with external gills; clings to submerged vegetation with sucker

Tail bud

Sucker

Development produces an embryo at 4 days with tail bud and early muscular movement; embryo living on yolk packed in gut

First cleavage occurs in 3-12 hours, depending on temperature; successive cleavages occur more rapidly

Three jelly coats of each egg swell with water, enclosing egg; egg rotates, bringing dark animal pole up and light, yolky vegetal pole down

Clasping by male stimulates female to lay 500 to 5000 eggs in one or more masses; male fertilizes eggs as they shed; egg laying takes about 10 minutes and occurs at night or early dawn, usually in March or April

Hind limbs appear first; then forelimbs emerge; internal gills replaced by lungs (75+ days)

Tail shortens by resorption and metamorphosis nearly complete at 90+ days; functional lungs; juvenile frog for 1 to 2 years

Sexually mature frog at 3 years

Amplexus
(Doggie Style)

Figure 24-21

Life cycle of a frog.

After fertilization the jelly layers absorb water and swell (Fig. 24-20). The eggs are laid in large masses, usually anchored to vegetation.

Development of the fertilized egg (zygote) begins almost immediately (Fig. 24-21). By repeated division (cleavage) the egg is converted into a hollow ball of cells (blastula). This undergoes continued differentiation to form an embryo with a tail bud. At 6 to 9 days, depending on the temperature, a tadpole hatches from the protective jelly coats that had surrounded the original fertilized egg.

At the time of hatching, the tadpole has a distinct head and body with a compressed tail. The mouth is located on the ventral side of the head and is provided with horny jaws for scraping off vegetation from objects for food. Behind the mouth is a ventral adhesive disc for clinging to objects. In front of the mouth are two deep pits, which later develop into the nostrils. Swellings are found on each side of the head, and these later become external gills. There are finally three pairs of external gills, which are later replaced by three pairs of internal gills within the gill slits. On the left side of the neck region is an opening, the **spiracle** (L., *spiraculum*, air hole), through which water flows after entering the mouth and passing the internal gills. The hindlegs appear first, while the forelimbs are hidden for a time by the folds of the operculum. During metamorphosis the tail is resorbed, the intestine becomes much shorter, the mouth undergoes a transformation into the adult condition, lungs develop, and the gills are resorbed. The leopard frog usually completes its metamorphosis within 3 months; the bullfrog takes 2 or 3 years to complete the process.

Migration of frogs and toads is correlated with their breeding habits. Males usually return to a pond or stream in advance of the females, which they then attract by their calls. Some salamanders are also known to have a strong homing instinct, returning year after year to the same pool for reproduction guided by olfactory cues. The initial stimulus for migration in many cases is attributable to a seasonal cycle in the gonads plus hormonal changes that increase the frogs' sensitivity to temperature and humidity changes.

Summary

The Amphibia are a transitional group, neither fully aquatic nor fully terrestrial. Although the group enjoyed a lengthy period of prominence in the late Paleozoic era, their aquatic mode of reproduction prevented a successful conquest of land. Most amphibians must return to water to lay their eggs, and their larvae are clearly fishlike. Direct development that omits the aquatic larval stage is not uncommon, however. Despite their insignificance as a group today, the amphibians made several important contributions to vertebrate evolution, which include a shift from gill to lung breathing, separation of pulmonary and systemic circulations, development of tetrapod limbs, restructuring of the skeleton to support the body in air, and redesigning of the senses of vision, smell, and hearing for use on land.

The modern amphibians consist of three evolutionary lines. The caecilians (order Gymnophiona) are a small tropical group of highly specialized, wormlike forms. The salamanders and newts (order Urodela) are tailed amphibians that have retained the generalized four-legged body plan of their Paleozoic ancestors. Fertilization is internal following spermatophore transfer from male to female. Some urodeles are paedomorphic, becoming sexually mature while retaining gills and other larval characteristics.

Longtail salamander *Eurycea longicauda,* a common plethydontid salamander.
Photograph by C.P. Hickman, Jr.

The most successful of the modern amphibians are the frogs and toads (order Salientia). All are specialized for a jumping mode of locomotion. Most inhabit wet habitats, but many toads and tree frogs are tolerant of arid environments. The integument is moist and contains numerous glands, some of which produce a poisonous irritant as protection against predators. Frogs are lung breathers, but the skin and mouth cavity are important supplementary avenues of gas exchange. A pulmonary circulation serves the lungs, and the heart is partly divided to keep pulmonary and systemic blood circuits mostly separated. All regions of the brain except the cerebellum are better developed in frogs and toads than in fishes. Most frogs have well-developed vocal cords, used principally by males to attract females. Fertilization is external. The eggs hatch into tadpole larvae that undergo a dramatic metamorphosis to the adult body form.

Selected references

Barbour, R.W. 1971. Amphibians and reptiles of Kentucky. Lexington, University of Kentucky Press. *Usefulness of this excellent survey of species, habitats, and life histories extends well beyond Kentucky.*

Cochran, D.H., and C.J. Goin. 1978. The new field book of reptiles and amphibians. New York, G.P. Putnam's Sons. *One of the most useful of several field guides available for identification of reptiles and amphibians. Other popular guides listed are those of Conant, King and Behler, Smith, and Stebbins.*

Conant, R. 1975. A field guide to reptiles and amphibians of Eastern and Central North America, ed. 2. (Peterson Field Guide Series.) Boston, Houghton Mifflin Co.

Ecker, A. 1889. The anatomy of the frog. (Translated from the original German by G. Haslam.) Oxford, Eng., Clarendon Press. (1971 reprint, Amsterdam, A. Asher and Co.) *Classical detailed anatomy.*

Goin, C.J., and O.B. Goin. 1978. Introduction to herpetology, ed. 3. San Francisco, W.H. Freeman & Co. Publishers. *Basic introductory text for the study of amphibians and reptiles.*

King, F.W., and J. Behler. 1979. The Audubon Society field guide to North American reptiles and amphibians. New York, Alfred A. Knopf, Inc.

Moore, J. (ed.). (Vols. 2 and 3 edited by B. Lofts.) 1960-1976. Physiology of the Amphibia. New York, Academic Press, Inc. *Valuable reference on the Amphibia for the advanced student.*

Noble, G.K. 1931. Biology of the Amphibia. New York, McGraw-Hill Book Co. *A dated but invaluable classic containing information to be found nowhere else.*

Oliver, J.A. 1955. The natural history of North American amphibians and reptiles. New York, D. Van Nostrand Co. *A good introduction to classification, distribution, and behavior of reptiles and amphibians.*

Porter, G. 1967. The world of the frog and the toad. Philadelphia, J.B. Lippincott Co. *Illustrated natural history.*

Porter, K.R. 1972. Herpetology. Philadelphia, W.B. Saunders Co. *Textbook of general biology of amphibians and reptiles.*

Smith, H.M. 1978. Amphibians of North America. (Golden Field Guide Series.) Racine, Wis., Western Publishing Co., Inc.

Stahl, B.J. 1974. Vertebrate history: problems in evolution. New York, McGraw-Hill Book Co. *A contemporary treatment of vertebrate paleontology. Good account of amphibian beginnings.*

Stebbins, R.C. 1966. A field guide to Western reptiles and amphibians. (Peterson Field Guide Series.) Boston, Houghton Mifflin Co.

Taylor, D.H., and S.I. Guttman (eds.). 1977. The reproductive biology of the amphibians. New York, Plenum Publishing Corp. *Symposium volume with contributed chapters on life history patterns and courtship, acoustic, and mating behavior.*

Twitty, V.C. 1966. Of scientists and salamanders. San Francisco, W.H. Freeman & Co. Publishers. *Delightfully written account of the author's personal study of the experimental biology of salamanders and newts.*

Wright, A.H., and A.A. Wright. 1949. Handbook of frogs of the United States and Canada, ed. 3. Ithaca, N.Y., Comstock Publishing Associates. *A volume that has, with time, become a standard reference work for the study of frogs.*

CHAPTER 25

THE REPTILES

Phylum Chordata
Class Reptilia

A chameleon snares a dragonfly. After cautiously edging close to its target, the chameleon suddenly lunges forward, anchoring its tail and feet to a branch. A split second later, it launches its sticky-tipped, foot-long tongue to trap the prey. The eyes of this common European chameleon *(Chamaeleo chamaeleon)* are swiveled forward to provide binocular vision and excellent depth perception.

Photograph by J. Andrada.

The class Reptilia (rep-til'e-a) (L., *repere,* to creep) are the first truly terrestrial vertebrates. With some 7000 species (approximately 300 species in the United States and Canada) occupying a great variety of aquatic and terrestrial habitats, they are clearly a successful group. Nevertheless, reptiles are perhaps remembered best for what they once were, rather than for what they are now. The age of reptiles, which lasted 100 million years, encompassing the Jurassic and Cretaceous periods of the Mesozoic era, saw the appearance of a great radiation of reptiles, many of huge stature and awesome appearance, that completely dominated life on land. Then they suddenly declined.

Of the dozen or so principal groups of reptiles that evolved, four remain today. The most successful of these are the lizards and snakes of the order Squamata. A second group is the crocodilians; having survived for 200 million years, they may finally be made extinct by humans. To a third group belong the turtles of the order Testudines, an ancient group that has somehow survived and remained mostly unchanged from its early reptile ancestors. The last group is a relic stock represented today by a sole survivor, the tuatara of New Zealand.

Reptiles are easily distinguished from amphibians by several adaptations that permit them to live in arid regions and in the sea: habitats barred to amphibians by their reproductive requirements. Reptiles have a dry, scaly skin, almost free of glands, that resists desiccation. Most important, reptiles lay their eggs on land; amphibians must lay their eggs in fresh water or in moist places. This seemingly simple difference was, in fact, a remarkable evolutionary achievement that was to have a profound impact on subsequent vertebrate evolution. To abandon totally an aquatic life, there evolved a sophisticated internally fertilized egg containing a complete set of life support systems. This **shelled egg** (known also as an **amniotic** egg because of the membranous amnion that encloses the embryo) could be laid on dry land. Within, the embryo floats and develops in an aquatic environment. It is provided with a yolk sac containing its food supply; another membrane, the allantois, serves as a surface for gas exchange through the calcareous or parchmentlike shell; the allantoic membrane also encloses a chamber for storing toxic wastes that accumulate during development.

The early reptiles that developed this "land egg" must certainly have enjoyed an immediate advantage over the amphibians. They could hide their eggs in a protected situation away from water—and away from the numerous creatures that fed freely on the eggs provided by amphibians each spring. With the evolution of this ultimate adaptation, conquest of land by the vertebrates was possible.

ORIGIN AND ADAPTIVE RADIATION OF REPTILES

Biologists generally agree that reptiles arose from the labyrinthodont amphibians sometime before the Permian period, which began approximately 280 million years ago. The oldest "stem reptiles" were the captorhinomorphs (Gr., *kaptō,* to gulp down, + *rhinē,* file, + *morphē,* form) (Fig. 25-1). These were small, lizard-like animals that probably fed mainly on insects, which were undergoing an adaptive radiation at the same time and were already numerous. Early in their evolution, the captorhinomorphs rather quickly (in geological time sense) diverged into several specialized lineages and entered a long and spectacular evolutionary history that carried them to the present. Their descendants included the dinosaurs,

Figure 25-1

Evolution of the reptiles. The transition from certain labyrinthodont amphibians to reptiles occurred in the late Paleozoic to Mesozoic eras. This transition was effected by the development of an amniotic egg that made land existence possible, although this egg may well have developed before the earliest reptiles had ventured far on land. Explosive radiation by the reptiles may have been due partly to the increased variety of ecological habitats into which they could move. The fossil record shows that lines arising from stem reptiles led to marine reptiles, dinosaurs, pterosaurs, crocodilians, turtles, lizards and snakes, and rhynchosaurs. Another radiation led to the mammals. Of this great assemblage, the only reptiles now in existence belong to four orders: Testudines, Crocodilia, Squamata, and Rhynchocephalia. How are the mighty fallen!

Classical views of the dinosaurs and other Mesozoic reptiles as witless, cold-blooded beasts with inferior adaptability have recently been undergoing revision. Many biologists believe that the dinosaurs were alert creatures showing complex behavior equal to that of today's lizards and crocodilians. Some certainly traveled in organized family groups. Speculations drawn from ecological and paleontological data that the dinosaurs were warm blooded (endothermic) have generally been discounted, although because of their large size the dinosaurs probably enjoyed fairly stable body temperatures.

Perhaps the most exotic hypothesis offered to explain the great extinction of animals at the end of the Mesozoic era is the recent suggestion of Alvarez and colleagues (1980) that the earth was struck by a large asteroid, perhaps 10 km (6 miles) in diameter. The impact of such a large object would inject an enormous quantity of rock dust into the stratosphere where it would circle the globe for months, turning day into night. The absence of sunlight would shut off photosynthesis and attack food chains at their base. Both marine algae and land plants would die, and all herbivorous and carnivorous animals would become extinct except those feeding on insects or decaying vegetation. The hypothesis is supported by the discovery of significant deposits of extraterrestrial iridium in sedimentary rocks at the precise Mesozoic-Cenozoic boundary 63 million years ago. Moreover, the fossil record reveals that many groups of marine microorganisms that depended directly or indirectly on photosynthesis, as well as all animals larger than 25 kg, became extinct at this time.

marine reptiles, flying reptiles (pterosaurs [Gr., *pteron*, wing, + *sauros*, lizard]), and mammal-like reptiles (therapsids [Gr., *theraps*, attendant, + *ida*, suffix]), which produced the ancestral stock of the mammals. All were highly successful groups.

The adaptive radiation of reptiles, especially pronounced in the Triassic period (which followed the Permian), corresponded to the appearance of new ecological habitats. These were provided by the climatic and geological changes that were taking place at that time, such as a variable climate from hot to cold, mountain building and terrain transformations, and a varied assortment of plant life.

The Mesozoic era was the age of the great ruling reptiles. Then suddenly they disappeared near the close of the Cretaceous period approximately 65 to 80 million years ago. What caused their demise? Many changes were occurring during the Cretaceous period: Modern flowering plants were spreading rapidly, as were the aggressive and intelligent mammals. The climate became cooler and much more variable. In general, the modern fauna and flora as we know them today were becoming well established, and the dinosaurs were not sufficiently adaptable to survive. Their extinction probably resulted from the combined effect of climatic and ecological factors, excessive specialization, and low reproductive potential. But this is speculation, and debate continues among paleontologists. Why did some reptiles survive against the fierce competition of the mammals? Turtles had their protective shells; snakes and lizards evolved in habitats of dense forests and rocks where they could meet the competition of any tetrapod; and crocodiles, because of their size, stealth, and aggressiveness, had few enemies in their aquatic habitats.

CHARACTERISTICS

1. Body varied in shape, compact in some, elongated in others; **body covered with an exoskeleton of horny epidermal scales** with the addition sometimes of bony dermal plates; **integument with few glands**
2. Limbs paired, **usually with five toes,** and adapted for climbing, running, or paddling; absent in snakes and some lizards
3. Skeleton well ossified; ribs with sternum forming a complete thoracic basket; **skull with one occipital condyle**
4. Respiration by lungs; **no gills;** cloaca used for respiration by some; branchial arches in embryonic life
5. **Three-chambered heart; crocodiles with four-chambered heart;** usually one pair of aortic arches
6. Ectothermic; some lizards and snakes behaviorally thermoregulate
7. **Metanephric kidney (paired); uric acid main nitrogenous waste**
8. Nervous system with the optic lobes on the dorsal side of brain; **12 pairs of cranial nerves** in addition to nervus terminalis
9. Sexes separate; fertilization internal
10. **Eggs covered with calcareous or leathery shells;** extraembryonic membranes (**amnion, chorion, yolk sac,** and **allantois**) present during embryonic life

CLASSIFICATION

Order Testudines (tes-tu'din-eez) (L., *testudo*, tortoise) (**Chelonia**)—turtles (330 species). Body in a bony case of dermal plates with dorsal carapace and ventral plastron; jaws without teeth but with horny sheaths; quadrate immovable; vertebrae and ribs fused to shell; anus a longitudinal slit.

Suborder Cryptodira (krip'to-dy'ra) (Gr., *kryptos*, hidden, + *deirē*, neck). Hidden-necked turtles; head withdrawn into shell by flexing neck ventrally. Ten families: Chelydridae (snapping turtles), Platysternidae (big-headed turtle), Emydidae (common terrapins), Kinosternidae (musk and mud turtles), Testudinidae (tortoises), Cheloniidae (sea turtles), Trionychidae (soft-shelled turtles), Dermochelyidae (leatherback turtle), Dermatemydidae (river turtles), Carettochelyidae (pitted-shelled turtles).

 Suborder Pleurodira (ploor'o-dy'ra) (Gr., *pleura*, side, + *deirē*, neck). Side-necked turtles; head withdrawn into shell by bending neck sideways. Two families: Chelidae (snake-necked turtles), Pelomedusidae (pelomedusid turtles).

Order Squamata (squa-ma'ta) (L., *squamatus*, scaly, + *ata*, characterized by)—snakes (2700 species), lizards (3000 species), amphisbaenids (130 species). Skin of horny epidermal scales or plates, which is shed; teeth attached to jaws; quadrate freely movable; vertebrae usually concave in front; anus a transverse slit.

 Suborder Sauria (sawr'e-a) (Gr., *sauros*, lizard) (**Lacertilia**)—**lizards.** Body slender, usually with four limbs; rami of lower jaw fused; eyelids movable; copulatory organs paired. Nineteen families; major ones are Gekkonidae (geckos), Iguanidae (New World lizards), Agamidae (Old World lizards), Chamaeleontidae (chameleons), Lacertidae (Old World lizards), Scincidae (skinks), Helodermatidae (poisonous lizards), Anguidae (plated lizards).

 Suborder Serpentes (sur-pen'tes) (L., *serpere*, to creep) (**Ophidia**)—**snakes.** Body elongated; limbs and ear openings absent; mandibles jointed anteriorly by ligaments; eyes lidless and immovable; tongue bifid and protrusible; teeth conical and on jaws and roof of mouth. Eleven families; major ones are Leptotyphlopidae (blind snakes), Boidae (boas and pythons), Colubridae (common snakes), Elapidae (poisonous fixed-fang snakes), Viperidae (vipers and pit vipers).

 Suborder Amphisbaenia (am'fis-bee'nee-a) (L., *amphis*, on both sides, + *baina*, to walk)—**worm lizards.** Body elongate and of nearly uniform diameter; short tail; no legs (except one genus with short front legs); limb girdles vestigial; eyes hidden beneath skin; only one lung. Two families: Trogonophidae (ovoviviparous worm lizards), Amphisbaenidae (oviparous worm lizards).

Order Crocodilia (croc'o-dil'e-a) (L., *crocodilus*, crocodile, + *ia*, pl. suffix) (**Loricata**). Four-chambered heart; vertebrae usually concave in front; forelimbs usually with five digits, hindlimbs with four digits; quadrate immovable; anus a longitudinal slit. Two families: Crocodylidae (crocodiles, alligators, caimans), Gavialidae (gavial) (25 species).

Order Rhynchocephalia (rin'ko-se-fay'le-a) (Gr., *rhynchos*, snout, + *kephalē*, head). Vertebrae biconcave; quadrate immovable; parietal eye fairly well developed and easily seen; anus a transverse slit. *Sphenodon* only species existing.

—— Characteristics of Reptiles That Distinguish Them from Amphibians

 1. **Reptiles have tough, dry, scaly skin offering protection against desiccation and physical injury.** The skin consists of a thin **epidermis**, shed periodically, and a much thicker, well-developed **dermis**. The dermis is provided with **chromatophores**, the color-bearing cells that give many lizards and snakes their colorful hues. It is also the layer that, unfortunately for their bearers, is converted into alligator and snakeskin leather, so esteemed for expensive pocketbooks and shoes. The characteristic **scales** of reptiles are formed largely of keratin. They are derived mostly from the epidermis and thus are not homologous to fish scales, which are bony, dermal structures. In some reptiles, such as alligators, the scales remain throughout life, growing gradually to replace wear. In others, such as snakes and lizards, new scales grow beneath the old, which are then shed at intervals. Turtles add new layers of keratin under the old layers of the platelike scutes, which are modified scales. In snakes the old skin (epidermis and scales) is turned inside out when discarded; lizards split out of the old skin leaving it mostly intact and right side out, or it may slough off in pieces.

 2. **The shelled egg of reptiles contains food and protective membranes for supporting embryonic development on dry land.** The great significance of this

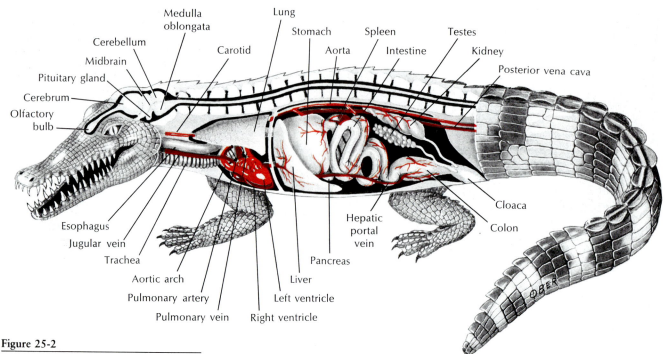

Medulla oblongata
Lung
Cerebellum
Stomach
Spleen
Testes
Midbrain
Carotid
Aorta
Intestine
Kidney
Pituitary gland
Cerebrum
Olfactory bulb
Posterior vena cava
Esophagus
Jugular vein
Trachea
Aortic arch
Pulmonary artery
Pulmonary vein
Liver
Left ventricle
Right ventricle
Pancreas
Hepatic portal vein
Cloaca
Colon

Figure 25-2

Internal structures of male crocodile.

adaptation was described earlier in this chapter. The shelled egg is illustrated and described in some detail on pp. 874 and 875. Amphibian eggs have a gelatinous covering and must be protected from drying. The appearance of the shelled egg marked a great division between amphibians and reptiles and, probably more than any other adaptation, contributed to the decline of amphibians and the ascendance of reptiles.

3. **Reptiles have some form of copulatory organ, permitting internal fertilization.** Internal fertilization is obviously a requirement for a shelled egg, since the sperm must reach the egg before the egg is enclosed. Sperm from the paired testes are carried by the vasa deferentia to the copulatory organ, which is an evagination of the cloacal wall. The female system consists of paired ovaries and oviducts. The glandular walls of the oviducts secrete albumin and shells for the large eggs.

4. **Reptiles have a more efficient circulatory system and higher blood pressures than amphibians.** In all reptiles the right atrium, which receives unoxygenated blood from the body, is completely partitioned from the left atrium, which receives oxygenated blood from the lungs. In the crocodilians there are two completely separated ventricles as well (Fig. 25-2); in other reptiles the ventricle is incompletely separated. The crocodilians are thus the first vertebrates with a four-chambered heart. Even in reptiles with incomplete separation of the ventricles, flow patterns within the heart prevent admixture of pulmonary (oxygenated) and systemic (unoxygenated) blood; all reptiles therefore have two functionally separate circulations.

5. **Reptile lungs are better developed than those of amphibians.** Reptiles depend almost exclusively on the lungs for gas exchange, supplemented by pharyngeal membrane respiration in some of the aquatic turtles. The lungs have a larger respiratory surface in reptiles than amphibians, and air is *sucked* into the lungs, as in higher vertebrates, rather than *forced* in by mouth muscles, as in the amphibians. Skin breathing, so important to most amphibians, has been completely abandoned by the reptiles.

Figure 25-3

Spotted turtle *Clemmys guttata*. This pond turtle of the eastern United States is most frequently sighted in the spring while basking on a log or rock and is seldom seen at other seasons. It is carnivorous.

Photograph by C.P. Hickman, Jr.

6. The reptilian kidneys are of the advanced metanephros type with their own passageways (ureters) to the exterior. The kidneys are very efficient in producing small volumes of urine, thus conserving precious water. Nitrogenous wastes are excreted as uric acid, rather than urea or ammonia. Uric acid has a low solubility and precipitates out of solution readily; as a result the urine of many reptiles is a semisolid paste.

7. All reptiles, except the limbless members, have better body support than the amphibians and more efficiently designed limbs for travel on land. Many of the dinosaurs walked on powerful hindlimbs alone.

8. The reptilian nervous system is considerably more advanced than the amphibian. Although the reptile's brain is small, the **cerebrum** is increased in size relative to the rest of the brain. The crocodilians have the first true cerebral cortex (neopallium). Central nervous system connections are more advanced, permitting complex kinds of behavior unknown in the amphibians. Sense organs in general are well developed. All reptiles have a middle and an inner ear, but the sense of hearing is poorly developed in most. The lateral line system is entirely lost. Jacobson's organ, a unique sense organ, is a separate part of the nasal sac and communicates with the mouth; it is especially well developed in snakes and lizards. It is innervated by a branch of the olfactory nerve and is used in smelling the food in the mouth cavity. This organ in some form is found in other groups, including the amphibians.

CHARACTERISTICS AND NATURAL HISTORY OF REPTILIAN ORDERS
Turtles—Order Testudines (Chelonia)

The turtles are an ancient group that has plodded on from the Triassic period to the present with very little change in their early basic morphology. They are enclosed in shells consisting of a dorsal **carapace** (Sp., *carapacho,* covering) and a ventral **plastron** (Fr., breastplate) (Fig. 25-3). Clumsy and unlikely as they appear to be within their protective shells, they are nonetheless a varied and successful group that seems able to accommodate to human presence. The shell is so much a part of the animal that it is built in with the thoracic vertebrae and ribs. The shell is composed of two layers: an outer horny layer of keratin and an inner layer of bone. New layers of keratin are laid down beneath the old as the turtle grows and ages.

The terms "turtle," "tortoise," and "terrapin" are applied variously to different members of the turtle order. In North American usage, they are all correctly called turtles. The term "tortoise" is frequently given to land turtles, especially the large forms. British usage of the terms is different: "tortoise" is the inclusive term, whereas "turtle" is applied only to the aquatic members.

Figure 25-4

Mating Galápagos tortoises. During copulation, males make loud grunting roars that may be heard for long distances.
Photograph by C.P. Hickman, Jr.

Figure 25-5

Florida softshell turtle *Trionyx spiniferus* laying eggs in freshly dug nest.
Photograph by C.P. Hickman, Jr.

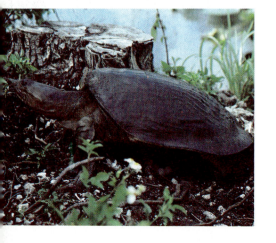

One consequence of living in a rigid shell with fused ribs is that a turtle cannot expand its chest to breathe. Turtles solved this problem in their own way, by employing certain of the abdominal and pectoral muscles as a "diaphragm." Air is drawn in by contracting limb flank muscles to make the body cavity larger. Exhalation is also active and is accomplished by drawing the shoulder girdle back into the shell, thus compressing the viscera and forcing air out of the lungs. Many water turtles gain enough oxygen by just pumping water in and out of the mouth cavity; this enables them to remain submerged for long periods when inactive. When active they must lung-breathe more frequently.

A turtle's brain, like that of other reptiles, is small, never exceeding 1% of the body weight. The cerebrum, however, is larger than that of an amphibian, and turtles are able to learn a maze about as quickly as a rat. Turtles have both a middle and an inner ear, but sound perception is poor. Not unexpectedly, therefore, turtles are virtually mute (the biblical "voice of the turtle" refers to the turtledove), although many tortoises utter grunting or roaring sounds during mating (Fig. 25-4). Compensating for poor hearing are a good sense of smell, acute vision, and color perception evidently as good as that of humans.

Turtles are oviparous. Fertilization is internal and all turtles, even the marine forms, bury their shelled, amniotic eggs in the ground (Fig. 25-5). Usually considerable care is exercised in constructing the nest, but once the eggs are deposited and covered, the female deserts them.

The great marine turtles, buoyed by their aquatic environment, may reach 2 m in length and 725 kg in weight. One is the leatherback. The green turtle, so named because of its greenish body fat, may exceed 360 kg, although most individuals of this economically valuable and heavily exploited species seldom live long enough to reach anything approaching this size. Some land tortoises may weigh several hundred kilograms, such as the giant tortoises of the Galápagos

Islands that so intrigued Darwin during his visit there in 1835. Most tortoises are rather slow moving; an hour of determined trudging carries a large Galápagos tortoise approximately 300 m. Their low metabolism probably explains their longevity, for some are believed to live more than 150 years.

Turtles are the Methuselahs of vertebrates, and individuals of five species are known to have lived a century or more. However, except for longevity records based on specimens in captivity, reports of vast life spans are of dubious value; a box tortoise captured some years ago with "1850" carved on its plastron is an example of evidence that should be accepted with a healthy measure of skepticism.

The shell, like a medieval coat of armor, offers obvious advantages. The head and appendages can be drawn in for protection. The familiar box tortoise (*Terrapene carolina*) has a plastron that is hinged, forming two movable parts that can be pulled up against the carapace so tightly that one cannot force a knife blade between the shells. Some turtles, such as the large eastern snapping turtle (*Chelydra serpentina*), have reduced shells, making complete withdrawal for protection quite impossible. Snappers, however, have another formidable defense, as their name implies (Fig. 25-6). Ferocious and short tempered, they are often referred to as the "tigers of the pond." They are entirely carnivorous, living on fish, frogs, waterfowl, or almost anything that comes within reach of their powerful jaws. The alligator snapper lures unwary fish into its mouth with a "bait" (Fig. 25-7). Snappers are wholly aquatic and come ashore only to lay their eggs.

Figure 25-6

Eastern snapper *Chelydra serpentina* demonstrates why it should be treated with respect.
Photograph by J.H. Gerard.

Lizards, Snakes, and Worm Lizards—Order Squamata

The lizards and snakes of the order Squamata are the most recent products of reptile evolution and by all odds the most successful, comprising approximately 95% of all known living reptiles. The modern lizards began their adaptive radiation during the Cretaceous period of the Mesozoic era when the great dinosaurs were at the climax of their dominance of land. Lizards were successful because of their adaptability, which allowed them to occupy a variety of habitats and adopt diverse body forms and functional specializations.

Snakes appeared during the late Cretaceous period, probably from a group of lizards whose descendants include the Gila monster and monitor lizards, although the fossil record of snakes is poor. Legless species have evolved in other reptile groups that took up a burrowing existence. But none has refined this specialized life-style as have the snakes, which have radiated into terrestrial, aquatic, and arboreal niches. Two adaptations in particular characterize all snakes. One is the extreme elongation of the body and accompanying displacement and rearrangement of the internal organs. The other is the highly mobile jaw apparatus that enables snakes to swallow prey much larger than the snake's own diameter.

The order Squamata is divided into suborders Sauria (Lacertilia), the lizards; Serpentes (Ophidia), the snakes; and Amphisbaenia, the worm lizards. Structural features are even more reduced in the amphisbaenians than they are in snakes. Most amphisbaenians are limbless and have both eyes and ears completely hidden beneath the skin.

Figure 25-7

Alligator snapping turtle *Macroclemys temmincki*, although larger than the eastern snapper, is less active—and for good reason. It lies on the bottom, mouth agape, luring its prey by undulating a wormlike protrusion from its tongue.
Photograph by P.C.H. Pritchard.

Figure 25-8

Tokay *(Gekko gecko)* of Southeast Asia may reach 35 cm (14 inches) in length and is the most aggressive of the geckos. This species has a true voice and is named after the strident, repeated *to-kay, to-kay* call.

Photograph by J.H. Gerard.

Figure 25-9

True iguana of tropical America, *Iguana iguana.* It prefers forested habitats near streams into which it may jump if disturbed.

Photograph by K. Sandved.

Figure 25-10

Marine iguanas *Amblyrhynchus cristatus* of the Galápagos Islands. This is the only marine lizard in the world. It has special salt-removing glands in the eye orbits and long claws that enable it to cling to the bottom while feeding on seaweed, its exclusive diet. It may dive to depths exceeding 10 m (35 feet) and remain submerged more than 30 minutes.

Photograph by C.P. Hickman, Jr.

Lizards—suborder Sauria

The lizards are an extremely diversified group, including terrestrial, burrowing, aquatic, arboreal, and aerial members. Among the more familiar groups in this varied suborder are the **geckos** (Fig. 25-8), small, agile, mostly nocturnal forms with adhesive toe pads that enable them to walk upside down and on vertical surfaces; the **iguanas** (Fig. 25-9), New World lizards, often brightly colored with ornamental crests, frills, and throat fans, a group that includes the remarkable marine iguana of the Galápagos Islands (Fig. 25-10); the **skinks,** with elongate bodies and reduced limbs; and the **chameleons,** a group of arboreal lizards, mostly of Africa and Madagascar. The chameleons are entertaining creatures that catch insects with the sticky-tipped tongue that can be flicked accurately and rapidly to a distance greater than their own body length.

Unlike turtles, snakes, and crocodilians, which have distinctive body forms

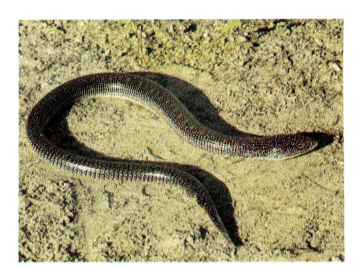

Figure 25-11

Glass lizard *Ophisaurus* sp. of the south-eastern United States. This legless lizard feels stiff and brittle to the touch and has an extremely long, fragile tail that readily fractures when the animal is struck or seized. Most specimens, such as this one, have only a partly regenerated tip to replace a much longer tail previously lost. Glass lizards can be readily distinguished from snakes by the deep, flexible groove running along each side of the body. They feed on worms, insects, spiders, birds' eggs, and small reptiles.
Photograph by L.L. Rue, III.

and ways of life, the lizards have radiated extensively into a variety of habitats and reveal a bewildering array of functional and behavioral specializations. The great majority of lizards have four limbs and relatively short bodies, but in many the limbs are degenerate, and a few such as the glass lizards (Fig. 25-11) are completely limbless.

Despite their diversity of form, lizards as a group bear a number of characteristics that distinguish them from snakes. One is the lower jaw. Even in limbless forms the two halves are firmly united at the mandibular symphysis. This makes it impossible for lizards to swallow oversize meals as can snakes, which have "floating" jaw elements. Most lizards have movable eyelids, whereas a snake's eyes are permanently covered with a transparent cap. Lizards have keen vision for daylight, although one group, the nocturnal geckos, has pure rod retinas. Most lizards have an external ear that snakes lack. The inner ear of lizards is variable in structure, but as with other reptiles, hearing does not play an important role in the lives of most lizards. Geckos are exceptions because the males are strongly vocal (to announce territory and discourage other males from approaching), and it is reasonable to assume that they can hear their own vocalizations. Other species of lizards vocalize in defensive behavior.

Lizards have teeth, but in no species are they developed into fangs, and only two species, the Gila monster and the Mexican bearded lizard, are known to be venomous. Many lizards, such as geckos, have instead evolved a novel defense tactic at the opposite end of the body: they drop their tails when seized by a predator. Tail-dropping lizards have a special adaptation of the tail vertebrae and surrounding musculature that allows a vertebra to simply break apart at a special fracture point. The predator is left with a wildly contorting tail while the owner escapes, or if the lizard itself has been caught, the predator may be so distracted by the whipping (and often brightly colored) appendage that it may in its confusion release the body and go after the tail. A gecko can completely regenerate its lost tail in about 7 weeks.

Many lizards live in the world's hot and arid regions, aided by several adaptations for desert life. Since their skin lacks glands, water loss by this avenue is much reduced. They produce a semisolid urine with a high content of crystalline uric acid. This is an excellent adaptation for conserving water and is found in other groups living successfully in arid habitats (birds, insects, and pulmonate snails). Some, such as the Gila monster of the southwestern United States deserts,

Figure 25-12

Gila monster *Heloderma suspectum* of southwestern United States desert regions. This lizard and the congeneric Mexican beaded lizard are the only venomous lizards known. These brightly colored, clumsy-looking lizards feed principally on birds' eggs, nestling birds and mammals, and insects. Unlike poisonous snakes, the gila monster secretes venom from glands in its lower jaw. The bite is painful to humans but seldom fatal.
Photograph by L.L. Rue, III.

Figure 25-13

Black rat snake *Elaphe obsoleta obsoleta* swallowing a chipmunk.
Photograph by L.L. Rue III.

store fat in their tails, which they draw on during drought to provide both energy and metabolic water (Fig. 25-12).

Especially interesting are the techniques by which desert lizards maintain a relatively constant body temperature, using what physiologists term "behavioral thermoregulation." Lizards, like other reptiles, are **ectothermic;** if a lizard is placed under constant temperature conditions in the laboratory, its body temperature soon becomes indistinguishable from that of its surroundings. But in their natural environment where surrounding temperatures vary widely, lizards modulate their body temperature by exploiting hour-to-hour changes in thermal flux from the sun. In the early morning they emerge from their burrows and bask in the sun with their bodies flattened to absorb the heat. As the day warms, they turn to face the sun to reduce the body area exposed, and they raise their bodies from the hot substrate. In the hottest part of the day they may retreat to their burrows. Later they emerge to bask as the sun sinks lower and the air temperature drops. These behavioral patterns help to maintain a relatively steady body temperature of 36° to 39° C while the air temperature is varying between 29° and 44° C. Some lizards can tolerate intense midday heat without shelter. The desert iguana of the southwestern United States prefers a body temperature of 42° C when active and can tolerate a rise to 47° C, a temperature that is lethal to all birds and mammals and most other lizards. The term "cold blooded" clearly does not apply to these animals!

Snakes—suborder Serpentes

Snakes are entirely limbless and lack both the pectoral and pelvic girdles (the latter persists as a vestige in pythons and boas). The numerous vertebrae of snakes, shorter and wider than those of tetrapods, permit quick lateral undulations through grass and over rough terrain. The ribs increase rigidity of the vertebral column, providing more resistance to lateral stresses. The elevation of the neural spine gives the numerous muscles more leverage.

The highly specialized skull and feeding apparatus of snakes, which enable them to eat prey several times their own diameter, are perhaps their most remarkable specialization. The two halves of the lower jaw (mandibles) are joined only by muscles and skin, allowing them to spread widely apart. Furthermore, many of the

Figure 25-14

Parrot snake *Leptophis ahaetulla*. The slender body of this Central American tree snake is an adaptation for sliding along branches without weighing them down.
Photograph by C.P. Hickman, Jr.

skull bones are so loosely articulated that the entire skull can flex asymmetrically to accommodate oversize prey (Fig. 25-13). Since the snake must keep breathing during the slow process of swallowing, the tracheal opening is thrust forward between the two mandibles.

The cornea of the snake's eye is permanently protected with a transparent membrane, which, together with a lack of eyeball mobility, gives snakes the cold, unblinking stare that most people find so unnerving. Most snakes have relatively poor vision, with the tree-living snakes of the tropical forest being a conspicuous exception (Fig. 25-14). Some arboreal snakes possess excellent binocular vision that helps them track prey through branches where scent trails would be impossible to follow.

It was mentioned earlier that snakes lack any superficial indication of an ear. This, together with the absence of any obvious response to aerial sounds, led to the widespread opinion that snakes are totally deaf. But snakes do have internal ears, and recent work has shown quite clearly that within a limited range of low frequencies (100 to 700 Hz), hearing in snakes compares favorably with that of most lizards. Snakes are also quite sensitive to vibrations carried in the ground.

Nevertheless, for most snakes it is the chemical senses and not vision and hearing that are employed to hunt their prey. In addition to the usual olfactory areas in the nose, which are not well developed, there are **Jacobson's organs,** a pair of pitlike organs in the roof of the mouth. These are lined with an olfactory epithelium and are richly innervated. The forked tongue, flicking through the air, picks up the scent particles and conveys them to the mouth; the tongue is then drawn past Jacobson's organs or the tips of the forked tongue are inserted directly into the organs (Fig. 25-15). Information is then transmitted to the brain where scents are identified.

As with lizards, the snake's body is entirely covered with a tough, impervious skin. The skin is not elastic, and when required to stretch, as it must after the snake has enjoyed a hefty meal, it does so in a novel manner. The hard scales are set together, sometimes overlapping like shingles on a roof, with the skin folded inward between the scales. When the snake swallows a large object, the skin folds are pulled out straight, leaving the scales separated like islands on the skin.

Locomotion is an obvious problem for the legless animal, and snakes have discovered several solutions. The most typical pattern of movement is **lateral**

Figure 25-15

Timber rattlesnake *Crotalus horridus* flicks its tongue to smell its surroundings. Scent particles trapped on the tongue's surface are transferred to Jacobson's organs, olfactory organs in the roof of the mouth. Note the heat-sensitive pit organ between the nostril and eye.

Photograph by L.L. Rue, III.

A

0 sec   1 sec   2 sec

Lateral undulation

Figure 25-16

Snake locomotion. **A,** Lateral undulation. **B,** Concertina motion. **C,** Rectilinear motion.

B

Concertina motion

C

Move Contract Fix Stretch Move

Rectilinear motion

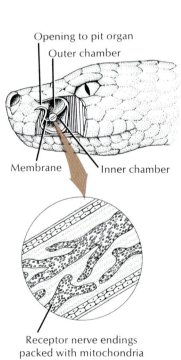

Opening to pit organ
Outer chamber
Membrane   Inner chamber

Receptor nerve endings packed with mitochondria

Figure 25-17

Pit organ of rattlesnake, a pit viper. Cutaway shows location of a deep membrane that divides the pit into inner and outer chambers. Heat-sensitive nerve endings are concentrated in the membrane.

Figure 25-18

Young cottonmouth, or water moccasin (*Agkistrodon piscivorus piscivorus*), venomous denizen of swamps, rivers, and ditches in the southeastern United States. Old adults lose the distinctive crossband coloration, becoming completely dark.
Photograph by C.P. Hickman, Jr.

undulation (Fig. 25-16, *A*). Movement follows an S-shaped path, with the snake propelling itself by exerting lateral force against surface irregularities. The snake seems to "flow," since the moving loops appear stationary with respect to the ground. Lateral undulatory movement is fast and efficient under most but not all circumstances. **Concertina movement** (Fig. 25-16, *B*) enables a snake to move in a narrow passage, as when climbing a tree by using the irregular channels in the bark. The snake extends forward while bracing S-shaped loops against the sides of the channel. To advance in a straight line as when stalking prey, many snakes use **rectilinear movement** (Fig. 25-16, *C*), a form of locomotion that utilizes the large abdominal scutes. Two or three zones of scutes make frictional contact with the ground, while the rest of the body is moved forward. This effective but slow movement requires very loose, flexible skin and special muscle and bone structure. **Sidewinding** is a fourth form of movement that enables desert vipers to move with surprising speed across loose, sandy surfaces with minimum surface contact. The sidewinder rattlesnake moves by throwing its body forward in loops with its body lying at an angle of about 60 degrees to its direction of travel.

Snakes of the subfamily Crotalinae within the family Viperidae are called **pit vipers** because of special heat-sensitive pits on their heads, between the nostrils and the eyes (Figs. 25-15 and 25-17). All of the best-known North American poisonous snakes are pit vipers, such as the several species of rattlesnakes, the water moccasin (Fig. 25-18), and the copperhead. The pits are supplied with a dense packing of free nerve endings from the fifth cranial nerve. They respond to radiant energy in the long-wave infrared (5000 to 15,000 nm) and are especially sensitive to the heat emitted by the warm-bodied birds and mammals that comprise their food (infrared wavelengths of about 10,000 nm). Some measurements suggest that the pit organs can distinguish temperature differences of only 0.003° C from a radiating surface. Pit vipers use the pit organs to track warm-blooded prey and to aim strikes with great accuracy, as effectively in total darkness as in daylight. Boa constrictors and pythons also have heat receptors, but the anatomy is quite different from that of pit vipers, suggesting that they probably evolved independently.

All pit vipers have a pair of teeth on the maxillary bones modified as fangs. These lie in a membrane sheath when the mouth is closed. When the viper strikes, a special muscle and bone lever system erects the fangs when the mouth opens

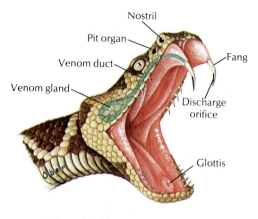

Nostril
Pit organ
Venom duct
Venom gland
Fang
Discharge orifice
Glottis

Figure 25-19

Head of rattlesnake showing the venom apparatus.

The LD₅₀ (median lethal dose) is a standardized procedure originally developed by pharmacologists for assaying the toxicity of drugs. In practice, small samples of laboratory animals, usually mice, are exposed to a graded series of doses of the drug or toxin. The dose that kills 50% of the animals in the test period is recorded as the LD_{50}.

(Fig. 25-19). The fangs are driven into the prey by the thrust, and venom is injected into the wound through a channel in the fangs.

A pit viper immediately releases its prey after the bite and follows it until it is paralyzed or dies. Then the snake swallows the prey whole. Approximately 1500 people are bitten by pit vipers each year in the United States, and of those, approximately 45 die.

The tropical and subtropical countries are the homes of most species of snakes, both of the venomous and nonvenomous varieties. Even there, less than one third of snakes are venomous. The nonvenomous snakes kill their prey by constriction or by biting and swallowing. Their diet tends to be restricted, many feeding principally on rodents, whereas others feed on fishes, frogs, and insects. Some African, Indian, and Neotropical snakes are egg eaters.

Poisonous snakes are usually divided into four groups based on the type of fangs. The vipers (family Viperidae) have highly developed tubular fangs at the front of the mouth; the group includes the American pit vipers previously mentioned and the Old World true vipers, which lack facial heat-sensing pits. Among the latter are the common European adder and the African puff adder. A second family of poisonous snakes (family Elapidae) has short, permanently erect fangs so that the venom must be injected by chewing. In this group are the cobras (Fig. 25-21), mambas, coral snakes, and kraits. The highly poisonous sea snakes are usually placed in a third family (Hydrophiidae). The very large family Colubridae, which contains most of the familiar (and nonvenomous) snakes, does include at least two poisonous snakes that have been responsible for human fatalities: the African boomslang and the African vine snake. Both are rear-fanged snakes that normally use their venom to quiet struggling prey.

The saliva of all harmless snakes possesses limited toxic qualities, and it is logical that evolution should have stressed this toxic tendency. Snake venoms have traditionally been divided into two types. The neurotoxic type acts mainly on the nervous systems, affecting the optic nerves (causing blindness) or the phrenic nerve of the diaphragm (causing paralysis of respiration). The hemolytic type breaks down the red blood corpuscles and blood vessels and produces extensive extravasation of blood into the tissue spaces. In fact, most snake venoms are complex mixtures of various fractions that attack different organs in specific ways; they seldom can be assigned categorically to one or the other of the two traditional types.

The toxicity of a venom is determined by the median lethal dose on laboratory animals (LD_{50}). By this standard the venoms of the Australian tiger snake and some of the sea snakes appear to be the most deadly of poisons drop for drop. However, several larger snakes are more dangerous. The aggressive king cobra, which may exceed 5.5 m in length, is the largest and probably the most dangerous of all poisonous snakes. In India, where snakes come in constant contact with people, cobra bites cause more than 10,000 deaths each year.

Most snakes are **oviparous** (L., *ovum*, egg, + *parere*, to bring forth) species that lay their shelled, elliptical eggs beneath rotten logs, under rocks, or in holes dug in the ground (Fig. 25-22). Most of the remainder, including all the American pit vipers, except the tropical bushmaster, are **ovoviviparous** (L., *ovum*, egg, + *vivus*, living, + *parere*, to bring forth), giving birth to well-formed young. A very few snakes are **viviparous** (L., *vivus*, living, + *parere*, to bring forth); a primitive placenta forms, permitting the exchange of materials between the embryonic and maternal bloodstreams. Snakes are able to store sperm and can lay several clutches of fertile eggs at long intervals after one mating.

Figure 25-20

Eastern hognose snake *Heterodon platyrhinos*. When approached, this harmless snake makes a courageous display of hostility, hissing and puffing up its head and neck. If its antagonist fails to retreat, it soon rolls over on its back, opens its mouth, gives a few convulsive quivers, and plays dead *(above right)*. If righted, it immediately flips over on its back again, undoing the deception.
Photographs by C.P. Hickman, Jr.

Figure 25-21

Yellow cobra *Naja flava* of Africa. Cobras erect the front of the body and flatten the neck as a threat display and before attacking. All cobras are extremely poisonous.
Photograph by L.L. Rue, III.

Figure 25-22

Milk snake *Lampropeltis doliata* with eggs. This distinctively banded snake feeds largely on rodents and is one of our most beneficial snakes.
Photograph by L.L. Rue, III.

Figure 25-23

American crocodilians (order Crocodilia). The American alligator *Alligator mississipiensis* is found along the southeastern coast of the United States from central Texas to the Atlantic. The American crocodile *Crocodylus acutus* is now limited to the Everglades National Park in Florida and is in danger of extinction. Enlargement of heads shows easily recognized differences between the two species. The crocodile has a more slender snout, and the fourth tooth from the front of the lower jaw fits *outside* the upper jaw and is visible when the mouth is closed. It is not true, as commonly believed, that there is a difference in the way the jaws are hinged in the two species.

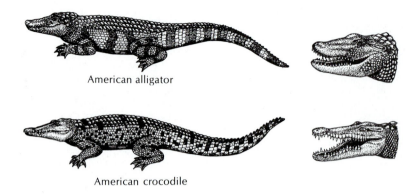

American alligator

American crocodile

Worm lizards—suborder Amphisbaenia

The somewhat inappropriate common name "worm lizards" describes a group of highly specialized, burrowing forms that are neither worms nor true lizards but certainly are related to the latter. The name of the suborder literally means "walk on both sides" (or both ends), in reference to their peculiar ability to move backward nearly as effectively as forward. They have elongate, cylindrical bodies of nearly uniform diameter, and most lack any trace of external limbs. The soft skin is divided into numerous rings, and these rings, combined with the absence of visible eyes and ears (both are hidden under the skin), make the amphisbaenians look like earthworms. The resemblance, although superficial, is the kind of structural convergence that not infrequently occurs when two totally unrelated groups come to occupy similar niches. The amphisbaenians have an extensive distribution in South America and tropical Africa. In the United States, one species, *Rhineura florida,* is found in Florida where it is known as the "graveyard snake."

Crocodiles and Alligators—Order Crocodilia

The modern crocodiles are the largest living reptiles. They are what remain of a group once abundant in the Jurassic and Cretaceous periods. Having managed to survive virtually unchanged for some 160 million years, the modern crocodilians face a forbidding, and perhaps short, future in a world dominated by humans.

Most crocodiles have relatively long slender snouts; alligators (Sp., *el lagarto,* lizard) have short and broader snouts (Fig. 25-23). With their powerful jaws and sharp teeth, they are formidable antagonists. The "man-eating" members of the group are found mainly in Africa and Asia. The estuarine crocodile *(Crocodylus porosus)* found in southern Asia and the Nile crocodile *(C. niloticus)* grow to great size (adults weighing 1000 kg have been reported) and are much feared. Both species are swift and aggressive, eating any bird or mammal they can drag from the shore to water where, by rapidly turning over and over, they violently tear the prey apart. They then gulp down the pieces. Crocodiles are known to attack animals as large as cattle.

Alligators are less aggressive than crocodiles and certainly far less dangerous to humans. Large alligators are powerful animals nevertheless, and adults have almost no enemies but humans. The chink in their formidable armor is the developmental stages. Nests left unguarded by the mother are almost certain to be discovered and raided by any of several mammals that relish eggs, and the young hatchlings may be devoured by large fish.

Figure 25-24

American alligator *Alligator mississipiensis,* an increasingly noticeable resident of the rivers, bayous, and swamps of the southeastern United States.
Photograph by C.P. Hickman, Jr.

Alligators and crocodiles are oviparous. Usually 20 to 50 eggs are laid in a mass of vegetation and guarded by the mother. The mother hears vocalizations from the hatching young and responds by opening the nest to allow the hatchlings to escape. An odd feature about alligator reproduction is that the incubation temperature of the eggs determines the sex ratio of the offspring. Low nest temperatures produce only females, whereas high nest temperatures produce only males. This results in highly unbalanced sex ratios in some areas. For example, in one Louisiana study area, female hatchlings outnumbered males five to one.

American alligators were nearing extinction in the southern United States, but now, under protection, they are increasing to the point of nuisance (Fig. 25-24).

___ The Tuatara—Order Rhynchocephalia

The order Rhynchocephalia is represented by a single living species, the tuatara (*Sphenodon punctatum* [Gr., *sphēnos,* wedge, + *odontos,* tooth]) of New Zealand (Fig. 25-25). This animal is the sole survivor of a group of primitive reptiles that otherwise became extinct 100 million years ago. The tuatara was once widespread on the North Island of New Zealand but is now restricted to islets of Cook Strait and off the northern coast of North Island where, under protection from the New Zealand government, it may recover.

The tuatara is a lizardlike form 66 cm long or less that lives in burrows often shared with petrels. They are slow-growing animals with a long life; one is recorded to have lived 77 years.

The tuatara has captured the interest of biologists because of its numerous primitive features that are almost identical to those of Mesozoic fossils 200 million years old. These features include a primitive skull structure found in early Permian reptiles that were ancestors to the modern lizards. Tuataras also bear a well-developed parietal eye, complete with evidences of a retina (Fig. 25-25), and a complete palate. They lack a copulatory organ. A specialized feature is the teeth, which are fused wedgelike to the edge of the jaws rather than being set in sockets. *Sphenodon* represents one of the slowest rates of evolution known among the vertebrates.

Figure 25-25

Tuatara *Sphenodon punctatum,* the only living representative of order Rhynchocephalia. This "living fossil" reptile has a well-developed parietal "eye" with retina and lens on top of the head. The eye is covered with scales and is considered nonfunctional but may have been an important sense organ in early reptiles. The tuatara is found only in New Zealand.

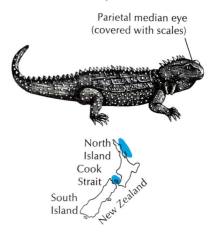

Parietal median eye (covered with scales)

North Island
Cook Strait
South Island
New Zealand

____ Summary

The reptiles evolved from labyrinthodont amphibians during the late Paleozoic era, some 300 million years ago. Their success as the first truly terrestrial vertebrates is attributed to the evolution of the shelled, amniotic egg, whose internal membranes provide the developing embryo with its own independent water and food supplies. Reptiles are also distinguished from amphibians by their dry, scaly skin that prevents water loss and by having internal fertilization and more advanced circulatory, respiratory, excretory, and nervous systems. Like amphibians, reptiles are ectotherms, but most exercise considerable behavioral control over their body temperature.

The modern reptiles are descendants of survivors of the Mesozoic age of reptiles when a burst of reptile evolution produced a worldwide fauna of great diversity. The turtles (order Testudines) with their distinctive shells have changed little in design since the Triassic period. Turtles are a small group of long-lived terrestrial, semiaquatic, aquatic, and marine species. They lack teeth. All are oviparous and all, including the marine forms, bury their eggs.

The lizards, snakes, and worm lizards (order Squamata) comprise 95% of all living reptiles. Lizards are a diversified and successful group adapted for walking, running, climbing, swimming, and burrowing. They are distinguished from snakes by typically having two pairs of legs (some species are legless), united lower jaw halves, movable eyelids, external ears, and absence of fangs. Some species are able to break off the tail when attacked. Many lizards maintain relatively steady, elevated body temperatures by behavioral thermoregulation. Snakes, in addition to being entirely limbless, are characterized by their elongate bodies and an elastic connection between the two halves of the lower jaw that permits the halves of the jaw to spread widely during swallowing. Most snakes rely on the chemical senses, especially Jacobson's organs, to hunt prey, rather than on the weakly developed visual and auditory senses. Two groups of snakes (pit vipers and boids) have unique infrared-sensing organs for tracking warm-bodied prey. Many snakes are venomous. The worm lizards (amphisbaenians) are a small tropical group of legless, burrowing forms with both eyes and ears hidden beneath the skin.

The crocodiles and alligators (order Crocodilia) are the largest living reptiles and have the most complex social behavior. Most are endangered species today.

The tuatara of New Zealand (order Rhynchocephalia) is a relic species and sole survivor of a group that otherwise disappeared 100 million years ago. It bears several primitive features that are almost identical to those of Mesozoic fossil reptiles.

Selected references

Alvarez, L.W., W. Alvarez, F. Asaro, and H.V. Michel. 1980. Extraterrestrial cause for the Cretaceous-Tertiary extinction. Science 208:1095-1108.

Barbour, R.W. 1971. Amphibians and reptiles of Kentucky. Lexington, University of Kentucky Press.

Bellairs, A. 1970. The life of reptiles, 2 vols. New York, Universe Books. *An accurate, well-written treatise that is primarily concerned with anatomy and evolution. Perhaps a bit advanced for the beginning student.*

Carr, A. 1963. The reptiles. New York, Life Nature Library, Time-Life Books. *There is a wealth of reptile lore in this superbly illustrated volume.*

Conant, R. 1975. A field guide to reptiles and amphibians of eastern and central North America, ed. 2. Boston, Houghton Mifflin Co. *Standard field guide.*

Ernst, C.H., and R.W. Barbour. 1972. Turtles of the United States. Lexington, University of Kentucky Press. *Authoritative monograph on identification, distribution, and detailed life histories of all turtles of the United States.*

Gans, C. (ed.). 1969-1982. Biology of the Reptilia, 13 vols. New York, Academic Press, Inc. *A work for the advanced student or researcher. The series consists of morphological, embryological and physiological, and ecological and behavioral portions. Specialists contribute chapters on topics that correspond to their research interests.*

Gans, C. 1974. Biomechanics: an approach to vertebrate biology. Philadelphia, J.B. Lippincott Co. *Many examples of interesting functional adaptations, especially of snakes.*

Goin, C.J., O.B. Goin, and G.R. Zug. 1978. Introduction to herpetology, ed. 3. San Francisco, W.H. Freeman & Co. Publishers. *Popular, basic text.*

Heatwole, H. 1978. Adaptations of marine snakes. Am. Sci. 66:594-604.

Klauber, L.M. 1973. Rattlesnakes, ed. 2, 2 vols. Berkeley and Los Angeles, University of California Press. *An excellent monograph on this group of reptiles.*

Pope, C.H. 1955. The reptile world: a natural history of the snakes, lizards, turtles, and crocodilians. New York, Alfred A. Knopf, Inc. *One of the best written and accurate of semipopular accounts, although dated.*

Schmidt, K.P., and R.F. Inger. 1975. Living reptiles of the world. New York, Doubleday & Co., Inc. *A magnificent volume with excellent illustrations of the various families of living reptiles.*

Smith, H.M. 1946. Handbook of lizards of the United States and Canada. Ithaca, N.Y., Comstock Publishing Associates. *A standard reference for those interested in the natural history and taxonomy of lizards.*

Spellerberg, I.F. 1982. Biology of reptiles: an ecological approach. Blackie & Son, Ltd., Glasgow. *Short and readable, undergraduate level.*

Thomas, R.D.K., and E.C. Olson (eds.). 1980. A cold look at the warm-blooded dinosaurs. Papers from a symposium. AAAS Selected Symposium Series, 28. Boulder, Colo., Westview Press, Inc. *Thorough examination of the somewhat battered argument that the dinosaurs were "warm blooded" (endothermic).*

Wright, A.H., and A.A. Wright. 1957. Handbook of snakes of the United States and Canada, 2 vols. Ithaca, N.Y., Comstock Publishing Associates. *These two volumes are indispensable and are probably the best available on snakes of the United States and Canada.*

Selected *Scientific American* articles

Bakker, R.T. 1975. Dinosaur renaissance. 232:58-78 (Apr.). *Interesting presentation of the argument that dinosaurs were endothermic.*

Bogert, C.M. 1959. How reptiles regulate body temperature. 200:105-120 (Apr.). *Many reptiles, especially lizards, achieve a remarkable degree of temperature regulation by behavioral responses.*

Buffetaut, E. 1979. The evolution of the crocodilians. 241:130-144 (Oct.). *The crocodiles and alligators are the last of the archosaurians, ruling reptiles of the Mesozoic era. Their evolution and present endangered status is detailed.*

Carr, A. 1965. The navigation of the green turtle. 212:78-86 (May). *These marine turtles make regular migrations over vast ocean routes.*

Crews, D. 1979. The hormonal control of the behavior in a lizard. 241:180-187 (Aug.). *Describes how the sex glands and the brain interact to guide sexual behavior in the green anole.*

Gamow, R.T., and J.E. Harris. 1973. The infrared receptors of snakes. 228:94-100 (May). *The anatomy and physiology of the remarkable "sixth sense" of snakes is described.*

Gans, C. 1970. How snakes move. 222:82-96 (June).

Langston, W., Jr. 1981. Pterosaurs 224:122-136 (Feb.). *These flying reptiles endured 135 million years and were the largest animals ever to fly.*

Minton, S.A., Jr. 1957. Snakebite. 196:114-122 (Jan.). *A survey of the world's most poisonous snakes and their venoms.*

Newman, E.A., and P.H. Hartline. 1982. The infrared "vision" of snakes. 246:116-127 (Mar.).

Pooley, A.C., and C. Gans. 1976. The Nile crocodile. 234:114-124 (Apr.). *The remarkably advanced social behavior of this large reptile is described.*

Russell, D.A. 1982. The mass extinctions of the late Mesozoic. 246:58-65 (Jan.). *Extinction 63 million years ago of many plants and animals may have been caused by the fall of an asteroid.*

Van Riper, W. 1953. How a rattlesnake strikes. 189:100-102 (Oct.). *The rattlesnake strike is examined with high-speed photography.*

T H E   B I R D S

Phylum Chordata

Class Aves

Covey of bobwhite quail. These familiar North American birds are gregarious during most of the year,
feeding and roosting together in coveys of 10 to 30 birds. Quail prefer open farmlands
where, in spring and summer, males perch on fences or in trees while uttering
their distinctive *bob-WHITE* call.

Photograph by C.P. Hickman, Jr.

Of the vertebrates, birds of the class Aves (ay′veez) (L., pl. of *avis*, bird) are the most studied, the most observable, the most melodious, and many think the most beautiful. With 8600 species distributed over nearly the entire earth, birds far outnumber all other vertebrates except the fishes. Birds are found in forests and deserts, in mountains and prairies, and on all the oceans. Four species are known to have visited the North Pole, and one, a skua, was seen at the South Pole. Some birds live in total blackness in caves, finding their way about by echolocation, and others dive to depths greater than 45 m to prey on aquatic life. The "bee" hummingbird of Cuba weighs only 1.8 g and is the smallest vertebrate endotherm.

The single unique feature that distinguishes birds from other animals is their feathers. If an animal has feathers, it is a bird; if it lacks feathers, it is not a bird. No other vertebrate group bears such an easily recognizable and foolproof identification tag.

There is great uniformity of structure among birds. Despite approximately 130 million years of evolution, during which they proliferated and adapted themselves to specialized ways of life, we have no difficulty recognizing a bird as a bird. In addition to feathers, all birds have forelimbs modified into wings (although they may not be used for flight); all have hindlimbs adapted for walking, swimming, or perching; all have horny beaks; and all lay eggs. Probably the reason for this great structural and functional uniformity is that birds evolved into flying machines. This fact greatly restricts diversity, so much more evident in other ver-

A

FOSSIL

Figure 26-1

Archaeopteryx, the 150 million year old ancestor of modern birds. **A,** Cast of the second and most nearly perfect fossil of *Archaeopteryx*, which was discovered in a Bavarian stone quarry. **B,** Reconstruction of *Archaeopteryx*.

A, Courtesy American Museum of Natural History.

B

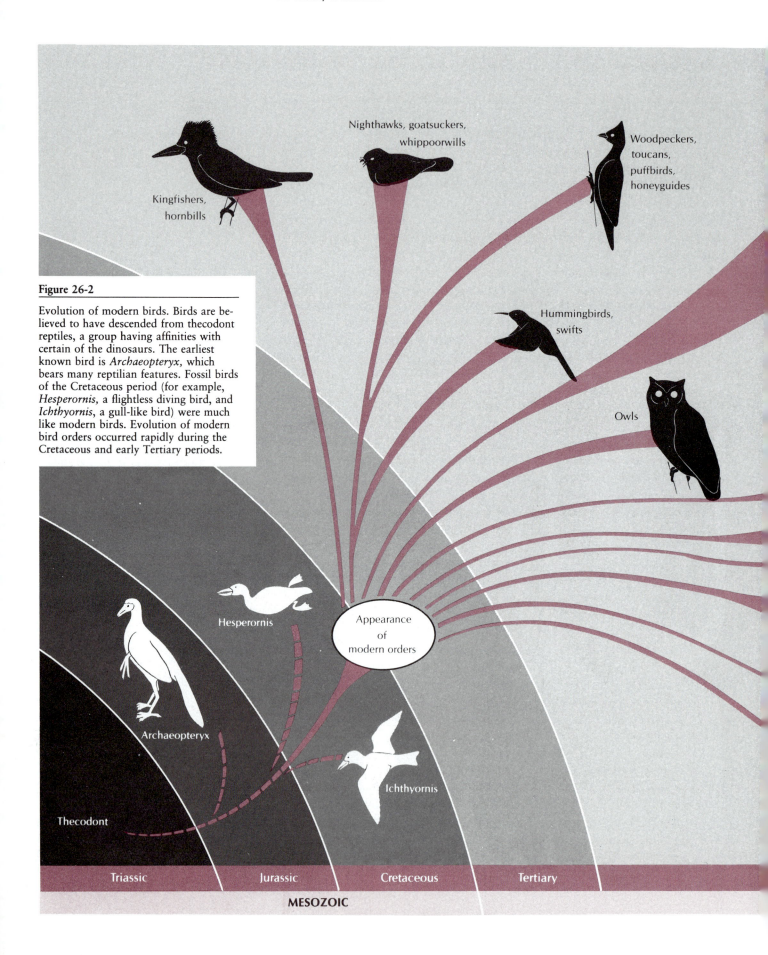

Kingfishers, hornbills

Nighthawks, goatsuckers, whippoorwills

Woodpeckers, toucans, puffbirds, honeyguides

Hummingbirds, swifts

Owls

Figure 26-2

Evolution of modern birds. Birds are believed to have descended from thecodont reptiles, a group having affinities with certain of the dinosaurs. The earliest known bird is *Archaeopteryx*, which bears many reptilian features. Fossil birds of the Cretaceous period (for example, *Hesperornis*, a flightless diving bird, and *Ichthyornis*, a gull-like bird) were much like modern birds. Evolution of modern bird orders occurred rapidly during the Cretaceous and early Tertiary periods.

Hesperornis

Appearance of modern orders

Archaeopteryx

Ichthyornis

Thecodont

Triassic   Jurassic   Cretaceous   Tertiary

MESOZOIC

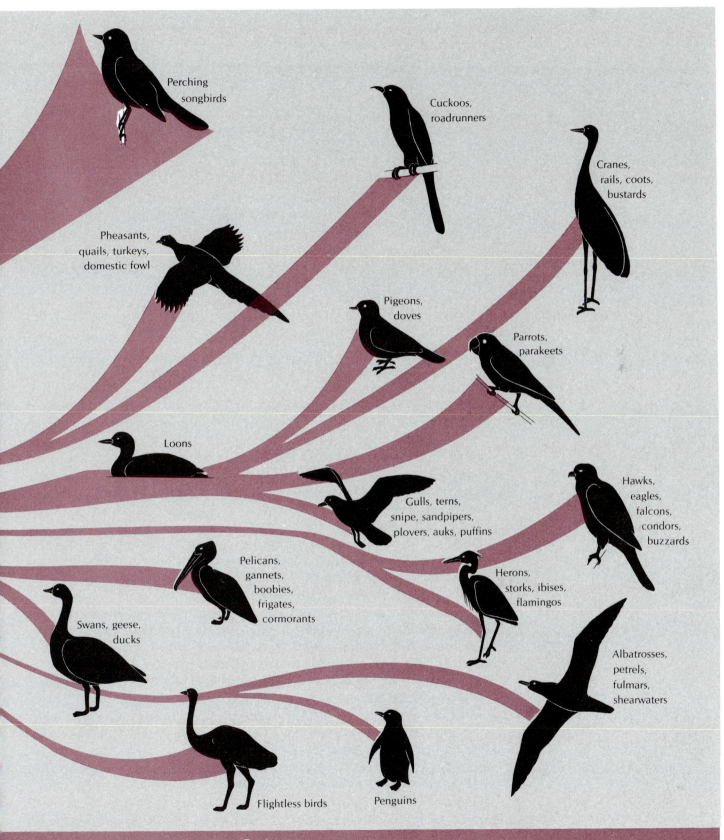

Perching songbirds

Cuckoos, roadrunners

Cranes, rails, coots, bustards

Pheasants, quails, turkeys, domestic fowl

Pigeons, doves

Parrots, parakeets

Loons

Gulls, terns, snipe, sandpipers, plovers, auks, puffins

Hawks, eagles, falcons, condors, buzzards

Pelicans, gannets, boobies, frigates, cormorants

Herons, storks, ibises, flamingos

Swans, geese, ducks

Albatrosses, petrels, fulmars, shearwaters

Flightless birds

Penguins

Quaternary

CENOZOIC

tebrate classes. For example, birds do not begin to approach the diversity seen in their warm-blooded evolutionary peers, the mammals, a group that includes forms as unlike as a whale, porcupine, bat, and giraffe.

Birds share with mammals the highest organ system development in the animal kingdom. But a bird's entire anatomy is designed around flight and its perfection. An airborne life for a large vertebrate is a highly demanding evolutionary challenge. A bird must, of course, have wings for support and propulsion. Bones must be light and hollow yet serve as a rigid airframe. The respiratory system must be highly efficient to meet the intense metabolic demands of flight and serve also as a thermoregulatory device to maintain a constant body temperature. A bird must have a rapid and efficient digestion to process an energy-rich diet; it must have a high metabolic rate; and it must have a high-pressure circulatory system. Above all, birds must have a finely tuned nervous system and acute senses, especially superb vision, to handle the complex problems of headfirst, high-velocity flight.

ORIGIN AND RELATIONSHIPS

Approximately 150 million years ago, a flying animal drowned and settled to the bottom of a tropical lake in what is now Bavaria, Germany. It was rapidly covered with a fine silt and eventually fossilized. There it remained until discovered in 1861 by a workman splitting slate in a limestone quarry. The fossil was approximately the size of a crow, with a skull not unlike that of modern birds except that the beaklike jaws bore small bony teeth set in sockets like those of reptiles (Fig. 26-1). The skeleton was decidedly reptilian with a long bony tail, clawed fingers, and abdominal ribs. It might have been classified as a reptile except that it carried the unmistakable imprint of **feathers,** those marvels of biological engineering that only birds possess. The finding was dramatic because it proved beyond reasonable doubt that birds had evolved from reptiles.

Archaeopteryx (ar-kee-op′ter-ix, meaning "ancient wing"), as the fossil was named, was an especially fortunate discovery because the fossil record of birds is disappointingly meager. The bones of birds are lightweight and quickly disintegrate, so that only under the most favorable conditions will they fossilize. Nevertheless, there are certain localities where bird fossils are relatively abundant. One of these is the famous Rancho La Brea tarpits in Los Angeles where in one pit alone were found 30,000 fossil birds representing 81 species. By 1952 over 780 different fossil species had been recorded. Although most of these are relatively recent fossils, enough intermediate forms are known to provide a reasonable picture of bird evolution from the Jurassic period, when *Archaeopteryx* lived, to recent times (Fig. 26-2). Two well-known fossil birds in particular deserve mention. One was *Ichthyornis* (ik-thee-or′nis), a small, ternlike sea bird that lived along the shores of North America's inland sea during the Cretaceous period about 100 million years ago, 50 million years after *Archaeopteryx*. The other was *Hesperornis,* a flightless, loonlike diving bird (Fig. 26-2). Both were essentially modern birds but still retained certain reptilian features, including toothed jaws and a reptilelike jaw articulation. Nevertheless, by the close of the Cretaceous period, about 63 million years ago, the characteristics of modern birds had been thoroughly molded. There remained only the emergence and proliferation of the modern orders of birds. Hundreds of thousands of bird species have appeared and nearly as many have disappeared, following *Archaeopteryx* to extinction. Only a minute fraction of these nameless species have been discovered as fossils.

Most paleontologists agree that the ancestors of both birds and dinosaurs were derived from a stem group of archosaurian reptiles called thecodonts (Fig. 25-1, pp. 580 and 581). Birds probably have a monophyletic origin (evolved from a single ancestor). However, existing birds are divided into two broad groups: (1) **ratite** (rat′ite) (L., *ratitus,* marked like a raft, from *ratis,* raft), the large flightless birds (ostriches, emus, rheas, cassowaries) and the kiwis, which have a flat sternum with poorly developed pectoral muscles, and (2) **carinate** (L., *carina,* keel), the flying birds, which have a keeled sternum on which powerful flight muscles insert. The division arose from the notion that the ratites represented a separate line of descent that never acquired the power of flight. This idea is not completely rejected; the ratites clearly have descended from a flying ancestor (or ancestors, since they may not be a monophyletic group). Furthermore, not all carinate birds can fly. The penguins are flightless, although their wing movements while swimming underwater are similar to those of flying birds. Nor do all carinate birds have keeled sternums! They are absent, for example, in the many species of flightless rails and in the flightless ibis of Hawaii, and keeled sternums have almost disappeared from the flightless cormorants of the Galápagos Islands (Fig. 26-3). Thus, the classical ratite-carinate distinction separates neither all flightless from all flying birds nor all keel-less from all keeled birds (emphasizing once again the difficulty of making absolute generalizations in biology). Flightlessness has appeared independently among many groups of birds; the fossil record reveals flightless wrens, pigeons, parrots, cranes, ducks, and auks and even a flightless owl. Flightlessness has almost always evolved on islands where few terrestrial predators are found. The only flightless birds living on continents today are the large ratites such as ostrich, rhea, cassowary, and emu, which have evolved great running speed for escaping predators (the ostrich can run 70 kilometers per hour).

It may seem paradoxical that birds with their agile, warm-blooded, colorful, and melodious way of life should have descended from lethargic, cold-blooded, and silent reptiles. Yet the numerous anatomical affinities of the two groups are abundant evidence of close kinship and led the great English zoologist Thomas Henry Huxley to call birds merely "glorified reptiles." This unflattering description has never pleased bird lovers, who answer, "But how wondrously glorified."

Ancient and modern birds are divided into two subclasses. (A complete classification of the orders of living birds appears on pp. 630 to 632.)

> **Subclass Archaeornithes** (ar′ke-or′ni-theez) (Gr., *archaios,* ancient, + *ornis, ornithos,* bird). Fossil birds. This included *Archaeopteryx* and possibly one or two other genera.
> **Subclass Neornithes** (ne-or′ni-theez) (Gr., *neos,* new, + *ornis,* bird). Modern birds are placed in this group. Some extinct species with teeth are also included here because of their likeness to modern forms.

CHARACTERISTICS

1. Body usually spindle shaped, with four divisions: head, neck, trunk, and tail; **neck disproportionately long** for balancing and food gathering
2. Limbs paired, with the **forelimbs usually adapted for flying;** posterior pair variously adapted for perching, walking, and swimming; foot with four toes (chiefly)
3. Epidermal **covering of feathers** and **leg scales;** thin integument of epidermis and dermis; no sweat glands; oil or preen gland at root of tail; **pinna of ear rudimentary**

The bodies of flightless birds are dramatically redesigned. All of the restrictions of flight are removed. The keel of the sternum is lost, and the heavy flight muscles (as much as 17% of the body weight of flying birds), as well as other specialized flight apparatus, disappear. Since body weight is no longer a restriction, flightless birds tend to become large. Several extinct flightless birds were enormous: the giant moas of New Zealand weighed more than 225 kg (500 pounds), and the elephantbird of Madagascar, the largest bird that ever lived, probably weighed nearly 450 kg (about 1000 pounds) and stood nearly 2 m tall.

Figure 26-3

One of the strangest birds in a strange land, the flightless cormorant of the Galápagos Islands *(Nannopterum harrisi)* dries its wings after a fishing forage. It is a superb swimmer, propelling itself through the water with its feet to catch fish and octopuses. The flightless cormorant is an example of a carinate bird (having a keeled sternum) that has lost the keel and the ability to fly.

Photograph by C.P. Hickman, Jr.

4. **Skeleton fully ossified with air cavities;** skull bones fused with **one occipital condyle;** jaws covered with **horny beaks;** small ribs; vertebrae tend to fuse, especially the terminal ones; sternum well developed with keel or reduced with no keel; **no teeth**
5. Nervous system well developed, with brain and 12 pairs of cranial nerves
6. Circulatory system of **four-chambered heart,** with the **right aortic arch persisting;** reduced renal portal system; nucleated red blood cells
7. **Endothermic**
8. Respiration by slightly expansible lungs, with thin **air sacs** among the visceral organs and skeleton; **syrinx (voice box)** near junction of trachea and bronchi
9. Excretory system of metanephric kidney; ureters open into cloaca; **no bladder;** semisolid urine; uric acid main nitrogenous waste
10. Sexes separate; testes paired, with the vas deferens opening into the cloaca; **females with left ovary and oviduct only;** copulatory organ in ducks, geese, ratites, and a few others
11. Fertilization internal; **amniotic eggs with much yolk and hard calcareous shells;** embryonic membranes in egg during development; **incubation external;** young active at hatching (**precocial**) or helpless and naked (**altricial**); sex determination by females (heterogametic)

▬ FORM AND FUNCTION

Just as an airplane must be designed and built according to rigid aerodynamic specifications if it is to fly, so too must birds meet stringent structural requirements if they are to stay airborne. All the special adaptations found in flying birds contribute to two things: more power and less weight. Flight by humans became possible when they developed an internal combustion engine and learned how to reduce the weight-to-power ratio to a critical point. Birds did this millions of years ago. But birds must do much more than fly. They must feed themselves and convert food into high-energy fuel; they must escape predators; they must be able to repair their own injuries; they must be able to air-condition themselves when overheated and heat themselves when too cool; and, most important of all, they must reproduce themselves.

▬ Feathers

A feather is very lightweight, yet possesses remarkable toughness and tensile strength. A typical **contour feather** consists of a hollow **quill,** or calamus, thrust into the skin and a **shaft,** or rachis, which is a continuation of the quill and bears numerous **barbs** (Fig. 26-4). The barbs are arranged in closely parallel fashion and spread diagonally outward from both sides of the central shaft to form a flat, expansive, webbed surface, the **vane.** There may be several hundred barbs in the vane.

If the feather is examined with a microscope, each barb appears to be a miniature replica of the feather, with numerous parallel filaments, called **barbules,** set in each side of the barb and spreading laterally from it. There may be 600 barbules on each side of a barb, adding up to more than 1 million barbules for the feather. The barbules of one barb overlap the barbules of a neighboring barb in a herringbone pattern and are held together with great tenacity by tiny hooks. Should two adjoining barbs become separated—and considerable force is needed to pull the vane apart—they are instantly zipped together again by drawing the feather through the fingertips. The bird, of course, does this with its bill, and much of a bird's time is occupied with preening to keep its feathers in perfect condition.

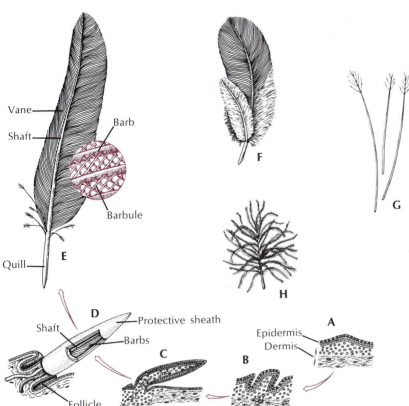

Figure 26-4

Types of bird feathers and their development. **A** to **E,** Successive stages in the development of a vaned, or contour, feather. Growth occurs within a protective sheath, **D,** that splits open when growth is complete, allowing the mature feather to spread flat. **F** to **H,** Other feather varieties, including a pheasant vane feather with aftershaft, **F,** filoplumes, **G,** and down feather, **H.**

Principally after Welty, J.C. 1982. The life of birds, ed. 3. Philadelphia, W.B. Saunders Co.

Types of feathers

There are different types of bird feathers, serving different functions. **Contour feathers** (Fig. 26-4, *E*) give the bird its outward form and are the type we have already described. Contour feathers that extend beyond the body and are used in flight are called **flight feathers. Down feathers** (Fig. 26-4, *H*) are soft tufts hidden beneath the contour feathers. They are soft because their barbules lack hooks. They are especially abundant on the breast and abdomen of water birds and on the young of game birds and function principally to conserve heat. **Filoplume feathers** (Fig. 26-4, *G*) are hairlike, degenerate feathers; each is a weak shaft with a tuft of short barbs at the tip. They are the "hairs" of a plucked fowl. They have no known function. The bristles around the mouths of flycatchers and whippoorwills are probably modified filoplumes. A fourth type of highly modified feather, called **powder-down feathers,** is found on herons, bitterns, hawks, and parrots. Their tips disintegrate as they grow, releasing a talclike powder that helps to waterproof the feathers and give them metallic luster.

Origin and development

Feathers are epidermal structures that evolved from the reptilian scale; indeed, a developing feather closely resembles a reptile scale when growth is just beginning. We can imagine that in its evolution, the scale elongated and its edges frayed outward until it became the complex feather of birds. Strangely enough, although modern birds possess both scales (especially on their feet) and feathers, no intermediate stage between the two has been discovered on either fossil or living forms.

Like a reptile's scale, a feather grows from a dermal papilla that pushes up against the overlying epidermis (Fig. 26-4, *A*). However, instead of flattening like a scale, the feather rolls into a cylinder or feather bud and is covered with epidermis. This feather bud sinks in slightly at its base and comes to lie in a feather follicle from which the feather will protrude. A layer of keratin is produced around the cylinder or bud and encloses the pulp cavity of blood vessels. This surface layer of keratin splits away from the deeper layer to form a sheath. The deeper layer becomes frayed distally to form parallel ridges, the median one of which grows large to form the shaft (contour feathers) and the others the barbs. The sheath bursts, and the barbs spread flat to form the vane (Fig. 26-4, *A* to *E*).

The pulp cavity of the quill dries up when growth is finished, leaving it hollow, with openings (umbilici) at its two ends. If the feather is to be a down feather, the sheath bursts and releases the barbs without the formation of a shaft or vane. Pigments (lipochromes and melanins) are added to the epidermal cells during growth in the follicle.

The vivid color of feathers is of two kinds: pigmentary and structural. Red, orange, and yellow feathers are colored by pigments, called lipochromes, deposited in the feather barbules as they are formed. Black, brown, red-brown, and gray colors are due to a different pigment, melanin. The blue feathers of blue jays, indigo buntings, and bluebirds depend not on pigment but on the scattering of shorter wavelengths of light by particles within the feather; these are structural colors. Blue feathers are usually underlain by melanin, which absorbs certain wavelengths, thus intensifying the blue. Such feathers look the same from any angle of view. Green colors are almost always a combination of yellow pigment and blue feather structure. Another kind of structural color is the beautiful iridescent color of many birds, which ranges from red, orange, copper, and gold to green, blue, and violet. Iridescent color is based on interference that causes light waves to reinforce, weaken, or eliminate each other. Iridescent colors may change with the angle of view; the quetzal, for example, looks blue from one angle and green from another. In the animal kingdom, only tropical reef fishes can vie with birds for intensity and vividness of color.

Molting

When fully grown, a feather, like mammalian hair, is a dead structure. The shedding, or molting, of feathers is a highly orderly process. Except in penguins, which molt all at once, feathers are discarded gradually to avoid the appearance of bare spots. Flight and tail feathers are lost in exact pairs, one from each side, so that balance is maintained (Fig. 26-18). Replacements emerge before the next pair is lost, and most birds can continue to fly unimpaired during the molting period; only ducks and geese are completely grounded during the molt. Nearly all birds molt at least once a year, usually in late summer after the nesting season. Many birds also undergo a second partial or complete molt just before breeding season, to equip them with their breeding finery, so important for courtship display.

—— Movement and Integration

Skeleton

One of the major adaptations that allows a bird to fly is its light skeleton (Fig. 26-5). Bones are phenomenally light, delicate, and laced with air cavities, yet they are strong. The skeleton of a frigate bird with a 2.1 m (7 foot) wingspan weighs only 114 grams (4 ounces), less than the weight of all its feathers. A pigeon skull weighs only 0.21% of its body weight; the skull of a rat by comparison weighs 1.25%. The bird skull is mostly fused into one piece. The braincase and orbits are large to accommodate a bulging brain and the large eyes needed for quick motor coordination and superior vision.

The anterior skull bones are elongated to form a beak. The lower mandible is a complex of several bones that hinge on two small movable bones, the quadrates. This provides a double-jointed action that permits the mouth to open wide. The upper mandible, consisting of premaxillae, maxillae, and other bones, is usually fused to the forehead, but in many birds—parrots, for instance—the upper jaw is hinged also. This adaptation allows greater flexibility of the beak in food manipulation and provides insect-catching species with a wider gap for successful feeding on the wing.

The vertebral column of birds is highly specialized for flight. Its most distinctive feature is its rigidity. Most of the vertebrae except those of the neck are

Figure 26-5

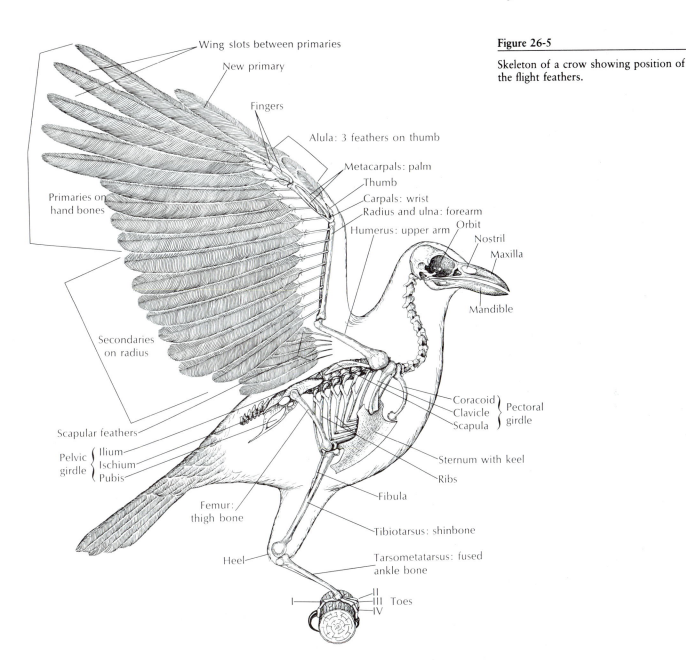

Skeleton of a crow showing position of the flight feathers.

Wing slots between primaries

New primary

Fingers

Alula: 3 feathers on thumb

Metacarpals: palm

Thumb

Carpals: wrist

Radius and ulna: forearm

Primaries on hand bones

Humerus: upper arm

Orbit

Nostril

Maxilla

Mandible

Secondaries on radius

Coracoid
Clavicle
Scapula
} Pectoral girdle

Scapular feathers

Pelvic girdle {
Ilium
Ischium
Pubis

Sternum with keel

Ribs

Fibula

Femur: thigh bone

Tibiotarsus: shinbone

Heel

Tarsometatarsus: fused ankle bone

I
II
III
IV
Toes

fused together and with the pelvic girdle to form a stiff but light framework to support the legs and provide rigidity for flight. To assist in this rigidity, the ribs are mostly fused with the vertebrae, pectoral girdle, and sternum. Except in the flightless birds, the sternum bears a large, thin keel that provides for the attachment of the powerful flight muscles. Of the body box, only the eight to 24 (according to the species) vertebrae of the neck remain fully flexible.

The bones of the forelimbs have become highly modified for flight. They are hollow (for lightness) and reduced in number, and several are fused together. Despite these alterations, the bird wing is clearly a rearrangement of the basic vertebrate tetrapod limb from which it arose, and all the elements—upper arm, forearm, wrist, and fingers—are represented in modified form (Fig. 26-5). The birds' legs have undergone less pronounced modification than the wings, since they are still designed principally for walking, as well as for perching and occasionally for swimming, as were those of their reptilian ancestors.

Figure 26-6

Perching mechanism of a bird. When a bird settles on a branch, tendons automatically tighten, closing the toes around the perch.

Perching tendons

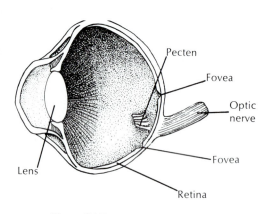

Pecten

Fovea

Optic nerve

Fovea

Lens

Retina

Figure 26-7

Hawk eye has all the structural components of the mammalian eye, plus a peculiar pleated structure, the pecten, believed to provide nourishment to the retina. The extraordinarily keen vision of the hawk is attributed to the extreme density of cone cells in the foveae: 1.5 million per fovea compared with 0.2 million for humans. Each hawk eye has two foveae as opposed to one in humans, meaning that each hawk eye focuses on two objects simultaneously—the better to select its next meal!

Muscular system

The locomotor muscles of the wings are relatively massive to meet the demands of flight. The largest of these is the **pectoralis,** which depresses the wings in flight. Its antagonist is the **supracoracoideus** muscle, which raises the wing. Surprisingly, perhaps, this latter muscle is not located on the backbone (anyone who has been served the back of a chicken knows that it offers little meat) but is positioned under the pectoralis on the breast. It is attached by a tendon to the upper side of the humerus of the wing so that it pulls from below by an ingenious "rope-and-pulley" arrangement. Both of these muscles are anchored to the keel. Thus, with the main muscle mass low in the body, aerodynamic stability is improved.

The main leg muscle mass is located in the thigh, surrounding the femur, and a smaller mass lies over the tibiotarsus (shank, or "drumstick"). Strong but thin tendons extend downward through sleevelike sheaths to the toes. Consequently the feet are nearly devoid of muscles, explaining the thin, delicate appearance of the bird leg. This arrangement places the main muscle mass near the bird's center of gravity and at the same time allows great agility to the slender, lightweight feet. Since the feet are made up mostly of bone, tendon, and tough, scaly skin, they are highly resistant to damage from freezing. When a bird perches on a branch, an ingenious toe-locking mechanism (Fig. 26-6) is activated, which prevents the bird from falling off its perch when asleep. The same mechanism causes the talons of a hawk or owl to automatically sink deeply into its victim as the legs bend under the impact of the strike. The powerful grip of a bird of prey was described by L. Brown*:

> When an eagle grips in earnest, one's hand becomes numb, and it is quite impossible to tear it free, or to loosen the grip of the eagle's toes with the other hand. One just has to wait until the bird relents, and while waiting one has ample time to realize that an animal such as a rabbit would be quickly paralyzed, unable to draw breath, and perhaps pierced through and through by the talons in such a clutch.

*Brown, L. 1970. Eagles. New York, Arco Publishing Co., Inc.

Birds have lost the long reptilian tail, still fully evident in *Archaeopteryx*, and have substituted a pincushion-like muscle mound into which the tail feathers are rooted. It contains a bewildering array of tiny muscles, as many as 1000 in some species, which control the crucial tail feathers. But the most complex muscular system of all is found in the neck of birds; the thin and stringy muscles, elaborately interwoven and subdivided, provide the bird's neck with the ultimate in vertebrate flexibility.

Nervous and sensory system

A bird's nervous and sensory system accurately reflects the complex problems of flight and a highly visible existence, in which it must gather food, mate, defend territory, incubate and rear young, and correctly distinguish friend from foe. The brain of a bird has well-developed **cerebral hemispheres, cerebellum,** and **midbrain tectum** (optic lobes) (Fig. 32-12, p. 770). The **cerebral cortex**—the portion in mammals that becomes the chief coordinating center—is thin, unfissured, and poorly developed in birds. But the core of the cerebrum, the **corpus striatum,** has enlarged into the principal integrative center of the brain, controlling such activities as eating, singing, flying, and all the complex instinctive reproductive activities. Relatively intelligent birds, such as crows and parrots, have larger cerebral hemispheres than do less intelligent birds such as chickens and pigeons. The **cerebellum** is a crucial coordinating center where muscle-position sense, equilibrium sense, and visual cues are all assembled and used to coordinate movement and balance. The **optic lobes,** laterally bulging structures of the midbrain, form a visual association apparatus comparable to the visual cortex of mammals.

Except in flightless birds and in ducks, the senses of smell and taste are poorly developed in birds. This deficiency, however, is more than compensated by good hearing and superb vision, the keenest in the animal kingdom. As in mammals, the bird ear consists of three regions: (1) the **external ear,** a sound-conducting canal extending to the eardrum, (2) the **middle ear,** containing a rodlike **columella** that transmits vibrations, and (3) the **inner ear,** where the organ of hearing, the **cochlea,** is located. The bird cochlea is much shorter than the coiled mammalian cochlea, yet birds can hear roughly the same range of sound frequencies as humans. Actually, the bird ear far surpasses that of humans in capacity to distinguish differences in intensities and to respond to rapid fluctuations in pitch.

The bird eye resembles that of other vertebrates in gross structure but is relatively larger, less spherical, and almost immobile; instead of turning their eyes, birds turn their heads with their long and flexible necks to scan the visual field. The light-sensitive **retina** (Fig. 26-7) is elaborately equipped with rods (for dim night vision) and cones (for color vision). Cones predominate in day birds, and rods are more numerous in nocturnal birds. A distinctive feature of the bird eye is the **pecten,** a highly vascularized organ attached to the retina near the optic nerve and jutting out into the vitreous humor (Fig. 26-7). Because the retina is devoid of blood vessels and retinal metabolism is primarily anaerobic, the pecten is thought to sweep out acid metabolites that would otherwise accumulate.

The position of a bird's eyes in its head is correlated with its life habits. Vegetarians that must avoid predators have eyes placed laterally to give a wide view of the world; predaceous birds such as hawks and owls have eyes directed to the front. In birds of prey and some others, the **fovea,** or region of keenest vision on the retina, is placed in a deep pit, which makes it necessary for the bird to focus exactly on the source. Many birds, moreover, have two sensitive spots (foveae) on

Recent research showing that the vision of at least some birds extends into the near ultraviolet range may surprise people accustomed to assuming that human color vision approaches evolutionary perfection. In humans, ultraviolet light below 400 nm is filtered out by pigments in the lens and the macula, an adaptation that reduces chromatic aberration, which becomes severe at short wavelengths. Birds also possess ultraviolet-filtering pigments in their eyes, but these are located within the retinal cones rather than the lens. Recently it was shown that several species of hummingbirds can see in the near ultraviolet range down to 370 nm. This may help attract them to flowers having "nectar guides," which are striking patterns, visible only in the ultraviolet part of the spectrum, that have evolved to guide pollinating insects to these flowers.

Figure 26-8

Great horned owl *Bubo virginianus virginianus* (order Strigiformes) with gray squirrel after a successful forage. Owls possess eyes incredibly sensitive to light, enabling them to see prey in light one-hundredth to one-tenth the intensity required by humans (0.000,000,73 footcandle). But this particular ultrasensitivity is traded off for relatively poor visual acuity, narrow visual field, and weak accommodation (ability to focus on near objects).

Photograph by L.L. Rue, III.

the retina (Fig. 26-7): the central one for sharp monocular views and the posterior one for binocular vision. Woodcocks can probably see binocularly both forward and backward. Bitterns, in their freezing stance of bill pointing up, can also see binocularly. The visual acuity of a hawk is believed to be eight times that of a human (enabling it to see clearly a crouching rabbit more than a mile away), and an owl's ability to see in dim light is more than 10 times that of a human (Fig. 26-8). Birds have good color vision, especially toward the red end of the spectrum.

Food, Feeding, and Digestion

Birds have evolved along with food resources in nearly every environment on earth. In their early evolution, most birds were carnivorous, feeding principally on insects. Insects were well established on the earth's surface in both variety and numbers long before birds made their appearance, and they presented an enormously valuable food resource only partly exploited by amphibians and reptiles. With the advantage of flight, birds could hunt insects on the wing and carry their assault to insect refuges mostly inaccessible to their earthbound tetrapod peers. Today, there is a bird to hunt nearly every insect; they probe the soil, search the bark, scrutinize every leaf and twig, and drill into insect galleries hidden in tree trunks.

Other animal foods—worms, molluscs, crustaceans, fish, frogs, reptiles, mammals, as well as other birds—all found their way into the diet of birds. Fruit- and seed-eating birds are more recent additions, appearing during the Miocene epoch 10 to 15 million years ago. A very large group, nearly one fifth of all birds, feeds on nectar (Fig. 26-9). Thus, as a group, birds eat almost anything, and this is one important reason for their success. Some are omnivores, showing little specialization, while others have become adapted to highly restricted diets. Each extreme offers its own advantage. The opportunistic diet of an omnivore (often termed a **euryphagous,** or "wide-eating" species) allows it to eat whatever is seasonally abundant. However, it must compete with numerous other omnivores for the same broad spectrum of food. The specialist, on the other hand, by refining feeding adaptations, may eliminate most competition for a particular food item. Such a **stenophagous** ("narrow-eating") species has the pantry to itself—but at a price. Should its food specialty be reduced or destroyed for some reason (disease, adverse climate, and the like), its very survival as a species may be jeopardized. In fact, few birds cling to a single feeding habit throughout their lives. More typically, a bird may be stenophagous during one season or one period of its life and euryphagous at other times.

The beaks of birds are strongly adapted to specialized food habits—from generalized types, such as the strong, pointed beaks of crows, to grotesque, highly specialized ones in flamingoes, hornbills, and toucans (Fig. 26-10). The beak of a woodpecker is a straight, hard, chisel-like device. Anchored to a tree trunk with its tail serving as a brace, the woodpecker delivers powerful, rapid blows to build nests or expose the burrows of wood-boring insects (Fig. 26-11). It then uses its long, flexible, barbed tongue to seek out insects in their galleries. The woodpecker's skull is especially thick to absorb shock.

How much do birds eat? By a peculiar twist of reality, the commonplace "to eat like a bird" is supposed to signify a diminutive appetite. Yet birds, because of their intense metabolism, are voracious feeders. Small birds eat relatively more than large birds because their metabolic rate is greater. This happens because the

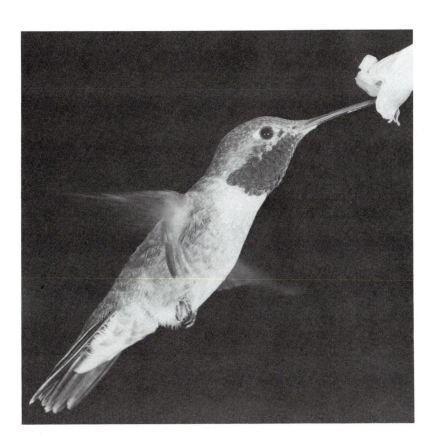

Figure 26-9

A male broad-tailed hummingbird *Selasphorus platycerus* drinks nectar from a flower. This is one of about 50 species of hummingbirds distributed in the western United States and Mexico. Although nectar satisfies the intense energy demands of these small birds, they must supplement their diet with insects and spiders to provide the protein required for growth.

Photograph by L.L. Rue, III.

Seizing and crushing
(toucan)

Seed eating
(sparrow)

Tearing
(hawk)

Probing
(woodcock)

Scooping
(pelican)

Figure 26-10

Some bills of birds showing variety of adaptations.

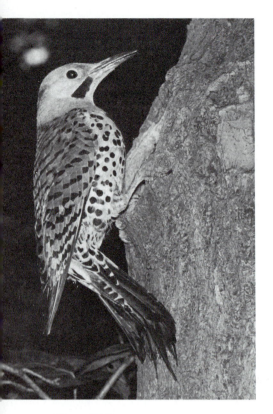

Figure 26-11

Adaptations for chopping holes in wood. This yellow-shafted flicker *Colaptes auratus*, in common with other woodpeckers, has a heavy skull, chisel-edged beak, strong feet with two opposing toes (instead of the more common one), and stiff tail feathers that serve as a third, bracing leg. The black "mustache" mark beneath the eye of this male is the only visible difference between the sexes. Order Piciformes.

Photograph by L.L. Rue, III.

oxygen consumption increases only about three fourths as rapidly as body weight. For example, the resting metabolic rate (oxygen consumed per gram of body weight) of a hummingbird is 12 times that of a pigeon and 25 times that of a chicken. A 3 g hummingbird may eat 100% of its body weight in food each day, an 11 g blue tit about 30%, and a 1880 g domestic chicken, 3.4%. Obviously the weight of food consumed also depends on water content of the food, since water has no nutritive value. A 57 g Bohemian waxwing was estimated to eat 170 g of watery *Cotoneaster* berries in one day—three times its body weight! Seed-eaters of equivalent size might eat only 8 g of dry seeds per day.

Birds rapidly process their food with efficient digestive equipment. A shrike can digest a mouse in 3 hours, and berries will pass completely through the digestive tract of a thrush in just 30 minutes. Furthermore, birds utilize a very high percentage of the food they eat. There are no teeth in the mouth, and the poorly developed salivary glands mainly secrete mucus for lubricating the food and the slender, horn-covered tongue. There are few taste buds, although all birds can taste to some extent. Hummingbirds and some others have sticky tongues, and woodpeckers have tongues that are barbed at the end. From the short **pharynx** a relatively long, muscular, elastic **esophagus** extends to the **stomach.** Many birds have an enlargement (**crop**) at the lower end of the esophagus that serves as a storage chamber.

In pigeons, doves, and some parrots the crop not only stores food but also produces milk by the breakdown of epithelial cells of the lining. This "bird milk" is regurgitated by both male and female into the mouth of the young squabs. It has a much higher fat content than cow's milk.

The stomach proper consists of a **proventriculus,** which secretes gastric juice, and the muscular **gizzard,** which is lined with horny plates that serve as millstones for grinding the food. To assist in the grinding process, birds swallow coarse, gritty objects or pebbles, which lodge in the gizzard. Certain birds of prey such as owls form pellets of indigestible materials, for example, bones and fur, in the proventriculus and eject them through the mouth. At the junction of the intestine with the rectum are paired **ceca,** which may be well developed in some birds. Two **bile ducts** from the **gallbladder** or liver and two or three **pancreatic ducts** empty into the duodenum, or first part of the intestine. The **liver** is relatively large and bilobed. The terminal part of the digestive system is the **cloaca,** which also receives the genital ducts and ureters; in young birds the dorsal wall of the cloaca bears the **bursa of Fabricius,** which produces immune bodies.

Body Temperature Regulation

Birds and mammals are **homeothermic.** They are the only animals that generally maintain a nearly constant body temperature, independent of large variations in environmental temperature. They are also **endothermic;** that is, their metabolism is the source of body heat. This distinguishes them from the reptiles, whose body temperature can be elevated above that of their surroundings under the influence of an external heat source, principally the sun. Such reptiles are **ectothermic.**

The body temperature of birds is high, ranging between 40° and 42° C as compared with 36° to 39° C for mammals. Some thrushes have normal body temperatures of 43.5° C (110.5° F), well past the lethal limit for most mammals and only about 2.5° C below the upper lethal temperature for these birds. Small birds tend to have rather more variable body temperatures than do large birds; for example, the body temperature of a house wren may fluctuate 8° C over 24 hours.

Body temperature is a balance between metabolic heat production and heat loss through physical means. If a bird begins to overheat, heat loss is accelerated by dilating blood vessels in the skin (to increase radiant heat loss) and by increasing the breathing rate (to increase evaporative cooling). Many species pant in extreme heat. In cold weather, birds ruffle their feathers to form a blanket of warm, insulative air next to the skin. They vasoconstrict peripheral blood vessels to reduce radiant heat loss. If these physical mechanisms are not sufficient to prevent a drop in body temperature in very cold weather, a bird will shiver. As in mammals, this muscular movement creates needed heat. But it also increases food and oxygen consumption. A sparrow will consume twice as much oxygen and eat twice as much food at 0° C (32° F) as at 37° C (98° F). What person living in a northern climate has not marveled at the ability of the tiny chickadee, a minute furnace of cheerful activity, to survive exposure to the coldest winter weather?

____ Circulation, Respiration, and Excretion

Circulatory system

The general plan of bird circulation is not greatly different from that of mammals. The four-chambered heart is large, with strong ventricular walls; thus, birds share with mammals a complete separation of the respiratory and systemic circulations. However, the right aortic arch, instead of the left as in the mammals, leads to the dorsal aorta. The two jugular veins in the neck are connected by a cross vein, an adaptation for shunting the blood from one jugular to the other as the head is turned around. The brachial and pectoral arteries to the wings and breast are unusually large.

The heartbeat is extremely fast, and, as in mammals, there is an inverse relationship between heart rate and body weight. For example, a turkey has a heart rate at rest of about 93 beats per minute, a chicken has 250 beats per minute, and a black-capped chickadee has 500 beats per minute when asleep, which may increase to a phenomenal 1000 beats per minute during exercise. Blood pressure in birds is roughly equivalent to that in mammals of similar size.

Bird's blood contains nucleated, biconvex red corpuscles that are somewhat larger than those of mammals. The phagocytes, or mobile ameboid cells, of the blood are unusually active and efficient in birds in the repair of wounds and in destroying microbes.

Respiratory system

The respiratory system of birds differs radically from the lungs of reptiles and mammals and is marvelously adapted for meeting the high metabolic demands of flight. The lungs, which are relatively inexpansible because of their direct attachment to the body wall, are filled with numerous tiny **air capillaries** instead of alveoli of the mammalian type. Also unique is the extensive system of nine interconnecting **air sacs** that are located in pairs in the thorax and abdomen and are even extended by tiny tubes into the centers of the long bones (Fig. 26-12). The air sacs are connected to the lungs in such a way that perhaps 75% of the inspired air bypasses the lungs and flows directly into the posterior air sacs, which serve as

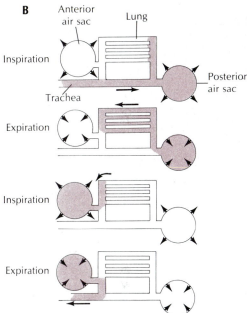

Figure 26-12

Respiratory system of a bird. **A,** Lungs and air sacs. One side of the bilateral air sac system is shown. **B,** Movement of a single volume of air through the bird's respiratory system. Two full respiratory cycles are required to move the air through the system.

B, From Schmidt-Nielsen, K. 1979. Animal physiology: adaptation and environment. New York, Cambridge University Press.

Secretory
tubule

Central
canal

Figure 26-13

Salt glands of a marine bird (gull). One salt gland is located above each eye. Each gland consists of several lobes arranged in parallel. One lobe is shown in cross section, much enlarged. Salt is secreted into many radially arranged tubules, then flows into a central canal that leads into the nose.

reservoirs for fresh air. On expiration, this oxygenated air is shunted through the lung and collected in the anterior air sacs. From there it flows directly to the outside. The air flow sequence is shown in Fig. 26-12. The advantage of such a system is obvious: the lungs receive fresh air during both inspiration and expiration. An almost continuous stream of fully oxygenated air is passed through a system of richly vascularized air capillaries. Although many details of the bird's respiratory system are not yet understood, it is clearly the most efficient of any vertebrate system.

In addition to performing its principal respiratory function, the air sac system helps to cool the bird during vigorous exercise. A pigeon, for example, produces about 27 times more heat when flying than when at rest. The air sacs have numerous diverticula that extend inside the larger pneumatic bones of the pectoral and pelvic girdles, wings, and legs. Because they contain warmed air, they provide considerable buoyancy to the bird.

Excretory system

The relatively large paired metanephric kidneys are attached to the dorsal wall in a depression against the sacral vertebrae and pelvis. Urine passes by way of **ureters** to the **cloaca.** There is no urinary bladder. The kidney is composed of many thousands of **nephrons,** each consisting of a renal corpuscle and a nephric tubule. Urine is formed in the usual way by glomerular filtration followed by selective modification of the filtrate in the tubule (the details of this sequence are described on pp. 730 to 735).

The urine of birds differs from that of mammals in having a high concentration of uric acid, rather than urea. This is a strikingly useful adaptation for birds, many of which function on a water-poor economy, eating dry seeds and drinking little or no water. Uric acid can be excreted using far less water than is required for urea because of uric acid's low solubility. A bird can excrete 1 g of uric acid in only 1.5 to 3 ml of water, whereas a mammal may require 60 ml of water to excrete 1 g of urea. The concentration of uric acid occurs almost entirely in the cloaca, where it is combined with fecal material, and the water is reabsorbed to form a white paste. Thus, despite having kidneys that are much less effective in true concentrative ability than mammalian kidneys, birds can excrete uric acid nearly 3000 times more concentrated than that in the blood. Even the most effective mammalian kidneys—those of certain desert rodents—can excrete urea only about 25 times the plasma concentration. This paradox is explained by the insoluble nature of uric acid, which allows it to crystallize out of solution without contributing to the osmotic pressure of the urine.

Marine birds (also marine turtles) have evolved a unique solution for excreting the large loads of salt eaten with their food and in the seawater they drink. Seawater contains about 3% salt and is three times saltier than a bird's body fluids. Yet the bird kidney cannot concentrate salt in urine above about 0.3%. The problem is solved by special **salt glands,** one located above each eye (Fig. 26-13). These glands are capable of excreting a highly concentrated solution of sodium chloride—up to twice the concentration of seawater. The salt solution runs out the internal or external nostrils, giving gulls, petrels, and other sea birds a perpetual runny nose. The development of the salt gland in some birds depends on how much salt the bird takes in its diet. For example, a race of mallard ducks living a semimarine life in Greenland has salt glands 10 times larger than those of ordinary freshwater mallards.

___ Flight

What prompted the evolution of flight in birds, the ability to rise free of earth-bound concerns, as almost every human has dreamed of doing? Much as we may envy birds their conquest of the air, we also recognize that evolution of flight was the pragmatic result of complex selective pressures; certainly the forerunners of birds did not take up flight just to enjoy a new experience. The air was a relatively unexploited habitat stocked with flying insects for food. Flight also offered escape from terrestrial predators and opportunity to travel rapidly and widely to establish new breeding areas and to benefit from year-round favorable climate by migrating north and south with the seasons.

Birds unquestionably evolved from reptilian ancestors, but not directly from the membrane-winged flying reptiles (pterosaurs) as one might innocently suppose. They appear to have descended instead from a small group of thecodont reptiles (Pseudosuchia) that gave rise to both dinosaurs and birds. The fossil evidence is far too meager to provide us with a recorded history of the origin of flight, but it must have happened in one of two ways. Birds began to fly either by climbing up to a high place and gliding down or by flapping their way into the air from the ground. The principal advocate of the "ground up" or **cursorial model** is J.H. Ostrom, who suggests that the earliest birds were ground-dwelling runners that used their primitive wings as aerodynamic stabilizers and as aids in snaring insects. With continued enlargement the protowings eventually provided sufficient support to enable the running animal to flap its way into the air.

The alternative and more widely favored "trees down" or **arboreal model** proposes that proavian reptiles passed through a sequence of quadrupedal to bipedal locomotion, climbing into trees, leaping between trees, parachute gliding, and, finally, powered flight. Many adaptations of birds, such as the perching mechanism and active climbing habits, indicate such an arboreal apprenticeship. Natural selection favored the swifter and more agile, and eventually wings became strong enough to support the bird in air. One thing seems certain: feathers were an absolute requirement for flight and the evolution of flight and of feathers must have progressed together. There is absolutely no support for the idea that bird ancestors were originally membrane-winged flyers, like bats, that later developed feathers.

Bird wing as a lift device

Bird flight, especially the familiar flapping flight of birds, is complex. Despite careful analysis by conventional aerodynamic techniques and high-speed photography, it is not well understood. Nevertheless, we know that the bird wing is an airfoil that is subject to recognized laws of aerodynamics. It is adapted for high lift at low speeds, and, not surprisingly perhaps, it resembles the wings of early low-speed aircraft. The bird wing is streamlined in cross section, with a slightly concave (cambered) lower surface and with small, tight-fitting feathers where the leading edge meets the air (Fig. 26-14). Air slips efficiently over the wing, creating lift with minimum drag. Some lift is produced by positive pressure against the undersurface of the wing. But on the upper side, where the airstream must travel farther and faster over the convex surface, a negative pressure is created that provides more than two thirds of the total lift.

The lift-to-drag ratio of an airfoil is determined by the angle of tilt (angle of

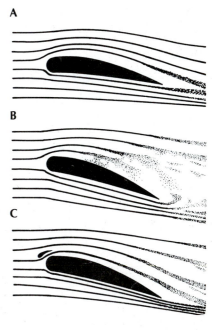

Figure 26-14

Air patterns formed by the airfoil, or wing, moving from right to left. **A,** Normal flight with a low angle of attack. As air moves smoothly over the wing, areas of negative pressure on the upper wing surface and high pressure on the lower wing surface create lift. **B,** Appearance of lift-destroying turbulence on the upper wing surface when the angle of attack becomes too great. Stalling occurs. **C,** Prevention of stalling by directing a layer of rapidly moving air over upper surface with a wing slot.

From Welty, J.C. 1982. The life of birds, ed. 3. Philadelphia, W.B. Saunders Co.

Figure 26-15

Elliptical wing of the black-billed magpie *Pica pica* in slow flight. Note well-developed alula and separation (slotting) between primaries, typical of wings adapted for high maneuverability and low-speed flight. This member of the crow family is a familiar feature of the western North American landscape. Order Passeriformes.

Photograph by C.G. Hampson.

Figure 26-16

High-speed wing of arctic tern *Sterna paradisaea*. Sweepback, taper, and absence of wing slotting adapt the tern for high speeds during its incredibly long migrations from the Arctic to the Antarctic and back each year, with some logging as much as 24,000 miles. Order Charadriiformes.

Photograph by B. Tallmark.

attack) and the airspeed (Fig. 26-14). A wing carrying a given load can pass through the air at high speed and small angle of attack or at low speed and larger angle of attack. But as speed decreases, a point is reached at which the angle of attack becomes too steep; turbulence appears on the upper surface, lift is destroyed, and stalling occurs. Stalling can be delayed or prevented by placing a **wing slot** along the leading edge so that a layer of rapidly moving air is directed across the upper wing surface. Wing slots were and still are used in aircraft traveling at a low speed. In birds, two kinds of wing slots have developed: (1) the **alula,** or group of small feathers on the thumb (Fig. 26-5), which provides a midwing slot, and (2) **slotting between the primary feathers,** which provides a wing-tip slot. In a number of songbirds, these together provide stall-preventing slots for nearly the entire outer (and aerodynamically more important) half of the wing.

Basic forms of bird wings

Bird wings vary in size and form because the successful exploitation of different habitats has imposed special aerodynamic requirements. Four types of bird wings are easily recognized (Savile, 1957).

Elliptical wings

Birds that must maneuver in forested habitats, such as sparrows, warblers, doves, woodpeckers, and magpies (Fig. 26-15), have elliptical wings. This type has a **low aspect ratio** (ratio of length to width). The outline of a sparrow wing is almost identical to that of the British Spitfire fighter plane of World War II fame—also a highly maneuverable flyer. Elliptical wings are highly slotted between the primary feathers (Fig. 26-15); this helps prevent stalling during sharp turns, low-speed flight, and frequent landing and takeoff. Each separated primary behaves as a narrow wing with a high angle of attack, providing high lift at low speed. The high maneuverability of the elliptical wing is exemplified by the tiny chickadee, which, if frightened, can change course within 0.03 second.

High-speed wings

Birds that feed on the wing, such as swallows, hummingbirds, and swifts, or that make long migrations, such as plovers, sandpipers, terns (Fig. 26-16), and gulls, have wings that sweep back and taper to a slender tip. They are rather flat in section, have a moderately high aspect ratio, and lack the wing-tip slotting characteristic of the preceding group. Sweepback and wide separation of the wing tips reduce "tip vortex," a drag-creating turbulence that tends to develop at wing tips. The fastest birds, such as sandpipers, clocked at 175 km (109 miles) per hour, belong to this group.

Soaring wings

The oceanic soaring birds have **high–aspect ratio** wings resembling those of sailplanes. This group includes albatrosses (Fig. 26-17), frigate birds, and gannets. Such long, narrow wings lack wing slots and are adapted for high speed, high lift, and dynamic soaring. They have the highest aerodynamic efficiency of all wings but are less maneuverable than the wide, slotted wings of land soarers. Dynamic soarers have learned how to exploit the highly reliable sea winds, using adjacent air currents of different velocities.

Figure 26-17

Soaring wing of waved albatross *Diomedea irrorata*. The long, high-aspect wing, like that of a sailplane, has great aerodynamic efficiency and lift but is relatively weak and lacking in maneuverability. Order Procellariiformes.
Photograph by C.P. Hickman, Jr.

Figure 26-18

High-lift wings of the osprey *Pandion haliaetus* (order Falconiformes), landing on nest. Note alulas *(top arrows)* and new primary feathers *(side arrows)*. Feathers are molted in sequence in exact pairs so that balance is maintained during flight.

Photograph by B. Tallmark.

High-lift wings

Vultures, hawks, eagles, owls, and ospreys (Fig. 26-18)—predators that carry heavy loads—have wings with slotting, alulas, and pronounced camber, all of which promote high lift at low speed. Many of these birds are land soarers, with broad, slotted wings that provide the sensitive response and maneuverability required for static soaring in the capricious air currents over land.

MIGRATION AND NAVIGATION

Perhaps it was inevitable that birds, having mastered the art of flight, would use this ability to make the long, arduous seasonal migrations that have captured human wonder and curiosity. The term **migration** refers to the regular, extensive, seasonal movements that birds make between their summer breeding regions and their wintering regions. The chief advantage seems obvious: it enables birds to live in an optimal climate all the time, where abundant and unfailing sources of food are available to sustain their intense metabolism. Migrations also provide optimal conditions for rearing young when demands for food are especially great. Broods are largest in the far north where the long summer days and the abundance of insects combine to provide parents with ample food-gathering opportunity. Predators are relatively rare in the north, and the brief, once-a-year appearance of vulnerable young birds does not encourage the buildup of predator populations. Migration also vastly increases the amount of space available for breeding and reduces aggressive territorial behavior. Furthermore, migration favors homeostasis by allowing birds to avoid climatic extremes.

Origin of Migration

Migration has become so firmly established in the behavior of birds that it long ago became a hereditary instinct. But what prompted the origin of migration? Undoubtedly, it was ecological pressures. We must suppose that birds, like other animals, will move only when compelled by some necessity. One hypothesis of migration suggests that birds spread over the Northern Hemisphere when the climate was warm and food conditions were favorable all through the year. The arrival of the glacial era forced the birds to go south for survival. When the Ice Age receded, they came back in the spring, only to be forced south again in winter because of the sharp establishment of the winter and summer seasons. This led in time to the firm fixing of the habit. Another hypothesis is that the ancestral home of birds was in the tropics and that some went north to avoid congestion and competition during the breeding season, returning after raising their young.

Migration Routes

Most migratory birds have well-established routes trending north and south. Since most birds (and other animals) live in the Northern Hemisphere, where most of the earth's land mass is concentrated, most birds are south-in-winter and north-in-summer migrants. Of the 4000 or more species of migrant birds (a little less than half the total bird species), most breed in the more northern latitudes of the hemisphere; the percentage of migrants in Canada is far higher than the percentage of migrants in Mexico, for example. Some use different routes in the fall and spring (Fig. 26-19). Some, especially certain aquatic species, complete their migratory routes in a very short time. Others, however, make the trip in a leisurely manner, often stopping here and there to feed. Some of the warblers are known to take 50 to 60 days to migrate from their winter quarters in Central America to their summer breeding areas in Canada.

Not all members of a species migrate at the same time; there is a great deal of straggling so that some members do not reach the summer breeding grounds until others are well along with their nesting. Some birds, such as robins, are "weather migrants" that move northward as the winter retreats. Others, such as purple martins and catbirds, are "instinctive migrants" that are little influenced by year-to-year weather changes. Records kept of catbirds in a certain eastern state reveal that the birds arrived in the particular locality about the middle of April and did not vary more than a day in a period of 5 years.

Many of the smaller species migrate at night and feed by day; others migrate chiefly in the daytime; and many swimming and wading birds migrate by either day or night. The height at which they fly varies greatly. Although some passerines (perching birds) have been observed as high as 6400 m (nearly 4 miles) by means of radar, the great majority (90%) fly below 1500 m. Migrants tend to fly higher over water than land and higher at night than during the day.

Many birds are known to follow landmarks, such as rivers and coastlines, but others do not hesitate to fly directly over large bodies of water in their routes. Some birds have very wide migration lanes, whereas others, such as certain sandpipers, are restricted to very narrow ones, keeping well to the coastlines because of their food requirements.

Some species are known for their long-distance migrations. The arctic tern (Fig. 26-16), greatest globe spanner of all, breeds north of the Arctic Circle and in winter is found in the Antarctic regions. This species is also known to take a circuitous route in migrations from North America, passing over to the coastlines of Europe and Africa and then to their winter quarters, a trip that may exceed 18,000 km (11,200 miles). Other birds that breed in Alaska follow a more direct line down the Pacific coast of North and South America.

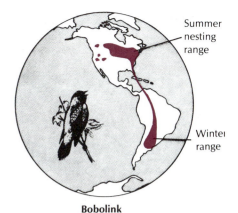

Bobolink

Golden plover

Figure 26-19

Migrations of the bobolink and golden plover. The bobolink commutes 22,500 km (14,000 miles) each year between nesting sites in North America and its wintering range in Argentina, a phenomenal feat for such a small bird. Although the breeding range has extended to colonies in western areas, these birds take no shortcuts but adhere to the ancestral eastern seaboard route. The golden plover flies a loop migration, striking out across the Atlantic in its southward autumnal migration but returning in the spring via Central America and the Mississippi Valley because ecological conditions are more favorable at that time.

Figure 26-20

Part of a colony of Australian gannets *Sula serrator*. Order Pelecaniformes.
Photograph by C.P. Hickman, Jr.

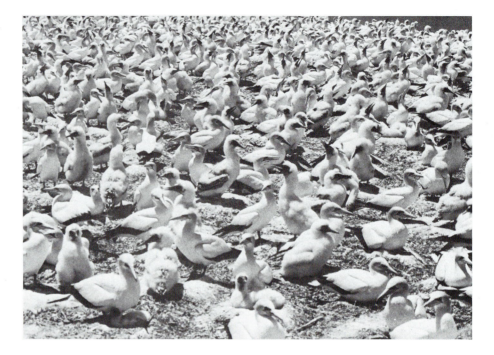

Many small songbirds also make great migration treks (Fig. 26-19). Africa is a favorite wintering ground for European birds, and many fly there from Central Asia as well.

___ Stimulus for Migration

Humans have known for centuries that the onset of the reproductive cycle of birds is closely related to season. Only within the last 50 years, however, has it been proved that the lengthening days of late winter and early spring stimulate the development of the gonads and accumulation of fat—both important internal changes that predispose birds to migrate northward. There is evidence that increasing day length stimulates the anterior lobe of the pituitary into activity. The release of pituitary gonadotropic hormone in turn sets in motion a complex series of physiological and behavioral changes, resulting in gonadal growth, fat deposition, migration, courtship and mating behavior, and care of the young.

___ Direction Finding in Migration

Numerous experiments suggest that most birds navigate chiefly by sight. Birds recognize topographical landmarks and follow familiar migratory routes—a behavior assisted by flock migration, during which navigational resources and experience of older birds can be pooled. But in addition to visual navigation, birds make use of a variety of orientation cues at their disposal. Birds have an innate time sense, a built-in clock of great accuracy; they have an innate sense of direction; and very recent work adds credence to an old, much debated theory that birds can detect and navigate by the earth's magnetic field. All of these resources are inborn and instinctive, although a bird's navigational abilities may improve with experience.

Recent experiments by German ornithologists G. Kramer and E. Sauer and American ornithologist S. Emlen have demonstrated convincingly that birds can

In the early 1970s, W.T. Keeton showed that the flight bearings of homing pigeons were significantly disturbed by magnets attached to the birds' heads, or by minor fluctuations in the geomagnetic field. But until recently the nature and position of a magnetic receptor in pigeons remained a mystery. Deposits of a magnetic substance called magnetite (Fe_3O_4) have now been discovered in the neck musculature of pigeons and migratory white-crowned sparrows. If this material were coupled to sensitive muscle receptors, as has been proposed, the structure could serve as a magnetic compass that would enable birds to detect and orient their migrations to the earth's magnetic field.

Figure 26-21

Cooperative feeding behavior of white pelicans *Pelecanus onocrotalus*. **A,** Pelicans on Lake Nakuru, East Africa, form a horseshoe to drive fish together. **B,** Then they plunge simultaneously to scoop up fishes in their huge bills. Pelicans were attracted to the lake in mid-1960s to feed on fish *(Tilapia grahami)* introduced to control malaria by eating mosquito larva. (The pictures were taken 2 seconds apart.) Order Pelecaniformes. Photographs by B. Tallmark.

navigate by celestial cues: the sun by day and the stars by night. Using special circular cages, Kramer concluded that birds possess a built-in time sense that enables them to maintain compass direction by referring to the sun, regardless of time of day. This is called **sun-azimuth orientation** (*azimuth,* compass bearing of the sun). Sauer's and Emlen's ingenious planetarium experiments strongly suggest that some birds, probably many, learn to use the constellations to navigate at night.

Some of the remarkable feats of bird navigation still defy rational explanation. Most birds undoubtedly use a combination of environmental and innate cues to migrate. Migration is a rigorous undertaking; the target is often small, and natural selection relentlessly prunes off individuals making errors in migration, leaving only the best navigators to propagate the species.

REPRODUCTION AND BEHAVIOR

The adage says "birds of a feather flock together," and birds are indeed highly social creatures. Especially during the breeding season, sea birds gather, often in enormous colonies, to nest and rear young (Fig. 26-20). Land birds, with some conspicuous exceptions (such as starlings and rooks), tend to be less gregarious than sea birds during breeding and to seek isolation for rearing their brood. But these same species that covet separation from their kind during breeding may aggregate for migration or feeding. Togetherness offers advantages: mutual protection from enemies, greater ease in finding mates, less opportunity for individual straying during migration, and mass huddling for protection against low night temperatures during migration. Certain species, such as pelicans (Fig. 26-21), may use highly organized cooperative behavior to feed. At no time are the highly organized social interactions of birds more evident than during the breeding season, as they stake out territorial claims, select mates, build nests, incubate and hatch their eggs, and rear their young.

Reproductive System

In the male the paired **testes** and accessory ducts are similar to those in many other forms. From the **testes** the **vasa deferentia** run to the cloaca. Before being discharged, the sperm are stored in the **seminal vesicle,** the enlarged distal end of the vas deferens. This seminal vesicle may become so large with stored sperm during the breeding season that it causes a cloacal protuberance. The high body temper-

Figure 26-22

Figure 26-22

Culmination of courtship activities is copulation, shown here in a pair of waved albatrosses *Diomedea irrorata*. Order Procellariiformes.
Photograph by C.P. Hickman, Jr.

ature, which tends to inhibit spermatogenesis in the testes, is probably counteracted by the cooling effect of the abdominal air sacs. The testes of birds undergo a great enlargement at the breeding season, as much as 300 fold, and then shrink to tiny bodies afterward. Some birds, including ducks and geese, have a large, well-developed **copulatory organ** (penis), provided with a groove on its dorsal side for the transfer of sperm. However, in the more advanced birds, copulation is a matter of bringing the cloacal surfaces into contact, usually while the male stands on the female's back (Fig. 26-22). Some swifts copulate in flight.

In the female of most birds, only the left ovary and oviduct develop; those on the right dwindle to vestigial structures. Eggs discharged from the ovary are picked up by the expanded end of the oviduct, the **ostium** (Fig. 26-23). The oviduct runs posteriorly to the cloaca. While the eggs are passing down the oviduct, **albumin,** or egg white, from special glands is added to them; farther down the oviduct, the shell membrane, shell, and shell pigments are also secreted about the egg. Fertilization takes place in the upper oviduct several hours before the layers of albumin, shell membranes, and shell are added. Sperm remain alive in the female oviduct for many days after a single mating. Hen eggs show good fertility for 5 or 6 days after mating, but then fertility drops rapidly. However, the occasional egg will be fertile as long as 30 days after separation of the hen from the rooster.

___ Mating Systems

The two most common types of mating system in animals are **monogamy,** in which an individual mates with only one partner each breeding season, and **polygamy,** in which an individual mates with two or more partners each breeding period. Monogamy is rare in most animal groups, but in birds it is the general rule: more than 90% of the birds are monogamous. In a few bird species such as swans and geese, partners are chosen for life and often remain together throughout the year. Seasonal monogamy is more common, however, in the great majority of

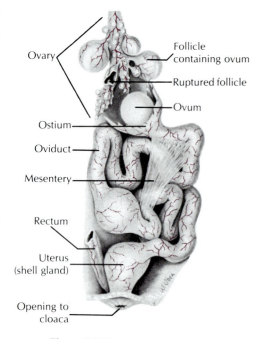

Ovary
Follicle containing ovum
Ruptured follicle
Ovum
Ostium
Oviduct
Mesentery
Rectum
Uterus (shell gland)
Opening to cloaca

Figure 26-23

Reproductive system of female bird.

Figure 26-24

Dominant male sage grouse surrounded by several hens that have been attracted by his "booming" display. Order Galliformes.
Photograph by L.L. Rue, III.

migrant birds, which pair up during the breeding season but lead independent lives the rest of the year.

One reason that monogamy is much more common among birds than among mammals is that female birds are not equipped, as mammals are, with a built-in food supply for the young. Thus, the ability of the two sexes to provide parental care, especially food for the young, is more equal in birds than in mammals. A female bird will choose a male whose parental investment in their young is apt to be high and avoid a male that has mated with another female. If the male had mated with another female, he could at best divide his time between his two mates and might even devote most of his attention to the alternate mate. Thus, females enforce monogamy.

Monogamy in birds is also encouraged by the need for the male to secure and defend a territory before he can attract a mate. The male may sing a great deal to announce his presence to females and to discourage rival males from entering his territory. The female wanders from one territory to another, seeking a male with foraging territory that offers the best chances for reproductive success. Usually a male is able to defend an area that provides just enough resources for one nesting female.

Polygyny does occur in birds, however, usually in habitats that are particularly rich in food resources such as marshes. A male red-winged blackbird may defend a "superterritory" so favorable that he can gather a harem of as many as 10 nesting females, all of whom enjoy reproductive success that is the same as or higher than monogamous females in less favored territories. This is known as **resource defense polygyny.** The females are in some way able to assess their reproductive chances in different territories and choose polygyny when it clearly will benefit them.

A kind of polygyny known as **dominance polygyny** is common in many species of grouse (Fig. 26-24) and pheasants. The male birds gather in a collective display ground, called a **lek,** which typically is composed of individually owned courts (territories), each aggressively defended by a displaying male. There is nothing of value in the lek to the female except the male, and all he can offer are his genes, for only the females care for the young. Usually there are a dominant male and several males subordinate to him in the lek. Competition among males for females is intense, but the females appear to choose the dominant male for mating because, presumably, social rank correlates with genetic quality.

The term "polygamy" ("many marriages") is used when the sex of the individual possessing a plurality of mates is not specified. The most common form of polygamy is polygyny ("many females"), in which a male mates with more than one female. Much less common is polyandry ("many males"), in which a female mates with more than one male per breeding season.

___ Nesting and Care of the Young

All birds are oviparous, laying eggs that with rare exceptions must be incubated by one or both parents. The exceptions are found among the mound-builders (megapodes) of Australia and the East Indies, which lay their eggs in huge mounds. Fermenting vegetation or solar radiation provides enough heat to incubate the eggs. Viviparity did not evolve in birds, probably because flight would be difficult while carrying around the young.

Most birds build some form of nest in which to rear their young. Some birds simply lay their eggs on the bare ground or rocks and make no pretense of nest building. Others build elaborate nests, such as the pendant nests constructed by orioles, the neat lichen-covered nests of hummingbirds (Fig. 26-25) and flycatchers, the chimney-shaped mud nests of cliff swallows, the floating nests of red-necked grebes, and the huge brush pile nests of Australian brush turkeys. Most birds take considerable pains to conceal their nests from enemies. Woodpeckers, chickadees, bluebirds, and many others place their nests in tree hollows or other cavities; kingfishers excavate tunnels in the banks of streams for their nests; and birds of prey build high in lofty trees or on inaccessible cliffs. A few birds such as the American cowbird and the European cuckoo build no nests at all but simply lay their eggs in the nests of birds smaller than themselves. When the eggs hatch, the foster parents care for the young.

Most American songbirds lay from three to six eggs, but the number of eggs laid in a clutch varies from one or two (some hawks and pigeons) to 18 to 20 (quail). Some birds (such as the herring gull) are **determinate layers** and lay only a fixed number (clutch) of eggs in a season. If any of the eggs of a set are removed, the deficit is not made up by additional laying. **Indeterminate layers** (such as flickers, ducks, and domestic poultry), however, will continue to lay additional eggs for a long time if some of the first-laid eggs are continually removed. Most birds are probably determinate layers. Many birds such as songbirds lay an egg a day until the clutch is completed; others stagger their egg laying and lay every other day or so. Domestic geese usually lay every other day, which also is probably the pattern for the large birds of prey.

The eggs of most songbirds require approximately 14 days for hatching; those of ducks and geese require at least twice that long. Most of the duties of incubation fall to the female, although in many instances both parents share the task, and occasionally only the male performs this work.

Nesting success is very low with many birds, especially in altricial species (see the following paragraph). One investigation of 170 altricial bird nests reported that only 21% produced at least one young. Of the many causes of nesting failures, predation by snakes, skunks, chipmunks, blue jays, crows, and others is by far the chief factor. Birds of prey probably have a much higher percentage of reproductive success.

Newly hatched birds are of two types: **precocial** and **altricial.** The precocial young, such as quail, fowl, ducks, and most water birds, are covered with down when hatched and can run or swim as soon as their plumage is dry (Fig. 26-26). The altricial ones, on the other hand, are naked and helpless at birth and remain in the nest for a week or more. The young of both types require care from parents for some time after hatching. They must be fed, guarded, and protected against rain and sun. The parents of altricial species must carry food to their young almost constantly, for most young birds will eat more than their weight each day. This enormous food consumption explains the rapid growth of the young and their

How do eggs breathe? The answer, in a word, is diffusion. Oxygen diffuses in and carbon dioxide diffuses out through thousands of pores in the egg shell. The position of the pores can be seen by placing the egg in a jar of water and pumping out the air with a vacuum pump; bubbles of air stream out of the pores all over the egg. The pores also are avenues of water loss, and all eggs, whether large or small or with short or long incubation periods, lose relatively the same amount of water, about 15% of the initial egg weight. Losing just the right amount of water is critical because the embryo will drown if water loss is too little and will desiccate if it is too great. Thus, the number and size of the pores in an egg shell are determined by the necessity for a fixed water loss, rather than for gas exchange, but they serve both functions equally well.

Figure 26-25

Ruby-throated hummingbird *Archilochus colubris* in nest built of plant down and spider webs and decorated on the outside with lichens. The female builds the nest, incubates the two pea-sized eggs, and rears the young with no assistance from the male. These frail-looking but pugnacious little birds make arduous seasonal migrations between Canada and Mexico. Order Apodiformes.

Photograph by L.L. Rue, III.

Altricial
One-day-old meadow lark

Precocial

Figure 26-26

Comparison of 1-day-old altricial and precocial young. The altricial meadowlark *(top)* is born nearly naked, blind, and helpless. The precocial ruffed grouse *(bottom)* is covered with down, alert, strong legged, and able to feed itself.

Figure 26-27

Robin *Turdus migratorius* feeds its altricial young. They have phenomenal appetites and develop rapidly. These young have opened their eyes and have learned to gape toward the parent. The parents will supply all the food until the young are nearly adult size. Order Passeriformes.

Photograph by L.L. Rue, III.

quick exit from the nest (Fig. 26-27). The food of the young, depending on the species, includes worms, insects, seeds, and fruit. Pigeons and doves are peculiar in feeding their young "pigeon milk," the sloughed-off epithelial lining of the crop.

BIRD POPULATIONS

Bird populations, like those of other animal groups, vary in size from year to year. Snowy owls, for example, are subject to population cycles that closely follow cycles in their food supply, mainly rodents. Voles, mice, and lemmings in the north have a fairly regular 4-year cycle of abundance; at population peaks, predator populations of foxes, weasels, and buzzards, as well as snowy owls, increase because there is abundant food for rearing their young. After a crash in the rodent population, snowy owls move south, seeking alternative food supplies. They occasionally appear in large numbers in southern Canada and the northern United States, where their total absence of fear of humans makes them easy targets for thoughtless hunters.

Occasionally the activities of people bring about spectacular changes in bird distribution. Both starlings (Fig. 26-28) and house sparrows have been accidentally or deliberately introduced into numerous countries, and they have become the two most abundant bird species on earth, with the exception of domestic fowl.

Figure 26-28

A, Starling with insect larva. Starlings are omnivorous. They eat mostly insects in spring and summer and shift to wild fruits in fall. **B,** Colonization of North America by starlings *Sturnus vulgaris* (order Passeriformes) after the introduction of 120 birds into Central Park in New York City in 1890. There are now perhaps 100 million starlings in the United States alone, testimony to the great reproductive potential of birds.

A, Photograph by L.L. Rue, III; **B,** modified from Fisher, J., and R.T. Peterson. 1971. Birds. London, Aldus Books Ltd.

A

B

Humans also are responsible for the extinction of many bird species. More than 80 species of birds have, since 1695, followed the last dodo to extinction. Many died naturally, victims of changes in their habitat or competition with better-adapted species. But several have been hunted to extinction, among them the passenger pigeon (Fig. 26-29), which only a century ago darkened the skies over North America in incredible numbers estimated in the billions (Fig. 26-30). Hunters kill millions of game birds annually, as well as many nongame birds that happen to make convenient targets. An even greater number of game birds die indirectly as the result of eating lead pellets (which they mistake for seeds) or from the crippling effects of embedded pellets. One survey in Wisconsin revealed that the average hunter required 36 shots to kill one goose. Of the Canada geese that survived the barrage to fly as far south as the Mississippi Valley, 44% contained embedded lead shot.

Our most destructive effects on birds are usually unintentional. The draining of marshes—more than 99% of Iowa's once extensive marshland is now farmland—has destroyed waterfowl nesting. Deforestation has likewise had great impact on tree-nesting species. The vertical appendages of civilization, such as television towers, monuments, tall buildings, and electrical transmission towers and lines, take a fearful toll during bird migration in bad weather. Most birds, through their impressive reproductive potential, can replace in numbers those that become victims of human activities. Someone has calculated that a single pair of robins, producing two broods of four young a season, would leave 19,500,000 descendants in 10 years, should all survive that long. But, although many birds have accommodated to the heavy-handed influence of humans on their environment, and some such as robins, house sparrows, and starlings even thrive on it, most birds find it adverse, and to some species it is lethal.

Figure 26-29

"Martha," the last passenger pigeon *Ectopistes migratorius,* died in the Cincinnati Zoo in 1914. Passenger pigeons traveled and roosted in huge masses, with nesting areas exceeding 80 sq km (about 30 square miles). In 1869, hunters shot 7.5 million pigeons from a single nesting site.

Courtesy Smithsonian Institution, Washington, D.C.

Figure 26-30

Shooting passenger pigeons for sport in Louisiana during the nineteenth century. Relentless sport and market hunting eventually dropped the population too low to sustain colonial breeding.

Courtesy Culver Pictures.

Figure 26-31

Male rhea *(Rhea americana)* displays to a female *(foreground)*. Order Rheiformes.
Photograph by L.L. Rue, III.

CLASSIFICATION

Class Aves (birds) is made up of about 27 orders of living birds and a few fossil orders. More than 8600 species and many subspecies have been described. Probably only a relatively few species remain to be discovered and named, but many subspecies are added yearly. With their powers of flight and wide distribution, most species of birds are more easily detected than are many animals. Only those that are solitary, shy, and restricted to remote regions have a chance of remaining undiscovered for any length of time. Altogether, the species are grouped into 170 families. Of the 27 recognized orders, 20 are represented by North American species.

The first four orders in this classification are the **ratite,** or flightless, birds, although as noted earlier, flightlessness is not restricted to these orders. The remaining orders are the **carinate** birds (birds with a keeled sternum).

Order Struthioniformes (stroo'thi-on-i-for'meez) (L., *struthio,* ostrich, + *forma,* form)—ostriches. The flightless ostrich of Africa *(Struthio camelus)* is the largest of living birds, with some specimens being 2.4 m tall and weighing 135 kg. The feet are provided with only two toes of unequal size covered with pads, which enable the birds to travel rapidly through sandy country.

Order Rheiformes (re'i-for'meez) (Gr. mythology, *Rhea,* mother of Zeus, + form)—rheas (Fig. 26-31). These flightless birds are restricted to South America and are often called the American ostrich.

Order Casuariiformes (kazh'u-ar'ee-i-for'meez) (N.L., *Casuarius,* type genus, + form)—cassowaries, emus. This is a group of flightless birds found in Australia, New Guinea, and a few other islands. Some specimens may reach a height of 1.5 m.

Order Apterygiformes (ap'te-rij'i-for'meez) (Gr., *a,* not, + *pteryx,* wing, + form)—kiwis. Kiwis are flightless birds about the size of the domestic fowl, found only in New Zealand. The three species belong to the genus *Apteryx.* Only the merest vestige of a wing is present. The egg is extremely large for the size of the bird.

Order Tinamiformes (tin-am'i-for'meez) (N.L., *Tinamus,* type genus, + form)—tinamous. These are flying birds found in South America and Mexico. They resemble the ruffed grouse and are classed as game birds. There are more than 60 species in this order.

Order Sphenisciformes (sfe-nis'i-for'meez) (Gr., *sphēniskos*, dim. of *sphen*, wedge, from the shortness of the wings, + form)—**penguins**. Penguins are web-footed, marine swimmers of the southern seas, from Antarctica to the Galápagos Islands. Although carinate birds, they use their wings as paddles rather than for flight. The largest penguin is the emperor penguin (*Aptenodytes forsteri*) of the Antarctic, which breeds in enormous rookeries on the shores of that region.

Order Gaviiformes (gay'vee-i-for'meez) (L., *gavia*, bird, probably sea mew, + form)—**loons**. Loons are remarkable swimmers and divers with short legs and heavy bodies. They live exclusively on fish and small aquatic forms. The familiar great northern diver (*Gavia immer*) is found mainly in northern waters of North America and Eurasia.

Order Podicipediformes (pod'i-si-ped'i-for'meez) (L., *podex*, rump, + *pes, pedis*, foot)—**grebes**. These are short-legged divers with lobate-webbed toes. The pied-billed grebe (*Podilymbus podiceps*) is a familiar example of this order. Grebes are most common in old ponds where they build their raftlike floating nests. Worldwide distribution.

Order Procellariiformes (pro-sel-lar'ee-i-for'meez) (L., *procella*, tempest, + form)—**albatrosses, petrels, fulmars, shearwaters**. All are marine birds with tubular nostrils. In wingspan (more than 3.6 m in some), albatrosses are the largest of flying birds. *Diomedea* is a common genus of albatrosses. Worldwide distribution.

Order Pelecaniformes (pel'e-can-i-for'meez) (Gr., *pelekan*, pelican, + form)—**pelicans** (Fig. 26-32), **cormorants, gannets, boobies**, and so on. These are fish-eaters with throat pouch and all four toes of each foot included within the web. Mostly colonial nesters. Worldwide distribution, especially in the tropics.

Order Ciconiiformes (si-ko'nee-i-for'meez) (L., *ciconia*, stork, + form)—**herons, bitterns, storks, ibises, spoonbills, flamingoes**. These are long-necked, long-legged, mostly colonial waders. A familiar eastern North American representative is the great blue heron (*Ardea herodias*), which frequents marshes and ponds. Worldwide distribution.

Order Anseriformes (an'ser-i-for'meez) (L., *anser*, goose, + form)—**swans, geese, ducks**. The members of this order have broad bills with filtering ridges at their margins, a foot web restricted to the front toes, and a long breastbone with a low keel. The common domestic mallard duck is *Anas platyrhynchos*. Worldwide distribution.

Order Falconiformes (fal'ko-ni-for'meez) (L., *falco*, falcon, + form)—**eagles, hawks, vultures, falcons, condors, buzzards**. These are the great diurnal birds of prey. All are strong fliers with keen vision. Worldwide distribution.

Order Galliformes (gal'li-for'meez) (L., *gallus*, cock, + form)—**quail, grouse** (Fig. 26-33), **pheasants, ptarmigan, turkeys, domestic fowl**. These are chickenlike vegetarians with strong beaks and heavy feet. Some of the most desirable game birds are in this order. The bobwhite quail (*Colinus virginianus*) is found all over the eastern half of the United States. The ruffed grouse (*Bonasa umbellus*), or partridge, is found in about the same region, but in the woods instead of the open pastures and grain fields, which the bobwhite frequents. Worldwide distribution.

Order Gruiformes (groo'i-for'meez) (L., *grus*, crane, + form)—**cranes, rails, coots, gallinules**. These are prairie and marsh breeders. Worldwide distribution.

Order Charadriiformes (ka-rad'ree-i-for'meez) (N.L., *Charadrius*, genus of plovers, + form)—**gulls, oyster catchers, plovers, sandpipers, terns, woodcocks, turnstones, lapwings, snipe, avocets, phalaropes, skuas, skimmers, auks, puffins**. All are shorebirds. They are strong fliers and are usually colonial. Worldwide distribution.

Order Columbiformes (co-lum'bi-for'meez) (L., *columba*, dove, + form)—**pigeons, doves**. All have short necks, short legs, and a short, slender bill. Worldwide distribution.

Order Psittaciformes (sit'ta-si-for'meez) (L., *psittacus*, parrot, + form)—**parrots, parakeets**. These have a hinged and movable upper mandible. Pantropical distribution.

Order Cuculiformes (ku-koo'li-for'meez) (L., *cuculus*, cuckoo, + form)—**cuckoos, roadrunners**. The common cuckoo (*Cuculus canorus*) of Europe lays its eggs in the nests of smaller birds, which rear the young cuckoos. The American cuckoos, black billed and yellow billed, usually rear their own young. Worldwide distribution.

Order Strigiformes (strij'i-for'meez) (L., *strix*, screech owl, + form)—**owls**. Owls are nocturnal predators with large eyes, powerful beaks and feet, and silent flight. Worldwide distribution.

Figure 26-32

Brown pelican *Pelecanus occidentalis*. Pelicans catch fish by diving from the air. Order Pelecaniformes.

Photograph by C.P. Hickman, Jr.

Figure 26-33

Ruffed grouse *Bonasa umbellus* "drumming" to attract a female. Order Galliformes.

Photograph by N. Bolen.

Figure 26-34

Female nighthawk *Chordeiles minor* broods two 1-day-old young, their down barely visible under her breast. Nighthawks originally nested on beaches and in old stumps, but with the spread of civilization they discovered building roofs to be ideal nesting sites. Their nasal "peent" is a familiar summer evening sound above city streets. Order Caprimulgiformes.

Photograph by C.P. Hickman, Jr.

Figure 26-35

Kookaburra *Dacelo novaeguineae,* the wood kingfisher of Australia, famous for its cry that resembles demented laughter. Order Coraciiformes.

Photograph by C.P. Hickman, Jr.

Order Caprimulgiformes (kap′ri-mul′ji-for′meez) (L., *caprimulgus,* goatsucker, + form)—**goatsuckers, nighthawks** (Fig. 26-34), **whippoorwills.** The birds of this group are night and twilight feeders with small, weak legs and wide mouths fringed with bristles. The whippoorwills *(Antrostomus vociferus)* are common in the woods of the eastern states, and the nighthawk *(Chordeiles minor)* is often seen and heard in the evening flying around city buildings. Worldwide distribution.

Order Apodiformes (up-pod′i-for′meez) (Gr., *apous,* sandmartin; footless, + form)—**swifts, hummingbirds.** These are small birds with short legs and rapid wingbeat. The familiar chimney swift *(Chaetura pelagica)* fastens its nest in chimneys by means of saliva. A swift found in China *(Collocalia)* builds a nest of saliva that is used by the Chinese for soup making. Most species of hummingbirds are found in the tropics, but there are 14 species in the United States, of which only one, the ruby-throated hummingbird, is found in the eastern part of the country. Most hummingbirds live on nectar, although some also catch insects. Worldwide distribution.

Order Coliiformes (ka-ly′i-for′meez) (Gr., *kolios,* green woodpecker, + form)—**mousebirds.** These are small birds of uncertain relationship. Restricted to southern Africa.

Order Trogoniformes (tro-gon′i-for′meez) (Gr., *trōgon,* gnawing, + form)—**trogons.** Richly colored birds. Pantropical distribution.

Order Coraciiformes (ka-ray′see-i-for′meez or kor′uh-sigh′uh-for′meez) (N.L., *coracii* from Gr., *korakias,* a kind of chough [akin to *korax,* raven or crow], + form)—**kingfishers** (Fig. 26-35), **hornbills, and so on.** These birds have strong, prominent bills and colorful plumage. In the eastern half of the United States, the belted kingfisher *(Megaceryle alcyon)* is common along most waterways of any size. It makes a nest in a burrow in a high bank or cliff along a water course. Worldwide distribution.

Order Piciformes (pis′i-for′meez) (L., *picus,* woodpecker, + form)—**woodpeckers, toucans, puffbirds, honeyguides.** Birds of this order have two of the toes extending forward and two backward and a highly specialized bill (chisel-like in woodpeckers). All nest in cavities. There are many species of woodpeckers in North America, the most common of which are the flickers and the downy, hairy, red-bellied, redheaded, and yellow-bellied woodpeckers. The largest is the pileated woodpecker, which is usually found in deep and remote woods. Worldwide distribution.

Order Passeriformes (pas′er-i-for′meez) (L., *passer,* sparrow, + form)—**perching songbirds.** This is the largest order of birds, containing 56 families and 60% of all birds. Most have a highly developed syrinx. Their feet are adapted for perching on thin stems and twigs. The young are altricial. To this order belong many birds with beautiful songs such as the skylark, nightingale, hermit thrush, mockingbird, meadowlark, robin, and hosts of others. Others of this order, such as the swallow, magpie, starling, crow, raven, jay, nuthatch, and creeper, have no songs worthy of the name. Worldwide distribution.

___ Summary

The 8600 species of living birds are egg-laying, endothermic vertebrates covered with feathers and having the forelimbs modified as wings. Birds have evolved from archosaurian reptiles during the Mesozoic era and bear numerous reptilian morphological characters. The oldest known fossil bird, *Archaeopteryx* from the Jurassic period of the Mesozoic era, was even more reptilelike than modern birds.

The adaptations of birds for flight are of two basic kinds: those reducing body weight and those promoting more power for flight. Feathers, the hallmark of birds, are complex derivatives of reptilian scales and combine lightness with strength, water repellency, and high insulative value. Body weight is further reduced by elimination of some bones, fusion of others (to provide rigidity for flight), and the presence in many bones of hollow, air-filled spaces. The light, horny bill, replacing the heavy jaws and teeth of reptiles, serves as both hand and mouth for all birds and is variously adapted for different feeding habits.

Adaptations that provide power for flight include a high metabolic rate and body temperature coupled with an energy-rich diet; a highly efficient respiratory system consisting of a system of air sacs arranged to pass air through the lungs during both inspiration and expiration; powerful flight and leg muscles arranged to place muscle weight near the bird's center of gravity; and an efficient, high-pressure circulation.

Birds have keen eyesight, good hearing, poorly developed sense of smell, and superb coordination for flight. The metanephric kidneys produce uric acid as the principal nitrogenous waste.

Birds fly by applying the same aerodynamic principles as an airplane, and using similar equipment: wings for lift and support, a tail for steering and landing control, and wing slots for control at low flight speed. Flightlessness in birds is unusual but has evolved independently in several bird orders, usually on islands where terrestrial predators are absent; all are derived from flying ancestors.

Bird migration refers to regular movements between summer nesting places and wintering regions. Spring migration to the north where more food is available for nestlings enhances reproductive success. Many cues are used for direction finding in migration, including innate sense of direction and ability to navigate by the sun, the stars, or the earth's magnetic field.

The highly developed social behavior of birds is manifested in vivid courtship displays, mate selection, territorial behavior, and incubation of eggs and care of the young.

Selected references

Aidley, D.J. (ed.). 1981. Animal migration. Cambridge, Eng., Cambridge University Press. *Several chapters deal with bird migration.*

Baker, R. (ed.). 1981. The mystery of migration. New York, The Viking Press. *Handsomely illustrated, popularized account.*

Bent, A.C. 1919-1968. Life histories of North American birds. United States National Museum Bulletins. *More than a score of monographs in this outstanding series provide a wealth of information on birds. Dover reprints of the entire series are available.*

Farner, D.S., and J.R. King (eds.). 1971-1975. Avian biology, 5 vols. New York, Academic Press, Inc. *Advanced treatise composed of contributed chapters.*

Feduccia, A. 1980. The age of birds. Cambridge, Mass., Harvard University Press. *Semipopular but authoritative account of bird evolution. Excellent text and illustrations.*

Fisher, J., and R.T. Peterson, 1971. An introduction to general ornithology. London, Aldus Books, Ltd. *Beautifully illustrated general biology of birds by two famous ornithologists.*

Gould, J.L. 1980. The case for magnetic sensitivity in birds and bees (such as it is). Am. Sci. **68**:256-267.

Griffin, D.R. 1974. Bird migration. New York, Dover Publications, Inc. *Interesting semipopular account of the subject.*

Keeton, W.T. 1979. Avian orientation and navigation. Ann. Rev. Physiol. **41**:353-366. *Review emphasizing the amazing flexibility of bird navigational systems.*

Lorenz, K.Z. 1952. King Solomon's ring. New York, Thomas Y. Crowell Co., Publishers. *A deservedly popular account of animal (especially bird) behavior by a great ethologist.*

Ostrom, J.H. 1979. Bird flight: how did it happen? Am. Sci. **67**:46-56. *The author argues his cursorial theory of the origin of bird flight.*

Peterson, R.T. 1980. Field guide to the birds (east of the Rockies), ed. 2. Boston, Houghton Mifflin Co. *This popular field guide was completely reillustrated for this edition.*

Regal, P.J. 1975. The evolutionary origin of feathers. Q. Rev. Biol. **50**:35-66. *Reviews the problems of deriving a branched feather from an elongate reptilian scale.*

Robbins, C.S., B. Brunn, H. Zim, and A. Singer. 1966. Birds of North America: a guide to field identification. Racine, Wis., Western Publishing Co., Inc. *Excellent full-color illustrations of all species with range maps on opposite page.*

Rue, L.L., III. 1974. Game birds of North America. New York, Harper & Row, Publishers, Inc. *Comprehensive description of 75 game birds with fine bird paintings by nature artist Douglas Allen.*

Rüppell, G. 1975. Bird flight. New York, Van Nostrand Reinhold Co. *Clear descriptions and illustrations.*

Savile, B.D.O. 1957. Adaptive evolution in the avian wing. Evolution **11**:212-224.

Terres, J.K. 1980. The Audubon Society encyclopedia of North American birds. New York, Alfred A. Knopf, Inc. *Comprehensive, authoritative, and richly illustrated.*

Tinbergen, N. 1960. The herring gull's world. New York, Basic Books, Inc., Publishers. *A superb account of bird behavior by a renowned ethologist. Excellent illustrations by the author.*

Welty, J.C. 1982. The life of birds, ed. 3. Philadelphia, W.B. Saunders Co. *Among the best of the ornithology texts; lucid style and excellent illustrations.*

Selected *Scientific American* articles

Calder, W.A., III. 1978. The kiwi. **239**:132-142 (July). *This flightless bird of New Zealand has developed mammal-like characteristics.*

Cone, C.D., Jr. 1962. The soaring flight of birds. **206**:130-140 (Apr.). *The nature of air currents and patterns of soaring flight are analyzed.*

Eklund, C.R. 1964. The Antarctic skua. **210**:94-100 (Feb.). *Discusses the biology of this large, aggressive, and cold-adapted bird.*

Emlen, J.E., and R.L. Penny. 1966. The navigation of penguins. **215**:104-113 (Oct.). *Penguins depend on an innate biological clock and the sun's direction to guide them across hundreds of miles of featureless Antarctic landscape.*

Emlen, S.T. 1975. The stellar-orientation system of a migratory bird. **233**:102-111 (Aug.). *Describes fascinating research with indigo buntings, revealing their ability to orient by the stars.*

Greenewalt, C.H. 1969. How birds sing. **221**:126-139 (Nov.). *The mechanism of bird song is quite different from that of musical instruments or the human voice.*

Keeton, W.T. 1974. The mystery of pigeon homing. **231**:96-107 (Dec.). *Birds use several compass systems in navigation.*

Nicoli, J. 1974. Mimicry in parasitic birds. **231**:92-98 (Oct.).

Peakall, D.B. 1970. Pesticides and the reproduction of birds. **222**:72-78 (Apr.). *Pesticides threaten the survival of several species of birds of prey. The reasons are explained.*

Pennycuick, C.J. 1973. The soaring flight of vultures. **229**:102-109 (Dec.). *Patterns of soaring flight are studied with the aid of powered glider.*

Sauer, E.G.F. 1958. Celestial navigation by birds. **199**:42-47 (Aug.). *The author describes his ingenious planetarium experiments to demonstrate that migratory birds navigate by the stars.*

Schmidt-Nielsen, K. 1959. Salt glands. **200**:109-116 (Jan.). *The anatomy and physiology of this special salt-excretory organ of marine birds are described.*

Schmidt-Nielsen, K. 1971. How birds breathe. **225**:72-79 (Dec.).

Shettleworth, S.J. 1983. Memory in food-hoarding birds. **248**:102-110 (Mar.). *Birds that hide and later recover seeds have excellent spatial memory.*

Stettner, L.J., and K.A. Matyniak. 1968. The brain of birds. **218**:64-76 (June).

Tickell, W.L.N. 1970. The great albatrosses. **223**:84-93 (Nov.). *Describes the reproductive behavior and movements of the largest of oceanic birds.*

Tucker, V.A. 1969. The energetics of bird flight. **220**:70-78 (May).

Welty, C. 1955. Birds as flying machines **192**:88-96 (Mar.). *A description of the remarkable adaptations that fit birds for flight.*

Williams, T.C., and J.M. Williams. 1978. An oceanic mass migration of land birds. **239**:166-176 (Oct.). *Tracing bird migration with radar.*

CHAPTER 27

THE MAMMALS

Phylum Chordata
Class Mammalia

The alert expression of this red fox suggests a principal reason why mammals, as a group, dominate the animal world: their exceptional intelligence.

Photograph by I. Vandermolen, Leonard Rue Enterprises.

Mammals, with their highly developed nervous system and numerous ingenious adaptations, occupy almost every environment on earth that supports life. Although not a large group (4500 species as compared with 8600 species of birds, approximately 21,000 species of fishes, and 800,000 species of insects), the class Mammalia (mam-may′lee-a) (L., *mamma*, breast) is overall the most biologically successful group in the animal kingdom, with the possible exception of the insects. Many potentialities that dwell more or less latently in other vertebrates are highly developed in mammals. Mammals are exceedingly diverse in size, shape, form, and function. They range in size from the diminutive pigmy shrew, which has a body length of less than 4 cm and a weight of only a few grams, to the whales, some of which exceed 100 tons in weight.

Yet, despite their adaptability and in some instances because of it, mammals have been influenced by the presence of humans more than any other group of animals. We have domesticated numerous mammals for food and clothing, as beasts of burden, and as pets. We use millions of mammals each year in biomedical research. We have introduced alien mammals into new habitats, occasionally with benign results but more frequently with unexpected disaster. Although history provides us with numerous warnings, we continue to overcrop valuable wild stocks of mammals. The whale industry threatens itself with total collapse by exterminating its own resource—a classic example of self-destruction in the modern world, in which competing segments of an industry are intent only on reaping all they can today as though tomorrow's supply were of no concern whatever. In some cases destruction of a valuable mammalian resource has been deliberate, such as the officially sanctioned (and tragically successful) policy during the Indian wars of exterminating the bison to drive the Plains Indians into starvation. Although commercial hunting has declined, the ever-increasing human population with the accompanying destruction of wild habitats has harassed and disfigured the mammalian fauna. We are becoming increasingly aware that our presence on this planet as the most powerful product of organic evolution makes us responsible for the character of our natural environment. Since our welfare has been and continues to be closely related to that of the other mammals, it is clearly in our interest to preserve the natural environment of which all mammals, ourselves included, are a part. We need to remember that nature can do without us but we cannot exist without nature.

ORIGIN AND RELATIONSHIPS

In the early Mesozoic era, long before the great dinosaurs had reached the peak of their evolutionary success, a group of reptiles with mammal-like characteristics appeared. These were **therapsids** (Fig. 27-1). The evolution of the therapsids and their descendants was accompanied by several structural changes that brought them ever closer to full mammalian status. The clumsy limbs of the reptile that stuck out laterally were replaced by straight legs held close to the body, which provided speed and efficiency for hunting. Since reptilian stability was sacrificed by raising the animal from the ground, the muscular coordination center of the brain, the cerebellum, took on a greatly expanded role. Among the many changes in the bony structure of the head was the separation of air and food passages in the mouth. This enabled the animal to breathe while holding prey in its mouth. A stronger jaw joint made possible prolonged chewing and some predigestion of food. And at some point, probably in the late Permian period, the premammals

Figure 27-1

Evolution of the mammals. Mammals take their origin from the therapsid reptiles, which were probably warm blooded. The most primitive mammals are the monotremes, which lay reptilelike eggs. They may have arisen from a group of therapsid reptiles distinct from those from which the viviparous therians, or "true" mammals, arose. The pouched marsupials probably arose in the Jurassic period, although some authorities believe they separated from the placental eutherians in the Cretaceous period. The great radiation of modern mammal orders occurred during the Cretaceous and Tertiary periods.

acquired those two most characteristic of all mammalian identification tags: hair and mammary glands.

Most of the living mammals belong to the subclass Theria and have descended from a common ancestor of the Jurassic period, some 150 million years ago. However, monotremes (subclass Prototheria), the egg-laying mammals of Australia, Tasmania, and New Guinea, are so different from the others and possess so many reptilian characters that they are believed to have descended from an entirely different mammal-like reptile. The separation of Prototheria and Theria probably occurred approximately 50 million years earlier in the Triassic period. The geological record during the Jurassic and Cretaceous periods is fragmentary, in large part because the mammals of these periods were creatures the size of a rat or smaller, with fragile bones that fossilized only under the most ideal circumstances.

When the dinosaurs vanished near the beginning of the Cenozoic era, the mammals suddenly expanded. This point, about 70 million years ago, marks the beginning of the age of mammals. This is partly attributable to the numerous ecological niches vacated by the reptiles, into which the mammals could move as their divergent adaptations fitted them. There were other reasons for their success. Mammals were agile, warm blooded, and insulated with hair; they had developed placental reproduction and suckled their young, thus dispensing with vulnerable eggs and nests; and they were more intelligent than any other animal alive. During the Eocene and Oligocene epochs of the Tertiary period (55 to 30 million years ago), the mammals flourished and reached their peak. In terms of number of species, this was the golden age of mammals. They have declined somewhat in numbers since then, especially within the last million years, because humans became formidable adversaries of wildlife. Nevertheless, mammals as a whole are a secure group, dominating the land environment now as they did 50 million years ago.

CHARACTERISTICS

1. **Body covered with hair,** but reduced in some
2. **Integument with sweat, scent, sebaceous,** and **mammary glands**
3. Skeletal features of skull with **two occipital condyles, seven cervical vertebrae** (usually), and often an elongated tail
4. Mouth with **diphyodont teeth** on both jaws
5. **Movable eyelids** and **fleshy external ears**
6. Four limbs (reduced or absent in some) adapted for many forms of locomotion
7. Circulatory system of a four-chambered heart, **persistent left aorta,** and **nonnucleated, biconcave red blood corpuscles**
8. Respiratory system of lungs and a voice box
9. **Muscular partition (diaphragm) between thorax and abdomen**
10. Excretory system of metanephros kidneys and ureters that usually open into a bladder
11. Brain highly developed, especially **neocerebrum;** 12 pairs of cranial nerves
12. Endothermic and homeothermic
13. Cloaca present only in monotremes
14. Separate sexes; reproductive organs of a penis, testes (usually in a scrotum), ovaries, oviducts, and vagina
15. Internal fertilization; **eggs develop in a uterus** with **placental attachment** (except in monotremes); **fetal membranes (amnion, chorion, allantois);** sex determination by males (heterogametic)
16. Young nourished by **milk from mammary glands**

Since mammals and birds both evolved from reptiles, there are many structural similarities among the three groups. It is, in fact, much easier to point to

Figure 27-2

American beaver *Castor canadensis* (order Rodentia, family Castoridae) cutting up a trembling aspen tree. This second largest rodent has a heavy, waterproof pelage consisting of long, tough guard hairs overlying the thick, silky underhair so valued in the fur trade. Other adaptations for an aquatic life are nostrils and ear canals provided with valves, webbed hindfeet, flexible forefeet for gripping branches, a flat and broad paddlelike tail for swimming, diving, and signaling, and a mouth that closes behind the incisors to permit gnawing underwater.
Photograph by L.L. Rue, III.

numerous resemblances between the mammals and the reptiles than to point to characteristics that are unique to mammals. **Hair** is the most obvious mammalian characteristic, although it is vastly reduced in some (such as whales), and although reptilian scales, from which hair is derived, may persist (such as on tails of rats and beavers). A second unique characteristic of mammals is the method of nourishing their young with **milk-secreting glands;** reptiles have nothing remotely similar. Although less obvious, several important differences are present in cranial and jaw structure and jaw articulation. Placental mammals have **diphyodont teeth** (milk teeth replaced by a permanent set of teeth) rather than reptilian **polyphyodont teeth** (successive sets of teeth). But the single most important factor contributing to the success of mammals is the remarkable development of the **neocerebrum,** permitting a level of adaptive behavior, learning, curiosity, and intellectual activity far beyond the capacity of any reptile.

Class Mammalia is divided into two subclasses: Prototheria and Theria. Subclass **Prototheria** includes the monotremes, or egg-laying mammals. Subclass **Theria** includes two infraclasses, the **Metatheria,** with one order (marsupials), and the **Eutheria,** with 16 orders, all of which are placental mammals. A complete classification is found on pp. 659 to 663.

STRUCTURAL AND FUNCTIONAL ADAPTATIONS OF MAMMALS
Integument and Its Derivatives

The mammalian skin and its modifications especially distinguish mammals as a group. As the interface between the animal and its environment, the skin is strongly molded by the animal's way of life. In general the skin is thicker in mammals than in other classes of vertebrates, although as in all vertebrates it is made up of **epidermis** and **dermis** (see Fig. 28-1, p. 671). Among the mammals the dermis becomes much thicker than the epidermis. The epidermis is relatively thin where it is well protected by hair, but in places subject to much contact and use, such as the palms or soles, its outer layers become thick and cornified with keratin.

Hair

Hair is especially characteristic of mammals, although humans are not very hairy creatures, and in whales hair is reduced to only a few sensory bristles on the snout. A hair grows out of a hair follicle which, although an epidermal structure, is sunk into the dermis of the skin (Fig. 28-1, p. 671). The hair grows continuously by rapid proliferation of cells in the follicle. As the hair shaft is pushed upward, new cells are carried away from their source of nourishment and die, turning into the same dense type of keratin that constitutes nails, claws, hooves, and feathers.

Mammals characteristically have two kinds of hair forming the **pelage** (fur coat): (1) dense and soft **underhair** for insulation and (2) coarse and longer **guard hair** for protection against wear and to provide coloration. The underhair traps a layer of insulating air; in aquatic animals, such as the fur seal, otter, and beaver, it is so dense that it is almost impossible to wet it. In water the guard hairs become wet and mat down over the underhair, forming a protective blanket (Fig. 27-2). A quick shake when the animal emerges flings off the water and leaves the outer guard hair almost dry.

A hair is more than a strand of keratin. It consists of three layers: the medulla or pith in the center of the hair, the cortex with pigment granules next to the medulla, and the outer cuticle composed of imbricated scales. The hair of different mammals shows a considerable range of structure. It may be deficient in cortex, such as the brittle hair of deer, or it may be deficient in medulla, such as the hollow, air-filled hairs of the wolverine, so favored by northerners for trimming the hoods of parkas because it resists frost accumulation. The hairs of rabbits and some others are scaled to interlock when pressed together. Curly hair, such as that of sheep, grows from curved follicles.

A

B

Figure 27-3

Snowshoe, or varying, hare *Lepus americanus* (order Lagomorpha) in brown summer coat, **A**, and white winter coat, **B**. In winter, extra hair growth on the hindfeet broadens the animal's support in snow. Snowshoe hares are common residents of the taiga (northern coniferous forests) and are an important food for lynxes, foxes, and other carnivores. Population fluctuations of hares and their predators are closely related.
Photographs by L.L. Rue, III.

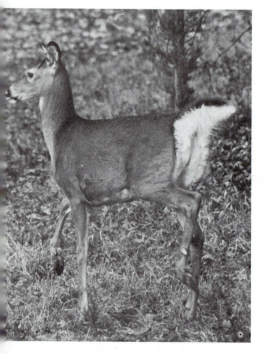

Figure 27-4

Alarmed white-tailed deer *Odocoileus virginianus* (order Artiodactyla) lifts its tail to expose conspicuous white underside. This mild alarm signal serves two functions: (1) silently warning other deer of impending danger and (2) communicating to the predator that it has been seen and thus would be wasting its effort to chase an alerted prey.
Photograph by L.L. Rue, III.

When a hair reaches a certain length, it stops growing. Normally it remains in the follicle until a new growth starts, whereupon it falls out. In humans, hair is shed and replaced throughout life. But in most mammals, there are periodic molts of the entire coat.

In the simplest cases, such as foxes and seals, the coat is shed once each year during the summer months. Most mammals have two annual molts, one in the spring and one in the fall. The summer coat is always much thinner than the winter coat and is usually a different color. Several of the northern mustelid carnivores, such as the weasel, have white winter coats and colored summer coats. It was once believed that the white inner pelage of arctic animals conserves body heat by reducing radiation loss, but recent research has shown that dark and white pelages radiate heat equally well. The winter white of arctic animals is simply camouflage in a land of snow. The varying hare of North America has three annual molts: the white winter coat is replaced by a brownish gray summer coat, and this is replaced in autumn by a grayer coat, which is soon shed to reveal the winter white coat beneath (Fig. 27-3). The white fur of arctic mammals in winter (leukemism) is not to be confused with albinism, caused by a recessive gene that blocks pigment formation. Albinos have red eyes and pinkish skin, whereas arctic animals in their winter coats have dark eyes and often dark-colored ear tips, noses, and tail tips.

Outside the Arctic, most mammals wear somber colors that are protective. Often the species is marked with "salt-and-pepper" coloration or a disruptive pattern that helps to make it inconspicuous in its natural surroundings. Examples are the spots of leopards and fawns and the stripes of tigers. Other mammals, such as skunks, advertise their presence with conspicuous warning coloration.

An interesting aspect of color is seen in the pair of rump patches of the pronghorn antelope, which are composed of long white hairs erected by special muscles. When alarmed, the animal can flash these patches in a manner visible for a long distance. They may be used as a warning signal to other members of the herd. The well-known "flag" of the white-tailed deer, visible when the animal raises its tail, serves a similar purpose (Fig. 27-4).

The hair of mammals has become modified to serve many purposes. The bristles of hogs, vibrissae on the snouts of most mammals, and spines of porcupines and their kin are examples.

Vibrissae, commonly called "whiskers," are really sensory hairs that provide a sensitive tactile sense to many mammals. The bulb at the base of each follicle is provided with a large sensory nerve. The slightest movement of a vibrissa generates impulses in the nerve endings that travel to a special sensory area in the brain. The vibrissae are especially long in nocturnal and burrowing animals. In seals they apparently serve as a "distance touch" sensitive to pressure waves and turbulence in the water caused by objects or passing fishes. Vision is of little use to seals hunting in turbid water, where they are frequently found; investigators have noted that blind seals remain as fat and healthy as normal seals.

Porcupines, hedgehogs, echidnas, and a few other mammals have developed an effective and dangerous spiny armor; the spines of the common North American porcupine break off at the bases when struck and, aided by backward-pointing hooks on the tips, work deeply into their victims. To assist slow learners, such as dogs, in understanding what they are dealing with, porcupines rattle the spines and prominently display the white markings on the quills toward their tormentors.

Horns and antlers

Three kinds of horns or hornlike substances are found in mammals. **True horns,** found in ruminants such as sheep and cattle, are hollow sheaths of keratinized epidermis that embrace a core of bone arising from the skull. Horns are not normally shed, are not branched (although they may be greatly curved), and are found in both sexes. The horns of North American pronghorn antelope are unique in that they are shed each year after the breeding season. But, unlike the shedding of deer antlers, the new horn replaces the old by growing up inside and pushing off the outer sheath.

Antlers of the deer family are entirely bone when mature. During their annual growth, antlers develop beneath a covering of highly vascular soft skin called **"velvet"** (Fig. 27-5). When growth of the antlers is complete just before the breeding season, the blood vessels constrict and the stag tears off the velvet by rubbing the antlers against trees. The antlers are dropped after the breeding season. New buds appear a few months later to herald the next set of antlers. For several years each new pair of antlers is larger and more elaborate than the previous set. The annual growth of antlers places a strain on the mineral metabolism, since during the growing season a large moose or elk must accumulate 50 or more pounds of calcium salts from its vegetable diet.

The **rhinoceros horn** is the third kind of horn. Hairlike horny fibers arise from the dermal papillae and are cemented together to form a single horn.

Glands

Of all vertebrates, mammals have the greatest variety of integumentary glands. Most fall into one of four classes: sweat, scent, sebaceous, and mammary. All are derivatives of the epidermis.

Sweat glands are simple, tubular, highly coiled glands that occur over much of the body in most mammals. They are not present in other vertebrates. Two

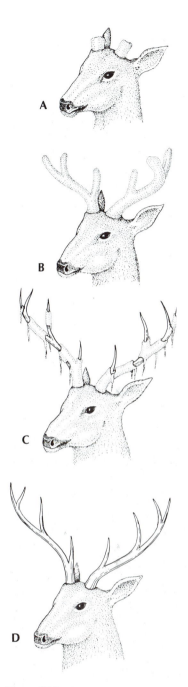

Figure 27-5

Annual growth of deer antlers. **A,** Antlers begin growth in late spring, stimulated by pituitary gonadotropins. **B,** The bone grows very rapidly until halted by a rapid rise in testosterone production by the testes. **C,** The skin (velvet) dies and sloughs off. **D,** Testosterone levels peak during the fall breeding season. The antlers are shed in January as testosterone levels subside.

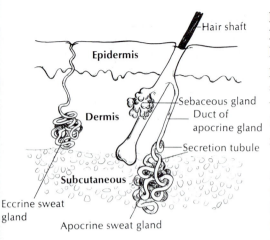

Figure 27-6

Sweat glands (eccrine and apocrine). Phylogenetically, apocrine glands are older. Eccrine glands, best developed in primates, play an important role in temperature regulation. Most glands in dogs, pigs, cows, horses, and others are apocrine, but these have declined in humans, along with hair, for they develop from follicular epithelium. Apocrine glands are not involved in temperature regulation, but their odorous secretions play a part in sexual attraction.

Milk varies in composition. Human milk is composed of 1% to 2% protein, 3% to 5% fat, 6% to 8% carbohydrate, 0.2% salts, and the remainder water. Cows' milk has more protein, about the same amount of fat, and less carbohydrate. In marine mammals (whales and seals) and arctic mammals (polar bears and caribou), where rapid growth of the young is important for species survival, the milk may contain 30% to 40% fat.

kinds of sweat glands may be distinguished: eccrine and apocrine (Fig. 27-6). **Eccrine glands** secrete a watery sweat that functions mainly in temperature regulation (evaporative cooling). They occur in hairless regions, especially the foot pads, in most mammals, although in horses, some apes, and humans they are scattered all over the body. They are much reduced or absent in rodents, rabbits, whales, and others. Dogs are now known to have sweat glands all over the body. In humans, racial differences are pronounced. Black people, who have more sweat glands than white people, can tolerate warmer temperatures.

Apocrine glands, the second type of sweat gland, are larger than eccrine glands and have longer and more winding ducts. Their secretory coil is in the subdermis. They always open into the follicle of a hair or where a hair has been. Black people have more apocrine glands than do white people, and women have twice as many as men. They develop approximately at sexual puberty and are restricted (in the human species) to the axillae (armpits), mons pubis, breasts, external auditory canals, prepuce, scrotum, and a few other places. Their secretion is not watery, like ordinary sweat (eccrine gland), but is a milky, whitish or yellow secretion that dries on the skin to form a plasticlike film. Apocrine glands are not involved in heat regulation, but their activity is known to be correlated with certain aspects of the sex cycle, among other possible functions.

Scent glands are present in nearly all mammals. Their location and functions vary greatly. They are used in communication with members of the same species (Fig. 27-7), to mark territorial boundaries, for warning, or for defense. Scent-producing glands are located in orbital, metatarsal, and interdigital regions (deer); behind the eyes and on the cheek (pica and woodchuck); preputial regions on the penis (muskrats, beavers, and many canines); base of the tail (wolves and foxes); back of the head (dromedary); and anal region (skunks, minks, and weasels). These last, the most odoriferous of all glands, open by ducts into the anus; their secretions can be discharged forcefully for several feet. During the mating season many mammals give off strong scents for attracting the opposite sex. Humans also are endowed with scent glands. But civilization has taught us to dislike our own scent, a concern that has stimulated a lucrative deodorant industry to produce an endless output of soaps and odor-masking compounds.

Sebaceous glands are intimately associated with hair follicles, although some are free and open directly onto the surface. The cellular lining of the gland itself is discharged in the secretory process and must be renewed for further secretion. These gland cells become distended with a fatty accumulation, then die and are expelled as a greasy mixture called sebum into the hair follicle. Called a "polite fat" because it does not turn rancid, it serves as a dressing to keep the skin and hair pliable and glossy. Most mammals have sebaceous glands all over the body; in humans they are most numerous in the scalp and on the face.

Mammary glands, which provide the name for mammals, are probably modified apocrine glands, although recent studies suggest that they may have been derived from sebaceous glands. Whatever their evolutionary origin, they occur on all female mammals and in a rudimentary form on all male mammals. They develop by the thickening of the epidermis to form a milk line along each side of the abdomen in the embryo. On certain parts of these lines the mammae appear, while the intervening parts of the ridge disappear.

In the human female the mammary glands begin to increase in size at puberty because of fat accumulation and reach their maximum development in approximately the twentieth year. The breasts (or mammae) undergo additional development during pregnancy. In other mammals the breasts are swollen only peri-

Figure 27-7

Olfactory exploration during courtship in thirteen-lined ground squirrels *Citellus tridecemlineatus* (order Rodentia, family Sciuridae). Scent is by far the most important means of communication in mammals. Each produces an odor characteristic of the species; the same species may vary its scent for different communicative purposes. Anal glands, as in these two ground squirrels, are especially common. This species lives on the prairies of western Canada and United States and feeds on grains, other vegetation, and insects.

Photograph by C.G. Hampson.

odically when they are distended with milk during pregnancy and subsequent nursing of the young.

___ Food and Feeding

Mammals have exploited an enormous variety of food sources; some mammals require highly specialized diets, whereas others are opportunistic feeders that thrive on diversified diets. In all, food habits and physical structure are inextricably linked. A mammal's adaptations for attack and defense and its specializations for finding, capturing, reducing, swallowing, and digesting food all determine a mammal's shape and habits.

Teeth, perhaps more than any other single physical characteristic, reveal the life-style of a mammal (Fig. 27-8). It has been claimed that, if all mammals except humans were extinct and represented only by fossil teeth, we could still construct a classification nearly as correct as the one we have now, which is based on all anatomical features. All mammals have teeth, except certain whales, monotremes, and anteaters, and their modifications are correlated with what the mammal eats.

Typically, mammals have a **diphyodont** dentition, that is, two sets of teeth: a set of deciduous, or milk, teeth that is replaced by a set of permanent teeth. In any given species, mammalian teeth are modified to perform specialized tasks such as cutting, nipping, gnawing, seizing, tearing, grinding, or chewing. Teeth differentiated in this manner in the individual are called **heterodont**, in contrast to the uniform, **homodont** dentition characteristic of lower vertebrates.

Usually four types of teeth are recognized. **Incisors**, with simple crowns and slightly sharp edges, are mainly for snipping or biting; **canines**, with long conical crowns, are specialized for piercing; **premolars**, with compressed crowns and one or two cusps, are suited for shearing and slicing; and **molars**, with large bodies and variable cusp arrangement, are for crushing and mastication. Molars always belong to the permanent set.

Carnivorous animals have teeth with sharp edges for tearing and piercing. They have well-developed canines, but some of the molars are poorly developed. In the herbivores the canines are suppressed, whereas the molars are broad, with enamel ridges for grinding. Such teeth are also usually high crowned, in contrast to the low-crowned teeth of carnivores.

The incisors of rodents have enamel only on the anterior surface so that the softer dentin behind wears away faster, resulting in chisel-shaped teeth that are always sharp. Moreover, rodent incisors grow throughout life and must be worn

Wolf

Deer

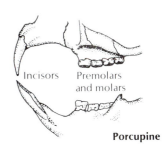

Porcupine

Figure 27-8

Adaptations of mammal tooth patterns for different kinds of diet. Sharp canines of the wolf are adapted for stabbing, and premolars and molars are for cutting rather than grinding. Browsing deer has predominantly grinding teeth; lower incisors and canines bite against a horny pad in the upper jaw. Porcupine has no canines; self-sharpening incisors are used for gnawing.

Modified from Carrington, R. 1968. The mammals. New York, Life Nature Library, Time-Life Books, Inc.

Figure 27-9

Malocclusion in the woodchuck *Marmota monax* (order Rodentia, family Sciuridae). Teeth of rodents are two pairs of deeply implanted incisors that grow throughout life to keep pace with wear. Should incisors not meet correctly, continued growth prevents feeding and the animal starves to death. Natural selection often works harshly to remove genetic defects! Woodchucks (also called groundhogs) are hibernators.
Photograph by L.L. Rue, III.

away to keep pace with growth. The failure of two opposing incisors to meet results in serious consequences to the animal (Fig. 27-9).

The **tusks** of the elephant and the wild boar are modifications of teeth. The elephant tusk is a modified upper incisor and may be present in both males and females; in the wild boar the tusk is a modified canine present only in the male. Both are formidable weapons.

The number and arrangement of permanent teeth are expressed by a **dental formula.** The figures above the horizontal line represent the number of incisors, canines, premolars, and molars on half of the upper jaw; the figures below the line indicate the corresponding teeth in half of the lower jaw.

Human	Rabbit	Dog	White-tailed deer
$\dfrac{2\text{-}1\text{-}2\text{-}3}{2\text{-}1\text{-}2\text{-}3}$	$\dfrac{2\text{-}0\text{-}3\text{-}3}{1\text{-}0\text{-}2\text{-}3}$	$\dfrac{3\text{-}1\text{-}4\text{-}2}{3\text{-}1\text{-}4\text{-}3}$	$\dfrac{0\text{-}0\text{-}3\text{-}3}{3\text{-}1\text{-}3\text{-}3}$

On the basis of food habits, animals may be divided into herbivores, carnivores, omnivores, and insectivores.

Herbivorous animals that feed on grasses and other vegetation form two main groups: **browsers** or **grazers,** such as the ungulates (horses, swine, deer, antelope, cattle, sheep, and goats), and the **gnawers** and **nibblers,** such as the rodents (Fig. 27-10) and rabbits. In herbivores the canines are suppressed, whereas the molars are broad and high crowned and bear enamel ridges for grinding. Rodents have chisel-shaped incisors that grow throughout life and must be worn away to keep pace with their continual growth.

Herbivorous mammals have a number of interesting adaptations for dealing with their massive diet of plant food. **Cellulose,** the structural carbohydrate of plants, is a potentially nutritious foodstuff, comprised of long chains of glucose units. However, the glucose molecules in cellulose are linked by a type of chemical bond that few enzymes can attack. No vertebrates synthesize cellulose-splitting enzymes. Instead, the herbivorous vertebrates harbor a microflora of anaerobic bacteria in huge fermentation chambers in the gut. These bacteria break down and metabolize the cellulose, releasing a variety of fatty acids, sugars, and starches that the host animal can absorb and use.

In some herbivores, such as horses and rabbits, the gut has a capacious sidepocket, or diverticulum, called a **cecum,** which serves as a fermentation chamber and absorptive area. Hares, rabbits, and some rodents often eat their fecal pellets (**coprophagy**), giving the food a second pass through the fermenting action

Figure 27-10

Eastern chipmunk *Tamias striatus* with cheek pouches stuffed with seeds that it will carry to an underground cache. It will try to store at least a half bushel of food for the winter. It hibernates but awakens periodically to eat some of its cached food. Order Rodentia, family Sciuridae.
Photograph by L.L. Rue, III.

of the intestinal bacteria. Coprophagy may also provide an opportunity for the animal to obtain vitamins produced by the cecal bacteria.

The **ruminants** (cattle, bison, buffalo, goats, antelopes, sheep, deer, giraffes, and okapis) have a huge **four-chambered stomach** (Fig. 27-11). When a ruminant feeds, grass passes down the esophagus to the **rumen,** where it is broken down by the rich microflora and then formed into small balls of cud. At its leisure the ruminant returns the cud to its mouth where the cud is deliberately chewed at length to crush the fiber. Swallowed again, the food returns to the rumen where it is digested by the cellulolytic bacteria. The pulp passes to the **reticulum,** then to the **omasum,** and finally to the **abomasum** ("true" stomach), where proteolytic enzymes are secreted and normal digestion takes place.

Herbivores in general have large, long digestive tracts and must eat a considerable amount of plant food to survive. A large African elephant weighing 6 tons must consume 135 to 150 kg (300 to 400 pounds) of rough fodder each day to obtain sufficient nourishment for life.

Carnivorous mammals feed mainly on herbivores. This group includes foxes, weasels, cats, dogs, wolverines, fishers, lions, and tigers. Carnivores are well equipped with biting and piercing teeth and powerful clawed limbs for killing their prey. Since their protein diet is much more easily digested than is the woody food of herbivores, their digestive tract is shorter and the cecum small or absent. Carnivores eat separate meals and have much more leisure time for play and exploration.

In general, carnivores lead more active—and by human standards more interesting—lives than do the herbivores. Since a carnivore must find and catch its prey, there is a premium on intelligence; many carnivores, such as the cats, are noted for their stealth and cunning in hunting prey (Fig. 27-12). Although evolution seems to have favored the carnivores, their success has led to a selection of herbivores capable either of defending themselves or of detecting and escaping carnivores. Thus, for the herbivores, there has been a premium on keen senses and agility. Some herbivores, however, survive by virtue of their sheer size (for example, elephants) or by defensive group behavior (for example, muskoxen).

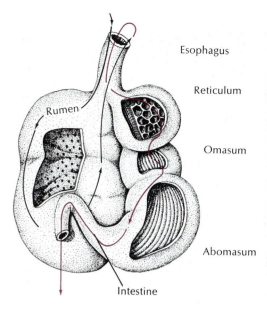

Figure 27-11

Ruminant's stomach. Food passes first to the rumen (sometimes through the reticulum) and then is returned to mouth for chewing (chewing the cud, or rumination) *(black arrow)*. After reswallowing, food returns to the rumen or passes directly to reticulum, omasum, and abomasum for final digestion *(red arrow)*.

Figure 27-12

Lioness *Panthera leo* with Thompson gazelle she killed. Lions stalk prey, then charge suddenly to surprise the victim. They lack stamina for a long chase. Lions will gorge themselves with the kill, then sleep and rest for periods as long as a week before eating again. Order Carnivora, family Felidae.
Photograph by L.L. Rue, III.

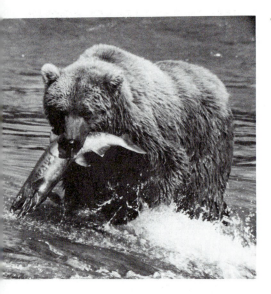

Figure 27-13

Alaskan brown bear *Ursus arctos* (order Carnivora) with a large salmon captured during the spawning run. All bears are opportunistic omnivores that take advantage of any seasonally abundant resource. They are highly dependent on vegetable food but also kill small mammals, scavenge, and rob all bees' nests they can find and enter. Bears are the least carnivorous of the carnivores.

Photograph by L.L. Rue, III.

Humans have changed the rules in the carnivore-herbivore contest. Carnivores, despite their intelligence, have suffered much from human presence and have been virtually exterminated in some areas. Herbivores, on the other hand, especially the rodents with their potent reproductive ability, have consistently defeated our most ingenious efforts to banish them from our environment. The problem of rodent pests in agriculture has intensified; we have removed carnivores, which served as the herbivores' natural population control, but have not been able to devise a suitable substitute.

Omnivorous mammals live on both plant food and animals. Examples are pigs, raccoons, rats, bears (Fig. 27-13), humans, and most other primates. Many carnivorous forms also eat fruits, berries, and grasses when hard pressed. The fox, which usually feeds on mice, small rodents, and birds, eats frozen apples, beechnuts, and corn when its normal food sources are scarce.

Insectivorous mammals subsist chiefly on insects and grubs. Examples are moles, shrews, anteaters, and most bats. The insectivorous category is not a sharply distinguished one, however, because many omnivores, carnivores, and even some herbivores eat insects on occasion (sometimes by accident).

For most mammals, searching for food and eating occupy most of their active life. Seasonal changes in food supplies are considerable in temperate zones. Living may be easy in the summer when food is abundant, but in winter many carnivores must range far and wide to eke out a narrow existence. Some migrate to regions where food is more abundant. Others hibernate and sleep the winter months away.

But there are many provident mammals that build up food stores during periods of plenty. This habit is most pronounced in rodents, such as squirrels, chipmunks, gophers, and certain mice. All tree squirrels—red, fox, and gray—collect nuts, conifer seeds, and fungi and bury these in caches for winter use. Often each item is hidden in a different place (scatter hoarding) and marked by a scent to assist relocation in the future. The chipmunk (Fig. 27-10) is one of the greatest providers because it spends the autumn months collecting nuts and seeds. Some of its caches may exceed a bushel in size.

Body weight and food consumption

The relationship between body size and metabolic rate has been discussed in relation to food consumption of birds (p. 612) and will be treated again in Chapter 36 (p. 885). The smaller the animal, the greater is its metabolic rate and the more it must eat relative to its body size. This happens because the metabolic rate of an animal—and therefore the amount of food it must eat to sustain this metabolic rate—varies in rough proportion to the surface area rather than to the body weight. Surface area is proportional to a 0.7 power of body weight, and the amount of food a mammal (or bird) eats is also roughly proportional to a 0.7 power of its body weight. This means that as the size of animals gets smaller, their metabolic rate (usually measured as oxygen consumption per gram of body weight) becomes more intense. A 3 g mouse will consume *per gram body weight* five times more food than does a 10 kg dog and about 30 times more food than does a 50,000 kg elephant. One can easily see why small mammals (shrews, bats, mice) must spend much more time hunting and eating food than do large mammals. The smallest shrews weighing only 2 g may eat more than their body weight each day and will starve to death in a few hours if deprived of food (Fig. 27-14). In contrast, a large carnivore can remain fat and healthy with only one meal every few days. The mountain lion is known to kill an average of one deer a week, although it will kill more frequently when game is abundant.

___ Body Temperature Regulation

Mammals share with birds the ability to regulate their body temperature physiologically. Both groups are commonly called "warm-blooded" animals to distinguish them from all other animals, which are "cold blooded." It is true that the body temperature of mammals is usually (although not always) warmer than the ambient temperature, but a "cold-blooded" animal is not necessarily cold. Tropical fishes and insects, and reptiles basking in the sun, may have body temperatures equaling or surpassing those of mammals. Moreover, when many "warm-blooded" mammals hibernate, their body temperatures approach the freezing point of water. Thus, the terms "warm blooded" and "cold blooded" are hopelessly subjective and nonspecific but are so firmly entrenched in our vocabulary that most biologists find it easier to accept the usage than try to change people's perceptions.

The term **homeothermic** (constant body temperature) is frequently applied to mammals and birds, and the term **poikilothermic** (variable body temperature) to all other animals. Again, these terms offer difficulties, since, for example, deep-sea fishes live in an environment having no perceptible temperature change. Even though their body temperature is absolutely stable, day in and day out, few would argue that they are homeotherms. Furthermore, among the homeothermic birds and mammals are many whose body temperatures fluctuate diurnally, or, as with hibernators, seasonally. For these reasons, many physiologists prefer to call birds and mammals **endothermic;** that is, they maintain a high body temperature by *internal* (metabolic) heat production. Animals that depend on an *external* heat source are termed **ectothermic.** Unfortunately, none of the existing terminology can be applied without qualification to large groups of animals. Nevertheless, it is convenient and usually correct to say that mammals are both endothermic and homeothermic, keeping in mind that the latter term is imprecise in some situations.

Homeothermy allows mammals to stabilize their internal temperature so that biochemical processes and nervous function can proceed at steady high levels of activity. Thus, they can remain active in winter and exploit habitats unavailable to the poikilotherms. Most mammals have body temperatures between 36° and 38° C (somewhat lower than those of birds, which range between 40° and 42° C). This constant temperature is maintained by a delicate balance between heat production and heat loss—not a simple matter when mammals are constantly alternating between periods of rest and bursts of activity.

Heat is produced by the animal's metabolism, which includes the oxidation of foodstuffs, basal cellular metabolism, and muscular contraction. Heat is lost by radiation and conduction to a cooler environment and by the evaporation of water. The mammal can control both processes of heat production and heat loss within rather wide limits. If the animal becomes too cool, it can increase heat production by increasing muscular activity (exercise or shivering) and by decreasing heat loss by increasing its insulation. If the mammal becomes too warm, it decreases heat production and increases heat loss. We will examine these processes in the following examples.

Figure 27-14

The masked (common) shrew *Sorex cincereus* (order Insectivora) feeding on a deer mouse it has killed. Note small size of shrew relative to much larger mouse. This tiny but fierce mammal, with a prodigious appetite for insects, mice, snails, and worms, spends most of its time underground and so is seldom seen by humans. Shrews are a primitive group believed to closely resemble the insectivorous ancestors of placental mammals. Photograph by C.G. Hampson.

A

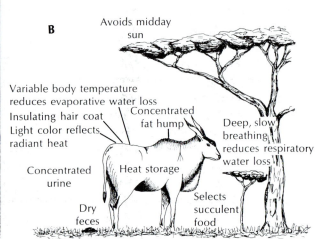

B

Avoids midday sun

Variable body temperature reduces evaporative water loss

Insulating hair coat

Light color reflects radiant heat

Concentrated fat hump

Concentrated urine

Heat storage

Deep, slow breathing reduces respiratory water loss

Dry feces

Selects succulent food

Figure 27-15

A, The common eland *Taurotragus oryx* (order Artiodactyla), inhabitant of the arid, open savanna of central Africa. It is one of 72 species of African antelopes that occupy a variety of habitats including open savanna, bush savanna, marshes, and flooded grassland. Special food preferences reduce competition between different species. **B,** Physiological and behavioral adaptations of the eland for maintaining a constant body temperature in a hot environment.

A, Photograph by C.G. Hampson; **B,** from Tallmark, B. 1972. Fauna och Flora (Stockholm) **67:**163-175; modified from Taylor, C.P. 1969. Sci. Am. **220:**88-95.

Figure 27-16

The long, sparsely insulated ears of the black-tailed jackrabbit *Lepus californicus* of the American Southwest serve as thermal "windows" for the removal of heat by convection and conduction to the air and by radiation to cool spots in the environment (such as the animal's own shadow). The large ears of elephants perform the same function. Order Lagomorpha, family Leporidae.

Photograph by L.L. Rue, III.

Adaptations for hot environments

Despite the harsh conditions of deserts—intense heat during the day, cold at night, and scarcity of water, vegetation, and cover—many kinds of animals live there successfully. The smaller desert mammals are mostly fossorial (fitted for digging burrows) and nocturnal. The lower temperature and higher humidity of burrows help to reduce water loss by evaporation. Water loss is replaced by free water in food or by drinking water if it is available. Water is also formed in the cells by the metabolic oxidation of foods. This gain from **oxidation water,** as it is called, can be very significant, since water is not always available for drinking. In fact, some desert mammals, such as the kangaroo rats and ground squirrels of American deserts, can if necessary derive all the water they need from their dry food without drinking any water at all. Such animals produce a highly concentrated urine and form nearly solid feces.

The large desert ungulates obviously cannot escape the desert heat by living in burrows. Animals such as camels and desert antelopes (gazelle, oryx, and eland) possess a number of adaptations for coping with heat and dehydration. Those of the eland are shown in Fig. 27-15. The mechanisms for controlling water loss and preventing overheating are closely linked. The glossy, pallid color of the fur reflects direct sunlight, and the fur itself is an excellent insulation that works to keep heat out. Heat is lost by convection and conduction from the underside of the eland where the pelage is very thin. Fat tissue of the eland, an essential food reserve, is concentrated in a single hump on the back, instead of being uniformly distributed under the skin where it would impair heat loss by radiation. The eland avoids evaporative water loss—the only means an animal has for cooling itself when the environmental temperature is higher than that of the body—by permitting its body temperature to decrease during the cool night and then increase slowly during the day as the body stores heat. Only when the body temperature reaches 41° C must the eland prevent further rise through **evaporative cooling** by sweating and panting. Water is also conserved by means of concentrated urine and dry feces. All of these adaptations are also found developed to a similar or even greater degree in camels, the most perfectly adapted of all large desert mammals.

Adaptations for cold environments

In cold environments mammals use two major mechanisms to maintain homeothermy: (1) **decreased conductance,** that is, reduction of heat loss by increasing the effectiveness of the insulation, and (2) **increased heat production.**

The excellent insulation of the thick pelage of arctic animals is familiar. In all mammals living in cold regions of the earth fur thickness increases in winter, sometimes by as much as 50%. As described earlier, the thick underhair is the major insulating layer, whereas the longer and more visible guard hair serves as protection against wear and for protective coloration.

But the body extremities (legs, tail, ears, nose) of arctic mammals cannot be insulated as well as can the trunk. To prevent these parts from becoming major avenues of heat loss, they are allowed to cool to low temperatures, often approaching the freezing point. As warm arterial blood passes into a leg, for example, heat is shunted directly from artery to vein and carried back to the core of the body (Fig. 27-17). This device prevents the loss of valuable body heat through the poorly insulated distal regions of the leg. A consequence of this

Figure 27-17

Countercurrent heat exchange in the leg of an arctic wolf. The upper diagram shows how the extremities cool when the animal is exposed to low air temperatures. The lower diagram depicts a portion of the front leg artery and vein, showing how heat is exchanged between outflowing arterial and inflowing venous blood.

Figure 27-18

Barren-ground caribou *Rangifer tarandus groenlandicus* of Canada. **A,** Caribou moving southwest in autumn toward forest winter range. Two males in foreground in autumn pelage and velvet-covered antlers. Adult females in background. Cows and younger animals normally lead the herd; males follow. Caribou feed while moving, grazing on low ground vegetation, principally although not exclusively lichens. **B,** Summer and winter ranges of the barren-ground caribou of Canada. The principal spring migration routes are indicated by arrows; routes vary considerably from year to year. Caribou in Alaska have similar migrations.

A, Photograph by D. Thomas; B, modified from Kelsall, J.P. 1968. The migratory barren-ground caribou of Canada. Ottawa, Canadian Wildlife Service, Queens Printers.

peripheral (**countercurrent**) **heat exchange system** is that the legs and feet must operate at low temperatures. The temperatures of the feet of the arctic fox and barren-ground caribou are just above the freezing point; in fact, the temperature may be below 0° C in the footpads and hooves. To keep feet supple and flexible at such low temperatures, fats in the extremities have very low melting points, perhaps 30° C lower than ordinary body fats.

In severely cold conditions all mammals can produce more heat by **augmented muscular activity** through exercise or shivering. We are all familiar with the effectiveness of both activities. A person can increase heat production as much as 18 fold by violent shivering when maximally stressed by cold. Another source of heat is the increased oxidation of foodstuffs, especially brown fat stores. This mechanism is called **nonshivering thermogenesis.**

Small mammals the size of lemmings, voles, and mice meet the challenge of cold environments in a different way. Small mammals are not as well insulated as large mammals because there is an obvious practical limit to how much pelage a mouse, for example, can carry before it becomes an immobile bundle of fur. Consequently these forms have successfully exploited the excellent insulating qualities of snow by living under it in runways on the forest floor, where incidentally their food is also located. In this **subnivean environment** the temperature seldom drops below $-5°$ C even though the air temperature above may fall to $-50°$ C. The snow insulation decreases thermal conductance from small mammals in the same way that pelage does for large mammals. Living beneath the snow is really a type of avoidance response to cold.

We will now look at two additional ways in which mammals may survive low temperatures: migration and hibernation.

___ Migration

Migration is a much more difficult undertaking for mammals than for birds; not surprisingly, few mammals make regular seasonal migrations, preferring instead to center their activities in a defined and limited home range. Nevertheless, there are some striking examples of mammalian migrations. More migrators are found in North America than on any other continent.

An example is the barren-ground caribou of Canada and Alaska, which undertakes direct and purposeful mass migrations spanning 160 to 1100 km (100 to 700 miles) twice annually (Fig. 27-18). From winter ranges in the boreal forests (taiga), they migrate rapidly in late winter and spring to calving ranges on the barren grounds (tundra). The calves are born in mid-June. Harassed by warble and nostril flies that bore into their flesh, the caribou move southward in July and August, feeding little along the way. In September they reach the forest, feeding there almost continuously on low ground vegetation. Mating (rut) occurs in October.

The caribou have suffered a drastic decline in numbers. In primitive times there were several million of them; by 1958 they numbered less than 200,000. The decline has been caused by excessive hunting, poor calf crops, and destruction of the vulnerable forested wintering areas caused by fires accidentally started during recent exploration and exploitation activities in the north. However, the population has increased slowly since 1958 under protection (Kelsall, 1968).

The plains bison, before its deliberate near extinction by white people, made huge circular migrations to separate summer and winter ranges.

The longest mammal migrations are made by the oceanic seals and whales. One of the most remarkable migrations is that of the fur seal, which breeds on the Pribilof Islands approximately 300 km (190 miles) off the coast of Alaska and north of the Aleutian Islands. From wintering grounds off southern California the females journey 4800 km (3000 miles) across open ocean, arriving in the spring at the Pribilofs where they congregate in enormous numbers (Fig. 27-19). The young are born within a few hours or days after arrival of the cows. Then the bulls, having already arrived and established territories, collect harems of cows, which they guard with vigilance. After the calves have been nursed for approximately 4 months, cows and juveniles leave for their long migration southward. The bulls do not follow but remain in the Gulf of Alaska during the winter.

Although we might expect the only winged mammals, bats, to use their gift of flight to migrate, few of them do. Most spend the winter in hibernation. The four species of American bats that do migrate, the red bat (Fig. 27-22), silver-

Figure 27-19

Breeding colony of fur seals *Callorhinus ursinus* on the Pribilof Islands. A harem master is seen surrounded by part of his harem. Two pups are visible in the foreground. Order Carnivora, suborder Pinnipedia.

Photograph by L.L. Rue, III.

haired bat, hoary bat, and Brazilian free-tailed bat, spend their summers in the northern or western states and their winters in the southern United States or Mexico.

Hibernation

Many small and medium-sized mammals in northern temperate regions solve the problem of winter scarcity of food and low temperature by entering a prolonged and controlled state of dormancy. True hibernators, such as ground squirrels, jumping mice, marmots, and woodchucks (Fig. 27-20), prepare for hibernation by building up large amounts of body fat. Entry into hibernation is gradual. After a series of "test drops" during which body temperature decreases a few degrees and then returns to normal, the animal cools to within a degree or less of the ambient temperature. Metabolism decreases to a fraction of normal. In the ground squirrel, for example, the respiratory rate decreases from a normal rate of 200 per minute to four or five per minute, and the heart rate from 150 to five beats per minute. During arousal the hibernator both shivers violently and employs non-shivering thermogenesis to produce heat.

Some mammals, such as bears, badgers, raccoons, and opossums, enter a state of prolonged sleep in winter with little or no decrease in body temperature. This is not true hibernation. Bears of the northern forest den-up for several months. A bear's heart rate may decrease from 40 to 10 beats per minute, but body temperature remains normal and the bear is awakened if sufficiently disturbed. One intrepid but reckless biologist learned how lightly a bear sleeps when he crawled into a den and attempted to measure the bear's rectal temperature with a thermometer!

Flight and Echolocation

Mammals have not exploited the skies to the same extent that they have the terrestrial and aquatic environments. However, many mammals scamper about in trees with amazing agility; some can glide from tree to tree, and one group, the bats, is capable of full flight. Gliding and flying evolved independently in several groups of mammals, including the marsupials, rodents, flying lemurs, and bats. Anyone who has watched a gibbon perform in a zoo realizes there is something akin to flight in this primate, too. Among the arboreal squirrels, all of which are nimble acrobats, by far the most efficient is the flying squirrel (Fig. 27-21). These forms actually glide rather than fly, using the gliding skin that extends from the sides of the body.

Bats, the only group of flying mammals, are nocturnal insectivores and thus occupy a niche left vacant by birds (Fig. 27-22). Their outstanding success is attributed to two things: flight and the capacity to navigate by echolocation. Together these adaptations enable bats to fly and avoid obstacles in absolute darkness, to locate and catch insects with precision, and to find their way deep into caves (another habitat largely ignored by both mammals and birds) where they sleep away the daytime hours.

Research has been concentrated on members of the family Vespertilionidae, to which most of the common North American bats belong. When in flight, these bats emit short pulses 5 to 10 msec in duration in a narrow directed beam from the mouth. Each pulse is frequency modulated; that is, it is highest at the beginning, up to 100,000 Hertz (Hz, cycles per second), and drops to perhaps 30,000 Hz at

Figure 27-20

Hibernating woodchuck *Marmota monax* (order Rodentia) in den exposed by road-building work sleeps on, unaware of the intrusion. Woodchucks begin hibernation in late September while the weather is still warm and may sleep 6 months. The animal is rigid and decidedly cold to the touch. Breathing is imperceptible, as slow as one breath every 5 minutes. Although it appears to be dead, it will awaken if the den temperature drops dangerously low.

Photograph by L.L. Rue, III.

Figure 27-21

Flying squirrel *Glaucomys sabrinus* coming in for a landing, photographed with stroboscopic flash. Area of undersurface is nearly trebled when gliding skin is spread. Glides of 40 to 50 m are possible; good maneuverability during flight is achieved by adjusting the position of the gliding skin with special muscles. Flying squirrels are nocturnal and have superb night vision. Order Rodentia, family Sciuridae.

Photograph by C.G. Hampson.

Figure 27-22

Red bat *Lasiurus borealis* (order Chiroptera) in flight with four young. This species is unusual in giving birth to three or four young; most bats have one or two. The mother carries the young until their combined weight may exceed her own weight; then they are left in the roost, usually a tree. Mortality among the young is rather high. These medium-sized bats are distributed over all the eastern and southern United States. They are strong fliers, migrating northward in spring and southward in autumn.

Photograph by L.L. Rue, III.

the end. Sounds of this frequency are ultrasonic to the human ear, which has an upper limit of about 20,000 Hz. The pulses are produced at a rate of 30 to 40 a second, increasing to perhaps 50 a second as the bat nears an object. Furthermore, the pulses are spaced so that the echo of each is received before the next pulse is emitted, an adaptation that prevents jamming. Since the transmission-to-reception time decreases as the bat approaches an object, it can increase the pulse frequency to obtain more information about the object. The pulse length is also shortened as the bat nears the object.

The external ears of bats are large, like hearing trumpets, and shaped variously in different species. Less is known about the bat's inner ear, but it obviously is capable of receiving the ultrasonic sounds emitted. Biologists believe that bat navigation is so refined that the bat builds up a mental image of its surroundings from echo scanning that is virtually as complete as the visual image from eyes of diurnal animals.

Bats have undergone some adaptive radiation, yet for reasons not fully understood, all are nocturnal, even the fruit-eating bats that use vision and olfaction to find their food instead of sonar. The tropics and subtropics have many nectar-feeding bats that are important pollinators for a wide variety of chiropter-

Figure 27-23

African lions *Panthera leo* (order Carnivora, family Felidae) mating. Lions breed at any season, although predominantly in spring and summer. During the short period a female is receptive, she may mate repeatedly. Three or four cubs are born after gestation of 100 days. Once the mother introduces the cubs into the pride, they are treated with affection by both adult males and females. Cubs go through an 18- to 24-month apprenticeship learning how to hunt and then are frequently driven from the pride to manage for themselves.

Photograph by L.L. Rue, III.

ophilous ("bat-loving") plants. The flowers of these plants open at night, are white or light in color, and emit a musky, batlike odor that the nectar-feeding bats find attractive.

The famed tropical vampire bat has razor-sharp incisors that it uses to shave away the epidermis of its prey, exposing underlying capillaries. After infusing an anticoagulant to keep the blood flowing, it laps up its meal and stores it in a specially modified stomach. It is said that dogs can hear an approaching vampire's sonar and thus awaken and escape.

Reproduction

Most mammals have definite mating seasons, usually in the winter or spring and timed to coincide with the most favorable time of the year for rearing the young after birth. Many male mammals are capable of fertile copulation at any time, but the female mating function is restricted to a time during a periodic cycle, known as the **estrous cycle.** The female receives the male only during a relatively brief period known as **estrus,** or heat (Fig. 27-23).

The estrous cycle is divided into stages marked by characteristic changes in the ovary, uterus, and vagina. **Proestrus,** or period of preparation, when new ovarian follicles grow, is followed by **estrus,** when mating occurs. Almost simultaneously the ovarian follicles burst, releasing the eggs (**ovulation**), which are fertilized. In all placental mammals the fertilized egg then implants itself in the uterine wall and pregnancy follows. However, should mating and fertilization not occur, estrus is followed by **metestrus,** a period of repair. This stage is followed by **diestrus,** during which the uterus becomes small and anemic. The cycle then repeats itself, beginning with proestrus.

How often females are in heat varies greatly among the different mammals. Animals that have only a single estrus during the breeding season are called **monestrous;** those that have a recurrence of estrus during the breeding season are called **polyestrous.** Dogs, foxes, and bats belong to the first group; field mice and squirrels are all polyestrous, as are many mammals living in the more tropical regions of the earth. The Old World monkeys and humans have a somewhat different cycle in which the postovulation period is terminated by **menstruation,** during which the lining of the uterus (endometrium) collapses and is discharged with some blood. This is called a **menstrual cycle** and is described in Chapter 35.

There are three different patterns of reproduction in mammals. One pattern is represented by the egg-laying mammals, the monotremes. The duck-billed platypus (Fig. 27-24, *A*) has one breeding season each year. The ovulated eggs, usually two, are fertilized in the oviduct. As they continue down the oviduct, various glands add albumin and then a thin, leathery shell to each egg. When laid, the eggs are about the size of a robin's egg. The platypus lays its eggs in a burrow nest where they are incubated for about 12 days. After hatching, the young are fed milk (which they obtain by licking, not suckling) for a prolonged period. Thus, in monotremes there is no gestation (period of pregnancy) and the developing embryo draws on nutrients stored in the egg, much as do the embryos of reptiles and birds. But in common with all other mammals, the monotremes rear their young on milk.

The pouched mammals (marsupials) (Fig. 27-24, *C*) exhibit a second pattern of reproduction. The physiology of gestation and lactation may be complicated in members of this group, which have a brief gestation period. In red kangaroos the first pregnancy of the season is followed by a 33-day gestation, after which the young ("joey") is born, crawls to the pouch without assistance from the mother, and attaches to a nipple. The mother immediately becomes pregnant again, but the presence of a suckling young in the pouch arrests development of the new embryo in the uterus at about the 100-cell stage. This period of arrest, called embryonic diapause, lasts approximately 235 days during which time the first joey is growing in the pouch. When the joey leaves the pouch, the uterine embryo resumes development and is born about a month later. The mother again becomes pregnant, but because the second joey is suckling, once again development of the new embryo is arrested. Meanwhile, the first joey returns to the pouch from time to time to suckle. At this point the mother has three young of different ages dependent on her: a joey on foot, a joey in the pouch, and a diapause embryo in the uterus. There are variations on this remarkable sequence—not all marsupials have developmental delays like kangaroos, and some do not even have pouches—but in all the young are born at an extremely early stage of development and undergo prolonged development while dependent on a teat.

The third pattern of reproduction is that of the placental mammals, the eutherians. In this most successful of the mammal groups, the reproductive investment is in gestation. The embryo remains in the mother's uterus, nourished by food supplied through the placenta, an intimate connection between mother and young. The length of gestation varies greatly. In general, the larger the mammal, the longer the gestation time. For example, mice have a gestation period of 21 days; rabbits and hares, 30 to 36 days; cats and dogs, 60 days; cattle, 280 days; and elephants, 22 months. But there are important exceptions (nature seldom offers perfect correlations). Baleen whales, the largest mammals, carry their young for only 12 months, while bats, no larger than mice, have gestation periods of 4 to 5 months. The condition of the young at birth also varies. An antelope bears its young well furred, eyes open, and able to run about. Newborn mice, however, are blind, naked, and helpless. We all know how long it takes a human baby to gain its footing. Human growth is in fact slower than that of any other mammal, and this is one of the distinctive attributes that sets us apart from other mammals (p. 885).

A

B

C

Figure 27-24

Mammals without placentas. The duck-billed platypus, *A*, and echidna, *B*, of Australia and New Guinea are egg-laying monotremes. The platypus lays her eggs in damp vegetation in a burrow, whereas the echidna deposits her eggs in a pouch. The gray kangaroo with her joey, *C*, is a marsupial.

Photographs by C.P. Hickman, Jr.

The renowned fecundity of meadow mice, and the effect of removing the natural predators from rodent populations, is felicitously expressed in this excerpt from Thornton Burgess's "Portrait of a Meadow Mouse":

He's fecund to the nth degree
In fact this really seems to be
His one and only honest claim
To anything approaching fame.
In just twelve months, should all survive,
A million mice would be alive—
His progeny. And this, 'tis clear,
Is quite a record for a year.

Quite unsuspected, night and day
They eat the grass that would be hay.
On any meadow, in a year,
The loss is several tons, I fear.
Yet man, with prejudice for guide,
The checks that nature doth provide
Destroys. The meadow mouse survives
And on stupidity he thrives.

The number of young produced by mammals in a season depends on many factors. Usually the larger the animal, the smaller the number of young in a litter. One of the greatest factors involved is the number of enemies a species has. Small rodents, which serve as prey for many carnivores, usually produce more than one litter of several young each season. Meadow mice are known to produce as many as 17 litters of four to nine young in a year. Most carnivores have but one litter of three to five young per year. Large mammals, such as elephants and horses, give birth to a single young with each pregnancy. An elephant produces, on the average, four calves during her reproductive life of perhaps 50 years.

___ Territory and Home Range

Many mammals have territories—areas from which individuals of the *same* species are excluded. In fact, many wild mammals, like many people, are basically unfriendly to their own kind, especially so to their own sex during the breeding season. If the mammal dwells in a burrow or den, this area forms the center of its territory. If it has no fixed address, the territory is marked out, usually with the highly developed scent glands described earlier in this chapter. Territories vary greatly in size, of course, depending on the size of the animal and its feeding habits. The grizzly bear has a territory of several square miles, which it guards zealously against all other grizzlies.

Mammals usually use natural features of their surroundings in staking their claims. These are marked with secretions from the scent glands or by urinating or defecating. When an intruder knowingly enters another's marked territory, it is immediately placed at a psychological disadvantage. Should a challenge follow, the intruder almost invariably breaks off the encounter in a submissive display characteristic for the species.

A beaver colony is a family unit, and beavers are among several mammalian species in which the male and female form a strong monogamous bond that lasts a lifetime. Because beavers invest considerable time and energy in constructing a lodge and dam and storing food for winter (Fig. 27-25), the family, especially the adult male, vigorously defends its real estate against intruding beavers. Most of the work of building dams and lodges is undertaken by male beavers, but the females help when not occupied with their young.

An interesting exception to the strong territorial nature of most mammals is the prairie dog, which lives in large, friendly communities called prairie dog "towns" (Fig. 27-26). When a new litter has been reared, the adults relinquish the old home to the young and move to the edge of the community to establish a new home. Such a practice is totally antithetical to the behavior of most mammals, which drive off the young when they are self-sufficient.

The **home range** of a mammal is a much larger foraging area surrounding a

Figure 27-25

Each beaver colony constructs its own lodge in a pond it creates by damming a stream. Each year the mother bears four or five young; when the third litter arrives, the 2-year-olds are driven out of the colony. They will establish new colonies elsewhere.

Figure 27-26

Family of prairie dogs *Cynomys ludovicianus* (order Rodentia). These highly social prairie dwellers are plant eaters that provide an important source of food to many animals. They live in elaborate tunnel systems so closely interwoven that they form "towns" of as many as 1000 individuals. Towns are subdivided into wards, in turn divided into coteries, the basic family unit, containing one or two adult males, several females, and their litters. Although prairie dogs display ownership of burrows with territorial calls, they are friendly with inhabitants of adjacent burrows. The name "prairie dogs" derives from the sharp, doglike bark they make when danger threatens.
Photograph by L.L. Rue, III.

defended territory. Home ranges are not defended in the same way as is a territory; home ranges may, in fact, overlap, producing a neutral zone used by the owners of several territories for seeking food.

Mammal Populations

A population of animals includes all the members of a species that interbreed and share a particular space (Chapter 41). All mammals (like other organisms) live in communities, each composed of numerous populations of different animal and plant species. Each species is affected by the activities of other species and by other changes, especially climatic, that occur. Thus, populations are always changing in size. Populations of small mammals are lowest before the breeding season and greatest just after the addition of the new members. Beyond these expected changes in population size, animal populations may fluctuate from other causes.

Irregular fluctuations are commonly produced by variations in climate, such as unusually cold, hot, or dry weather, or by natural catastrophes, such as fires, hailstorms, and hurricanes. These are density-independent causes, since they affect a population whether it is crowded or dispersed. However, the most spectacular fluctuations are density dependent; that is, they are correlated with population crowding (p. 1038). Cycles of abundance are common among many rodent species.

The population peaks and mass migrations of the Scandinavian and arctic North American lemmings are well known. Lemmings breed all year round, although more in the summer than in winter. The gestation period is only 21 days; young born at the beginning of the summer are weaned in 14 days and are capable of reproducing by the end of the summer. At the peak of their population density, having devastated the vegetation by tunneling and grazing, they begin long, mass migrations to find new undamaged habitats for food and space. They swim across streams and small lakes as they go but cannot distinguish these from large lakes, rivers, and the sea, in which they drown. Since lemmings are the main diet of many carnivorous mammals and birds, any change in lemming population density affects all their predators as well.

In his book *The Arctic* (1974. Montreal, Infacor, Ltd.), Canadian naturalist Fred Bruemmer describes the growth of lemming populations in arctic Canada:

"After a population crash one sees few signs of lemmings; there may be only one to every 10 acres. The next year, they are evidently numerous; their runways snake beneath the tundra vegetation, and frequent piles of rice-sized droppings indicate the lemmings fare well. The third year one sees them everywhere. The fourth year, usually the peak year of their cycle, the populations explode. Now more than 150 lemmings may inhabit each acre of land and they honeycomb it with as many as 4000 burrows. Males meet frequently and fight instantly. Males pursue females and mate after a brief but ardent courtship. Everywhere one hears the squeak and chitter of the excited, irritable, crowded animals. At such times they may spill over the land in manic migrations."

Figure 27-27

Changes in population of varying hare
and lynx in Canada as indicated by pelts
received by the Hudson's Bay Company.
The abundance of lynx (predator) follows
that of the hare (prey).

From Fundamentals of ecology, ed. 3, by Eugene P. Odum.
Copyright © 1971 by W.B. Saunders Company. Reprinted
by permission of Holt, Rinehart and Winston, CBS College
Publishing.

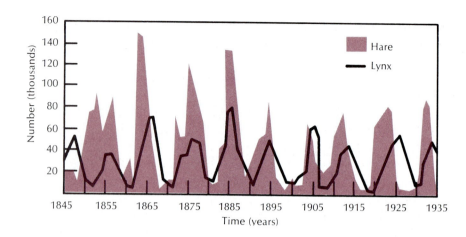

The varying hare (snowshoe rabbit) of North America shows 10-year cycles
in abundance. The well-known fecundity of rabbits enables them to produce litters of three or four young as many as five times per year. The density may
increase to 4000 hares competing for food in each square mile of northern forest.
Predators (owls, minks, foxes, and especially lynxes) also increase (Fig. 27-27).
Then the population crashes precipitously, for reasons that have long been a puzzle to scientists. Rabbits die in great numbers, not from lack of food or from an
epidemic disease (as was once believed) but evidently from some density-dependent psychogenic cause. As crowding increases, hares become more aggressive,
show signs of fear and defense, and stop breeding. The entire population reveals
symptoms of pituitary–adrenal gland exhaustion, an endocrine imbalance called
"shock disease," which results in death. These dramatic crashes are not well
understood. Whatever the causes, population crashes that follow superabun-
dance, although harsh, are clearly advantageous to the species because the vegetation is allowed to recover, providing the survivors with a much better chance for
successful breeding.

HUMANS AND MAMMALS

Some 10,000 years ago, at the time people developed agricultural methods, they
also began the domestication of mammals. Dogs were certainly among the first to
be domesticated, probably entering voluntarily into their human dependence. The
dog is an extremely adaptable and genetically plastic species derived from wolves.
Much less genetically variable and certainly less social than dogs is the domestic
cat, probably derived from an African race of wildcat. Wildcats look like over-
sized domestic cats and are still widespread in Africa and Eurasia. The domestication of cattle, buffaloes, sheep, and pigs probably came much later. It is believed
that the beasts of burden—horses, camels, oxen, and llamas—probably were subdued by early nomadic peoples. Certain domestic species no longer exist as wild
animals—for example, the one-humped Arabian camel and the llama and the
alpaca of South America. All of the truly domestic animals breed in captivity and
have become totally dependent on humans; many have been molded by selective
breeding to yield characteristics that are desirable for our purposes.

Some mammals hold special positions as "domestic" animals. The elephant
has never been truly domesticated because it will not breed in captivity. In Asia,
adults are captured and submit to a life of toil with astonishing docility. The

reindeer of northern Scandinavia are domesticated only in the sense that they are "owned" by nomadic peoples who continue to follow them in their seasonal migrations. The eland of Africa (Fig. 27-15) is undergoing experimental domestication in several places. It is placid, gentle, and immune to native diseases and produces excellent meat.

We should not leave the subject of domestication without mentioning the albino rat, a domesticated brown rat. It has been suggested that the gentle nature of the albino, which has contributed so much to medical and psychological research, is the result of a small defect in the amygdaloid nucleus of the brain. Fierce and intractable wild rats can be converted to docile, easily handled, tame rats by destroying a small part of the amygdala in an operation.

In the introduction to this chapter we alluded to the senseless human exploitation of the great marine whales, the largest animals that have ever lived. The International Whaling Commission voted in 1982 to phase out whaling altogether by 1986, but there is no certainty that the major whaling nations, Japan and the Soviet Union, will adhere to the ban. In the meantime whaling continues.

The whale tragedy is just one example of our inability to reconcile progress with the preservation of wildlife, a dilemma that is explored in the final chapter of this book. The extermination of a species for commercial gain is so totally indefensible that no debate is required. Once a species is extinct, no amount of scientific or technical ingenuity will bring it back. What has taken millions of years to evolve can be destroyed in a decade of thoughtless exploitation. Many people are concerned with the awesome impact we have on wildlife, and there is more determination today to reverse a regrettable trend than ever before. If given a chance, mammals will usually make spectacular recoveries from human depredations, as have the sea otter and the saiga antelope, both once in danger of extinction and now numerous. Paradoxically, in Africa where conservationists wage a seesaw battle with opposing interests, it appears that the commercial gain of tourism and game cropping will do more to save the fauna than the outraged concern of preservationists.

Mammals can of course be enemies of humans. Rodents and rabbits are capable of inflicting staggering damage to growing crops and stored food (Fig. 27-28). We have provided an inviting forage for rodents with our agriculture and convenienced them further by removing their natural predators. Rodents also carry various diseases. Bubonic plague and typhus are carried by house rats. Tularemia, or rabbit fever, is transmitted to humans by the wood tick carried by rabbits, woodchucks, muskrats, and other rodents. Rocky Mountain spotted fever is carried to humans by ticks from ground squirrels and dogs. Trichina worms and tapeworms are acquired by humans who eat the meat of hogs, cattle, and other mammals.

CLASSIFICATION

The classification given here recognizes 18 living orders of mammals, although some mammalogists remove the aquatic carnivores (seals, sea lions, and walruses) from the order Carnivora and place them in a distinct order Pinnipedia. Fourteen extinct orders are not included in this classification.

> **Subclass Prototheria** (pro'to-thir'e-a) (Gr., *prōtos*, first, + *thēr*, wild animal). The egg-laying mammals.
>> **Order Monotremata** (mon'o-tre'ma-tah) (Gr., *monos*, single, + *trēma*, hole)— **egg-laying mammals: duck-billed platypus** (Fig. 27-29), **spiny anteater.** The representatives of this order are from Australia, Tasmania, and New Guinea.

Figure 27-28

Brown rat *Rattus norvegicus* (order Rodentia, family Murridae). Living all too successfully beside human habitations, the brown rat not only causes great damage to food stores but also spreads disease, including bubonic plague (a disease carried by infected fleas that greatly influenced human history in medieval Europe), typhus, infectious jaundice, *Salmonella* food poisoning, and rabies.
Photograph by L.L. Rue, III.

Figure 27-29

Duck-billed platypus, an egg-laying monotreme of Australia and Tasmania. Order Monotremata.
Photograph by C.P. Hickman, Jr.

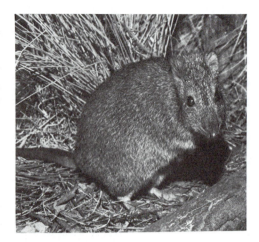

Figure 27-30

Long-nosed potoroo, a nocturnal rat kangaroo. Order Marsupialia.

Photograph by C.P. Hickman, Jr.

The most noted member of the order is the duck-billed platypus *(Ornithorhynchus anatinus).* The spiny anteater, or echidna *(Tachyglossus),* has a long, narrow snout adapted for feeding on ants, its chief food. Monotremes represent the only order that is oviparous, and there is no known group of extinct mammals from which they can be derived. Their fossils date from the Pleistocene epoch.

Subclass Theria (thir′e-a) (Gr., *thēr,* wild animal).

Infraclass Metatheria (met′a-thir′e-a) (Gr., *meta,* after, + *thēr,* wild animal). The marsupial mammals.

Order Marsupialia (mar-su′pe-ay′le-a) (Gr., *marsypion,* little pouch)—**pouched mammals: opossums, kangaroos, koalas, Tasmanian wolves, wombats, bandicoots, numbats, and others** (Fig. 27-30). These are primitive mammals characterized by an abdominal pouch, the **marsupium,** in which they rear their young. Although the young are nourished in the uterus for a short time, there is rarely a placenta present. This order has many representatives; only the opossum is found in the Americas, but the order is the dominant group of mammals in Australia.

Infraclass Eutheria (yu-thir′e-a) (Gr., *eu,* true, + *thēr,* wild animals). The placental mammals.

Order Insectivora (in-sec-tiv′o-ra) (L., *insectum,* an insect, + *vorare,* to devour)—**insect-eating mammals: shrews, hedgehogs** (Fig. 27-31), **tenrecs, moles.** The principal food of animals in this order is insects. The most primitive of placental mammals, they are widely distributed over the world except Australia and New Zealand. Placental mammals and marsupials are believed to have arisen independently from common ancestors during the Cretaceous period, but in time the placentals became dominant in most parts of the world because of their superior intelligence. Insectivora are small, sharp-snouted animals that spend a great part of their lives underground. The shrews are the smallest of the group; some of them are the smallest mammals known.

Order Chiroptera (ky-rop′ter-a) (Gr., *cheir,* hand, + *pteron,* wing)—**bats.** The wings of bats, the only true flying mammals, are modified forelimbs in which the second to fifth digits are elongated to support a thin integumental membrane for flying. The first digit (thumb) is short with a claw. There are many families and species of bats the world over. The common North American forms are the little brown bat *(Myotis),* the free-tailed bat *(Tadarida),* which lives in the Carlsbad Caverns, and the large brown bat *(Eptesicus).* In the Old World tropics the fruit bats, or "flying foxes," *(Pteropus)* are the largest of all bats, with a wingspread of 1.2 to 1.5 m; they live chiefly on fruits.

Order Dermoptera (der-mop′ter-a) (Gr., *derma,* skin, + *pteron,* wing)—**flying lemurs.** These are related to the true bats and consist of the single genus *Galeopithecus.* They are found in the Malay peninsula in the East Indies. They are not lemurs (which are primates) and cannot fly in the strict sense of the word, but glide like flying squirrels.

Order Carnivora (car-niv′o-ra) (L., *caro,* flesh, + *vorare,* to devour)—**flesh-eating mammals: dogs, wolves, cats, bears, weasels.** To this extensive order belong some of the strongest and most intelligent of animals. They all have predatory habits, and their teeth are especially adapted for tearing flesh. They are divided among two suborders: Fissipedia, whose feet contain toes, and Pinnipedia, with limbs modified for aquatic life.

Suborder Fissipedia (fi-se-peed′e-a) (L., *fissus,* cleft, + *ped,* foot). Consists of the well-known carnivores—wolves, tigers, dogs, cats, foxes, weasels, skunks, and many others. They vary in size from certain tiny weasels to the mammoth Alaskan bear and Bengal tiger. They are distributed all over the world except in the Australian and Antarctic regions, where there are no native forms. This suborder is divided into certain familiar families, among which are **Canidae** (the dog family), consisting of dogs, wolves, foxes, and coyotes; **Felidae** (the cat family), whose members include the domestic cats, tigers, lions, cougars, and lynxes; **Ursidae** (the

Figure 27-31

The European hedgehog is a primitive placental mammal related to shrews and moles. Order Insectivora.

Photograph by I. Vandermolen, Leonard Rue Enterprises.

bear family), made up of bears; and **Mustelidae** (the fur-bearing family), containing the martens, skunks, weasels, otters, badgers, minks, and wolverines.

Suborder Pinnipedia (pi-ni-peed′e-a) (L., *pinna*, feather, + *ped*, foot). Includes the aquatic carnivores, sea lions, seals, sea elephants, and walruses. Their limbs have been modified as flippers for swimming. They are all saltwater forms, and their food is mostly fish.

Order Tubulidentata (tu′byu-li-den-ta′ta) (L., *tubulus*, tube, + *dens*, tooth)—**aardvark.** The name "aardvark" is Dutch for earth pig, a peculiar animal with a piglike body found in Africa. The order is represented by a single species.

Order Rodentia (ro-den′che-a) (L., *rodere*, to gnaw)—**gnawing mammals: squirrels, rats, woodchucks.** The rodents are the most numerous of all mammals. Most of them are small. They are found on all continents and many of the large islands. They have no canine teeth, but their chisel-like incisors (never more than four) grow continually. Their basic adaptive feature therefore is gnawing. This adaptation has been largely responsible for the evolution of a very active and diversified group. Some rodents are useful for their fur. The beaver *(Castor)*, the largest rodent in the United States, has a valuable pelt. Many rodents are used as food by carnivores and by humans. Important families of this order are **Sciuridae** (squirrels and woodchucks), **Muridae** (rats and house mice), **Castoridae** (beavers), **Erethizontidae** (porcupines), **Geomyidae** (pocket gophers), and **Cricetidae** (hamsters, deer mice, gerbils, voles, lemmings).

Order Pholidota (fol′i-do′ta) (Gr., *pholis*, horny scale)—**pangolins.** In this order there is one genus *(Manis)* with eight species. They are an odd group of animals whose bodies are covered with overlapping horny scales that have arisen from fused bundles of hair. Their home is in tropical Asia and Africa.

Order Lagomorpha (lag′o-mor′fa) (Gr., *lagos*, hare, + *morphē*, form)—**rabbits, hares, pikas.** The chief difference between this order and Rodentia is the presence of four upper incisors, one pair of which is small and the other large, with enamel on the posterior as well as the anterior surface of the tooth.

Order Edentata (ee′den-ta′ta) (L., *edentatus*, toothless)—**toothless mammals: sloths, anteaters, armadillos.** These forms either are toothless or have degenerate peglike teeth without enamel. Most of them live in South and Central America, although the nine-banded armadillo *(Dasypus novemcinctus)* occurs in the southern United States. The sloths are very sluggish animals that have the queer habit of hanging upside down on branches. The hairs of sloths have tiny pits in which green algae grow, rendering them invisible against a background of mosses and lichens. The extinct ground sloths were represented by some members as large as small elephants.

Order Cetacea (see-tay′she-a) (L., *cetus*, whale)—**fishlike mammals: whales, dolphins** (Fig. 27-32), **porpoises.** This order is well adapted for aquatic life. Their anterior limbs are modified into broad flippers; the posterior limbs are absent. Some have a fleshy dorsal fin, and the tail is divided into transverse fleshy flukes. The nostrils are represented by a single or double blowhole on top of the head. They have no hair except a few hairs on the muzzle, no skin glands except the mammary and those of the eye, no external ear, and small eyes. The order is divided into two suborders.

Suborder Odontoceti (o-don-te-see′tie) (Gr., *odont*, tooth, + *cete*, whales)—**toothed whales.** Made up of toothed members and represented by the sperm whales, porpoises, and dolphins. The killer whale *(Orcinus)* does not hesitate to attack the larger whales and is destructive to seal rookeries. The sperm whale *(Physeter)* is the source of sperm oil, which is obtained from the head. A peculiar substance, ambergris, is sometimes formed in its stomach and is used in perfumes. Porpoises and dolphins are only about 2 m long and feed mainly on fish.

Suborder Mysticeti (mis-te-see′tie) (Gr., *mystikētos*, whale)—**whalebone whales.** Includes many species, some of which are the largest animals that have ever lived. Instead of teeth, they have a peculiar straining device of

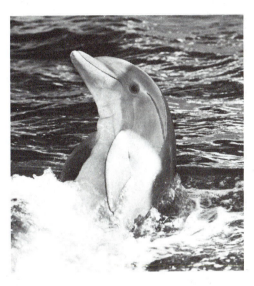

Figure 27-32

Bottle-nosed, or common, dolphin. Order Cetacea.
Photograph by L.L. Rue, III.

Figure 27-33

Rock hyrax, a colonial mammal widely distributed in Africa. Order Hyracoidea.
Photograph by B. Tallmark.

IV   II

III

Rhinoceros   **Horse**

III

III

V   II

IV   III

Hippopotamus

V   II

IV   III

Deer

Figure 27-34

Odd- and even-toed ungulates. The rhinoceros and horse (order Perissodactyla) are odd toed; the hippopotamus and deer (order Artiodactyla) are even toed. The lighter, faster animals run on only one or two toes.

whalebone (baleen) attached to the palate, used to filter floating and weakly swimming animals (plankton) out of the water. The largest of the whales is the blue whale *(Balaenoptera),* which may grow 30 m long and weigh 125 tons.

Order Proboscidea (pro′ba-sid′e-a) (Gr., *proboskis,* elephant's trunk, from *pro,* before, + *boskein,* to feed)—**proboscis mammals: elephants.** These are the largest of living land animals. The two upper incisors are elongated as tusks, and the molar teeth are well developed. There are two species of elephants: the Indian *(Elephas maximus),* with relatively small ears, and the African *(Loxodonta africana),* with large ears. The Asiatic or Indian elephant has long been domesticated and is trained to do heavy work. The taming of the African elephant is more difficult but was done extensively by the ancient Carthaginians and Romans, who employed them in their armies. Barnum's famous "Jumbo" was an African elephant.

Order Hyracoidea (hy′ra-coi′de-a) (Gr., *hyrax,* shrew)—**hyraxes (coneys)** (Fig. 27-33). Coneys are herbivores that are restricted to Africa and Syria. They have some resemblance to short-eared rabbits but have teeth like rhinoceroses, with hoofs on their toes and pads on their feet. They have four toes on the front feet and three toes on the back.

Order Sirenia (sy-re′ne-a) (Gr., *seiren,* sea nymph)—**sea cows (manatees).** Sea cows, or manatees, are large, clumsy aquatic animals. They have a blunt muzzle covered with coarse bristles, the only hairs these queer animals possess. They have no hindlimbs, and their forelimbs are modified into swimming flippers. The tail is broad with flukes but is not divided. They live in the bays and rivers along the coasts of tropical and subtropical seas. There are only two genera living at present: *Trichechus,* found in the rivers of Florida, West Indies, Brazil, and Africa, and *Halicore,* the dugong of India and Australia.

Order Perissodactyla (pe-ris′so-dak′ti-la) (Gr., *perissos,* odd, + *dactylos,* toe)—**odd-toed hoofed mammals: horses, asses, zebras, tapirs, rhinoceroses.** The odd-toed hoofed mammals have an odd number (one or three) of toes, each with a cornified hoof (Fig. 27-34). Both the Perissodactyla and the Artiodactyla are often referred to as **ungulates** (L., *ungula,* hoof), or hoofed mammals, with teeth adapted for chewing. The horse family (Equidae), which also includes asses and zebras, has only one functional toe. Tapirs have a short proboscis formed from the upper lip and nose. The rhinoceros *(Rhinoceros)* includes several species found in Africa and Southeast Asia. All are herbivorous.

Order Artiodactyla (ar′te-o-dak′ti-la) (Gr., *artios,* even, + *dactylos,* toe)—**even-toed hoofed mammals: swine, camels, deer, hippopotamuses, antelopes, cattle, sheep, goats.** Most of these ungulates have two toes, although the hippopotamus and some others have four (Fig. 27-34). Each toe is sheathed in a cornified hoof. Many, such as the cow, deer, and sheep, have horns. Many are ruminants, that is, animals that chew the cud. Like Perissodactyla, they are strictly herbivorous. The group is divided into nine living families and many extinct ones and includes some of the most valuable domestic animals. This extensive order is commonly divided into three suborders: the **Suina** (pigs, peccaries, hippopotamuses), the **Tylopoda** (camels), and the **Ruminantia** (deer, giraffes, sheep, cattle, and so on).

Order Primates (pry-may′teez) (L., *prima,* first)—**highest mammals: lemurs, monkeys, apes, humans, and others.** This order stands first in the animal kingdom in brain development, possessing especially large cerebral hemispheres. Most of the species are arboreal, apparently derived from tree-dwelling insectivores. The primates represent the end product of a line that branched off early from other mammals and have retained many primitive characteristics. It is believed that their tree-dwelling habits of agility in capturing food or avoiding enemies were largely responsible for their advances in brain structure. As a group, they are generalized, with five digits (usually provided with flat nails) on both forelimbs and hindlimbs. All have their bodies covered with hair except humans. Forelimbs are often adapted for grasping, as are the hindlimbs sometimes. The group is singularly lacking in claws, scales, horns, and hoofs. There are two suborders.

Suborder Prosimii (pro-sim'ee-i) (Gr., *pro*, before, + *simia*, ape)—lemurs, tree shrews, tarsiers, lorises, pottos. These are primitive arboreal primates, with their second toe provided with a claw and a long nonprehensile tail. They look like a cross between squirrels and monkeys. They are found in the forests of Madagascar, Africa, the Malay peninsula, and the Philippines. Their food is both plants and small animals.

Suborder Anthropoidea (an'thro-poi'de-a) (Gr., *anthropos*, man)—monkeys, gibbons, apes, humans. There are three superfamilies.

Superfamily Ceboidea (se-boi'de-a) (Gr., *kebos*, long-tailed monkey) (Platyrhinii). These are New World monkeys, characterized by the broad flat nasal septum, nonopposable thumb, prehensile tail, and the absence of ischial callosities and cheek pouches. Familiar members of this superfamily are the capuchin monkey *(Cebus)* of the organ grinder, the spider monkey *(Ateles)*, and the howler monkey *(Alouatta)*.

Superfamily Cercopithecoidea (sur'ko-pith'e-koi'de-a) (Gr., *kerkos*, tail, + *pithekos*, monkey) (Catarrhini). These Old World monkeys have the external nares close together, and many have internal cheek pouches. They never have prehensile tails, there are callused ischial tuberosities on their buttocks, and their thumbs are opposable. Examples are the savage mandrill *(Cynocephalus)*, the rhesus monkey *(Macaca)* (Fig. 27-35), widely used in biological investigation, and the proboscis monkey *(Nasalis)*.

Superfamily Hominoidea (hom'i-noi'de-a) (L., *homo, hominis*, man). The higher (anthropoid) apes and humans make up this superfamily. Their chief characteristics are lack of a tail and lack of cheek pouches. There are two families: Pongidae and Hominidae. The Pongidae family includes the higher apes, gibbon *(Hylobates)*, orangutan *(Simia)*, chimpanzee *(Pan)*, and gorilla *(Gorilla)*. The other family, Hominidae, is represented by a single living species *(Homo sapiens)*, modern humans. Humans differ from the members of family Pongidae in being more erect, in having shorter arms and larger thumbs, and in having lighter jaws with smaller front teeth. Most of the apes also have much more prominent ridges over the eyes. Many human differences from the anthropoid apes are associated with higher human intelligence, human speech centers in the brain, and the fact that humans are no longer arboreal animals.

Figure 27-35

Rhesus monkey *Macaca mulatta*. Order Primates, superfamily Cercopithecoidea. Photograph by I. Vandermolen, Leonard Rue Enterprises.

___ Summary

The 4600 living mammals are descended from a mammal-like reptile (therapsid) of the Jurassic period of the Mesozoic era. They diversified rapidly during the Tertiary period of the Cenozoic era to become the most intelligent and advanced animals on earth. Mammals are named for the glandular organs of the female (rudimentary in the male) that secrete milk for the nourishment of the young after their birth. An even more obvious mammalian characterisic is the presence of hair, an integumentary outgrowth that covers most mammals. Hair serves variously for mechanical protection, thermal insulation, protective coloration, and waterproofing. Mammalian skin is rich in glands: sweat glands that function in evaporative cooling, scent glands used in social interactions, and sebaceous glands that secrete lubricating skin oil. All placental mammals have deciduous teeth that are replaced by permanent teeth (diphyodont dentition). The four groups of teeth—incisors, canines, premolars, and molars—may be highly modified in different mammals for specialized feeding tasks, or they may be absent.

The food habits of mammals strongly influence their body form and physiology. Herbivorous mammals have special adaptations for harboring the intestinal microflora that breaks down cellulose of the woody diet, and they have developed adaptations for detecting and escaping predators. Carnivorous mammals feed mainly on herbivores, have a simple digestive tract, and have developed adaptations for a predatory life. Omnivores feed on both plant and animal foods. Insectivores feed mainly on insects.

Mammals are endothermic homeotherms, although in many species body temperatures fluctuate daily or seasonally. Adaptations for hot environments include behavioral avoidance of heat, relaxation of body temperature control, evaporative cooling, and several adaptations for conserving body water. The major adaptations for life in cold environments are increased heat production and control of heat loss by insulative adjustments. Some mammals migrate to separate summer and winter ranges, and others have met the problem of winter survival by hibernation.

Mammals with true flight, the bats, are nocturnal and thus avoid direct competition with birds. Most employ ultrasonic echolocation to navigate and feed in darkness.

The most primitive living mammals are the egg-laying monotremes, a remnant group today. All other mammals are viviparous. Embryos of marsupials are born underdeveloped and complete their early growth in the mother's pouch, nourished by milk. The largest and most successful mammals are the placentals in which the embryo undergoes an extensive development in the uterus, nourished by the placenta, a specialization of the embryonic membranes. The unqualified success of mammals as a group cannot be attributed to greater organ system perfection, but rather to their impressive overall adaptability—the capacity to fit more perfectly in total organization to environmental conditions and thus exploit virtually every habitat on earth.

Selected references

Asdell, S.A. 1964. Patterns of mammalian reproduction, ed. 2. Ithaca, N.Y., Cornell University Press. *Authoritative and thorough synthesis of information on mammalian reproductive habits.*

Carrington, R. 1975. The mammals. New York, Life Nature Library, Time-Life Books, Inc. *Well-written, beautifully illustrated, semipopular treatment.*

Chapman, J.A., and G.A. Feldhamer (eds.). 1982. Wild mammals of North America: biology, management, and economics. Baltimore, The Johns Hopkins University Press. *Major reference work on most North American mammals.*

Eisenberg, J.F. 1981. The mammalian radiations: an analysis of trends in evolution, adaptation, and behavior. Chicago, University of Chicago Press. *Wide-ranging, authoritative synthesis of mammalian evolution and behavior.*

Ewer, R.F. 1973. The carnivores. Ithaca, N.Y., Cornell University Press. *Thorough synthesis.*

Griffiths, M. 1978. The biology of the monotremes. New York, Academic Press, Inc. *Comprehensive treatment of this fascinating remnant group.*

Gunderson, H.L. 1976. Mammalogy. New York, McGraw-Hill Book Co. *Comprehensive text emphasizing adaptations.*

Hall, E.R., and K.R. Kelson. 1959. The mammals of North America, 2 vols. New York, The Ronald Press Co. *Full descriptions of species and subspecies with distribution maps. Taxonomic keys, records, and revealing line drawings of skull characteristics are included in this authoritative work.*

Halstead, L.B. 1978. The evolution of the mammals. London, Eurobook, Ltd. *Richly illustrated, semipopular account.*

Hamilton, W.J., and J.O. Whitaker. 1979. Mammals of the eastern United States, ed. 2. Ithaca, N.Y., Cornell University Press. *Habits and distribution of mammals found east of the Mississippi.*

Kelsall, J.D. 1968. The migratory barren-ground caribou of Canada. Ottawa, Canadian Wildlife Service, Queen's Printers.

Kirseh, J.A.W. 1977. The six-percent solution: second thoughts on the adaptedness of the Marsupialia. Am. Sci. 65:276-288. *An argument against a persistent opinion that marsupials are less well adapted than placental mammals.*

Matthews, L.H. 1969. The life of mammals, 2 vols. New York, Universe Books. *The first volume of this excellent set treats the origins, structure, and adaptations of mammals; the second volume reviews the orders and families of mammals.*

Rue, L.L., III. 1967. Pictorial guide to the mammals of North America. New York, Thomas Y. Crowell Co. *Characteristics, habits, and life cycles of mammals with a wealth of animal lore.*

Sanderson, I.T. 1955. Living mammals of the world. New York, Garden City Books (Hanover House). *A beautiful and informative work with many photographs and concise text material. It is a delight to any zoologist regardless of specialized interest.*

Scheffer, V.B. 1958. Seals, sea lions, and walruses: a review of the Pinnipedia. Stanford, Calif., Stanford University Press. *Treats the group's evolution, characteristics, and classification. Many fine photographs and a good bibliography are included.*

Schmidt-Nielsen, K. 1964. Desert animals: physiological problems of heat and water. New York, Oxford University Press (Dover Publications reprint, 1979). *Classic treatise on the functional adaptations of desert animals, especially mammals.*

Stonehouse, B., and D. Gilmore (eds.). 1977. The biology of marsupials. London, the Macmillan Press, Ltd. *Contributed chapters on origins, ecology, anatomy, and metabolic aspects of marsupials.*

Tyndale-Biscoe, H. 1973. Life of marsupials. New York, American Elsevier Publishers, Inc. *Comprehensive general biology of marsupials with emphasis on functional adaptations.*

Vaughan, T.A. 1978. Mammalogy, ed. 2. Philadelphia, W.B. Saunders Co. *This basic text takes a systematic approach to the subject.*

Walker, E.P. 1975. Mammals of the world, 2 vols., ed. 3. Baltimore, The Johns Hopkins University Press. *The only single compendium of information on all known and living mammalian genera. A valuable reference work.*

Young, J.Z., and M.J. Hobbs. 1975. The life of mammals: their anatomy and physiology, ed. 2. New York, Oxford University Press. *This is a well-known work about mammals, especially their anatomy, histology, physiology, and embryology. Classification is not treated.*

Selected *Scientific American* articles

Bartholomew, G.A., and J.W. Hudson. 1961. Desert ground squirrels. **205**:107-116 (Nov.). *Two species living in California's Mojave Desert have developed interesting adaptations for survival in desert heat and aridity.*

Bekoff, M., and M.C. Wells. 1980. The social ecology of coyotes. **242**:130-148 (Apr.). *Social behavior is determined by the nature of the food supply.*

Dawson, T.J. 1977. Kangaroos. **237**:78-89 (Aug.). *These marsupials have several adaptations fitting them for life on the Australian grasslands.*

Degabriele, R. 1980. The physiology of the koala. **243**:110-117 (July). *These endearing marsupials eat eucalyptus leaves, which are toxic to other animals.*

Griffin, D.R. 1958. More about bat "radar." **199**:40-44 (July).

Irving, L. 1966. Adaptations to cold. **214**:94-101 (Jan.). *The homeothermic birds and mammals have evolved several adaptations that permit them to survive in cold environments.*

Kanwisher, J.W., and S.H. Ridgeway. 1983. The physiological ecology of whales and porpoises. **248**:110-120 (June). *Their adaptations for deep dives are described.*

King, J.A. 1959. The social behavior of prairie dogs. **201**:128-140 (Oct.).

Kooyman, G.L. 1969. The Weddell seal. **221**:100-106 (Aug.). *This antarctic seal swims for miles under shelf ice on one breath of air, returning unerringly to its breathing hole.*

Modell, W. 1969. Horns and antlers. **220**:114-122 (Apr.). *Their differences, growth, and structure are described.*

Montagna, W. 1965. The skin. **212**:56-66 (Feb.). *The structure and diverse functions of mammalian skin are described.*

Mrosovsky, N. 1968. The adjustable brain of hibernators. **218**:110-118 (Mar.). *Hibernation is preceded by a remarkable series of changes and a resetting of the hypothalamic thermostat.*

Myers, J.H., and C.J. Krebs. 1974. Population cycles in rodents. **230**:38-46 (June). *Population fluctuations appear to be associated with periodic changes in genetic makeup.*

Mykytowycz, R. 1968. Territorial marking by rabbits. **218**:116-126 (May). *Describes the use of odor-producing glands by Australian colonial rabbits to mark territories.*

Pruitt, W.O., Jr., 1960. Animals in the snow. **202**:60-68 (Jan.). *Describes the adaptations of the many homeotherms that live where snow persists for more than half the year.*

Schmidt-Nielsen, K., and B. Schmidt-Nielsen. 1953. The desert rat. **189**:73-78 (July). *The kangaroo rat possesses several adaptations that enable it to live in hot, arid regions, eating only dry food and drinking no water at all.*

Scholander, P.F. 1963. The master switch of life. **209**:92-106 (Dec.). *Diving vertebrates are obviously specialized for making prolonged dives without breathing. One of the most important adaptations is the capacity to grossly redistribute the circulation.*

Taylor, C.R. 1969. The eland and the oryx. **220**:88-95 (Jan.). *These large African antelopes thrive in desert or near desert regions without drinking water. Their adaptations for heat and aridity are described.*

Wursig, B. 1979. Dolphins. **240**:136-148 (Mar.). *Discusses the behavior and intelligence of these large-brained aquatic mammals.*

PART THREE

Mature bull elk foraging for grass in a wintering area of Yellowstone National Park.

ACTIVITY OF LIFE

Courtesy U.S. Soil Conservation Service.

Motility, nutrition, respiration, internal transport, excretion, irritability, and integration are necessary activities of animal life. These and the metabolic processes that provide energy for them are functional activities inherent in the simplest to the most complex animals. Animals have evolved various ways to perform these common tasks. Not all animals have specialized systems for carrying out specific functions; specialization of organ systems seems to be correlated with increase in body size and overall complexity. Higher forms exercise finer control over physiological processes and exhibit greater internal constancy. Regardless of the degree of specialization, however, all animals possess integrative systems for coordinating internal activities and for relating the animal's behavior to its external environment.

CHAPTER 28

SUPPORT, PROTECTION, AND MOVEMENT

Skeletal muscle of killifish *Fundulus*. This electron micrograph shows three myofibrils, each composed of numerous myofilaments. The sliding filament hypothesis is a widely accepted model that explains how the myofilaments interact to produce muscle shortening. (×50,000.)

Electron micrograph by F.A. Pepe, University of Pennsylvania/BPS.

INTEGUMENT AMONG VARIOUS GROUPS OF ANIMALS

The integument is the outer covering of the body, a protective wrapping that includes the skin and all structures derived from or associated with the skin, such as hair, setae, scales, feathers, and horns. In most animals it is tough and pliable, providing mechanical protection against abrasion and puncture and forming an effective barrier against the invasion of bacteria. It may provide moisture proofing against fluid loss or gain. The skin helps protect the underlying cells against the damaging action of the ultraviolet rays of the sun. In addition to being a protective cover, the skin serves a variety of important regulatory functions. For example, in warm-blooded (homeothermic) animals, it is vitally concerned with temperature regulation, since most of the body's heat is lost through the skin; it contains mechanisms that cool the body when it is too hot and slow heat loss when the body is too cold. The skin contains sensory receptors that provide essential information about the immediate environment. It has excretory functions and in some forms respiratory functions as well. Through skin pigmentation the organism can make itself more or less conspicuous. Skin secretions can make the animal sexually attractive or repugnant or provide olfactory cues that influence behavioral interactions between individuals.

Invertebrate Integument

Many protozoa have only the delicate cell or plasma membranes for external coverings; others, such as *Paramecium*, have developed a protective pellicle. Most multicellular invertebrates, however, have more complex tissue coverings. The principal covering is a single-layered **epidermis.** Some invertebrates have added a secreted noncellular **cuticle** over the epidermis for additional protection.

The molluscan epidermis is delicate and soft and contains mucous glands, some of which secrete the calcium carbonate of the shell. Cephalopod molluscs (squids and octopuses) have developed a more complex integument, consisting of cuticle, simple epidermis, layer of connective tissue, layer of reflecting cells (iridocytes), and thicker layer of connective tissue.

Arthropods have the most complex of invertebrate integuments, providing not only protection but also skeletal support. The development of a firm exoskeleton and jointed appendages suitable for the attachment of muscles has been a key feature in the extraordinary evolutionary success of this phylum, the largest of animal groups. The arthropod integument consists of a single-layered **epidermis** (also called more precisely **hypodermis**), which secretes a complex cuticle of two zones (Fig. 28-1, *A*). The inner zone, the **procuticle,** is composed of protein and chitin. Chitin is a polysaccharide comprised of *N*-acetylglucosamine units. The strength of the cuticle is contributed principally by a tough protein called **sclerotin.** The outer zone of cuticle, lying on the external surface above the procuticle, is the thin **epicuticle.** The epicuticle is a nonchitinous complex of proteins and lipids that provides a protective moisture-proofing barrier to the integument.

The arthropod cuticle may remain as a tough but soft and flexible layer, or it may be hardened by one of two ways. In the decapod crustaceans, for example, crabs and lobsters, the cuticle is stiffened by **calcification,** the deposition of calcium carbonate. In insects hardening is achieved by a process called **sclerotization,** in which protein molecules form stabilizing cross-linkages. Arthropod cuticle is one of the toughest materials synthesized by animals; it is strongly resistant to

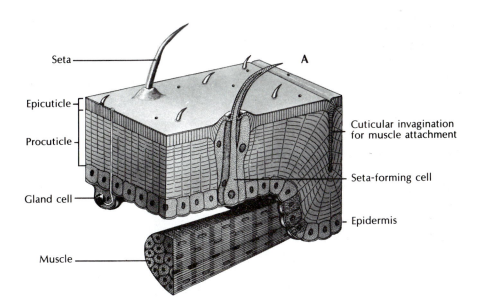

Seta

Epicuticle

Procuticle

Gland cell

Muscle

A

Cuticular invagination
for muscle attachment

Seta-forming cell

Epidermis

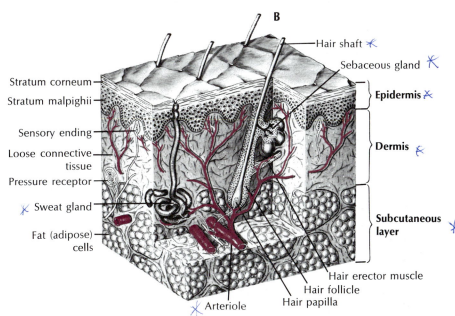

B

Stratum corneum
Stratum malpighii

Sensory ending
Loose connective
tissue
Pressure receptor

Sweat gland

Fat (adipose)
cells

Hair shaft
Sebaceous gland

Epidermis

Dermis

**Subcutaneous
layer**

Hair erector muscle
Hair follicle
Hair papilla
Arteriole

Figure 28-1

A, Structure of insect integument. This
reconstruction shows block of integument
drawn at point where cuticle invaginates
to provide exoskeletal muscle attachment.
B, Structure of human skin.

pressure and tearing and can withstand boiling in concentrated alkali, yet it is
light, having a specific mass of only 1.3 (1.3 times the weight of water).

When arthropods molt, the epidermal cells first divide by mitosis. Enzymes
secreted by the epidermis dissolve most of the procuticle; the digested materials
are then absorbed and consequently are not lost to the body. Then in the space
beneath the old cuticle a new epicuticle and procuticle are formed. After the old
cuticle is shed, the new cuticle is thickened and calcified or sclerotized.

___ Vertebrate Integument

The basic plan of the vertebrate integument, as exemplified by human skin (Fig.
28-1, *B*), includes a thin, outer stratified epithelial layer, the **epidermis,** derived
from ectoderm and an inner, thicker layer, the **dermis,** or true skin, which is of
mesodermal origin.

The reptiles were the first to exploit the adaptive possibilities of the remarkably tough protein keratin. The reptilian epidermal scale that develops from keratin is a much lighter and more flexible structure than the bony, dermal scale of fishes, yet it provides excellent protection from abrasion and desiccation. Scales may be overlapping structures, as in snakes and some lizards, or develop into plates, as in turtles and crocodilians. In birds, keratin found new uses. Feathers, beaks, and claws, as well as scales, are all epidermal structures composed of dense keratin. Mammals continued to capitalize on keratin's virtues by turning it into hair, hooves, claws, and nails. As a result of its keratin content, hair is by far the strongest material in the body. It has a tensile strength comparable to that of rolled aluminum and is nearly twice as strong, weight for weight, as the strongest bone.

Although the epidermis is thin and appears simple in structure, it gives rise to most derivatives of the integument, such as hair, feathers, claws, and hooves. The dermis, containing blood vessels, collagenous fibers, nerves, pigment cells, fat cells, and fibroblasts, supports, cushions, and nourishes its overlying partner, which is devoid of blood vessels.

The epidermis consists usually of several layers of cells. The basal part is made up of columnar cells that undergo frequent mitosis to renew the layers that lie above. As the outer layers of cells are displaced upward by new generations of cells beneath, an exceedingly tough, fibrous protein called **keratin** accumulates in the interior of the cells. Gradually, keratin replaces all metabolically active cytoplasm. The cell dies and is eventually shed, lifeless and scalelike. Such is the origin of dandruff as well as a significant fraction of household dust. This process is called **keratinization,** and the cell, thus transformed, is said to be "**cornified.**" Cornified cells, highly resistant to abrasion and water diffusion, comprise the stratum corneum. This epidermal layer becomes especially thick in areas exposed to persistent pressure or friction, such as calluses and the human palms and soles.

The **dermis,** as already mentioned, mainly serves a supportive role for the epidermis. Nevertheless, true bony structures, where they occur in the integument, are always dermal derivatives. Heavy bony plates were common in primitive ostracoderms and placoderms of the Paleozoic era but occur in few living fishes. Scales of contemporary fishes are bony dermal structures that have evolved from the bony armor of the Paleozoic fishes but are much smaller and more flexible. Although of dermal origin, fish scales are intimately associated with the thin, overlying epidermis; in some species the scales protrude through the epidermis, but typically the epidermis forms a continuous sheath that is reflected under the overlapping scales (Fig. 28-2). Dermal bone also forms the flat bones of the skull and gives rise to antlers, which are outgrowths of dermal frontal bone.

Color

Nearly all vertebrates are colored. The colors may be subdued and cryptic when serving protective functions, or vivid and dramatic when serving as important recognition marks. Integumentary color is usually caused by **pigments,** but in some vertebrates, especially birds, some colors are produced by the physical structure of the surface tissue, which reflects certain light wavelengths and eliminates others. Colors produced this way are called **structural color,** and they are responsible for the most beautifully iridescent and metallic hues to be found in the animal kingdom. Many butterflies and beetles and a few fishes thus share with birds the distinction of being the earth's most resplendent animals. Certain structural colors of feathers are caused by minute, air-filled spaces or pores that reflect white light (white feathers) or some portion of the spectrum (for example, Tyndall blue coloration produced by scattering of light [see marginal note, p. 608]). Iridescent colors are produced when light passes through several layers of thin, transparent film on the feather barbules and is diffracted into its component parts, much as a film of oil on a puddle breaks up sunlight into a rainbowlike spectrum.

Pigment color is caused by **chromatophores,** specialized cells located usually in the dermis but occasionally in the epidermis. Pigments are large molecules that reflect light rays. In fishes, amphibians, and reptiles the expansion and contraction of pigments within the chromatophores are under hormonal or nervous control

(p. 568). When expanded, the pigment is visible; when contracted, it concentrates into a central aggregate too small to be visible. The animal then pales or assumes the color of a deeper pigment normally masked by the overlying chromatophores. Some reptiles and fishes can shift their color and color patterns in remarkable ways.

Melanophores contain the pigment **melanin.** This is by far the most widespread animal pigment and is responsible for the various earth-colored shades— black, browns, and grays—that most animals wear. Yellow and red colors are often caused by **carotenoid** pigments, which are frequently contained within special pigment cells called **xanthophores.** Most vertebrates are incapable of synthesizing their own carotenoid pigments but must obtain them directly or indirectly from plants. Two entirely different classes of pigments called ommochromes and pteridines are usually responsible for the yellow pigments of molluscs and arthropods. Green colors are rare; when they occur, they are usually produced by yellow pigment overlying blue structural color. **Iridophores,** a third type of chromatophore, contain crystals of guanine or some other purine, rather than pigment. They produce a silvery or metallic effect by reflecting light.

By vertebrate standards, the mammals are a somber-colored group. Most mammals are more or less color blind, a deficiency that is doubtless connected with the lack of bright colors in the group. Exceptions are the brilliantly colored skin patches of some baboons and mandrills. Significantly, the primates have color vision and thus can appreciate such eye-catching ornaments. The muted colors of mammals are caused by melanin, which is deposited in growing hair by dermal melanophores.

Sunburning and tanning

In general, humans lack the special body coverings that protect other land vertebrates from the damaging action of ultraviolet rays of the sun; we must depend on thickening of the outer layer of the epidermis (**stratum corneum**) and on epidermal pigmentation for protection from the sun's spectrum. Sunburn and suntanning are caused largely by exposure to the ultraviolet area of the sun's spectrum (wavelength 300 to 390 nm). This spectral band acts almost entirely on epidermis; very little penetrates to the dermis beneath. The ultraviolet rays photochemically decompose nucleoproteins within the nuclei of cells of the deeper layer of the epidermis. Blood vessels then enlarge and other tissue changes occur, producing the red coloration of sunburn. Light skins suntan through the formation of the pigment **melanin** in the deeper epidermis and by "pigment darkening," that is, the photooxidative blackening of bleached pigment already present in the epidermis. Regrettably, white Americans pay dearly for their sun worship with approximately 300,000 cases of skin cancer each year.

▬ SKELETAL SYSTEMS

Skeletons are supportive systems that provide rigidity to the body, surfaces for muscle attachment, and protection for vulnerable body organs. The familiar bone of the vertebrate skeleton is only one of several kinds of supportive and connective tissues serving various binding and weight-bearing functions, which are described in this discussion.

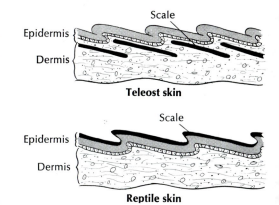

Figure 28-2

Integument of bony fishes and reptiles. Bony (teleost) fishes have bony scales from dermis, and reptiles have horny scales from epidermis. Dermal scales of fishes are retained throughout life. Epidermal scales of reptiles are shed periodically.

Hydrostatic Skeletons

Not all skeletons are rigid; many invertebrate groups use their body fluids as an internal hydrostatic skeleton. The muscles in the body wall of the earthworm, for example, have no firm base for attachment but develop muscular force by contracting against the coelomic fluids, which are enclosed within a limited space and are incompressible, much like the hydraulic brake system of an automobile.

Alternate contractions of the circular and longitudinal muscles of the body wall enable the worm to thin and thicken, setting up backward-moving waves of motion that propel the animal forward. Earthworms and other annelids are helped by the septa that separate the body into more or less independent compartments. An obvious advantage is that if a worm is punctured or even cut into pieces, each part can still develop pressure and move. Worms that lack internal compartments, for example, the lugworm *Arenicola,* are rendered helpless if the body fluid is lost through a wound.

Rigid Skeletons

Rigid skeletons differ from hydrostatic skeletons in one fundamental way: rigid skeletons consist of rigid elements, usually jointed, to which muscles can attach. Muscles can only contract; to be lengthened they must be extended by the pull of an antagonistic set of muscles. Rigid skeletons provide the anchor points required by opposing sets of muscles, such as flexors and extensors.

There are two principal types of rigid skeletons: the **exoskeleton,** typical of molluscs and arthropods, and the **endoskeleton,** characteristic of echinoderms and vertebrates. The invertebrate exoskeleton may be mainly protective, but it may also perform a vital role in locomotion. An exoskeleton may take the form of a shell, a spicule, or a calcareous, proteinaceous, or chitinous plate. It may be rigid, as in molluscs, or jointed and movable, as in arthropods. Unlike the endoskeleton, which grows with the animal, the exoskeleton is often a limiting coat of armor that must be periodically shed (molted) to make way for an enlarged replacement. Some invertebrate exoskeletons, such as the shells of snails and bivalves, grow with the animal.

The vertebrate endoskeleton is formed inside the body and is composed of bone and cartilage, which, as we have seen earlier in this chapter, are forms of dense connective tissue. Bone not only supports and protects but is also the major body reservoir for calcium and phosphorus. In higher vertebrates the red blood cells and certain white blood cells are formed in the bone marrow.

Cartilage

Cartilage and bone are the characteristic vertebrate supportive tissues. The **notochord,** the semirigid axial rod of protochordates and vertebrate larvae and embryos, is also a primitive vertebrate supportive tissue. Except in the most primitive chordates, for example, amphioxus and the cyclostomes, the notochord is surrounded or replaced by the backbone during embryonic development. The notochord is composed of large, vacuolated cells and is surrounded by layers of elastic and fibrous sheaths. It is a stiffening device, preserving body shape during locomotion (p. 498).

Cartilage is the major skeletal element of primitive vertebrates. The jawless fishes (agnathans) and elasmobranchs have purely cartilaginous skeletons, which

From the viewpoint of structural mechanics, the arthropod-type exoskeleton is perhaps a better arrangement for small animals than a vertebrate-type endoskeleton because a hollow cylindrical tube can support much more weight without collapsing than can a solid cylindrical rod of the same material and weight. Arthropods can thus enjoy both protection and structural support from their exoskeleton. But for larger animals the hollow tube loses its advantage, because the rigidity of a cylinder decreases rapidly as the radius is increased. For a very large animal the hollow cylinder would be completely impractical. If made thick enough to support the body weight, it would be too heavy to lift; but if kept thin and light, it would be extremely sensitive to buckling or shattering on impact. Finally, can you imagine the sad plight of a large animal when it shed its exoskeleton to molt?

strangely enough is a degenerative feature, since their Paleozoic ancestors had bony skeletons. Higher vertebrates as adults have principally bony skeletons with some cartilage interspersed. Cartilage is a soft, pliable, characteristically deeply-lying tissue. Unlike most connective tissues, which are quite variable in form, cartilage is basically the same wherever it is found. The basic form, **hyaline cartilage,** has a clear, glassy appearance (Fig. 6-12, *B*, p. 136). It is composed of cartilage cells (**chondrocytes**) surrounded by firm complex protein gel interlaced with a meshwork of collagenous fibers. Blood vessels are virtually absent. In addition to forming the cartilaginous skeleton of the primitive vertebrates and that of all vertebrate embryos, hyaline cartilage makes up the articulating surfaces of many bone joints of higher adult vertebrates and the supporting tracheal, laryngeal, and bronchial rings.

Bone

Bone is a living tissue that differs from other connective and supportive tissues by having significant deposits of inorganic calcium salts laid down in an extracellular matrix. Its structural organization is such that bone has nearly the tensile strength of cast iron, yet is only one third as heavy. Most bones develop from cartilage (**endochondral bone**) by a complex replacement of embryonic cartilage with bone tissue.

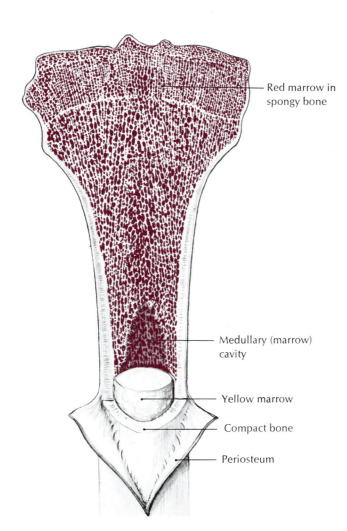

Red marrow in spongy bone

Medullary (marrow) cavity

Yellow marrow

Compact bone

Periosteum

Figure 28-3

Cutaway section of a long bone, showing appearance of spongy and compact bone.
From Anthony, C.P., and G.A. Thibodeau. 1983. Textbook of anatomy and physiology, ed. 11. St. Louis, The C.V. Mosby Co.

Canaliculi (passages interconnecting lacunae)

Lacunae (containing bone cells)

Peri-osteum

Canal

Blood vessel

Osteon

Figure 28-4

Structure of bone, showing dense calcified matrix and bone cells arranged into osteons. Bone cells are entrapped within cell-like lacunae but receive nutrients from the circulatory system via tiny canaliculi that interlace the calcified matrix. Bone cells were known as osteoblasts when they were building bone, but, in mature bone shown here, they become resting osteocytes. Bone is covered with compact connective tissue called periosteum.

A second type of bone is **membrane bone,** which develops directly from sheets of embryonic cells. In higher vertebrates membrane bone is restricted to bones of the face and cranium; the remainder of the skeleton is endochondral bone. Despite differences in origin, endochondral bone and membrane bone are not distinguishable histologically. In the fishes the dermal scales and plates that may cover most of the body are formed from membrane bone.

Two kinds of bone structure are distinguishable: **spongy** (or **cancellous**) and **compact** (or **dense**) (Fig. 28-3). Spongy bone (so named for its appearance) consists of an open, interlacing framework of bony tissue, oriented to give maximum strength under the normal stresses and strains that the bone receives. Compact bone is dense, appearing absolutely solid to the naked eye. Both structural kinds of bone are found in the typical long bones of the body, such as the humerus (upper arm bone) (Fig. 28-3).

Microscopic structure of bone

Compact bone is composed of a calcified bone matrix arranged in concentric rings. The rings contain cavities (**lacunae**) filled with bone cells (**osteocytes**) that are interconnected by many minute passages (**canaliculi**). These serve to distribute nutrients throughout the bone. This entire organization of lacunae and canaliculi is arranged into an elongated cylinder called an **osteon** (**haversian system**) (Fig. 28-4). Bone consists of bundles of osteons cemented together and interconnected with blood vessels.

Bone growth is a complex restructuring process, involving both its destruction internally by bone-resorbing cells (**osteoclasts**) and its deposition externally by bone-building cells (**osteoblasts**). Both processes occur simultaneously so that the marrow cavity inside grows larger by bone resorption while new bone is laid down outside by bone deposition. Bone growth responds to several hormones, in particular **parathyroid hormone,** which stimulates bone resorption, and **calcitonin,** which inhibits bone resorption. These two hormones, together with a derivative of vitamin D, are responsible for maintaining a constant level of calcium in the blood (p. 804).

Plan of the vertebrate skeleton

The vertebrate skeleton is composed of two main divisions: the **axial skeleton,** which includes the skull, vertebral column, sternum, and ribs, and the **appendicular skeleton,** which includes the limbs (or fins or wings) and the pectoral and pelvic girdles (Fig. 28-5). Not surprisingly, the skeleton has undergone extensive remodeling in the course of vertebrate evolution. The move from water to land forced dramatic changes in body form. With cephalization, that is, the concentration of brain, sense organs, and food-gathering and respiratory apparatus in the head, the skull became the most intricate portion of the skeleton. The lower vertebrates have a larger number of skull bones than the more advanced vertebrates. Some fish have 180 skull bones (a source of frustration to paleontologists); amphibians and reptiles, 50 to 95; and mammals, 35 or fewer. Humans have 29.

The numerous elements of the head skeleton belong to three structural and functional components: (1) the **neurocranium,** which is the original, primitive skull that encloses the brain and sense organs, (2) the **splanchnocranium,** which supports the respiratory and food-gathering equipment (gill apparatus and jaws), and (3) the **dermatocranium,** which arose from ancient, superficial head armor *[handwritten annotations: "cranium", "mandible" near Skull; "2 pts of attachment 1st one" near Atlas/Axis; circled Cervical vertebrae (7); circled Thoracic vertebrae (12); circled Lumbar vertebrae (5); circled Sacrum; circled Coccyx; "wrist", "inthand" near Carpals/Metacarpals; circled foot bones at Tarsals/Metatarsals/Phalanges of toes]*

A

Skull
Clavicle
Coracoid process
Scapula
Ribs(12)
Humerus
Sternum
Ilium
Pubis
Ischium
Ulna
Radius
Carpals
Metacarpals (5)
Phalanges of fingers (14)
Femur
Patella
Tibia
Fibula
Tarsals (7)
Metatarsals (5)
Phalanges of toes (14)

B

Parietal
Occipital
Atlas
Axis
Cervical vertebrae (7)
Thoracic vertebrae (12)
Lumbar vertebrae (5)
Sacrum
Coccyx

Figure 28-5

Human skeleton. **A,** Ventral view. **B,** Dorsal view. Numbers in parentheses indicate number of bones in that unit. In comparison with other mammals, the human skeleton is a patchwork of primitive and specialized parts. Erect posture, brought about by specialized changes in legs and pelvis, enabled the primitive arrangement of arms and hands (arboreal adaptation of human ancestors) to be used for manipulation of tools. Development of the skull and brain followed as a consequence of the premium natural selection put on dexterity, better senses, and ability to appraise environment.

and serves to protect deep-lying delicate tissues (Fig. 28-6). In the lower vertebrates these three skull components are more or less separated from each other; in higher forms they are all fused together or incorporated into a single unit—the vertebrate skull. There is a basic plan of homology in the skull elements of vertebrates from fish to human beings; evolution has meant reduction in numbers of bones through loss and fusion in accordance with size and functional changes.

The vertebral column is the main stiffening axis of the postcranial skeleton. In fishes it serves much the same function as the notochord from which it is derived; that is, it provides points for muscle attachment and prevents telescoping of the body during muscle contraction. Since fish musculature is similar throughout the trunk and tail, fish vertebrae are differentiated only into trunk and caudal vertebrae.

With the evolution of tetrapods, the vertebral column became structurally adapted to withstand new regional stresses transmitted to the column by the two paired appendages. In the higher tetrapods, the vertebrae are differentiated into **cervical** (neck), **thoracic** (chest), **lumbar** (back), **sacral** (pelvic), and **caudal** (tail)

Dermatocranium
Neurocranium
Splanchnocranium

Figure 28-6

Head skeleton of the bowfin (*Amia calva*), showing the three structural components: neurocranium *(light red)*, splanchnocranium *(deeper red)*, and overlying dermatocranium *(gray)*.

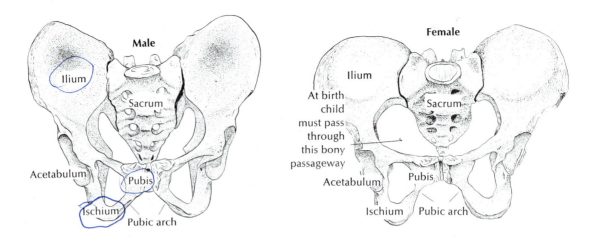

Figure 28-7

The chief difference between male and female skeletons is the structure of the pelvis. The female pelvis has less depth with broader, less sloping ilia, a more circular bony ring (pelvic canal), a wider and more rounded pubic arch, and a shorter and wider sacrum. Most structures of the female pelvis are correlated with childbearing functions. In the evolution of the human skeleton, the pelvis has changed more than any other part because it has to support the weight of the erect body. (Anterior view.)

vertebrae. In birds and also in humans the caudal vertebrae are reduced in number and size, and the sacral vertebrae are fused. The number of vertebrae varies among the different animals. The python seems to lead the list with 435. In humans (Fig. 28-5) there are 33 in the child, but in the adult five are fused to form the **sacrum** and four to form the **coccyx.** Besides the sacrum and coccyx, humans have seven cervical, 12 thoracic, and five lumbar vertebrae. The number of cervical vertebrae (seven) is constant in nearly all mammals.

The first two cervical vertebrae, the **atlas** and the **axis,** are modified to support the skull and permit pivotal movements. The atlas bears the globe of the head much as the mythological Atlas bore the earth on his shoulders. The axis, the second vertebra, permits the head to turn from side to side.

Ribs are long or short skeletal structures that articulate medially with vertebrae and extend into the body wall. Primitive forms have a pair of ribs for every vertebra; they serve as stiffening elements in the connective tissue septa that separate the muscle segments and thus improve the effectiveness of the muscle contractions. Many fishes have both dorsal and ventral ribs, and some have numerous riblike intermuscular bones as well—all of which increase the difficulty and reduce the pleasure of eating certain kinds of fish. Higher vertebrates have a reduced number of ribs, and some, such as the familiar leopard frog, have no ribs at all. Others, such as elasmobranchs and some amphibians, have very short ribs. Humans have 12 pairs of ribs, but approximately one person in 20 has a thirteenth pair. In mammals the ribs together form the thoracic basket, which supports the chest wall and prevents collapse of the lungs.

Most vertebrates, fishes included, have paired appendages. All fishes except the agnathans have thin pectoral and pelvic fins that are supported by the pectoral and pelvic girdles, respectively. Forms above the fishes (except snakes and limbless lizards) have two pairs of **pentadactyl** (five-toed) limbs, also supported by girdles. The pentadactyl limb is similar in all tetrapods, alive and extinct; even when highly modified for various modes of life, the elements are rather easily homologized.

Modifications of the basic pentadactyl limb for life in different environments involve the distal elements much more frequently than the proximal, and it is far more common for bones to be lost or fused than for new ones to be added. Horses and their relatives developed a foot structure for fleetness by elongation of the third toe. In effect, a horse stands on its third fingernail (hoof), much like a ballet dancer standing on the tips of the toes (Fig. 27-34, p. 662). The bird wing is a good example of distal modification. The bird embryo bears 13 distinct wrist and hand bones (carpals and metacarpals), which are reduced to three in the adult. Most of the finger bones (phalanges) are lost, leaving four bones in three digits (see p. 609). The proximal bones (humerus, radius, and ulna), however, are little modified in the bird wing.

In nearly all tetrapods the pelvic girdle (Fig. 28-7) is firmly attached to the axial skeleton, since the greatest locomotory forces transmitted to the body come from the hindlimbs. The pectoral girdle, however, is much more loosely attached to the axial skeleton, providing the forelimbs with greater freedom for manipulative movements.

In humans the pectoral girdle is made up of two scapulae and two clavicles; the arm is made up of the humerus, ulna, radius, eight carpals, five metacarpals, and 14 phalanges. The pelvic girdle consists of three fused bones—ilium, ischium, and pubis; the leg is made up of the femur, patella, tibia, fibula, seven tarsals, five metatarsals, and 14 phalanges. Each bone of the leg has its counterpart in the arm with the exception of the patella. This correspondence between anterior and posterior parts is another example of **serial homology.**

ANIMAL MOVEMENT

Movement is a unique characteristic of animals. Plants may show movement, but this usually results from changes in turgor pressure or growth rather than from specialized contractile proteins as in animals. Animal movement occurs in many forms in animal tissues, ranging from barely discernible streaming of cytoplasm to frank movements of powerful striated muscles of vertebrates. It has become evident that virtually all animal movement depends on a single fundamental mechanism: **contractile proteins,** which can change their form to elongate or contract. This contractile machinery is always composed of ultrafine fibrils—fine filaments, striated fibrils, or tubular fibrils (microtubules)—arranged to contract when powered by **ATP.** By far the most important protein contractile system is the **actomyosin system,** composed of two proteins, **actin** and **myosin.** This is an almost universal biomechanical system found from protozoa to vertebrates; it performs a long list of diverse functional roles. In this discussion we examine the three principal kinds of animal movement: ameboid, ciliary, and muscular.

Ameboid Movement

Ameboid movement is a form of movement especially characteristic of amebas and other protozoa; it is also found in many wandering cells of higher animals, such as white blood cells, embryonic mesenchyme, and numerous other mobile cells that move through the tissue spaces. Ameboid cells change their shape by sending out and withdrawing **pseudopodia** (false feet) from any point on the cell surface. Such cells are surrounded by a delicate, highly flexible membrane called **plasmalemma** (Fig. 8-3, p. 174). Beneath this lies a nongranular layer, the gel-like **ectoplasm,** which encloses the more liquid **endoplasm.**

Optical studies of an ameba in movement suggest that the outer layer of ectoplasm surrounds a rather fluid core of endoplasm. As the pseudopod extends, the inner endoplasm fountains out to the periphery, changing from the sol to the gel state. The newly formed ectoplasm then slips posteriorly under the plasmalemma and is changed to endoplasm at the rear to begin another cycle. Although no completely satisfactory analysis exists, it seems certain that ameboid move-

Figure 28-8

Flagellum beats in wavelike undulation, propelling water parallel to the main axis of the flagellum. Cilium propels water in direction parallel to the cell surface.

With permission from Sleigh, M.A. 1974. Cilia and flagella. Copyright by Academic Press, Inc. (London), Ltd.

ment is based on the same fundamental contractile system that powers vertebrate muscles: an actomyosin machinery driven by ATP.

___ Ciliary Movement

Cilia are minute, hairlike, motile processes that extend from the surfaces of the cells of many animals. They are a particularly distinctive feature of ciliate protozoa, but except for the nematodes in which motile cilia are absent and the arthropods in which they are rare, cilia are found in all major groups of animals. Cilia perform many roles either in moving small animals such as protozoa through their aquatic environment or in propelling fluids and materials across the epithelial surfaces of larger animals.

Cilia are of remarkably uniform diameter (0.2 to 0.5 μm) wherever they are found. The electron microscope has shown that each cilium contains a peripheral circle of nine double microtubules and an additional two microtubules in the center (Fig. 8-2, p. 173). (Exceptions to the 9 + 2 arrangement have been noted; sperm tails of flatworms have but one central fibril.) A **flagellum** is a whiplike structure longer than a cilium and usually present singly or in small numbers at one end of a cell. They are found in members of flagellate protozoa, in animal spermatozoa, and in sponges. The main difference between a cilium and a flagellum is in their beating pattern rather than in their structure, since both look alike internally. A flagellum beats symmetrically with snakelike undulations so that the water is propelled parallel to the long axis of the flagellum. A cilium, in contrast, beats asymmetrically with a fast power stroke in one direction followed by a slow recovery during which the cilium bends as it returns to its original position. The water is propelled parallel to the ciliated surface (Fig. 28-8).

According to the currently favored theory of ciliary movement, the fibrils behave as "sliding filaments" that move past one another much like the sliding filaments of vertebrate skeletal muscle that is described in the next discussion. During contraction, fibrils on the concave side slide outward past fibrils on the convex side to increase curvature of the cilium; during the recovery stroke, fibrils on the opposite side slide outward to bring the cilium back to its starting position. For such a system to work, the fibrils must be interconnected by molecular bridges, which, if present, are too small to be seen with the electron microscope.

___ Muscular Movement

Contractile tissue is most highly developed in muscle cells called **fibers**. Although muscle fibers themselves can do work only by contraction and cannot actively lengthen, they can be arranged in so many different configurations and combinations that almost any movement is possible.

Types of vertebrate muscle

Vertebrate muscle is broadly classified on the basis of the appearance of muscle cells (fibers) when viewed with a light microscope. **Striated muscle** appears transversely striped (striated), with alternating dark and light bands (Fig. 28-9). We can recognize two types of striated muscle: **skeletal** and **cardiac muscle.** A third kind of vertebrate muscle is **smooth** (or visceral) **muscle,** which lacks the characteristic alternating bands of the striated type.

Figure 28-9

Skeletal muscle, showing several striated fibers lying side by side.

Photomicrograph courtesy J.W. Bamberger.

Skeletal muscle is typically organized into sturdy, compact bundles or bands (Fig. 28-9). It is called skeletal muscle because it is attached to skeletal elements and is responsible for movements of the trunk, appendages, respiratory organs, eyes, mouthparts, and so on. Skeletal muscle **fibers** are extremely long, cylindrical, multinucleate cells that may reach from one end of the muscle to the other. They are packed into bundles called **fascicles** (L., *fasciculus,* small bundle), which are enclosed by tough connective tissue. The fascicles are in turn grouped into a discrete **muscle** surrounded by a thin connective tissue layer. Most skeletal muscles taper at their ends, where they connect by tendons to bones. Other muscles, such as the ventral abdominal muscles, are flattened sheets.

In most fishes, amphibians, and to some extent reptiles, there is a segmented organization of muscles alternating with the vertebrae. The skeletal muscles of higher vertebrates, by splitting, fusion, and shifting, have developed into specialized muscles best suited for manipulating the jointed appendages that have evolved for locomotion on land. Skeletal muscle contracts powerfully and quickly but fatigues more rapidly than does smooth muscle. Skeletal muscle is sometimes called **voluntary muscle** because it is stimulated by motor fibers and is under conscious cerebral control.

Smooth muscle lacks the striations typical of skeletal muscle (Fig. 28-10). The cells are long, tapering strands, each containing a single nucleus. Smooth muscle cells are organized into sheets of muscle circling the walls of the alimentary canal, blood vessels, respiratory passages, and urinary and genital ducts. Smooth muscle is typically slow acting and can maintain prolonged contractions with very little energy expenditure. It is under the control of the autonomic nervous system; thus, unlike skeletal muscle, its contractions are involuntary and unconscious. The principal functions of smooth muscles are to push the material in a tube, such as the intestine, along its way by active contractions or to regulate the diameter of a tube, such as a blood vessel, by sustained contraction.

Cardiac muscle, the seemingly tireless muscle of the vertebrate heart, combines certain characteristics of both skeletal and smooth muscle (Fig. 28-11). It is fast acting and striated like skeletal muscle, but contraction is under involuntary autonomic control like smooth muscle. Actually the autonomic nerves serving the heart can only speed up or slow down the rate of contraction; the heartbeat originates within specialized cardiac muscle, and the heart continues to beat even after all autonomic nerves are severed. Until recently, cardiac muscle was believed to be **syncytial** (a tissue with many nuclei not separated into discrete cells by cell membranes) with branching, interconnected fibers. Histologists, their understanding vastly increased by the electron microscope, now consider cardiac muscle to be comprised of closely opposed, but separate, uninucleate cell fibers.

Types of invertebrate muscle

Smooth and striated muscles are also characteristic of invertebrate animals, but there are many variations of both types and even instances in which the structural and functional features of vertebrate smooth and striated muscle are combined in the invertebrates. Striated muscle appears in invertebrate groups as diverse as the primitive cnidarians and the advanced arthropods. The thickest muscle fibers known, approximately 3 mm in diameter and 6 cm long, are those of giant barnacles and of Alaska king crabs living along the Pacific coast of North America. These cells are so large that they can be readily cannulated for physiological studies and are understandably popular with muscle physiologists.

Figure 28-10

Myofilaments within a smooth muscle cell. The myofilaments are the contractile units. Smooth muscle lacks the striations characteristic of skeletal and cardiac muscle. (×40,000.)
Electron micrograph courtesy M.E. Todd.

Figure 28-11

Cardiac muscle, showing the bifurcating network and the intercalated discs, dark vertical lines where separate cells join end to end.
Photomicrograph courtesy J.W. Bamberger.

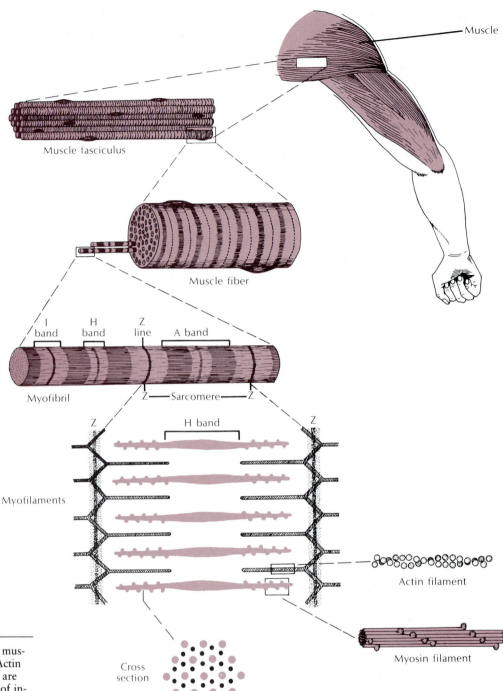

Muscle

Muscle fasciculus

Muscle fiber

I band
H band
Z line
A band

Myofibril
Z — Sarcomere — Z

Z   H band   Z

Myofilaments

Actin filament

Myosin filament

Cross section

Figure 28-12

Organization of vertebrate skeletal muscle from gross to molecular level. Actin (thin) and myosin (thick) filaments are enlarged to show supposed shapes of individual molecules and probable positioning of cross bridges (shown as knobs) on myosin molecules that serve to link thick and thin filaments during contraction. Cross section shows that each thick filament is surrounded by six thin filaments and that each thin filament is surrounded by three thick filaments.

From Bloom, W., and D.W. Fawcett. 1975. A textbook of histology, ed. 10. Philadelphia, W.B. Saunders Co.; modified from Fawcett, D.W. 1952. J. Morphol. **90:**363.

It is not possible in this short space to describe adequately the tremendous diversity of muscle structure and function in the vast assemblage of invertebrates. We will mention only two functional extremes.

Bivalve molluscan muscles contain fibers of two types. One kind is striated muscle that can contract rapidly, enabling the bivalve to snap shut its valves when disturbed. Scallops use these "fast" muscle fibers to swim in their awkward manner (Fig. 13-21, *B*, p. 320). The second muscle type is smooth muscle, capable of slow, long-lasting contractions. Using these fibers, a bivalve can keep its valves tightly shut for hours or even days. Obviously these are no ordinary muscle fibers!

It has been discovered that such retractor muscles use very little metabolic energy and receive remarkably few nerve impulses to maintain the activated state. The contracted state has been likened to a "catch mechanism" involving some kind of stable cross-linkage between the contractile proteins within the fiber. However, despite considerable research, there is still much uncertainty about how this retractor mechanism works.

Insect flight muscles are virtually the functional antithesis of the slow, holding muscles of bivalves. The wings of some of the small flies operate at frequencies greater than 1000 per second. The so-called **fibrillar muscle,** which contracts at these incredible frequencies—far greater than even the most active of vertebrate muscles—shows unique characteristics. It has very limited extensibility; that is, the wing leverage system is arranged so that the muscles shorten hardly at all during each downbeat of the wings. Furthermore, the muscles and wings operate as a rapidly oscillating system in an elastic thorax (Fig. 17-13, p. 414). Since the muscles rebound elastically during flight, they receive impulses only periodically rather than one impulse per contraction; one reinforcement impulse for every 20 or 30 contractions is enough to keep the system active.

Structure of striated muscle

As we pointed out earlier, striated muscle is so named because of the periodic bands, plainly visible under the light microscope, that pass across the widths of the muscle cells. Each cell, or **fiber,** contains numerous **myofibrils** packed together and invested by the cell membrane, the **sarcolemma** (Fig. 28-12). Also present in each fiber are several hundred nuclei usually located along the edge of the fiber, numerous mitochondria (sometimes called **sarcosomes**), a network of tubules called the **sarcoplasmic reticulum** (to be discussed later), and other cell inclusions typical of any living cell. Most of the fiber, however, is packed with the unique **myofibrils,** each 1 to 2 μm in diameter.

The characteristic banding of the muscle fiber represents the fine structure of the myofibrils that make up the fiber. In the resting fiber are alternating light-staining and dark-staining bands called the **I bands** and **A bands,** respectively (Fig. 28-12). The functional unit of the myofibril, the **sarcomere,** extends between successive **Z** lines. The myofibril is actually an aggregate of much smaller parallel units called **myofilaments.** These are of two kinds: thick filaments, 11 nm in diameter and composed of the protein **myosin,** and thin filaments, 5 nm in diameter and composed of the protein **actin** (Fig. 28-12). These are the actual contractile proteins of muscle. The thick myosin filaments are confined to the A-band region. The thin actin filaments are located mainly in the light I bands but extend some distance into the A band as well. In the relaxed muscle, they do not quite meet in the center of the A band. The **Z** line is a dense protein different from either actin or myosin, which serves as the attachment plane for the thin filaments and keeps them in register. These relationships are diagrammed in Fig. 28-12.

Sliding filament model of muscle contraction

In the 1950s the English physiologists A.F. Huxley and H.E. Huxley independently proposed the **sliding filament model** to explain striated muscle contraction. According to this model, the thick and thin filaments become linked together by molecular cross bridges, which act as levers to pull the filaments past each other. During contraction, the cross bridges on the thick filaments swing rapidly back

Figure 28-13

Sliding filament model, showing how thick and thin filaments interact during contraction. **A,** Muscle relaxed. **B,** Muscle contracted.

Figure 28-14

Molecular structure of thick and thin filaments of skeletal muscle. **A,** The myosin molecule is composed of two peptides coiled together and expanded at their ends into a globular head. **B,** The thick filament is composed of a bundle of myosin molecules with the globular heads extended outward. **C,** The thin filament consists of a double strand of actin surrounded by two tropomyosin strands. A globular protein complex, troponin, occurs in pairs at every seventh actin unit. Troponin is a calcium-dependent switch that controls the interaction between actin and myosin.

and forth, alternately attaching and releasing to special receptor sites on the thin filaments, and drawing the thin filaments past the thick in a kind of ratchet action. As contraction continues, the **Z** lines are pulled closer together (Fig. 28-13).

At the time the sliding filament model was proposed, the nature of the mechanism that pulled the thin filaments past the thick was largely a mystery. In the intervening years, however, there have been important improvements in biochemical techniques and in the technology of electron microscopy and X-ray diffraction; these advances have permitted much better visualization of the complex architecture of the contractile machinery.

Each myosin molecule, shown in Fig. 28-14, *A,* is composed of two polypeptide chains, each having a club-shaped "head." Lined up as they are in a bundle to form a thick filament (Fig. 28-14, *B*), the double heads of each myosin molecule face outward from the center of the filament. These heads act as the molecular cross bridges that interact with the thin filaments during contraction.

The thin filaments are more complex because they are composed of three different proteins. The backbone of the thin filament is a double strand of the protein actin, twisted into a double helix. Surrounding the actin filament are two thin strands of another protein, **tropomyosin,** that lie near the grooves between the actin strands. Each tropomyosin strand is itself a double helix as shown in Fig. 28-14, C.

The third protein of the thin filament is **troponin,** a complex of three globular proteins located at intervals along the filament. Troponin is a calcium-dependent switch that acts as the control point in the contraction process.

For shortening to occur, the cross bridges must attach, swivel, detach, and reattach at a point farther along the thin filament. The attach-pull-release cycle occurs in a series of steps (Fig. 28-15). First, myosin binds and then splits a molecule of ATP. The release of bond energy from ATP activates the myosin head, which attaches to the adjacent actin strand and swings 45 degrees, at the same time releasing the ADP molecule. This is the power stroke that pulls the actin filament a distance of about 10 nm, and it comes to an end when another ATP molecule binds to the myosin head, inactivating the site. Thus, each cycle requires the expenditure of energy in the form of ATP.

As long as the muscle is stimulated and new ATP becomes available, the attach-pull-release cycle can repeat again and again, 50 to 100 times per second, pulling the thick and thin filaments past each other. While the distance each sarcomere can shorten is very small, this distance is multiplied by the thousands of sarcomeres lying end to end in a muscle fiber. Thus, a strongly contracted muscle may shorten as much as one-third its resting length.

Stimulation of contraction

To contract, skeletal muscle must of course be stimulated. If the nerve supply to a muscle is severed, the muscle **atrophies,** or wastes away. Skeletal muscle fibers are arranged in groups of approximately 100, each group under the control of a single motor nerve fiber. Such a group is called a **motor unit.** As the nerve fiber approaches the muscle fibers, it splays out into many terminal branches. Each branch attaches to a muscle fiber by a special structure, called a **synapse,** or **myoneural junction** (Fig. 28-16). At the synapse is a tiny gap, or cleft, that thinly separates nerve fiber and muscle fiber. In the synapse is stored a chemical, **acetylcholine,** which is released when a nerve impulse reaches the synapse. This substance is a chemical mediator that diffuses across the narrow junction and acts on the muscle fiber membrane to generate an electrical depolarization. The depolarization spreads rapidly through the muscle fiber, causing it to contract. Thus, the synapse is a special chemical bridge that couples together the electrical activities of nerve and muscle fibers.

For a long time physiologists were puzzled as to how the depolarization at the myoneural junction could spread quickly enough through the fiber to cause simultaneous contraction of all the densely packed filaments within. Then it was discovered that vertebrate skeletal muscle contains an elaborate communication system that performs just this function. This is the endoplasmic reticulum (called the **sarcoplasmic reticulum** in muscle), a system of fluid-filled channels running parallel to the myofilaments and communicating with the sarcolemma that surrounds the fiber (Fig. 28-17). The system is ideally arranged for speeding the electrical depolarization from the myoneural junction to the myofilament within.

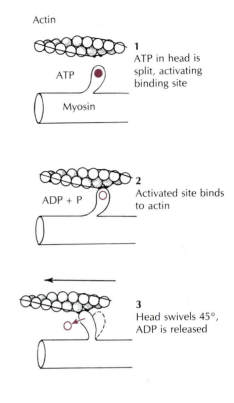

Actin

1 ATP in head is split, activating binding site

ATP · Myosin

2 Activated site binds to actin

ADP + P

3 Head swivels 45°, ADP is released

4 Another ATP enters head, inactivating site, which detaches from actin and swivels to 90° position

Figure 28-15

Successive steps in the attach-pull-release cycle that pulls actin past myosin and shortens the filament length.

Figure 28-16

Nerve-muscle synapse (myoneural junction). Slender terminations of the motor nerve extend along depressions in the muscle fiber. Terminations are covered by extension of a Schwann cell but lack insulating myelin sheath. The nerve terminal contains synaptic vesicles packed with molecules of acetylcholine. When the nerve impulse arrives at the synapse, vesicles fuse with the terminal membrane, releasing acetylcholine into the synaptic cleft. These transmitter molecules diffuse rapidly across the cleft and bind with receptors on the muscle fiber membrane. Here, biochemical changes trigger a muscle impulse.

Figure 28-17

Three-dimensional representation of vertebrate striated muscle showing distribution of sarcoplasmic reticulum and connecting transverse tubules (T system). In the frog muscle shown here, the transverse tubules are positioned at the Z regions where they serve to conduct electrical depolarizations and energy-rich supplies to the myofibrils via the sarcoplasmic reticulum.

From Bloom, W., and D.W. Fawcett. 1975. A textbook of histology, ed. 10. Philadelphia, W.B. Saunders Co.

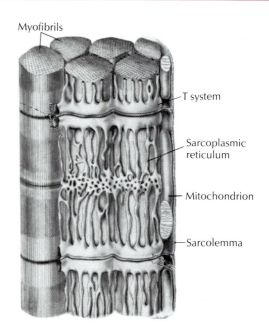

How does the electrical depolarization activate the contraction process? In the resting, unstimulated muscle, shortening does not occur because the thin tropomyosin strands lie in a position on the actin filament that prevents the myosin heads from attaching to actin. When the muscle is stimulated and the electrical depolarization arrives at the sarcoplasmic reticulum surrounding the fibrils, calcium ions are released. Some of the calcium binds to the control protein troponin. Troponin immediately undergoes conformational changes that allow tropomyosin to move out of its blocking position, and the attach-pull-release cycle is set in motion. Shortening will continue as long as nerve impulses arrive at the neuromuscular junction and free calcium remains available around the microfilament. But when stimulation stops, the calcium is quickly pumped back into the sarcoplasmic reticulum. Troponin resumes its original shape, tropomyosin moves back into its blocking position on actin, and the muscle relaxes.

Energy for contraction

ATP is the immediate source of energy for muscle, but the amount present will sustain contraction for only a fraction of a second. However, vertebrate muscle contains a much larger reservoir of high-energy phosphate, creatine phosphate. This compound contains even more free bond energy than ATP (p. 103) and thus can readily transfer its bond energy to ADP to form ATP.

$$\text{Creatine phosphate} + \text{ADP} \rightleftharpoons \text{ATP} + \text{Creatine}$$

The reserves of creatine phosphate are soon depleted in rapidly contracting muscle and must be restored by the oxidation of carbohydrate. The major store of carbohydrate in muscle is glycogen. In fact, about three fourths of all the glycogen in the body is stored in muscle (most of the rest is stored in the liver). Glycogen can be readily converted into glucose-6-phosphate, the first stage of glycolysis that leads into mitochondrial respiration and the generation of ATP (p. 107).

If muscular contraction is not too vigorous or too prolonged, glucose can be completely oxidized to carbon dioxide and water by **aerobic metabolism.** During prolonged or heavy exercise, however, the blood flow to the muscles, although greatly increased above the resting level, is insufficient to supply oxygen as rapidly as required for the complete oxidation of glucose. When this happens, the contractile machinery receives its energy largely by **anaerobic glycolysis,** a process that does not require oxygen (p. 114). The ability to take advantage of this anaerobic pathway, although not nearly as efficient as the aerobic one, is of great importance; without it, all forms of heavy muscular exertion would be impossible.

During anaerobic glycolysis, glucose is degraded to lactic acid with the release of energy. This is used to resynthesize creatine phosphate, which in turn passes the energy to ADP for the resynthesis of ATP. Lactic acid accumulates in the muscle and diffuses rapidly into the general circulation. If the muscular exertion continues, the buildup of lactic acid causes enzyme inhibition and fatigue. Thus, the anaerobic pathway is a self-limiting one, since continued heavy exertion leads to exhaustion. The muscles incur an **oxygen debt** because the accumulated lactic acid must be oxidized by extra oxygen. After the period of exertion, oxygen consumption remains elevated until all of the lactic acid has been oxidized or resynthesized to glycogen.

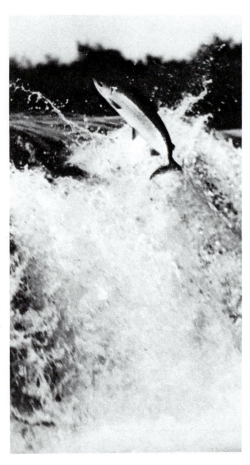

Salmon leaping falls.
Courtesy G.B. Kelez, U.S. Fish and Wildlife Service.

___ Summary

An animal is wrapped in a protective covering, the integument, which may be as simple as the delicate plasma membrane of a protozoan or as complex as the skin of a mammal. Vertebrate integument consists of two layers: the epidermis, which gives rise to various derivatives such as hair, feathers, and claws; and the dermis, which supports and nourishes the epidermis. It also is the origin of bony derivatives such as fish scales and the antlers of deer.

Integument color is of two kinds: structural color, produced by refraction or scattering of light by particles in the integument, and pigmentary color, produced by pigments that are usually confined to special pigment cells (chromatophores).

Skeletons are supportive systems that may be hydrostatic or rigid. The hydrostatic skeletons of several soft-walled invertebrate groups depend on body wall muscles that contract against a noncompressible internal fluid of constant volume. Rigid skeletons have evolved with attached muscles that act with the supportive skeleton to produce movement. In higher animals, two forms of skeleton have appeared. Arthropods have an external skeleton, which must be periodically shed to make way for an enlarged replacement. The vertebrates developed an internal skeleton, a framework formed of cartilage or bone, that can grow with the animal, while, in the case of bone, additionally serving as a reservoir of calcium and phosphate.

Animal movement, whether in the form of cytoplasmic streaming, ameboid movement, or the contraction of an organized muscle mass, depends on specialized contractile proteins. The most important of these is the actomyosin system, which in higher animals is usually organized into elongate thick and thin filaments that slide past one another during contraction. When a muscle is stimulated, an electrical depolarization is conducted into the muscle fibers through the sarcoplasmic reticulum, causing the release of calcium. Calcium binds to a protein troponin complex associated with the thin actin filament. This causes tropomyosin to shift out of its blocking position and allows the myosin heads to cross-bridge with the actin filament. Powered by ATP, the myosin heads swivel back and forth to pull the thick and thin filaments past each other. Phosphate bond energy for contraction is supplied by carbohydrate fuels through a storage intermediate, creatine phosphate.

Selected references

See also general references for Part Three, p. 837.

Alexander, R.M. 1968. Animal mechanics. London, Sidgwick & Jackson.

Alexander, R.M., and G. Goldspink. 1977. Mechanics and energetics of animal locomotion. London, Chapman & Hall, Ltd.

Bagnara, J.T., and M.E. Hadley. 1973. Chromatophores and color change. Englewood Cliffs, N.J., Prentice-Hall, Inc.

Bendall, J.R. 1969. Muscles, molecules and movement. New York, American Elsevier Publishing Co., Inc. *Contains a wealth of well-organized information on muscle structure and physiology, pitched at the advanced undergraduate level.*

Bloom, W., and D.W. Fawcett. 1975. A textbook of histology, ed. 10. Philadelphia, W.B. Saunders Co. *Authoritative human histology text.*

Bourne, G.H. (ed.). 1972-1977. The structure and function of muscle, 4 vols. New York, Academic Press, Inc.

Fogden, M., and P. Fogden. 1979. Animals and their colors: camouflage, warning coloration, courtship and territorial display, mimicry. New York, Crown Publishers, Inc. *Semipopular treatment, lavishly illustrated.*

Fox, D.L. 1976. Animal biochromes and structural colors, ed. 2. Berkeley, University of California Press. *Advanced monograph.*

Gray, J. 1968. Animal locomotion. London, Weidenfeld & Nicholson.

Hancox, N.M. 1972. Biology of bone. Cambridge, Eng., Cambridge University Press. *Morphology and function of bone clearly described.*

Keynes, R.D., and D.J. Aidley. 1981. Nerve and muscle. Cambridge, Eng., Cambridge University Press. *Chapters 8 and 9 provide a concise account of skeletal muscle anatomy and function.*

Maderson, P.F.A. (ed.). 1972. The vertebrate integument. Symposium Am. Zool. **12:**12-171.

Montagna, W., and P.F. Parakkal. 1974. The structure and function of the skin, ed. 3. New York, Academic Press, Inc.

Romer, A.S., and T.S. Parsons. 1977. The vertebrate body. Philadelphia, W.B. Saunders Co.

Sokolov, V.E. 1983. Mammal skin. Berkeley, University of California Press. *Comprehensive, authoritative, comparative survey dealing with structure, physiology, and adaptations of the skin within the different orders of mammals.*

Spearman, R.I.C. 1973. The integument: a textbook of skin biology. London, Cambridge University Press. *Concise, comparative treatment.*

Spearman, R.I.C. (ed.). 1977. Comparative biology of skin. (Symposium Zool. Soc. London No. 39.) New York, Academic Press, Inc. *Recent advances in skin research, covering flatworms to mammals.*

Squire, J. 1981. The structural basis of muscular contraction. New York, Plenum Press. *Detailed account of muscle structure and the techniques employed in current research.*

Stein, R.B. 1980. Nerve and muscle: membranes, cells, and systems. New York, Plenum Press. *Advanced undergraduate and graduate level; considerable mathematical notation used.*

Trueman, E.R. 1975. The locomotion of soft-bodied animals. New York, American Elsevier Publishing Co., Inc. *Hydrostatic skeletons as applied to invertebrate locomotion.*

Tucker, V.A. 1975. The energetic cost of moving about. Am. Sci. **63:**413-419. *Muscle efficiency and the cost of different forms of locomotion.*

Wilkie, D.R. 1976. Muscle, ed. 2. London, Edward Arnold, Ltd. *Concise, undergraduate-level primer.*

Selected *Scientific American* articles

Chapman, C.B., and J.H. Mitchell, 1965. The physiology of exercise. **212:**88-96 (May). *Muscular activity mobilizes several adaptive nervous, respiratory, circulatory, and metabolic responses.*

Cohen, C. 1975. The protein switch of muscle contraction. **233:**36-45 (Nov.). *The roles of calcium and regulatory proteins in muscle contraction are described.*

Hoyle, G. 1958. The leap of the grasshopper. **198:**30-35 (Jan.). *The powerful muscle system of the grasshopper's hindleg can propel the animal 20 times its body length.*

Hoyle, G. 1970. How is muscle turned on and off? **222:**84-93 (Apr.). *Calcium plays a crucial role in muscle contraction.*

Huxley, H.E. 1965. The mechanism of muscular contraction. **213:**18-27 (Dec.). *The sliding filament theory is described.*

Lester, H.A. 1977. The response to acetylcholine. **236:**106-118 (Feb.). *Action of acetylcholine on cell receptors at the myoneural junction is described.*

McLean, F.C. 1955. Bone **192:**84-91 (Feb.). *Structure and physiology of bone.*

Merton, P.A. 1972. How we control the contraction of our muscles. **226:**30-37 (May). *Voluntary movements of skeletal muscle are controlled by a sensitive feedback mechanism.*

Murray, J.M., and A. Weber. 1974. The cooperative action of muscle proteins. **230:**58-71 (Feb.). *Describes the interactions of muscle proteins in contraction.*

Satir, P. 1974. How cilia move. **231:**44-52 (Oct.).

CHAPTER 29

INTERNAL FLUIDS

Circulation, Immunity, and

Gas Exchange

Smooth-walled, biconcave erythrocytes (red blood cells) and rough-surfaced leukocytes
(white blood cells) lie in the opened arteriole of a mammal. Mammalian erythrocytes
lack nuclei and are little more than bags of hemoglobin. Leukocytes are variable
in shape. Many are phagocytes, and all play important roles in the body's
defense against infection. (×5000.)

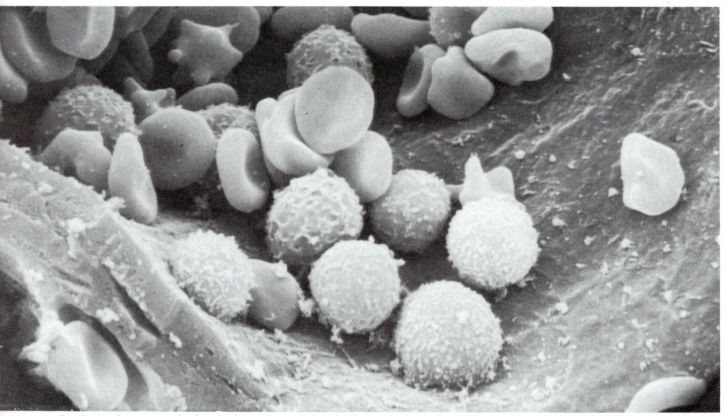

From Tissues and organs: a text-atlas of scanning electron microscopy by Richard G. Kessel and Randy H. Kardon. W.H. Freeman and Company. Copyright © 1979.

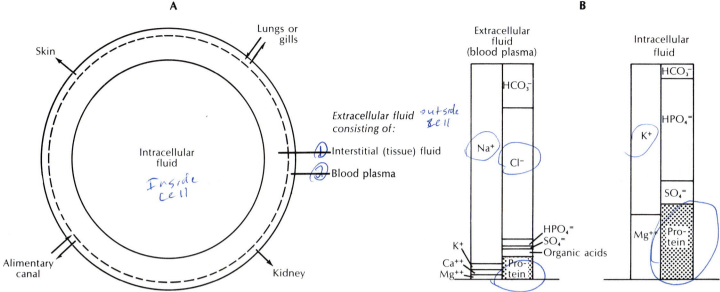

A

Skin

Lungs or
gills

Intracellular
fluid

*Inside
cell*

Extracellular fluid *outside cell*
consisting of:

(1) Interstitial (tissue) fluid

(2) Blood plasma

Alimentary
canal

Kidney

B

Extracellular
fluid
(blood plasma)

HCO_3^-

Na^+

Cl^-

$HPO_4^=$
$SO_4^=$
Organic acids

K^+
Ca^{++}
Mg^{++}

Pro-
tein

Intracellular
fluid

HCO_3^-

$HPO_4^=$

K^+

$SO_4^=$

Mg^{++}

Pro-
tein

Figure 29-1

Fluid compartments of the body. **A,** All body cells can be represented as belonging to a single large fluid compartment that is completely surrounded and protected by extracellular fluid *(milieu intérieur)*. This fluid is further subdivided into plasma and interstitial fluid. All exchanges with the environment occur across the plasma compartment. **B,** Electrolyte composition of extracellular and intracellular fluids. Total equivalent concentration of each major constituent is shown. Equal amounts of anions (negatively charged ions) and cations (positively charged ions) are in each fluid compartment. Sodium and chloride, the major plasma electrolytes, are virtually absent from intracellular fluid (actually they are present in low concentration). Note the much higher concentration of protein inside the cells.

Single-celled organisms live a contact existence with their environment. Nutrients and oxygen are obtained, and wastes are released, directly across the cell surface. These animals are so small that no special internal transport system, beyond the normal streaming movements of the cytoplasm, is required. Even some primitive multicellular forms such as sponges, cnidarians, and flatworms have such a simple internal organization and low rate of metabolism that no circulatory system is needed. Most of the more advanced multicellular organisms, because of their size, activity, and complexity, require a specialized circulatory, or vascular, system to transport nutrients and respiratory gases to and from all tissues of the body.

In addition to serving these primary transport needs, circulatory systems have acquired additional functions. Hormones are moved about, finding their way to target organs where they assist the nervous system to integrate body function. Water, electrolytes, and the many other constituents of the body fluids are distributed and exchanged between different organs and tissues. The body's defenses against microbial invasion are centered in the vascular system. The warm-blooded birds and mammals depend heavily on the blood circulation to conserve or dissipate heat as required for the maintenance of constant body temperature.

INTERNAL FLUID ENVIRONMENT

The body fluid of a single-celled animal is the cellular cytoplasm, a fluid substance in which the various membrane systems and organelles of the cell are suspended. In multicellular animals the body fluids are divided into two main phases, the **intracellular** and the **extracellular.** The intracellular phase (also called intracellular fluid) is the fluid inside all the body's cells. The extracellular phase (or fluid) is the fluid outside and surrounding the cells (Fig. 29-1, *A*). Thus, the cells, the sites of the body's crucial metabolic activities, are bathed by their own aqueous environment, the extracellular fluid that buffers them from the often harsh physical and chemical changes occurring outside the body. The importance of the extracellular fluid was first emphasized by the great French physiologist Claude Bernard (Fig. 29-2).

In animals having closed circulatory systems (vertebrates, annelids, and a few other invertebrate groups), the extracellular fluid is further subdivided into **blood plasma** and **interstitial fluid** (Fig. 29-1, *A*). The blood plasma is contained within the blood vessels, whereas the interstitial fluid, or tissue fluid as it is sometimes called, occupies the space immediately around the cells. Nutrients and gases passing between the vascular plasma and the cells must traverse this narrow fluid separation. The interstitial fluid is constantly formed from the plasma by filtration through the capillary walls.

Composition of the Body Fluids

All these fluid spaces—plasma, interstitial, and intracellular—differ from one another in solute composition, but all have one feature in common: they are mostly water. Despite their firm appearance, animals are 70% to 90% water. Humans, for example, are about 70% water by weight: of this, 50% is cell water, 15% is interstitial fluid water, and the remaining 5% is in the blood plasma. As Fig. 29-1, *A*, shows, it is the plasma space that serves as the pathway of exchange between the cells of the body and the outside world. This exchange of respiratory gases, nutrients, and wastes is accomplished by specialized organs (kidney, lung, gill, alimentary canal), as well as by the integument.

The body fluids contain many inorganic and organic substances in solution. Principal among these are the inorganic electrolytes and proteins. Fig. 29-1, *B*, shows that **sodium, chloride,** and **bicarbonate** are the chief extracellular electrolytes, whereas **potassium, magnesium, phosphate,** and **proteins** are the major intracellular electrolytes. These differences are dramatic; they are always maintained despite the continuous flow of materials into and out of the cells of the body. The two subdivisions of the extracellular fluid—plasma and interstitial fluid—have similar compositions except that the plasma has more proteins, which are too large to filter through the capillary wall into the interstitial fluid.

Composition of blood

Among the lower invertebrates that lack a circulatory system (such as flatworms and cnidarians), it is not possible to distinguish a true "blood." These forms possess a clear, watery tissue fluid containing some primitive phagocytic cells, a little protein, and a mixture of salts similar to seawater. The "blood," or **hemolymph,** of higher invertebrates is more complex. Invertebrates with closed circulatory systems maintain a clear separation between blood contained within blood vessels and tissue (interstitial) fluid surrounding the vessels.

In vertebrates, blood is a complex liquid tissue composed of plasma and formed elements, mostly corpuscles, suspended in the plasma. When the red blood corpuscles and other formed elements are separated from the fluid components by centrifugation, the blood is found to be approximately 55% plasma and 45% formed elements.

The composition of mammalian blood is as follows:

Plasma
1. Water 90%
2. Dissolved solids, consisting of the plasma proteins (albumin, globulins, fibrinogen), glucose, amino acids, electrolytes, various enzymes, antibodies, hormones, metabolic wastes, and traces of many other organic and inorganic materials
3. Dissolved gases, especially oxygen, carbon dioxide, and nitrogen

Figure 29-2

French physiologist Claude Bernard (1813-1878), one of the most influential of nineteenth-century physiologists. Bernard believed in the constancy of the *milieu intérieur* ("internal environment"), which is the extracellular fluid bathing the cells. He pointed out that it is through the *milieu intérieur* that foods and wastes and gases are exchanged and chemical messengers are distributed.

From Fulton, J.F., and L.G. Wilson. 1966. Selected readings in the history of physiology. Springfield, Ill., Charles C Thomas, Publisher.

A   B

Figure 29-3

Mammalian and amphibian red blood corpuscles. **A,** The erythrocytes of a gerbil are biconcave discs containing hemoglobin and surrounded by a tough stroma. **B,** The frog erythrocytes are convex discs, each containing a nucleus, which is plainly visible in the scanning electron micrograph as a bulge in the center of each cell. (Magnifications, mammalian erythrocytes, ×6300, frog erythrocytes, ×2400.)

Courtesy P.P.C. Graziadei.

Formed elements (Fig. 29-4)
1. Red blood cells (erythrocytes), containing hemoglobin for the transport of oxygen and carbon dioxide
2. White blood cells (leukocytes), serving as scavengers and as defensive cells
3. Platelets (thrombocytes), functioning in blood coagulation

The plasma proteins are a diverse group of large and small proteins that perform numerous functions. The major protein groups are (1) **albumin,** the most abundant plasma protein, which constitutes 60% of the total; (2) the **globulins** (α_1, α_2, β, and γ), a diverse group of high–molecular weight proteins (35% of total) that includes immunoglobulins and various metal-binding proteins; and (3) **fibrinogen,** a very large protein that functions in blood coagulation.

Red blood cells, or **erythrocytes,** are present in enormous numbers in the blood, approximately 5.4 billion per milliliter of blood in an adult man and 4.8 billion in women. They are formed continuously from large nucleated **erythroblasts** in the red bone marrow. Here hemoglobin is synthesized and the cells divide several times. In mammals the nucleus shrinks during development to a small remnant and eventually disappears altogether. Many other characteristics of a typical cell also are lost: ribosomes, mitochondria, and most enzyme systems. What is left is a biconcave disc consisting of a baglike membrane, the **stroma,** packed with about 280 million molecules of the blood-transporting pigment **hemoglobin.** Approximately 33% of the erythrocyte by weight is hemoglobin. The biconcave shape (Fig. 29-3, *A*) is a mammalian innovation that provides a larger surface for gas diffusion than would a flat or spherical shape. All other vertebrates have nucleated erythrocytes that are usually ellipsoidal rather than round discs (Fig. 29-3, *B*).

The erythrocyte enters the circulation for an average life span of approximately 4 months. During this time it may journey 700 miles, squeezing repeatedly through the capillaries, which are sometimes so narrow that the erythrocyte must bend to get through. At last it fragments and is quickly engulfed by large scavenger cells called **macrophages,** located in the liver, bone marrow, and spleen. The iron

RED BLOOD CELLS

PLATELETS

WHITE BLOOD CELLS

Granular leukocytes

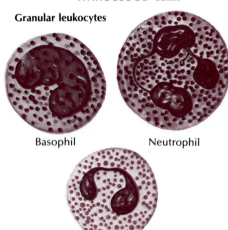

Basophil   Neutrophil

Eosinophil

Nongranular leukocytes

Lymphocyte

Monocyte

Figure 29-4

Formed elements of human blood. Hemoglobin-containing red blood cells of humans and other mammals lack nuclei, but those of all lower vertebrates have nuclei. Various leukocytes provide a wandering system of protection for the body. Platelets participate in the body's clotting mechanism.

From Anthony, C.P., and G.A. Thibodeau. 1983. Textbook of anatomy and physiology, ed. 11. St. Louis, The C.V. Mosby Co.

from the hemoglobin is salvaged to be used again; the rest of the heme is converted to **bilirubin,** a bile pigment. It is estimated that 10 million erythrocytes are produced and another 10 million destroyed every second in the human body.

The white blood cells, or **leukocytes,** form a wandering system of protection for the body. In adults they number only approximately 7.5 million per milliliter of blood, a ratio of one white cell to 700 red cells. There are several kinds of white blood cells: **granulocytes** (subdivided into neutrophils, basophils, and eosinophils), **lymphocytes,** and **monocytes** (Fig. 29-4). The role of the leukocytes in the body's defense mechanisms will be discussed later.

CIRCULATION

The circulatory system of vertebrates is made up of a system of tubes, the **blood vessels,** and a propulsive organ, the **heart.** This is a **closed circulation** because the circulating medium, the **blood,** is confined to vessels throughout its journey from the heart to the tissues and back again. Many invertebrates have an **open circulation;** the blood is pumped from the heart into blood vessels that open into tissue spaces. The blood circulates in direct contact with the tissues and then reenters open blood vessels to be propelled forward again. In invertebrates having open circulatory systems, there is no clear separation of the extracellular fluid into plasma and interstitial fluids, as there must be in closed systems. Closed systems are more suitable for large and active animals because the blood can be moved rapidly to the tissues needing it. In addition, flow to various organs can be readjusted to meet changing needs by varying the diameters of the blood vessels.

The closed circulatory system of vertebrates works with the **lymphatic system.** This is a fluid "pickup" system. It re-collects tissue fluid (lymph) that has been squeezed out through the walls of the capillaries and returns it to the blood circulation. In a sense "closed" circulatory systems are not absolutely closed because fluid is constantly leaking out into the tissue spaces. However, this leakage is but a small fraction of the total blood flow.

Although it seems obvious to us today that blood flows in a circuit, the first correct description of blood flow by the English physician William Harvey initially received vigorous opposition when published in 1628. Centuries before, Galen had taught that air enters the heart from the windpipe and that blood is able to pass from one ventricle to the other through "pores" in the interventricular septum. He also believed that blood first flows out of the heart into all vessels, arteries, and veins alike and then returns to the heart by these same vessels—an idea of ebb and flow of the blood.

Even though almost nothing about this theory was right, it was still doggedly trusted at the time of Harvey's publication. Harvey's conclusions were based on sound experimental evidence. He used a variety of animals for his experiments, including a little snake found in English meadows. By tying ligatures on arteries, he noticed that the region between the heart and ligature swelled up. When veins were tied off, the swelling occurred beyond the ligature. When blood vessels were cut, blood flowed in arteries from the cut end nearest the heart; the reverse happened in veins. By means of such experiments, Harvey worked out a correct scheme of blood circulation, even though he could not see the capillaries that connected the arterial and venous flows.

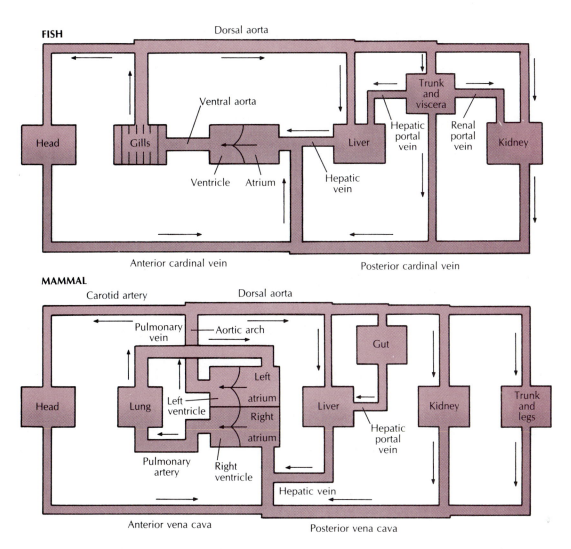

Figure 29-5

Plan of circulatory system of fish *(top)* and mammal *(bottom)*. *Red,* Oxygenated blood. *Dark red,* Deoxygenated blood.

Plan of the Circulatory System

All vertebrate vascular systems have certain features in common. A **heart** pumps the blood into **arteries** that branch and narrow into **arterioles** and then into a vast system of **capillaries.** Blood leaving the capillaries enters **venules** and then **veins** that return the blood to the heart. Fig. 29-5 compares the circulatory systems of fish and mammals. The principal differences in circulation involve the heart in the transformation from gill to lung breathing.

The fish heart contains two main chambers in series: the **atrium** (or **auricle**) and the **ventricle.** There are also two subsidiary chambers (not shown in Fig. 29-5): the **sinus venosus,** which precedes the atrium, and the **conus arteriosus,** which follows the heart and contains valves that prevent backward flow of the blood when the heart is relaxed. Blood makes a single circuit through the fish's vascular system; it is pumped from the heart to the gills, where it is oxygenated, and then flows into the dorsal aorta to be distributed to the body organs. After passing through the capillaries of the body organs and musculature, it returns by veins to the heart. In this circuit the heart must provide sufficient pressure to push the blood through two sequential capillary systems, one in the gills and the other in the organ tissues. The principal disadvantage of the single-circuit system is that

Figure 29-6

Human heart. Deoxygenated blood *(black arrows)* enters right side of heart and is pumped to the lungs. Oxygenated blood *(red arrows)* returning from the lungs enters left side of the heart and is pumped to the body.

the gill capillaries offer so much resistance to blood flow that the pressure drops considerably before entering the dorsal aorta. This system can never provide high and continuous blood pressure to the body organs.

The evolution of land forms with lungs and their need for highly efficient blood delivery resulted in the introduction of a **double** circulation. One **systemic** circuit with its own pump provides oxygenated blood to the capillary beds of the body organs; another **pulmonary** circuit with its own pump sends deoxygenated blood to the lungs. Rather than actually developing two separate hearts, the existing two-chambered heart was divided down the center into four chambers—really two two-chambered hearts lying side-by-side.

Such a great change in the vertebrate circulatory plan, involving not only the heart but the attendant plumbing as well, took many millions of years to evolve. The partial division of the atrium and ventricle began with the ancestors of present-day lungfishes. The complete separation of the atrium occurred in the amphibians, but the ventricle is still undivided in this group. In some reptiles the ventricle is completely divided, and the four-chambered heart appears for the first time. All birds and mammals have the four-chambered heart and the two separate circuits—one through the lungs (pulmonary) and the other through the body (systemic). The course of the blood through this double circuit is shown in the lower diagram of Fig. 29-5.

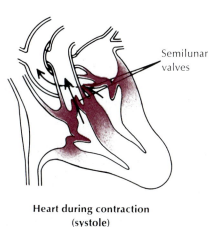

**Heart at rest
(diastole)**

**Heart during contraction
(systole)**

Figure 29-7

Human heart in systole and diastole.

Heart

The vertebrate heart (Fig. 29-6) is a muscular organ located in the thorax and covered by a tough, fibrous sac, the **pericardium.** As we have seen, the higher vertebrates have a four-chambered heart. Each half consists of a thinner-walled atrium and a thicker-walled ventricle. Heart (cardiac) muscle is a unique type of muscle found nowhere else in the body. It resembles striated muscle, but the cells are branched, and the dense end-to-end attachments between the cells are called intercalated discs.

There are two sets of valves. **Atrioventricular (A-V) valves** separate the cavities of the atrium and ventricle in each half of the heart. These permit blood to flow from atrium to ventricle but prevent backflow. Where the great arteries, the **pulmonary** from the right ventricle and the **aorta** from the left ventricle, leave the heart, **semilunar valves** prevent backflow.

The contraction of the heart is called **systole** (sis′to-lee), and the relaxation, **diastole** (dy-as′to-lee) (Fig. 29-7). The rate of the heartbeat depends on age, sex, and especially exercise. Exercise may increase the **cardiac output** (volume of blood forced from either ventricle each minute) more than fivefold. Both the heart **rate** and the **stroke volume** increase. Heart rates among vertebrates vary with the general level of metabolism and the body size. The cold-blooded codfish has a heart rate of approximately 30 beats per minute; a warm-blooded rabbit of about the same weight has a rate of 200 beats per minute. Small animals have higher heart rates than do large animals. The heart rate in an elephant is 25 beats per minute, in a human 70 per minute, in a cat 125 per minute, and in a mouse 400 per minute. In the tiny 4 g shrew, the smallest mammal, the heart rate approaches a prodigious 800 beats per minute. We must marvel that the shrew's heart can sustain such a frantic pace throughout this animal's life, brief as it is.

The heart rests only during the short interval between contractions. The mammalian heart does an amazing amount of work during a lifetime. Someone has calculated that the heart of a human approaching the end of a normal lifetime has beat some 2.5 billion times and pumped 300,000 tons of blood!

Excitation of the heart

The vertebrate heartbeat originates in embryonic-type muscle tissue, called the **sinus node,** located where the large caval veins enter the right atrium (Fig. 29-8).

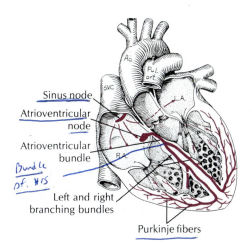

Figure 29-8

Neuromuscular mechanisms controlling heartbeat. Arrows indicate spread of excitation from the sinus node, across the atria, to the atrioventricular node (A-V). Wave of excitation is then conducted very rapidly to ventricular muscle over the specialized bundle of His and Purkinje fiber system.

This tissue serves as the pacemaker of the heart. The wave of contraction spreads rapidly across the two atria to the atrioventricular (A-V) node, located in the mammalian heart near the partition between the right atrium and the ventricles. From this point the electrical activity is conducted quickly through specialized fibers called the **atrioventricular bundle** to the apex of the ventricle and then through fine fibers (Purkinje fibers) into the heart muscle. This arrangement allows the contraction to begin at the apex or "tip" of the ventricles and spread upward to squeeze off the blood in the most efficient way; it also ensures that both ventricles contract simultaneously.

Regulation of the heartbeat

The vertebrate heart has the capacity to beat spontaneously. Even if removed from the body, a fish or amphibian heart may continue beating for hours in a balanced saline solution. Because the heartbeat originates spontaneously in muscle tissue, the vertebrate heart is said to be **myogenic** ("muscle-origin"). Most invertebrate hearts are myogenic, but some, especially the tubular hearts of crustaceans and spiders, are controlled by a separate nerve ganglion, or series of ganglia, external to the heart. Such hearts are referred to as **neurogenic** ("nerve-origin") because the stimulus for the beat originates in true nervous tissue.

While the contraction of the vertebrate heart starts spontaneously in the pacemaker, the rate of the heartbeat is normally under nervous control. The control (cardiac) center is located in the medulla and sends out two sets of motor nerves. Impulses sent along one set, the **vagus** (parasympathetic) nerves, apply a brake action to the heart rate, and impulses sent along the other set, the **accelerator** (sympathetic) nerves, speed it up. Both sets of nerves terminate in the sinus node, thus guiding the activity of the pacemaker.

The cardiac center in turn receives sensory information about a variety of stimuli. Pressure receptors (sensitive to blood pressure) and chemical receptors (sensitive to carbon dioxide and pH) are located at strategic points in the vascular system. This information is used by the cardiac center to increase or reduce the heart rate and cardiac output in response to activity or changes in body position. The heart is thus controlled by a series of feedback mechanisms that keep its activity constantly attuned to body needs.

Coronary circulation

It is no surprise that an organ as active as the heart needs a good blood supply of its own. The heart muscle of the frog and other amphibians is so thoroughly channeled with spaces between the muscle fibers that sufficient oxygenated blood is squeezed through by the heart's own pumping action. In birds and mammals, however, the heart muscle is very thick and has such a high rate of metabolism that it must have its own vascular (**coronary**) circulation. The coronary arteries branch into an extensive capillary network surrounding the muscle fibers and provide them with oxygen and nutrients. Heart muscle has an extremely high oxygen demand, removing 80% of the oxygen from the blood, in contrast to most other body tissues, which remove only approximately 30%.

Arteries

All vessels leaving the heart are called arteries whether they carry oxygenated blood (aorta) or deoxygenated blood (pulmonary artery). To withstand high, pounding pressures, arteries are invested with layers of both elastic and tough

Coronary heart disease takes a severe social and economic toll, accounting for two thirds of all cardiovascular deaths and nearly one half of *all* deaths in the United States. Coronary disease is caused by narrowing of the coronary vessels by fatty cholesterol deposits in the vessel lining and walls and is often associated with chest pains (angina pectoris). A sudden heart attack (a "coronary") results from a small blood clot (thrombosis) that blocks the coronary arteries.

Artery

Vein

Tunica externa
(adventitia)

Tunica media
(muscularis)

Tunica intima

Endothelial
cell layer

Tunica externa

Tunica media

Tunica intima

Figure 29-9

Artery and vein, showing layers. Note greater thickness of the muscularis layer (tunica media) in the artery.

inelastic connective tissue fibers. The elasticity of the arteries allows them to yield to the surge of blood leaving the heart during systole and then to squeeze down on the fluid column during diastole. This smooths out the blood pressure. Thus, the normal arterial pressure in humans varies only between a high of 120 mm Hg (systole) and a low of 80 mm Hg (diastole) (usually expressed as 120/80 or 120 over 80), rather than dropping to zero during diastole as we might expect in a fluid system with an intermittent pump.

As the arteries branch and narrow into **arterioles,** the walls become mostly smooth muscle (Fig. 29-9). Contraction of this muscle narrows the arterioles and reduces the flow of blood. The arterioles thus control the blood flow to body organs, diverting it to where it is needed most. The blood requires a hydrostatic pressure sufficient to overcome the resistance of the narrow passages through which the blood must flow. Consequently, large animals tend to have higher blood pressure than do small animals.

Blood pressure was first measured in 1733 by Stephen Hales, an English clergyman with unusual inventiveness and curiosity. He tied his mare, which was "to have been killed as unfit for service," on her back and exposed the femoral artery. This he cannulated with a brass tube, connecting it to a tall glass tube with the windpipe of a goose. The use of the windpipe was both imaginative and practical; it gave the apparatus flexibility "to avoid inconveniences that might arise if the mare struggled." The blood rose 8 feet in the glass tube and bobbed up and down with the systolic and diastolic beats of the heart. The weight of the 8-foot column of blood was equal to the blood pressure. We now express this as the height of a column of mercury, which is 13.6 times heavier than water. Hales's figures, expressed in millimeters of mercury, indicate that he measured a blood pressure of 180 to 200 mm Hg, about normal for a horse.

Capillaries

The Italian Marcello Malpighi was the first to describe the capillaries in 1661, thus confirming the existence of the minute links between the arterial and venous systems that Harvey knew must be there but could not see. Malpighi studied the capillaries of the living frog's lung, which incidentally is still one of the simplest and most vivid preparations for demonstrating capillary blood flow.

The capillaries are present in enormous numbers, forming extensive networks in nearly all tissues (Fig. 29-10). In muscle there are more than 2000 per square millimeter (1,250,000 per square inch), but not all are open at once. Indeed, perhaps less than 1% are open in resting skeletal muscle. But when the

Blood pressure in humans is most commonly and easily measured with an instrument called a sphygmomanometer. Air is used to inflate a cuff on the upper arm to a pressure sufficient to close the arteries in the arm. As air is slowly released from the cuff, a person with a stethoscope held over the brachial artery (in the crook of the elbow) can hear the first spurts of blood through the artery when the pressure in the cuff allows the artery to open slightly. This is equivalent to the systolic pressure. As the pressure in the cuff is decreased, the sound heard with the stethoscope finally disappears when the blood is running smoothly through the artery. The pressure at which the sound disappears is the diastolic pressure.

Figure 29-10

Capillary bed. Precapillary sphincters control blood flow through the capillaries.

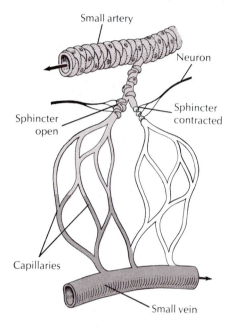

Small artery

Neuron

Sphincter open

Sphincter contracted

Capillaries

Small vein

The actual situation is a bit more complicated because there is a small hydrostatic pressure in the interstitial fluid, and a small amount of protein does leak through the capillary wall. The protein tends to accumulate at the venule end of the capillary, building up a small osmotic pressure there. Although actual calculation of the pressure differences must take into account the interstitial fluid hydrostatic and osmotic pressures, the principle of the capillary fluid shift is as we have presented it.

Water movement

Hydrostatic pressure	40	30	20	15
Protein osmotic pressure	25	25	25	25

Direction of blood flow

Arterial end   Venous end

Figure 29-11

Fluid movement across the wall of a capillary. At the arterial end of the capillary, hydrostatic (blood) pressure exceeds protein osmotic pressure contributed by plasma proteins, and a plasma filtrate (shown as "water movement") is forced out. At the venous end, protein osmotic pressure exceeds the hydrostatic pressure, and fluid is drawn back in.

muscle is active, all the capillaries may open to bring oxygen and nutrients to the working muscle fibers and to carry away metabolic wastes.

Capillaries are extremely narrow, averaging less than 10 μm in diameter in mammals, which is hardly any wider than the red blood cells that must pass through them. Their walls are formed of a single layer of thin **endothelial** cells, held together by a delicate basement membrane and connective tissue fibers. Capillaries have a built-in leakiness that allows water and most dissolved substances except proteins to filter through into the interstitial space.

Because of the low permeability of the capillaries to protein, the solute concentration in the blood is higher than in the interstitial fluid; therefore there is a net osmotic pressure difference, because of the protein, of about 25 mm Hg in mammals. The hydrostatic pressure of the blood at the arteriole end of the capillaries is about 40 mm in humans. Thus, there is a **net filtration pressure** (the hydrostatic pressure, which tends to force fluid out, less the osmotic pressure, which tends to draw water back in) of about 15 mm Hg at the arteriole end of the capillaries (Fig. 29-11). Water and dissolved materials are forced out of the capillaries and circulate through the tissue space. As the blood proceeds through the narrow capillary, the blood pressure decreases steadily to perhaps 15 mm Hg. At this point the hydrostatic pressure is less than the osmotic pressure because of the plasma proteins, still approximately 25 mm Hg, and water is drawn back into the capillaries.

Thus, it is the balance between hydrostatic pressure and protein osmotic pressure that determines the direction of capillary fluid shift. Normally, water is forced out of the capillary at the arteriole end, where hydrostatic pressure exceeds osmotic pressure, and is drawn back into the capillary at the venule end, where osmotic pressure exceeds hydrostatic pressure. Any fluid left behind is picked up and removed by the **lymph capillaries.**

Veins

The venules and veins into which the capillary blood drains for its return journey to the heart are thinner walled, less elastic, and of considerably larger diameter than their corresponding arteries and arterioles (Fig. 29-9). Blood pressure in the venous system is low, from approximately 10 mm Hg, where capillaries drain into venules, to approximately zero in the right atrium. Because pressure is so low, the venous return gets assists from valves in the veins, muscles surrounding the veins, and the rhythmical pumping action of the lungs. If it were not for these mechanisms, the blood might pool in the lower extremities of a standing animal—a very real problem for people who must stand for long periods. Veins that lift blood from the extremities to the heart contain valves that divide the long column of blood into segments. When the muscles around the veins contract, as in even slight activity, the blood column is squeezed upward and cannot slip back because of the valves. The well-known risk of fainting while standing at stiff attention in hot weather can usually be prevented by deliberately pumping the leg muscles. The negative pressure created in the thorax by the inspiratory movement of the lungs also speeds the venous return by sucking the blood up the large vena cava into the heart.

Lymphatic system

The lymphatic system is an extensive network of thin-walled vessels that is separate from the circulatory system. The system arises as blind-ended lymph capillaries in most tissues of the body. These unite to form larger and larger lymph vessels, which finally drain into veins in the lower neck (Fig. 29-12).

The lymphatic system is an accessory drainage system for the body. As we have seen, the blood pressure in the arteriole end of the capillaries forces a plasma filtrate through the capillary walls and into the interstitial space. This tissue fluid bathing the cells is a clear, nearly colorless liquid. Tissue fluid and plasma are nearly identical except that tissue fluid contains very little protein, which was screened out as the plasma was squeezed through the capillary walls. Most of the tissue fluid returns to the vascular system at the venous end of the capillaries by the capillary fluid-shift mechanism described earlier. Usually, however, outflow from the capillaries slightly exceeds backflow. This difference is gathered up and returned to the circulatory system by lymphatic vessels (Fig. 29-12, B). Tissue fluid that has entered the lymph vessels is referred to as **lymph.** The rate of lymph flow is very low, a minute fraction of the blood flow.

Located at strategic intervals along the lymph vessels are **lymph nodes** that have several defense-related functions. They are effective filters, removing foreign particles, especially bacteria, that might otherwise enter the general circulation. They are also germinal centers for immune cells that produce immunoglobulin **antibodies**—essential components of the body's defense mechanisms.

____ Hemostasis: Prevention of Blood Loss   *Read*

Animals must have ways of preventing the rapid loss of body fluids after an injury. Since blood is flowing and is under considerable hydrostatic pressure, it is especially vulnerable to hemorrhagic loss.

When a vessel is damaged, smooth muscle in the wall contracts, which causes the vessel lumen to narrow, sometimes so strongly that blood flow is completely stopped. This primitive but highly effective means of preventing hemorrhage is used by invertebrates and vertebrates alike. Beyond this first defense against blood loss, all vertebrates, as well as some of the larger, active invertebrates with high blood pressures, have special cellular elements and proteins in the blood that are capable of forming plugs, or clots, at the injury site.

In higher vertebrates **blood coagulation** is the dominant hemostatic defense.

Figure 29-12

Human lymphatic system, showing major vessels, **A,** and a detail of the blood and lymphatic capillaries, **B.**

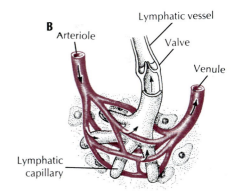

Blood clots form as a tangled network of fibers from one of the plasma proteins, **fibrinogen.** The transformation of fibrinogen into a **fibrin** meshwork (Fig. 29-13) that entangles blood cells to form a gel-like clot is catalyzed by the enzyme thrombin. Thrombin is normally present in the blood in an inactive form called **prothrombin,** which must be activated for coagulation to occur.

The blood platelets (Fig. 29-4) play a vital role in this process. Platelets—minute, colorless, incomplete cells lacking nuclei—are present in large numbers in the blood. When the normally smooth inner surface of a blood vessel is disrupted, either by a break or by deposits of a cholesterol-lipid material, the platelets rapidly adhere to the surface and release a variety of substances. These factors, along with factors released from damaged tissue and with calcium ions, initiate the conversion of prothrombin to the active thrombin. Thrombin, in turn, converts soluble fibrinogen to the gel form of the protein, fibrin. The stages in the formation of fibrin are summarized below.

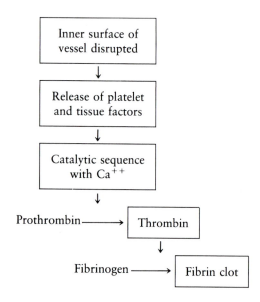

The catalytic sequence in this scheme is unexpectedly complex, involving a series of plasma protein factors, each normally inactive until activated by a previous factor in the sequence. The sequence behaves like a "cascade" with each reactant in the sequence leading to a large increase in the amount of the next reactant. At least 13 different plasma coagulation factors have been recognized. A deficiency of a single factor can delay or prevent the clotting process. Why has such a complex clotting mechanism evolved? Probably it is necessary to provide a fail-safe system that is capable of responding to any kind of internal or external hemorrhage that might occur and yet cannot be activated into forming dangerous intravascular clots unless injury has occurred.

Several kinds of clotting abnormalities in humans are known. One of these, hemophilia, is a condition characterized by the failure of the blood to clot, so that even insignificant wounds can cause continuous severe bleeding. It is due to a rare mutation (about one in 10,000) on the X sex chromosome, resulting in an inherited lack of one of the platelet factors in males and in homozygous females. Called the "disease of kings," it once ran through several interrelated royal families of Europe, apparently having originated from a mutation in one of Queen Victoria's parents.

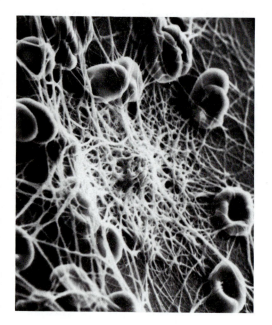

Figure 29-13

Human red blood cells entrapped in fibrin clot. Clotting is initiated after tissue damage by the disintegration of platelets in the blood, resulting in a complex series of intravascular reactions that end with the conversion of a plasma protein, fibrinogen, into long, tough, insoluble polymers of fibrin. Fibri   and entangled erythrocytes form the   d clot, which arrests bleeding. An a   ation of platelets probably underlies   raised mass of fibrin in center.

Photomicrograph courtesy N.F.   chman.

Hemophilia is one of the best-known cases of sex-linked inheritance in humans. Actually two different loci on the X chromosome are involved. Classical hemophilia (hemophilia A) accounts for about 80% of persons with the condition, and the remainder are due to Christmas disease (hemophilia B). The allele at each locus results in the deficiency of a different platelet factor.

IMMUNE SYSTEM

Real

Immunity is mediated through all the physiological mechanisms that enable animals to defend themselves against foreign invaders, such as bacteria, viruses, fungi, and parasites. All multicellular animals have defenses against microbes that would otherwise quickly swamp their cellular machinery. Cells and tissue fluids have nutrients that provide an ideal culture medium for microbes. Without host immune defenses, invasive organisms would use these vital cellular components for growth, preventing normal host cell function.

Every animal's first line of defense is the integument that is exposed to the external environment. Few microbes can penetrate this barrier when it is intact. Many animals increase the effectiveness of the integument by secreting mucus or other glandular materials that contain chemical substances toxic to bacteria. Some secretions contain lysozyme, an enzyme particularly effective in preventing bacterial growth. Bacteria that adhere to sticky mucus are simply swept away as old mucus is replaced with new. Other animals that lack surface mucous secretions harbor a "friendly" microbial flora on the integument that suppresses the growth of more virulent microorganisms.

Despite such physical and chemical defenses, microbes do frequently breach the external barrier through small breaks and injuries; some viruses even gain entry through intact integument. Once inside, the body's second line of defense, the immune system, responds to the assault. The lower invertebrates have a primitive but effective immune system: ameboid phagocytic cells that move through the tissues and circulating fluids, recognizing and engulfing (phagocytizing) foreign material when it is encountered. By migrating into injured areas, these wandering cells also initiate tissue repair. In more advanced invertebrates, phagocytic cells become organized into distinct reticular networks through which the blood filters on its way to the heart. Such structures are not unlike the more highly organized lymphatic systems of birds and mammals.

In the vertebrates the immune system is far more elaborate. In addition to the innate, nonspecific phagocytic cell system inherited from the invertebrates, the vertebrates have evolved an *acquired* immune response that provides a **specific** reaction to a particular infection. Acquired (specific) immunity differs from innate (nonspecific) immunity in (1) being highly specific for the foreign body it recognizes, (2) requiring time to develop, and (3) having memory, that is, the ability to respond more effectively to a subsequent invasion by the foreign body. We will consider both systems—nonspecific and specific—in this section.

Nonspecific Defense Mechanisms   *Real*

Should a foreign body or microorganism penetrate the body's first lines of defense, it is important that the invader be recognized as "nonself"; the cells of an animal must "know" that the substance does not belong in that animal. **Phagocytosis** (Gr., *phago,* to eat, + *kytos,* hollow vessel, cell) is one response to nonself recognition. It is found in all metazoa and is a feeding mechanism in protozoa. A cell with this capacity is a **phagocyte.** Phagocytosis is a process of engulfment of the invading particle with an invagination of the phagocyte's cell membrane (Fig. 29-14). The invagination becomes pinched off, enclosing the particle in an intracellular vacuole. Lysosomes empty digestive enzymes into the vacuole to destroy the particle. In metazoan invertebrates the cells performing this function are

Figure 29-14

Phagocytosis. A macrophage is ingesting two worn-out erythrocytes. Thin cytoplasmic extensions of the macrophage are surrounding the erythrocyte surface.
Photograph by J.P. Revel, California Institute of Technology.

Specific Immune Mechans

Thymus

① **Cell-mediated immunity** *Circulate in Blood & Lymph*

T lymphocyte

Sensitized T cell *Viruses Fungi Parasites*

Erythrocytes

Stem cells

Granulocytes

Monocytes

B site (adult bone marrow)

② **Humoral immunity** *Major defense against Bacteria*

B lymphocyte *Bone*

Plasma cell

Antibodies *immune globulins Gam globins*

Lymphocytes *~ produced in lymph glands*

Figure 29-15

Stimulation of an immune response by an antigen. When antigen molecules bind with a lymphocyte that bears receptors for a specific antigen on its surface, the lymphocyte is stimulated to undergo numerous mitoses. There are two kinds of lymphocytes. T lymphocytes, which effect cellular responses, become sensitized by contact with an antigen. Some T cells destroy foreign cells by direct cell-to-cell contact. A B lymphocyte makes antibodies. Its surface receptors are samples of the antibody it can synthesize. When it is stimulated by contact with a specific antigen, the B lymphocyte transforms into a plasma cell, which produces large amounts of antibodies for the antigen. A subclass of T cells known as regulators interacts with B cells to enhance or suppress antibody production.

known as **amebocytes** (or another name, depending on the group of animals). If the particle is too large for phagocytosis, the amebocytes may gather around it and wall it off. In humans there are **fixed** and **mobile** phagocytes. The fixed phagocytes, found in the liver, spleen, lymph nodes, and other tissues, together form the **reticuloendothelial system** (**RE system**). The bloodstream circulates through the organ systems collecting particles and dead cells. This cellular debris is trapped in the RE system where phagocytic cells engulf and destroy it, as well as infective organisms. The ease with which a particle or an organism is phagocytized depends on the nature of its membrane or outer surface. Organisms bearing a mucous-like capsule, such as some encapsulated bacteria, are not easily phagocytized. However, if proteins called antibodies (discussed later in the chapter) are present in the host, phagocytosis of the organism is greatly enhanced.

The mobile phagocytic cells that circulate in the blood are of two types: **polymorphonuclear** (multiform nucleus) **leukocytes** and **monocytes**. The polymorphonuclear leukocytes are responsible for most of the nonspecific phagocytic activity in the circulation. These granulocytic leukocytes have "granules" full of enzymes and substances, which are toxic to most bacteria and fungi. Some of the substances in these granules signal the activation of cells involved in the specific immune response. The types of cells present in this group include neutrophils, eosinophils, and basophils. When monocytes move from the blood into the tissues in response to infection, they become activated and differentiate into active phagocytes termed **macrophages.**

Inflammation

Inflammation is a vital process in the mobilization of the body defenses against an invading organism and in the repair of damage thereafter. Although inflammation is a nonspecific process, it is greatly influenced by the host's degree of immunity to the invader. Also, a more noxious foreign substance will produce more intense inflammation. Tissue damage initiates release of pharmacologically active substances (such as histamine) from mast cells in the area. These substances increase the permeability of local capillaries and increase blood flow to the area. The area becomes red and swollen ("inflamed"). Neutrophils accumulate in enormous numbers in the area and set about engulfing the invading organisms and foreign debris. Later, macrophages (either fixed or differentiated from monocytes) predominate in the inflamed area. The battle is not all one sided, however. Should the infection be large or the bacteria especially virulent, the white blood cells may themselves be killed in large numbers by bacterial toxins and accumulate as pus in the infection site. Occasionally an abscess, or walled-off bag of pus, is formed that will not heal spontaneously. However, the great majority of minute invasions, which are always occurring and of which we are seldom aware, are quickly and efficiently countered. Once the infection is destroyed, the tissue repairs by cellular regeneration. If tissue damage has been severe, a scar (fibrous connective tissue) will form in the area.

Some years ago, a substance named **interferon** was discovered that has proved to be a potent natural inhibitor of virus multiplication in cells. It is a low—molecular weight protein that is rapidly produced by cells in response to viral infection. Unlike antibodies, which we will consider later in this discussion, interferon is a nonspecific defense. Once it is produced, the cell becomes resistant to many kinds of viruses. Interferon acts to destroy viruses inside the infected cell. Antibodies cannot pass the cell's plasma membrane and thus are ineffective against intracellular viral invasions.

Interferon's most important role may be its effect on the host's immune system. Interferon stimulates the activity of **natural killer cells,** special blood cells that function to protect the body against tumor virus infections. Natural killer cells require no prior exposure to the tumor or tumor virus for their killing activity.

Specific Immune Mechanisms

Specific immunity is produced in the body following exposure to a specific foreign substance or antigen (Gr., *anti*, against, + *genos*, birth). An antigen is any of a variety of substances, most commonly proteins, that will stimulate an immune response.

Two separate immune systems are involved. One is **cell-mediated immunity,** which is important in the defense against parasites, viruses, and fungi, and the other is **humoral immunity,** which protects the body against pathogens through the production of antibodies (Fig. 29-15). Both kinds of immunity are centered on lymphocytes, a small, unpigmented type of white blood cell. All lymphocytes are derived from the same blood-forming tissue in bone marrow but later develop into two separate lines, B cells and T cells, which are responsible for humoral and cellular immune responses, respectively.

Humoral immunity

Humoral immunity is based on **antibodies** (Gr., *anti*, against, + A.S., *bodig,* body). Antibodies belong to a class of proteins called **immunoglobulins** (or γ-globulins). There are five subclasses of antibodies, of which immunoglobulin G (IgG) is the most common. An antibody is made of four polypeptide chains, paired in such a way that the molecule consists of two long ("heavy") chains and two short ("light") chains in a Y configuration. Each antibody has two identical antigen-binding sites, one at the end of each arm of the Y (Fig. 29-16). The two arms

Because interferon attacks tumors and viral diseases such as hepatitis, herpes, influenza, and the common cold, it has been in great demand for research and clinical use. In the past, it was extremely expensive and scarce because its extraction from human blood was costly. The recent introduction of gene-splicing techniques in which bacteria are programmed to produce interferon with inserted segments of human DNA has changed all this. It is now being produced in relatively large quantities. Basic research and clinical trials with interferon are being carried out around the world. Although the prediction that interferon would soon become the "magic bullet" for cancer treatment was premature, great progress has been made in defining interferon's chemistry, actions, and cellular origin.

A major problem of immunology is understanding how the mammalian genome could contain the information needed to produce at least a million different antibodies. The recently discovered answer seems to be that antibody genes occur in pieces, rather than as continuous stretches of DNA, and that the antigen-recognizing sites (variable regions) of the heavy and light chains of the antibody molecules are pieced together from information supplied by separate DNA sequences, which can be shuffled to vastly increase diversity of the gene products. The immense repertoire of antibodies is achieved in part by complex gene rearrangements (the exact mechanism of DNA switching is not yet clear) and in part by frequent somatic mutations that produce additional variation in protein structure of the variable regions of the heavy and light antibody chains.

Many aspects of immunology have been greatly assisted by the recent discovery of a method for producing stable clones of cells that will produce only one kind of antibody. Such monoclonal antibodies will bind to only *one kind* of antigenic determinant (most proteins bear many different antigenic determinants and thus stimulate the body to produce complex mixtures of antibodies). Monoclonal antibodies are made by fusing normal antibody-producing plasma cells with a continuously growing plasma cell line, producing a hybrid of the normal cell with one that can divide indefinitely in culture. This is called a hybridoma. Clones are grown from the hybrids, becoming "factories" that produce almost unlimited quantities of one specific antibody. Although clinical trials with monoclonal antibodies in cancer detection and therapy are only beginning, the hybridoma techniques discovered in 1975 have already become one of the most important research tools for the immunologist.

are joined at the stem of the Y by a hinge that allows the angle of the arms to vary; this flexibility permits the antibody to cross-link two antigenic sites having variable spacing between them.

Antibodies are produced by lymphocytes that differentiate into **B cells** after leaving the bone marrow. B cells are produced from stem cells (Fig. 29-15). In birds, differentiation of the B cells occurs in the bursa of Fabricius (hence the name "B" cell), a lymphoid organ attached to the intestine near the cloaca. In mammals the equivalent of the bursa is the fetal liver and the adult bone marrow. When the B cell matures, it becomes a **plasma cell,** the antibody-producing cell (Fig. 29-15).

During a life span of several days, plasma cells elaborate enormous numbers of antibodies, some 2000 molecules per second. Following the first introduction of an antigen into the animal, the antibody level is low or undetectable until the specific population of plasma cells rises. The antibody level in the blood then typically increases to a plateau and subsequently falls as the plasma cells die and the antibodies are degraded in the system. If the antigen is again introduced, however, the antibody level usually rises quickly to 10 to 100 times the previous level. This is called the **secondary response.** It occurs because not all of the originally sensitized lymphocytes gave rise to plasma cells; some of them produced long-lived **memory cells,** which can respond immediately to the antigen challenge.

By attaching to an antigen, antibodies may attack it in different ways. First, antibodies can coat the surfaces of the invasive organism to increase nonspecific phagocytosis. Second, antibodies can cause a "stitching together" or agglutination of cells, preventing cell growth. Finally, antibodies can attach to the surface of the organism and activate the attack by a group of plasma enzymes collectively called complement. The 11 proteins of the complement system circulate in the plasma all the time in an inactive state. When activated, complement binds to antigen-antibody complexes at special sites (Fig. 29-16), coating the foreign substance (antigen) and making it much easier for phagocytes to engulf the foreigner. Complement can also directly destroy microbes without the assistance of phagocytes by forming lesions on the microbes' lipid-membrane surface.

Cell-mediated immunity

Cell-mediated immunity is conferred by T cells, so called because they are processed in the thymus, a gland that in mammals lies in the chest beneath the sternum. T cells look just like B cells, but unlike B cells they do not synthesize antibodies or differentiate into antibody-producing plasma cells. Nevertheless, T cells are very much involved in most immune reactions. Several different kinds of T cells are recognized, but they all may be grouped into one or the other of two categories. There are **effector** T cells that destroy target cells by direct cell-to-cell contact. These may include the body's own cells when they have been infected with viruses or if they display characteristics of tumorlike cells. Other T cells act as **regulators** that interact with B cells in the production of antibodies (they both enhance and suppress reactions by B cells). If such responses were unregulated, the immune response to infection would be too slow at the critical time when infection is overpowering the host, and then, after the critical time of infection is over, would be too slow in stopping the response to that particular infection. T cells also enhance the effectiveness of the body's nonspecific defense system mediated by phagocytic cells.

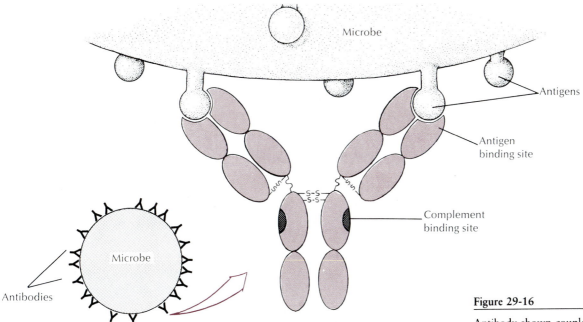

Microbe

Antigens

Antigen
binding site

—S—S—
—S—S—

Complement
binding site

Microbe

Antibodies

Figure 29-16

Antibody shown coupled to two antigenic sites on a microbe. The most common
type of antibody, immunoglobulin G
(IgG), consists of four polypeptide
chains—two long, central chains and two
short, peripheral chains—arranged in a Y
configuration. The two long chains are
held together by disulfide bonds (—S—
S—). Each antibody couples through two
receptors, which are antigen-binding sites
having geometrical and chemical specificity for the antigens. Antibodies, together
with attached plasma enzymes called
complement, modify the surface of the
invading microorganisms *(lower left)*,
making it easier for white blood cells to
engulf and destroy it.

Immune response   *Read*

Having introduced all the main components and stated their roles in the body's
specific defense system, let us summarize their interactions during an infection.
When a foreign antigen enters the body for the first time, it is immediately
attacked by phagocytes (neutrophils and monocytes) and by antigen-specific regulator T cells. At the same time the antigen triggers antibody synthesis by B cells.
For this to happen, the antigen must be transported, usually by lymph vessels, to
lymph nodes, the spleen, or other lymphoid cell aggregates where the B cells are
located. There the antigen stimulates a small number of B cells, assisted by regulator T cells, to divide and mature rapidly into plasma cells, which begin producing antibodies against the antigen. It usually requires several days for the plasma
cells to build up to full-scale antibody production. In doing so, a fraction of the
undifferentiated B cells becomes a "memory bank" for the antigen, ready to
respond immediately should the same antigen appear a second time.

In the meantime, while the B cells are "tooling up" for antibody production,
the phagocytes are fighting the infection. If they are immediately successful, the
antibodies may never enter combat. But if the infection persists for several days,
new antibodies activate complement, which directly destroys the microbes and
amplifies phagocytic activity. Whether the infection is short lived or more persistent, the specific immune system has been alerted, and any subsequent invasion by
the antigen will be met with much greater force. The animal now bears an **active
immunity** against the antigen.

Until recently, suffering a disease or infection was the only way to obtain an
active immunity. Now it may be achieved safely from the injection of vaccines
(living or weakened microbes) or microbial derivatives, such as a bacterial toxin.
The purpose is to provoke an antibody response, which will leave the antibody-
synthesizing machinery poised to respond immediately to a future invasion by that
organism.

Passive immunity is gained by directly injecting preformed antibodies from one person or animal to another person. This is the kind of protective immunity passed from mother to fetus across the placenta. Passive immunity is short lived; the antibodies are soon destroyed and cannot be naturally replaced because the antibody-synthesizing machinery has not been set in motion.

Transplantation and Blood Antigens
Histocompatibility antigens

When a piece of skin or other tissue is grafted from one individual to another, the transplant seldom survives unless the two individuals are genetically identical. Within a few days the graft becomes inflamed, eventually dies, and drops away, having been rejected by the recipient's tissues. This occurs because protein molecules on the graft, called **histocompatibility antigens,** are recognized as foreign by the recipient. The cells involved in the recognition are T cells. Histocompatibility antigens are surface proteins that are present on almost every nucleated cell and give the animal bearing those cells its own chemical identity.

Invertebrates have genetic systems that permit the recognition of tissues from other individuals as foreign, or nonself. This genetic diversification reaches its highest expression in the **major histocompatibility complex** (MHC) of higher vertebrates, where many genetic systems that code protein diversity are concentrated in one region of one chromosome. The MHC enables the immune system to distinguish between self and nonself. Recognition develops gradually during the early development of the organism, and all substances present at the time the capacity develops are recognized as self in later life.

Unfortunately, the system of self and nonself recognition sometimes breaks down, and an animal may begin to produce antibodies against some part of its own body. This leads to one of several known autoimmune diseases, such as rheumatoid arthritis, systemic lupus erythematosus, some hemolytic anemias, and encephalitis.

In 1980 the Nobel Prize was awarded to Baruj Benacerraf, Jean Dausset, and George Snell for their many years of research on the identification and action of the histocompatibility antigens.

Blood group antigens
ABO blood types

Blood differs chemically from person to person, and when two different (incompatible) blood types are mixed, **agglutination** (clumping together) results. The basis of these chemical differences is naturally occurring antigens on the membranes of red blood cells. The best known of these inherited immune systems is the ABO blood group. The antigens A and B are inherited as dominant genes. Thus, as shown in Table 29-1, an individual with, for example, genes *A/A* or *A/O* develops A antigen (blood type A). The presence of a B gene produces B antigens (blood type B), and for the genotype *A/B* both A and B antigens develop on the erythrocytes (blood type AB).

The ABO system has an odd feature. Normally we would expect that a type A individual would develop antibodies against type B blood only if B cells were introduced into the body. In fact, type A persons always have anti-B antibodies in their blood, even without prior exposure to type B blood. Similarly, type B individuals carry anti-A antibodies. Type AB blood has neither anti-A nor anti-B antibodies (if it did, it would destroy its own blood cells), and type O blood has both anti-A and anti-B antibodies.

Table 29-1 Major Blood Groups

Blood type	Genotype	Antigens on red blood cells	Antibodies in serum	Possible recipients	Possible donors	Frequency in United States (%)		
						Whites	Blacks	Orientals
O	O/O	None	Anti-A and anti-B	All	O	45	38	46
A	A/A, A/O	A	Anti-B	A, AB	O, A	41	27	28
B	B/B, B/O	B	Anti-A	B, AB	O, B	10	21	23
AB	A/B	AB	None	AB	All	4	4	13

We see then that the blood group names identify their *antigen* content. Persons with type O blood are called universal donors because, lacking antigens, their blood can be infused into a person with any blood type. Even though it contains anti-A and anti-B antibodies, these are so diluted during transfusion that they do not react with A or B antigens in a recipient's blood. In practice, however, clinicians match blood types to prevent any possibility of incompatibility.

Rh factor

It is difficult to think of another area of physiology as totally linked with the name of a single man as blood grouping is with the name Karl Landsteiner. This Austrian—later American—physician discovered the ABO blood groups in 1900. The great importance of his work became abundantly clear during World War I when blood transfusion was first attempted on a large scale. In 1927 Landsteiner in collaboration with Philip Levine in the United States discovered the MN blood group, also present in all mankind. This classification is not important in transfusions but may be crucial in determining relationship in paternity cases.

In 1940, 10 years after receiving the Nobel Prize in recognition of contributions that were more than adequate for the lifetime of any scientist, Landsteiner made still another famous discovery. This new group was called the Rh factor, named after the rhesus monkey, in which it was first found. Approximately 85% of white individuals in the United States have the factor (positive) and the other 15% do not (negative). Landsteiner also found that Rh-positive and Rh-negative bloods are incompatible; shock and even death may follow their mixing when Rh-positive blood is introduced into an Rh-negative person who has been sensitized by an earlier transfusion of Rh-positive blood.

For practical purposes, we can regard inheritance of the Rh factor as a single dominant gene, yielding an Rh-positive phenotype in the homozygous dominant or the heterozygous genotype. This accounts for a peculiar and often fatal form of anemia of newborn infants called **erythroblastosis fetalis.** Although the fetal and maternal bloods are separated by the placenta, this separation is not perfect. Some seepage of the fetal blood into the maternal blood may occur, especially right after birth when the placenta ("afterbirth") separates from the uterine wall. This admixture of blood, normally of no consequence, can be serious *if* the father is Rh positive, the mother Rh negative, and the fetus Rh positive (by inheriting the factor from the father). The fetal blood, containing the Rh antigen, can stimulate the formation of Rh-positive antibodies in the blood of the mother. The mother is permanently immunized against the Rh factor. During the second pregnancy these antibodies may diffuse back into the fetal circulation and produce agglutination and destruction of fetal red blood cells. Because the mother is usually sensitized at the end of the first pregnancy, subsequent babies are more severely threatened than is the first.

Erythroblastosis fetalis can now be prevented by giving an Rh-negative mother anti-Rh antibodies just after the birth of her first child. These antibodies remain long enough to neutralize any Rh-positive fetal blood cells that may have entered her circulation, thus preventing her own antibody machinery from being stimulated to produce the Rh-positive antibodies. Active, permanent immunity is blocked. If the mother has already developed an immunity, however, the baby may be saved by an immediate, massive transfusion of blood free of antibodies.

GAS EXCHANGE

The energy bound up in food must be released by **respiration,** or aerobic energy metabolism. In this cellular process, described in some detail in Chapter 5, oxygen is consumed by the body cells and carbon dioxide is released. In this section we examine **gas exchange:** those activities that exchange oxygen and carbon dioxide between the organism and its environment.

Small aquatic animals such as the one-celled protozoa obtain what oxygen they need by direct diffusion from the environment. Carbon dioxide, the gaseous waste of metabolism, is also lost by diffusion to the environment. Such a simple solution to the problem of gas exchange is really possible only for very small animals (less than 1 mm in diameter) that have a large surface relative to their volume or for those having very low rates of metabolism.

As animals became larger and evolved a waterproof covering, specialized devices such as lungs and gills developed that greatly increased the effective surface for gas exchange. But, because gases diffuse so slowly through protoplasm, a circulatory system was necessary to distribute the gases to and from the deep tissues of the body. Even these adaptations were inadequate for advanced animals with their high rates of cellular respiration. The solubility of oxygen in the blood plasma is so low that plasma alone could not carry enough to satisfy metabolic demands. With the evolution of special oxygen-transporting blood proteins such as hemoglobin, the oxygen-carrying capacity of the blood was greatly increased. Thus, what began as a simple and easily satisfied requirement resulted in the evolution of several complex and essential respiratory and circulatory adaptations.

Problems of Aquatic and Aerial Breathing

How an animal respires is largely determined by the nature of its environment. The two great arenas of animal evolution—water and land—are vastly different in their physical characteristics. The most obvious difference is that air contains far more oxygen—at least 20 times more—than does water. Atmospheric air contains oxygen (approximately 21%), nitrogen (approximately 78%), carbon dioxide (0.03%), a variable amount of water vapor, argon (0.93%), and very small amounts of other inert gases (helium, neon, and others). These gases are variably soluble in water. The amount of oxygen dissolved depends on the concentration of oxygen in the air and on the water temperature. Water at 5° C fully saturated with air contains approximately 9 ml of oxygen per liter. (In comparison, air contains approximately 210 ml of oxygen per liter.) The solubility of oxygen in water decreases as the temperature rises. For example, water at 15° C contains approximately 7 ml of oxygen per liter, and at 35° C, only 5 ml of oxygen per liter. The relatively low concentration of oxygen dissolved in water is the greatest respiratory problem facing aquatic animals. Unfortunately, it is not the only one. Oxygen diffuses much more slowly in water than in air, and water is much denser and more viscous than air. All of this means that successful aquatic animals must have evolved very efficient ways of removing oxygen from water. Yet even the most advanced fishes with highly efficient gills and pumping mechanisms may use as much as 20% of their energy just extracting oxygen from water. In comparison, a mammal uses only 1% to 2% of its resting metabolism to breathe.

Respiratory surfaces must be thin and always kept wet to allow diffusion of gases between the environment and the underlying circulation. This is hardly a problem for aquatic animals, immersed as they are in water, but it is a very real problem for air breathers. To keep the respiratory membranes moist and protected from injury, air breathers have in general developed invaginations of the body surface and then added pumping mechanisms to move air in and out. The lung is the best example of a successful solution to breathing on land. In general, **evaginations** of the body surface, such as gills, are most suitable for aquatic respiration; **invaginations,** such as lungs, are best for air breathing. We can now consider the specific kinds of respiratory organs employed by animals.

Cutaneous respiration

Protozoa, sponges, cnidarians, and many worms respire by direct diffusion of gases between the organism and the environment. We have noted that this kind of **integumentary respiration** is inadequate when the mass of living protoplasm exceeds approximately 1 mm in diameter. But, by greatly increasing the surface of the body relative to the mass, many multicellular animals respire in this way. Integumentary respiration frequently supplements gill or lung breathing in larger animals such as amphibians and fishes. For example, an eel can exchange 60% of its oxygen and carbon dioxide through its highly vascular skin. During their winter hibernation, frogs exchange all their respiratory gases through the skin while submerged in ponds or springs.

Gills

Gills of various types are more effective respiratory devices for life in water. Gills may be simple external extensions of the body surface, such as the **dermal papulae** of starfish or the **branchial tufts** of marine worms and aquatic amphibians. Most efficient are the **internal** gills of fishes (p. 541) and arthropods. Fish gills are thin filamentous structures, richly supplied with blood vessels arranged so that blood flow is opposite to the flow of water across the gills. This arrangement, called **countercurrent flow,** provides for the greatest possible extraction of oxygen from water. Water flows over the gills in a steady stream, pushed and pulled by an efficient branchial pump, and often assisted by the fish's forward movement through the water.

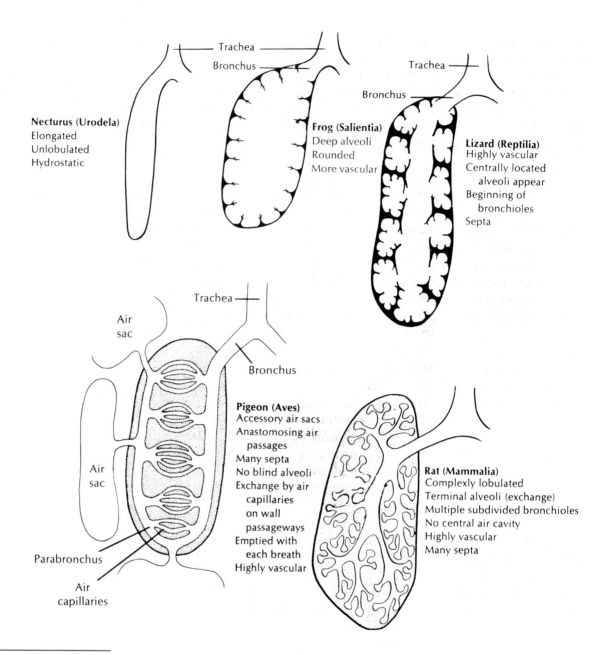

Necturus (Urodela)
Elongated
Unlobulated
Hydrostatic

Trachea

Bronchus

Frog (Salientia)
Deep alveoli
Rounded
More vascular

Trachea

Bronchus

Lizard (Reptilia)
Highly vascular
Centrally located
   alveoli appear
Beginning of
   bronchioles
Septa

Trachea

Air
sac

Bronchus

Air
sac

Parabronchus

Air
capillaries

Pigeon (Aves)
Accessory air sacs
Anastomosing air
   passages
Many septa
No blind alveoli
Exchange by air
   capillaries
   on wall
   passageways
Emptied with
   each breath
Highly vascular

Rat (Mammalia)
Complexly lobulated
Terminal alveoli (exchange)
Multiple subdivided bronchioles
No central air cavity
Highly vascular
Many septa

Figure 29-17

Internal structures of lungs among vertebrate groups. In general, the evolutionary trend has been from simple sacs with little exchange surface between blood and air spaces to complex, lobulated structures of complex divisions and extensive exchange surfaces.

Lungs

Gills are unsuitable for life in air because, when removed from the buoying water medium, the gill filaments collapse and stick together; a fish out of water rapidly asphyxiates despite the abundance of oxygen around it. Consequently, air-breathing vertebrates possess lungs, highly vascularized internal cavities. Lungs of a sort are found in certain invertebrates (pulmonate snails, scorpions, some spiders, some small crustaceans), but these structures cannot be very efficiently ventilated.

Lungs that can be ventilated more efficiently are characteristic of the terrestrial vertebrates. The most primitive vertebrate lungs are those of lungfishes (Dipneusti), which use them to supplement, or even replace, gill respiration during periods of drought. Although of simple construction, the lungfish is supplied with a capillary network in its largely unfurrowed walls, a tubelike connection to the pharynx, and a primitive ventilating system for moving air in and out of the lung.

Amphibians also have simple baglike lungs, whereas in higher forms the inner surface area is vastly increased by numerous lobulations and folds (Fig. 29-17). This increase is greatest in the mammalian lung, which is complexly divided into many millions of small sacs (**alveoli**), each veiled by a rich vascular network. It has been estimated that human lungs have a total surface area of from 50 to 90 m²—50 times the area of the skin surface—and contain 1000 miles of capillaries.

Moving air into and out of lungs was an evolutionary design problem that has been, of course, solved. However, we wonder whether an imaginative biological engineer, if given the proper resources, could not come up with a better design. Unlike the efficient one-way flow of water across fish gills, air must enter and exit a lung through the same channel. Furthermore, a tube of some length—the bronchi, trachea, and mouth cavity—connects the lungs to the outside. This is a "dead-air space" containing a volume of air that shuttles back and forth with each breath, adding to the difficulty of properly ventilating the lungs. In fact, lung ventilation is so inefficient that in normal breathing only approximately one sixth of the air in the lungs is replenished with each inspiration.

One group of vertebrates, the birds, vastly improved lung efficiency by adding an extensive system of air sacs (Fig. 29-17) that serve as air reservoirs during ventilation. On inspiration, some 75% of the incoming air bypasses the lungs to enter the air sacs. At expiration, some of this fresh air passes directly through the lung passages. Thus, the air capillaries receive nearly fresh air during both inspiration and expiration (Fig. 26-12, p. 615). The beautifully designed bird lung is the result of selective pressures during the evolution of flight and its high metabolic demands.

Frogs force air into the lungs by first lowering the floor of the mouth to draw air into the mouth through the external nares (nostrils); then they close the nares and raise the floor of the mouth to drive air into the lungs. Much of the time, however, frogs rhythmically ventilate only the mouth cavity, which serves as a kind of auxiliary "lung" (Fig. 24-16, p. 571). Amphibians therefore employ a **positive-pressure** action to fill their lungs, unlike most reptiles, birds, and mammals, which breathe by sucking air into the lungs (**negative-pressure** action).

Tracheae

Insects and certain other terrestrial arthropods (centipedes, millipedes, and some spiders) have a highly specialized type of respiratory system; in many respects it is the simplest, most direct, and most efficient respiratory system found in active animals. It consists of a system of tubes (**tracheae**) that branch repeatedly and extend to all parts of the body (Fig. 17-17, p. 417). The smallest end channels (**air capillaries**), less than 1 μm in diameter, sink into the plasma membranes of the body cells. Air enters the tracheal system through valvelike openings (**spiracles**) on each side of the body, and oxygen diffuses directly to all cells of the body. Carbon dioxide diffuses out in the opposite direction. Some insects can ventilate the tracheal system with body movements; the familiar telescoping movement of the bee abdomen is an example. The tracheal system is simple because blood is not needed to transport the respiratory gases; the cells have a direct pipeline to the outside.

The student will notice that the same word (trachea, pl., tracheae) is used for certain respiratory structures in vertebrates as in some arthropods. However, they are entirely different in evolutionary origin and morphology. About the only thing they have in common is that they are tubes through which air passes.

Figure 29-18

A, Human lungs. B, Terminal portion of lung, showing bronchiole and air sacs with their blood supply. Arrows show direction of blood flow. (Approximately ×90.)

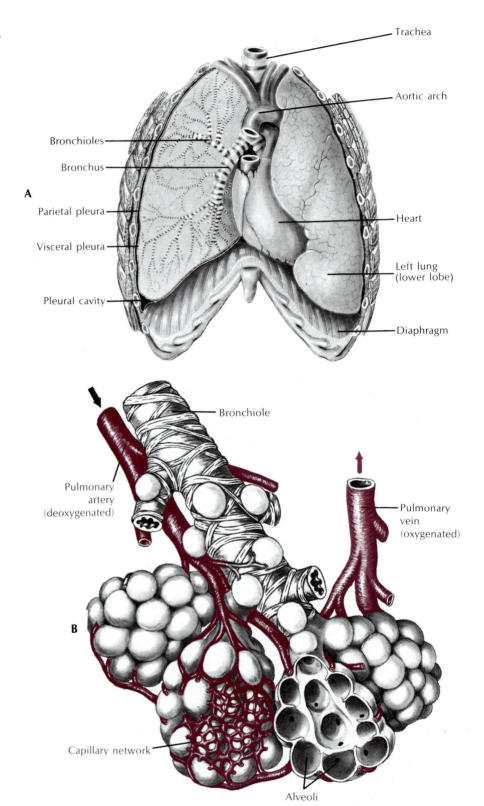

Trachea

Aortic arch

Bronchioles

Bronchus

A

Parietal pleura

Visceral pleura

Heart

Left lung (lower lobe)

Pleural cavity

Diaphragm

Bronchiole

Pulmonary artery (deoxygenated)

Pulmonary vein (oxygenated)

B

Capillary network

Alveoli

___ Respiration in Humans

In mammals the respiratory system is made up of the following: the nostrils (external nares); the **nasal chamber,** lined with mucus-secreting epithelium; the **posterior nares,** which connect to the **pharynx** where the pathways of digestion and respiration cross; the **epiglottis,** a flap that folds over the **glottis** (the opening to the larynx) to prevent food from going the wrong way in swallowing; the **larynx,** or voice box; the **trachea,** or windpipe; and the two **bronchi,** one to each lung (Fig. 29-18). Within the lungs each bronchus divides and subdivides into small tubes (**bronchioles**) that lead to the air sacs (**alveoli**) (Fig. 29-19). The walls of the alveoli are thin and moist to facilitate the exchange of gases between the air sacs and the adjacent blood capillaries. Air passageways are lined with mucus-secreting ciliated epithelium, which plays an important role in conditioning the air before it reaches the alveoli. There are partial cartilage rings in the walls of the tracheae, bronchi, and even some of the bronchioles to prevent those structures from collapsing.

In its passage to the air sacs the air undergoes three important changes: (1) it is filtered free from most dust and other foreign substances, (2) it is warmed to body temperature, and (3) it is saturated with moisture.

The lungs consist of a great deal of elastic connective tissue and some muscle. They are covered by a thin layer of tough epithelium known as the **visceral pleura.** A similar layer, the **parietal pleura,** lines the inner surface of the walls of the chest (Fig. 29-18). The two layers of the pleura are in contact and slide over one another as the lungs expand and contract. The "space" between the pleura, called the **pleural cavity,** contains a partial vacuum, which helps keep the lungs expanded to fill the pleural cavity. Therefore no real pleural space exists; the two pleura rub together, lubricated by tissue fluid (lymph). The chest cavity is bounded by the spine, ribs, and breastbone, and floored by the **diaphragm,** a dome-shaped, muscular partition between the chest cavity and abdomen.

Mechanism of breathing

The chest cavity is an airtight chamber. In **inspiration** the ribs are pulled upward, the diaphragm is contracted and flattened, and the chest cavity is enlarged. The resultant increase in volume of chest cavity and lungs causes the air pressure in the lungs to fall below atmospheric pressure; air rushes in through the air passageways to equalize the pressure. **Expiration** is a less active process than inspiration. When the muscles relax, the ribs and diaphragm return to their original positions and the chest cavity size decreases. The elastic lungs then deflate and force the air out.

Composition of inspired, expired, and alveolar airs

The composition of expired and alveolar airs is not identical. Air in the alveoli contains less oxygen and more carbon dioxide than does the air that leaves the lungs. Inspired air has the composition of atmospheric air. Expired air is really a mixture of alveolar and inspired airs. The composition of the three kinds of air is shown in Table 29-2.

The water given off in expired air depends on the relative humidity of the external air and the activity of the person. At ordinary room temperature and with a relative humidity of approximately 50%, an individual performing light work loses approximately 350 ml of water from the lungs each day.

Figure 29-19

A, Scanning electron micrograph of mammalian lung. ($\times 35$.) **B,** Resin cast of lung, showing the extensive capillary network surrounding each alveolus. ($\times 150$.)

A, Courtesy E.E. Morrison; B, from Tissues and organs: a text-atlas of scanning election microscopy, by Richard G. Kessel and Randy H. Kardon. W.H. Freeman and Company. Copyright © 1979.

Table 29-2 Composition of Respired Air

	Inspired air (vol%)	Expired air (vol%)	Alveolar air (vol%)
Oxygen	20.96	16	14.0
Carbon dioxide	0.04	4	5.5
Nitrogen	79.00	80	80.5

Because of the weight of water, the hydrostatic pressure increases the equivalent of 1 atmosphere for every 10 m of depth in seawater, and the air supply to a diver must be increased correspondingly so that it can be drawn into the lungs in breathing. However, the increase in pressure of the air also increases the partial pressure of its components. At a depth of 61 m (200 feet), the partial pressure of oxygen in dry air would be 1113 mm Hg. Going deeper than this, the diver breathing compressed air is in grave danger of oxygen poisoning because cellular metabolism becomes deranged at very high oxygen partial pressures. Can you recognize the danger of a diver breathing pure oxygen at only a 10 m depth (a total of 2 atmospheres)? Conversely, breathing pure oxygen at very high altitudes can be vital to life; at an atmospheric pressure of 159 mm Hg (altitude about 12,000 m), the partial pressure of oxygen in air would be only about 33 mm Hg, but the partial pressure of pure oxygen at that atmospheric pressure would be 159 mm Hg—the same as at sea level. Incidentally, the diver descending to depths greater than about 61 m is also in danger of a condition known as nitrogen narcosis ("rapture of the deep"), because nitrogen at such high partial pressures has a narcotic effect on the nervous system.

Gaseous exchange in lungs

The diffusion of gases takes place in accordance with the laws of physical diffusion; that is, the gases pass from regions of high pressure to those of low pressure. The partial pressure of a gas refers to pressure that the gas exerts in a mixture of gases, in other words, the part of the total pressure made up of that component. If the atmospheric pressure at sea level is equivalent to 760 mm Hg, the partial pressure of oxygen is 21% (percentage of oxygen in air) of 760, or 159 mm Hg in dry air. The partial pressure oxygen in the lung alveoli is greater (100 mm Hg pressure) than it is in venous blood of lung capillaries (40 mm Hg pressure) (Fig. 29-20). Oxygen then naturally diffuses into the capillaries. In a similar manner the carbon dioxide in the blood of the lung capillaries has a higher concentration (46 mm Hg) than has this same gas in the lung alveoli (40 mm Hg), so that carbon dioxide diffuses from the blood into the alveoli.

In the tissues respiratory gases also move according to their concentration gradients (Fig. 29-20). The concentration of oxygen in the blood (100 mm Hg pressure) is greater than in the tissues (0 to 30 mm Hg pressure), and the carbon dioxide concentration in the tissues (45 to 68 mm Hg pressure) is greater than that in blood (40 mm Hg pressure). The gases in each case go from a high to a low concentration.

Coordination of breathing

Respiration must adjust itself to changing requirements of the body for oxygen. Breathing is normally involuntary and automatic but comes under voluntary control for talking, singing, coughing, eating, and numerous other activities. Normal, quiet breathing is regulated by neurons centered in the medulla oblongata of the brain. These neurons spontaneously produce rhythmical bursts that travel over the phrenic and intercostal nerves and lead to contraction of the diaphragm and the intercostal muscles between the ribs. The rhythm and depth of breathing are precisely regulated by the amount of carbon dioxide in the blood. Exercise raises the carbon dioxide level, and the breathing rate increases. Even small increases in carbon dioxide may double or triple the ventilation volume. Actually, the effects of carbon dioxide increase are due to the increase in blood hydrogen ion concentration that it causes. Carbon dioxide in solution behaves as follows:

$$CO_2 + H_2O \rightleftharpoons \underset{\substack{\text{Carbonic} \\ \text{acid}}}{H_2CO_3} \rightleftharpoons \underset{\substack{\text{Bicarbonate} \\ \text{ion}}}{HCO_3^-} + \underset{\substack{\text{Hydrogen} \\ \text{ion}}}{H^+}$$

Atmospheric air
O_2 = 159 mm Hg
CO_2 = 0.3 mm Hg

Alveolar air
O_2 = 100
CO_2 = 40

O_2 = 40
CO_2 = 46

O_2 = 100
CO_2 = 40

O_2
O_2
CO_2

O_2
CO_2

O_2 = 40
CO_2 = 46

O_2 = 100
CO_2 = 40

Body cells
O_2 = 30
CO_2 = 50

CO_2
O_2

O_2 = 40
CO_2 = 46

Figure 29-20

Exchange of respiratory gases in lungs and tissue cells. Numbers present partial pressures in millimeters of mercury (mm Hg).

Any increase in carbon dioxide drives this reaction to the right, releasing more hydrogen ions. The increase in hydrogen ions stimulates the respiratory center in the medulla oblongata, leading to increased rate and depth of respiration.

It may seem odd that respiration is not tuned to oxygen levels in the blood rather than to the waste product of metabolism, carbon dioxide. The fact is that in lung breathers, arterial blood is almost always nearly saturated with oxygen, even during exercise. It is true that the venous oxygen becomes depleted during exercise, but the respiratory center receives arterial blood and thus cannot respond to changes in venous oxygen.

There are, however, instances when respiration is regulated by lowered arterial oxygen. At high altitude, oxygen availability is severely reduced, and the arterial oxygen levels drop. At 5500 m (18,000 feet), the highest human habitation, there is only about half as much oxygen as at sea level. Fortunately, the body is equipped to deal with the problem. Oxygen-sensitive chemoreceptors respond to reduced oxygen by increasing lung ventilation.

In fish, crustaceans, and many other aquatic animals, unlike lung breathers, lack of oxygen is the primary stimulus to respiration. The reason is that carbon dioxide levels are low in natural waters and carbon dioxide is quickly removed from the blood as it is produced. Thus, aquatic animals cannot depend on carbon dioxide as a respiratory stimulant.

Transport of gases in blood

In some invertebrates the respiratory gases are simply carried dissolved in the body fluids. However, the solubility of oxygen is so low in water that it is adequate only for animals with low rates of metabolism. For example, only approx-

It is well known that swimmers can remain submerged much longer if they vigorously hyperventilate first to blow off carbon dioxide from the lungs. This delays the overpowering urge to surface and breathe. The practice is dangerous because blood oxygen is depleted just as rapidly as without prior hyperventilation, and the swimmer may lose consciousness when the oxygen supply to the brain drops below a critical point. Several documented drownings among swimmers attempting long underwater swimming records have been caused by this practice.

Figure 29-21

Oxygen dissociation curves, showing how the amount of oxygen that can bind to hemoglobin is related to oxygen partial pressure. **A,** Small animals have blood that gives up oxygen more readily than does the blood of large animals. **B,** Hemoglobin is also sensitive to carbon dioxide partial pressure. As carbon dioxide enters blood from the tissues, it shifts the curve to the right, decreasing the affinity of hemoglobin for oxygen. Thus, the hemoglobin unloads more oxygen in the tissues where carbon dioxide concentration is higher.

Although hemoglobin is the only vertebrate respiratory pigment, several other respiratory pigments are known among the invertebrates. Hemocyanin, a blue, copper-containing protein, is present in the crustaceans and most molluscs. Among other pigments is chlorocruorin (klor-a-croo′o-rin), a green, iron-containing pigment found in four families of polychaete tubeworms. Its structure and oxygen-carrying capacity are very similar to those of hemoglobin, but it is carried free in the plasma rather than being enclosed in blood corpuscles. Hemerythrin is a red pigment found in some polychaete worms. Although it contains iron, this metal is not present in a heme group (despite the name of the pigment!), and its oxygen-carrying capacity is poor.

imately 1% of a human's oxygen requirement can be transported in this way. Consequently, in many invertebrates and in the vertebrates, special colored proteins, or **respiratory pigments,** in the blood transport nearly all the oxygen and a significant amount of the carbon dioxide. In most animals (all vertebrates) these respiratory pigments are packaged into blood cells. This is necessary because, if this amount of respiratory pigment were free in blood, the blood would have the viscosity of syrup and would hardly flow through the blood vessels at all.

The most widespread respiratory pigment in the animal kingdom is **hemoglobin,** a red, iron-containing protein present in all vertebrates and many invertebrates. Each molecule of hemoglobin is made up of 5% **heme,** an iron-containing compound giving the red color to blood, and 95% **globin,** a colorless protein. The heme portion of the hemoglobin has a great affinity for oxygen; each gram of hemoglobin (there are approximately 15 g of hemoglobin in each 100 ml of human blood) can carry a maximum of approximately 1.3 ml of oxygen; each 100 ml of fully oxygenated blood contains approximately 20 ml of oxygen. Of course, for hemoglobin to be of value to the body it must hold oxygen in a loose, reversible chemical combination so that it can be released to the tissues. The actual amount of oxygen with which hemoglobin can combine depends on small structural changes in the hemoglobin molecule. These structural changes result from variation in the oxygen partial pressure surrounding the blood cells and in certain other conditions. When the oxygen concentration is high, as it is in the capillaries of the lung alveoli, the hemoglobin can actually combine with more oxygen than it can when the oxygen concentration is low, as it is in the systemic capillaries in the body tissues. Thus, when the blood enters regions of low oxygen partial pressure, it is forced to give up or unload its oxygen because of its structural change under these conditions. The relationship of carrying capacity to surrounding oxygen concentration is shown by oxygen dissociation curves (Fig. 29-21). As these curves show, the lower the surrounding oxygen tension, the greater the quantity of oxygen released. This is an important characteristic because it allows more oxygen to be released to those tissues that need it most (have the lowest partial pressure of oxygen). More oxygen is loaded in the lungs and more unloaded in the tissues than if the combination and release depended on concentration gradients alone.

Another characteristic facilitating the release of oxygen to the tissues is the sensitivity of oxyhemoglobin to carbon dioxide. Carbon dioxide shifts the oxygen dissociation curve to the right (Fig. 29-21, *B*), a phenomenon that has been called the **Bohr effect** after the Danish scientist who first described it. Therefore, as carbon dioxide enters the blood from the respiring tissues, it encourages the release of additional oxygen from the hemoglobin. The opposite event occurs in the lungs; as carbon dioxide diffuses from the venous blood into the alveolar space, the oxygen dissociation curve shifts back to the left, allowing more oxygen to be loaded onto the hemoglobin.

Transport of carbon dioxide by the blood

The same blood that transports oxygen to the tissues from the lungs must carry carbon dioxide back to the lungs on its return trip. However, unlike oxygen, which is transported almost exclusively in combination with hemoglobin, carbon dioxide is transported in three major forms.

1. Most of the carbon dioxide, approximately 67%, is converted in the red blood cells into bicarbonate and hydrogen ions by undergoing the following reaction:

$$CO_2 + H_2O \rightleftharpoons H_2CO_3$$

Carbonic
acid

This reaction would normally proceed very slowly, but an enzyme in the red blood cells, **carbonic anhydrase,** catalyzes the reaction, enabling it to proceed almost instantly. As soon as carbonic acid forms, it instantly and almost completely ionizes as follows:

$$H_2CO_3 \rightleftharpoons HCO_3^- + H^+$$

Carbonic   Bicarbonate   Hydrogen
acid   ion   ion

The hydrogen ion is buffered by several buffer systems in the blood, thus preventing a severe decrease in blood pH. The bicarbonate ion remains in solution in the plasma and red blood cell water since, unlike carbon dioxide, bicarbonate is extremely soluble.

2. Another fraction of the carbon dioxide, approximately 25%, combines reversibly with hemoglobin. It is carried to the lungs where the hemoglobin releases it in exchange for oxygen.

3. A third small fraction of the carbon dioxide, approximately 8%, is carried as the physically dissolved gas in the plasma and red blood cells.

Unfortunately for humans and other higher animals, hemoglobin has an affinity for carbon monoxide that is about 200 times greater than its affinity for oxygen. Consequently, even when carbon monoxide is present in the atmosphere at lower concentrations than oxygen, it tends to displace oxygen from hemoglobin to form a stable compound called carboxyhemoglobin. Air containing only 0.2% carbon monoxide may be fatal. Because of their higher respiratory rate, children and small animals are poisoned more rapidly than adults. Carbon monoxide is becoming an atmospheric contaminant of ever-increasing proportions as the world's population and industrialization continue to increase rapidly.

_____ Summary

The fluid in the body, whether intracellular, plasma, or interstitial, is mostly water, but it has many substances dissolved in it, including electrolytes and proteins. Mammalian blood consists of the fluid plasma and the formed elements, including red and white blood cells and platelets. The plasma has many dissolved solids, as well as dissolved gases. Mammalian red blood cells lose their nucleus during their development and contain the oxygen-carrying pigment hemoglobin. White blood cells are important defensive elements. Platelets are vital in the process of clotting, necessary to prevent excess blood loss when the blood vessel is damaged. They release a series of factors that activate prothrombin to thrombin, an enzyme that causes fibrinogen to be changed to the gel form, fibrin.

In a closed circulatory system, the heart pumps blood into arteries, then into arterioles of smaller diameter, through the bed of fine capillaries, through venules, and finally through the veins, which lead back to the heart. In fishes, which have a two-chambered heart with a single atrium and a single ventricle, the blood is pumped to the gills and then directly to the systemic capillaries throughout the body without first returning to the heart. The four-chambered heart of birds and mammals is more efficient than the two-chambered heart of fishes because the blood is pumped through the capillary bed of the lungs by one ventricle, then returned to the heart and pumped through the systemic circulation by another ventricle. One-way flow of blood during the heart's contraction (systole) and relaxation (diastole) is ensured by valves between the atria and the ventricles and between the ventricles and the pulmonary arteries and the aorta. Although the heart can beat spontaneously, its rate is controlled by parasympathetic and sympathetic nerves from the central nervous system. The heart muscle uses a great deal of oxygen and has a well-developed coronary blood circulation.

The walls of arteries are thicker than those of veins, and the connective tissue in the walls of arteries allows them to expand during systole and contract during diastole. Normal arterial blood pressure (hydrostatic) of humans is 120 mm Hg in systole and 80 mm Hg in diastole. It decreases to about 40 mm Hg at the arteriolar end of the capillaries, about 15 mm Hg at the venule end of the capillaries, 10 mm Hg in the veins, and finally near zero at the right atrium. Because the capillary walls are permeable to water, and there is a net osmotic pressure owing to proteins in the plasma, water enters the surrounding tissue at the arteriole end and reenters the blood at the venule end of the capillaries. Not all the fluid reenters the blood at this point, but the remainder is collected by the lymphatic system and is returned to the blood through the thoracic duct.

Phagocytosis is one of the most important defense mechanisms in humans and most other animals. This process and the overall process of inflammation may be regarded as nonspecific defense mechanisms, but they are greatly influenced by the specific immune responses of vertebrates. The immune response depends on the sensitization of T and B lymphocytes by antigens. B lymphocytes give rise to plasma cells, which secrete large amounts of antibody into the blood (humoral immunity), while the antibody is retained in the cell membrane of T lymphocytes, giving rise to cell-mediated immunity. People have genetically determined antigens in the surfaces of their red blood cells (ABO blood groups and others); blood types must be compatible in transfusions, or the transfused blood will be agglutinated by antibodies in the recipient.

Very small animals can depend on diffusion between the external environment and their tissues or cytoplasm for transport of respiratory gases, but larger animals require specialized organs, such as gills, tracheae, or lungs, for this function. Gills and lungs provide an increased surface area for exchange of respiratory gases between the blood and the environment. Since simple solution of gases in the blood may be insufficient for respiratory needs, many animals have special respiratory pigments and other mechanisms to help transport oxygen and carbon dioxide. The pigment in vertebrates, hemoglobin, undergoes small structural changes that enable it to combine with more oxygen at higher oxygen concentrations than it can at lower oxygen concentrations. This makes it possible for hemoglobin to load up more oxygen in the lungs and unload more in the tissues than if the process depended on concentration gradients alone. Carbon dioxide is carried from the tissues to the lungs in the blood as the bicarbonate ion, in combination with hemoglobin, and as the dissolved gas.

Selected references

See also general references for Part Three, p. 837.

Baglioni, C., and T.W. Nilsen. 1981. The action of interferon at the molecular level. Am. Sci. 69:392-399.

Barrett, J.T. 1978. Textbook of immunology: an introduction to immunochemistry and immunobiology, ed. 3. St. Louis, The C.V. Mosby Co.

Bellanti, J.A. (ed.). 1979. Immunology: basic processes. Philadelphia, W.B. Saunders Co. *Eleven contributors; direct and factual account.*

Bier, O.G., W.D. da Silva, D. Gotze, and I. Mota. 1981. Fundamentals of immunology. New York, Springer-Verlag, Inc. *Comprehensive text.*

Brooks, S.M. 1973. Basic facts of body water and ions, ed. 3. New York, Springer Publishing Co., Inc. *An excellent elementary account of the fluid and electrolyte balance in the body.*

Chapman, G. 1967. The body fluids and their function. Institute of Biology's Studies in Biology No. 8. New York, St. Martin's Press, Inc. *Brief, comparative treatment of body fluids, their transport, and regulation.*

Clark, W.R. 1980. The experimental foundations of modern immunology. New York, John Wiley & Sons, Inc.

Comroe, J.H. 1974. Physiology of respiration, ed. 2. Chicago, Year Book Medical Publishers, Inc. *Standard, respected text on human respiration.*

Gowans, J.L. 1977. Cellular immunology. Carolina Biology Reader. Burlington, N.C., Carolina Biological Supply Co.

Mill, P.J. 1972. Respiration in the invertebrates. London, The Macmillan Press, Ltd. *Anatomy and physiology of respiratory systems, circulation, respiratory pigments, and control mechanisms. Comprehensive, amply illustrated.*

Negus, V. 1965. The biology of respiration. Edinburgh, E. & S. Livingstone, Ltd. *Comparative account of gas exchange with numerous interesting, often unique, illustrations.*

Randall, D.J., W.W. Burggren, A.P. Farrell, and M.S. Haswell. 1981. The evolution of air breathing in vertebrates. Cambridge, Eng., Cambridge University Press. *Traces the physiology of air breathing from aquatic ancestors.*

Selected *Scientific American* articles

Adolph, E.F. 1967. The heart's pacemaker. 216:32-37 (Mar.).

Buisseret, P.D. 1982. Allergy. 247:86-95 (Aug.). *Allergies occur when immune regulatory systems fail.*

Capra, J.D., and A.B. Edmundson. 1977. The antibody combining site. 236:50-59 (Jan.). *The details of the site on the antibody molecule that binds to the antigen have been worked out.*

Clarke, C.A. 1968. The prevention of "rhesus" babies. 217:46-52 (Nov.).

Comroe, J.H., Jr. 1966. The lung. 215:56-68 (Feb.). *Physiology of the human lung.*

Cooper, M.D., and A.R. Lawton, III. 1974. The development of the immune system. 231:58-72 (Nov.). *Review of the origin of cell-mediated and humoral immunity.*

Cunningham, B.A. 1977. The structure and function of histocompatability antigens. 237:96-107 (Oct.). *Histocompatability antigens are proteins on the cell surface that cause a grafted tissue to stimulate an immune reaction and be rejected.*

Doolittle, R.F. 1981. Fibrinogen and fibrin. 245:126-135 (Dec.). *Clot formation may be understood in the structure of proteins forming them.*

Jerne, N.K. 1973. The immune system. 229:52-59 (July).

Leder, P. 1982. The genetics of antibody diversity. 246:102-115 (May).

Mayer, M.M. 1973. The complement system. 229:54-66 (Nov.). *The complex series of reactions of the components of complement with bound antibody to produce lysis of cells is described.*

Mayerson, H.S. 1963. The lymphatic system. 208:80-90 (June). *The lymphatics are a crucial "second" circulatory system that picks up fluids leaking from the bloodstream.*

McKusick, V.A. 1965. The royal hemophilia. 213:88-95 (Aug.). *Hemophilia and the gene that causes it are traced through the descendants of Queen Victoria.*

Milstein, C. 1980. Monoclonal antibodies. 243:66-74 (Oct.). *What they are and how they are produced.*

Perutz, M.F. 1978. Hemoglobin structure and respiratory transport. 240:92-125 (Dec.). *Hemoglobin transports oxygen and carbon dioxide between the lungs and tissues by clicking back and forth between two structures. Perutz and J.C. Kendrew won the Nobel Prize in 1962 for discovering the structure of hemoglobin.*

Rose, N.R. 1981. Autoimmune diseases. 244:80-103 (Feb.).

Schmidt-Nielsen, K. 1971. How birds breathe. 225:73-79 (Dec.).

Wiggers, C.J. 1957. The heart. 196:74-87 (May). *The development, structure, and function of a remarkable organ.*

Wood, J.E. 1968. The venous system. 218:86-96 (Jan.).

Zucker, M.B. 1980. The functioning of the blood platelets. 242:86-103 (June). *The small blood elements that act to stop blood flow from a wound also perform complex roles in health and disease.*

Zweifach, B.W. 1959. The microcirculation of the blood. 200:54-60 (Jan.). *Describes the anatomy and function of the capillary bed that serves the body's tissues.*

CHAPTER 30

INTERNAL FLUIDS
Homeostasis and Excretion

Scanning electron micrograph of the microcirculation of a mammalian kidney. Several spherical glomeruli, the kidney's pressure filters where urine formation begins, are evident. Each glomerulus is a coiled tuft of capillaries, which in the living animal is enclosed within a double-walled Bowman's capsule. This preparation is a cast that was prepared by infusing a resin compound into the circulation and allowing it to polymerize and harden. The surrounding tissues were then dissolved away to reveal a replica of the circulation. (×230.)

At the beginning of the preceding chapter we described the double-layered environment of the body's cells: the extracellular fluid, which immediately surrounds the cells, and the external environment of the outside world.

The life-supporting metabolic activities that occur within a body's cells can proceed only as long as they are bathed by a protective extracellular fluid of relatively constant composition. Yet there are many activities that threaten to throw the system out of balance. On the inside, metabolic activities within the cell require a steady supply of materials, and these activities turn out a continuous flow of products and wastes. On the outside, materials are constantly being exchanged between the plasma and the external environment.

Obviously body composition is a dynamic rather than a static thing; it operates as a **dynamic steady state.** This means that fixity of composition is maintained despite the continuous shifting of components within the system. This kind of internal regulation is called **homeostasis** (Fig. 30-1). The internal environment is not kept absolutely constant, however, but rather is held within limits of fluctuations that the body can tolerate without disruption of function.

Homeostasis is maintained by the coordinated activities of numerous body systems, such as the nervous system, the endocrine system, and especially the organs that serve as sites of exchange with the external environment, which include the kidneys, lungs or gills, alimentary canal, and skin. Through these organs oxygen, foodstuffs, minerals, and other constituents of the body fluids enter, water is exchanged, and metabolic wastes are eliminated.

The kidney is the chief regulator of the body fluids. It is popularly regarded strictly as a sanitation system that serves to rid the body of assorted metabolic wastes. But, in fact, it is as much a regulatory organ as an excretory organ. It is responsible for individually monitoring and regulating the concentrations of body water, salt ions in the blood, and other major and minor body fluid constituents. In its task of fine-tuning the composition of the internal environment, the kidney is assisted by the other organs of exchange, such as the lungs, skin, and digestive tract, as well as by many internal mechanisms.

Several other specialized structures have evolved among the vertebrates that assist in body fluid regulation in various environments, for example, the salt-secreting cells of fish gills and the salt glands of birds and reptiles.

We will look first at the problems of controlling the internal environment of animals living in aquatic habitats. Then we will briefly examine how these problems are solved by terrestrial animals. Finally, we will look at the excretory organs themselves and consider how they function.

Figure 30-1

Walter Bradford Cannon (1871-1945), Harvard professor of physiology who coined the term "homeostasis" and developed the concept originated by French physiologist Claude Bernard.

From Fulton, J.F., and L.G. Wilson. 1966. Selected readings in the history of physiology. Springfield, Ill., Charles C Thomas, Publisher.

WATER AND OSMOTIC REGULATION
How Aquatic Animals Meet Problems of Salt and Water Balance

Marine invertebrates

Most marine invertebrates are in osmotic equilibrium with their seawater environment. They have body surfaces that are permeable to salts and water so that their body fluid concentration rises or falls in conformity with changes in concentrations of seawater. Because such animals are incapable of regulating their body fluid osmotic pressure, they are referred to as **osmotic conformers.** Invertebrates living in the open sea are seldom exposed to osmotic fluctuations because the

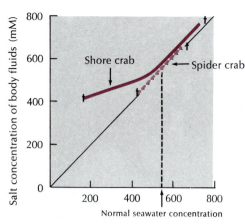

Figure 30-2

Salt concentration of body fluids of two crabs as affected by variations in the seawater concentration. The 45-degree line represents equal concentration between body fluids and seawater. Since the spider crab cannot regulate its body-fluid salt concentration, it conforms to whatever changes happen in the external seawater environment. The shore crab, however, can regulate osmotic concentration of its body fluids to some degree because in dilute seawater it can hold its body-fluid concentration above the seawater concentration. For example, when seawater is 200 mM, the shore crab's body fluids are approximately 430 mM. Crosses at ends of lines indicate tolerance limits of each species.

ocean is a highly stable environment. Oceanic invertebrates have, in fact, very limited abilities to withstand osmotic change. If they should be exposed to dilute seawater, they die quickly because their body cells cannot tolerate dilution and are helpless to prevent it. These animals are restricted to living in a narrow salinity range and are said to be **stenohaline** (Gr., *stenos*, narrow, + *hals*, salt). An example is the marine spider crab, represented in Fig 30-2.

Conditions along the coasts and in estuaries and river mouths are much less constant than those of the open ocean. Here animals must be able to withstand large and often abrupt salinity changes as the tides move in and out and mix with fresh water draining from rivers. These animals are referred to as **euryhaline** (Gr., *eurys*, broad, + *hals*, salt), meaning that they can survive a wide range of salinity change. Most coastal invertebrates also show varying powers of **osmotic regulation.** For example, the brackish-water shore crab can resist body fluid dilution by dilute (brackish) seawater (Fig. 30-2). Although the body fluid concentration falls, it does so less rapidly than the fall in seawater concentration. This crab is a **hyperosmotic regulator** because in a dilute environment it can maintain the concentration of its blood above that of the surrounding water.

What is the advantage of hyperosmotic regulation over osmotic conformity, and how is this regulation accomplished? The advantage is that by regulating against excessive dilution, thus protecting the body cells from extreme changes, these crabs can successfully live in the physically unstable but biologically rich coastal environment. Their powers of regulation are limited, however, since if the water is highly diluted, their regulation fails and they die.

To understand how the brackish-water shore crab and other coastal invertebrates achieve hyperosmotic regulation, let us examine the problems they face. First, the salt concentration of the internal fluids is greater than in the dilute seawater outside. This causes a steady osmotic influx of water. As with the membrane osmometer placed in a sugar solution (p. 85), water diffuses inward because it is more concentrated outside than inside. The shore crab is not nearly as permeable as a membrane osmometer—most of its shelled body surface is, in fact, almost impermeable to water—but the thin respiratory surfaces of the gills are highly permeable. Obviously the crab cannot insulate its gills with an impermeable hide and still breathe. The problem is solved by removing the excess water through the action of the kidney (the antennal gland located in the crab's head).

The second problem is salt loss. Again, because the animal is saltier than its environment, it cannot avoid loss of ions by outward diffusion across the gills. Salt is also lost in the urine. This problem is solved by special salt-secreting cells in the gills that can actively remove ions from the dilute seawater and move them into the blood, thus maintaining the internal osmotic concentration. This is an **active transport** process that requires energy because ions must be transported against a concentration gradient, that is, from a lower salt concentration (in the dilute seawater) to an already higher one (in the blood).

Invasion of fresh water

Some 400 million years ago, during the Silurian and Lower Devonian periods, the major groups of jawed fishes began to penetrate brackish-water estuaries and then gradually freshwater rivers. Before them lay a new, unexploited habitat already stocked with food in the form of insects and other invertebrates, which had preceded them into fresh water. However, the advantages of this new habitat were traded off for a tough physiological challenge: the necessity of developing effective osmotic regulation.

Freshwater animals must keep the salt concentration of their body fluids higher than that of the water. Water enters their bodies osmotically, and salt is lost by diffusion outward. Their problems are similar to those of the brackish-water crab, but more severe and unremitting. Fresh water is much more dilute than are coastal estuaries, and there is no retreat, no salty sanctuary into which the freshwater animal can retire for osmotic relief. It must and has become a permanent and highly efficient hyperosmotic regulator.

The scaled and mucus-covered body surface of a fish is about as waterproof as any flexible surface can be. The water that inevitably enters by osmosis across the gills is pumped out by the kidney. Although the kidney is able to make a very dilute urine, some salt is lost; this is replaced by salt in food and by active absorption of salt (primarily sodium and chloride) across the gills. The bony fishes that inhabit lakes and streams today are so well adapted to their dilute surroundings that they need expend little energy to regulate themselves osmotically. Osmotic regulation in fishes is described on p. 542 and illustrated in Fig. 23-27, p. 543.

Crayfishes, aquatic insect larvae, mussels, and other freshwater animals are also hyperosmotic regulators and face the same hazards as freshwater fishes; they tend to gain too much water and lose too much salt. Not surprisingly, all of these forms solved these problems in the same direct way that fishes did. They excrete the excess water as urine, and they actively absorb salt from the water by some salt-transporting mechanism on the body surface.

Amphibians, when they are living in water, also must compensate for salt loss by actively absorbing salt from the water (Fig. 30-3). They use their skin for this purpose. Physiologists learned some years ago that pieces of frog skin continue to transport sodium and chloride actively for hours when removed and placed in a specially balanced salt solution. Fortunately for biologists, but unfortunately for frogs, these animals were so easily collected and maintained in the laboratory that frog skin became a favorite membrane system for studies of ion-transport phenomena.

Marine fishes

The great families of marine bony fishes maintain the salt concentration of their body fluids at approximately one-third that of seawater (body fluids = 0.3 to 0.4 M; seawater = 1 M). Obviously they are osmotic regulators. Bony fishes living in the oceans today are descendants of earlier freshwater bony fishes that moved back into the sea during the Triassic period approximately 200 million years ago. The return to their ancestral sea was probably prompted by unfavorable climatic conditions on land and the deterioration of freshwater habitats, but we can only guess at the reasons. During the many millions of years that the freshwater fishes were adapting themselves so well to their environment, they established a body fluid concentration equivalent to approximately one-third that of seawater, thus setting the pattern for all the vertebrates that were to evolve later, whether aquatic, terrestrial, or aerial. The ionic composition of vertebrate body fluid is remarkably similar to that of dilute seawater too, a fact that is undoubtedly related to their marine heritage.

When some of the freshwater bony fishes of the Triassic period ventured back to the sea, they encountered a new set of problems. Having a much lower internal osmotic concentration than the seawater around them, they lost water

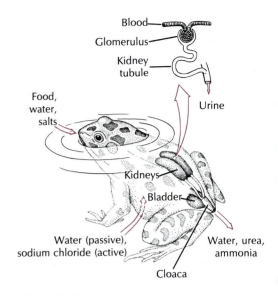

Figure 30-3

Water and solute exchange in a frog. Water enters the highly permeable skin and is excreted by the kidney. The skin also actively transports ions (sodium chloride) from the environment. The kidney forms a dilute urine by reabsorbing sodium chloride. Urine flows into the urinary bladder, where, during temporary storage, most of the remaining sodium chloride is removed and returned to the blood.

Modified from Webster, D., and H. Webster. 1974. Comparative vertebrate morphology. New York, Academic Press, Inc.

When we express seawater or body fluid concentration in molarity, we are saying that the osmotic strength is equivalent to the molar concentration of an ideal solute having the same osmotic strength. In fact, seawater and animal body fluids are not ideal solutions because they contain electrolytes that dissociate in solution. A 1 M solution of sodium chloride (which dissociates in solution) has a much greater osmotic strength than a 1 M solution of glucose, an ideal solute that does not dissociate in solution. Consequently, biologists usually express the osmotic strength of a biological solution in osmolarity rather than in molarity. A 1 osmolar solution exerts the same osmotic pressure as a 1 M solution of a nonelectrolyte.

Table 30-1   Water Balance in the Human and the Kangaroo Rat, a Desert Rodent

	Human (%)	Kangaroo rat (%)
Gains		
Drinking	48	0
Free water in food	40	10
Metabolic water	12	90
Losses		
Urine	60	25
Evaporation (lungs and skin)	34	70
Feces	6	5

Data in part from Schmidt-Nielsen, K. 1972. How animals work. New York, Cambridge University Press.

The high concentration of urea in the blood of sharks and their kin—more than 100 times as high as in mammals—could not be tolerated by most other vertebrates. In the latter, such high concentrations of urea disrupt the peptide bonds of proteins, altering protein configuration. Sharks have adapted biochemically to the presence of the urea that permeates all their body fluids, even penetrating freely into the cells. So accommodated are the elasmobranchs to urea that their tissues cannot function without it, and the heart will stop beating in its absence. Certain other vertebrates retain urea. In the lungfish *Protopterus,* which can estivate for months in a cocoon during the dry season, urea builds up to a level approaching that of sharks. The crab-eating frog of Southeast Asia, which lives in an unfroglike manner in salty habitats, has solved its osmotic problem like sharks by allowing urea to accumulate to very high levels.

and gained salt. Indeed the marine body fish literally risks drying out, much like a desert mammal deprived of water. Osmotic regulation of the marine bony fishes is described on p. 542.

In brief, to compensate for water loss, the marine teleost drinks seawater. This is absorbed from the intestine, and the major sea salt, sodium chloride, is carried by the blood to the gills, where specialized salt-secreting cells transport it back into the surrounding sea. The ions remaining in the intestinal residue, especially magnesium, sulfate, and calcium, are voided with the feces or excreted by the kidney. In this roundabout way, marine fishes rid themselves of the excess sea salts they have drunk, resulting in a net gain of water, which replaces the water lost by osmosis. Samuel Taylor Coleridge's ancient mariner, surrounded by "water, water, everywhere, nor any drop to drink" would undoubtedly have been tormented even more had he known of the marine fishes' simple solution for thirst. A marine fish carefully regulates the amount of seawater it drinks, consuming only enough to replace water loss and no more.

The cartilaginous sharks and rays (elasmobranchs) solve their water balance problems in a completely different way. This primitive group is almost totally marine. The salt composition of shark's blood is similar to that of the bony fishes, but the blood also carries a large content of organic compounds, especially urea and trimethylamine oxide. Urea is, of course, a metabolic waste that most animals quickly excrete in the urine. The shark kidney, however, conserves urea, causing it to accumulate in the blood. The blood urea, added to the usual blood electrolytes, raises the blood osmotic pressure to slightly exceed that of seawater. In this way the sharks and their kin turn an otherwise useless waste material into an asset, eliminating the osmotic problem encountered by the marine bony fishes.

How Terrestrial Animals Maintain Salt and Water Balance

The problems of living in an aquatic environment seem small indeed compared with the problems of life on land. Since our bodies are mostly water, all metabolic activities proceed in water, and life itself originated in water, it seems that animals were meant to stay in water. Yet many animals, like the plants preceding them, moved onto land, carrying their watery composition with them. Once on land, the terrestrial animals continued their adaptive radiation, undaunted by the threat of desiccation, until they became abundant even in some of the most arid parts of the earth.

Terrestrial animals lose water by evaporation from the lungs and body surface, excretion in the urine, and elimination in the feces. Such losses are replaced by water in the food, drinking water if it is available, and formation of **metabolic water** in the cells by the oxidation of foodstuffs, especially carbohydrates. In some desert rodents, metabolic water may constitute most of the animals' water gain.

Particularly revealing is a comparison of water balance in the human being, a nondesert mammal that drinks water, with that of the kangaroo rat, a desert rodent that may drink no water at all (Table 30-1).

The kangaroo rat gains all of its water from its food (90% as metabolic water derived from the oxidation of foodstuffs, 10% as free moisture in the food). Even though humans eat foods with a much higher water content than the dry seeds that comprise much of the kangaroo rat's diet, people must still drink half their total water requirement.

The excretion of wastes presents a special problem in water conservation. The primary end product of protein breakdown is ammonia, a highly toxic material. Fishes can easily excrete ammonia across their gills, since there is an abundance of water to wash it away. The terrestrial insects, reptiles, and birds have no convenient way to rid themselves of toxic ammonia; instead they convert it into uric acid, a nontoxic, almost insoluble compound. This enables them to excrete a semisolid urine with little water loss. The use of uric acid has another important benefit. The reptiles and birds lay amniotic eggs enclosing the embryos, their stores of food and water, and whatever wastes accumulate during development. By converting ammonia to uric acid, the developing embryo's waste can be precipitated into solid crystals, which are stored harmlessly within the egg until hatching.

Marine birds and turtles have evolved a unique solution for excreting the large loads of salt eaten with their food. Located above each eye is a special **salt gland** capable of excreting a highly concentrated solution of sodium chloride—up to twice the concentration of seawater. In birds the salt solution runs out the nares (see p. 616). Marine lizards and turtles, like Alice in Wonderland's Mock Turtle, shed their salt gland secretion as salty tears. Salt glands are important accessory organs of salt excretion in these animals because their kidney cannot produce a concentrated urine, as can the mammalian kidney.

INVERTEBRATE EXCRETORY STRUCTURES

In such a variety of groups as make up the invertebrates, it is hardly surprising that there is a great variety of morphological structures serving as excretory organs. Many protozoa and some freshwater sponges have special excretory organelles called contractile vacuoles. The more advanced invertebrates have excretory organs that are basically tubular structures, forming urine by first producing an ultrafiltrate or fluid secretion of the blood. This enters the proximal end of the tubule and is modified continuously as it flows down the tubule. The final product is urine.

Given ample water to drink, humans can tolerate extremely high temperatures while preventing a rise in body temperature. Our ability to keep cool by evaporation was impressively demonstrated more than 200 years ago by a British scientist who remained for 45 minutes in a room heated to 260° F (126° C). A steak he carried in with him was thoroughly cooked, but he remained uninjured and his body temperature did not rise. Sweating rates may exceed 3 liters of water per hour under such conditions and cannot be long tolerated unless the lost water is replaced by drinking. Without water, a human continues to sweat unabated until the water deficit exceeds 10% of the body weight, when collapse occurs. With a water deficit of 12% a human is unable to swallow even if offered water, and death occurs when the water deficit reaches about 15% to 20%. Few people can survive more than a day or two in a desert without water. Thus, people are not physiologically well adapted for desert climates but prosper there nonetheless by virtue of their technological culture.

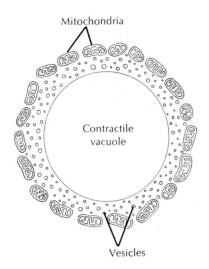

Figure 30-4

Contractile vacuole of *Amoeba proteus*, surrounded by a layer of tiny vesicles that fill with fluid, then empty into the vacuole. The layer of vesicles is bounded by mitochondria that probably provide energy for adjusting the salt content of the tiny vesicles.

Contractile Vacuole

The tiny, spherical, intracellular vacuole of protozoa and freshwater sponges is not a true excretory organ, since ammonia and other nitrogenous wastes of metabolism readily leave the cell by direct diffusion across the cell membrane into the surrounding water. The contractile vacuole is really an organ of water balance. Because the cytoplasm of freshwater protozoa is considerably saltier than their freshwater environment, they tend to draw water into themselves by osmosis. In *Amoeba proteus* this excess water collects in numerous tiny vesicles surrounding the single thin membrane of the contractile vacuole (Fig. 30-4). These vesicles then fuse with the vacuolar membrane, emptying their contents (a weak salt solution) into the contractile vacuole. This grows larger as water accumulates within it. Finally the vacuole is emptied through a pore on the surface, and the cycle is rhythmically repeated. Although the mechanism for filling is not fully understood, it is noteworthy that a layer of mitochondria surrounds the contractile vacuole. These are believed to provide energy for reabsorbing salts from the tiny vesicles as they are formed. This mechanism would create a hypoosmotic solution for excretion, while conserving valuable salts.

In *Paramecium* the contractile vacuole is a more complex structure, having a permanent pore to the exterior and several ampullae and canals radiating out from the contractile vacuole (Fig. 8-21, p. 193).

Contractile vacuoles are common in freshwater protozoa but rare or absent in marine protozoa, which are isosmotic with seawater and consequently neither lose nor gain too much water.

Nephridium

The nephridium is the most common type of invertebrate excretory organ. All nephridia are tubular structures, but there are large differences in degree of complexity. One of the simplest arrangements is the flame cell system (or **protonephridia**) of the acoelomate and several pseudocoelomate phyla.

In *Planaria* and other flatworms the protonephridium takes the form of two highly branched systems of tubules distributed throughout the body (Fig. 30-5). Fluid enters the system through specialized "flame" cells, moves slowly into and down the tubules, and is excreted through pores that open at intervals on the body surface. It is believed that fluid containing wastes enters the flame bulb from the surrounding tissues by **pinocytosis** ("cell drinking"). In this process fluid-filled vesicles are formed just under the outer cell surface. The vesicles are transported across the cell and set free into the ciliated lumen of the flame cell. Here, the rhythmical beat of the ciliary tuft (the "flame") creates a negative fluid pressure that drives the fluid into the tubular portion of the system. It is probable that, as the fluid passes down the tubules, the tubular epithelial cells add certain waste materials to the tubular fluid (secretion) and withdraw valuable materials from it (reabsorption) to complete the formation of urine.

The flame cell system, like the contractile vacuole of protozoa, is primarily a water balance system, since it is best developed in free-living freshwater forms. Branched flame cell systems are typical of acoelomate and pseudocoelomate invertebrates that lack circulatory systems. Since there is no circulation to carry wastes to a compact excretory organ such as the kidney of higher invertebrates and vertebrates, the flame cell system must be distributed to reach the cells directly.

The protonephridium just described is a **closed** system; that is, the urine is formed from a fluid that must first enter the tubule by being transported across the flame cells. Another type of nephridium, typical of coelomate invertebrate phyla such as the annelids, molluscs, sipunculids, brachiopods, and phoronids, is the **open,** or "true," nephridium (**metanephridium**). The earthworm *Lumbricus* has paired nephridia in every segment of the body, except the first three and the last one (Fig. 14-5, p. 346). Each nephridium occupies parts of two successive segments. In the earthworm each nephridium is a tiny, self-contained "kidney" that drains to the outside through pores (**nephridiopores**) in the body wall.

Coelomic fluid containing wastes to be excreted is swept into a ciliated, funnel-like opening (**nephrostome**) of the nephridium and carried through a long, twisted tubule of increasing diameter. It then enters a bladder and is finally expelled through a nephridiopore to the outside. The nephridial tubule is surrounded by an extensive network of blood vessels. Solutes, especially sodium and chloride, are reabsorbed from the formative urine during its travel through the tubule. The addition of the blood-vascular network to the annelid nephridium makes it a much more versatile and effective system than the flame cell system. However, the basic process of urine formation is the same: fluid flows continuously through a tubule while materials are added here and taken away there, until urine is formed.

Arthropod Kidney

The **antennal glands** of crustaceans form a single, paired tubular structure located in the ventral part of the head. Their structure and function are described on p. 388. These excretory devices are an advanced design of the basic nephridial organ. However, they lack open nephrostomes. Instead, a protein-free filtrate of the blood (ultrafiltrate) is formed in the end sac by the hydrostatic pressure of the blood. In the tubular portion of the gland, the filtrate is modified by the selective reabsorption of certain salts and the active secretion of others. Thus, crustaceans have excretory organs that are basically vertebrate like in the functional sequence of urine formation.

Insects and spiders have a unique excretory system consisting of **malpighian tubules** that operate in conjunction with specialized glands in the wall of the rectum (Fig. 17-18, p. 418). The thin, elastic, blind malpighian tubules are closed and lack an arterial supply. Consequently, urine formation cannot be initiated by blood ultrafiltration as in the crustaceans and vertebrates. Instead, salts, largely potassium, are actively secreted into the tubules. This primary secretion of ions creates an osmotic drag that pulls water, solutes, and waste materials into the tubule. The fluid, or "urine," then drains from the tubules into the intestine, where specialized rectal glands actively reabsorb most of the potassium and water, leaving behind wastes such as uric acid. This unique excretory system is ideally suited for life in dry environments. We must assume that it has contributed to the success of insects, the most abundant and widespread group of land animals.

VERTEBRATE KIDNEY

The ancestral vertebrate kidney is believed to have extended the length of the coelomic cavity and to have been made up of segmentally arranged uriniferous tubules. Each tubule opened at one end into the coelom by a nephrostome and at the other end into a common archinephric duct. Such a kidney has been called an

Figure 30-5

Flame cell system of *Planaria*.

archinephros, or **holonephros,** and is found in the embryos of hagfishes (Fig. 30-6).

Kidneys of higher vertebrates developed from this primitive plan. During embryonic development of vertebrates, there is a succession of three developmental stages of kidneys: **pronephros, mesonephros,** and **metanephros.** In all vertebrate embryos, the pronephros is the first and most primitive kidney to appear. As its name implies, it is located anteriorly in the body. It becomes the persistent kidney of adult hagfishes. In all other vertebrates it degenerates during development and is replaced by a more centrally located and more structurally advanced kidney, the mesonephros. The mesonephros becomes the persistent kidney of adult fishes and amphibians. But in the developing embryos of amniotes (reptiles, birds, and mammals), the mesonephros is replaced in turn by the metanephros. The metanephros develops behind the mesonephros and is structurally and functionally the most advanced of the three kidney types. Thus, three kidneys are formed in succession, each more advanced and each located more caudally than its predecessor.

___ Vertebrate Kidney Function

The kidneys of humans and other vertebrates play a critical role in the body's economy. Their failure means death; in this respect they are neither more nor less important than are the heart, lungs, and liver. The kidney is a part of many interlocking mechanisms that maintain **homeostasis**—constancy of the internal environment. However, the kidney's share in this regulatory council is an especially large one. It must individually monitor and regulate most of the major constituents of the blood and several minor constituents as well. In addition, it labors to remove a variety of potentially harmful substances that animals deliberately or unconsciously eat, drink, or inhale.

Perhaps even more remarkable is the way in which the kidney does its job. These small organs, which in humans weigh less than 0.5% of the body weight, receive nearly 25% of the total cardiac output, amounting to approximately 2000 liters of blood per day! This vast blood flow is channeled to approximately 2 million **nephrons,** which comprise the bulk of the two human kidneys. Each nephron is a tiny excretory unit consisting of a pressure filter (**glomerulus**) and a long **nephric tubule.** Urine formation begins in the glomerulus where an ultrafiltrate of the blood is squeezed into the nephric tubule by the hydrostatic blood pressure. The ultrafiltrate then flows steadily down the twisted tubule. During its travel some substances are added to the ultrafiltrate and others are subtracted from it. The final product of this process is urine.

All mammalian kidneys are paired structures that lie embedded in fat, anchored against the dorsal abdominal wall. The two **ureters,** 25 to 30 cm (10 to 12 inches) long in humans, extend from the **renal pelvis** to the dorsal surface of the **urinary bladder.** Urine is discharged from the bladder by way of the single **urethra** (Fig. 30-7). In the male the urethra is the terminal portion of the reproductive system as well as of the excretory system. In the female the urethra is solely excretory in function, opening to the outside just anterior to the vagina.

Since each of the thousands of nephrons in the kidney forms urine independently, each is in a way a tiny, self-contained kidney that produces a minuscule amount of urine—perhaps only a few nanoliters per hour. This amount, multiplied by the number of nephrons in the kidney, produces the total urine flow. The

Pronephros: Functional kidney in adult hagfish and embryonic fishes and amphibians: fleeting existence in embryonic reptiles, birds, and mammals

Archinephros: Ancestral prototype of vertebrate kidney and kidney found in embryo of hagfish; from prototype, three successive kidneys evolved during vertebrate evolution

Gonad

Tubules with open nephrostomes

Nephrogenic plate

Archinephric duct

no conection

Pronephros: Functional kidney in adult hagfish and embryonic fishes and amphibians: fleeting existence in embryonic reptiles, birds, and mammals

Pronephros

Gonad

Pronephric tubules with nephrostomes

Pronephric duct

Figure 30-6

Evolution of male vertebrate kidney from archinephric prototype. *Red,* Functional structures. *Light red,* Degenerative or undeveloped parts.

Mesonephros: Functional kidney of adult lampreys, fishes, and amphibians; transient function *of hagfish* in embryonic reptiles, birds, and mammals

inferior vena cava *aorta*

Adrenal glands

renal arteries & vein on each kidney

Kidney

Ureter

Figure 30-7

Urinary system of the human male.

Bladder

Urethra

Degenerative pronephric tubules

Testis

Epididymis (derived from mesonephric tubules)

Mesonephric tubules with glomeruli

conects

area of genital system

Metanephros: Functional kidney of adult reptiles, birds, and mammals

Testis

Epididymis

Degenerative pronephric and mesonephric tubules

Metanephric kidney

Ureter

Vas deferens (wolffian duct)

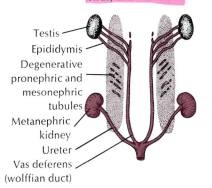

kidney is an "in parallel" system of independent units. However, these "independent" nephrons actually work together to create large osmotic gradients in the kidney medulla. This makes it possible for the mammalian kidney to concentrate urine whose salt concentration is well above that of the blood.

As previously indicated, the nephron, with its pressure filter and tubule, is intimately associated with the blood circulation (Fig. 30-8). Blood from the aorta is delivered to the kidney by way of the large **renal artery,** which breaks up into a branching system of smaller arteries. The arterial blood flows to each nephron through an **afferent arteriole** to the **glomerulus** (glo-mer′ yoo-lus), which is a tuft of blood capillaries enclosed within a thin, cuplike **Bowman's capsule.** Blood leaves the glomerulus via the **efferent arteriole.** This vessel immediately branches into an extensive system of capillaries, the **peritubular capillaries,** which completely surround the nephric tubules. Finally the blood from these many capillaries is collected by veins that unite to form the **renal vein.** This vein returns the blood to the vena cava.

Bowman's capsule

Glomerulus

Efferent arteriole

Afferent arteriole

Juxtaglomerular apparatus

Intralobular artery and vein (connect to renal artery and vein)

Proximal convoluted tubule

Distal convoluted tubule

Capillaries surrounding tubules

Ascending limb of Henle's loop

Descending limb of Henle's loop

Collecting tubule

Figure 30-8

Structure of a nephron and collecting duct of human kidney.

Glomerular filtration

Let us now return to the glomerulus, where the process of urine formation begins. The glomerulus acts as a specialized mechanical filter in which a protein-free filtrate resembling plasma is driven by the blood pressure across the capillary walls and into the fluid-filled space of Bowman's capsule. As shown in Fig. 30-9, the net filtration pressure is the difference between the blood pressure in the glomerular capillaries, believed to be approximately 45 mm Hg, and the opposing colloid osmotic and hydrostatic back pressures. Most important of these negative pressures is the colloid (protein) osmotic pressure, which is created because the proteins are too large to pass the glomerular membrane. The unequal distribution of protein causes the water concentration of the plasma to be less than the water concentration of the ultrafiltrate in Bowman's capsule. The osmotic gradient created, approximately 25 mm Hg, opposes filtration. Although small, a net filtration pressure of 10 mm Hg is sufficient to force the ultrafiltrate that is formed down the nephric tubule.

The nephric tubule consists of several segments. The first segment, the **proximal convoluted tubule,** leads into a long, thin-walled, hairpin loop called the **loop of Henle** (Fig. 30-8). This loop drops deep into the medulla of the kidney and then returns to the cortex to join the third segment, the **distal convoluted tubule.** The collecting duct empties into the kidney **pelvis,** a cavity that collects the urine before it passes into the **ureter,** on its way to the **urinary bladder** (Fig. 30-7).

Tubular modification of the formative urine

The ultrafiltrate that enters this complex tubular system must undergo extensive modification before it becomes urine. Approximately 200 liters of filtrate is formed each day by the average person's kidneys. Obviously the loss of this volume of body water, not to mention the many other valuable materials present in the filtrate, cannot be tolerated. How does tubular action convert the plasma filtrate into urine?

Two general processes are involved: **tubular reabsorption** and **tubular secretion.** Since the nephric tubules are at all points in close contact with the peritubular capillaries, materials can be transferred from the tubular lumen to the capillary blood plasma (tubular reabsorption) or from the blood plasma to the tubular lumen (tubular secretion).

Tubular reabsorption

The plasma contains a great variety of ions and molecules. With the exception of the plasma proteins, which are too large to pass the glomerular filter, all the plasma components are filtered and most are reabsorbed. Some vital materials, such as glucose and amino acids, are completely reabsorbed. Others, such as sodium, chloride, and most other minerals, undergo variable reabsorption. That is, some are strongly reabsorbed and others weakly reabsorbed, depending on the body's need to conserve each mineral. Much of this reabsorption is by **active transport,** in which cellular energy is used to transport materials from the tubular fluid, across the cell, and into the peritubular blood that returns them to the general circulation.

For most substances there is an upper limit to the amount of substance that can be reabsorbed. This upper limit is termed the **transport maximum** for that substance. For example, glucose is normally completely reabsorbed by the kidney because the transport maximum for the glucose reabsorptive mechanism is well above the amount of glucose normally present in the plasma filtrate.

Unlike glucose, most of the mineral ions are excreted in the urine in variable amounts. Their excretion is regulated. The reabsorption of sodium, the dominant cation in the plasma, illustrates the flexibility of the reabsorption process. Approximately 600 g of sodium is filtered by the human kidneys every 24 hours. Nearly all of this is reabsorbed, but the exact amount is precisely matched to sodium intake. With a sodium chloride intake of 4 g a day, the kidney excretes 4 g and reabsorbs 596 g each day. A person on a low-salt diet of 0.3 g of sodium chloride a day still maintains salt balance because only 0.3 g escapes reabsorption. With a very high salt intake, above 10 g a day, the kidney cannot excrete sodium

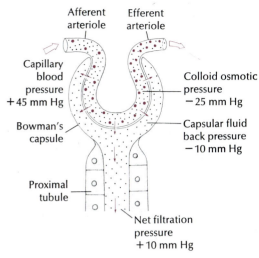

Figure 30-9

Pressures determining the net filtration pressure in a glomerulus. The net filtration pressure is the blood hydrostatic pressure, less the blood osmotic pressure resulting from plasma proteins, less the capsular hydrostatic pressure.

In the disease diabetes mellitus ("sweet running through"), glucose rises to abnormally high concentrations in the blood plasma (hyperglycemia) because the hormone insulin, which enables the body cells to take up glucose, is deficient. As the blood glucose rises above a normal level of about 100 mg/100 ml of plasma, the concentration of glucose in the filtrate also rises, and more glucose must be reabsorbed by the proximal tubule. Eventually a point is reached (about 300 mg/100 ml of plasma) at which the reabsorptive capacity of the tubular cells is saturated. This is the transport maximum for glucose. Should the plasma glucose continue to rise, glucose spills over into the urine. In untreated diabetes the victim's urine tastes sweet, thirst is unrelenting, and the body wastes away despite a large food intake. In England the disease for centuries was appropriately called the "pissing evil."

as fast as it enters. The unexcreted sodium chloride holds additional water in the body fluids, and the person begins to gain weight. (The salt intake of the average American is about 10 g a day, approximately 20 times more than the body really needs, and three times more than is considered acceptable for those predisposed to high blood pressure.)

It may seem odd that the kidney can excrete only 10 g of sodium chloride per day when approximately 600 g is filtered. It would appear that more sodium could be excreted by simply allowing more to escape tubular reabsorption. Unfortunately for salt lovers, however, the reabsorption of salt is not completely flexible. Some 80% to 85% of the salt and water filtered is reabsorbed in the proximal tubule; this is an **obligatory reabsorption** because it is governed entirely by a physical process (the osmotic pressure of the solutes) and cannot be controlled physiologically. In the distal tubule, however, sodium reabsorption is controlled by **aldosterone**, a steroid hormone of the adrenal cortex. This is called **facultative reabsorption,** meaning that the reabsorption can be adjusted physiologically according to need. We can say that proximal reabsorption is involuntary and distal reabsorption is voluntary, although, of course, we are not aware of the adjustments the kidney is performing on our behalf. The flexibility of distal reabsorption varies considerably in different animals: it is restricted in humans but very broad in many rodents. These differences have appeared because selective pressures during evolution have resulted in rodents adapted for dry environments. They must conserve water and at the same time excrete considerable sodium. Humans, however, were not designed to accommodate the large salt appetites many have. Our closest relatives, the great apes, are vegetarians with an average salt intake of less than 0.5 g a day.

As mentioned previously, salt reabsorption is controlled by the steroid hormone aldosterone. But what regulates the release of aldosterone from the adrenal cortex? Experiments performed to answer this question have revealed a remarkable system of delicate homeostatic control. The secretion of aldosterone is regulated mainly by the enzyme **renin,** produced by the **juxtaglomerular apparatus,** a complex of cells located in the afferent arteriole at its junction with the glomerulus (Fig. 30-8). Renin is released in response to a low blood sodium level or to low blood pressure (which can occur if the blood volume drops too low). Renin then initiates a series of events that culminate in the production of **angiotensin,** a blood protein that has several related effects. First, it stimulates the release of aldosterone, which acts in turn to increase sodium reabsorption by the distal tubule. Second, it increases the secretion of ADH (vasopressin, discussed later in the chapter), a hormone that promotes water conservation by the kidney. Third, it increases the blood pressure. Finally, it stimulates thirst. These actions of angiotensin tend to reverse the circumstances (low blood sodium and low blood pressure and/or blood volume) that triggered the secretion of renin. Sodium and water are conserved, and blood volume and blood pressure are restored to normal.

Tubular secretion

In addition to reabsorbing large amounts of materials from the plasma filtrate, the kidney tubules are able to secrete certain substances into the tubular fluid. This process, which is the reverse of tubular reabsorption, enables the kidney to build up the urine concentrations of materials to be excreted, such as hydrogen and potassium ions, drugs, and various foreign organic materials. The distal tubule is the site of most tubular secretion.

In the kidney of bony marine fishes, reptiles, and birds, tubular secretion is a

The medical profession is in agreement that too much dietary salt causes high blood pressure (hypertension) in humans, but why it does so has been a mystery. Since angiotensin is a potent vasoconstrictor, it has long been suspected that a derailment of the renin-angiotensin system is responsible for some forms of hypertension. However, according to new findings, excess salt in the diet may indirectly produce hypertension by causing the release of a natriuretic (salt-releasing) hormone. This hormone has two effects: it increases sodium excretion and it constricts arterioles, leading to increased blood pressure.

Figure 30-10

Mechanism of urine concentration in humans. Sodium chloride is actively pumped from the ascending limb of loop of Henle and passively reenters the descending limb, building up the osmotic concentration to approximately four times that of blood. This creates an osmotic gradient for the controlled reabsorption of water from the collecting duct. Many rodent and desert mammals have relatively longer loops of Henle and can produce much more concentrated urine than humans.

much more highly developed process than it is in mammalian kidneys. Marine bony fishes actively secrete large amounts of magnesium and sulfate, which are by-products of their mode of osmotic regulation (p. 542). Reptiles and birds excrete uric acid instead of urea as their major nitrogenous waste. This material is actively secreted by the tubular epithelium. Since uric acid is nearly insoluble, it forms crystals in the urine and requires little water for excretion. Thus, the excretion of uric acid is an important adaptation for water conservation.

Water excretion

The osmotic pressure of the blood is closely regulated by the kidney. When fluid intake is high, the kidney excretes a dilute urine, saving salts and excreting water. When fluid intake is low, the kidney conserves water by forming a concentrated urine. A dehydrated person can concentrate urine to approximately four times blood osmotic concentration.

The capacity of the kidney of mammals and some birds to produce a concentrated urine involves the loop of Henle, the long hairpin loop between the proximal and distal tubules that extends into the renal medulla. Although the loop of Henle was believed to be the locus for urine concentration, the mechanism has only recently been satisfactorily explained. The loops of Henle constitute a **countercurrent multiplier system.** Flow is in opposite directions in the two limbs, hence the name "countercurrent."

The functional characteristics of this system are as follows. Sodium chloride is actively transported out of the ascending limb and into the surrounding tissue fluid (Fig. 30-10). The ascending limb is relatively impermeable to both sodium

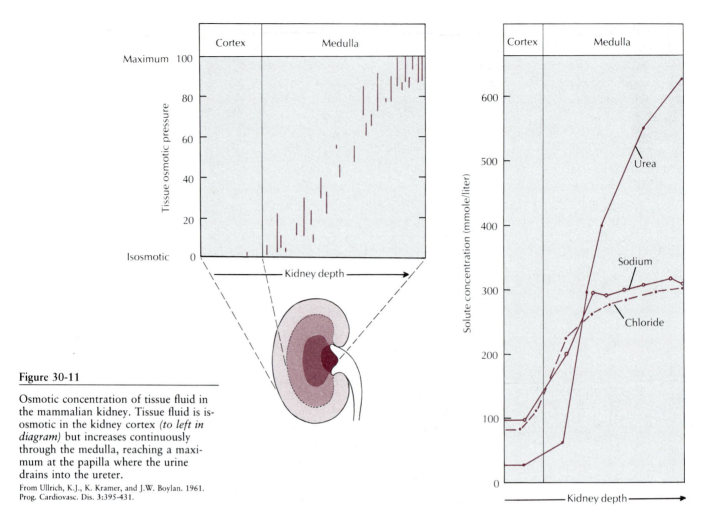

Figure 30-11

Osmotic concentration of tissue fluid in the mammalian kidney. Tissue fluid is isosmotic in the kidney cortex (*to left in diagram*) but increases continuously through the medulla, reaching a maximum at the papilla where the urine drains into the ureter.

From Ullrich, K.J., K. Kramer, and J.W. Boylan. 1961. Prog. Cardiovasc. Dis. 3:395-431.

chloride and water, so there is minimal passive reentry of sodium chloride or water into this limb. However, the descending limb, which does not transport sodium chloride, is permeable to sodium chloride and water. Consequently, the sodium chloride that has been actively pumped out the ascending limb tends to passively enter the descending limb from the tissue fluid. By cycling sodium between the two opposing limbs, the concentrations of both the urine within the loop and the tissue fluid surrounding it become multiplied at the bottom of the loop. Tissue fluid osmotic concentration is greatest at the bottom of the loop deep in the medulla and lowest at the top of the loop in the cortex (Fig. 30-11).

The final adjustment of urine concentration does not occur in the loops of Henle, but in the collecting ducts that lie parallel to the loops of Henle. As the urine flows down the collecting duct into regions of increasing osmotic concentration, water is osmotically withdrawn from the urine. The amount of water saved and the final concentration of the urine depend on the permeability of the walls of the collecting duct. This is controlled by the **antidiuretic hormone** (ADH, or vasopressin), which is released by the posterior pituitary gland (neurohypophysis). The release of this hormone is governed in turn by special receptors in the brain that constantly sense the osmotic pressure of the blood. When the blood osmotic pressure increases, as during dehydration, the secretion of ADH is increased. ADH increases the permeability of the collecting duct, probably by expanding the pore size in the duct membrane. The result is that water diffuses out of the collecting duct into the surrounding interstitial fluid as the fluid in the collecting duct passes through the hyperosmotic region (Fig. 30-10). The urine loses water and becomes more concentrated. Given this sequence of events for dehydration, we can readily imagine the response of this system to overhydration. ADH secretion decreases, the collecting ducts become relatively impermeable, and urine flow and water content are high.

The varying ability of different mammals to form a concentrated urine is closely correlated with the length of the loops of Henle. The beaver, which has no need to conserve water in its aquatic environment, has short loops and can concentrate its urine to only approximately twice that of the blood plasma. Humans, with relatively longer loops, can concentrate urine 4.2 times that of the blood. As we would anticipate, desert mammals have much greater urine-concentrating powers. The camel can produce a urine eight times the plasma concentration, the gerbil 14 times, and the Australian hopping mouse 22 times. In this creature, the greatest urine concentrator of all, the loops of Henle extend to the tip of a long renal papilla that pushes out into the mouth of the ureter.

Summary

Throughout life, matter and energy pass through the body, producing perturbations of the internal physiological state. Homeostasis, an organism's ability to maintain internal stability despite such perturbations, is a characteristic of all living systems. Homeostasis involves the coordinated activity of several physiological and biochemical mechanisms, and it is possible to relate major advances in animal evolution to increasing internal independence from the consequences of environmental change. In this chapter we have examined one aspect of homeostasis, the varying ability of animals to stabilize the osmotic and chemical composition of the blood.

Most marine invertebrates either must depend on the stability of the ocean to which they conform osmotically or must be able to tolerate wide fluctuations in environmental salinity. Some organisms with the latter ability show limited powers of osmotic regulation, that is, the capacity to resist internal osmotic change, through the evolution of specialized regulatory organs. All animals living in fresh water are hyperosmotic to their environment and have developed mechanisms for recovering salt from the environment and pumping out excess water that enters the body osmotically.

All vertebrate animals except the primitive hagfishes show excellent osmotic homeostasis. The marine bony fishes maintain their body fluids distinctly hypoosmotic to their environment by drinking seawater and physiologically distilling it. The elasmobranchs (sharks and their kin) have adopted a strategy of near osmotic conformity by retaining urea in the blood.

The kidney is the most important organ for regulating the chemical and osmotic composition of the blood. In all metazoa the kidney is some variation on a basic theme: a tubular structure that forms urine by introducing a fluid secretion or ultrafiltrate of the blood into a tubule in which it is selectively modified to form urine. The terrestrial vertebrates have especially sophisticated kidneys, since they must be able to regulate closely the water content of the blood by balancing gains and expenditures. All mammals and some birds can produce a concentrated urine by means of a countercurrent multiplier system localized in the loop of Henle, a specialization not found in lower vertebrates.

Scanning electron micrograph of podocyte processes surrounding and supporting the glomerular capillaries of the kidney. (×8800.)
Courtesy W.A. Weber, University of British Columbia.

Selected references

See also general references for Part Three, p. 837.

Brooks, S.M. 1973. Basic facts of body water and ions, ed. 3. New York, Springer Publishing Co., Inc. *Useful elementary account.*

Deetjen, P., J.W. Boylan, and K. Kramer. 1975. Physiology of the kidney and of water balance. New York, Springer-Verlag, Inc. *A primer designed for medical students; balanced treatment of mammalian kidney function.*

Edney, E.B. 1957. The water relations of terrestrial arthropods. New York, Cambridge University Press.

Harvey, R.J. 1974. The kidneys and the internal environment. London, Chapman & Hall. *Stresses basic physical and chemical principles that underlie kidney function, especially dissociation and acid-base balance.*

Lockwood, A.P.M. 1963. Animal body fluids and their regulation. Cambridge, Mass., Harvard University Press. *This concise volume deals with the physiology of body fluid regulation in both invertebrates and vertebrates.*

Pitts, R.F. 1974. Physiology of the kidney and body fluids: an introductory text, ed. 3. Chicago, Year Book Medical Publishers, Inc. *Authoritative standard text.*

Potts, W.T.W., and G. Parry. 1964. Osmotic and ionic regulation in animals. New York, Macmillan, Inc. *An excellent treatise on concepts of homeostatic mechanisms, with special emphasis on osmoregulation and fluid balance.*

Rankin, J.C., and J. Davenport. 1981. Animal osmoregulation. New York, John Wiley & Sons, Inc. *Up-to-date concise volume, selective treatment.*

Riegel, J.A. 1972. Comparative physiology of renal excretion. New York, Hafner Publishing Co., Inc. *Useful review of animal excretion, beginning with vertebrates and ending with the simplest invertebrate systems and a helpful closing chapter on theory of fluid movement.*

Smith, H.W. 1953. From fish to philosopher. Boston, Little, Brown & Co. *Vertebrate kidney evolution.*

Selected *Scientific American* articles

Smith, H.W. 1953. The kidney. **188:**40-48 (Jan.). *Structure, physiology, and evolution of the vertebrate kidney.*

Solomon, A.K. 1962. Pumps in the living cell. **207:**100-108 (Aug.). *Active transport processes in kidney tubules are described.*

CHAPTER 31

DIGESTION AND NUTRITION

Scanning electron micrograph of the folded epithelium of the human stomach. Epithelial cells, resembling cobblestone paving, cover the stomach surface and line gastric glands, which secrete hydrochloric acid and pepsinogen; the opening of one gland is indicated by the arrow. (×315.)

From Pfeiffer, C.J. 1970. J. Ultrastruct. Res. 33:252.

All organisms require energy to maintain their highly ordered and complex structures. This energy is chemical energy that is released by transforming complex compounds acquired from the organism's environment into simpler ones. Obviously, if living organisms must depend on the breakdown of complex foodstuffs to build and maintain their own complexity, these foodstuffs must somehow be synthesized in the first place. Most of the energy for this synthesis is provided by the powerful radiations of the sun, the one great source of energy reaching our planet, which is otherwise a virtually isolated system.

At this point it may be helpful to summarize discussions appearing elsewhere in this book (Chapters 3 and 41) on energy flow through living communities. Organisms capable of capturing the sun's energy by the process of photosynthesis are of course the green plants. Green plants are **autotrophic organisms** capable of synthesizing all the essential organic compounds needed for life. Autotrophic organisms need only inorganic compounds absorbed from their surroundings to provide the raw materials for synthesis and growth. Most autotrophic organisms are the chlorophyll-bearing **phototrophs,** although some, the chemosynthetic bacteria, are **chemotrophs;** they gain energy from inorganic chemical reactions.

Almost all animals are **heterotrophic organisms** that depend on already synthesized organic compounds of plants and other animals to obtain the materials they will use for growth, maintenance, and reproduction of their kind. Since the food of animals, normally the complex tissues of other organisms, is usually too bulky to be absorbed directly by the body cells, it must be broken down, or digested, into soluble molecules that are small enough to be used.

Animals may be divided into a number of categories on the basis of dietary habits. **Herbivorous** animals feed mainly on plant life. **Carnivorous** animals feed mainly on herbivores and other carnivores. **Omnivorous** forms eat both plants and animals. A fourth category sometimes included is the **insectivorous** animals, which are those animals subsisting chiefly on insects.

The ingestion of foods and their simplification by digestion are only initial steps in nutrition. Foods reduced by digestion to soluble, molecular form are **absorbed** into the circulatory system and are **transported** to the tissues of the body. There they are **assimilated** into the protoplasm of the cells. Oxygen is also

Figure 31-1

Some filter feeders and their feeding mechanisms. **A,** The marine fan worm (class Polychaeta, phylum Annelida) has a crown of tentacles. Numerous cilia on the edges of the tentacles draw water *(solid arrows)* between pinnules where food particles are entrapped in mucus; the particles are then carried down a "gutter" in the center of the tentacle to the mouth *(broken arrows).* **B,** Bivalve molluscs (class Bivalvia, phylum Mollusca) use their gills as feeding devices, as well as for respiration. Water currents created by cilia on the gills carry food particles into the inhalant siphon and between slits in the gills where they are entangled in a mucous sheet covering the gill surface. The particles are then transported by ciliated food grooves to the mouth (not shown). Arrows indicate direction of water movement. **C,** Whalebone whales (class Mammalia, phylum Chordata) filter out plankton, principally large crustaceans called "krill," with whalebone, or baleen. Water enters the swimming whale's open mouth by the force of the animal's forward motion and is strained out through the more than 300 horny baleen plates that hang down like a curtain from the roof of the mouth. Krill and other plankters caught in the baleen are periodically wiped off with the huge tongue and swallowed. **D,** Herring and other filter-feeding fishes (class Osteichthyes, phylum Chordata) use gill rakers, which project forward from the gill bars into the pharyngeal cavity to strain out plankters. Herring swim almost constantly, forcing water and suspended food into the mouth; food is strained out by the gill rakers, and the water passes on out the gill openings.

transported by the blood to the tissues, where food products are **oxidized,** or burned to yield energy and heat. Much food is not immediately used but is **stored** for future use. Then the wastes produced by oxidation must be **excreted.** Food products unsuitable for digestion are rejected by the digestive system and are **egested** in the form of feces.

The sum total of all these nutritional processes is called **metabolism.** Metabolism includes both constructive and tearing-down processes. When smaller molecules are formed into larger molecules and built into new tissues or stored for later use, such processes are called **synthetic** or **anabolic reactions.** The processes of breaking down complex materials into simpler ones, usually for the release of energy, are called **degradative** or **catabolic reactions.** Both processes occur simultaneously in all living cells.

In this chapter we will first examine the feeding adaptations of animals. Next we will discuss digestion and absorption of foodstuffs. We will close with a consideration of nutritional requirements of animals.

FEEDING MECHANISMS

Only a few animals can absorb nutrients directly from their external environment. Some blood parasites and intestinal parasites may derive all their nourishment as primary organic molecules by surface absorption; some aquatic invertebrates may soak up part of their nutritional needs directly from the water. For most animals, however, working for their meals is the main business of living, and the specializations that have evolved for food procurement are almost as numerous as the species of animals. In this brief discussion we consider some of the major food-gathering devices.

Feeding on Particulate Matter

Drifting microscopic particles are found in the upper hundred meters of the ocean. Most of this multitude is **plankton,** plant and animal microorganisms too small to do anything but drift with the ocean's currents. The rest is organic debris, the disintegrating remains of dead plants and animals. Although this oceanic swarm of plankton forms a rich life domain, it is unevenly distributed. The heaviest plankton growth occurs in estuaries and areas of upwelling, where there is an abundant nutrient supply. It is preyed on by numerous larger animals, invertebrates and vertebrates, using a variety of feeding mechanisms. Some protozoa, such as the ameboid sarcodines, ingest particulate food by phagocytosis (p. 177). The animal, stimulated by the proximity of food, pushes out armlike extensions of the plasmalemma (cell membrane) and engulfs the particle into a food vacuole, in which it is digested. Other protozoa have specialized openings, called cytostomes, through which the food passes to be enclosed in a food vacuole.

One of the most important methods for feeding to have evolved is **filter feeding** (Fig. 31-1). It is a primitive but immensely successful and widely employed mechanism. The majority of filter feeders use ciliated surfaces to produce currents that draw drifting food particles into their mouths. Most filter-feeding invertebrates, such as the tube-dwelling worms and bivalve molluscs, entrap the particulate food in mucous sheets that convey the food into the digestive tract. In the freshwater developmental stages of certain insect orders, the organisms use fanlike arrangements of setae or spin silk nets to entrap food. Filter feeding is character-

Gums called Gerbavee

Grown

nick

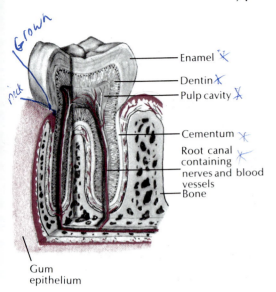

— Enamel ✗
— Dentin ✗
— Pulp cavity ✗

— Cementum ✗
Root canal
containing
nerves and blood
vessels
— Bone

Gum
epithelium

Figure 31-2

Structure of a human molar tooth. The tooth is built of three layers of calcified tissue covering: enamel, which is 98% mineral and the hardest material in the body; dentin, which composes the mass of the tooth and is approximately 75% mineral; and cementum, which forms a thin covering over the dentin in the root of the tooth and is very similar to dense bone in composition. The pulp cavity contains loose connective tissue, blood vessels, nerves, and tooth-building cells. The roots of the tooth are anchored to the wall of the socket by a fibrous connective tissue layer called the periodontal membrane.

Modified from Netter, F.H. 1959. The CIBA collection of medical illustrations, vol. 3. Summit, N.J., CIBA Pharmaceutical Products, Inc.

istic of a sessile way of life; the ciliary currents bring the food to the immobile or slow-moving animal. However, actively swimming animals such as tiny copepod crustaceans and herring are also filter feeders, as are immense baleen (whalebone) whales. The vital importance of one component of the plankton, the diatoms, in supporting a great pyramid of filter-feeding animals is stressed by N.J. Berrill*:

> A humpback whale . . . needs a ton of herring in its stomach to feel comfortably full—as many as five thousand individual fish. Each herring, in turn, may well have 6000 or 7000 small crustaceans in its own stomach, each of which contains as many as 130,000 diatoms. In other words, some 400 billion yellow-green diatoms sustain a single medium-sized whale for a few hours at most.

Filter feeding uses the abundance and extravagance of life in the sea. Filter feeders are as a rule nonselective (except as to the size of a particle) and omnivorous. Sessile filter feeders take what they can get, but many have mechanisms that allow some selectivity of particle size. Active filter feeders, however, such as fish and baleen whales, are much more selective in their feeding.

___ Feeding on Food Masses

Some of the most interesting animal adaptations are those for procuring and manipulating solid food. Such adaptations and the animals bearing them are partly shaped by what the animal eats.

Predators must be able to locate, capture, hold, and swallow prey. Most vertebrates use teeth for this purpose. Although teeth are variable in size, shape, and arrangement, vertebrates as different as fish and mammals sometimes have remarkably similar tooth arrangements for seizing the prey and cutting it into pieces small enough to swallow.

Mammals characteristically have four different types of teeth, each adapted for specific functions. **Incisors** are designed for biting, cutting, and stripping; **canines** are for seizing, piercing, and tearing; **premolars** and **molars,** at the back of the jaw, are for grinding and crushing. This basic pattern, well illustrated in human dentition (Figs. 31-2 and 31-3), is often greatly modified in animals having specialized food habits (Fig. 27-8, p. 643). Herbivores have suppressed canines but well-developed molars with enamel ridges for grinding. The well-developed, self-sharpening incisors of rodents grow throughout life and must be worn away by gnawing to keep pace with growth. Some teeth have become so highly modified that they are no longer useful for biting or chewing food. An elephant's tusk is a modified upper incisor used for defense, attack, and rooting, and the male wild boar has modified canines that are used as weapons.

Many carnivores among the fishes, amphibians, and reptiles swallow their prey whole. Snakes and some fishes can swallow enormous meals. This, together with the absence of limbs, is associated with some striking feeding adaptations in these groups: recurved teeth for seizing and holding the prey and distensible jaws and stomachs to accommodate their large and infrequent meals.

Teeth are not vertebrate innovations; biting, scraping, and gnawing devices are common in the invertebrates. Insects, for example, have three pairs of appendages on their heads that serve variously as jaws, teeth, chisels, tongues, or sucking tubes. Usually the first pair serves as crushing teeth; the second, grasping jaws; and the third, a probing and tasting tongue.

*Berrill, N.J. 1958. You and the universe. New York, Dodd, Mead & Co.

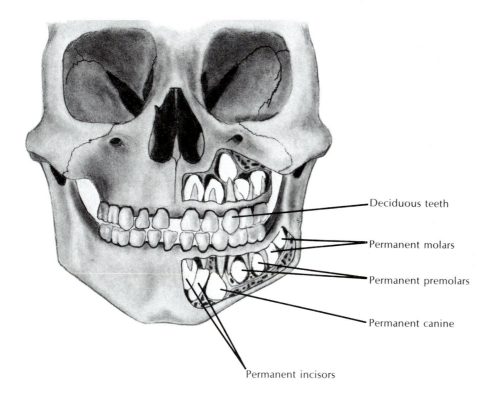

Deciduous teeth

Permanent molars

Permanent premolars

Permanent canine

Permanent incisors

Figure 31-3

Human deciduous and permanent teeth. Partly dissected skull of a 5-year-old child, showing milk (deciduous) teeth and permanent teeth. Milk teeth begin to erupt at 6 months and are gradually replaced by the permanent teeth beginning at about 6 years of age. There are 20 deciduous teeth, 5 on each side of each jaw, and 32 permanent teeth, 8 on each side of each jaw. These 8 are arranged as follows: 2 incisors, 1 canine (also called cuspid), 2 premolars (bicuspids), 3 molars. The last molar, known as the wisdom tooth, erupts between ages of 17 and 25 or not at all. Upper permanent molars are not seen in this frontal view. Modified from Arey, L.B. 1965. Developmental anatomy. Philadelphia, W.B. Saunders Co.

Herbivorous, or plant-eating, animals, whether vertebrate or invertebrate, have evolved special devices for crushing and cutting plant material. Despite its abundance on earth, the woody cellulose that encloses plant cells is to many animals an indigestible and useless material; some herbivores, however, make use of intestinal microoganisms to digest cellulose, once it is ground up. One highly specialized group, the ruminants, is described on p. 645. Certain invertebrates such as snails have rasplike, scraping mouthparts. Insects such as locusts have grinding and cutting mandibles; herbivorous mammals such as horses and cattle use wide, corrugated molars for grinding. All these mechanisms disrupt the tough cellulose cell wall to accelerate its digestion by intestinal microorganisms, as well as to release the cell contents for direct enzymatic breakdown.

_____ Feeding on Fluids

Fluid feeding is especially characteristic of parasites, but it is certainly practiced among free-living forms as well. Some internal parasites (endoparasites) simply absorb the nutrient surrounding them, unwittingly provided by the host, whereas others bite and rasp off host tissue, suck blood, and feed on the contents of the host's intestine. External parasites (ectoparasites) such as leeches, lampreys, parasitic crustaceans, and insects use a variety of efficient piercing and sucking mouthparts to feed on blood or other body fluid. Unfortunately for humans and other warm-blooded animals, the ubiquitous mosquito excels in its bloodsucking habit. Alighting gently, the mosquito sets about puncturing its prey with an array of six needlelike mouthparts (Fig. 17-16, p. 416). One of these is used to inject an anticoagulant saliva (responsible for the irritating itch that follows the "bite" and serving as a vector for microorganisms causing malaria, yellow fever, encephalitis, and other diseases); another mouthpart is a channel through which the blood is

Figure 31-4

Peristalsis. Food is pushed along before a wave of circular muscle contraction.

From Schottelius, B.A., and D.D. Schottelius. 1978. A textbook of physiology, ed. 18. St. Louis, The C.V. Mosby Co.

sucked. It is of little comfort that only the female of the species dines on blood. Far less annoying to people are the free-living butterflies, moths, and aphids that suck up plant fluids with long, tubelike mouthparts.

DIGESTION

In the process of digestion, which means literally "carrying asunder," organic foods are mechanically and chemically broken down into small units for absorption. Even though food solids consist principally of carbohydrates, proteins, and fats, the very components that make up the body of the consumer, these components must nevertheless be reduced to their simplest molecular units before they can be used. Each animal reassembles some of these digested and absorbed units into organic compounds of the animal's own unique pattern. Cannibals enjoy no special metabolic benefit from eating their own kind; they digest their victims just as thoroughly as they do food of another species.

Movement of food through the digestive tract is either by **cilia** or by **musculature.** In general, the filter feeders that use cilia to feed, such as bivalve molluscs, also use cilia to propel the food through the gut. Animals feeding on bulky foods rely on well-developed gut musculature. As a rule the gut is lined with two opposing layers of muscle: a longitudinal layer, in which the smooth muscle fibers run parallel with the length of the gut, and a circular layer, in which the muscle fibers embrace the circumference of the gut. This arrangement is ideal for mixing and propelling foods. The most characteristic gut movement is **peristalsis** (Fig. 31-4). In this movement a wave of circular muscle contraction sweeps down the gut for some distance, pushing the food along before it. The peristaltic waves may start at any point and move for variable distances. Also characteristic of the gut are **segmentation** movements that divide and mix the food.

Intracellular versus Extracellular Digestion

Humans and other vertebrates and the higher invertebrates digest their food **extracellularly** by secreting digestive juices into the intestinal lumen. There, foodstuffs are enzymatically split into molecular units small enough to be selectively absorbed by the intestinal epithelium, transported by the circulation, and used by all body cells. Digestion, then, occurs outside the body's tissues.

Intracellular digestion is a primitive process typical of the lower invertebrates. This type of digestion is practiced by many multicellular invertebrates, especially filter-feeding marine animals such as brachiopods, rotifers, bivalves, and cephalochordates, as well as the cnidarians and flatworms. In these forms the food particle, phagocytized by the cell, is enclosed within a membrane as a food vacuole (Fig. 31-5). Digestive enzymes are then added. The products of digestion, the simple sugars, amino acids, and other molecules, are absorbed into the cell

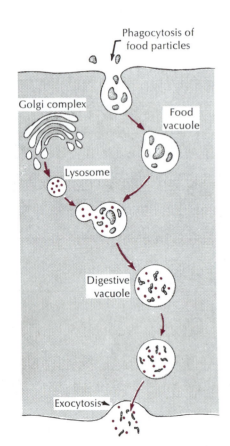

Phagocytosis of food particles

Golgi complex

Food vacuole

Lysosome

Digestive vacuole

Exocytosis

Figure 31-5

Intracellular digestion. Lysosomes containing digestive enzymes (lysozymes) are produced within the cell, possibly by the Golgi complex. Lysosomes fuse with food vacuoles and release enzymes that digest the enclosed food. Usable products of digestion are absorbed into the cytoplasm, and indigestible wastes are expelled.

Villi

Lumen

Muscle
layers

Figure 31-6

Scanning electron micrograph of a rat intestine showing the numerous fingerlike
villi that project into the lumen and vastly increase the effective absorptive and
secretory surface of the intestine. (×21.)
From Tissues and organs: a text-atlas of scanning electron
microscopy, by Richard G. Kessel and Randy H. Kardon.
W.H. Freeman and Company. Copyright © 1979.

cytoplasm where they may be used directly or may be transferred to other cells.
The inevitable food wastes are extruded from the cell.

The big limitation of intracellular digestion is that only small particles of
food can be handled. This limitation was probably responsible for shaping the
evolution of extracellular digestion. Extracellular digestion offers several advantages: bulky foods may be ingested; the digestive tract can be smaller, more specialized, and more efficient; and food wastes are more easily discarded. Only with
extracellular digestion could the enormous variation in feeding methods of the
higher animals have evolved.

Vertebrate Digestion

The vertebrate digestive plan is similar to that of the higher invertebrates. Both
have a highly differentiated alimentary canal with devices for increasing the surface area, such as increased length, inside folds, and diverticula. The more primitive fishes (lampreys and sharks) have longitudinal or spiral folds in their intestines. Higher vertebrates have developed elaborate folds and minute fingerlike
projections called **villi,** some 10 to 40/mm^2, that give fresh intestinal tissue the
appearance of velvet (Fig. 31-6). Also the electron microscope reveals that each
cell lining the intestinal cavity is bordered by hundreds of short, delicate processes
called **microvilli** (Fig. 31-7). These processes, together with larger villi and intestinal folds, may make the internal surface of the intestine more than a million
times greater than a smooth cylinder of the same diameter. The total surface area
of the human intestine is approximately 300 m^2. The absorption of food molecules is enormously facilitated as a result.

Action of digestive enzymes

We have already pointed out that digestion involves both mechanical and chemical alterations of food. Mechanical processes of cutting and grinding by teeth and
muscular mixing by the intestinal tract are important in digestion. However, the

reduction of foods to small, absorbable units relies principally on chemical break-down by **enzymes.** Enzymes are the highly specific organic catalysts essential to the orderly progression of virtually all life processes.

It must be stated that, although digestive enzymes are probably the best known and most studied of all enzymes, they represent but a small fraction of the numerous enzymes, perhaps thousands, that ultimately regulate all processes in the body. The digestive enzymes are **hydrolytic** enzymes or **hydrolases,** so called because food molecules are split by the process of **hydrolysis,** that is, the breaking of a chemical bond by adding the components of water across it:

$$R\text{---}R + H_2O \xrightarrow[\text{enzyme}]{\text{Digestive}} R\text{---}OH + H\text{---}R$$

In this general enzymatic reaction, R—R represents a food molecule that is split into two products, R—OH and R—H. Usually these reaction products must in turn be split repeatedly before the original molecule is reduced to its numerous subunits. Proteins, for example, are composed of hundreds, or even thousands, of interlinked amino acids, which must be completely separated before the individual amino acids can be absorbed. Similarly, carbohydrates must be reduced to simple sugars. Fats (lipids) are reduced to molecules of glycerol and fatty acids, although some fats, unlike proteins and carbohydrates, may be absorbed without being completely hydrolyzed first. There are specific enzymes for each class of organic compounds. These enzymes are located in various regions of the alimentary canal in a sort of "enzyme chain," in which one enzyme may complete what another has started; the product moves along posteriorly for still further hydrolysis.

Digestion in the human, an omnivore
Oral cavity

In the mouth, food is reduced mechanically by the teeth and is moistened with saliva from the salivary glands. In addition to **mucin,** which helps to lubricate the food for swallowing, saliva contains the enzyme **amylase.** Salivary amylase is a

Figure 31-7

A, Human digestive system. **B,** Portion of mucosa lining of intestine, showing fingerlike villi. **C,** Section of single mucosal lining cell. **D,** Microvilli on surface of mucosal cell, rat intestine. (×16,400.)

D, Electron micrograph courtesy J.D. Berlin.

Labels for A: Salivary gland, Pharynx, Trachea, Esophagus, Liver, Gallbladder, Pancreas, Stomach, Large intestine, Small intestine, Rectum

Labels for B: Blood capillaries, Lacteal, Villus, Blood vessels, Lymph vessel, Intestinal gland

Labels for C: Endoplasmic reticulum, Microvilli, Nucleus, Mitochondrion carbohydrate-splitting enzyme that begins the hydrolysis of plant and animal starches (Fig. 31-8). Starches are long polymers of glucose. Salivary amylase does not completely hydrolyze starch but breaks it down mostly into two glucose fragments called **maltose.** Some free glucose, as well as longer fragments of starch, is also produced. When the food mass (bolus) is swallowed, salivary amylase continues to act for some time, digesting perhaps half of the starch before the enzyme is inactivated by the acid environment of the stomach. Further starch digestion resumes beyond the stomach in the intestine.

Swallowing

Swallowing is a reflex process involving both voluntary and involuntary components. Swallowing begins with the tongue pushing the moistened food bolus toward the pharynx. The nasal cavity is reflexively closed by raising the soft palate. As the food slides into the pharynx, the epiglottis is tipped down over the windpipe, nearly closing it. Some particles of food may enter the opening of the windpipe but are prevented from going farther by contraction of laryngeal muscles. Once in the esophagus, the bolus is forced smoothly toward the stomach by peristaltic contraction of the esophageal muscles.

Digestion in the stomach

When food reaches the stomach, the **cardiac sphincter** opens reflexively to allow entry of the food, then closes to prevent regurgitation back into the esophagus. The stomach is a combination storage, mixing, digestion, and release center. Gentle peristaltic waves pass over the filled stomach at the rate of approximately three

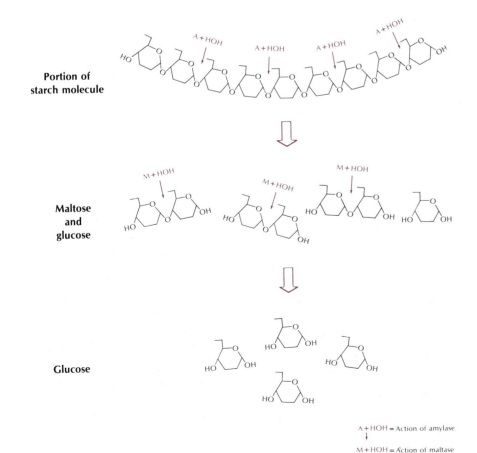

Figure 31-8

Digestion (hydrolysis) of starch. Starch is composed of long chains of glucose units. They are first cleaved into disaccharide residues (maltose) by the salivary enzyme amylase. Some glucose may also be split off at the ends of starch chains. The intestinal enzyme maltase then completes the hydrolysis by cleaving the maltose molecules into glucose. A molecule of water is inserted into each enzymatically split bond.

The stomach contains both a strong acid, having a concentration some 4 million times that found in the blood, and a powerful proteolytic enzyme. Thus, it seems remarkable that the stomach mucosa is not digested by its own secretions. That it is not is a result of another gastric secretion, mucin, a highly viscous organic compound that coats and protects the mucosa from both chemical and mechanical injury. We should note that, despite the popular misconception of an "acid stomach" being unhealthy, a notion carefully nourished in media advertising, stomach acidity is normal and essential. Sometimes, however, the protective mucous coating fails, allowing the gastric juices to begin digesting the stomach. The result is a peptic ulcer.

each minute; churning is most vigorous at the intestinal end where food is steadily released into the duodenum, the first region of the intestine. Approximately 2 liters of **gastric juice** is secreted each day by deep, tubular glands in the stomach wall. Two types of cells line these glands: **chief cells,** which secrete **pepsin,** and **parietal cells,** which secrete **hydrochloric acid.** Pepsin is a **protease** (protein-splitting enzyme) that acts only in an acid medium—pH 1.6 to 2.4. It is a highly specific enzyme that splits large proteins by preferentially breaking down certain peptide bonds scattered along the peptide chain of the protein molecule. Although pepsin, because of its specificity, cannot completely degrade proteins, it effectively breaks them up into a number of small polypeptides. Protein digestion is completed in the intestine by other proteases that can together split all peptide bonds.

Rennin is another enzyme found in the stomachs of the suckling newborn of many mammals, although not humans. Rennin is a milk-curdling enzyme that transforms the proteins of milk into a finely flocculent form that is more readily attacked by pepsin. Rennin extracted from the stomachs of calves is used in cheese making. Human infants, lacking rennin, digest milk proteins with acidic pepsin, the same as adults do.

The secretion of the gastric juices is intermittent. Although a small volume of gastric juice is secreted continuously, even during prolonged periods of starvation, secretion is normally increased by the sight and smell of food, the presence of food in the stomach, and emotional states such as anxiety and anger.

The most unique and classic investigation in the field of digestion was made by U.S. Army surgeon William Beaumont during the years 1825 to 1833. His subject was a young, hard-living French Canadian voyageur, named Alexis St. Martin, who in 1822 had accidentally shot himself in the abdomen with a musket, the blast "blowing off integuments and muscles of the size of a man's hand, fracturing and carrying away the anterior half of the sixth rib, fracturing the fifth, lacerating the lower portion of the left lobe of the lungs, the diaphragm, and perforating the stomach." Miraculously the wound healed, but a permanent opening, or fistula, was formed that permitted Beaumont to see directly into the stomach (Fig. 31-9). St. Martin became a permanent, although temperamental, patient in Beaumont's care, which included food and housing. Over a period of 8 years, Beaumont was able to observe and record how the lining of the stomach changed under different psychological and physiological conditions, how foods changed during digestion, the effect of emotional states on stomach motility, and many other facts about the digestive processes of his famous patient.

Digestion in the small intestine

The major part of digestion occurs in the small intestine. Two secretions are poured into this region: **pancreatic juice** and **bile.** Both of these secretions have a high bicarbonate content, especially the pancreatic juice, which effectively neutralizes the gastric acid, raising the pH of the liquefied food mass, now called **chyme,** from 1.5 to 7 as it enters the duodenum. This change in pH is essential because all the intestinal enzymes are effective only in a neutral or slightly alkaline medium.

Pancreatic enzymes

Approximately 2 liters of pancreatic juice is secreted each day. The pancreatic juice contains several enzymes of major importance in digestion. Two powerful proteases, **trypsin** and **chymotrypsin,** continue the enzymatic digestion of proteins

Figure 31-9

Dr. William Beaumont at Fort Mackinac, Michigan Territory, collecting gastric juice from Alexis St. Martin.
From Myer, J.S. 1939. Life and letters of Dr. William Beaumont. St. Louis, The C.V. Mosby Co.

begun by pepsin, which is now inactivated by the alkalinity of the intestine. Trypsin and chymotrypsin, like pepsin, are highly specific proteases that split apart peptide bonds deep inside the protein molecule. The hydrolysis of the peptide linkage may be shown as:

Pancreatic juice also contains **carboxypeptidase,** which splits amino acids off the carboxyl ends of polypeptides; **pancreatic lipase,** which hydrolyzes fats into fatty acids and glycerol; **pancreatic amylase,** which is a starch-splitting enzyme identical to salivary amylase in its action; and **nucleases,** which degrade RNA and DNA to nucleotides.

Membrane enzymes

The cells lining the intestine have digestive enzymes embedded in their surface membrane that continue the digestion of carbohydrates, proteins, and phosphate compounds. Until recently it was thought that these enzymes were secreted into the intestinal lumen as an intestinal "juice." Now it is known that the enzymes are

Cells of the intestinal mucosa, like those of the stomach mucosa, are subjected to considerable wear and tear and are undergoing constant replacement. Cells deep in the crypt between adjacent villi divide rapidly and migrate up the villus. In mammals the cells reach the tip of the villus in about 2 days. There they are shed, along with their membrane enzymes, into the lumen at the rate of some 17 billion a day along the length of the human intestine. Before they are shed, however, these cells differentiate into absorptive cells that transport nutrients into the network of blood and lymph vessels, once digestion is complete.

Although milk is the universal food of newborn mammals and one of the most complete human foods, most adult humans cannot digest milk because they are deficient in lactase, the enzyme that hydrolyzes lactose (milk sugar). Lactose intolerance is genetically determined. It is characterized by abdominal bloating, cramps, flatulence, and watery diarrhea, all appearing within 30 to 90 minutes after ingesting milk or its unfermented by-products. (Fermented dairy products, such as yogurt and cheese, create no intolerance problems.)

Northern Europeans and their descendants, which include the majority of North American whites, are most tolerant of milk. Many other ethnic groups are generally intolerant to lactose, including the Japanese, Chinese, Jews in Israel, Eskimos, South American Indians, and most African blacks. Only about 30% of North American blacks are tolerant; those who are tolerant are mostly descendants of slaves brought from east and central Africa where dairying is traditional and tolerance to lactose is high. The widespread intolerance to lactose is a matter of concern to international agencies that are planning food distribution programs in developing countries, as well as in school lunch programs in developed countries.

actually a part of the microvillus membrane (Fig. 31-7, *D*) where, as attached glycoproteins, they accomplish much of the work of digestion. Among the membrane digestive enzymes is **aminopeptidase.** It splits terminal amino acids from the amino end of short peptides; its action is similar to that of the pancreatic enzyme carboxypeptidase. Several **disaccharidases** (enzymes that split 12-carbon sugar molecules into 6-carbon units) are also part of the microvillus membrane. These include **maltase,** which splits maltose into two molecules of glucose (Fig. 31-8); **sucrase,** which splits sucrose to fructose and glucose; and **lactase,** which breaks down lactose (milk sugar) into glucose and galactose. Also present is **alkaline phosphatase,** which attacks a variety of phosphate compounds.

Bile

Bile is secreted by the cells of the liver into the **bile duct,** which drains into the upper intestine (duodenum). Between meals the bile is collected in the **gallbladder,** an expansible storage sac that releases the bile when stimulated by the presence of fatty food in the duodenum. Bile contains no enzymes. It is made up of water, bile salts, and pigments. The bile salts (mainly sodium taurocholate and sodium glycocholate) are essential for the complete absorption of fats, which, because of their tendency to remain in large, water-resistant globules, are especially resistant to enzymatic digestion. **Bile salts** reduce the surface tension of fats, so that they are broken up into small droplets by the churning movements of the intestine. This greatly increases the total surface exposure of fat particles, giving the fat-splitting lipases the opportunity to hydrolyze them. The golden yellow color of bile is produced by the **bile pigments,** which are breakdown products of hemoglobin from worn-out red blood cells. The bile pigments also give the feces its characteristic color.

The great versatility of the liver should be emphasized. Bile production is only one of the liver's many functions; it is a storehouse for glycogen, production center for the plasma proteins, site of protein synthesis and detoxification of protein wastes, destruction of worn-out red blood cells, center for metabolism of fat, amino acids, and carbohydrates, and many others.

Function of the large intestine

The liquefied material, called **chyle,** reaching the large intestine, or **colon,** is low in nutrients, since most important food materials have already been absorbed into the bloodstream from the small intestine. The main function of the colon is the absorption of water and some minerals from the intestinal chyle that enters. In removing more than half the water from the chyle, the colon forms semisolid feces consisting of undigested food residue, bile pigments, secreted heavy metals, and bacteria. The feces are eliminated from the rectum by the process of **defecation,** a coordinated muscular action that is part voluntary and part involuntary.

The colon contains enormous numbers of bacteria that enter the sterile colon of the newborn infant. In the adult approximately one third of the dry weight of feces is bacteria; these include harmless bacilli as well as cocci that can cause serious illness if they should escape into the abdomen or bloodstream. Normally the body's defenses prevent invasion of such bacteria. The bacteria break down organic wastes in the feces and provide some nutritional benefit by synthesizing certain vitamins (vitamin K and small quantities of some of the B vitamins), which are absorbed by the body.

Absorption

Most digested foodstuffs are absorbed from the small intestine, where the numerous finger-shaped **villi** provide an enormous surface area through which materials can pass from the intestinal lumen into the circulation (Fig. 31-7). Little food is absorbed in the stomach because digestion is still incomplete and because of the limited surface exposure. Some materials, however, such as drugs and alcohol, are absorbed in part there, which explains their rapid action.

Carbohydrates are absorbed almost exclusively as simple sugars (for example, glucose, fructose, and galactose) because the intestine is virtually impermeable to polysaccharides. Proteins, too, are absorbed principally as their amino acid subunits, although it is believed that small amounts of small proteins or peptide fragments may sometimes be absorbed. Simple sugars and amino acids are transferred across the intestinal epithelium by both passive and active processes.

Immediately after a meal these materials are in such high concentration in the gut that they readily diffuse into the blood, where their concentration is initially lower. However, if absorption were passive only, we would expect transfer to cease as soon as the concentrations of a substance became equal on both sides of the intestinal epithelium. This would permit much of the valuable foodstuff to be lost in the feces. In fact, very little is lost because passive transfer is supplemented by an **active transport** mechanism located in the epithelial cells that picks up the food molecules and transfers them into the blood. Materials are thus moved *against* their concentration gradient, a process that requires the expenditure of energy. Although not all food products are actively transported, those that are, such as glucose, galactose, and most of the amino acids, are handled by transport mechanisms that are specific for each kind of molecule.

As already described, fat droplets are emulsified by bile salts and then digested by pancreatic lipase. Triglycerides are thus broken down into fatty acids and monoglycerides, which are absorbed by simple diffusion. However, free fatty acids never enter the blood. Instead, during their passage through the intestinal epithelial cells, the fatty acids are resynthesized into triglycerides that pass out of the cells and into the lacteals. From the lacteals, the fat droplets enter the lymph system and eventually get into the blood by way of the thoracic duct. After a fatty meal, even a peanut butter sandwich, the presence of numerous fat droplets in the blood imparts a milky appearance to the blood plasma.

▬ REGULATION OF FOOD INTAKE

Most animals unconsciously adjust food intake to balance energy expenditure. If energy expenditure is increased by, for example, increased physical activity, food intake is increased accordingly. Most vertebrates, from fish to mammals, eat for calories rather than bulk because, if the diet is diluted with fiber, they respond by eating more. Similarly, intake is adjusted downward following a period of several days when caloric intake is too high.

Food intake is regulated in large part by a "hunger" center located in the hypothalamus region of the brain. Blood sugar level has an important influence on this center because hunger pangs coincide with decreasing levels of blood glucose. While most animals seem able to stabilize their weight at normal levels with ease, many humans cannot. It is becoming clear that many obese people do not in fact

Brown fat, the tissue that mediates nonshivering thermogenesis, is brown because it is packed with mitochondria containing large quantities of iron-bearing cytochrome molecules. In ordinary body cells, ATP is generated by a gradient of hydrogen ions produced during the flow of electrons down the respiratory chain (chemiosmotic hypothesis of oxidative phosphorylation, p. 111). This ATP is then used to power various cellular processes. In brown fat cells, the hydrogen ions bypass the coupling of oxidation with ATP production and generate heat instead. Thermogenesis is activated by the sympathetic nervous system, which responds to signals from the hypothalamus.

eat more food than thin people. Rather they have a reduced capacity to burn off excess calories by "nonshivering thermogenesis." The defect has been traced to **brown fat,** a diffuse tissue located in adults in the chest, upper back, and near the kidneys (newborn mammals, including human infants, have much more brown fat than adults). In normal people an increased caloric intake induces brown fat tissue to dissipate the excess energy as heat. This is referred to as "diet-induced thermogenesis." The capacity is diminished in people tending toward obesity because they have less brown fat or because their brown fat does not respond to hypothalamic signals as it should. There are other reasons for obesity in addition to the fact that many people simply eat too much. Fat stores are supervised by the hypothalamus, which is set at a point that may be higher or lower than the population norm. A high setpoint can be lowered somewhat by exercise, but as dieters are painfully aware, the body defends its fat stores with remarkable efficiency.

NUTRITIONAL REQUIREMENTS

The food of animals must include carbohydrates, proteins, fats, water, mineral salts, and vitamins. Carbohydrates and fats are required as fuels for energy demands of the body and for the synthesis of various substances and structures. Proteins (actually the amino acids of which they are composed) are needed for the synthesis of the body's specific proteins and other nitrogen-containing compounds. Water is required as the solvent for the body's chemistry and as the major component of all the body fluids. The inorganic salts are required as the anions and cations of body fluids and tissues and form important structural and physiological components throughout the body. The vitamins are accessory food factors that are often built into the structure of many of the enzymes of the body.

All animals require these broad classes of nutrients, although there are differences in the amounts and kinds of food required. Of these basic food classes some nutrients are used principally as fuels (carbohydrates and lipids), whereas others are required principally as structural and functional components (proteins, minerals, and vitamins). Any of the basic foods (proteins, carbohydrates, and fats) can serve as fuel to supply energy requirements, but no animal can thrive on fuels alone. A **balanced diet** must satisfy all metabolic requirements of the body—requirements for energy, growth, maintenance, reproduction, and physiological regulation.

The recognition years ago that many diseases of humans and domesticated animals were caused by or associated with dietary deficiencies led biologists to search for specific nutrients that would prevent such diseases. These studies eventually yielded a list of "essential" nutrients for humans and other animal species studied. The essential nutrients are those that are needed for normal growth and maintenance and that *must* be supplied in the diet. In other words, it is "essential" that these nutrients be in the diet because the animal cannot synthesize them from other dietary constituents. Nearly 30 organic compounds (amino acids and vitamins) and 21 elements have been established as essential. If we consider that the body contains thousands of different organic compounds, the list given in the margin is remarkably short. Animal cells have marvelous powers of synthesis, enabling them to build compounds of enormous variety and complexity from a small, select group of raw materials.

In the average diet of Americans and Canadians, approximately 50% of the total calories (energy content) comes from carbohydrates and 40% comes from lipids. Proteins, essential as they are for structural needs, supply only a little more than 10% of the total calories of the average North American's diet. Carbohydrates are widely consumed because they are more abundant and cheaper than proteins or lipids. Actually humans and many other animals can subsist on diets devoid of carbohydrates, provided sufficient total calories and essential nutrients are present. Eskimos, before the decline of their native culture, lived on a diet that was high in fat and protein and very low in carbohydrate.

Lipids are needed principally to provide energy. However, at least three fatty acids are essential for humans because they cannot be synthesized. Much interest and research have been devoted to lipids in our diets because of the association between fatty diets and the disease **atherosclerosis** (narrowing of the arteries). The matter is complex, but evidence suggests that atherosclerosis may occur when the diet is high in saturated lipids (lipids with few or no double bonds in the carbon chains of the fatty acids) but low in polyunsaturated lipids (numerous double bonds in the carbon chains). Eskimos who live along the western shores of Greenland and whose diet consists largely of fish have a remarkably low incidence of heart attacks and cerebrovascular accidents. Fish oils are high in polyunsaturated fats. Most North Americans, however, prefer a diet high in saturated fats. Such diets promote a high blood level of cholesterol, which may be deposited in plate-like formations in the lining of the major arteries. For this reason the polyunsaturated fatty acids are often considered necessary nutrients for humans. Generally, animal fat is more saturated, whereas fat from plants is more unsaturated.

Proteins are expensive foods and restricted in the diet. Proteins, of course, are not themselves the essential nutrients, but rather contain essential amino acids. Of the 20 amino acids commonly found in proteins, nine and possibly 11 are essential to humans (see marginal note). The rest can be synthesized. We must keep in mind that the terms "nonessential" and "essential" relate only to dietary requirements and to which amino acids can and cannot be synthesized by the body. All 20 amino acids are essential for the various cellular functions of the body. In fact, some of the so-called nonessential amino acids participate in more crucial metabolic activities than the essential amino acids.

Generally, animal proteins have more of the essential amino acids than do proteins of plant origin. An adult man would require approximately 67 g of whole wheat bread each day to meet his amino acid requirement, but only 19 g of beefsteak to meet these same requirements. One reason that many plants have lower protein scores than animal foods is that plant proteins are often low in certain essential amino acids. All nine of the essential amino acids must be present simultaneously in the diet for protein synthesis. If one or more are missing, the use of the other amino acids will be reduced proportionately; they cannot be stored and are broken down for energy. Thus, heavy reliance on a single plant source will inevitably lead to protein deficiency. This problem can be corrected if two kinds of plant proteins having complementary strengths in essential amino acids are ingested together. For example, when wheat flour, which is poor only in lysine, is mixed with a legume (peas or beans), which is a good source of lysine but deficient in methionine and cystine, a balanced diet with respect to protein results. Each plant complements the other by having adequate amounts of those amino acids that are deficient in the other.

Because animal proteins are so nutritious, they are in great demand in all

Human nutrient requirements*
Amino acids

Phenylalanine	Methionine
Lysine	Cystine
Isoleucine	Tryptophan
Leucine	Threonine
Valine	

Polyunsaturated fatty acids
  Arachidonic
  Linoleic
  Linolenic
Water-soluble vitamins
  Thiamine (B_1)
  Riboflavin (B_2)
  Niacin
  Pyridoxine (B_6)
  Pantothenic acid
  Folacin
  Vitamin B_{12}
  Biotin
  Choline
  Ascorbic acid (C)
Fat-soluble vitamins
  A, D, E, and K
Minerals

Calcium	Silicon
Phosphorus	Vanadium
Sulfur	Tin
Potassium	Nickel
Chlorine	Selenium
Sodium	Manganese
Magnesium	Iodine
Iron	Molybdenum
Fluorine	Chromium
Zinc	Cobalt
Copper	

*Modified from Scrimshaw, N.S., and V.R. Young. 1976. Sci. Am. 235:50-64.

By genetic manipulation, plant breeders have been able to produce cereal proteins having much higher nutritional quality than the parent cereals. An example is triticale, an intergeneric cross between wheat and rye, which has more protein and a much higher lysine content than either of its parents.

countries. North Americans eat far more animal proteins than do Asians and Africans; on the average a North American eats 66 g of animal protein a day, supplemented by milk, eggs, cereals, and legumes. In the Middle East the individual consumption of protein is 14 g, in Africa 11 g, and in Asia 8 g.

Undernourishment and malnourishment are the world's major health problems today. The United Nations Food and Agricultural Organization estimates that 450 million people are chronically undernourished. The World Bank, using different calculations, has placed the figure at 1 billion—nearly one fourth of the human population. Growing children and pregnant and lactating women are especially vulnerable to the devastating effects of malnutrition. Cell proliferation and growth in the human brain are most rapid in the terminal months of pregnancy and the first year after birth. Adequate protein for neuron development is a requirement during this critical time to prevent neurological dysfunction. The brains of children who die of protein malnutrition during the first year of life have 15% to 20% fewer brain cells than those of normal children (Fig. 31-10). Malnourished children who survive this period suffer permanent brain damage and cannot be helped by later corrective treatment (Fig. 31-11).

The major cause of the world's precarious food situation is recent rapid population growth. The world population was 2 billion in 1930, reached 3 billion in 1960, is 4 billion today, and probably will be 6 billion in less than 20 years. Eighty million people are added each year. The equivalent of the total U.S. population is added to the world every 30 months. Thus, the search for new ways to increase food production and distribution takes on a desperate urgency.

It was fitting that the 1970 Nobel Prize for Peace should go to Dr. Norman Borlaug, who developed several of the new wheat varieties that ushered in the Green Revolution of the 1960s. The Green Revolution has enabled developing countries to avoid catastrophic hunger and starvation by introducing improved plant varieties, chemical fertilizers, irrigation, and mechanization. However, all of these elements depend mainly on the availability of fossil fuels. Research is now focusing on less energy-intensive technology, such as improved biological nitrogen fixation, greater photosynthetic efficiency, more efficient nutrient and water uptake, and the development of genetic resistance to pests. To be successful, this promising approach will require collaborative genetic research by Western scientists and the developing countries; this seems essential to the building of self-reliant food systems in the energy-poor developing world. However, Dr. Borlaug himself emphasizes that, despite our best efforts to develop more productive grains, mass famine seems inevitable unless the human population is stabilized.

Vitamins

A vitamin is a relatively simple organic compound that is not a carbohydrate, fat, protein, or mineral and that is required in very small amounts in the diet for some specific cellular function. Vitamins are not sources of energy but are often associated with the activity of important enzymes that have vital metabolic roles. Plants and many microorganisms synthesize all the organic compounds they need; animals, however, have lost certain synthetic abilities during their long evolution and depend ultimately on plants to supply these compounds. Vitamins therefore represent synthetic gaps in the metabolic machinery of animals.

Vitamins are usually classified as fat soluble (soluble in fat solvents such as ether) or water soluble. The water-soluble ones include the B complex and vitamin

---

Two different types of severe food deficiency are recognized: marasmus, general undernourishment from a diet low in both calories and protein, and kwashiorkor, protein malnourishment from a diet adequate in calories but deficient in protein. Marasmus (Gr., *marasmos*, to waste away) is common in infants weaned too early and placed on low-calorie–low-protein diets; these children are listless, and their bodies waste away. Kwashiorkor is a West African word describing a disease a child gets when displaced from the breast by a newborn sibling. This disease is characterized by retarded growth, anemia, weak muscles, a bloated body with typical pot belly, acute diarrhea, susceptibility to infection, and high mortality. Ten million children the world over are seriously undernourished or malnourished, and 1 million children die of hunger each year in India alone.

DNA (mg)

Figure 31-10

Effect of early malnutrition on cell number (measured as total DNA content) in the human brain.
From Winick, M. 1976. Malnutrition and brain development. New York, Oxford University Press.

Figure 31-11

Biafran refugee child suffering severe malnutrition.
From Hosp. Tribune 8:1, 1974.

C. The family of B vitamins, so grouped because the original B vitamin was subsequently found to consist of several distinct compounds, tends to be found together in nature. Almost all animals, vertebrate and invertebrate, require the B vitamins; they are "universal" vitamins. The dietary need for vitamin C and the fat-soluble vitamins A, D, E, and K tends to be restricted to the vertebrates, although some are required by certain invertebrates. Even within groups of close relationship, vitamin requirements are relative, not absolute. A rabbit does not require vitamin C, but guinea pigs and humans do. Some songbirds require vitamin A, but others do not.

Lipid-soluble vitamins

Vitamin A, unlike most other vitamins, exists in several different isomeric forms with different potentials for biological activity. Vitamin A consists of half of a β-carotene molecule; carotenes are a class of organic compounds synthesized only by plants. Animals convert the plant carotenoid to vitamin A; therefore many animal foods, especially butter, eggs, and milk, are sources of the vitamin precursor, as are green leafy and yellow vegetables. Vitamin A functions in visual photochemistry and is also necessary for normal cell growth. A deficiency causes night blindness and growth retardation.

Vitamin A deficiency afflicts millions of people in the Western Pacific, Far East, semiarid zones of Africa, and parts of Latin America. Night blindness is an early sign of deficiency. Severe deficiencies lead to xerophthalmia, a disease of the eye in which the cornea and conjunctiva become dry and infected. If the disease is untreated, the cornea softens and perforates, resulting in total blindness (keratomalacia). Worldwide, 50,000 to 100,000 children become blind each year from this disease.

Vitamin D is derived from eggs, fish oils, and beef fat. The two forms of vitamin D are vitamin D_2 (ergocalciferol) and vitamin D_3 (cholecalciferol). The latter is synthesized from a precursor in the skin by ultraviolet irradiation in sunlight. Vitamin D is converted in the liver and kidneys to a hormonal derivative, 1,25-dihydroxyvitamin D, which promotes absorption of calcium in the intestine. A deficiency of vitamin D causes rickets, a disease characterized by defective bone formation.

Vitamin E is a poorly understood group of tocopherols found in grains, meat, milk, and green leafy vegetables. It is essential for cellular respiration, probably as a cofactor in a Krebs cycle enzyme system. A deficiency causes sterility, defective embryonic growth, muscular weakness, and anemia. Vitamin E's current popularity with food faddists as a panacea for nearly all ailments is largely wishful thinking.

Vitamin K belongs to a group of compounds known as quinones. It is necessary for the synthesis of prothrombin in the liver. Its deficiency causes failure of blood to clot. It is scarce in the normal diet but is synthesized by bacteria in the colon.

Water-soluble vitamins
B-complex vitamins

Thiamine (vitamin B$_1$) is an essential coenzyme in pyruvate metabolism. Thiamine is synthesized by plants and is found in beans, grain, yeast, and roots. It is also present in eggs and lean meat. A deficiency causes beriberi, nervous system degeneration, and cessation of growth.

Riboflavin (vitamin B$_2$) is a part of the oxidative flavoprotein coenzyme (FAD). It is present in many foods such as green beans, eggs, liver, and milk. A deficiency, rare in humans, causes nonspecific digestive disturbances and certain kinds of dermatitis.

Nicotinic acid (niacin) is converted in the body to hydrogen donor-acceptor coenzymes (NAD and NADP). It is found in green leaves, egg yolk, wheat germ, and liver. A deficiency leads to depressed oxidative metabolism, producing a complex of symptoms called pellagra.

Vitamin B$_6$ is a vitamin complex found in nature in three forms: pyridoxine, pyridoxal, and pyridoxamine. All are biologically active in mammals. Vitamin B$_6$ is a coenzyme that functions in amino acid metabolism. It is widely distributed in foods, especially meat, eggs, yeast, and cereals. A dietary deficiency is rare in humans but causes a variety of symptoms (dermatitis, growth retardation, anemia) in experimental animals.

Pantothenic acid is part of coenzyme A that functions in carbohydrate and lipid metabolism. It is present in many foods, and a deficiency is not known in humans. In experimental animals its lack causes dermatitis, growth retardation, graying of hair, and other abnormalities.

Folic acid is essential for growth and blood cell formation. It is found in green leaves, soybeans, yeast, and egg yolk. A deficiency causes anemia and kidney hemorrhage.

Biotin (vitamin H) functions in fatty-acid oxidation and synthesis. It is found in liver, egg yolk, meat, and many other sources. A deficiency is very rare in humans. In experimental animals a lack causes dermatitis.

Vitamin B$_{12}$ (cyanocobalamin) is essential for red blood cell formation. It is a unique vitamin in that it is synthesized only by bacteria. Chief sources are milk, egg yolk, liver, and oysters. A deficiency causes pernicious anemia.

Vitamin C

Vitamin C (ascorbic acid) is necessary for the formation of intercellular material. It is found in citrus fruits, tomatoes, and other fresh vegetables. A deficiency causes scurvy, perhaps the most famous deficiency disease of humans. Scurvy was the scourge of sailors and soldiers who subsisted for long periods on dried meats and grains. Scurvy is characterized by capillary bleeding and defective wound healing.

____ Summary

Autotrophic organisms (mostly green plants), using inorganic compounds as raw materials, capture the energy of sunlight through photosynthesis and produce complex organic molecules. Heterotrophic organisms (bacteria, fungi, and animals) use the organic compounds synthesized by plants, and the chemical bond energy stored therein, for their own nutritional and energy needs.

Most animals procure their food by filter feeding or selective feeding. Many invertebrate groups, as well as animals as large as baleen whales, are filter feeders; all strain small particulate food from the water. Selective feeders, on the other hand, usually have mechanisms for capturing food, such as the jaws and teeth of vertebrates.

Digestion, the process of breaking down food mechanically and chemically into molecular subunits for absorption, occurs in sequential stages. Food is received in the mouth and mixed with saliva, which begins starch digestion. Passed to the stomach, the highly acid gastric secretion destroys bacteria and initiates protein digestion. Most digestion occurs in the small intestine. Enzymes from the pancreas and membrane enzymes embedded in the intestinal mucosal cells hydrolyze proteins, carbohydrates, fats, nucleic acids, and various phosphate compounds. The liver secretes bile, containing salts that emulsify fats. Once foodstuffs are digested, they are absorbed as molecular subunits (monosaccharides, amino acids, and fatty acids) into the blood or lymph vessels of the villi of the small intestine. The large intestine (colon) serves mainly to absorb water and minerals from the food wastes as they pass through. It also contains symbiotic bacteria that produce certain vitamins.

Most animals balance food intake with energy expenditure. Food intake is regulated primarily by a hunger center located in the hypothalamus. In mammals, should caloric intake exceed energy requirements, the excess calories normally are dissipated as heat in specialized brown fat tissue. A deficiency in this response is one cause of human obesity.

All animals require a balanced diet containing both fuels (mainly carbohydrates and lipids) and structural and functional components (proteins, minerals, and vitamins). For every multicellular animal, certain amino acids, lipids, vitamins, and minerals are "essential" dietary factors that cannot be produced by the animal's own synthetic machinery. Animal proteins are better-balanced sources of amino acids than are plant proteins, which tend to lack one or more essential amino acids. Undernourishment (marasmus) and protein malnourishment (kwashiorkor) are among the world's major health problems, afflicting millions of people.

Vitamins are simple organic compounds required for specific cellular functions. Most are associated with metabolic enzyme systems.

Wild turkey jumping to feed on berries.
Photograph by N. Bolen.

Selected references

See also general references for Part Three, p. 837.

Brooks, F.P. 1970. Control of gastrointestinal function. New York, Macmillan, Inc. *A concise, well-illustrated summary of human digestive physiology.*

Chrispeels, M.J., and D. Sadava. 1977. Plants, food, and people. San Francisco, W.H. Freeman & Co. Publishers. *Well-written overview of the human nutrition problem, plants and agriculture, and the Green Revolution.*

Hegstead, D.M. 1978. Protein-calorie malnutrition. Am. Sci. **66:**61-65. *Its causes are still poorly understood.*

Jennings, J.B. 1973. Feeding, digestion and assimilation in animals, ed. 2. New York, St. Martin's Press, Inc. *A general, comparative approach. Excellent account of feeding mechanisms in animals.*

Keesey, R.E., and T.L. Powley. 1975. Hypothalamic regulation of body weight. Am. Sci. **63:**558-565. *Experiments with rats indicate that body fat deposition is determined by a hypothalamic "set point."*

Lloyd, L.W., B.E. McDonald, and E.W. Crampton. 1978. Fundamentals of nutrition, ed. 2. San Francisco, W.H. Freeman & Co. Publishers. *Integrated approach to what nutrients are and how they are metabolized.*

Madge, D.S. 1975. The mammalian alimentary system: a functional approach. London, Edward Arnold (Publishers) Ltd. *Undergraduate-level textbook.*

Pivorunas, A. 1979. The feeding mechanism of baleen whales. Am. Sci. **67:**432-440.

Winick, M. 1976. Malnutrition and brain development. New York, Oxford University Press, Inc.

Selected *Scientific American* articles

Davenport, H.W. 1972. Why the stomach does not digest itself. **226:**86-93 (Jan.).

Jones, J.C. 1978. The feeding behavior of mosquitoes. **238:**138-148 (June).

Kretchmer, N. 1972. Lactose and lactase. **227:**70-78 (Oct.). *Most adult mammals, humans included, lack lactase, the enzyme that breaks down lactose, or milk sugar.*

Mayer, J. 1976. The dimensions of human hunger. **235:**40-49 (Sept.). *Excellent description of the worsening world nutritional situation.*

Merritt, R.W., and J.B. Wallace. 1981. Filter-feeding insects. **244:**132-144 (Apr.). *Certain larval insects gather food with nets, brushes, and other filters.*

Moog, F. 1981. The lining of the small intestine. **245:**154-176 (Nov.). *Describes how the mucosal cells actively process foods.*

Neurath, H. 1964. Protein-digesting enzymes. **211:**68-79 (Dec.). *Describes studies of enzyme structure and how these digestive enzymes exert their catalytic effect.*

Rogers, T.A. 1958. The metabolism of ruminants. **198:**34-38 (Feb.). *How cellulose is digested in the four-chambered stomach of cows and other ruminants.*

Scrimshaw, N.S., and V.R. Young. 1976. The requirements of human nutrition. **235:**50-64 (Sept.). *Describes the difficulties of arriving at recommended energy and nutrient allowances for humans.*

Spain, D.M. 1966. Atherosclerosis. **215:**48-56 (Aug.). *How dietary factors contribute to increasing prevalence of this disease.*

Trowell, H.C. 1954. Kwashiorkor. **191:**46-50 (Dec.). *The most severe and widespread nutritional disease known to medical science is described.*

Young, V.R., and N.S. Schrimshaw. 1971. The physiology of starvation. **225:**14-21 (Oct.). *Studies with human volunteers have helped to clarify the body's nutritional needs.*

C H A P T E R   3 2

N E R V O U S   C O O R D I N A T I O N
Nervous System and Sense Organs

Scanning electron micrograph of rod and cone photoreceptor cells from the retina of a mudpuppy *Necturus maculosus*. The rods, adapted for high sensitivity in dim light, are square ended. The cones, adapted for color vision, have more pointed, somewhat tilted ends. (×1500.)

Courtesy Dr. M. Hollenberg.

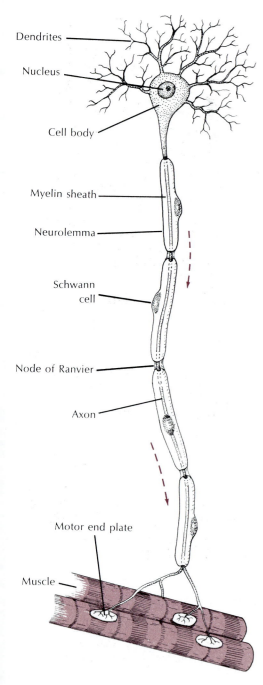

Figure 32-1

Structure of a motor (efferent) neuron.

The nervous system originated in a fundamental property of protoplasm: irritability. Each cell responds to stimulation in a manner characteristic of that type of cell. But certain cells have become highly specialized for receiving stimuli and for conducting impulses to various parts of the body. Through evolutionary changes, these cells have become organized into a vast communications network, and the most complex of all body systems. Indeed, the human brain is unparalleled in complexity among structures known to humans. The endocrine system is also part of the body's communication network and interacts continuously with the nervous system in the control of body function. Functionally, the nervous system differs from the endocrine system in its capacity to monitor external as well as internal changes and to respond immediately to such changes. Nervous responses are measured in milliseconds, whereas the fastest endocrine responses are measured in seconds.

The evolution of the nervous system has been correlated with the development of bilateral symmetry and cephalization. Along with this development, animals acquired exteroceptors and associated ganglia. The basic plan of the nervous system is to code sensory information and transmit it to regions of the central nervous system, where it is processed into appropriate action. This action may be any of several types, such as simple reflexes, automatic behavior patterns, conscious perception, or learning processes.

NERVOUS SYSTEMS OF INVERTEBRATES

The various metazoan phyla reveal a progressive increase in nervous system complexity that probably reflects in a general way the stages in the evolution of the nervous system. The simplest pattern of invertebrate nervous system is the **nerve net** of cnidarians, which, although primitive, is nonetheless a quantum leap in complexity beyond the protozoa, which lack any organized nervous network. The nerve net contains bipolar and multipolar cells (protoneurons). These may be separated from each other by synaptic junctions, but they form an extensive network that is found in and under the epidermis over the entire body. An impulse starting in one part of this net is conducted in all directions, since the synapses do not restrict transmission to one-way movement, as they do in higher animals. There are no differentiated sensory, motor, or connector components in the strict meaning of those terms. Branches of the nerve net connect to receptors in the epidermis and to epitheliomuscular cells. Most responses tend to be generalized, yet many are astonishingly complex for so simple a nervous system. It is interesting that this type of nervous system is found among higher animals in the form of nerve plexuses located, for example, in the intestinal wall, where they govern generalized intestinal movements such as peristalsis.

Flatworms are provided with two anterior **ganglia** of nerve cells from which two main nerve trunks run posteriorly, with lateral branches extending to the various parts of the body (Fig. 11-4, *B*, p. 258). This is the true beginning of a differentiation into a **peripheral nervous system** (a communications network extending to all parts of the body) and a **central nervous system,** which coordinates everything. It is also the first appearance of the **linear** type of nervous system, which is more developed in higher invertebrates. Higher invertebrates have a more centralized nervous system, with the two longitudinal nerve cords fused (although still recognizable) and many ganglia present. The annelids have a well-developed nervous system consisting of distinctive **afferent** (sensory) and **efferent** (motor) neurons. At the anterior end the ventral nerve cord divides and passes upward around the digestive tract to join the bilobed brain. In each segment the double nerve cord bears a double ganglion, each with two pairs of nerves. Arthropods have a system similar to that of earthworms, except that the ganglia are larger and the sense organs better developed.

Molluscs have a system of three pairs of ganglia; one pair is near the mouth, another pair at the base of the foot, and the third pair in the viscera. The ganglia are joined by connectives. The molluscs also have a number of sense organs; they are especially well developed in the cephalopods. Among the echinoderms the nervous system is radially arranged (Fig. 20-18, *A*, p. 480).

The nerve cord in all invertebrates is ventral to the alimentary canal and is solid. This arrangement is in pronounced contrast to the nerve cord of vertebrates, which is dorsal to the digestive system, single, and hollow.

NERVOUS SYSTEMS OF VERTEBRATES

Vertebrates have, as a rule, a brain much larger than the spinal cord. In lower vertebrates this difference is not significant, but higher in the vertebrate subphylum the brain increases in size, reaching its maximum in mammals, especially humans. Along with this enlargement has come an increase in complexity, bringing better patterns of coordination, integration, and intelligence. The nervous system is commonly divided into central and peripheral parts. The **central nervous system** is housed within the skull and vertebral column and is concerned with integrative activity. The **peripheral nervous system** consists of nerve cells or extensions of nerve cells that lie outside the skull and vertebral column. It is a communications system for the conduction of sensory and motor information to all parts of the body.

Neurons and Associated Cells

The neuron: functional unit of the nervous system

The neuron is a cell body with all its processes. Although neurons assume many shapes, depending on their function and location, a typical kind is shown diagrammatically in Fig. 32-1. From the nucleated cell body extends an **axon**, which carries impulses *away* from the cell body. Typically several branching **dendrites** extend from the cell body. These carry impulses *toward* the cell body. Axons are typically much longer than dendrites (often many feet in length in a large animal) and are usually covered with a soft, white, lipid-containing material called **myelin.** This insulating material is often laid down in concentric rings by specialized **Schwann cells** to form a **myelin sheath** (Figs. 32-2 and 32-3). This is enclosed by an outer membrane called the **neurolemma.**

Neurons are commonly classified as **afferent,** or sensory; **efferent,** or motor; and **association** (interneurons). Afferent and efferent neurons lie mostly outside the skull and vertebral column; association neurons, which in humans comprise 99% of all the nerve cells in the body, lie entirely within the central nervous system. Afferent neurons are connected to receptors. When these respond to some environmental change, they generate **action potentials** in the afferent neurons,

Nucleus

Schwann cell

Axon

Figure 32-2

Development of the myelin sheath. The Schwann cell grows around the axon, then rotates around it, enclosing the axon in a tight, multilayered, insulating myelin sheath.

Figure 32-3

Cross section of nerve showing cut ends of nerve processes *(small white circles)*. Such a trunk may contain thousands of both afferent and efferent fibers.

Figure 32-4

Nerve bundle, showing a myelinated fiber surrounded by several unmyelinated fibers. The inset shows an enlargement of the myelin sheath with its successive layers of Schwann cell plasma membrane. (×13,600.)

Electron micrograph courtesy M.E. Todd.

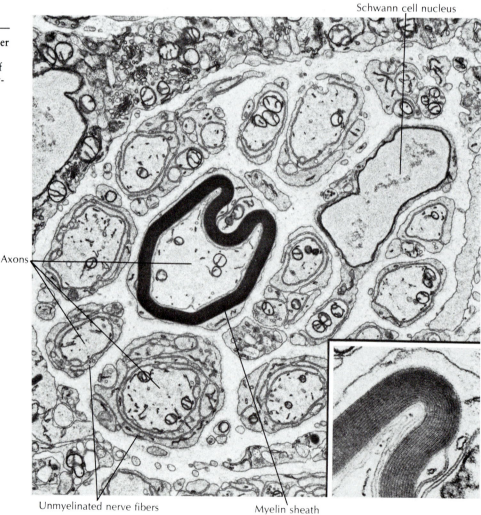

Schwann cell nucleus

Axons

Unmyelinated nerve fibers

Myelin sheath

which are carried into the central nervous system. Here the impulses may be perceived as conscious sensation. The impulses also move to efferent neurons, which carry them out by the peripheral system to **effectors** (muscles or glands).

Nerves (not to be confused with neurons) are actually made up of many neuronal processes—axons or dendrites or both—bound together with connective tissue (Figs. 32-3 and 32-4). The cell bodies of these nerve processes are located either in ganglia or somewhere in the central nervous system (brain or spinal cord).

Satellite cells in the nervous system

Surrounding the neurons are nonnervous satellite cells that have a special relationship to the nerve cells. Satellite cells are of two kinds: (1) Schwann cells in the peripheral nervous system that, as mentioned previously, provide an insulating sheath around axons, and (2) **neuroglial cells** in the brain. Neuroglial cells (or "glial" cells as they are often called) outnumber nerve cells 10 to 1 and make up almost half the volume of the brain. Some glial cells form intimate sheaths of insulating myelin around central axons, just as Schwann cells insulate peripheral axons. The functional roles of other glial cells remain to be clarified. Since many glial cells lie between blood vessels and nerve cells, they may nourish the nerve cells metabolically. It is certain that glial cells serve in regenerative processes that follow injury and disease. Recently, some neurobiologists have attributed important information-processing functions to the neuroglia, although strong experimental support for this possibility is still lacking.

Nature of the Nerve Impulse

The nerve impulse is the chemical-electrical message of nerves, the common functional denominator of all nervous system activity. Despite the incredible complexity of the nervous system of advanced animals, nerve impulses are basically alike in all nerves and in all animals. It is an "all-or-none" phenomenon; either the fiber is conducting an impulse, or it is not. Because all impulses are alike, the only way a nerve fiber can vary its effect on the tissue it innervates is by changing the frequency of impulse conduction. Frequency change is the language of a nerve fiber. A fiber may conduct no impulses at all or very few per second up to a maximum approaching 1000 per second. The higher the frequency (or rate) of conduction, the greater is the level of excitation.

Resting potential

To understand what happens when an impulse is conducted down a fiber, we need to know something about the resting, undisturbed fiber. Nerve cell membranes, like all cell membranes, have special permeability properties that create ionic imbalances. The interstitial fluid surrounding nerve cells contains relatively high concentrations of sodium (Na^+) and chloride (Cl^-) ions, but a low concentration of potassium ions (K^+). Inside the neuron, the ratio is reversed: the potassium concentration is high, but the sodium and chloride concentrations are low (Fig. 32-5; see also Fig. 29-1, *B,* p. 691). These differences are quite dramatic; there is approximately 10 times more sodium outside than in and 25 to 30 times more potassium inside than out. However, the nerve cell membrane is 50 to 70 times

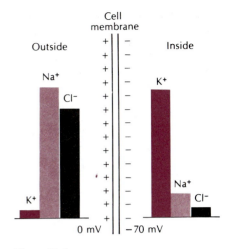

Figure 32-5

Ionic composition inside and outside a resting nerve cell. An active sodium pump located in the cell membrane drives sodium to the outside, keeping its concentration low inside. Potassium concentration is high inside, and although the membrane is "leaky" to potassium, this ion is held inside by the repelling positive charge outside the membrane.

Membrane potential
(mV)

Figure 32-6

Action potential of a nerve impulse. The electrical event, moving from left to right, is associated with rapid changes in membrane permeability to sodium ions. The trace at the top is that recorded by an electrode with the tip inside the axon membrane. When the impulse arrives at a point, sodium ions suddenly rush in, making the axon positive inside and negative outside. Potassium ions can now penetrate the membrane and restore the normal resting potential. Impermeability to sodium ions returns. (Although the impulse is moving from left to right, it is easier to follow the time course of the sequence of voltage and ionic changes by reading the graph from right to left.)

more permeable (or "leaky") to potassium than to sodium. As a result, potassium ions tend to leak out of the cell, following their concentration gradient. This movement gives rise to an electrical potential, with the outside of the membrane positive with respect to the inside.

If the membrane is highly permeable to potassium, why does not all of the potassium escape from the cell, allowing the potential to disappear? This does not happen because the potential difference created by outward movement of potassium begins to influence this movement. Since potassium ions are positively charged, they are attracted by the negatively charged inside membrane and repelled by the positively charged outside membrane. As potassium flows outward, the electrical force across the membrane becomes large enough to prevent any further net outward movement of potassium. This membrane potential is called an **equilibrium potential** because it is a permanent bioelectrical potential produced by a balance between a concentration force favoring the outward flow of potassium and an electrical force that opposes it.

This is the origin of the **resting transmembrane potential**, which is positive outside and negative inside. It is created, as we have seen, by two important characteristics of the living nerve cell: (1) the potassium concentration is much greater inside the cell than outside and (2) the cell membrane is far more permeable to potassium than to sodium. The resting potential is usually -70 mV (millivolts), with the inside of the membrane negative to the outside.

Action potential

The nerve impulse is a rapidly moving change in electrical potential called the **action potential** (Fig. 32-6). It is a very rapid and brief depolarization of the nerve fiber membrane; in fact, not only is the resting potential abolished, but in most nerve fibers the potential actually reverses for an instant so that the outside becomes negative as compared to the inside. Then, as the action potential moves ahead, the membrane returns to its normal resting potential ready to conduct another impulse. The entire event occupies approximately a millisecond. Perhaps the most significant property of the nerve impulse is that it is self-propagating; once started, the impulse moves ahead automatically, much like the burning of a fuse.

What causes the reversal of polarity in the cell membrane during passage of an action potential? We have seen that the resting potential depends on the high membrane permeability (leakiness) to potassium, some 50 to 70 times greater than the permeability to sodium. When the action potential arrives at a given point, the permeability of the membrane to sodium is significantly changed. The membrane suddenly becomes approximately 600 times more permeable to sodium, whereas potassium permeability changes very little. Sodium rushes in.

Actually only an extremely small amount of sodium traverses the membrane in that instant—less than one millionth of the sodium outside—but this brief shift of positive ions inward causes the membrane potential to disappear, even reverse. An electrical "hole" is created. Potassium, finding its electrical barrier gone, begins to move out. Then, as the action potential passes on, the membrane quickly regains its resting properties. It becomes once again practically impermeable to sodium, and the outward movement of potassium is checked.

The rising phase of the action potential is associated with the rapid influx (inward movement) of sodium (Fig. 32-6). When the action potential reaches its peak, the sodium permeability is restored to normal, and potassium permeability briefly increases above the resting level. This causes the action potential to decrease rapidly toward the resting membrane level.

Sodium pump

The resting cell membrane has a very low permeability to sodium. Nevertheless some sodium ions leak across, even in the resting condition. When the axon is active, sodium flows inward with each passing impulse, and, although the amount is very small, it is obvious that the ionic gradient would eventually disappear if the sodium ions were not moved back out again. This is accomplished by the sodium pump, a complex of protein subunits embedded in the plasma membrane of the axon. Each sodium pump uses the energy stored in ATP to transport sodium from the inside to the outside of the membrane. The name of the pump is something of a misnomer, since, as in several other cell membranes, it carries potassium in as it pumps sodium out. The exchange of sodium for potassium is not equal because three sodium ions on the inside are pumped out for every two potassium ions pumped in. An average neuron contains 100 to 200 sodium pumps per square micrometer of membrane surface. When working near capacity, each pump can transport about 200 sodium ions and 130 potassium ions per second (the actual rate is adjusted to meet the needs of the cell). Since more sodium ions are moved out of the axon than potassium ions are moved in, the sodium pump produces a net outward movement of positive charges. This of course helps to maintain the transmembrane polarity, which is positive outside.

—— Synapses: Junction Points between Nerves

A synapse is a tiny gap at the end of a nerve axon where it connects to the dendrites or cell body of the next neuron. Neurons bringing impulses toward synapses are called **presynaptic neurons;** those carrying impulses away are **postsynaptic neurons.** At the synapse the membranes are separated by a narrow gap, the synaptic cleft, having a very uniform width of approximately 20 nm.

The axon of most nerves divides at its end into many branches, each of which bears a synaptic knob that sits on the dendrites or cell body of the next nerve (Fig. 32-7). The axon terminations of several nerves may almost cover a nerve cell body and its dendrites with thousands of synaptic clefts. Because a single impulse coming down a nerve axon splays out into the many branches and synaptic endings on the next nerve cell, many impulses therefore converge at the cell body at one instant.

The 20 nm fluid-filled gap between presynaptic and postsynaptic membranes prevents impulses from spreading directly to the postsynaptic neuron. Instead the synaptic knobs secrete a specific transmitter substance that communicates chemically with the postsynaptic cell. Inside the synaptic knobs are numerous tiny vesicles, each containing several thousand molecules of the chemical transmitter. When an impulse arrives at the terminal knob, some of the vesicles discharge their contents into the synaptic cleft. Once released from the vesicles, the transmitter molecules diffuse rapidly across the gap to bind with protein receptor molecules embedded in the postsynaptic membrane (Fig. 32-7). The interaction between chemical transmitter and receptor produces a small postsynaptic potential.

Acetylcholine is the most common neurotransmitter in the peripheral nervous system. The sequence of its release, receptor interaction, inactivation, and

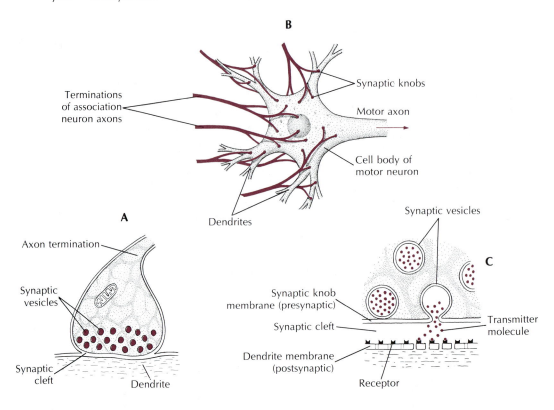

Figure 32-7

Transmission of impulses across nerve synapses. **A,** The cell body of a motor nerve is shown covered with the terminations of association neurons. Each termination ends in a synaptic knob; hundreds of synaptic knobs may be on a single nerve cell body and its dendrites. **B,** A synaptic knob enlarged 60 times more than in **A.** An impulse traveling down the axon causes some synaptic vesicles to move down to the synaptic cleft and rupture, releasing transmitter molecules into the cleft. **C,** A synaptic cleft as it might appear under a high-resolution electron microscope. Transmitter molecules from a ruptured synaptic vesicle move quickly across the gap to bind with receptor molecules in the postsynaptic membrane. An electrical potential is produced in the postsynaptic membrane.

resynthesis is summarized in Fig. 32-8. Each vesicle contains some 10,000 molecules of acetylcholine. When discharged from the vesicle following the arrival of a nerve impulse at the synapse, the molecules of acetylcholine diffuse across the gap in a fraction of a millisecond and bind to receptor molecules. The receptor molecules are also ion channels that are opened by acetylcholine for a brief instant (about 1 millisecond), allowing thousands of sodium and potassium ions to pass through. This results in a voltage change in the postsynaptic membrane. Whether the voltage change is large enough to trigger an action potential in the postsynaptic cell depends on how many acetylcholine molecules are released and how many channels are opened. The acetylcholine molecules are rapidly destroyed by the enzyme acetylcholinesterase. This is important because, if not inactivated in this way, the transmitter would continue to stimulate indefinitely. The organophosphate insecticides and certain nerve gases developed for military use are poisonous for precisely this reason.

Several different chemical transmitters have been identified. These include (in addition to acetylcholine) norepinephrine (Fig. 32-9), epinephrine, serotonin, and γ-aminobutyric acid (GABA). Other chemicals suspected of behaving as neurotransmitters have been identified, but it is often very difficult to verify that a substance is a natural transmitter. In the brain the chemical identity of the transmitter at many synapses is unknown.

The synapse is of great functional importance because it acts as a one-way valve that allows nerve impulses to move in one direction only. It is also part of the decision-making equipment of the central nervous system because it is here that information is modulated from one nerve to the next. If many synapses are activated at one time, they can reduce the membrane voltage enough in the postsynaptic cell to fire an impulse. Some synapses, however, are inhibitory, causing the membrane voltage to increase rather than decrease. Thus, it is the net effect of all the excitatory and inhibitory inputs that determines whether the postsynaptic cell will fire or remain silent.

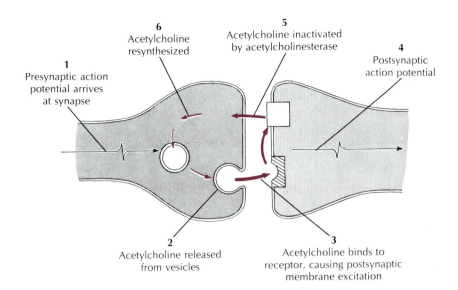

6
Acetylcholine
resynthesized

5
Acetylcholine inactivated
by acetylcholinesterase

4
Postsynaptic
action potential

1
Presynaptic action
potential arrives
at synapse

2
Acetylcholine released
from vesicles

3
Acetylcholine binds to
receptor, causing postsynaptic
membrane excitation

Figure 32-8

Sequence of events in synaptic transmission excitation and chemistry.

Smooth muscle cell

Synapse with synaptic
vesicles containing neurotransmitter

Extracellular material

Schwann cell nucleus

Figure 32-9

Nerve fiber synapse on a vascular smooth muscle cell. Note the numerous synaptic vesicles; these contain norepinephrine. (×16,500.)

Electron micrograph courtesy M.E. Todd.

___ Components of the Reflex Arc

Many neurons work in groups called **reflex arcs** (Fig. 32-10). There must be at least two neurons in a reflex arc, but usually there are more. The parts of a typical reflex arc consist of (1) a **receptor,** a sense organ in the skin, muscle, or other organ; (2) an **afferent** or sensory neuron, which carries the impulse toward the central nervous system; (3) a **nerve center,** where synaptic junctions are made between the sensory neurons and the association neurons; (4) the **efferent** or

Figure 32-10

Reflex arc. Impulse generated in the receptor is conducted over an afferent (sensory) nerve to the spinal cord, relayed by an association neuron to an efferent (motor) nerve cell body and by the efferent axon to an effector.

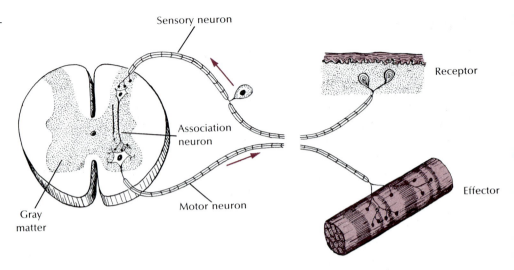

motor neuron, which makes synaptic junction with the association neuron and carries impulses out from the central nervous system; and (5) the **effector,** by which the animal responds to its environmental changes. Examples of effectors are muscles, glands, cilia, nematocysts of the cnidarians, electric organs of fish, and chromatophores.

A reflex arc at its simplest consists of only two neurons: a sensory (afferent) neuron and a motor (efferent) neuron. Usually, however, association neurons are interposed (Fig. 32-10). Association neurons may connect afferent and efferent neurons on the same side of the spinal cord, or on opposite sides, or connect them on different levels of the spinal cord, on either the same or opposite sides. In almost any reflex act a number of reflex arcs are involved. For instance, a single afferent neuron may make synaptic junctions with many efferent neurons. In a similar way an efferent neuron may receive impulses from many afferent neurons. In the latter case the efferent neuron is referred to as the **final common path.**

A **reflex act** is the response to a stimulus acting over a reflex arc. It is **involuntary** and may involve the cerebrospinal or autonomic nervous divisions of the nervous system. Many of the vital processes of the body, such as control of breathing, heartbeat, diameter of blood vessels, and sweat gland secretion, are reflex actions. Some reflex acts are inherited and innate; others are acquired through learning processes (conditioning).

___ Organization of the Vertebrate Nervous System

The basic plan of the vertebrate nervous system is a dorsal longitudinal hollow nerve cord that runs from head to tail. During early embryonic development, the central nervous system begins as an ectodermal **neural groove,** which by folding and enlarging becomes a long, hollow **neural tube.** The cephalic end enlarges into the brain vesicles, and the rest becomes the spinal cord. The spinal nerves (31 pairs in humans) have a dual origin. The **spinal ganglia** (Fig. 32-11) containing the sensory neurons differentiate from specialized cells, called **neural crest cells,** that pinch off from the edges of the neural groove as it closes to form a tube. The ventral roots contain motor fibers that originate in the spinal cord. Both dorsal (sensory) and ventral (motor) roots meet some distance beyond the cord to form a mixed **spinal nerve** (Fig. 32-11).

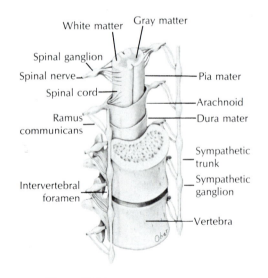

Figure 32-11

Spinal cord and meninges with relation to spinal nerves, sympathetic system, and vertebrae. Three coats of meninges have been partly cut away to expose the spinal cord. Only two vertebrae are shown in position.

Central nervous system

The central nervous system is composed of the spinal cord and brain.

Spinal cord

The spinal cord is enclosed by the vertebral canal and additionally protected by three layers collectively called the **meninges** (men-in'jeez). The three layers are a tough outer **dura mater,** a thin spider web–like **arachnoid,** and a delicate innermost sheath, the **pia mater** (Fig. 32-11). Between the arachnoid and the pia mater is a space containing **cerebrospinal fluid,** discussed later in this chapter. The meninges and cerebrospinal fluid blanket are continuous with those covering the brain.

In cross section the cord shows two zones. An inner H-shaped zone of **gray matter** is made up of association neurons and cell bodies of motor neurons (Fig. 32-10). The outer zone of **white matter** contains nerve bundles of axons and dendrites linking different levels of the cord with each other and with the brain. The fibers are bundled into **ascending tracts,** carrying impulses to the brain, and **descending tracts,** carrying impulses away from the brain. The sensory (ascending) tracts are located mainly in the dorsal part of the cord; the motor (descending) tracts are found ventrally and laterally in the cord. Fibers also cross over from one side of the cord to the other, with the sensory fibers crossing at a higher level than the motor fibers. Although the different tracts cannot be distinguished in a sectioned cord even with a microscope, their position is known from painstaking mapping experiments.

Brain

Unlike the spinal cord, which has changed little in structure during vertebrate evolution, the brain has changed dramatically. From the primitive linear brain of fishes and amphibians, it has expanded into the deeply fissured, enormously complex brain of mammals. It reaches its highest level in the human brain, which contains some 10 billion nerve cells, each connected, on the average, to about 1000 others. The ratio between the weight of the brain and that of the spinal cord affords a fair criterion of an animal's intelligence. In fish and amphibians this ratio is approximately 1:1, but in humans it is 55:1—in other words, the brain is 55 times heavier than the spinal cord. Although the human brain is not the largest (the sperm whale's brain is seven times heavier) nor the most convoluted (that of the porpoise is even more wrinkled), it is by all odds the best. This "great ravelled knot," as the British physiologist Sir Charles Sherrington called the human brain, in fact may be so complex that it will never be able to understand its own function.

The primitive three-part brain is made up of prosencephalon, mesencephalon, and rhombencephalon (forebrain, midbrain, and hindbrain) (Fig. 32-12; Table 32-1). The prosencephalon and rhombencephalon each divide again to form the five-part brain characteristic of the adults of all vertebrates. The five-part brain includes the telencephalon, diencephalon, mesencephalon, metencephalon, and myelencephalon. From these divisions the different functional brain structures arise.

The impressive evolutionary improvement of the vertebrate brain has accompanied the increased powers of locomotion and greater environmental awareness of the more advanced vertebrates. In the primitive vertebrate brain,

Although the large size of their brain undoubtedly makes humans the wisest of animals, it is apparent that they can do without much of it and still remain wise. Recent brain scans of persons with hydrocephalus (enlargement of the head resulting from pressure disturbances that cause the brain ventricles to enlarge many times their normal size) show that although many of them are functionally disabled, others are nearly normal. The cranium of one person with hydrocephalus was nearly filled with cerebrospinal fluid, and the only remaining cerebral cortex was a thin layer of tissue, 1 mm thick, pressed against the cranium. Yet this young man, with only 5% of his brain, had achieved first-class honors in mathematics at a British university and was socially normal. This and other similarly dramatic observations suggest that there is enormous redundancy and spare capacity in corticocerebral function. It also suggests that the deep structures of the brain, which are relatively spared in hydrocephalus, may carry out functions once believed to be performed solely by the cortex.

Table 32-1 Divisions of the Vertebrate Brain

Embryonic vesicles	Main components in adults
Prosencephalon (forebrain)	
Telencephalon	Olfactory bulbs Cerebral hemispheres Lateral ventricles
Diencephalon	Thalamus Hypothalamus Infundibulum Third ventricle
Mesencephalon (midbrain)	
Mesencephalon	Optic lobes (tectum) Cerebral peduncles Red nucleus Aqueduct of Sylvius
Rhombencephalon (hindbrain)	
Metencephalon	Cerebellum Pons Fourth ventricle
Myelencephalon	Medulla

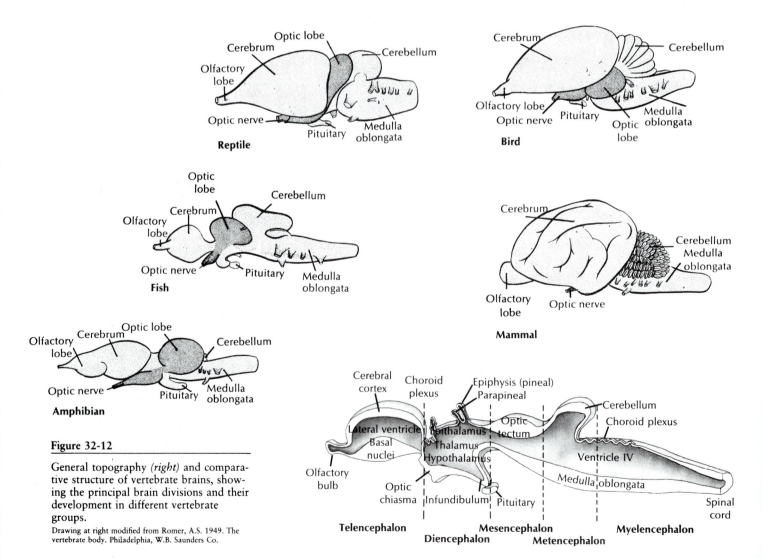

Figure 32-12

General topography *(right)* and comparative structure of vertebrate brains, showing the principal brain divisions and their development in different vertebrate groups.

Drawing at right modified from Romer, A.S. 1949. The vertebrate body. Philadelphia, W.B. Saunders Co.

each of the three parts was concerned with one or more special senses: the prosencephalon with the sense of smell, the mesencephalon with vision, and the rhombencephalon with hearing and balance. These primitive but very fundamental concerns of the brain have been in some instances amplified and in others reduced or overshadowed during continued evolution as sensory priorities were shaped by the animal's habitat and way of life.

The brain is made up of both white and gray matter, with the gray matter on the outside (in contrast to the spinal cord in which the gray matter is inside). The gray matter of the brain is mostly in the convoluted **cortex.** In the deeper white matter of the brain, myelinated bundles of nerve fibers connect the cortex with lower centers of the brain and spinal cord or connect one part of the cortex with another. Also in deeper portions of the brain are clusters of nerve cell bodies (gray matter) that provide synaptic junctions between the neurons of higher centers and those of lower centers.

The **medulla,** the most posterior division of the brain, is really a conical continuation of the spinal cord. The medulla, together with the more anterior midbrain, constitutes the "brain stem," an area in which numerous vital and largely subconscious activities are controlled, such as heartbeat, respiration, vasomotor tone, and swallowing. The brain stem contains the roots of all the cranial nerves except the first and is traversed by many sensory and motor fiber tracts. Although it is small in size and largely hidden from view by the much enlarged "higher" centers, it is, in fact, the most vital brain area; whereas damage to higher centers may result in severely debilitating loss of sensory or motor function, damage to the brain stem usually results in death.

The **pons,** between the medulla and the midbrain, is made up of a thick bundle of fibers that carry impulses from one side of the cerebellum to the other.

The **cerebellum,** lying above the medulla, is concerned with equilibrium, posture, and movement (Fig. 32-13). Its development is directly correlated with

Figure 32-13

Human brain. **A,** External view of the left side of the brain showing lobes of the cerebrum, cerebellum, and brain stem. **B,** Localization of function on the left cerebral cortex and cerebellum.

the animal's mode of locomotion, agility of limb movement, and balance. It is usually weakly developed in amphibians and reptiles, which are relatively clumsy forms that stay close to the ground, and is well developed in the more agile bony fishes. It reaches its apogee in birds and mammals in which it is greatly expanded and folded. The cerebellum does not initiate movements but operates as a precision error-control center, or servomechanism, that programs a movement initiated somewhere else, such as in the motor cortex. Primates and especially humans, who possess a manual dexterity far surpassing that of other animals, have the most complex cerebellum of all, since hand and finger movements may involve the simultaneous contraction and relaxation of hundreds of individual muscles.

Between the medulla and diencephalon is the **midbrain.** This is the anterior portion of the brain stem. The white matter of the midbrain consists of ascending and descending tracts that go to the thalamus and cerebrum. On the upper side of the midbrain are the rounded **optic lobes,** serving as centers for visual and auditory reflexes. The midbrain has undergone little evolutionary change in size among vertebrates but has changed in function. It mediates the most complex behavior of fishes and amphibians. Such integrative functions were gradually assumed by the forebrain in higher vertebrates, and in mammals the midbrain is mainly a reflex center for eye muscles and a relay and analysis center for auditory information.

The **thalamus,** above the midbrain, contains masses of gray matter surrounded by the cerebral hemispheres on each side. This is the relay center for the sensory tracts from the spinal cord. Centers for the sensations of pain, temperature, and touch are supposedly located in the thalamus. In the **hypothalamus** are "housekeeping" centers that regulate body temperature, water balance, sleep, appetite, and a few other body functions. The hypothalamus also has neurosecretory cells that produce pituitary-regulating neurohormones.

The anterior region of the brain, the **cerebrum** (Fig. 32-13), can be divided into two anatomically distinct areas, the **paleocortex** and **neocortex.** As its name implies, the paleocortex is the ancient telencephalon. Originally concerned with smell, it became well developed in the advanced fishes and early terrestrial vertebrates, which depend on this special sense. In mammals and especially in primates, the paleocortex is a deep-lying area called the rhinencephalon ("nose brain"), which actually has little to do with the sense of smell. Instead it seems to have acquired a variety of ill-defined functions concerned with consciousness, sleep, memory, emotional control, and sex. Together with a portion of the midbrain, it is often called the **limbic-midbrain system.**

Although a late arrival in vertebrate evolution, the neocortex completely overshadows the paleocortex and has become so expanded that it envelops the diencephalon and midbrain (Fig. 32-13). Almost all the integrative activities primitively assigned to the midbrain were transferred to the neocortex, or cerebral cortex as it is usually called.

Thus, mammals, and especially humans, have two brains, a primitive and an advanced, that mediate quite separate functions. The deep primitive brain, all of the brain but the cerebral cortex, governs the numerous vital functions that are removed from conscious control: respiration, blood pressure, heart rate, hunger, thirst, temperature balance, salt balance, sexual drive, and basic (sometimes irrational) emotions. It is also a complex endocrine gland that regulates the body's subservient endocrine system. This primitive brain is the *unconscious* mind. The other brain is the "new" brain, the cerebral cortex, wherein are seated intellect and reason. This governing brain is the *conscious* mind.

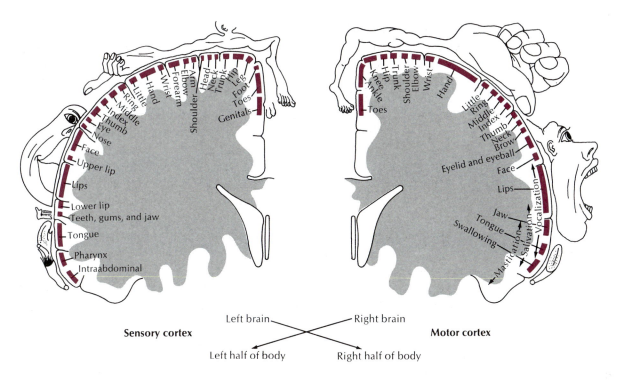

Sensory cortex
Left brain — Right brain
Left half of body   Right half of body
Motor cortex

The brain of course operates as a whole, and both the primitive and the advanced brains are intimately interconnected. Unconscious disturbances are communicated to the conscious brain, and the conscious brain may have powerful effects on the unconscious. Memory appears to transcend all brain levels rather than being a property of any particular part of the brain, as was once believed.

It has been possible to localize function in the cerebrum by direct stimulation of exposed brains of people and experimental animals, postmortem examination of persons suffering from various lesions, and surgical removal of specific brain areas in experimental animals. The cortex contains discrete motor and sensory areas (Figs. 32-13 and 32-14) as well as large "silent" regions, called **association areas,** concerned with memory, judgment, reasoning, and other integrative functions. These regions are not directly connected to sense organs or muscles.

Hemispheric specialization

The cerebral cortex is incompletely divided into two hemispheres by a deep longitudinal fissure. The right and left hemispheres are bridged through the **corpus callosum,** a neural mass lying between and connecting the hemispheres. Through the corpus callosum the two hemispheres are able to transfer information and coordinate mental activities.

Until recently it was believed that one hemisphere, almost always the left, becomes functionally dominant over the other during childhood. This concept is now recognized as misleading. It is now known that the left and right brain hemispheres are specialized for entirely different functions: the left brain hemisphere (controlling the right side of the body) for language development, mathematical and learning capabilities, and sequential thought processes; and the right brain hemisphere (controlling the left side of the body) for spatial, musical, artistic, intuitive, and perceptual activities. It has long been known that even extensive damage to the right hemisphere may cause varying degrees of left-sided paralysis but has little effect on intellect. Conversely, damage to the left hemisphere usually has disastrous effects on intellect. Since these differences in brain symmetry and

Figure 32-14

Arrangement of sensory and motor cortices. The location of sensory terminations from different parts of the body is shown at left; the sensory pattern is repeated as a mirror image on the right side. The origin of descending motor pathways to different parts of the body is shown at right. This pattern is repeated on the left brain. The motor cortex lies in front of the sensory, so the two are not superimposed. Ascending and descending tracts from each hemisphere connect to the opposite side of the body.

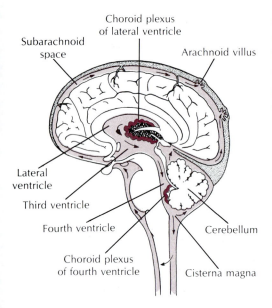

Figure 32-15

Circulation of cerebrospinal fluid (CSF). CSF is secreted by the choroid plexus and by capillaries in the brain. It circulates through all spaces and is drained into the venous system through the arachnoid villi.

function exist at birth, they appear to be inborn rather than the result of developmental or environmental effects as previously believed. Specialization of the left hemisphere for language skills and the right hemisphere for visual-spatial skills is true as a generalization only for right-handed (and right-eyed and right-legged) people who of course are the majority. Handedness is determined separately, since it is not always related to left cerebral speech dominance.

Fluid circulation in the brain

To sustain its unceasing activity, the brain depends on a copious blood supply. Nearly one fifth of the cardiac output is sent to the brain, which in the human amounts to some 800 ml of blood per minute. An uninterrupted supply of oxygen is crucial to brain cells, which are highly intolerant to anoxia. Should the oxygen supply be cut off by cardiac arrest or strangulation, consciousness would be lost within 8 to 12 seconds. If the interruption lasts longer than 8 to 10 minutes (longer at low temperatures), brain cells are usually irreversibly damaged. The blood circulation must also deliver an unfailing supply of glucose to the brain because the nerve cells derive their energy almost exclusively from the aerobic metabolism of glucose.

Paradoxically, despite a dense network of brain capillaries, brain neurons are not directly bathed by a filtrate of blood plasma as are most other body cells. Instead, they are surrounded by a specially secreted, clear, colorless, **cerebrospinal fluid,** which differs significantly in composition from both blood plasma and extracellular fluid. The 125 ml or so of cerebrospinal fluid in the average human adult central nervous system circulates around the brain, cushioning it from shocks. The brain actually floats in the cerebrospinal fluid. Cerebrospinal fluid also surrounds all the nerve and glial cells of the brain and spinal cord as an ultrathin layer; it is the immediate environment of all brain cells.

The cerebrospinal fluid is secreted by two systems: the endothelial cells that form the capillary walls and the epithelial cells of the **choroid plexus.** The choroid plexus is a rich capillary network that protrudes into the brain ventricles (Fig. 32-15). Cerebrospinal fluid is secreted continuously by these two systems and circulates slowly through the brain spaces before entering the systemic blood circulation. The fact that brain neurons are bathed by a special *secreted* fluid rather than by a plasma filtrate has important functional consequences. Only ions, molecules, and nutrients in the cerebrospinal fluid can reach and be exchanged with the neurons and glial cells. Many native and foreign substances do not pass through the blood capillary walls into brain tissue, even though they diffuse easily from the blood into other body tissues. There is, in effect, a **blood-brain barrier** between cerebral blood vessels and the surrounding cerebrospinal fluid that discriminates against certain materials in the blood. In this way the brain keeps its environment more closely controlled and protected than do other body organs. The cost of keeping such narrow tolerances, however, is that brain cells are quickly starved if the blood supply is interrupted.

Peripheral nervous system

The peripheral nervous system, the nerve processes connecting the central nervous system to receptors and effectors, can be broadly subdivided into afferent and efferent components. As shown in the following outline, the efferent system is considerably more complex, consisting of a somatic nervous system and an autonomic nervous system:

A. Afferent system (sensory)
B. Efferent system (motor)
  1. Somatic nervous system
  2. Autonomic nervous system
    a. Sympathetic nervous system
    b. Parasympathetic nervous system

Afferent system

Afferent (sensory) neurons carry signals from receptors in the periphery of the body to the central nervous system. The afferent neuron of a reflex arc (Fig. 32-10) is representative of all afferent pathways in the peripheral nervous system. One long nerve process extends from the cell body in the dorsal root ganglion just outside the spinal cord to innervate receptors; another process passes from the cell body into the central nervous system where it connects with other neurons.

Efferent system
Somatic nervous system

Nerve fibers of the somatic division of the peripheral nervous system pass from the brain or the spinal cord to skeletal muscle fibers. These are called motor neurons because they control muscle movement. They release acetylcholine as the transmitter substance at the nerve endings. Motor neurons in the reflex arc (Fig. 32-10) are representative of the functional position of the somatic nervous system. The somatic nervous system is a "voluntary" system because the movement of skeletal muscles is normally under cerebral control.

Autonomic nervous system

The autonomic nerves govern the involuntary functions of the body that do not ordinarily affect consciousness. The cerebrum has no direct control over autonomic nerves as it has over the somatic nervous system; thus we cannot by volition stimulate or inhibit their action. Autonomic nerves control the movements of the alimentary canal and heart, the contraction of the smooth muscle of the blood vessels, urinary bladder, iris of eye, and others, and the secretions of various glands.

Autonomic nerves originate in the brain or spinal cord as do the nerves of the somatic nervous system, but unlike the latter, the autonomic fibers synapse once after leaving the cord and before arriving at the effector organ. These synapses are located outside the spinal cord in clusters of cells called ganglia. Fibers passing from the cord to the ganglia are called preganglionic autonomic fibers; those passing from the ganglia to the effector organs are called postganglionic fibers. Thus, the autonomic is a *two-neuron* efferent system. These relationships are illustrated in Fig. 32-16.

Subdivisions of the autonomic system are the **parasympathetic** and the **sympathetic** systems. Most organs in the body are innervated by both sympathetic and parasympathetic fibers, and their actions are antagonistic (Fig. 32-17). If one fiber speeds up an activity, the other slows it down. However, neither kind of nerve is exclusively excitatory or inhibitory. For example, parasympathetic fibers inhibit heartbeat but excite peristaltic movements of the intestine; sympathetic fibers increase heartbeat but slow down peristaltic movement.

The **parasympathetic** system consists of motor nerves, some of which emerge from the brain stem by certain cranial nerves and others from the sacral (pelvic) region of the spinal cord by certain spinal nerves. It sometimes is referred to as the **craniosacral division** of the autonomic nervous system. Many parasympathetic

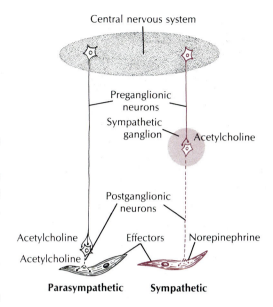

Figure 32-16

Arrangement of the preganglionic and postganglionic neurons of the sympathetic and parasympathetic divisions of the autonomic nervous system, and their neurotransmitters.

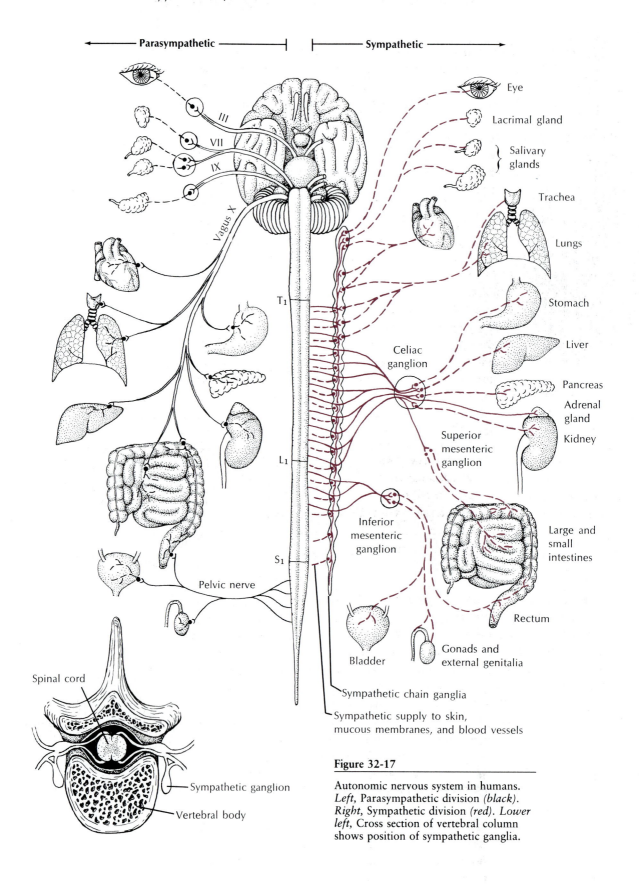

Parasympathetic — **Sympathetic** —

III
VII
IX
Vagus X

Eye
Lacrimal gland
Salivary glands
Trachea
Lungs
Stomach
Liver
Pancreas
Adrenal gland
Kidney

Celiac ganglion
Superior mesenteric ganglion
Inferior mesenteric ganglion

T₁
L₁
S₁

Pelvic nerve

Large and small intestines
Rectum

Bladder
Gonads and external genitalia

Sympathetic chain ganglia
Sympathetic supply to skin, mucous membranes, and blood vessels

Spinal cord
Sympathetic ganglion
Vertebral body

Figure 32-17

Autonomic nervous system in humans. *Left*, Parasympathetic division *(black)*. *Right*, Sympathetic division *(red)*. *Lower left*, Cross section of vertebral column shows position of sympathetic ganglia.

axons run in the vagus nerve from the brain stem to organs in the thorax and abdomen (Fig. 32-17). Parasympathetic fibers *excite* the stomach and intestine, urinary bladder, bronchi, constrictor of the iris, salivary glands, and coronary arteries. They *inhibit* the heart, intestinal sphincters, and sphincter of the urinary bladder.

In the **sympathetic** division the nerve cell bodies of the preganglionic fibers are located in the thoracic and upper lumbar areas of the spinal cord. It may be referred to as the **thoracicolumbar division** of the autonomic nervous system. The fibers pass out through the ventral roots of the spinal nerves, separate from these, and go to the sympathetic ganglia, which are paired and form a chain on each side of the spinal column. From these ganglia some of the postganglionic fibers run through spinal nerves to the limbs and body wall, where they innervate the blood vessels of the skin, the smooth muscles of the hair follicles, the sweat glands, and so on; other fibers run to the abdominal organs as the splanchnic nerves. Sympathetic fibers *excite* the heart, blood vessels, sphincters of the intestines, urinary bladder, dilator muscles of the iris, and others. They *inhibit* the stomach, intestine, and bronchial muscles and coronary arterioles.

All preganglionic fibers, whether sympathetic or parasympathetic, release **acetylcholine** at the synapse with the postganglionic cells. The terminations of the parasympathetic and sympathetic nervous systems release different types of chemical transmitter substances (Fig. 32-16). The parasympathetic postganglionic fibers release **acetylcholine** at their endings, whereas the sympathetic fibers release **norepinephrine** (also called noradrenaline). This difference is another important characteristic distinguishing the two parts of the autonomic nervous system.

SENSE ORGANS

Animals require a constant inflow of information from the environment to regulate their lives. Sense organs are specialized receptors designed for detecting environmental status and change. An animal's sense organs are its first level of environmental perception; they are data input channels for the brain.

A **stimulus** is some form of energy—electrical, mechanical, chemical, or radiant. The sense organ transforms the energy form of the stimulus it receives into nerve impulses, the common language of the nervous system. In a very real sense, then, sense organs are biological transducers. A microphone, for example, is a transducer that converts mechanical (sound) energy into electrical energy. Like the microphone that is sensitive only to sound, sense organs are, as a rule, specific for one kind, or modality, of stimulus energy. Eyes respond only to light, ears to sound, pressure receptors to pressure, and chemoreceptors to chemical molecules. All of these different forms of energy are converted into nerve impulses.

Since all nerve impulses are qualitatively alike, how do animals perceive and distinguish the different **sensations** of varying stimuli? The answer is that the real perception of sensation is done in localized regions of the brain, where each sense organ has its own hookup. Impulses arriving at a particular sensory area of the brain can be interpreted in only one way. This is why pressure on the eye causes us to see "stars" or other visual patterns; the mechanical distortion of the eye initiates impulses in the optic nerve fibers that are perceived as light sensations. Although such an operation probably could never be done, a deliberate surgical switching of optic and auditory nerves would cause the recipient to literally see thunder and hear lightning!

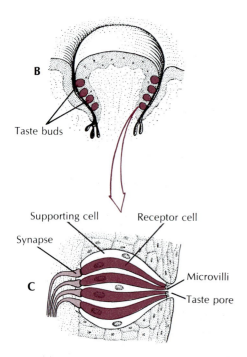

Figure 32-18

Taste receptors. **A,** Surface of human tongue showing regions of maximum sensitivity to the four primary taste sensations. **B,** Position of taste buds on a taste papilla. **C,** Structure of a taste bud.

Classification of Receptors

Receptors are traditionally classified on the basis of their location. Those near the external surface, called **exteroceptors,** keep the animal informed about the external environment. Internal parts of the body are provided with **interoceptors,** which pick up stimuli from the internal organs. Muscles, tendons, and joints have **proprioceptors,** which are sensitive to changes in the tension of muscles and provide the organism with a sense of body position.

Another way of classifying receptors is based on the form of energy to which the receptors respond, such as **chemical, mechanical, photo,** or **thermal.**

Chemoreception

Chemoreception is the most primitive and most universal sense in the animal kingdom. It probably guides the behavior of animals more than any other sense. The most primitive animals, protozoa, use **contact chemical receptors** to locate food and adequately oxygenated water and to avoid harmful substances. These receptors elicit an orientation behavior toward or away from the chemical source called **chemotaxis.** More advanced animals have specialized **distance chemical receptors.** These are often developed to a truly amazing degree of sensitivity. Distance chemoreception, usually referred to as sense of smell or olfactory sense, guides feeding behavior, location and selection of sexual mates, territorial and trail marking, and alarm reactions of numerous animals.

The social insects produce species-specific compounds, called **pheromones,** which comprise a highly developed chemical language. Pheromones are organic compounds released by an animal that affect the physiology or behavior of another individual. Examples are attracting mates or marking trails (releaser pheromones), or triggering metamorphosis (primer pheromones). Insects have a variety of chemoreceptors on the body surface for sensing specific pheromones, as well as other, nonspecific odors.

In all vertebrates and in insects as well, the senses of **taste** and **smell** are clearly distinguishable. Although there are similarities between taste and smell receptors, in general the sense of taste is more restricted in response and is less sensitive than the sense of smell. Taste and smell centers are also located in different parts of the brain.

In higher forms, **taste buds** are found in the mouth cavity and especially on the tongue (Fig. 32-18) where they provide a means for judging foods before they are swallowed. A taste bud consists of a cluster of several receptor cells surrounded by supporting cells and is provided with a small external pore through which the slender tips of the sensory cells project. Because they are subject to the wear and tear of abrasive and spicy foods, taste buds have a short life of only about 5 days and are continually being replaced.

The four basic taste sensations possessed by humans—sour, salt, bitter, and sweet—are each attributable to a different kind of taste bud. The tastes for salt and sweet are found mainly at the tip of the tongue, bitter at the base of the tongue, and sour along the sides of the tongue. Of these, the bitter taste is by far the most sensitive, since it serves as an early warning system against potentially dangerous foods, many of which are bitter.

The sense of smell is more complex than taste, and the basic nature of odor reception is still unknown. The olfactory endings are located in a special epithelium covered with a sheet of mucus, positioned deep in the nasal cavity (Fig.

32-19). There are perhaps 20 million olfactory receptors in the human nose, each ending in several projecting, cilia-like filaments. It is believed that the terminal cilia are the receptor sites, but they are so small that it has been difficult to obtain electrophysiological recordings from single cells.

Even humans, a species not renowned for detecting smells, can discriminate perhaps 10,000 different odors. The human nose can detect one 25 millionth of 1 mg of mercaptan, the odoriferous principle of the skunk. This averages out to approximately 1 molecule per sensory ending.

Smells are distinctive, identifiable, and memorable, and yet nearly impossible to describe to another person except in vague, nonspecific terms. This difficulty of defining odor qualities objectively is another reason why olfactory research has lagged behind other areas of sensory physiology.

Although our olfactory abilities have been overshadowed by other sense organs, vision especially, many animals rely on olfaction for their very survival. A dog explores new surroundings with its nose in the same way we do with our eyes. A dog's sense of smell is justifiably renowned; with some odorous sources a dog's nose is at least a million times as sensitive as ours. Of course, a dog's nose is located close to the ground where odors from passing creatures tend to linger. A human too can detect a fresh human foot trail on a firm floor if he or she is willing to crawl after it on the stomach.

Since flavor of food depends a great deal on odors reaching the olfactory epithelium through the throat passage, taste and smell are easily confused. All the various "tastes" other than the four basic ones (sweet, sour, bitter, salt) are really the result of the flavors reaching the sense of smell in this manner. Food loses its appeal during a common cold because a stuffy nose blocks off odors rising from the mouth cavity.

Of the many theories that have been proposed to explain olfaction, the favored ones today postulate a **physical interaction** between the odor molecule and a protein receptor site on a cell membrane. This interaction somehow alters membrane permeability and results in depolarization in the receptor cell, which triggers a nerve impulse. One hypothesis (J.E. Amoore) proposes that odor molecules have specific stereochemical shapes and that the range of detectable odors is attributable to differences in the way the smelled molecule fits the receptor site.

Mechanoreception

Mechanoreceptors are sensitive to quantitative forces such as touch, pressure, stretching, sound, and gravity. Many receptors in and on the body constantly monitor information about conditions within the body (muscle position, body equilibrium, blood pressure, pain, and so on) and conditions in the environment (sound and other vibrations such as water currents).

Touch and pain

Although superficial touch receptors are distributed over all the body, they tend to be concentrated in the few areas especially important in exploring and interpreting the environment. In most vertebrates these areas are on the face and limb extremities. Of the more than half a million separate sensitive spots on the human body surface, most are found on the lips, tongue, and fingertips. Many touch receptors are bare nerve-fiber terminals, but there is an assortment of other kinds of receptors of varying shapes and sizes. Each hair follicle is crowded with receptors that are sensitive to touch.

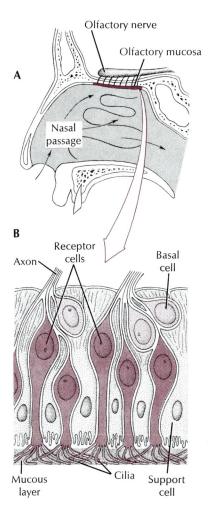

Figure 32-19

Human olfactory epithelium. **A,** The epithelium is patch of tissue positioned in the roof of the nasal cavity. **B,** It is composed of supporting cells, basal cells, and olfactory receptor cells with cilia protruding from their free ends.

Pain is a distress call from the body signaling some noxious stimulus or internal disorder. Although there is no cortical pain center, discrete nuclei have been located in the brain stem where pain messages from the periphery terminate. These nuclei contain two kinds of recently discovered small peptides, called endorphins and enkephalins, that have morphinelike or opium-like activity. When released, they bind with specific opiate receptors in the midbrain. They are the body's own analgesics. Acupuncture, long an enigma to Western science, seems to be based on the principle that by stimulating certain peripheral nerve fibers, the naturally occurring opiates are released, producing an analgesia that is referred to specific organs. Still, the basis of the acupuncture effect remains largely a mystery.

The sensation of deep touch and pressure is registered by relatively large receptors called **pacinian corpuscles.** They are common in deep layers of skin (Fig. 28-1, *B*, p. 671), connective tissue surrounding muscles and tendons, and the abdominal mesenteries. Each corpuscle consists of a nerve terminus surrounded by a capsule of numerous, concentric, onionlike layers of connective tissue (Fig. 32-20). Pressure at any point on the capsule distorts the nerve ending, producing a graded **generator potential.** This is a local flow of electric current. Progressively stronger stimuli lead to correspondingly stronger generator potentials until a **threshold current** is produced; this initiates an action potential in the sensory nerve fiber. Stronger stimuli will produce a burst of action potentials. If, however, the pressure applied is sustained, the corpuscle quickly adjusts to the new shape and no longer responds. This is referred to as **adaptation** and is characteristic of many kinds of touch receptors, which are admirably suited to detecting a sudden mechanical change but readily adapt to new conditions. We are aware of new pressures when we put on our shoes in the morning, but we are glad not to be reminded all day long that we have them on.

Pain receptors are relatively unspecialized nerve fiber endings that respond to a variety of stimuli signaling possible or real tissue damage. It is still uncertain whether pain fibers respond directly to injury or indirectly to some substance such as histamine, which is released by damaged cells.

Just as pain is a sign of danger, sensory pleasure is a sign of a stimulus useful to the subject. Pleasure depends on the internal state of the animal and is judged with reference to homeostasis and some physiological set point.

Lateral line system of fishes

The lateral line is a distant touch reception system for detecting wave vibrations and currents in water. The receptor cells, called **neuromasts,** are located free on the body surface in primitive fishes and aquatic amphibians, but in the advanced fishes they are located within canals running beneath the epidermis; these open at intervals to the surface (Fig. 32-21). Each neuromast is a collection of hair cells with the sensory hairs embedded in a gelatinous, wedge-shaped mass known as a **cupula.** This projects into the center of the lateral line canal so that it bends in response to any disturbance of water on the body surface. The lateral line system is one of the principal sensory systems that guide fishes in their movements and advise them about other animals in the vicinity.

Hearing

The ear is a specialized receptor for detecting sound waves in the surrounding environment. Because sound communication and reception are an integral part of the lives of higher vertebrates, we may be surprised to discover that most invertebrates inhabit a silent world. Only certain arthropod groups—crustaceans, spiders, and insects—have developed true sound organs. Even among the insects, only the locusts, cicadas, crickets, grasshoppers, and most moths possess ears, and these are of simple design: a pair of air pockets, each enclosed by a tympanic membrane that passes sound vibrations to sensory cells. Despite their spartan construction, insect ears are beautifully designed to detect the sound of a potential mate or a rival male.

Especially interesting are the ultrasonic detectors of certain nocturnal moths. These have evolved specifically to detect approaching bats and thus lessen the moth's chance of becoming a bat's evening meal (echolocation in bats is described on p. 652). Each moth ear possesses just two receptors (Fig. 32-22). One of these,

Pressure applied   Capsule   Myelin sheath   Nerve fiber   Action potential

Action potential   mV   msec   Generator potentials

Figure 32-20

Response of pacinian corpuscle to applied pressure. Progressively stronger pressure produces stronger generator potentials. When the threshold stimulus is reached, an all-or-none action potential is fired in the afferent nerve fiber.

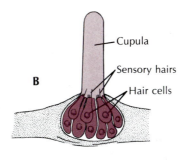

Figure 32-21

Lateral line system. **A,** Lateral line of a bony fish with both exposed and hidden neuromasts. **B,** Structure of a neuromast (lateral line organ).

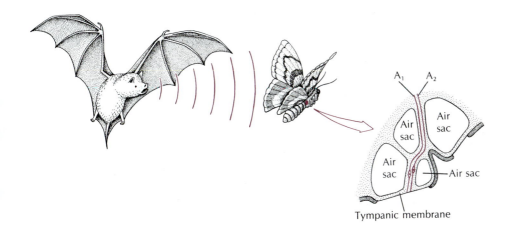

Figure 32-22

Ear of a moth used to detect approaching bats. See text for explanation.

known as the A_1 receptor, will respond to the ultrasonic cries of a bat that is still too far away to detect the moth. As the bat approaches and its cries increase in intensity, the receptor fires more rapidly, informing the moth that the bat is coming nearer. Since the moth has two ears, its nervous system can determine the bat's position by comparing firing rates from the two ears. The moth's strategy is to fly away before the bat detects it. But if the bat continues its approach, the second (A_2) receptor in each ear, which responds only to high-intensity sounds, will fire. The moth responds immediately with an evasive maneuver, usually making a power dive to a bush or the ground where it is safe because the bat cannot distinguish the moth's echo from those of the surroundings.

In its evolution, the vertebrate ear originated as a balance organ, the labyrinth, which itself was probably an outgrowth of the lateral line system of primitive fishes. In all jawed vertebrates, from fishes to humans, the labyrinth has a similar structure, consisting of two small chambers called the saccule and the utricle and three semicircular canals. In fish the base of the saccule is extended into a tiny flap called the lagena, which, in the course of evolution, became enlarged and elaborated into the cochlea, the hearing receptor of tetrapod vertebrates.

The structure of the human ear is illustrated in Fig. 32-23. The outer, or external, ear collects the sound waves and funnels them through the auditory canal to the tympanic membrane (eardrum) lying next to the middle ear. The middle ear is an air-filled chamber containing a remarkable chain of three tiny bones: **malleus** (hammer), **incus** (anvil), and **stapes** (stirrup). These bones conduct the sound waves across the middle ear (Fig. 32-23, *B*). The bridge of bones is so arranged that the force of sound waves pushing against the tympanic membrane is amplified as much as 90 times where the stapes contacts the oval window of the

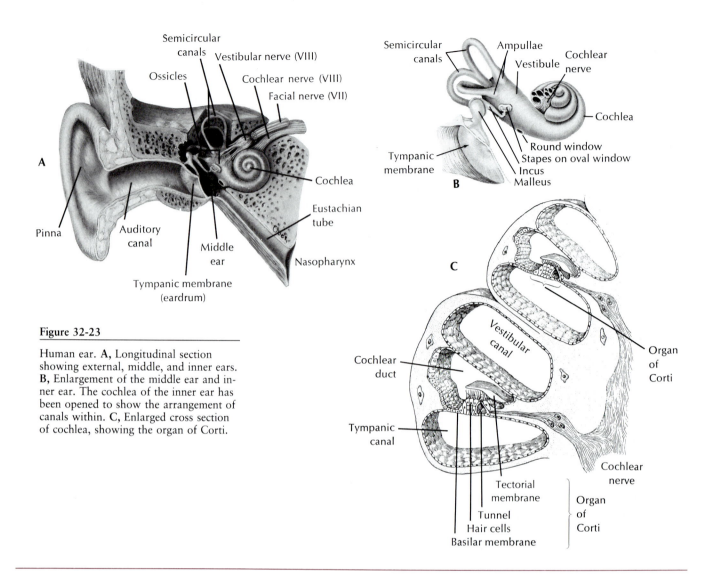

Figure 32-23

Human ear. **A,** Longitudinal section showing external, middle, and inner ears. **B,** Enlargement of the middle ear and inner ear. The cochlea of the inner ear has been opened to show the arrangement of canals within. **C,** Enlarged cross section of cochlea, showing the organ of Corti.

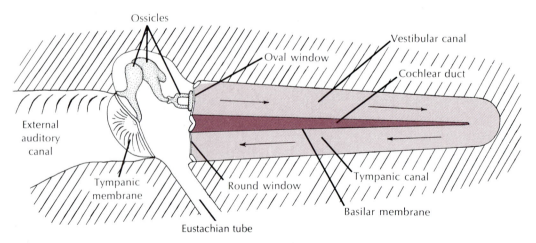

Figure 32-24

Mammalian ear as it would appear with the cochlea stretched out. Sound waves transmitted to the oval window produce vibration waves that travel down the basilar membrane. High-frequency vibrations cause the membrane to resonate at the end near the oval window before dying out; low-frequency tones travel farther down the basilar membrane.

inner ear. Muscles attached to the middle ear bones contract when the ear receives very loud noises, thus protecting the inner ear from damage. However, these muscles cannot contract quickly enough to protect the inner ear from the damaging effects of a sudden blast, nor can they indefinitely protect the ear from sustained loud sounds such as highly amplified music. The middle ear connects with the pharynx by means of the eustachian tube, which acts as a safety device to equalize pressure on both sides of the tympanic membrane.

The inner ear consists essentially of two labyrinths, one within the other. The inner one is called the **membranous labyrinth** and is a closed ectodermal sac filled with a fluid, **endolymph.** The part involved with hearing (**cochlea**) is coiled like a snail's shell, making two and a half turns in humans (Fig. 32-23, *B*). Surrounding the membranous labyrinth is the **bony labyrinth,** which is a hollowed-out part of the temporal bone and conforms to the shape and contours of the membranous labyrinth.

The cochlea is divided longitudinally into three tubular canals running parallel to one another. This relationship is indicated in Fig. 32-24, in which the cochlea is shown stretched out. These canals become progressively smaller from the base of the cochlea to the apex. One of these canals is called the **vestibular canal;** its base is closed by the oval window. The **tympanic canal,** which is in communication with the vestibular canal at the tip of the cochlea, has its base closed by the round window. Between these two canals is the **cochlear duct,** which contains the organ of Corti, the actual sensory apparatus. Within the organ of Corti are fine rows of hair cells that run lengthwise from the base to the tip of the cochlea. There are at least 24,000 of these hair cells in the human ear, each cell with many hairs projecting into the endolymph of the cochlear canal and each connected with neurons of the auditory nerve. The hair cells rest on the **basilar membrane,** which separates the tympanic canal and cochlear duct, and are covered over by the **tectorial membrane** found directly above them.

When a sound wave strikes the ear, its energy is transmitted through the chain of bones of the middle ear to the oval window, which oscillates back and forth, driving the fluid of the vestibular and tympanic canals before it. Because these fluids are noncompressible, an inward movement of the oval window produces a corresponding outward movement of the round window. The fluid oscillations also cause the basilar membrane with its hair cells to vibrate simultaneously.

According to the place hypothesis of pitch discrimination formulated by von Békésy, different areas of the basilar membrane respond to different frequencies; that is, for every sound frequency, there is a specific "place" on the basilar membrane where the hair cells respond to that frequency. The initial displacement of the basilar membrane starts a wave traveling down the membrane, much as flipping a rope at one end starts a wave moving down the rope (Fig. 32-25). The

Sounds with frequencies above 20,000 Hz (Hertz, cycles per second) are usually considered ultrasonic, since this is the practical limit perceived by humans with unimpaired hearing. Most vertebrates have much lower high-frequency limits: fish about 6000 Hz, amphibians 3500 Hz, reptiles 5000 Hz, and birds up to 29,000 Hz, although few birds can hear above 18,000 Hz. Only some mammals and a few birds among vertebrates can hear ultrasonic sounds. The limit for dogs is 44,000 Hz, for rats 72,000 Hz, and for bats 115,000 Hz. For a very large mammal such as an elephant, the high-frequency limit is 10,000 Hz. High-frequency limits are roughly related to body size but even more to the distance between the ears. Thus, mammals with the smallest heads, and therefore having close-set ears, hear the highest sounds!

Figure 32-25

Traveling waves along the basilar membrane. The oval window is at left, and the cochlear apex at right. The two wave formations (*solid and dashed black lines*) occur at separate instants of time. The curves in color represent the extreme displacements of the membrane because of traveling waves.

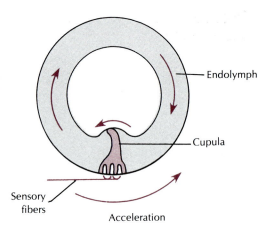

Endolymph

Cupula

Sensory
fibers

Acceleration

Figure 32-26

Semicircular canal, showing bending of
cupula on ampulla during angular acceleration.

displacement wave increases in amplitude as it moves from the oval window
toward the apex of the cochlea, reaching a maximum at the region of the basilar
membrane where the natural frequency of the membrane corresponds to the
sound frequency. Here, the membrane vibrates with such ease that the energy of
the traveling wave is completely dissipated. Hair cells in that region are stimulated
and the impulses conveyed to the fibers of the auditory nerve. Impulses carried by
certain fibers of the auditory nerve are interpreted by the hearing center as particular tones. The **loudness** of a tone depends on the number of hair cells stimulated, whereas the **timbre,** or quality, of a tone is produced by the pattern of the
hair cells stimulated by sympathetic vibration. This latter characteristic enables
us to distinguish between different human voices and different musical instruments, even though the notes in each case may be the same pitch and loudness.

Sense of equilibrium

As already noted, the inner ear contains both the cochlea and the labyrinth, the
latter consisting of the **saccule** and **utricle,** and three **semicircular canals.** Like the
cochlea, the sacs and canals are filled with endolymph. They are concerned with
the sense of balance and rotation. They are well developed in all vertebrates, and
in some lower forms they represent about all there is of the internal ear, since the
cochlea is absent in fishes. They are innervated by the nonacoustic branch of the
auditory nerve.

The utricle and saccule are hollow sacs lined with sensitive hairs on which is
deposited a mass of minute calcium carbonate crystals called **otoconia.** In bony
fishes, these crystals are formed into compact stonelike structures, the **otoliths.**
Similar stony accretions are found within statocysts, the balance organs of many
invertebrates. Although the anatomical nature of these static balance organs varies in different groups, they all function in the same basic way. The weight of the
stony accretion presses on the hair cells to give information about the position of
the head (or entire body) relative to the force of gravity. As the head is tilted in one
direction or another, different groups of hair cells are stimulated; conveyed to the
brain, this information is interpreted with reference to head position.

The semicircular canals of vertebrates are designed to respond to **rotational
acceleration** and are relatively insensitive to linear acceleration. The three semicircular canals are at right angles to each other, one for each axis of rotation. They
are filled with fluid (endolymph), and within each canal is a bulblike enlargement,
the **ampulla,** which contains hair cells. The hair cells are embedded in a gelatinous
membrane, the **cupula,** which projects into the fluid. When the head is rotated, the
fluid in the canal at first tends not to move because of inertia (Fig. 32-26). Since
the cupula is attached, its free end is pulled in the direction opposite to the direction of rotation. Bending of the cupula distorts and excites the hair cells embedded
in it, and this stimulation increases the discharge rate over the afferent nerve fibers
leading from the ampulla to the brain. This produces the sensation of rotation.
Since the three canals of each ear are in different planes, angular acceleration in
any direction stimulates at least one ampulla.

Photoreception
Vision

Light-sensitive receptors are called **photoreceptors.** These receptors range all the
way from simple light-sensitive cells scattered randomly on the body surface of the
lowest invertebrates (dermal light sense) to the exquisitely developed vertebrate

Figure 32-27

Section through human eye.

Upper lid
Ciliary muscle
Suspensory ligament
Anterior chamber
Cornea
Pupil
Iris
Posterior chamber
Lower lid
Conjunctiva

Eye muscle (superior rectus)
Retina
Choroid layer
Sclera
Vitreous body
Optic nerve
Retinal artery and vein
Fovea
Eye muscle (inferior rectus)

eye. Although dermal light receptors contain little photochemical substance and are far less sensitive than optic receptors, they are important in locomotory orientation, pigment distribution in chromatophores, photoperiodic adjustment of reproductive cycles, and other behavioral changes in many of the lower invertebrates.

The arthropods, however, have **compound** eyes composed of many independent visual units called **ommatidia.** The eye of a bee contains about 15,000 of these units, each of which views a separate narrow sector of the visual field. Such eyes form a mosaic of images from the separate units. The compound eye probably does not produce a very distinct image of the visual field, but it is extremely well suited to picking up motion, as anyone knows who has tried to swat a fly.

The vertebrate eye is built like a camera—or rather we should say a camera is modeled somewhat after the vertebrate eye. It contains a light-tight chamber with a lens system in front, which focuses an image of the visual field on a light-sensitive surface (the retina) in back (Fig. 32-27). Because eyes and cameras are based on the same laws of optics, we can wear glasses to correct optical defects in our eyes. But here the similarity between eye and camera ends.

The human eye is actually replete with optical shortcomings; projected on the retina of the normal eye are more colored fringe halos, apparitions, and distortions than would be produced by even the cheapest camera lens. Yet our brain corrects for this "poor design" so completely that we perceive a perfect image of the visual field. It is in the retina and the optic center of the brain that the marvel of vertebrate vision can be understood.

The spherical eyeball is built of three layers: (1) a tough outer white **sclerotic** coat (sclera) that provides support and protection, (2) the middle **choroid** coat containing blood vessels for nourishment, and (3) the light-sensitive **retinal** coat (Fig. 32-27). The **cornea** is a transparent modification of the sclera. A circular curtain, the **iris,** regulates the size of the light opening, the **pupil.** Just behind the iris is the **lens,** a transparent, elastic ball that bends the rays and focuses them on the retina. In land vertebrates the cornea actually does most of the bending of light rays, whereas the lens adjusts the focus for near and far objects. Between the cornea and the lens is the outer chamber filled with the watery **aqueous humor**; between the lens and the retina is the much larger inner chamber filled with the viscous **vitreous humor**. Surrounding the margin of the lens and holding it in place is the **suspensory ligament**. This, together with the **ciliary muscle**, a ring of radiating muscle fibers attached to the suspensory ligament, makes possible the stretching and relaxing of the lens for close or distant vision (accommodation).

The **retina** is composed of photoreceptors, the **rods** and **cones**. Approximately 125 million rods and 7 million cones are present in each human eye. Cones are primarily concerned with color vision in ample light; rods, with colorless vision in dim light. The retina is actually made up of three sets of neurons in series with each other: (1) photoreceptors (rods and cones), (2) intermediate neurons, and (3) ganglionic neurons whose axons form the optic nerve (Fig. 32-28).

The **fovea centralis**, the region of keenest vision, is located in the center of the retina, in direct line with the center of the lens and cornea. It contains only cones. The acuity of an animal's eyes depends on the density of cones in the fovea. The human fovea and that of a lion contain approximately 150,000 cones per square millimeter. But many water and field birds have up to 1 million cones per square millimeter. Their eyes are as good as human eyes would be if aided by eight-power binoculars.

At the peripheral parts of the retina only rods are found. This is why we can see better at night by looking out of the corners of our eyes; the rods, adapted for high sensitivity with dim light, are brought into use.

Chemistry of vision

Each rod contains a light-sensitive pigment known as **rhodopsin**. Each rhodopsin molecule consists of a large, colorless protein, **opsin**, and a small carotenoid molecule, **retinal** (formerly called retinene), a derivative of vitamin A. When a quantum of light strikes a rod and is absorbed by the rhodopsin molecule, the latter undergoes a chemical bleaching process that causes it to split into separate opsin and retinal molecules. This change triggers the discharge of a nerve impulse in the receptor cell, but there is as yet no uniform agreement on how the receptor potential is produced. The impulse is relayed to the optic center of the brain. Rhodopsin is then enzymatically resynthesized so that it can respond to a subsequent light signal.

The amount of intact rhodopsin in the retina depends on the intensity of light reaching the eye. The dark-adapted eye contains much rhodopsin and is very sensitive to weak light. Conversely most of the rhodopsin is broken down in the light-adapted eye. It takes approximately half an hour for the light-adapted eye to accommodate to darkness, while the rhodopsin level is gradually built up. The remarkable ability of the eye to adapt to darkness and light vastly increases the versatility of the eye; it enables us to see by starlight and also by the noonday sun, 10 billion times brighter.

The composition of the cone pigments has not yet been completely clarified, but they are believed to be similar to rhodopsin, containing retinal combined with a special protein, **cone opsin**. Cones function to perceive color and require 50 to 100 times more light for stimulation than do rods. Consequently, night vision is almost totally rod vision; this is why the landscape illuminated by moonlight appears in shades of black and white only. Unlike humans, who have both day and night vision, some vertebrates specialize for one or the other. Strictly nocturnal animals, such as bats and owls, have pure rod retinas. Purely diurnal forms, such

One of several marvels of the vertebrate eye is its capacity to compress the enormous range of light intensities presented to it into a narrow range that can be handled by the optic nerve fibers. Light intensity between a sunny noon and starlight differs more than 10 billion to 1. Rods quickly saturate with high light intensity, but the cones do not; they shift their operating range with changing ambient light intensity so that a high-contrast image is perceived over a broad range of light conditions. This is made possible by complex interactions among the network of nerve cells that lie between the cones and the ganglion cells that generate the retinal output to the brain.

A

Rod   Rod   Cone   Cone

Outer segment

Inner segment

Mitochondria

Direction of light entering eye ↑

C

Chromatophore

Cone

Rod

Horizontal cell

Bipolar cell

Amacrine cell

Ganglion cell

Optic nerve

Light source

B

Choroid

Pigment cells

Outer segment of cones

Inner segment of cones

Interconnecting nerve cell layer

Ganglion cell layer

Optic nerve fibers

Direction of light entering eye ↑

Figure 32-28

A, Scanning electron micrograph of photoreceptor cells of the guinea pig's retina. (×3500.) Rods can be distinguished from cones by the thin inner segment of the former and the swollen inner segments (resulting from more numerous mitochondria) of the latter. The photosensitive pigments are located in the outer segments of both types of cells. **B,** Photomicrograph of a section of the retina of a turtle. Turtles have almost pure cone retinas. Light entering the eye must pass through the nerve network of the retina before striking the outer segment of the photoreceptor cells (cones). (×230.) **C,** Structure of the primate retina, showing the organization of intermediate neurons that connect the photoreceptor cells to the ganglion cells of the optic nerve.

A, Courtesy A. Spira and M. Patten.

as the common gray squirrel and some birds, have only cones. They are of course virtually blind at night.

Color vision

How does the eye see colors? According to the trichromatic theory of color vision, there are three different types of cones, each reacting most strongly to red, green, or violet light. Colors are perceived by comparing the levels of excitation of the three different kinds of cones. This comparison is made both in nerve circuits in the retina and in the visual cortex of the brain. Color vision is present in some members of all vertebrate groups with the possible exception of the amphibians. Bony fishes and birds have particularly good color vision. Surprisingly, most mammals are color blind; exceptions are primates and a few other species such as squirrels.

___ Summary

The nervous system is a rapid communications system that interacts continuously with the endocrine system in the control and coordination of body function. The basic unit of nervous integration is the neuron, a highly specialized cell having dendrites, which receive impulses; a cell body; and an axon, which conducts impulses to other cells. The nerve impulse is a nondecremental, self-propagating, rapidly moving depolarization of the nerve membrane and is associated with rapid changes in membrane permeability to sodium and potassium. The nerve impulse is transmitted from one nerve to another across synapses. The thin gap between nerves at these junction points is bridged by a chemical transmitter, which is released from the synaptic knob. Acetylcholine, the most common neurotransmitter in the peripheral nervous system, is excitatory, but many other neurotransmitters, both excitatory and inhibitory, have been identified.

The most primitive organization of neurons into a system is the nerve net of cnidarians, basically a plexus of nerve cells that, with additions, comprises the basis of the nervous systems of several primitive invertebrate phyla. With the appearance of ganglia (nerve centers) in the flatworms, nervous systems became differentiated into central and peripheral divisions. In vertebrates the central nervous system consists of the brain and spinal cord. In its remarkable evolutionary history, the vertebrate brain has developed from a primitive, three-part, linear brain to a complex multicomponent structure. In mammals the cerebral cortex has become vastly enlarged and has assumed the most important integrative activities of the nervous system. It completely overshadows the primitive brain, which is consigned to the role of relay center and to serving numerous unconscious but nonetheless vital functions such as breathing, blood pressure, and heart rate.

In humans the left cerebral hemisphere is usually specialized for language and mathematical skills while the right hemisphere is specialized for visual-spatial and musical skills.

Brain cells are bathed by cerebrospinal fluid, which is secreted by capillary endothelial cells and by the choroid plexus. The blood-brain barrier protects brain cells from many blood-borne substances that diffuse easily into other tissues.

The peripheral nervous system connects the central nervous system to receptors and effector organs. It is divided broadly into an afferent system, which conducts sensory signals to the central nervous system, and an efferent system, which conveys motor impulses to effector organs. The autonomic nervous system is a motor system with its own separate set of fibers. It is subdivided into anatomically distinct sympathetic and parasympathetic systems, each of which sends fibers to most body organs. Generally the sympathetic system governs excitatory activities and the parasympathetic system governs maintenance and restoration of body resources.

Sense organs are receptors designed especially to respond to internal or environmental change. The most primitive and ubiquitous sense in the animal kingdom is chemoreception. Chemoreceptors may be contact receptors, such as the vertebrate sense of taste, or distance receptors such as smell, which detects airborne molecules. Most theories of olfaction postulate some kind of molecular integration between odorant and receptor, but the mechanism of odor reception remains unknown.

The receptors for touch, pain, equilibrium, and hearing are all mechanical force receptors. Touch and pain receptors are characteristically simple structures, but hearing and equilibrium are highly specialized senses based on special hair cells that respond to mechanical deformation. Sound waves received by the ear are mechanically amplified and transmitted to the inner ear where different areas of the cochlea respond to different sound frequencies. Equilibrium receptors, also located in the inner ear, consist of two saclike static balance organs and three semicircular canals that detect movement.

Vision receptors (photoreceptors) are associated with special pigment molecules that photochemically decompose in the presence of light and, in doing so, trigger nerve impulses in optic fibers. The advanced compound eye of arthropods is especially well suited to detecting motion in the visual field. Vertebrates have a camera eye with focusing optics. The photoreceptor cells of the retina are of two kinds: rods, designed for high sensitivity with dim light, and cones, primarily concerned with color vision. Cones predominate in the fovea centralis of the human eye, the area of keenest vision. Rods are more abundant in the peripheral areas of the retina.

Selected references

See also general references for Part Three, p. 837.

Bullock, T.H., R. Orkand, and A. Grinnell. 1977. Introduction to nervous systems. San Francisco, W.H. Freeman & Co. Publishers. *Excellent comparative treatment.*

Burton, M. 1972. The sixth sense of animals. New York, Taplinger Publishing Co., Inc. *Wide-ranging comparative account of animal senses. Undergraduate level.*

Dethier, V.G. 1977. The taste of salt. Am. Sci. **65:**744-751. *Salt receptors of mammals and insects are described.*

Dröscher, V.B. 1969. The magic of the senses. New York, E.P. Dutton & Co., Inc. *Readable comparative account of the senses, ending with consideration of animal migration and navigation. Undergraduate level.*

Eccles, J.C. 1977. The understanding of the brain, ed. 2. New York, McGraw-Hill Book Co.

Kuffler, S.W., and J.G. Nicholls. 1976. From neuron to brain: a cellular approach to the function of the nervous system. Sunderland, Mass., Sinauer Associates, Inc. *Authoritative neurobiology text.*

Lythgoe, J.N. 1979. The ecology of vision. Oxford, Eng., Oxford University Press. *Comprehensive and broadly comparative biology of animal vision.*

Milne, L., and M. Milne. 1972. The senses of animals and men. New York, Atheneum Publishers. *Beautifully written account of animal senses by these prolific authors. Undergraduate level.*

Nathan, P. 1982. The nervous system, ed. 2. Oxford, Eng., Oxford University Press. *One of the best of several semipopular accounts of the nervous system.*

Schmidt, R.F. (ed.). 1978. Fundamentals of neurophysiology. New York, Springer-Verlag. *Undergraduate text.*

Schmidt, R.F. (ed.). 1978. Fundamentals of sensory physiology. New York, Springer-Verlag. *Clear explanations of the human senses, good diagrams.*

Springer, S.P., and G. Deutsch. 1981. Left brain, right brain. San Francisco, W.H. Freeman & Co. Publishers. *Research in brain asymmetry.*

Stoddart, D.M. 1980. The ecology of vertebrate olfaction. London, Chapman & Hall, Ltd. *How vertebrates use olfaction in feeding, reproduction, behavior, warning and defense, and navigation.*

Selected *Scientific American* articles

Alkon, D.L. 1983. Learning in a marine snail. **249:**70-84 (July). *The nerve circuits that mediate associative learning have been traced.*

Amoore, J.E., J.W. Johnston, Jr., and M. Rubin. 1964. The stereochemical theory of odor. **210:**42-49 (Feb.).

Axelrod, J. 1974. Neurotransmitters. **230:**58-71 (June).

Bloom, F.E. 1981. Neuropeptides. **245:**148-168 (Oct.). *Recent advances in brain chemistry.*

Hodgson, E.S. 1961. Taste receptors. **204:**135-144 (May). *The mechanism of taste reception is studied with blowflies.*

Hubel, D.H. 1979. The brain. **241:**44-53 (Sept.). *The methods and challenges of neurobiological research are discussed.*

Hudspeth, A.J. 1983. The hair cells of the inner ear. **248:**54-64 (Jan.). *How these biological transducers work.*

Iversen, L.L. 1979. The chemistry of the brain. **241:**134-149 (Sept.). *A diverse array of chemical transmitters have been discovered in the brain. Their functions are now being elucidated.*

Jerison, H.J. 1976. Paleoneurology and the evolution of mind. **234:**90-101 (Jan.). *The relationship between brain size and body size during animal evolution provides insight into intelligence.*

Katz, B. 1961. How cells communicate. **205:**209-220 (Sept.). *Nervous communication and the nature of nerve impulses.*

Kennedy, D. 1967. Small systems of nerve cells. **216:**44-52 (May). *The simple nervous systems of invertebrates facilitate studies of nervous integration.*

Keynes, R.D. 1979. Ion channels in the nerve-cell membrane. **240**:126-135 (Mar.). *Recent research on the nature and functioning of ion channels that regulate the flow of sodium and potassium.*

Llinás, R.R. 1975. The cortex of the cerebellum. **232**:56-71 (Jan.). *The pattern of neuronal connections in the cerebellum can now be related to its role in motor coordination.*

Luria, A.R. 1970. The functional organization of the brain. **222**:66-78 (Mar.).

Miller, W.H., F. Ratliff, and H.K. Hartline. 1961. How cells receive stimuli. **205**:222-238 (Sept.). *Structure and functional properties of receptor cells.*

Morell, P., and W.T. Norton. 1980. Myelin. **242**:88-118 (May). *Development, structure, and function of a nerve fiber's myelin sheath are explained.*

Nathanson, J.A., and P. Greengard. 1977. "Second messengers" in the brain. **237**:108-119 (Aug.). *A survey of the various neurotransmitters of the vertebrate nervous system and how their chemical messages are translated into physiological actions.*

Nauta, W.J.H., and M. Feirtag. 1979. The organization of the brain. **241**:88-111 (Sept.). *Description of the brain's complex circuitry.*

Parker, D.E. 1980. The vestibular apparatus. **243**:118-135 (Nov.). *Functioning of the inner ear and other sense organs of balance and orientation.*

Rushton, W.A.H. 1975. Visual pigments and color blindness. **232**:64-74 (Mar.). *There are three types of cone cell, each with one of three visual pigments; color blindness may be caused by a lack of one of the pigments.*

Schwartz, J.H. 1980. The transport of substances in nerve cells. **242**:152-171 (Apr.). *The axon carries a busy traffic between the cell body and nerve endings.*

Stent, G.S. 1972. Cellular communication. **227**:43-51 (Sept.). *Information processing and communication are discussed with particular emphasis on vision.*

Stent, G.S., and D.A. Weisblat. 1982. The development of a simple nervous system. **246**:136-146 (Jan.). *Development of nerve cells in leeches.*

Stevens, C.F. 1979. The neuron. **241**:54-65 (Sept.). *Its function is detailed.*

Werblin, F.S. 1973. The control of sensitivity in the retina. **228**:70-79 (Jan.). *Recent studies of neuron interactions in the retina help to explain its versatility over wide-ranging light conditions.*

Young, R.W. 1970. Visual cells. **223**:80-91 (Oct.). *How rods and cones renew themselves.*

CHAPTER 33

CHEMICAL COORDINATION

Endocrine System

Uganda kob males fight for dominance. Male aggressiveness during the breeding season is associated with a rising blood level of the male sex hormone testosterone. The entire sex cycle is controlled by changing activity of endocrine glands, all orchestrated by neurosecretory centers in the brain.

Photograph by L.L. Rue, III.

── HORMONAL INTEGRATION

The endocrine system is the second great integrative system controlling the body's activities. Endocrine glands secrete **hormones** (Gr., *hormon*, to excite), chemical compounds that are transported by the blood to some part of the body where they initiate definite physiological responses.

Endocrine glands are small, well-vascularized ductless glands composed of groups of cells arranged in cords or plates. Since the endocrine glands have no ducts, their only connection with the rest of the body is by the bloodstream; they must capture their raw materials from the blood and secrete their finished hormonal products into it. Consequently, it is not surprising that the endocrine glands receive enormous blood flows. The thyroid gland is said to have the highest blood flow per unit of tissue weight of any organ in the body. **Exocrine glands,** in contrast, are provided with ducts for discharging their secretions onto a free surface. Examples of exocrine glands are sweat glands and sebaceous glands of skin, salivary glands, and the various enzyme-secreting glands lining the walls of the stomach and intestine.

The classical definition of a hormone given in the first paragraph, like so many other generalizations in biology, may have to be altered as new information appears. For one thing, some hormones, such as certain neurosecretions, may never enter the general circulation at all. Furthermore, there is good evidence that many of the traditional hormones, such as insulin, are synthesized in minute amounts in a variety of nonendocrine tissues (nerve cells, for example) where they may function as local **tissue factors:** substances that stimulate cell growth or some biochemical process. Most hormones, however, are blood borne and therefore diffuse into every tissue space in the body. This is quite unlike the discrete action of the nervous system with its network of cablelike nerve fibers that selectively send messages to specific points.

The ubiquitous distribution of hormones makes it possible for certain hormones, such as the growth hormone of the pituitary gland, to affect most if not all cells during specific stages of cellular differentiation. However, the circulatory distribution of hormones everywhere creates a potential communications jam, since most hormones must produce highly specific responses at the right time and in the right cells. Confusion is avoided because the cell "selects" the hormone with which it will interact by having a specific receptor on its surface or in its cytoplasm that binds to that hormone and no other.

For example, only certain stomach cells respond to the hormone gastrin, even though gastrin penetrates throughout the body. These particular cells of the stomach bear receptors that selectively bind gastrin; other cells are insensitive to the hormone's presence because they lack gastrin-specific receptors. Cells that respond to a specific hormone are called **target-organ cells** for that hormone.

Compared to the nervous system, the endocrine system is slow acting because of the time required for a hormone to reach the appropriate tissue, cross the capillary endothelium, and diffuse through tissue fluid to, and sometimes into, cells. Thus, the minimum response time is a matter of seconds and may be much longer. Furthermore, hormone responses in general are much longer lasting than those under nervous control. Where a sustained effect is required, as in many metabolic and growth processes, or where some concentration or secretion rate must be maintained at a particular level, we expect to find endocrine control.

However, the nervous and endocrine systems really function as a single, united system. There is no sharp separation between the two. As we shall see, the

Figure 33-1

Founders of endocrinology. **A,** Sir William M. Bayliss (1860-1924). **B,** Ernest H. Starling (1866-1927).

From Fulton, J.F., and L.G. Wilson. 1966. Selected readings in the history of physiology. Springfield, Ill., Charles C Thomas, Publisher.

nervous system is itself an endocrine organ that controls most endocrine function. Conversely, several hormones act on the nervous system and may significantly affect many kinds of animal behavior.

Endocrinology is a comparatively young division of animal physiology. Its birthdate is usually given as 1902, the year two English physiologists, W.M. Bayliss and E.H. Starling, demonstrated the action of an internal secretion (Fig. 33-1). They were interested in determining how the pancreas secreted its digestive juice into the small intestine at the proper time of the digestive process. In an anesthetized dog they tied off a section of the small intestine beyond the duodenum (the part of the intestine next to the stomach) and removed all nerves leading to this tied-off loop, but left its blood vessels intact. Bayliss and Starling found that the injection of hydrochloric acid into the blood serving this intestinal loop had no effect on the secretion of pancreatic juice, but when they introduced 0.4% hydrochloric acid directly inside the intestinal loop, a pronounced flow of pancreatic juice into the duodenum occurred through the pancreatic duct. When they scraped off some of the mucous membrane lining of the intestine and mixed it with acid, they found the injection of this extract into the blood caused an abundant flow of pancreatic juice.

They concluded that when the partly digested and slightly acid food from the stomach arrives in the small intestine, the hydrochloric acid reacts with something in the mucous lining to produce an internal secretion, or chemical messenger, which is conveyed by the bloodstream to the pancreas, causing it to secrete pancreatic digestive juices. They called this messenger **secretin**. In a 1905 Croonian lecture at the Royal College of Physicians, Starling first used the word "hormone," a general term to describe all such chemical messengers, since he correctly surmised that secretin was only the first of many hormones that remained to be described.

Mechanisms of Hormone Action

How do hormones exert their effects? Obviously, it is much easier to observe the physiological effect of a hormone than to determine what the hormone does to produce the effect. Recently, however, progress has been made toward understanding the specificity of hormones: it seems to depend on specific receptor sites on or in target cells.

Cell surface receptors

In many hormone actions, when the hormone arrives at its target cell, it binds to a receptor site on the membrane. The combination of hormone and receptor causes activation of an enzyme, adenylate cyclase, which is coupled to the membrane receptor (Fig. 33-2). Adenylate cyclase converts ATP in the cytoplasm to cyclic AMP. This compound is formed when two of three phosphate groups are split from ATP and the remaining phosphate combines with a carbon atom of the adjacent ribose molecule of ATP to form a ring, making it "cyclic" (Fig. 33-3). The cyclic AMP thus generated acts as a "second messenger" that relays the hormone's message to the cell's biochemical machinery, where it alters (usually stimulates) some cellular process (Fig. 33-2). Since many molecules of cyclic AMP may be manufactured after a single hormone molecule has been bound, the message is amplified, perhaps many thousands of times.

Cyclic AMP mediates the actions of many hormones, including glucagon,

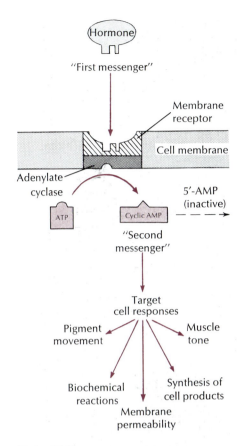

Figure 33-2

Second-messenger concept of hormone action. Many hormones act through cyclic AMP. The hormone is carried by the bloodstream from the endocrine gland to the target cell where it selectively combines with an immobile receptor in the plasma membrane. This interaction stimulates the enzyme adenylate cyclase to catalyze the formation of cyclic AMP (second messenger). Cyclic AMP acts intracellularly to initiate any of several changes, depending on the kind of cell.

Figure 33-3

Formation of cyclic AMP.

ATP   Cyclic AMP

epinephrine, adrenocorticotropic hormone (ACTH), thyrotropic hormone (TSH), melanophore-stimulating hormone (MSH), and vasopressin. With the exception of epinephrine, these are all peptides—small proteins but much too large to penetrate the cell membrane. All act *indirectly* through an immobile receptor on the cell surface.

Cytoplasmic receptors

Several hormones, including all of the steroids (for example, estrogen, testosterone, and aldosterone), diffuse into cells where they bind selectively to cytoplasmic receptor molecules found only in the target cells. The hormone-receptor complex can then diffuse into the nucleus where it binds directly to certain proteins (nonhistones) in the chromosomes. As a result, gene transcription is increased, and messenger RNA molecules are synthesized on specific sequences of DNA. Moving from the nucleus into the cytoplasm, the newly formed messenger RNA initiates the formation of new proteins, thus setting in motion the hormone's observed effect (Fig. 33-4). Thyroxine and the insect-molting hormone ecdysone are also believed to act through this mechanism.

As compared with hormones acting through the cyclic AMP mechanism, steroids have a more *direct* effect on protein synthesis because they combine with a mobile receptor and move with it into the nucleus to couple with chromosomal proteins.

All hormones are low-level signals. Even when an endocrine gland is secreting maximally, the hormone is so greatly diluted by the large volume of blood it enters that its plasma concentration seldom exceeds 10^{-9} M (or one billionth of a 1 M concentration). Since hormones have far-reaching and often powerful influences on cells, it is evident that their effects are vastly amplified at the cellular level.

How Hormone Secretion Rates Are Controlled

Hormones influence cell functions by altering the rates of a large range of biochemical processes. Some affect enzyme activity and thus alter cellular metabolism, some change membrane permeability, some regulate the synthesis of cellular proteins, and some stimulate the release of hormones from other endocrine glands. Since these are all dynamic processes that must adapt to changing metabolic demands, they must be regulated, not merely activated, by the appropriate hormones. This is achieved by varying hormone output from the gland. However, the concentration of hormone in the plasma depends on two factors: its rate of secretion and the rate at which it is inactivated and removed from the circulation. Consequently, an endocrine gland requires information about the level of its own hormone(s) in the plasma to control its secretion.

Many hormones, especially those of the pituitary gland, are controlled by negative feedback systems that operate between the glands secreting the hormones and the target cells. A feedback pattern is one in which the output is constantly compared with a set point. For example, ACTH, secreted by the pituitary, stimulates the adrenal gland (the target cells) to secrete cortisol. As the cortisol level in the plasma rises, it acts on the pituitary gland to inhibit the release of ACTH. Thus, any deviation from the set point (a specific plasma level of cortisol) leads to corrective action in the opposite direction. Such a system is highly effective in preventing extreme oscillations in hormone output. However, hormonal feedback systems are not identical to a rigid "closed-loop" system like the thermostat that controls the central heating system in a house, because they may be altered by input from the nervous system or by metabolites or other hormones.

INVERTEBRATE HORMONES

During the last half century physiologists have shown that many invertebrates have endocrine integrative systems that approach the complexity of the vertebrate endocrine system. Not surprisingly, however, there are few if any homologies between invertebrate and vertebrate hormones. The invertebrate phyla have different functional systems, growth patterns, and reproductive processes from vertebrates and have been separated from them phylogenetically for a vast span of time.

In many invertebrate phyla, the principal source of hormones is neurosecretory cells, specialized nerve cells capable of synthesizing and secreting hormones. Their products, called neurosecretions, or neurosecretory hormones, are discharged directly into the circulation. Neurosecretion is in fact important in vertebrates as well. It is an ancient physiological activity, and because it serves as a crucial link between the nervous and endocrine systems, we believe that hormones first evolved as nerve cell secretions. Later, nonnervous endocrine glands appeared, especially among the vertebrates, but remained chemically linked to the nervous system by the neurosecretory hormones.

Neurosecretory hormones have been found in all the larger invertebrate phyla, including the cnidarians, flatworms, nematodes, molluscs, annelids, arthropods, and echinoderms. Most extensively studied, however, have been the insects, and we will limit our discussion to that group.

In insects, as in other arthropods, growth is a series of steps in which the rigid, nonexpansible exoskeleton is periodically discarded and replaced with a new, larger one. Almost all insects undergo a process of metamorphosis, in which there is a series of juvenile stages, each requiring the formation of a new exoskeleton, and each ending with a molt. In some orders the change to the adult form is gradual. In others the adult is separated from the larval stages by a quiescent form, the pupa, and the change to the adult is abrupt. Hormonal control of both types is the same.

Insect physiologists have discovered that molting and metamorphosis are controlled by the interaction of two hormones, one favoring growth and the differentiation of adult structures and the other favoring the retention of juvenile structures. These two hormones are the **molting hormone** (also referred to as

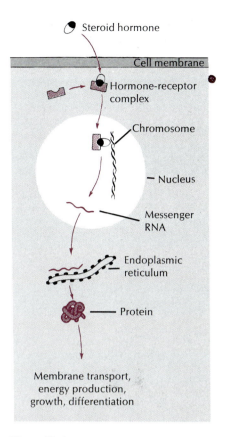

Figure 33-4

Concept of gene regulation by steroid hormones and thyroxine. The hormone penetrates the cell membrane to combine with a mobile cytoplasmic receptor. The complex enters the nucleus where it stimulates the transcription of messenger RNA. This is translated to specific proteins in the cytoplasm.

Figure 33-5

Endocrine control of molting in a moth. Moths mate in the spring or summer, and eggs soon hatch into the first of several larval stages (called instars). After the final larval molt, the last and largest larva (caterpillar) spins a cocoon in which it pupates. The pupa overwinters, and an adult emerges in the spring to start a new generation. Two hormones interact to control molting and pupation. The molting hormone, produced by the prothoracic gland and stimulated by a separate brain hormone (PTTH), favors molting and the formation of adult structures. These effects are inhibited, however, by the juvenile hormone, produced by the corpora allata. Juvenile hormone output declines with successive molts, and the larva undergoes adult differentiation.

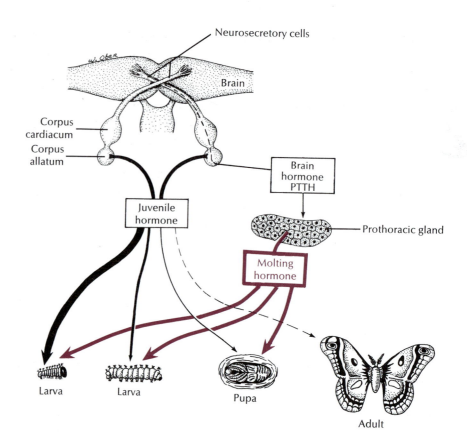

ecdysone [ek'duh-sone]), produced by the prothoracic gland, and the **juvenile hormone,** produced by the corpora allata (Fig. 33-5). The structure of both hormones has recently been determined. It required extraction from 1000 kg (about 1 ton) of silkworm pupae to show that the molting hormone is a steroid. The juvenile hormone has an entirely different structure.

Juvenile hormone of silkworm

Molting hormone (α-ecdysone) of silkworm

The molting hormone is under the control of the prothoracicotropic hormone (PTTH). This hormone is a polypeptide (molecular weight about 5000) that is produced by neurosecretory cells of the brain, transported down axons, and stored in the corpora allata, from where it is released into the blood. At intervals during juvenile growth, PTTH is released into the blood and stimulates the release of molting hormone. Molting hormone appears to act directly on the chromosomes to set in motion the changes resulting in a molt. The molting hormone favors the development of adult structures. It is held in check, however, by the juvenile hormone, which favors the development of juvenile characteristics. During juvenile life the juvenile hormone predominates and each molt yields another larger juvenile. Finally the output of juvenile hormone decreases and the final juvenile molt occurs.

Chemists have synthesized several potent analogs of the juvenile hormone, which hold great promise as insecticides. Minute quantities of these synthetic analogs induce abnormal final molts or prolong or block development. Unlike the usual chemical insecticides, they are highly specific and do not contaminate the environment.

The precise location of PTTH in the brain of pupal tobacco hornworms was recently revealed by N. Agui by delicate microdissection. Using a human eyebrow hair as a dissecting instrument, he was able to isolate the single cell in each brain hemisphere that contained PTTH activity. Thus, only two cells, each about 20 μm in diameter, produce this insect's total supply of PTTH. Agui also showed that the corpora allata are the storage-release sites for PTTH, not the corpora cardiaca as previously believed. In an age when sophisticated instrumentation has removed much of the tedium (and some of the creativity) from research, it is refreshing to learn that certain biological mysteries succumb only to skillful use of the human hand.

VERTEBRATE ENDOCRINE GLANDS AND HORMONES

In the remainder of this chapter we describe some of the best understood and most important of the vertebrate hormones. The hormones of reproduction are discussed in the next chapter. Space does not permit us to deal with all the hormones and hormonelike substances that have been discovered. The mammalian hormonal mechanisms are the best understood, since laboratory mammals and humans have always been the objects of the most intensive research. Research with the lower vertebrates has shown that all vertebrates share similar endocrine organs. All vertebrates have a pituitary gland, for example, and all have thyroid glands, adrenal glands (or the special cells of which they are composed), and gonads. Nevertheless, there are some important differences in the functional roles that the hormones of these glands have among the different vertebrates.

Hormones of the Pituitary Gland and Hypothalamus

The pituitary gland, or **hypophysis,** is a small gland (0.5 g in humans) lying in a well-protected position between the roof of the mouth and the floor of the brain (Fig. 33-6). It is a two-part gland having a double embryological origin. The **anterior pituitary** (adenohypophysis) is derived embryologically from the roof of the mouth. The **posterior pituitary** (neurohypophysis) arises from a ventral portion of the brain, the **hypothalamus,** and is connected to it by a stalk, the **infundibulum.** Although the anterior pituitary lacks any *anatomical* connection to the brain, it is nonetheless *functionally* connected to it by a special portal circulatory system. A portal circulation is one that delivers blood from one capillary bed to another (Fig. 33-6).

Anterior pituitary

The anterior pituitary consists of an **anterior lobe** (pars distalis) and an **intermediate lobe** (pars intermedia) as shown in Fig. 33-6. The anterior lobe, despite its minute dimensions, produces at least six protein hormones. All but one of these six are **tropic hormones** that regulate other endocrine glands (Table 33-1).

The **thyrotropic hormone** (TSH) regulates the production of thyroid hor-

Table 33-1 Hormones of the Vertebrate Pituitary and Hypothalamus—Chemical Nature and Actions

	Hormone	Chemical nature	Principal action
Adenohypophysis			
Anterior lobe	Thyrotropin (TSH)	Glycoprotein	Stimulates thyroid to secrete thyroid hormones
	Adrenocorticotropin (ACTH)	Polypeptide	Stimulates adrenal cortex to secrete steroid hormones
	Gonadotropins		
	1. Follicle-stimulating hormone (FSH)	Glycoprotein	Stimulates gamete production and secretion of sex hormones
	2. Luteinizing hormone (LH, ICSH)	Glycoprotein	Stimulates sex hormone secretion and ovulation
	Prolactin (LTH)	Protein	Stimulates mammary gland growth and secretion in mammals; various reproductive and nonreproductive functions in lower vertebrates
	Growth hormone (GH)	Protein	Stimulates growth
Intermediate lobe	Melanophore-stimulating hormone (MSH)	Polypeptide	Pigment dispersion in melanophores of ectotherms
Neurohypophysis			
Posterior lobe	Vasopressin (ADH)	Octapeptide	Antidiuretic effect on kidney
	Oxytocin	Octapeptide	Stimulates milk ejection and uterine contraction
	Vasotocin	Octapeptide	Antidiuretic activity
	Isotocin and three others in lower vertebrates	Octapeptide	Functions uncertain
Hypothalamus	Thyrotropin-releasing hormone (TRH)		
	Corticotropin-releasing hormone (CRH)		
	Follicle-stimulating hormone–releasing hormone (FSH-RH)		
	Luteinizing hormone–releasing hormone (LH-RH)		
	Prolactin release–inhibiting factor (PIF)	Probably all polypeptides	Control release of anterior and intermediate lobe hormones
	Prolactin-releasing factor (PRF)		
	Melanophore-stimulating hormone–releasing factor (MRF)		
	Melanophore-stimulating hormone–release-inhibiting factor (MIF)		
	Growth hormone–releasing factor (GH-RF)		
	Growth hormone release–inhibiting hormone (GHR-IF)		

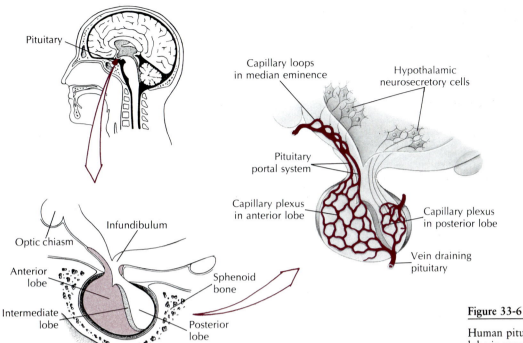

Figure 33-6

Human pituitary gland. The posterior lobe is connected directly to the hypothalamus by neurosecretory fibers. The anterior lobe is indirectly connected to the hypothalamus by a portal circulation beginning in the median eminence and ending in the anterior pituitary.

mones by the thyroid gland. The **adrenocorticotropic hormone** (ACTH) stimulates the adrenal cortex. Two of the tropic hormones are commonly called **gonadotropins** because they act on the gonads (ovary of the female, testis of the male). These are the **follicle-stimulating hormone** (FSH) and the **luteinizing hormone** (LH). (In the male the luteinizing hormone goes by a different name, interstitial cell stimulating hormone [ICSH], but it is the same hormone chemically.) A fifth tropic hormone is **prolactin,** which stimulates milk production by the female mammary glands and has a variety of other effects in the lower vertebrates. The functions of the two gonadotropins and prolactin are discussed in the next chapter in connection with the hormonal control of reproduction.

The sixth hormone of the anterior lobe is the **growth hormone** (also called somatotropic hormone). This hormone performs a vital role in governing body growth through its stimulatory effect on cellular mitosis and protein synthesis, especially in new tissue of young animals. If produced in excess, the growth hormone causes giantism. A deficiency of this hormone in the child or young animal causes dwarfism.

The intermediate lobe (Fig. 33-6) produces **melanophore-stimulating hormone** (MSH), which controls the dispersion of melanin within the melanophores of amphibians. In other vertebrates, MSH appears to perform no important physiological role, although it causes darkening of the skin in humans if injected into the circulation. MSH and ACTH are chemically very similar, and ACTH also causes skin darkening when it is secreted in abnormally large amounts.

Hypothalamus and neurosecretion

Because of the strategic importance of the pituitary in influencing most of the hormonal activities in the body, the pituitary was once called the body's "master gland." This description is not appropriate, however, since the tropic hormones

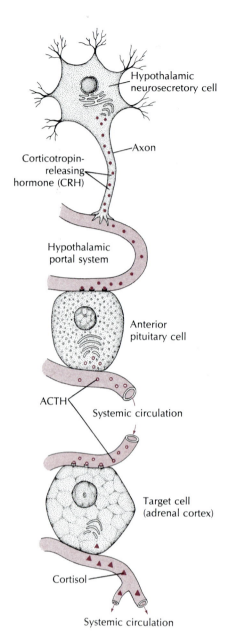

Figure 33-7

Relationship of hypothalamic, pituitary, and target-gland hormones. The hormone sequence controlling the release of cortisol from the adrenal cortex is used as an example.

are regulated by a higher council, the neurosecretory centers of the hypothalamus. The hypothalamus is itself under the ultimate control of the brain. The hypothalamus contains groups of neurosecretory cells, which are specialized giant nerve cells (Fig. 33-7). These cells manufacture polypeptide hormones, called releasing hormones (or "factors"), which then travel down the nerve fibers to their endings in the median eminence. Here they enter a capillary network to complete their journey to the anterior pituitary by way of a short pituitary portal system. The hypothalamic hormones then stimulate or inhibit the release of the various anterior pituitary hormones. Ten hypothalamic releasing hormones in all have been discovered since the demonstration in 1955 of a corticotropin-releasing hormone. There appear to be one or more releasing hormones regulating each of the six pituitary tropic hormones (Table 33-1). Several of the releasing hormones have now been isolated in pure state and characterized chemically. All are peptides.

Posterior pituitary

The hypothalamus is also the source of two hormones of the posterior lobe of the pituitary. They are formed in neurosecretory cells in the hypothalamus, then transported down the infundibular stalk and into the posterior lobe, ending in proximity to blood capillaries, which the hormones enter when released (Fig. 33-6). In a sense the posterior lobe is not a true endocrine gland, but a storage and release center for hormones manufactured entirely in the hypothalamus. The two posterior lobe hormones of mammals, oxytocin and vasopressin, are chemically very much alike; both are polypeptides consisting of eight amino acids and are referred to as octapeptides (Fig. 33-8). These hormones are among the fastest-acting hormones in the body, since they are capable of producing a response within seconds of their release from the posterior lobe.

Oxytocin has two important specialized reproductive functions in adult female mammals. It causes contraction of uterine smooth muscles during parturition (birth of the young). Physicians sometimes use oxytocin clinically to induce labor and facilitate delivery and to prevent uterine hemorrhage after birth. The second action of oxytocin is that of milk ejection by the mammary glands in response to suckling. Although present, oxytocin has no known function in the male.

Vasopressin, the second posterior lobe hormone, acts on the kidney to restrict urine flow, as already described on p. 736. It is therefore often referred to

Figure 33-8

Posterior lobe hormones of humans. Both oxytocin and vasopressin consist of eight amino acids (the two sulfur-linked cysteine molecules are considered to be a single amino acid, cystine). Oxytocin and vasopressin are identical except for amino acid substitutions in the red positions.

as the **antidiuretic hormone** (ADH). Vasopressin has a second, weaker effect of increasing the blood pressure through its generalized constrictor effect on the smooth muscles of the arterioles. Although the name "vasopressin" unfortunately suggests that the vasoconstrictor action is the hormone's major effect, it is probably of little physiological importance, except perhaps to help sustain the blood pressure during a severe hemorrhage.

All jawed vertebrates secrete two posterior lobe hormones that are quite similar to those of mammals. All are octapeptides, but there is some variation in structure because of amino acid substitutions in three of eight amino acid positions in the molecule.

Of all the posterior lobe hormones, **vasotocin** has the widest phylogenetic distribution and is believed to be the parent hormone from which the other octapeptides have evolved. It is found in all vertebrate classes except mammals. It is a water-balance hormone in amphibians, especially toads, in which it acts to conserve water by (1) increasing permeability of the skin (to promote water absorption from the environment), (2) stimulating water reabsorption from the urinary bladder, and (3) decreasing urine flow. The action of vasotocin is best understood in amphibians, but it appears to play some water-conserving role in birds and reptiles as well.

Brain neuropeptides

The blurred distinction between the endocrine and nervous systems is nowhere more evident than in the brain, where numerous hormonelike neuropeptides recently have been discovered. More than a dozen neuropeptides (short chains of amino acids) have been identified, and many are known to lead double lives. They are capable of behaving both as hormones, carrying signals from gland cells to their targets, and as neurotransmitters, relaying signals between nerve cells. For example, both oxytocin and vasopressin have been discovered at widespread sites in the brain by recently developed immunochemical methods. Apparently related to this is the fascinating observation that people and experimental animals injected with minute quantities of vasopressin experience enhanced learning and improved memory. As far as we can tell, this effect of vasopressin in brain tissue has nothing to do with its well-known antidiuretic function in the kidney (p. 736).

Just as amazing was the discovery in the cerebral cortex and hippocampus of several hormones, such as gastrin and cholecystokinin (p. 809), which long had been supposed to function only in the gut. We have a good idea of what these hormones do in the gastrointestinal tract, but what functional roles do they play in the brain?

Among the dramatic developments in this field was the discovery in 1975 of the endorphins and enkephalins, substances that bind with opiate receptors and are important in pain perception (see marginal note on p. 780). The endorphins and enkephalins are also found in brain circuits that modulate several other functions unrelated to pain, such as control of blood pressure, body temperature, and body movement. Even more intriguing, the endorphins are derived from the same chemical precursor that gives rise to the anterior pituitary hormones ACTH and MSH. It is clear that we have discovered in the brain a complex family of compounds whose functions and interrelationships are not yet clear. This is currently an extremely active area of biomedical research, and we seem to be on the threshold of some of the most exciting biological discoveries of the 1980s.

The radioimmunoassay technique developed by Solomon Berson and Rosalyn Yalow about 1960 after a decade of intensive study has revolutionized endocrinology and neurochemistry. First, antibodies to the hormone of interest (insulin, for example) are prepared by injecting guinea pigs or rabbits with the hormone. Then, a fixed amount of radioactively labeled insulin and unlabeled insulin antibodies is mixed with the sample of blood plasma to be measured. The native insulin in the blood plasma and the radioactive insulin compete for antibodies. The more insulin there is in the sample, the less radioactive insulin will bind to the antibodies. Bound and unbound insulin are then separated, and their radio-activities are measured together with those of appropriate standards to determine the amount of insulin present in the blood sample. The method is so incredibly sensitive that it can measure the equivalent of a cube of sugar dissolved in one of the Great Lakes. Yalow was awarded the Nobel Prize in 1977. Berson died in 1972; he did not receive the prize because it is never awarded posthumously.

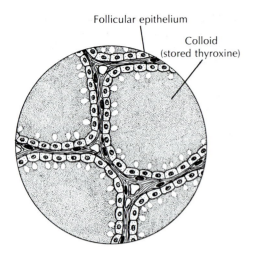

Follicular epithelium

Colloid
(stored thyroxine)

Inactive follicles

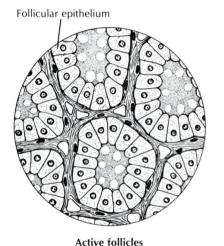

Follicular epithelium

Active follicles

Figure 33-9

Appearance of thyroid gland follicles viewed through the microscope. (About ×350.) When inactive, the follicles are distended with colloid, the storage form of thyroxine, and the epithelial cells are flattened. When active, the colloid disappears as thyroxine is secreted into the circulation, and the epithelial cells become greatly enlarged.

Hormones of Metabolism

Another important group of hormones adjusts the delicate balance of metabolic activities in the body. The rates of chemical reactions within cells are often regulated by long sequences of enzymes. Although such sequences are complex, each step in a pathway is mostly self-regulating, as long as the equilibrium between substrate, enzyme, and product remains stable. However, hormones may alter the activity of crucial enzymes in a metabolic process, thus accelerating or inhibiting the entire process. It should be emphasized that hormones never initiate enzymic processes. They simply alter their rate, speeding them up or slowing them down. The most important hormones of metabolism are those of the thyroid, parathyroid, and adrenal glands and the pancreas.

Thyroid hormones

The two thyroid hormones **thyroxine** and **triiodothyronine** are secreted by the thyroid gland. This largest of endocrine glands is located in the neck region of all vertebrates. The thyroid is made up of thousands of tiny spherelike units, called follicles, where thyroid hormone is synthesized, stored, and released into the bloodstream as needed. The size of the follicles, and the amount of stored thyroxine they contain, depends on the activity of the gland (Fig. 33-9).

One of the unique characteristics of the thyroid is its high concentration of **iodine;** in most animals this single gland contains well over half the body store of iodine. The epithelial cells of the thyroid follicles actively trap iodine from the blood and combine it with the amino acid tyrosine, creating the two thyroid hormones. Each molecule of thyroxine contains four atoms of iodine. Triiodothyronine is identical to thyroxine, except that it has three instead of four iodine atoms. Thyroxine is formed in much greater amounts than triiodothyronine, but both hormones have two important actions. One is to promote normal growth and development of the nervous system of growing animals. The other is to stimulate the metabolic rate.

$$HO-\underset{I}{\overset{I}{\bigcirc}}-O-\underset{I}{\overset{I}{\bigcirc}}-CH_2-\underset{NH_2}{\overset{|}{C}}H-COOH$$

Thyroxine

Undersecretion of thyroid hormone dramatically impairs growth, especially of the nervous system. The human **cretin,** a mentally retarded dwarf, is the tragic product of thyroid malfunction from a very early age. Conversely, the oversecretion of thyroid hormones causes precocious development, particularly in lower vertebrates. Frogs and toads undergo a dramatic metamorphosis from aquatic tadpole without lungs or legs to semiterrestrial or terrestrial adult with lungs, four legs, and a completely remodeled alimentary canal. This transformation occurs when the thyroid gland becomes active at the end of larval premetamorphosis. Stimulated by a rise in the blood thyroxine level, metamorphosis and climax occur (Fig. 33-10).

The control of oxygen consumption and heat production in birds and mammals is the best-known action of the thyroid hormones. The thyroid maintains metabolic activity of homeotherms (birds and mammals) at a normal level. Too

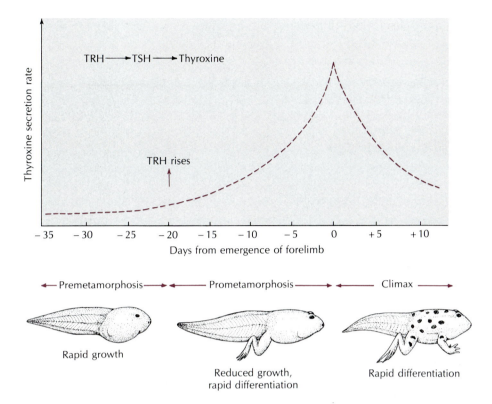

Days from emergence of forelimb

Thyroxine secretion rate

TRH ──▶ TSH ──▶ Thyroxine

TRH rises

◀──Premetamorphosis──▶ ◀──── Prometamorphosis ────▶ ◀─── Climax ───▶

Rapid growth

Reduced growth,
rapid differentiation

Rapid differentiation

Figure 33-10

Effect of thyroxine on frog growth and metamorphosis. The release of TRH from the hypothalamus at the end of premetamorphosis sets in motion the hormonal changes (increased TSH and thyroxine) leading to metamorphosis. Thyroxine levels are maximal at the time the forelimbs emerge.

Modified from Bentley, P.J. 1976. Comparative vertebrate endocrinology. Cambridge, Eng., Cambridge University Press.

much thyroid hormone will speed up body processes as much as 50%, resulting in irritability, nervousness, fast heart rate, intolerance of warm environments, and loss of body weight despite increased appetite. Too little thyroid hormone slows metabolic activities, which can result in loss of mental alertness, slowing of the heart rate, muscular weakness, increased sensitivity to cold, and weight gain. One important function of the thyroid gland is to help animals adapt to cold environments by increasing their heat production. Thyroxine in some way causes cells to produce more heat and store less chemical energy (ATP); in other words, thyroxine *reduces* the efficiency of the cellular oxidative phosphorylation system (p. 112). This is why many cold-adapted mammals have heartier appetites and eat more food in winter than in summer even though their activity is about the same in both seasons. In winter, a larger portion of the food is being converted directly into body-warming heat.

The synthesis and release of thyroxine and triiodothyronine are governed by **thyrotropic hormone** (TSH) from the anterior pituitary gland (Table 33-1). TSH controls the thyroid through a beautiful example of negative feedback. If the thyroxine level in the blood decreases, more TSH is released, which returns the thyroxine level to normal. Should the thyroxine level rise too high, it acts on the anterior pituitary to inhibit TSH release. With declining TSH output, the thyroid is less stimulated and the blood thyroxine level returns to normal. Such a system is obviously very effective in damping out oscillations in hormone output by the target gland. It can be overridden, however, by neural stimuli, such as exposure to cold, which can directly stimulate increased release of TSH.

The control of thyroid activity involves another component, the thyrotropin-releasing hormone (TRH) of the hypothalamus. As noted earlier, TRH is part of a higher regulatory council that controls the tropic hormones of the anterior pituitary. But, if the hypothalamus releasing hormone controls the anterior pituitary, what controls release of the releasing hormone? At present, there is no general agreement on the answer, although there is evidence that the thyroid hormones have a negative feedback effect on the hypothalamus as well as on the anterior pituitary.

Some years ago, a condition called **goiter** was common among people living in the Great Lakes region of the United States and Canada, as well as in other parts of the earth such as the Swiss Alps. Goiter is an enlargement of the thyroid gland caused by a deficiency of iodine in the food and water. In striving to produce thyroid hormone with not enough iodine available, the gland hypertrophies, sometimes so much that the entire neck region becomes swollen (Fig. 33-11). Goiter is seldom seen in North America because of the widespread use of iodized salt. However, it is estimated that even today 200 million people suffer from goiter worldwide, mostly in high mountain areas of Latin America, Europe, and Asia.

Hormonal regulation of calcium metabolism

Closely associated with the thyroid gland and often buried within it are the parathyroid glands. These tiny glands occur as two pairs in humans but vary in number and position in other vertebrates. They were discovered at the end of the nineteenth century when the fatal effects of "thyroidectomy" were traced to the unknowing removal of the parathyroid glands as well as the thyroid gland.

In many animals, including humans, removal of the parathyroid glands causes the blood calcium to decrease rapidly. This results in a serious increase in nervous system excitability, severe muscular spasms and tetany, and finally death.

The parathyroid glands are vitally concerned with the maintenance of the normal level of calcium in the blood. Actually, three hormones are involved in the stabilization of both calcium and phosphorus in the blood. They are **parathyroid hormone** (PTH), produced by the parathyroid gland; **calcitonin,** produced by specialized cells (C cells) in the thyroid gland; and a hormonal metabolite of vitamin D called **1,25-dihydroxyvitamin D** (1,25-[OH]$_2$D). Before considering how these factors interact, it will be helpful to summarize mineral metabolism in bone, a densely packed storehouse of both calcium and phosphorus.

Bone contains approximately 98% of the body calcium and 80% of the phosphorus. Although bone is second only to teeth as the most durable material in the body, as evidenced by the survival of fossil bones for millions of years, it is in a state of constant turnover in the living body. Bone-building cells (**osteoblasts**) withdraw calcium and phosphorus (as phosphate) from the blood and deposit them in a complex crystalline form around previously formed organic fibers. Bone-resorbing cells (**osteoclasts**), present in the same bone, tear down bone by engulfing it and releasing the calcium and phosphate into the blood. These opposing activities allow bone to constantly remodel itself, especially in the growing animal, for structural improvements to counter new mechanical stresses on the body. They additionally provide a vast and accessible reservoir of minerals that can be withdrawn as the body needs them for its general cellular requirements.

If the blood calcium should decrease slightly, the parathyroid gland increases its output of parathormone. This stimulates the osteoclasts to destroy bone adjacent to these cells, thus releasing calcium and phosphate into the bloodstream and returning the blood calcium level to normal. Should the calcium in the blood rise above normal, the parathyroid gland decreases its output of parathormone. The parathyroid hormone level varies inversely with blood calcium level, as shown in Fig. 33-12.

Figure 33-11

Thyroid goiter in a woman from western Colombia, an endemic goiter area of South America.

Courtesy Dr. Eduardo Gaitan, University of Mississippi Medical Center.

Figure 33-12

How parathyroid hormone (PTH) and calcitonin secretion rates respond to changes in blood calcium level in a mammal.

After Copp, D.H. 1969. J. Endocrinol. 43:137-161.

The second calcium-regulating hormone, calcitonin, is secreted when the blood level of calcium begins to rise too high (Fig. 33-12). Calcitonin lowers the blood calcium level by inhibiting bone resorption by the osteoclasts. It thus protects the body against a dangerous increase in the blood calcium level, just as parathormone protects it from a dangerous decrease in blood calcium. The two act together to smooth out oscillations in blood calcium (Fig. 33-13).

The third factor involved in calcium metabolism, 1,25-dihydroxyvitamin D, is an active hormonal form of vitamin D. Vitamin D, like all vitamins, is a dietary requirement. But unlike other vitamins, vitamin D may also be synthesized in the skin from a precursor by irradiation with ultraviolet light from the sun. Vitamin D is then converted in a two-step oxidation to 1,25-dihydroxyvitamin D. This steroid hormone is essential for active calcium absorption by the gut (Fig. 33-13). It also promotes the synthesis of a protein that transports calcium in the blood.

A deficiency of vitamin D causes rickets, a disease characterized by low blood calcium and weak, poorly calcified bones that tend to bend under postural and gravitational stresses. Rickets has been called a disease of northern winters, when sunlight is minimal. It was once common in the smoke-darkened cities of England and Europe.

Hormones of the adrenal cortex

The vertebrate adrenal gland is a double gland consisting of two very different kinds of tissue: **interrenal tissue,** called **cortex** in mammals, and **chromaffin** tissue, called **medulla** in mammals (Fig. 33-14). The mammalian terminology of cortex (meaning "bark") and medulla (meaning "core") arose because in this group of vertebrates the interrenal tissue completely surrounds the chromaffin tissue like a cover. Although in the lower vertebrates the interrenal and chromaffin tissues are usually separated, the mammalian terms "cortex" and "medulla" are so firmly fixed in our vocabulary that we commonly use them for all vertebrates instead of the more correct terms "interrenal" and "chromaffin."

Biochemists have found that the adrenal cortex contains at least 30 different compounds, all of them closely related lipoid compounds known as steroids. Only a few of these compounds, however, are true steroid *hormones;* most are various intermediates in the synthesis of steroid hormones from **cholesterol** (Fig. 33-15). The corticosteroid hormones are commonly classified into three groups, according to their function:

1. **Glucocorticoids,** such as **cortisol** (Fig. 33-15) and **corticosterone,** are concerned with food metabolism, inflammation, and stress. They cause the conver-

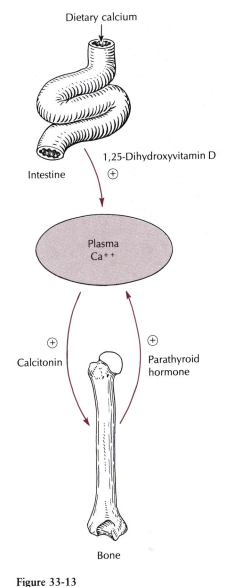

Figure 33-13

Regulation of blood calcium in birds and mammals.

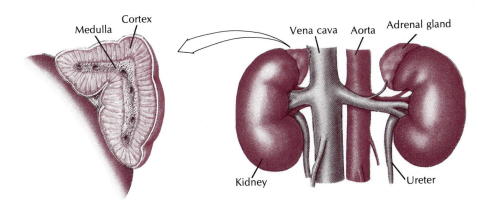

Figure 33-14

Paired adrenal glands of a human, showing gross structure and position on the upper poles of the kidneys. Steroid hormones are produced by the outer cortex. The sympathetic hormones epinephrine and norepinephrine are produced by the inner medulla.

Figure 33-15

Hormones of the adrenal cortex. Cortisol (a glucocorticoid) and aldosterone (a mineralocorticoid) are two of several steroid hormones synthesized from cholesterol in the adrenal cortex.

Aldosterone

Cholesterol

Cortisol

The adrenal steroid hormones, especially the glucocorticoids, are remarkably effective in relieving the *symptoms* of rheumatoid arthritis, allergies, and various connective tissue, skin, and blood disorders. Following the report in 1948 of Dr. P.S. Hench and his colleagues at the Mayo Clinic that cortisone dramatically relieved the pain and crippling effects of advanced arthritis, the steroid hormones were hailed by the media as "wonder drugs." Optimism was soon dimmed, however, when it became apparent that severe side effects (salt retention, high blood pressure, peptic ulcers, thinning of bones, and decreased resistance to infection) always attended long-term administration of the antiinflammatory steroids. Although more recently developed synthetic steroids cause less harmful side effects, they lull the adrenal cortex into inactivity and may permanently impair the body's capacity to produce its own steroids. Today steroid therapy is applied with caution, since it is realized that the inflammatory response is a necessary part of the body's defenses.

sion of nonglucose compounds, particularly amino acids and fats, into glucose. This process, called **gluconeogenesis,** is extremely important, since most of the body's stored energy reserves are in the form of fats and proteins that must be converted to glucose before they can be burned for energy. Cortisol, cortisone, and corticosterone are also **antiinflammatory.** Because several diseases of humans are inflammatory diseases (for example, allergies, hypersensitivity, and arthritis, p. 704), these corticosteroids have important medical applications. They must be used with great care, however, since, if administered in excess, they may suppress the body's normal repair processes and lower resistance to infectious agents.

2. **Mineralocorticoids,** the second group of corticosteroids, are those that regulate salt balance. **Aldosterone** (Fig. 33-15) and **deoxycorticosterone** are the most important steroids of this group. They promote the tubular reabsorption of sodium and chloride and the tubular excretion of potassium by the kidney. Since sodium usually is in short supply in the diet of many animals and potassium is in excess, it is obvious that the mineralocorticoids play vital roles in preserving the correct balance of blood electrolytes. We may also note that the mineralocorticoids *oppose* the antiinflammatory effect of cortisol and cortisone. In other words, they promote the *inflammatory* defense of the body to various noxious stimuli. Although these opposing actions of the corticosteroids seem self-defeating, they actually are not. They are necessary to maintain readiness of the body's defenses for any stress or disease threat, yet prevent these defenses from becoming so powerful that they turn against the body's own tissues.

3. **Sex hormones,** such as testosterone, estrogen, and progesterone, are produced primarily by the ovaries and testes (p. 856). The adrenal cortex is also a minor source of certain steroids that mimic the action of testosterone. These sex hormone–like secretions are of little physiological significance, except in certain disease states of humans.

The synthesis and secretion of the corticosteroids are controlled principally by ACTH of the anterior pituitary (Fig. 33-7). As with pituitary control of the thyroid, a negative feedback relationship exists between ACTH and the adrenal cortex: an increase in the level of corticosteroids suppresses the output of ACTH; a decrease in the blood steroid level increases ACTH output. ACTH is also controlled by the corticotropin-releasing hormone (CRH) of the hypothalamus.

Hormones of the adrenal medulla

The adrenal medulla secretes two structurally similar hormones: **epinephrine** (adrenaline) and **norepinephrine** (noradrenaline). Norepinephrine is also released at the endings of sympathetic nerve fibers throughout the body, where it serves as a "transmitter" substance to carry neural signals across the gap that separates the fiber and the organ it innervates. The adrenal medulla has the same embryological origin as sympathetic nerves; in many respects the adrenal medulla is nothing more than an overgrown sympathetic nerve ending.

Epinephrine

Norepinephrine

It is not surprising then that the adrenal medulla hormones have the same general effects on the body that the sympathetic nervous system has. These effects center on emergency functions of the body, such as fear, rage, fight, and flight, although they have important integrative functions in more peaceful times as well. We are all familiar with the increased heart rate, tightening of the stomach, dry mouth, trembling muscles, general feeling of anxiety, and increased awareness that attends sudden fright or other strong emotional states. These effects are attributable both to the rapid release into the blood of epinephrine from the adrenal medulla and to increased activity of the sympathetic nervous system.

Epinephrine and norepinephrine have many other effects of which we are not as aware, including constriction of the arterioles (which, together with the increased heart rate, increases the blood pressure), mobilization of liver glycogen and fat stores to release glucose and fatty acids for energy, increased oxygen consumption and heat production, hastening of blood coagulation, and inhibition of the gastrointestinal tract. All of these changes in one way or another tune up the body for emergencies.

Insulin from the islet cells of the pancreas

The pancreas is both an exocrine and an endocrine organ. The *exocrine* portion produces pancreatic juice, a mixture of digestive enzymes that is conveyed by ducts to the digestive tract. Scattered within the extensive exocrine portion of the pancreas are numerous small islets of tissue, called **islets of Langerhans.** This is the *endocrine* portion of the gland. The islets are without ducts and secrete their hormones directly into blood vessels that extend throughout the pancreas.

Figure 33-16

Insulin is synthesized in the beta cells of the pancreas as inactive proinsulin and is then converted to the hormone insulin by removal of the peptide that connects the A and B chains. **A,** The amino acid sequence of proinsulin. **B,** Chain folding as derived from x-ray analysis.

Connecting peptide

A chain

B chain

Figure 33-17

Charles H. Best and Sir Frederick Banting in 1921 with the first dog to be kept alive by insulin.

From Fulton, J.F., and L.G. Wilson. 1966. Selected readings in the history of physiology. Springfield, Ill., Charles C Thomas, Publisher.

Two polypeptide hormones are secreted by different cell types within the islets: **insulin** (Fig. 33-16), produced by the **beta cells,** and **glucagon,** produced by the **alpha cells.** Insulin and glucagon have antagonistic actions of great importance in the metabolism of carbohydrates and fats. Insulin is essential for the use of blood glucose by cells, especially skeletal muscle cells. Insulin somehow allows glucose in the blood to be transported into body cells. Without insulin, the cells cannot use glucose, even if there is an abnormally high blood glucose level (hyperglycemia), and sugar appears in the urine. Lack of insulin also inhibits the uptake of amino acids by skeletal muscle, and fats and muscle are broken down to provide energy. The body cells actually starve while the urine abounds in the very substance the body craves. The disease, called diabetes mellitus, afflicts nearly 5% of the human population in varying degrees of severity. If left untreated, it leads inexorably to emaciation, coma, and death.

The first extraction of insulin in 1921 by two Canadians, Frederick Banting and Charles Best, was one of the most dramatic and important events in the history of medicine. Many years earlier two German scientists, J. Von Mering and O. Minkowski, discovered that surgical removal of the pancreas of dogs invariably caused severe symptoms of diabetes, resulting in the animal's death within a few weeks. Many attempts were made to isolate the diabetes preventive factor, but all failed because powerful protein-splitting digestive enzymes in the exocrine portion of the pancreas destroyed the hormone during extraction procedures. Following a hunch, Banting, in collaboration with Best and his physiology professor J.J.R. Macleod, tied off the pancreatic ducts of several dogs. This caused the exocrine portion of the gland with its hormone-destroying enzyme to degenerate but left the islets' tissue healthy, since they were independently served by their own blood supply. Banting and Best then successfully extracted insulin from these glands. Injected into another dog, the insulin immediately lowered the blood sugar level (Fig. 33-17). Their experiment paved the way for the commercial extraction of insulin from slaughterhouse animals. It meant that millions of people with diabetes, previously doomed to invalidism or death, could look forward to more normal lives.

Glucagon, the second hormone of the pancreas, has several effects on carbohydrates and fat metabolism that are opposite to the effects of insulin. For example, glucagon raises the blood glucose level, whereas insulin lowers it. Glucagon and insulin do not have the same effects in all vertebrates, and in some glucagon is lacking altogether. Glucagon is an example of a hormone that operates through the cyclic AMP second-messenger system.

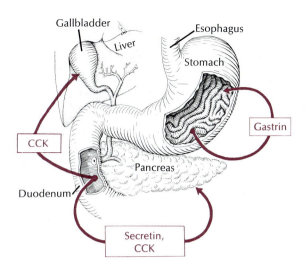

Figure 33-18

Three hormones of digestion. Arrows show source and target of three gastrointestinal hormones.

___ Hormones of Digestion

Gastrointestinal function is coordinated by a family of hormones produced by endocrine cells scattered through the gut. Although together they constitute the largest endocrine organ in the body, they have long been neglected by endocrinologists because it has been impossible to study them by applying the classical method of surgical removal of a gland, followed by examination of the effect of its absence. However, by the mid-1970s seven gut hormones had been chemically purified or defined. Recently several of these hormones were discovered in the nervous system, where they may serve as neurotransmitters. If this dual role of the gut hormones is confirmed by current research, it would be another example of nature's conservative capacity to put the same cellular products to completely different uses in unrelated systems.

The three best-understood gut hormones are gastrin, cholecystokinin (CCK), and secretin (Fig. 33-18). **Gastrin** is a small polypeptide hormone produced in the mucosa of the pyloric portion of the stomach. When food enters the stomach, gastrin stimulates the secretion of hydrochloric acid by the stomach wall. Gastrin is an unusual hormone in that it exerts its action on the same organ from which it is secreted. **CCK** is also a polypeptide hormone and has a striking structural resemblance to gastrin, suggesting that the two arose by duplication of ancestral genes. CCK has two distinct functions. It stimulates gallbladder contraction and thus increases the flow of bile salts into the intestine; it also stimulates an enzyme-rich secretion from the pancreas. The third gut hormone is **secretin**, the first hormone to be discovered (p. 793). Like CCK, it stimulates pancreatic secretion, but instead of being rich in enzymes, the secretion contains bicarbonate, which rapidly neutralizes stomach acid.

All of the gastrointestinal hormones are peptides that bind to surface receptors on target tissues and act through the second messenger, cyclic AMP.

___ Summary

Hormones are chemical messengers synthesized by special endocrine glands and transported by the bloodstream to target cells where they affect cell function by altering specific biochemical processes. Specificity of response is ensured by the presence of protein receptors on or in the target cells that bind only selected hormones. Hormone effects are vastly amplified in the target cells by acting through one or the other of two basic mechanisms. Many hormones, including epinephrine, glucagon, vasopressin, and some anterior pituitary hormones, cause production of cyclic AMP, a "second messenger" that relays the hormone's message from a surface receptor to the cell's biochemical machinery. The alternative mechanism relays the action of steroid hormones by operating through cytoplasmic receptors. A hormone-receptor complex is formed that moves into the cell's nucleus to induce protein synthesis by setting gene transcription in motion.

Most invertebrate hormones are products of neurosecretory cells. The best-understood invertebrate endocrine system is that controlling molting and metamorphosis in insects. An insect juvenile grows by passing through a series of molts under the control of two hormones, one (the molting hormone) favoring molting to an adult and the other (the juvenile hormone) favoring retention of juvenile characteristics. The molting hormone is under the control of a brain neurosecretory hormone called prothoracicotropic hormone.

The vertebrate endocrine system is orchestrated by the pituitary gland. The anterior lobe of the pituitary produces at least six hormones. Five of these are tropic hormones that regulate subservient endocrine glands: adrenocorticotropic hormone (ACTH), which stimulates the adrenal cortex; thyrotropic hormone (TSH); follicle-stimulating hormone (FSH) and luteinizing hormone (LH), which act on the ovaries and testes; and prolactin, which plays several diverse roles, including the stimulation of milk production. A sixth anterior pituitary hormone is the growth hormone that governs body growth. The intermediate lobe of the pituitary produces melanophore-stimulating hormone (MSH), which controls melanophore dispersion in amphibians. The release of all of the anterior and intermediate lobe hormones is regulated in part by hypothalamic neurosecretory products called releasing hormones. The hypothalamus also produces two neurosecretory hormones, oxytocin and vasopressin, which are stored and released from the posterior lobe of the pituitary.

The recent application of ultrasensitive radioimmunochemical techniques has revealed many neuropeptides in the brain, several of which behave as neurotransmitters in the brain but as hormones elsewhere in the body.

Several hormones play important roles in regulating cellular metabolic activities. The two thyroid hormones, thyroxine and triiodothyronine, promote normal growth and nervous system development, and they control the rate of cellular metabolism. Calcium metabolism is regulated principally by two antagonistic hormones: parathormone from the parathyroid glands and calcitonin from the thyroid gland. A hormonal derivative of vitamin D, 1,25-dihydroxyvitamin D, is essential for calcium absorption from the gut.

The steroid hormones of the adrenal cortex are glucocorticoids, which stimulate glucose formation from nonglucose sources; mineralocorticoids, which regulate blood electrolyte balance; and certain of the sex hormones. The adrenal medulla is the source of epinephrine and norepinephrine, which have many effects, including assisting the sympathetic nervous system in emergency responses.

Sugar metabolism is regulated by the antagonistic action of two pancreatic hormones. Insulin is needed for cellular use of blood glucose and the uptake of amino acids by muscle. Glucagon opposes the action of insulin.

Several gut hormones coordinate gastrointestinal function. They include gastrin, which stimulates acid secretion by the stomach, and CCK and secretin, which regulate gallbladder contraction and pancreatic secretion.

Selected references

See also general references for Part Three, p. 837.

Barrington, E.J.W. 1975. An introduction to general and comparative endocrinology, ed. 2. Oxford, Eng., Oxford University Press. *Thorough comparative treatment.*

Bentley, P.J. 1976. Comparative vertebrate endocrinology. Cambridge, Eng., Cambridge University Press. *Clearly written account relating endocrine function to the animal's ecology and evolutionary background.*

Goldstein, L. (ed.). 1977. Introduction to comparative physiology. New York, Holt, Rinehart & Winston. *This text contains an excellent chapter on endocrinology by P.J. Bentley.*

Goldsworthy, G.J., J. Robinson, and W. Mordue. 1981. Endocrinology. New York, John Wiley & Sons, Inc. *Concise comparative approach.*

Highnam, K.C., and L. Hill. 1977. The comparative endocrinology of the invertebrates, ed. 2. New York, American Elsevier Publishers, Co., Inc. *Clearly written, well-illustrated comparative account emphasizing hormonal action.*

Maurer, A.C. 1979. The therapy of diabetes. Am. Sci. 67:422-431. *Describes the management of the two basic forms of sugar diabetes.*

Norris, D.O. 1980. Vertebrate endocrinology. Philadelphia, Lea & Febiger. *Undergraduate textbook.*

Schally, A.V., A.J. Kastan, and A. Arimura. 1977. Hypothalamic hormones: the link between brain and body. Am. Sci. 65:712-719. *Review of functional interactions of the recognized hypothalamic hormones.*

Turner, C.L., and J.T. Bagnara. 1976. General endocrinology, ed. 6. Philadelphia, W.B. Saunders Co. *Undergraduate-level text.*

Yalow, R.S. 1978. Radioimmunoassay: a probe for the fine structure of biologic systems. Science 200:1236-1245. *The radioimmunoassay technique has revolutionized endocrinology. This is the text of Professor Yalow's Nobel Prize acceptance speech.*

Selected *Scientific American* articles

Bloom, F.E. 1981. Neuropeptides. 245:148-168 (Oct.).

Gillie, R.B. 1971. Endemic goiter. 224:92-101 (June). *In some parts of the world, many people still suffer from this thyroid disorder caused by insufficient iodine in the diet.*

Guillemin, R., and R. Burgus. 1972. The hormones of the hypothalamus. 227:24-33 (Nov.). *Describes the function of two of the brain's "releasing factors."*

Levine, R., and M.S. Goldstein. 1958. The action of insulin. 198:99-106 (May). *Describes insulin's role in promoting the passage of sugar across cell membranes.*

Li, C.H. 1963. The ACTH molecule. 209:46-53 (July). *Its composition and what it does.*

Loomis, W.F. 1970. Rickets. 223:76-91 (Dec.). *The role of vitamin D in preventing this oldest of air-pollution diseases.*

McEwen, B.S. 1976. Interactions between hormones and nerve tissue. 235:48-58 (July). *Steroid hormones secreted by gonads and adrenal cortex can be traced to target cells in the brain.*

Nathanson, J.A., and P. Greengard. 1977. "Second messengers" in the brain. 237:108-119 (Aug.). *Analogous messenger mechanisms underlie communication in the endocrine and nervous systems.*

Notkins, A.L. 1979. The cause of diabetes. 241:62-73 (Nov.). *The two major types of diabetes are described.*

O'Malley, B.W., and W.T. Schrader. 1976. The receptors of steroid hormones. 234:32-43 (Feb.). *The action of steroid hormones is mediated by receptor molecules that reside only in the target organs.*

Pastan, I. 1972. Cyclic AMP. 227:97-105 (Aug.). *The hormonal "second messenger" and some of the roles it plays.*

Rasmussen, H., and M.M. Pechet. 1970. Calcitonin. 223:42-50 (Oct.). *Discovery and action of this calcium-regulating hormone.*

Wilkins, L. 1960. The thyroid gland. 202:119-129 (Mar.). *How the gland is constructed, what it produces, and how it is controlled.*

Williams, C.M. 1958. The juvenile hormone. 198:67-74 (Feb.). *This insect hormone prevents metamorphosis of the larva into a pupa until growth is complete.*

A N I M A L   B E H A V I O R

Juvenile anubis baboon *(Papio anubis)* peers at a newborn clinging
to its mother's ventrum. Infants are a source of fascination
for all members of the troop.

Photograph by T.W. Ransom/BPS.

For as long as people have walked the earth, their lives have been touched by, indeed interwoven with, the lives of other animals. They hunted and fished for them, domesticated them, ate them and were eaten by them, made pets of them, revered them, hated and feared them, immortalized them in art, song, and verse, fought them, and loved them. The very survival of ancient peoples depended on knowledge of wild animals. To stalk them, people had to know the ways of the quarry. As the hunting society of primitive people gave way to agricultural civilizations, an awareness was retained of the interrelationship with other animals.

This is still evident today. Zoos attract more visitors than ever before; wildlife television shows are increasingly popular; game-watching safaris to Africa constitute a thriving enterprise; and millions of pet animals share the cities with us—more than a half million pet dogs live in New York City alone. Although ethology, the science of animal behavior, is a young discipline of zoology, people have always been behaviorists. Only recently, however, have we begun to understand how animal societies work.

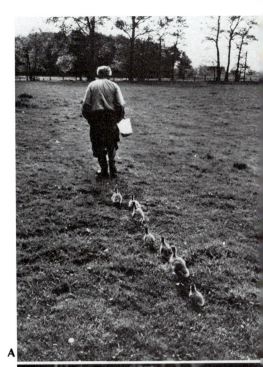

ETHOLOGY AND THE STUDY OF INSTINCT

In 1973 the Nobel Prize in physiology and medicine was awarded to three pioneering zoologists, Karl von Frisch, Konrad Lorenz, and Niko Tinbergen (Fig. 34-1). The citation stated that these three were the principal architects of the new science of ethology. It was the first time any contributor to the behavioral sciences was so honored, and it meant that the discipline of animal behavior, which is rooted in the work of Charles Darwin, had arrived.

The term "ethology," meaning literally "character study," was first used in the late eighteenth century to signify the interpretation of character through the study of gesture. It was an appropriate term for the new field of animal behavior, which had as its objective the study of motor patterns, that is, gestures of animals, with the anticipation that such study would reveal the true characters of animals just as the interpretation of human gestures might reveal the true characters of people. This decidedly restricted interpretation of ethology as a purely descriptive study of the "habits" of animals was considerably modified during the period in which ethology was established as a science, 1935 to 1950. Today we may define ethology as a discipline that involves the study of the total repertoire of the innate and the learned behavior that animals employ to resolve the problems of survival and reproduction.

The aim of ethologists has always been to describe the behavior of an animal in its *natural habitat*. From the beginning ethologists have been naturalists. Their laboratory has been the out-of-doors, and early ethologists gathered their data by field observation. They also conducted experiments, often with nature providing the variables, but increasingly ethologists have manipulated the variables for their own purposes by using animal models, playing recordings of animal vocalizations, altering the habitat, and so on. Modern ethologists also conduct many experi-

---

Figure 34-1

A, Konrad Lorenz. **B,** Karl von Frisch. **C,** Niko Tinbergen.

ments in the laboratory where they can test their predictions under closely controlled conditions. However, ethologists usually take pains to compare laboratory observations with observations of free-ranging animals in undisturbed natural environments. They recognize that it makes no more sense to try to study the natural behavior of an animal divorced from its natural surroundings than it does to try to interpret a structural adaptation of an animal apart from the function it serves.

With infinite patience Lorenz, Tinbergen, and their colleagues watched and catalogued the activities and vocalizations of animals during feeding, courtship, and nest building, as well as seemingly insignificant behavioral movements such as head scratching, stretching postures, and turning and shaking movements. These studies concentrated largely on innate motor patterns used for communication within a species.

One of the great contributions of Lorenz and Tinbergen was to demonstrate that behavioral traits are measurable entities like anatomical or physiological traits. This was to become the central theme of ethology: behavioral traits can be isolated and measured, and they have evolutionary histories. Lorenz and Tinbergen showed that behavior is not the wavering, transient, unpredictable phenomenon often depicted by earlier writers. In short, behavior is genetically mediated. It is apparent that, if behavior is determined by genes in the same way that genes determine morphological and physiological characters (ethologists have found abundant evidence that it is), then behavior evolves and is adaptive. Thus, modern behavioral study is founded on the recognition that the Darwinian view of evolution holds for behavioral traits, as well as for anatomical and functional characters.

STEREOTYPED BEHAVIOR

The European ethologists, through step-by-step analysis of the detailed behavior of animals in nature, especially of fishes and birds, focused on the invariant components of behavior. From such detailed studies emerged several concepts that were first made available to large numbers of American readers in Tinbergen's influential book *The Study of Instinct* (1951).

The basic concepts of ethological theory can be approached by considering the egg-rolling movement of the greylag goose, described by Lorenz and Tinbergen in 1938 (Fig. 34-2). If a greylag goose is presented with an egg a short distance from her nest, she reaches out with her bill until her lower beak touches the egg. Then, extending her bill just beyond the egg, she contracts her neck, pulling the egg carefully toward the nest with the underside of her bill. Since the egg naturally has a tendency to wander off course on the uneven terrain, the goose compensates for this by moving the bill from one side to the other, correcting the course of the egg until she has it in her nest.

If the egg is removed after the goose has begun her retrieval, the goose continues the egg-rolling behavior as though the egg were still there. The side-to-side movements cease, but the tucking movements continue as she slowly pulls her neck back in a straight line toward the nest with the invisible egg. If on another occasion the egg being retrieved slips completely away and rolls down the slope of the nest mound, the goose continues her retrieval movements without the egg until she is again settled comfortably on her nest. Then, seeing that the egg has not been retrieved, she begins the egg-rolling pattern all over again.

Figure 34-2

Egg-rolling movement of the greylag goose *Anser anser*.
From Lorenz, K., and N. Tinbergen. 1938. Zeit. Tierpsychol. 2:1-29.

Fixed Action Pattern

The egg-rolling movement of greylag geese is an example of a **fixed action pattern.** It is a motor act that is highly stereotyped and mostly invariable in its performance. Once the sequence is begun, it is completed whether or not the egg is actually being retrieved. The goose does not have to learn the movement; it is an innate, or instinctive, skill. The goose behaves as though an internal program had been triggered and must run its course before switching off.

Actually the egg-rolling movement can be separated into two components. The fixed action pattern represents the unvarying, straight retrieval movements that continue even in the absence of a stimulus (the egg). However, the lateral corrective movements that the goose makes to steer the egg past obstructions are orienting movements guided by external stimulation, in this case the changing tactile stimulation on the beak provided by the wandering egg. Fixed action patterns usually occur with orienting movements superimposed on them.

Figure 34-3

Oyster catcher *Haematopus ostralegus* attempts to roll a giant egg model into its nest while ignoring its own egg.
From Tinbergen, N. 1951. The study of instinct. Oxford, Eng., Oxford University Press.

Sign Stimuli

Much of an animal's behavior is triggered by a few key environmental stimuli. Such key signals, or **sign stimuli,** constitute only a small fraction of the total environmental information available. The egg placed outside the nest of the greylag goose is the specific stimulus that releases egg-retrieval behavior. However, at no time do releasers trigger a fixed action pattern in all members of a species. The animal must be in the proper motivational state. Only a *female* greylag goose *in a nest* responds to a wayward egg outside the nest. But, once she is properly motivated and in the "right" surroundings, the greylag goose is not terribly discriminating about what she retrieves. Lorenz and Tinbergen showed that almost any smooth and rounded object placed outside the nest would trigger the egg-retrieval behavior of this species; even a small toy dog and a large yellow balloon were dutifully retrieved.

Sometimes exaggerated sign stimuli release an exaggerated response. In one famous experiment, an oyster catcher tried mostly unsuccessfully to retrieve and incubate an egg four times the normal size while ignoring its own egg (Fig. 34-3). Such an exceptionally effective sign stimulus is called a **supernormal stimulus.**

Because sign stimuli are relevant to the animal's survival and reproduction, they are characteristically simple cues, a fact that reduces the chances of making a mistake or misunderstanding the cue. In every case the response is highly predictable. The alarm call of adult herring gulls releases a crouching freeze response in the chicks. Female frogs respond only to the courtship calls of males of their own species. Night-flying moths take evasive maneuvers or drop to the ground when they hear the ultrasonic cries of bats that feed on them; no other sound releases this response. Ethologists have described hundreds of such examples of sign stimuli.

Innate Releasing Mechanism

The sign stimulus, whether a sound, color, appropriate structure, odor, or movement, releases a predictable response. This strict correlation between stimulus and appropriate response led ethologists to conclude that the nervous system is organized into discrete "centers" capable of filtering the sensory input, correctly selecting the sign stimuli, and releasing an appropriate motor response. Lorenz called this organization the **innate releasing mechanism** (IRM). An IRM was considered to be an aggregation of nerve cells that, once triggered by the key stimulus, would direct motor neurons to fire in a programmed manner, causing the animal to perform a stereotyped fixed action pattern. Lorenz used an analogy to illustrate how an IRM operates: the sign stimulus is a key that unlocks only one of many possible doors; once the door (the IRM) is opened, the specific response inside is released.

More controversy surrounds the concept of the IRM than perhaps any other ethological concept. Physiologists are reluctant to believe that "centers" as visualized by Lorenz actually exist. The central nervous system operates as an integrated whole, rather than as a collection of nerve aggregates, each prewired to perform one and only one motor function. Thus, the IRM concept has been altered somewhat, but the idea seems to be fundamentally correct; brain "centers" as such probably do not exist, but the brain *works* as though they do. If not interpreted too strictly, the IRM is a useful tool to ethologists for understanding the sequence and coordination of stereotyped behavior.

___ Drive Concept

Animals are active because of internal motivation. It has been customary to refer to changes in responsiveness as drives. Thus, animals show hunger drives, thirst drives, courtship drives, mating drives, migration drives, and so on. Used in this context, a drive refers to a motivational change that results in the performance of certain usually predictable behaviors. A hungry animal searches for food in a manner characteristic of its species. The hunting behavior can be thought of as a search for a releasing situation that permits the discharge of prey-capturing behavior.

Ethologists recognize the following three stages in completing a stereotyped behavior:

1. *Appetitive behavior.* Appetitive behavior is the specific search for a releasing situation; it places an animal in a position to achieve a biological goal. A hungry fox becomes restless and begins a characteristic hunting behavior that is adapted to the situation; it knows the terrain, detours to make, habits of potential quarry, and location of a farmer's chicken yard. In lower animals, appetitive behavior is more predictable and less subject to variation from previous learning experience.

2. *Consummatory behavior.* The biological goal of appetitive behavior is the consummatory act. For the hungry fox, catching and eating a chicken is the climax of the hunger drive. Location of a mate by a songbird following a search (appetitive behavior) releases courtship behavior (consummatory act). A gravid tortoise locates a suitable nest site and lays her eggs. A blowfly's search for food ceases when it has discovered and eaten enough to comfortably fill the foregut. In each case, once the goal is achieved, the goal-directed activity ceases.

3. *Quiescence.* Following the consummatory act, appetitive behavior does not immediately resume. This is the period of quiescence. The sated animal does not hunt. Later, when the animal gets hungry, a new round of appetitive behavior, consummatory act, and quiescence follows.

Although use of the term **drive** is a convenient way to describe a positive motivation toward achieving some biological goal, the word is increasingly disfavored. Critics contend that it is vague and nonexplanatory and is used to embrace a variety of distantly related phenomena, having different neurophysio-

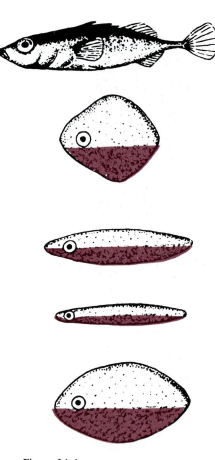

Figure 34-4

Stickleback models. The carefully made model of the stickleback *(top)* without a red belly is attacked much less frequently than the four simple red-bellied models.

From Tinbergen, N. 1951. The study of instinct. Oxford, Eng., Oxford University Press.

logical bases. Yet, the term persists in the absence of a completely acceptable substitute for expressing in a word the idea of motivation toward a biological goal.

_____ Instinct and Learning

The invariable and predictable nature of stereotyped behavior suggests that it is inherited, or innate, behavior. Many kinds of unpracticed stereotyped behavior appear suddenly in animals and are indistinguishable from similar behavior performed by older, experienced individuals. Newly emerged moths and butterflies fly perfectly as soon as their wings are dry. Orb-weaving spiders "know" how to build their webs without practice and without having watched other spiders build theirs. Newly hatched gull chicks crouch in the nest the first time they hear the alarm call of the parent.

To the observer, these behaviors have a mechanical, programmed appearance. This is even more evident when animals act out behaviors released in inappropriate situations. For example, a male stickleback fish vigorously attacks a plump lump of wax with a red underside placed in its tank by experimenters. The stickleback reacts to this unfishlike model as if it were another male stickleback with a red belly intruding into its territory. A carefully made model that closely resembles a stickleback but lacks the red belly is ignored·(Fig. 34-4). A male English robin will furiously attack a bundle of red feathers placed in its territory but ignore a stuffed juvenile robin without red feathers (Fig. 34-5). Male redwinged blackbirds attempt to copulate with a crude model consisting of rump and tail feathers of a female, if the tail is elevated in a precopulatory position.

In these and other examples of stereotyped behavior released by single sign stimuli, it is difficult to understand how the animal could have learned the response. These "built-in" or innate behavioral patterns are released in complete form and without practice the first time an animal of certain age and motivational state encounters the stimulus. To such behaviors the term **instinct,** meaning "driven from within," is applied. It is easy to understand why instinctive behavior is an important adaptation for survival, especially to lower forms that never know their parents. They must be equipped to respond immediately and correctly to their world as soon as they hatch. It is also evident that more advanced animals with longer lives and with parental care or other opportunities for social interactions have the opportunity to improve or change their behavior by learning.

Learning is the modification of behavior by experience. As a rule, behavioral modifications through learning are adaptive, since they improve the animal's fitness. The crouching behavior of gull chicks previously mentioned provides an excellent illustration of the adaptive value of learning. If the parent calls an alarm, the newly hatched chick crouches down—obviously a useful defensive response to overflying predators. After 2 or 3 days, the chick responds to the alarm call by running away before crouching. Later, it runs and hides in a chosen site before crouching.

As the chick grows stronger and more mobile, it also becomes more discriminating in its visual response to moving objects overhead. After several such experiences, it begins to lose its general fear of overflying birds. In other words, its sensitivity to this particular stimulus declines. This very simple kind of learning is called **habituation,** the reduction or elimination of a response in the absence of any reward or punishment. For the gull chick, habituation to overflying objects is clearly appropriate, since running and hiding from every passing shadow consume time and energy better applied to more productive activities.

Figure 34-5

Two models of the English robin. The bundle of red feathers is attacked by male robins, whereas the stuffed juvenile bird _(top)_ without a red breast is ignored.
From Tinbergen, N. 1951. The study of instinct. Oxford, Eng., Oxford University Press; after Lack, D. 1943. The life of the robin. Cambridge, Eng., Cambridge University Press.

Figure 34-6

Models used by Lorenz and Tinbergen for the study of predator reactions in young fowl. Young gull chicks crouch in alarm when hawk silhouettes *(red)* pass overhead but ignore shapes of harmless birds.

From Tinbergen, N. 1951. The study of instinct. Oxford, Eng., Oxford University Press.

However, gull chicks do not come to ignore *all* birds flying overhead. Absolute habituation in this instance would be even less appropriate than no habituation at all, since birds of prey are genuine predators of gull chicks. Chicks that fail to hide from an overflying hawk are less likely to survive than chicks that have retained a healthy fear of this predator.

Lorenz and Tinbergen discovered that chicks discriminate predatory birds from harmless songbirds and ducks on the basis of shape, especially the length of the head and neck. When chicks were presented with a silhouette having a hawk-like shape and a short neck such that the head protruded only slightly in front of the wings, they crouched in alarm. Long-necked silhouettes were ignored or aroused only mild interest (Fig. 34-6). In another experiment, a model was built having symmetrical wings, with the head and tail shaped so that either the front or the rear of the dummy could be regarded as the head or as the tail (Fig. 34-7). When sailed in the direction of the long-necked "head," the model resembled a goose and caused no alarm; when sailed in the direction of the short "head," however, it resembled a hawk and did cause alarm. Obviously both the shape of a bird and the direction of its motion are important in recognition.

Sometimes learning is demonstrated in surprising and amusing ways. Tinbergen describes one such incident.*

> In order to sail our models, which crossed a meadow where the birds were feeding or resting, at a height of about 10 yards along a wire, running from one tree to another 50 yards away, either Lorenz or I had to climb a tree and mount the dummy we wanted to test out. One family of geese (which also reacted to some of our dummies) very soon associated tree-climbing humans with something dreadful to come, and promptly called the alarm and walked off when one of us went up.

These observations with models might suggest incorrectly that gull chicks (as well as pheasant and turkey chicks that react similarly) have an innate ability to distinguish short-necked predators from harmless birds having longer necks. But, in fact, subsequent experiments demonstrated that newly hatched chicks, which are at first alarmed by anything that passes overhead—even a falling leaf— gradually become habituated to familiar objects. The chick learns that songbirds and shorebirds are common and harmless features of its world. They never become accustomed to short-necked predators because these are seldom seen. It is the unfamiliar that arouses fear.

The alarm response of herring gull chicks is an example of a simple behavior that becomes altered as the result of experience. As they grow, the chicks store information about their world and become increasingly selective in their alarm response. Animals are internally programmed to respond automatically to certain stimuli; however, this response requires adjustment from the environment to become efficient as the animal grows.

What can we say about the role of genes and that of environment in shaping instinctive and learned behavior? We tread into delicate territory because behaviorists do not all agree on just what constitutes innate behavior. The problem concerns the effects of the environment on the individual during its development. The idea that behavior must be fixed *either* by heredity *or* by environment has had a long history, resulting in what is termed the **nature versus nurture controversy.** It has proved to be a useless debate because *any* characteristic of an individual is determined by an interaction between information supplied in the genetic blueprint (nature) and that supplied by the environment (nurture). Let us examine

---

*Tinbergen, N. 1961. The herring gull's world; a study of the social behavior of birds. New York, Basic Books, Inc., Publishers.

once again our definitions of instinct and learning and then try to explain how gene-environment interactions contribute to each.

We defined an instinctive behavior as one that emerges in complete form the first time the animal reacts to the appropriate stimulus. It must have a genetic foundation because without genes there can be no behavior. Specifically, the animal's genotype contains instructions that result in the construction of specific neural organization, which permits certain types of behavior. We are not saying that an instinctive behavioral attribute is determined solely by information contained in specific chromosomal loci. The genetic code is an information-generating device that depends on an environment that supplies materials and provides order for embryonic development. A genotype remains just a genotype if the developing organism cannot obtain the substances required to form tissues, organs, and a nervous system.

Learning depends on experience encountered by the organism as it interacts with its environment. It also depends on internal programming because the things an organism learns to do best are determined by the genetic blueprint. The nervous system must be designed to facilitate the acquisition of learning at specific stages in the organism's development. In other words, through its genetically determined development, the brain possesses properties enabling it to "anticipate" its eventual use in the modification of behavior. Learned behavior, like instinctive behavior, contains both genetic and environmental components.

One kind of learned behavior that clearly illustrates the interaction of heredity and environment is **imprinting.** As soon as a newly hatched gosling or duckling is strong enough to walk, it follows its mother away from the nest. After it has followed the mother for some time, it follows no other animal (Fig. 34-8). But, if the eggs are hatched in an incubator or if the mother is separated from the eggs as they hatch, the goslings follow the first large, moving object they see. As they grow, the young geese prefer the artifical "mother" to anything else, including their true mother. The goslings are said to be imprinted on the artificial mother.

Imprinting was observed at least as early as the first century AD when the Roman naturalist Pliny the Elder wrote of "a goose which followed Lacydes as

←—''Goose'' profile —

—''Hawk'' profile →

Figure 34-7

Model that drew positive responses from gull chicks when sailed to the right (simulating a hawk) but none when sailed to the left (simulating a goose).

Figure 34-8

Canada goose *Branta canadensis* with her imprinted young.
Photograph by L.L. Rue, III.

KCS

Wild bird

5
4
3
2
1

Hand-reared bird

5
4
3
2
1

Figure 34-9

Sound spectrograms of songs of white-crowned sparrows *Zonotrichia leucophrys. Above,* Natural song of wild bird; *below,* abnormal song of isolated bird.

From Alcock, J. 1979. Animal behavior: an evolutionary approach, ed. 2. Sunderland, Mass., Sinauer Associates, Inc.

faithfully as a dog." Konrad Lorenz was the first to study the imprinting phenomenon objectively and systematically. When Lorenz hand-reared goslings, they formed an immediate and permanent attachment to him and waddled after him wherever he went (Fig. 34-1, *A*). They could no longer be induced to follow their own mother or another human being. Lorenz found that the imprinting period is confined to a brief *sensitive* period in the individual's early life and that once established the imprinted bond is retained for life.

What imprinting shows is that the goose or duck brain (or the brain of numerous other birds and mammals that show imprinting-like behavior) is designed to accommodate the imprinting experience. The animal's genotype is provided with an internal template that permits the animal to recognize its mother soon after hatching. Natural selection favors the evolution of animals having a brain structure that imprints in this way because following the mother and obeying her commands are important for survival. The fact that a gosling can be made to imprint to a mechanical toy duck or a human under artificial conditions is a cost to the system that can be tolerated; the disadvantages of the system's simplicity are outweighed by the advantages of its reliability.

Let us cite one final example to complete our consideration of instinct and learning. The males of many species of birds have characteristic territorial songs that identify the singers to other birds and announce territorial rights to other males of that species. Like many other songbirds, the male white-crowned sparrow must learn the song of its species by hearing the song of its father. If the sparrow is hand reared in acoustic isolation in the laboratory, it develops an abnormal song (Fig. 34-9). But if the isolated bird is allowed to hear recordings of normal white-crowned sparrow songs during a critical period of 10 to 50 days after hatching, it learns to sing normally. It even imitates the local dialect it hears.

It might appear from this that song characteristic is determined by learning alone. However, if during the critical learning period the isolated male white-crowned sparrow is played a recording of another sparrow species, even a closely related one, it does not learn the song. It learns only the song appropriate to its own species. Thus, although the song must be learned, the brain has been programmed in its development to recognize and learn vocalizations produced by males of its species alone. The sparrow *learns* by example, but its attention has been *innately* narrowed to focus on the appropriate example. Learning the wrong song would result in behavioral chaos, and natural selection quickly eliminates those genotypes that permit such mistakes to occur.

SOCIAL BEHAVIOR

When we think of "social" animals we are likely to think of highly structured honeybee colonies, herds of antelope grazing on the African plains (Fig. 34-10), schools of herring, or flocks of starlings. But social behavior is by no means limited to such obvious examples of animals *of the same species* living together in which individuals influence one another.

In the broad sense, any kind of interaction resulting from the response of one animal to another of the same species represents social behavior. Even a pair of rival males squaring off for a fight over the possession of a female is a social interaction, although our perceptual bias as people might encourage us to label it antisocial. Thus social aggregations are only one kind of social behavior, and indeed not all animal aggregations are social.

Clouds of moths attracted to a light at night, larval barnacles attracted to a common float, or trout gathering in the coolest pool of a stream are animal groupings responding to *environmental* signals. Social aggregations, on the other hand, depend on *animal* signals. They remain together and do things together by influencing one another.

Of course, not all animals showing sociality are social to the same degree. All sexually reproducing species must at least cooperate enough to achieve fertilization; but among most mammals, breeding is about the only adult sociality to occur. However, swans, geese, albatrosses, and beavers, to name just a few, form strong monogamous bonds that last a lifetime. Whether adult sociality is strongly or weakly developed, the most persistent social bonds usually form between mothers and their young, and these bonds for birds and mammals usually terminate at fledging or weaning.

Advantages of Sociality

Living together may be beneficial in many ways. Each species profits in its own particular way; what confers adaptive value to one species may not for another. One obvious benefit for social aggregations is defense, both passive and active, from predators. Musk-oxen that form a passive defensive circle when threatened by a wolf pack are much less vulnerable than an individual facing the wolves alone.

As an example of active defense, a breeding colony of gulls, alerted by the alarm calls of a few, attacks predators *en masse;* this is certain to discourage a predator more effectively than individual attacks. The members of a prairie dog town, although divided into social units called coteries, cooperate by warning

Figure 34-10

Wildebeest migration on the Serengeti Plain of Africa.
Photograph by B. Tallmark.

Figure 34-11

Yellow baboons resting and grooming. It is virtually impossible for a predator to approach such a group without being detected.

Courtesy Stuart and Jeanne Altmann.

The inhibiting effect of mass on predation was observed by ethologist P. Klopfer. He describes the behavior of a captive seal into whose tank a school of anchovies was released. "On previous occasions, when small numbers of the fish were released, the seal rapidly caught and devoured them. The larger number of anchovies, which formed a dense school whose outlines approximated the shape of an animal as large as a seal, not only inhibited pursuit but it also apparently frightened the seal out of its pool. Although anecdotal, the account does illustrate the power of masses" (Klopfer, 1974).

On the Galápagos Islands, hunting by humans in the last century had so greatly thinned the giant tortoise population on one island that the few surviving males and females seldom if ever met. Lichens grew on the females' backs because there were no males to scrub them off during mating! Research personnel saved the tortoise from inevitable extinction by collecting them in a pen, where they began to reproduce.

each other with a special bark when danger threatens. Thus, every individual in a social organization benefits from the eyes, ears, and noses of all other members of the group (Fig. 34-11).

Predators may also be distracted by the confusion effect created by large numbers of prey grouped together. A fish that can chase down and capture a lone crustacean may be unable to concentrate on a single individual in a large aggregation. Predators may even be frightened by a large aggregate of prey, which they would eat if encountered singly.

Sociality offers several benefits to animal reproduction. Social grouping helps to synchronize reproductive behavior through the mutual stimulation that individuals have on one another. In colonial birds the sounds and displays of courting individuals set in motion prereproductive endocrine changes in other individuals of the colony. Because there is more social stimulation, large colonies of gulls produce more young per nest than do small colonies. In colonial species a population size less than a certain minimum results in inadequate social stimulation and reproductive failure. This effect has been suggested as the cause of extinction of the passenger pigeon once heavy hunting had greatly thinned the population (p. 629).

Another benefit of social grouping to reproductive performance is that it facilitates encounters between males and females. For solitary animals, finding prospective mates may consume much time and energy. Should the population become depleted because of overhunting, habitat destruction, or severe weather, male-female encounters become increasingly rare.

Still another advantage of sociality to reproduction is care of the young. This is especially well developed in the vertebrates and social insects. Parental care, with direct provisioning of the young and food sharing, increases survival of the brood. Social living also provides opportunities for individuals to give aid to and share food with young other than their own. Such interactions in a social network have resulted in some intricate cooperative behavior among parents, their young, and their kin.

Of the many other advantages of social organization noted by ethologists, we may mention only a few in our brief treatment: cooperation in hunting for food; huddling for mutual protection from severe weather; opportunities for division of labor, which is especially well developed in the social insects with their caste systems; and the potential for learning and transmitting useful information through the society.

Observers of a seminatural colony of macaques (*Macaca fuscata*) in Japan recount an interesting example of passage of tradition in a society. The macaques were provisioned with sweet potatoes and wheat at a feeding station on the beach of an island colony. One day a young female named Imo was observed washing the sand off a sweet potato in seawater. Still later, when the young members of the troop became mothers, they waded into the sea to wash their potatoes; their offspring imitated them without hesitation. The tradition was firmly established in the troop.

Some years later Imo, an adult, discovered that she could separate wheat from sand by tossing a handful of sandy wheat in the water; allowing the sand to sink, she would scoop up the floating wheat to eat. Again, within a few years, wheat sifting became a tradition in the troop.

Imo's peers and social inferiors copied her innovations most readily. The adult males, her superiors in the social hierarchy, would not adopt the practice but continued laboriously to pick wet sand grains off their sweet potatoes and scour the beach for single grains of wheat.

If social living offers so many benefits, why have not all animals become social through natural selection? The answer is that a solitary existence offers its own set of advantages. In the diverse array of ecological situations in nature, species extract their own optimal ways of life. Species that survive by camouflage from potential predators profit by being well spaced out. Large predators benefit from a solitary existence for a different reason, their requirement for a large supply of prey. Thus, there is no overriding adaptive advantage to sociality that inevitably selects against the solitary way of life. It depends on the ecological situation.

Aggression and Dominance

Many animals species are social because of the numerous benefits that sociality offers. This requires cooperation. At the same time animals, like governments, tend to look out for their own interests. In short, they are in competition with one another because of limitations in the common resources that all require for life. Animals may compete for food, water, sexual mates, or shelter, when such requirements are limited in quantity and are therefore worth fighting over.

Much of what animals do to resolve competition is called **aggression,** which we may define as an offensive physical action, or threat, to force others to abandon something they own or might attain. Many ethologists consider aggression to be part of a somewhat more inclusive interaction called **agonistic** (Gr., contest) **behavior,** referring to any activity related to fighting, whether it be aggression, defense, submission, or retreat.

Contrary to the widely held notion that aggressive behavior aims at the destruction or at least defeat of an opponent, most aggressive encounters involve more saber rattling than real combat. Many species possess dangerous weapons such as teeth, beaks, claws, or horns, which could easily inflict serious injury or even kill an opponent; but such well-armed animals seldom use their weapons

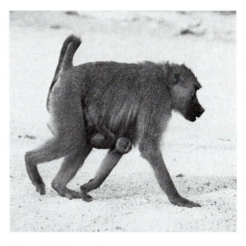

Figure 34-12

Adult male baboon gives an infant a ride on his ventrum. Most mother-infant pairs have a male associate, not always the infant's father, that provides a measure of protection from other group members. Older infants seek such protection by their "godfather."
Courtesy Stuart and Jeanne Altmann.

against members *of their own species*. However, no such inhibiting mechanism prevents their use in killing prey or in defense against attack from another species. A coyote that uses its teeth effectively in killing a prairie dog would never bite a rival coyote in an aggressive encounter over a mate or territory. A giraffe uses its short horns to fight rivals but uses its far more lethal hoofs in defense against predators (Fig. 34-13). Therefore, when biologists speak of aggression, they are usually (although not always) referring to encounters between conspecifics.

Animal aggression within the species seldom results in injury or death because animals have evolved many symbolical aggressive displays that carry mutually understood meanings. Fights over mates, food, or territory become ritualized jousts rather than bloody, no-holds-barred battles. When fiddler crabs spar for territory, their large claws usually are only slightly opened. Even in the most intense fighting when the claws are used, the crabs grasp each other in a way that prevents reciprocal injury. Rival male poisonous snakes engage in stylized bouts by winding themselves together; each attempts to butt the other's head with its own until one becomes so fatigued that it retreats. The rivals never bite each other. Many species of fish contest territorial boundaries with lateral display threats, the males puffing themselves up to look as threatening as possible. The encounter is usually settled when either animal perceives itself to be inferior, folds up its fins, and swims off.

Thus, animals fight as though programmed by rules that prevent serious injury. Fights between rival bighorn rams are spectacular to watch, and the sound of clashing horns may be heard for hundreds of yards (Fig. 34-14). But the skull is so well protected by the massive horns that injury occurs only by accident and death is almost unheard of.

The loser in such encounters may simply run away, or he may signal defeat by a specialized subordination ritual. If it becomes evident to him that he is going to lose anyway, he is better off communicating his submission as quickly as possible and avoiding the cost of a real thrashing. Such submissive displays that signal the end of a fight may be almost the opposite of threat displays (Fig. 34-15). Charles Darwin, whose book *Expression of the Emotions in Man and Animals* (1873) founded the science of ethology, described the seemingly opposite nature of threat and appeasement displays as the "principle of antithesis." The principle remains accepted by ethologists today.

Why does the victor of an aggressive contest not kill its opponent? A defeated wolf or dog presents its vulnerable neck to the victor as a sign of complete submission. Although the dominant wolf could easily kill the defeated foe and thus remove a competitor, it never does so. The display of submission has effectively inhibited further aggression by the winner. The best explanation for aggressive restraint is that the winner has little to gain by continuing the fight. His superiority is already ensured. By continuing the aggression he merely endangers himself, since a defeated opponent fighting for his life might inflict a wound. It is not difficult to see how natural selection would favor genes that induce aggressive restraint. Aggression that is inappropriate runs counter to the maximization of individual fitness. It is maladaptive and consequently is selected against.

The winner of an aggressive competition is dominant to the loser, the subordinant. For the victor, dominance means enhanced access to all the contested resources that contribute to reproductive success: food, mates, territory, and so on. In a social species, dominance interactions often take the form of a dominance hierarchy. One animal at the top wins encounters with all other members in the social group; the second in rank wins all but those with the top-ranking individual.

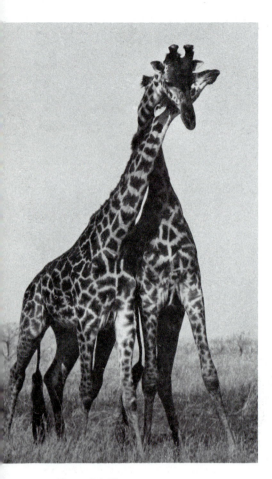

Figure 34-13

Male Masai giraffes *Giraffa camelopardalis* fight for social dominance. Such fights are largely symbolic, seldom resulting in injury.

Photograph by L.L. Rue, III.

Figure 34-14

Male bighorn sheep *Ovis canadensis* fight for social dominance during the breeding season.

Photograph by L.L. Rue, III.

Figure 34-15

Darwin's principle of antithesis as exemplified by the postures of dogs. **A,** A dog approaches another dog with hostile, aggressive intentions. **B,** The same dog is humble and conciliatory. The signals of aggressive display have been reversed.

From Darwin, C. 1873. Expression of the emotions in man and animals. New York, D. Appleton & Co.

Figure 34-16

Two yellow baboons fighting. Fights over social status and females frequently result in injuries, but seldom is either combatant killed in the encounter.

Courtesy Stuart and Jeanne Altmann.

Such a simple, linear hierarchy was first observed in chicken societies by Schjelderup-Ebbe, who called the hierarchy a "peck-order." Once social ranking is established, actual pecking diminishes and is replaced by threats, bluffs, and bows. Top hens and cocks get unquestioned access to feed and water, dusting areas, and the roost. The system works because it reduces the social tensions that would constantly surface if animals had to fight all the time over social position.

Still, life for the subordinates in any social order is likely to be hard. They are the expendables of the social group. They almost never get a chance to reproduce, and when times get difficult, they are the first to die. During times of food scarcity, the death of the weaker members helps to protect the resource for the stronger members. Rather than sharing food, the population excess is sacrificed. For the species, it is better for the weaker members to starve before the resources dwindle to crisis levels, rather than share the resource, thus denuding the countryside and risking ultimate starvation of the entire population.

___ Territoriality

Territorial ownership is another facet of sociality in animal populations. Just as an animal requires food for growth and maintenance and a mate with which to reproduce, it must also have space in which to carry out these activities. Since space, which an animal requires to satisfy its biological needs, is limited, it must somehow be divided among those who require it.

Territorial defense has been observed in numerous animals: insects, crustaceans, other invertebrates, fish, amphibians, lizards, birds, and mammals (including humans). A **territory** is an ecological area defended against intruders, usually of the same species. This involves announcing ownership, defending the area from intruders, and spending long periods of time on the site being conspicuous. Like every other competitive endeavor, there are both costs and advantages.

Holding exclusive rights to a piece of property is beneficial when it ensures access to limited resources, *unless* the territory boundaries cannot be maintained with a minimum of effort. The presumed benefits of a territory are, in fact, numerous: uncontested access to a foraging area; enhanced attractiveness to females, thus reducing the problems of pair bonding, mating, and rearing the young; reduced disease transmission; reduced vulnerability to predators. But the advantages of holding a territory begin to wane if the individual must spend most of the time in boundary disputes with neighbors.

For territoriality to work, the resources must be defensible, and, in fact, they usually are because natural selection relentlessly disposes of individuals with hopelessly unrealistic territorial appetites. Thus, in general, a territory must be large enough to provide the resources needed, but not so large that it cannot be economically defended.

Territory size tends to be flexible. When populations are low, territories are large. When resources, especially food, are abundant, territories tend to shrink, because no benefit is derived from defending large ones. On the other hand, in times of population crowding, defended territories may be abandoned altogether because the sheer numbers of individuals make boundary defense impossible.

Sometimes the space defended moves with the individual. This **individual distance**, as it is termed, is characteristic of the species. It can be observed as the spacing between swallows or pigeons on a wire, in gulls lined up on the beach, or in people queued up for a bus.

The need for individual distance or "personal space"—a sort of force field that surrounds the animal's head and moves with it—is as important for poultry and livestock as it is for wild animals. Overcrowded chickens lay fewer eggs, eat less, and suffer higher mortality than uncrowded chickens. The presence of too many steers or pigs in a pen produces stress and lowers production. Hauling cattle together in large trucks completely disrupts established social hierarchies because of constant invasion of each animal's personal space. Fighting erupts, resulting in injuries that can lead to considerable economic loss. These and many other lessons of animal behavior are now being applied to the farm industry, leading, we can hope, to more profit for the farmer and lower prices at the meat counter.

Most of the time and energy required for territoriality is expended when the territory is first established. Once the boundaries are located, they tend to be respected, and aggressive behavior diminishes as territorial neighbors come to recognize each other. Indeed, neighbors may look so peaceful that an observer who was not present when the territories were established may conclude (incorrectly) that the animals are not territorial. A "beachmaster" sea lion (that is, a dominant male with a harem) seldom quarrels with his neighbors who have their own territories to defend. However, he must be on constant vigilance against bachelor bulls who challenge the beachmaster for harem privileges.

Of all vertebrate classes, birds are the most conspicuously territorial. Most male songbirds establish territories in the early spring and defend these vigorously against all males of the same species during spring and summer when mating and nesting are at their height. A male song sparrow, for example, has a territory of approximately three fourths of an acre. In any given area, the number of song sparrows remains approximately the same year after year. The population remains stable because the young occupy territories of adults that die or are killed. Any surplus in the song sparrow population is excluded from territories and thus not able to mate or nest.

Sea birds such as gulls, gannets, boobies, and albatrosses occupy colonies that are divided into very small territories just large enough for nesting (Fig. 34-17). These birds' territories cannot include their fishing grounds, since they all forage in the sea where the food is always shifting in location and shared by all.

Territorial behavior is not as characteristic of mammals as it is of birds. Mammals are less mobile than birds, and this makes it more difficult for them to patrol a territory for trespassers. Instead, many mammals have **home ranges**. A home range is the total area an individual traverses in its activities. It is not an exclusive defended preserve but overlaps with the home ranges of other individuals of the same species.

For example, the home ranges of baboon troops overlap extensively, although a small part of each range becomes the recognized territory of each troop for its exclusive use. Home ranges may shift considerably with the seasons. A baboon troop may have to shift to a new range during the dry season to obtain water and better forage. Elephants, before their movements were restricted by humans, made long seasonal migrations across the African savanna to new feeding ranges. However, the home ranges established for each season were remarkably consistent in size.

Not surprisingly, the size of the home range increases with the body size of mammals, since larger animals require more foraging area to satisfy their energy requirements. Accordingly, the home range may be 1000 square meters for a field mouse, 40 hectares (about 100 acres) for a deer, 150 square kilometers for a grizzly bear, and 4000 square kilometers (about 1500 square miles) for an African hunting dog. In general, carnivores require more foraging space than herbivores, because any given area supports more plant food than animal food.

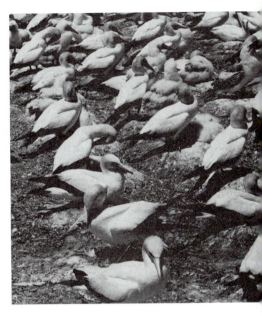

Figure 34-17

Gannet nesting colony. Note precise spacing of nests, with each occupant just beyond the pecking distance of its neighbors.

Photograph by C.P. Hickman, Jr.

_____ Communication

Social animals, like people, must be able to communicate with each other. Communication is the way in which one animal influences the behavior of another. Compared to the enormous communicative potential of human speech, nonhuman communication is severely restricted. Whereas human communication is

Figure 34-18

Waggle dance of the honeybee, used to communicate both the direction and the distance of a food source. The straight run of the waggle dance indicates direction according to the position of the sun.

based mainly, although by no means exclusively, on sounds, animals may communicate by sounds, scents, touch, and movement. Indeed any sensory channel may be used, and in this sense animal communication has richness and variety.

However, unlike our language, which is composed of words with definite meanings that may be rearranged to generate an almost infinite array of new meanings and images, communication of other animals consists of a limited repertoire of signals. Typically, each signal conveys one and only one message. These messages cannot be divided or rearranged to construct *new kinds* of information. A single message from the sender may, however, contain several bits of relevant information for the receiver.

The song of a cricket announces to an unfertilized female the species of the sender (males of different species have different songs), his sex (only males sing), his location (source of the song), and his social status (only a male able to defend the area around his burrow sings from one location). This is all crucial information to the female and accomplishes a biological goal. But there is no way for the male to alter his song to provide additional information concerning food, predators, or habitat, which might improve his mate's chances of survival and thus enhance his own fitness.

The limitations of communication are especially evident in the invertebrates and lower vertebrates. Signals are characteristically stereotyped, and the responses are highly predictable and constant throughout the species. This does not mean that such communication is always lacking in intensity and versatility, however. Of the two contrasting examples that follow, mate attraction in silkworm moths illustrates an extreme case of stereotyped, single-message communication that has evolved to serve a single biological goal: mating. Yet, in the same group, the insects, we find one of the most sophisticated and complex of all nonhuman communication systems, the symbolic language of bees.

Chemical sex attraction in moths

Virgin female silkworm moths have special glands that produce a chemical sex attractant to which the males are sensitive. Adult males smell with their large bushy antennae, covered with thousands of sensory hairs that function as receptors. Most of these receptors are sensitive to the chemical attractant (a complex alcohol called bombykol, from the name of the silkworm *Bombyx mori*) and to nothing else.

To attract the male, the female merely sits quietly and emits a minute amount of bombykol, which is carried downwind. When a few molecules reach the male's antennae, he is stimulated to fly upwind in search of the female. His search is at first random, but, when by chance he approaches within a few hundred yards of the female, he encounters a concentration gradient of the attractant. Guided by the gradient, he flies toward the female, finds her, and copulates with her.

In this example of chemical communication, the attractant bombykol, which is really a pheromone, serves as a signal to bring the sexes together. Its effectiveness is ensured because natural selection favors the evolution of males with antennal receptors sensitive enough to detect the attractant at great distances (several miles). Males with a genotype that produces a less sensitive sensory system fail to locate a female and thus are reproductively eliminated from the population.

Language of bees

Honeybees are able to communicate the location of food resources when these sources are too distant to be located easily by individual bees. Communication is done by dances, which are mainly of two forms. The form having the most communicative richness is the **waggle dance** (Fig. 34-18). Bees most commonly execute these dances when a forager has returned from a rich source, carrying either nectar in her stomach or pollen grains packed in basketlike spaces formed by hairs on her legs (p. 410). The waggle dance is roughly in the pattern of a figure-eight made against the vertical surface of the comb. One cycle of the dance consists of three components: (1) a circle with a diameter about three times the length of the bee, (2) a straight run while waggling the abdomen from side to side 13 to 15 times per second, and (3) another circle, turning in the opposite direction from the first. This dance is repeated many times with the circling alternating clockwise and counterclockwise.

The straight, waggle run is the important information component of the dance. Waggle dances are performed almost always in clear weather, and the direction of the straight run is related to the position of the sun. If the forager has located food directly toward the sun, she will make her waggle run straight upward over the vertical surface of the comb. If food was located 60 degrees to the right of the sun, her waggle run is 60 degrees to the right of vertical. We see then

The significance of the bee dances was discovered in the 1920s by the German zoologist Karl von Frisch, one of the recipients of the 1973 Nobel Prize. Despite detailed and extensive experiments by von Frisch that supported his original interpretations of the bee dances, the experiments have been criticized, especially by the American biologist A. Wenner, who suggested that the correlation between dance symbolism and food location is accidental. He argued that foraging bees bring back odors characteristic of the food source, and that recruits are stimulated by the dances to search for flowers bearing those odors. Few biologists were prepared to accept this interpretation, but Wenner's beneficial skepticism stimulated more rigorously controlled experiments (Gould, 1976), which established more conclusively than ever before that the bee dances communicate both distance and direction information and that the bees use this information in searching for food. The dances of bees are among the true wonders of the natural world.

that the waggle run points at the same angle relative to the vertical as the food is located relative to the sun.

Distance information about the food source is also coded into bee dances. If the food is close to the hive (less than 50 m), the forager employs a simpler dance called the **round dance**. The forager simply turns a complete clockwise circle, then turns, and completes a counterclockwise circle, a performance that is repeated many times. Other workers cluster around the scout and become stimulated by the dance as well as by the odor of nectar and pollen grains from flowers she has visited. The recruits then fly out and search in all directions but do not stray far. The round dance carries the message that food is to be found in the vicinity of the hive.

If the food source is farther away, the round dances become waggle dances, which provide both distance and direction information. The tempo of the waggle dance is inversely related to the food distance. If the food is about 100 m away, each figure-eight cycle lasts about 1.25 seconds; if 1000 m away, it lasts about 3 seconds; and if about 8 km away (5 miles), it lasts 8 seconds. When food is plentiful, the bees may not dance at all. But when food is scarce, the dancing becomes intense, and the other workers cluster about the returning scouts and follow them through the dance patterns.

Communication by displays

A display is a kind of behavior or series of behaviors that serves a communicative purpose. The release of sex attractant by the female moth and the dances of bees just described are examples of displays; so are the alarm calls of herring gulls, song of the white-crowned sparrow, courtship dance of the sage grouse, and "eyespots" of the hindwings of certain moths, which are quickly exposed to startle potential predators. Of course, just about anything an animal does communicates *something* to other animals that see, hear, or smell it. A true display, on the other hand, is a behavior pattern that has been modified through evolution to make it increasingly effective in serving a communicative function. This process is called **ritualization.** Through ritualization, simple movements or traits become more intensive, conspicuous, or precise, and their original undifferentiated function acquires signal value. The result of such intensification is to reduce the possibility of misunderstanding.

The elaborate pair-bonding behavior of the blue-footed boobies (Fig. 34-19) exemplifies this point. These displays are performed with maximum intensity when the birds come together after a period of separation. The male at right in the illustration is sky pointing: the head and tail are pointed skyward and the wings are swiveled forward in a seemingly impossible position to display their glossy upper surfaces to the female. This is accompanied by a high, piping whistle. The female at left, for her part, is parading. She goose steps with exaggerated slow deliberation, lifting each brilliant blue foot in turn, as if holding it aloft momentarily for the male to admire. Such highly personalized displays, performed with droll solemnity, appear comical, even inane to the observer. Indeed the boobies, whose name is derived from the Spanish word "bobo" meaning clown, presumably were so designated for their amusing antics.

Needless to say, for the birds, amusement plays no part in the ceremonies. The exaggerated nature of the displays ensures that the message is not missed or misunderstood. Such displays are essential to establish and maintain a strong pair bond between male and female. This requirement also explains the repetitious

Figure 34-19

Pair of Galápagos blue-footed boobies *Sula nebouxii* displays to each other. The male *(right)* is sky pointing; the female *(left)* is parading. Such vivid, stereotyped, communicative displays serve to maintain reciprocal stimulation and cooperative behavior during courtship, mating, nesting, and care of the young.

nature of the displays that follow one another throughout courtship and until egg laying. Redundancy of displays maintains a state of mutual stimulation between male and female, ensuring the degree of cooperation necessary for copulation and subsequent incubation and care of the young. A sexually aroused male has little success with an uninterested female.

DO ANIMALS HAVE MENTAL EXPERIENCES?

Most people, although aware of the enormous capabilities of the human brain that separate us from other animal species, take for granted that animals have feelings and awareness analogous to our own. As we watch animals interacting in behavior that resembles human behavior, we may conclude more or less intuitively that animals have humanlike mental experiences. However, most behavioral scientists have deep-seated objections to even considering such a possibility, believing that because mental experiences in animals cannot be observed, measured, or verified, it is consequently meaningless to suggest that they may exist. Strict behaviorists, who argue that even human mental experiences are unique qualities that cannot be objectively defined, rebel against the notion of animal awareness as anthropomorphic, that is, ascribing human characteristics to other species. Yet, as D.R. Griffin argues in his perceptive book *The Question of Animal Awareness,* "it is actually no more anthropomorphic . . . to postulate mental experiences in another species than to compare its bony structure, nervous system, or antibodies with our own." Griffin points to a curious duality in behavioral studies: rats, pigeons, and monkeys are used as models in behavioral investigations on the implicit assumption that principles revealed from such studies are applicable to human behavior, yet when the question of mental experiences arises, behaviorists reject evolutionary continuity between humans and other animals.

The reluctance of many behaviorists to acknowledge the existence of even simple mental experiences among animals stems in large part from the enormous difference in versatility and complexity that separates human language from any other known animal communication system. One criterion that we mentioned earlier as supposedly unique for human language is that words with discrete meanings and syllables, many of which are meaningless in themselves, can be arranged into almost endless combinations to generate a vast array of new meanings.

Until recently, it was accepted that this characteristic was absent from all nonhuman communication. However, in the early 1970s a female chimpanzee named Washoe was taught to employ *and combine* gestures, using words from the American Sign Language for the deaf, much as people use spoken words. The discovery that manual gestures and expressive motions were much more appropriate than vocalizations in communicating with apes was considered a major breakthrough in behavioral research. Since Washoe, sign-language studies have been extended to other chimpanzees and to gorillas; several have acquired "vocabularies" of several hundred reliable signs, some invented by the apes themselves.

Clearly, one problem in assessing the versatility of animal communication is understanding what sensory channel an animal is using. The signals may be visual displays, odors, vocalizations, tactile vibrations, or electrical currents (as, for example, among certain fishes). Even more difficult is establishing two-way communication between animals and humans, since the investigator must translate meanings into symbols the animal can understand. Furthermore, people are poor social partners for most animals. Nevertheless, when the appropriate communication channel is used, limited communication is possible.

The animal behaviorist Irven De Vore has reported how choosing the proper channel for dialogue can have more than academic interest*:

> One day on the savanna I was away from my truck watching a baboon troop when a young juvenile came and picked up my binoculars. I knew if the glasses disappeared into the troop they'd be lost, so I grabbed them back. The juvenile screamed. Immediately every adult male in the troop rushed at me—I realized what a cornered leopard must feel like. The truck was 30 or 40 feet away. I had to face the males. I started smacking my lips very loudly, a gesture that says as strongly as a baboon can, "I mean you no harm." The males came charging up, growling, snarling, showing their teeth. Right in front of me they halted, cocked their heads to one side—and started lip-smacking back to me. They lip-smacked. I lip-smacked, "I mean you no harm." "I mean *you* no harm." It was, in retrospect, a marvelous conversation. But while my lips talked baboon, my feet edged me toward the truck until I could leap inside and close the door.

We alluded earlier in this chapter to the stereotyped, mechanical nature of instinctive behavior. Yet in watching the interactions between mates during courtship, nest building, and care of the young, it is difficult for the observer to avoid anthropomorphic interpretations of behavior that resembles human behavior. It is natural and easy to describe animal behavior in terms of human behavior by using words such as "love," "deceit," "happiness," and "gentleness." This is not necessarily false, especially for the higher primates, but the ethologist must always take care to interpret every animal response by the simplest mechanism that is known to work.

Animals are capable of highly organized behavior in the absence of any

Whether apes are able to combine signals (that is, "words") to produce sentences—an ability that is crucial to true language—cannot be answered conclusively yet. Furthermore, although apes use signals for requests, commands, and pleas, they do not appear able to make statements aimed at changing the behavior or beliefs of the other party. Critics of the first ape-language studies charged that most of the signed utterances of apes were prompted by the teacher. They argued that the investigators had fallen victim to the "Clever Hans" error, after a horse prodigy of the turn of the century that appeared to do sums in his head and tap out answers with his hoof, but was in fact responding to subtle and inadvertent cues from the trainer. More recent studies appear to have dealt satisfactorily with this criticism by isolating the ape from the teacher during the training sessions.

*DeVore, I. 1972. In The marvels of human behavior. Washington, D.C., National Geographic Society.

Figure 34-20

Male baboon shows his white eyelids as an aggressive display. Although subtle, this display communicates a well-understood meaning to other baboons.
Photograph by B. Tallmark.

intelligent appreciation of its purpose. Sometimes instinctive behavior misfires, and such incidents often emphasize its stereotyped nature. The following excerpt contains a perfect example of the automatic release of inappropriate behavior in a gannet colony*:

> A male of an old pair flew into his nest. Normally he would bite his mate on the head with some violence and then go through a long and complicated meeting ceremony, an ecstatic display confined to members of a pair. Unfortunately, the female had caught her lower mandible in a loop of fish netting that was firmly anchored in the structure of the nest. Every time she tried to raise her head to perform the meeting ceremony with her mate she merely succeeded in opening her upper mandible whilst the lower remained fixed in the netting. So she apparently threatened the male with widely gaping beak and he immediately responded by attacking her. With each attack she lowered and turned away her bill (the way in which a female gannet appeases an aggressive male). At once the male stopped biting her and she again turned to greet him but simply repeated the beak-opening and drew another attack. And so it went on despite the fact that these two birds had been mated for years and that the netting, the cause of all the trouble, was clearly visible.

Despite such limitations to the adaptiveness of instinctive behavior, it obviously functions beautifully most of the time. In recognizing that reasoning and insight are not required for effective, highly organized behavior, we should not conclude that lower animals are little more than unintelligent machines acting out their lives like so many robots. Although the gannet in this example lacked the "intelligence" to free his mate by purposefully disentangling her beak from the netting, he was capable of appropriately analyzing the thousands of strategic choices he must make during his lifetime: how to find and hold a mate, where to build a nest and how to defend it, how to locate and catch evasive marine food, and what to do when the environment changes. All this and more requires endless behavioral adjustments to new situations. Conceivably this might be accomplished by a machine, but only by one of staggering complexity.

*Nelson, B. 1968. Galápagos: islands of birds. London, Longmans, Green & Co., Ltd.

Male ruffed grouse drumming to attract females.

Photograph by N. Bolen.

___ Summary

Ethology is the study of the behavior, both innate and learned, of animals in their natural habitat. Ethologists have shown that behavioral traits are genetically determined and thus are adaptive and evolve by natural selection.

Much innate (instinctive and inherited) behavior of animals is stereotyped; that is, it is highly predictable and invariable in performance. Ethologists have observed and catalogued many stereotyped motor acts, called fixed action patterns, which are triggered, or "released," by specific, and usually simple, environmental stimuli, called sign stimuli. Many kinds of stereotyped behavior are completed in three stages: appetitive behavior, the internal motivation or "drive" that causes an animal to search for a biological goal; consummatory behavior, an act that fulfills the goal; and quiescence, the period following the consummatory act when appetitive behavior is reduced or halted.

Innate behavior may be modified by learning through experience. A simple kind of learning behavior is habituation, which is the reduction or elimination of a behavioral response in the absence of any reward or punishment. The modification of the alarm response of herring gull chicks is an example of habituation. Another form of learning is imprinting, the lasting recognition bond that forms early in life between the young of many social animals and their mothers.

Social behavior is the behavior of a species when the members interact with one another. In social organizations, animals tend to remain together, communicate with each other, and usually resist intrusions by "outsiders." The advantages of sociality include cooperative defense from predators, improved reproductive performance and parental care of the young, cooperative searching for food, and transmission of useful information through the society. Because social animals compete with one another for common resources (such as food, sexual mates, and shelter), conflicts are often resolved by a form of overt hostility called aggression. Most aggressive encounters between conspecifics are stylized bouts involving more bluff than intent to injure or kill. Dominance hierarchies, in which a priority of access to common resources is established by aggression, are common in social organizations. Territoriality is related to dominance. A territory is a defended area from which intruders of the same species are excluded.

Communication, often considered the essence of social organization, is the means by which animals influence the behavior of other animals, using sounds, scents, visual displays, touch, or other sensory signals. As compared to the richness of human language, animals communicate with a very limited repertoire of signals. One of the most famous examples of animal communication is that of the symbolic dances of honeybees. Birds communicate by calls and songs and, especially, by visual displays. By ritualization, simple movements have evolved into conspicuous signals having definite meanings.

Selected references

Alcock, J. 1979. Animal behavior: an evolutionary approach, ed. 2. Sunderland, Mass., Sinauer Associates, Inc. *Well-written and well-illustrated discussion of the genetics, physiology, ecology, and history of behavior in an evolutionary perspective.*

Altmann, J. 1980. Baboon mothers and infants. Cambridge, Mass., Harvard University Press. *Detailed, long-term study, dealing with the costs of reproduction to females.*

Barnett, S.A. 1981. Modern ethology: the science of animal behaviour. Oxford, Eng., Oxford University Press.

Bramblett, C.A. 1976. Patterns of primate behavior. Palo Alto, Calif., Mayfield Publishing Co. *Behavior of primates with useful field descriptions of 15 best-known primates.*

Brown, J.L. 1975. The evolution of behavior. New York, W.W. Norton & Co., Inc. *Advanced text emphasizing social behavior.*

Clutton-Brock, T.H., F.E. Guinness, and S.D. Alton. 1982. Red deer: behavior and ecology of two sexes. Chicago, University of Chicago Press. *Deals with sexual selection and mating systems.*

Darwin, C. 1872. The expression of the emotions in man and animals. (Reprint 1965, University of Chicago Press.) *Early study of behavior, including observations of his own children.*

Dewsbury, D.A. 1978. Comparative animal behavior. New York, McGraw-Hill Book Co. *Ethology from the perspective of a comparative psychologist. Good coverage of principles.*

Eibl-Eibesfeldt, I. 1975. Ethology, the biology of behavior, ed. 2. New York, Holt, Rinehart & Winston, Inc. *Excellent general ethology text in the European tradition.*

Frings, H., and M. Frings. 1977. Animal communication, ed. 2. Norman, University of Oklahoma Press. *Comparative intermediate-level treatment.*

Gould, J.L. 1976. The dance-language controversy. Q. Rev. Biol. **51**:211-244.

Gould, J.L. 1982. Ethology: the mechanisms and evolution of behavior. New York, W.W. Norton & Company, Inc. *Introduction to ethology, written in lucid style.*

Griffin, D.R. 1981. The question of animal awareness, ed. 2. New York, The Rockefeller University Press. *An important and provocative book about a controversial question.*

Hahn, E. 1978. Look who's talking. New York, Thomas Y. Crowell Co., Inc. *A delightful account of the efforts people have made and are making to communicate with animals.*

Hinde, R.A. 1982. Ethology: its nature and relations with other sciences. Oxford, Eng., Oxford University Press. *Intermediate-level ethology text with good historical background.*

Klopfer, P.H. 1974. An introduction to animal behavior: ethology's first century, ed. 2. Englewood Cliffs, N.J., Prentice-Hall, Inc. *Historical approach.*

Krebs, J.R., and N.B. Davies. 1981. An introduction to behavioural ecology. Sunderland, Mass., Sinauer Associates. *This excellent textbook deals with the way in which ecological constraints affect an animal's behavior and reproductive success.*

Lehner, P.N. 1978. Handbook of ethological methods. New York, Garland Publishing, Inc. *Compilation of methods used in behavioral studies, a how-to-do-it book.*

Lorenz, K.Z. 1952. King Solomon's ring. New York, Thomas Y. Crowell Co., Inc. *One of the most delightful books ever written about the behavior of animals.*

McFarland, D. (ed.). 1981. The Oxford companion to animal behaviour. Oxford, Eng., Oxford University Press. *An alphabetical series of 227 articles on animal behavior. Although poorly indexed, it contains a wealth of valuable information.*

National Geographic Society. 1972. The marvels of animal behavior. Washington, D.C., National Geographic Society. *Superbly illustrated collection of essays by leading animal behaviorists. For the general reader.*

Nelson, B. 1968. Galápagos: islands of birds. London, Longmans, Green & Co., Ltd.

Savage-Rumbaugh, E.S., D.M. Rumbaugh, and S. Boysen. 1980. Do apes use language? Am. Sci. **68**:49-61. *A critical look at the ape-language controversy.*

Schaller, G.B. 1963. The mountain gorilla: ecology and behavior. Chicago, University of Chicago Press. *Exemplary, standard-setting field study. A personal and popularized version by the author, The Year of the Gorilla (1964), will be more appealing to the general reader.*

Sebeok, T.A. (ed.). 1977. How animals communicate. Bloomington, Indiana University Press. *Important collection of essays dealing with the evolution and mechanics of communication in animals.*

Smith, W.J. 1977. The behavior of communicating: an ethological approach. Cambridge, Mass., Harvard University Press. *A discussion of the meaning of the message an animal sends, in relation to message context.*

Thorpe, W.H. 1974. Animal nature and human nature. Garden City, N.Y., Anchor Press. *Comparison of animal and human behavior; especially useful sections on animal communication.*

Tinbergen, N. 1951. The study of instinct. New York, Oxford University Press, Inc. *Classic introduction to ethology.*

Tinbergen, N. 1961. The herring gull's world; a study of the social behavior of birds. New York, Basic Books, Inc., Publishers. *One of the most thorough studies of instinctive behavior ever made. Beautifully written.*

Tinbergen, N. 1965. Animal behavior. New York, Time-Life Books, Inc. *Popularized but still highly informative account. Fine illustrations.*

Tinbergen, N. 1966. Social behavior in animals with special reference to vertebrates, ed. 2. New York, Halsted Press.

von Frisch, K. 1971. Bees: their vision, chemical senses, and language, rev. ed. Ithaca, N.Y., Cornell University Press.

Wallace, R.A. 1979. Animal behavior: its development, ecology, and evolution. Santa Monica, Calif., Goodyear Publishing Co., Inc. *Introductory text.*

Wilson, E.O. 1975. Sociobiology: the new synthesis. Cambridge, Mass., Harvard University Press. *An important although controversial synthesis of facts and theories concerning the biological basis of social behavior.*

Wittenberger, J.F. 1981. Animal social behavior. Boston, Duxbury Press. *Evolutionary approach with emphasis on sociobiology.*

Selected *Scientific American* articles

Many important articles not listed separately are included in the *Scientific American* anthology edited by Eisner and Wilson.

Bekoff, M., and M.C. Wells. 1980. The social ecology of coyotes. **242:**130-148 (Apr.). *How patterns of behavior are determined by food supply.*

Bertram, B.C.R. 1975. The social system of lions. **232:**54-65 (May). *The social behavior of lions in their natural habitat.*

Burgess, J.W. 1976. Social spiders. **234:**100-106 (Mar.). *Contrary to the usual pattern of solitary behavior among spiders, some species are gregarious and build large communal webs.*

Crews, D. 1979. The hormonal control of behavior in a lizard. **241:**180-187 (Aug.). *How hormones interact with the nervous system to orchestrate sexual behavior.*

Eaton, G.G. 1976. The social order of Japanese macaques. **235:**96-106 (Oct.). *Long-term observations of a troop of macaques.*

Eisner, T., and E.O. Wilson (eds.). 1955-1975. Animal behavior. San Francisco, W.H. Freeman & Co. Publishers. *Collection of* Scientific American *articles with introductions by Eisner and Wilson.*

Esch, H. 1967. The evolution of bee language. **216:**96-104 (Apr.).

Hess, E.H. 1972. "Imprinting" in a natural laboratory. **227:**24-31 (Aug.). *Even before the egg hatches, a duckling and its parent interact in ways that will strengthen the juvenile-to-parent bond.*

Hölldobler, B. 1971. Communication between ants and their guests. **224:**86-93 (Mar.). *Some parasites learn the language of their ant hosts to gain free food and shelter.*

Ligon, J.D., and S.H. Ligon. 1982. The cooperative breeding behavior of the green woodhoopoe. **247:**126-134 (July). *Altruistic behavior in an East African bird.*

Pooley, A.C., and C. Gans. 1976. The Nile crocodile. **234:**114-124 (Apr.). *The remarkable social behavior of this large reptile includes parental protection of the young.*

Todd, J.H. 1971. The chemical language of fishes. **224:**98-108 (May). *Catfishes produce pheromones to label losers and winners of hierarchical fights.*

Topoff, H.R. 1972. The social behavior of army ants. **227:**70-79 (Nov.). *A complex social organization is described.*

Watts, C.R., and A.W. Stokes. 1971. The social order of turkeys. **224:**112-118 (June). *Describes a rigidly stratified society.*

Wilson, E.O. 1972. Animal communication. **227:**52-60 (Sept.). *The languages of animals and humans are compared.*

References to Part Three

The books listed in the following selection are mainly textbooks covering wide areas of physiology. They vary considerably in depth and in the level of background in biology and chemistry required of the reader for a full understanding, as indicated in the annotations.

Barrington, E.J.W. 1968. The chemical basis of physiological regulation. Glenview, Ill., Scott, Foresman & Co. *A selection of topics in comparative physiology, with emphasis on experimental approach. Clearly written.*

Beck, W.S. 1971. Human design: molecular, cellular, and systematic physiology. New York, Harcourt Brace Jovanovich, Inc. *Well-integrated treatment of human anatomy and physiology.*

Davson, H., and M.B. Segal. 1975-1980. Introduction to physiology, 5 vols. London, Academic Press, Ltd. *Advanced; mostly human physiology.*

Eckert, R., and D. Randall. 1982. Animal physiology, ed. 2. San Francisco, W.H. Freeman & Co. Publishers. *Special emphasis on general principles and on membrane, neural, and sensory physiology.*

Folk, G.E. 1974. Textbook of environmental physiology, ed. 2. Philadelphia, Lea & Febiger. *Stresses responses of mammals to heat, cold, light, and atmospheric pressure.*

Gordon, M.S. (ed.). 1982. Animal function: principles and adaptations, ed. 4. New York, Macmillan, Inc. *Graduate-level vertebrate physiology.*

Guyton, A.C. 1981. Textbook of medical physiology, ed. 6. Philadelphia, W.B. Saunders Co. *A detailed but readable treatment of medical physiology.*

Hill, R.W. 1976. Comparative physiology of animals: an environmental approach. New York, Harper & Row, Publishers. *Highly selective treatment, stressing environmental interactions.*

Hoar, W.S. 1983. General and comparative physiology, ed. 3. Englewood Cliffs, N.J., Prentice-Hall, Inc. *The best balanced of college comparative physiology texts.*

Marshall, P.T., and G.M. Hughes. 1980. Physiology of mammals and other vertebrates, ed. 2. Cambridge, Eng., Cambridge University Press. *Undergraduate comparative physiology; clearly presented and illustrated organ-system approach.*

Miller, J. 1978. The body in question. New York, Random House, Inc. *Selective, historically grounded view of human body function, based on a television series.*

Prosser, C.L. (ed.). 1973. Comparative animal physiology, ed. 3. Philadelphia, W.B. Saunders Co. *Advanced treatise.*

Schmidt-Nielsen, K. 1975. Animal physiology: adaptation and environment. New York, Cambridge University Press. *Interestingly written, selective treatment of comparative physiology, emphasizing physiological adaptations to the environment.*

Schottelius, B.A., and D.D. Schottelius. 1978. Textbook of physiology, ed. 18. St. Louis, The C.V. Mosby Co. *Intermediate-level college human physiology text. Clearly written and illustrated.*

Vander, A.J., J.H. Sherman, and D.S. Luciano. 1980. Human physiology: the mechanisms of body function, ed. 3. New York, McGraw-Hill Book Co. *Excellent intermediate-level human physiology text.*

Vertebrate structures and functions. Readings from *Scientific American* with introductions by N.K. Wessels. 1974. San Francisco, W.H. Freeman & Co. Publishers. *Excellent collection of articles on vertebrate structure and physiology with helpful introductions. Highly recommended supplementary reading.*

Wilson, J.A. 1979. Principles of animal physiology, ed. 2. New York, Macmillan, Inc. *Clearly written comparative physiology at the advanced undergraduate level.*

Young, J.Z. 1981. The life of vertebrates, ed. 3. Oxford, Eng., Oxford University Press. *The comprehensive treatment and trenchant writing style of this classic have been retained in this new edition, which has increased emphasis on physiology, ecology, and behavior.*

PART FOUR

Charles Darwin in 1881, 1 year
before his death.

CONTINUITY

AND EVOLUTION

OF ANIMAL LIFE

Since all living things are mortal, species perpetuation is a central activity in the lives of animals. To comprehend the continuity of life, it is necessary to understand how hereditary units are transmitted from parent to offspring, how such units direct the structural and functional differentiation of a fertilized egg into an adult organism, and how the capacity for evolutionary diversity has been built into the hereditary mechanism.

Organic evolution is the process through which existing animals and plants have attained their diversity of form and behavior by gradual, continuous change from previously existing forms.

Evolution comes about by natural selection acting on the inheritable variations of a population. It may be considered a descent in the course of time with modifications. It is an ongoing living process and is taking place today.

The following chapters deal with reproduction, development, and the principles of inheritance, with the evidences for and nature of the evolutionary process that comprises the framework of biology, and with the remarkable and recent divergence of the hominoid line, which gave rise to humans.

Chapter 35

THE REPRODUCTIVE PROCESS

Chapter 36

PRINCIPLES OF DEVELOPMENT

Chapter 37

PRINCIPLES OF INHERITANCE

Chapter 38

ORGANIC EVOLUTION

Chapter 39

HUMAN EVOLUTION

THE REPRODUCTIVE PROCESS

Section of a seminiferous tubule containing male germ cells. More than 200 long, highly coiled seminiferous tubules are packed in each human testis. As the germ cells differentiate into fertile sperm, they move inward from the periphery of the tubule toward its center. This scanning electron micrograph reveals numerous long tails of mature spermatozoa in the tubule's central cavity (lumen). The differentiation of sperm cells is the result of both mitotic and meiotic divisions. (×525.)

From Tissues and organs: a text-atlas of scanning electron microscopy, by Richard G. Kessel and Randy H. Kardon. W.H. Freeman and Company. Copyright © 1979.

All living organisms are capable of giving rise to new organisms similar to themselves (Principle 10, p. 14). If we admit that all living things are mortal, that every organism is endowed with a life span that must eventually end, we must acknowledge the indispensability of reproduction. Like Samuel Butler who concluded that a chicken is just an egg's way of making another egg, many biologists consider the ability to reproduce to be the ultimate objective of all life processes.

The word "reproduction" implies replication, and it is true that biological reproduction almost always yields a reasonable facsimile of the parent unit. However, sexual reproduction, practiced by the majority of animals, promotes the *diversity* needed for survival in a world of constant change. At least for multicellular animals sexual reproduction offers enormous advantages over asexual reproduction, as we shall explain later. The reproductive process, whether sexual or asexual, embodies a basic pattern: (1) the conversion of raw materials from the environment into the offspring or sex cells that develop into offspring of a similar constitution and (2) the transmission of a hereditary pattern or code (DNA) from the parents (Principle 17, p. 16).

NATURE OF THE REPRODUCTIVE PROCESS

The two fundamental types of reproduction are asexual and sexual. In **asexual** reproduction there is only one parent and there are no special reproductive organs or cells. Each organism is capable of producing genetically identical copies of itself as soon as it becomes an adult. The production of copies is marvelously simple and direct and typically rapid. **Sexual** reproduction (Fig. 35-1) as a rule involves two parents, each of which contributes special **sex cells,** or **gametes,** that in union develop into a new individual. The **zygote** formed from this union receives genetic material from *both* parents and accordingly is different from both. The combination of genes produces a genetically unique individual, still bearing the characteristics of the species but also bearing traits that make it different from its parents.

Sexual reproduction, by recombining the parental characters, tends to multiply variations and makes possible a richer and more diversified evolution. Mechanisms for interchange of genes between individuals are much more limited in organisms with only asexual reproduction. This would seem to explain why forms that can reproduce only asexually are unicellular; they can multiply rapidly enough to offset the disadvantages of repeated replication of identical products.

Of course, in asexual organisms such as fungi and bacteria that are haploid (bear only one set of genes), mutations are immediately expressed and evolution can proceed quickly. In sexual animals, on the other hand, a gene mutation is often not expressed immediately, since it may be masked by its normal partner on the homologous chromosome. (Homologous chromosomes are those that pair

Figure 35-1

Sexual reproduction usually involves two parents. Fertilization—union of the egg and sperm—may be external as in, **A,** amphibians (American toad), or internal as in, **B,** insects (gypsy moths) and, **C,** mammals (elk).

during meiosis and have genes controlling the same characteristics.) There is only a remote chance that both members of a gene pair will mutate in the same way at the same moment.

Asexual Reproduction

As pointed out previously, asexual reproduction is common only among the simpler forms of life, such as bacteria, protozoa, cnidarians, bryozoans, and a few others. It is absent among the higher invertebrates (molluscs and arthropods) and rare among the vertebrates. Even in the phyla in which it occurs, most of the members employ the sexual method of reproduction as well. In these groups, asexual reproduction ensures rapid increase in numbers when the differentiation of the organism has not advanced to the point of forming highly specialized gametes.

The forms of asexual reproduction are binary fission, budding (both internal and external), fragmentation, and multiple fission. **Binary fission** is common among bacteria and protozoa and to a limited extent among metazoa. In this method the body of the parent is divided into two approximately equal parts, each of which grows into an individual similar to the parent. Fission may be either transverse or longitudinal. **Budding** is an unequal division of the organism. The new individual arises as an outgrowth (bud) from the parent. This bud develops organs like those of the parent and then usually detaches itself. If the bud is formed on the surface of the parent, it is an external bud, but in some cases internal buds, or **gemmules,** are produced. Gemmules are collections of many cells surrounded by a dense covering in the body wall. When the body of the parent disintegrates, each gemmule gives rise to a new individual. External budding is common in the cnidarians, and internal budding in the freshwater sponges. Bryozoa also have a form of internal bud called statoblast. **Fragmentation** is a method in which an organism breaks into two or more parts, each capable of becoming a complete animal. This method is found among the Platyhelminthes, Rhynchocoela, and Echinodermata. In **multiple fission** the nucleus divides repeatedly before division of the cytoplasm, giving rise to many daughter cells almost simultaneously. Multiple fission occurs in a number of protozoan forms.

It would be a mistake to conclude that asexual reproduction is in any way a "defective" form of reproduction relegated to the minute forms of life that have not yet discovered the joys of sex. Given the facts of their abundance, that they have persisted on earth for 3.5 billion years, and that they form the roots of the food chain on which all higher forms depend, the single-celled asexual organisms are both resoundingly successful and supremely important. For these forms the advantages of asexual reproduction are its rapidity (many bacteria divide every half hour) and simplicity (no sex cells to produce and no time and energy expended in finding a mate).

Sexual Reproduction

In sexual reproduction there are usually, although not invariably, two parents that produce gametes (sex cells). These combine to create offspring having the mixed genetic identities of both parents. Only one sex, the female, can produce offspring, and this must depend on the intervention of the male. There are two kinds of gametes: the **ovum** (egg), produced by the female, and the **spermatozoon** (sperm), produced by the male. Ova are nonmotile, are produced in relatively small numbers, and may contain a large amount of yolk, the stored food material that sustains early development of the new individual. Sperm are motile, produced in enormous numbers, and small. The union of egg and sperm is called **fertilization,** and the resulting cell, known as a **zygote,** develops into a new individual. Sexual reproduction is the general rule in the animal kingdom.

There are two fundamental events that distinguish sexual from asexual reproduction: meiosis and fertilization. **Meiosis** is a distinctive type of gamete-producing nuclear division, actually a double division, that differs from ordinary cell division (mitosis) in an important way. (Unfortunately the terms "mitosis" and "meiosis" are confusingly similar.) As described later in this chapter, the chromosomes split once, but the cell divides *twice*, producing four cells, each with half the original number of chromosomes. Meiosis is followed by fertilization in which two gametes, each containing half the original number of chromosomes, are combined to restore the normal chromosome content of the species. The new cell (zygote) contains genetic material from both gametes. It is not difficult to understand why meiosis is required; if ordinary cells from each parent fused to form a zygote, the chromosome number would be doubled with each generation. Meiosis, followed by fertilization, keeps the chromosome number stable.

The zygote now begins to divide and grow by mitosis. The new individual has equal numbers of chromosomes from each parent and accordingly is different from each; it is a unique individual bearing a random assortment of parental characters. This is the great strength of sexual reproduction, the "master adaptation" that keeps introducing new varieties into the population. Neither meiosis nor fertilization ever occurs in asexual reproduction.

Sexual reproduction appears in many protozoa, although protozoa also reproduce asexually by fission. When sexual reproduction is found, it may involve the formation of male and female gametes that unite to form a zygote, or it may involve two mature sexual individuals that join together to exchange nuclear material or merge cytoplasm. In some cases it is difficult to distinguish sex, because although two parents are involved, they cannot be designated as male and female.

The male-female distinction is more clearly evident in the metazoa. Organs that produce the germ cells are known as **gonads**. The gonad that produces the sperm is called the **testis** (Fig. 35-2) and that which forms the egg, the **ovary** (Fig. 35-3). The gonads represent the **primary sex organs,** the only sex organs found in certain groups of animals. Most metazoa, however, have various **accessory sex organs** that transfer and receive sex cells (such as penis, vagina, oviducts, and uterus). In the primary sex organs the sex cells undergo many complicated changes during their development, the details of which are described in a later discussion. In our present discussion we will distinguish biparental reproduction from two alternatives: parthenogenesis and hermaphroditism.

Biparental reproduction

Biparental reproduction is the common and familiar method of sexual reproduction involving separate and distinct male and female individuals. Each has its own reproductive system and produces only one kind of sex cell, spermatozoon or ovum, but never both. Nearly all vertebrates and many invertebrates have separate sexes, and such a condition is called **dioecious** (Gr., *di-*, two, + *oikos*, house).

Parthenogenesis

Parthenogenesis is the development of an embryo without the participation of a spermatozoon. Spontaneous, or natural, parthenogenesis is known to occur in rotifers, some nematodes, crustaceans, insects, and several species of fish and desert lizards. Often several generations of parthenogenetic reproduction alternate with biparental reproduction in which the egg is fertilized. In some cases parthenogenesis appears to be the only form of reproduction.

The queen bee is fertilized only once by a male (drone) or sometimes by more than one drone. She stores the sperm in her seminal receptacles, and, as she lays her eggs, she can either fertilize the eggs or allow them to pass unfertilized. The fertilized eggs become females (queens or workers), and the unfertilized eggs become males (drones) (p. 428).

Hermaphroditism

Animals that have both male and female organs in the same individual are called hermaphrodites, and the condition is called hermaphroditism (from a combination of the names of the Greek god Hermes and goddess Aphrodite). In contrast to the dioecious state of separate sexes, hermaphrodites are **monoecious** (Gr., *monos*, single + *oikos*, house), meaning that both male and female organs are in the same organism. Many invertebrate animals (most flatworms, some hydroids, annelids, and crustaceans) are hermaphroditic. Most avoid self-fertilization by exchanging germ cells with each other. For example, although the earthworm bears both male and female organs, its eggs are fertilized by the copulating mate and vice versa (p. 348). Another way of preventing self-fertilization is by developing the eggs and sperm at different times.

_____ What Good Is Sex?

The question "What good is sex?" apppears to have an easy answer: it serves the purpose of reproduction. But if we rephrase the question to ask, "Why do so many animals reproduce sexually rather than asexually?" the answer is not so apparent. It is easier to list disadvantages to sex than advantages. Sexual reproduction takes more time and requires much more energy than does asexual reproduction, and it is anatomically and physiologically complicated. Mating partners must find each other and then cooperate to produce young. For most species there is a wastage in the production of males. Males of most species contribute little or nothing to the care of the young; having inseminated the female, the male fades into the sunset, leaving the female with the burden of incubating, nourishing, training, and protecting the young. Having accepted this burden, the female is further penalized by the cost of meiosis. Because male and female combine their sex cells, only 50% of her genes are transmitted to the next generation. If the female were to reproduce asexually, all of her genes would flow to the next generation.

Clearly, the costs of sexual reproduction are substantial. How are they offset? Biologists have wrestled with this question for years without producing an answer that satisfies everyone. Many biologists agree that a benefit of sexual reproduction is the *variability* of sexually produced offspring. Sexual reproduction, with its breakup and recombination of genotypes, keeps producing novel genotypes that in times of environmental change may survive and reproduce while most others die. Environments vary from place to place and from season to season. Animals that reproduce asexually may multiply rapidly when conditions are ideal but are severely disadvantaged when conditions change. It is a boom-or-bust strategy.

In his widely acclaimed book *Sex and Evolution*, George C. Williams argues that the sexual-asexual distinction is like a lottery in which one is offered a choice between several copies of the same ticket (asexual reproduction) and several different tickets (sexual reproduction). We would all choose to have different tickets

From time to time claims arise that spontaneous parthenogenetic development to term has occurred in humans. A British investigation of about 100 cases in which the mother denied having had intercourse revealed that in nearly every case the child possessed characters not present in the mother, and consequently must have had a father. Nevertheless, mammalian eggs very rarely will spontaneously start developing into embryos without fertilization. In certain strains of mice, such embryos will develop into fetuses and then die. The most remarkable instance of parthenogenetic development among the higher vertebrates has been found in turkeys in which certain strains, selected for their ability to develop without sperm, grow to reproducing adults.

Variety may make sexual reproduction a winning strategy for the unstable environment, but some biologists believe that for higher animals sexual reproduction is unnecessary and may even be maladaptive. In animals (humans, for example) in which most of the young survive to reproductive age, there is no demand for novel recombinations to cope with changing habitats. One offspring appears as successful as the next in each habitat. Significantly, asexual reproduction has evolved in several species of fish and in a few amphibians and reptiles. Such species are exclusively asexual, suggesting that where it has been possible to overcome the numerous constraints to making the transition, asexuality wins out. Would all vertebrates do better to live sexlessly, avoiding the costs of sex? Possibly, but despite the costs, it is unlikely that higher animals if given the choice would opt for sexless lives—especially the males, which would necessarily become extinct. Woody Allen has pointed out that bisexuality, if nothing else, doubles the chance of getting a date on Saturday night.

because they are more likely to produce a winner. For the female, it is better to have only one half her genes represented in the next generation of variable offspring, some of which have a good chance of survival, than to produce identical copies of herself with a low probability that any will survive. Fifty percent of something is better than 100% of nothing.

One approach to testing the validity of Williams's lottery analogy is to look at species that employ both sexual and asexual reproduction. Many parasites offer good examples. Within the host animal, where conditions are relatively constant, parasites reproduce rapidly, often explosively, by asexual reproduction. Sex is used to produce offspring that will leave the host for dispersal and invasion of new hosts in unpredictable environments. Another example is *Hydra*, which reproduces asexually throughout the spring and summer but begins producing eggs and sperm with the approach of winter. Fertilized eggs overwinter and hatch in the spring. The new combinations of genotypes are well suited to colonizing the spring pond, which may be very different from its condition the previous year. Other examples of alternating sexual and asexual reproduction (such as certain insects and crustaceans) appear to fit Williams's model. Thus, variety is the trump card of sexual reproduction, but where the need for each parent to diversify its own offspring is of little importance, the more efficient asexual system may prevail.

PLAN OF REPRODUCTIVE SYSTEMS

The basic plan of the reproductive systems is similar in all animals, although differences in reproductive habits, methods of fertilization, and so on have produced many variations. In vertebrate animals the reproductive and excretory systems are often referred to as the **urinogenital system** because of their close anatomical connection. This association is very striking during embryonic development.

The reproductive and excretory systems of the male are usually more intimately connected than they are in the female. For example, in male fishes and amphibians the duct that drains the kidney (**wolffian duct**) also serves as the sperm duct. In male reptiles, birds, and mammals in which the kidney develops its own independent duct (**ureter**) to carry away waste, the old wolffian duct becomes exclusively a sperm duct (**vas deferens**). In all these forms, with the exception of mammals, the ducts open into a **cloaca** (derived, appropriately, from the Latin meaning "sewer"), a common chamber into which the intestinal, reproductive, and excretory canals empty. Higher mammals have no cloaca; instead the urinogenital system has its own opening separate from the anal opening. The **oviduct** of the female is an independent duct that does, however, open into the cloaca in forms that have a cloaca.

The plan of the reproductive system in vertebrates includes (1) **gonads** that produce the sperm and eggs, (2) **ducts** to transport the gametes, (3) **accessory organs** for transferring and receiving gametes, (4) **accessory glands** (exocrine and endocrine) to provide secretions necessary to facilitate and synchronize the reproductive process, and (5) **organs** for storage before and after fertilization. This plan is modified among the various vertebrates, and some of the items may be lacking altogether.

Figure 35-2

Human male reproductive system.

Figure labels (Median section of male pelvis): Peritoneum, Vas deferens, Urinary bladder, Ureter, Seminal vesicle, Vertebral column, Pubic bone, Urethra, Penis, Glans penis, Prostate gland, Anus, Rectum, Ejaculatory duct, External urinary meatus, Cowper's glands, Testicle, Epididymis, Scrotum

secretion

Median section of male pelvis

Figure labels (Section of left testis): Testicle, Epididymis, Vasa efferentia, Rete testis, Ductus epididymis, Seminiferous tubule, Vas deferens

Section of left testis

Sequential stages in spermatogenesis

Spermatogonium → Primary spermatocyte → Secondary spermatocyte → Spermatid → Sperm cell

Figure labels (Cross section): Primary spermatocytes, Interstitial cells, Spermatozoa, Sertoli cell, Spermatogonium, Secondary spermatocytes, Blood vessel, Spermatids

Cross section of one seminiferous tubule, showing different stages in spermatogenesis

___ Human Reproductive System

Male reproductive system

The human male reproductive system (Fig. 35-2) includes testes, vasa efferentia, vasa deferentia, penis, and glands.

The paired **testes** are the locus of sperm production. Each testis is made up of numerous **seminiferous tubules,** in which the sperm develop (Fig. 35-2), and the **interstitial tissue** lying along the tubules, which produces the male sex hormone (testosterone). The two testes are housed in the scrotal sac, which in many mammals hangs down as an appendage of the body. This strange and seemingly insecure arrangement provides an environment of slightly lower temperature, since in at least some forms (including humans) sperm apparently do not form at temperatures maintained within the body.

The sperm are conveyed from the seminiferous tubules to the **vasa efferentia,** small tubes passing to a coiled **vas epididymis** (one for each testis). The epididymis is connected by a **vas deferens** to the **urethra.** From this point the urethra serves to carry both sperm and urinary products through the penis, or external intromittent organ.

Three pairs of glands open into the reproductive channels: **seminal vesicles, prostate glands,** and **Cowper's glands.** Fluid secreted by these glands furnishes food to the sperm, lubricates the passageways for the sperm, and counteracts the acidity of the urine so that the sperm are not harmed.

Most aquatic vertebrates have no need for a penis, since sperm and eggs are liberated into the water in close proximity to each other. However, in terrestrial (and some aquatic) vertebrates that bear their young alive or enclose the egg within a shell, sperm must be transferred to the female. In most birds, this is a rather haphazard process of simply presenting cloaca to cloaca. Only the reptiles and mammals have a true penis. In mammals the normally flaccid organ is erected when engorged with blood. Many mammals, although not humans, possess a bone in the penis (baculum), which presumably helps with rigidity. The baculum has a highly variable shape in different species and is a favored object for bewildering comparative anatomy students during practical examinations.

Figure 35-3

Human female reproductive system.

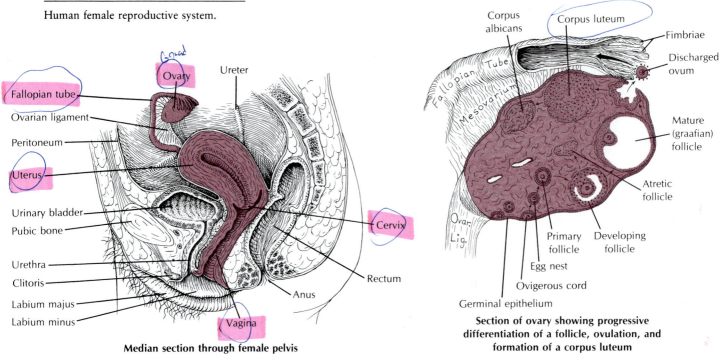

Median section through female pelvis

Section of ovary showing progressive
differentiation of a follicle, ovulation, and
formation of a corpus luteum

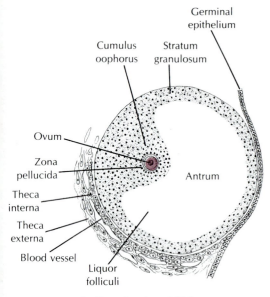

Section of mature follicle

Female reproductive system

The female reproductive system (Fig. 35-3) contains ovaries, oviduct, uterus, vagina, and vulva.

The paired ovaries, slightly smaller than the male testes, contain many thousands of eggs (ova). Each egg develops within a **graafian follicle** that enlarges and finally ruptures to release the mature egg (Fig. 35-3). During the fertile period of the woman, approximately 13 eggs mature each year, and usually the ovaries alternate in releasing an egg. Since the female is fertile for only some 30 years, only 300 to 400 eggs have a chance to reach maturity; the others degenerate and are absorbed.

The **oviducts,** or fallopian tubes, are egg-carrying tubes with funnel-shaped openings for receiving the eggs when they emerge from the ovary. The oviduct is lined with cilia for propelling the egg in its course. The two ducts open into the upper corners of the **uterus,** or womb, which is specialized for housing the embryo during the 9 months of its intrauterine existence. It is provided with thick muscular walls, many blood vessels, and a specialized lining: the **endometrium.** The uterus varies with different mammals. It was originally paired but tends to fuse in higher forms.

The **vagina** is a muscular tube adapted for receiving the male's penis and for serving as the birth canal during expulsion of the fetus from the uterus. Where the vagina and the uterus meet, the uterus projects down into the vagina to form the **cervix.**

The external genitalia of the female, or vulva, include folds of skin, the **labia majora** and **labia minora,** and a small erectile organ, the **clitoris.** The opening into the vagina is normally reduced in size in the virgin state by a membrane, the **hymen.**

FORMATION OF REPRODUCTIVE CELLS

The animal body has two basically different types of cells: the somatic cells, which are differentiated for specialized functions and die with the individual, and the germinal cells, some of which may contribute to the formation of a zygote and thereby to a new generation. The germinal cells are set aside at the beginning of embryonic development, usually in the endoderm, and migrate to the gonads. The germinal cells, or primordial germ cells, develop into eggs and sperm—nothing else. The other cells of the gonads are somatic cells. They cannot form eggs or sperm, but they are necessary aids in the development of the germinal cells (gametogenesis).

Origin and Migration of Germ Cells

The actual tissue from which the gonads arise appears in early development as a pair of ridges, or pouches, growing into the coelom from the dorsal coelomic lining on each side of the gut near the anterior end of the mesonephros.

Surprisingly perhaps, the primordial ancestors of the germ cells do not arise in the developing gonad but in the yolk-sac endoderm. From studies with frogs and toads, it has been possible to trace the germ cell line back to the fertilized egg, in which a localized area of "germinal cytoplasm" can be identified in the vegetal pole of the uncleaved egg mass. This material can be followed through subsequent cell divisions of the embryo until it becomes situated in primitive sex cells located deep in the endoderm of the yolk sac. From here they migrate to the developing gonads.

The primitive germ cells can be distinguished from somatic cells because they are larger and have large round nuclei with prominent nucleoli. In the human embryo the germ cells wander by ameboid movement from the yolk sac first into the gut mesentery, then to the kidney, and finally into the genital ridges. In some vertebrates, especially birds, the primitive sex cells travel passively through the bloodstream to the developing gonad. There is some evidence that the gonads release a chemical attractant that helps the germ cells to home in on the gonad. If, for example, the early gonad is removed from its normal position and implanted in some distant site, the primordial germ cells will still migrate to it.

The primordial germ cells are the future stock of gametes for the animal. Once in the gonad they begin to divide by mitosis, increasing their numbers from a few dozen to several thousand.

At first the gonad is sexually indifferent. It has been determined that in mammals the indifferent gonad has an inherent tendency to become an ovary. If the embryo is to become a male, male-determining genes on the sex chromosomes direct the primordial germ cells to grow into the central portion (medulla) of the gonad where, eventually, the seminiferous tubules of the testis develop. The inner walls of these tubules are lined with cells that have descended from the primordial germ cells. As the animal approaches sexual maturity, these develop into mature sperm.

If the animal is a genetic female, the *absence* of male-determining genes allows the gonad to follow its inherent tendency to become an ovary. In this alternative, the medullary tissue degenerates and the cortical (outer) tissue forms the substance of the ovary. The primordial germ cells, together with somatic cells in this area, differentiate into ovarian follicles with eggs (ova) (Fig. 35-3). We will return to this subject of sex determination in Chapter 37 (p. 903).

For every structure in the reproductive system of the male or female, there is a homologous structure in the other. This happens because during early development male and female characteristics begin to differentiate from the embryonic genital ridge and two duct systems that at first are identical in both sexes. Under the influence of the sex hormones, the genital ridge develops into the testes of the male and the ovaries of the female. One duct system (wolffian) becomes ducts of the testes in the male and a vestigial structure adjacent to the ovaries in the female. The other duct (müllerian) develops into the oviducts, uterus, and vagina of the female and into the small, vestigial appendix of the testes in the male. Similarly, the clitoris and labia of the female are homologous to the penis and scrotum of the male, since they develop from the same embryonic structures.

_____ Meiosis: Maturation Division of Germ Cells

Every body cell contains *two* chromosomes bearing genes for the same set of characteristics, and the two members of each pair usually, but not always, have the same size and shape. The members of such a pair are called **homologous** chromosomes. Thus, each cell normally has two genes coding for a given trait, one on each of the homologues. These may be alternative forms of the same gene, and if so they are **allelic genes,** or **alleles.** Sometimes only one of the alleles has an effect on the organism, although both are present in each cell, and either may be passed on to the progeny as a result of meiosis and subsequent fertilization.

During an individual's growth, all the chromosomes of the mitotically dividing cells are replicated during the S period of each cell cycle (Figure 4-23, p. 93), so that each new cell contains the double set of chromosomes. In the reproductive organs the germ cells are formed by a kind of maturation division, called meiosis, which *separates* the double sets of chromosomes. If it were not for this reductional division, the union of egg and sperm would produce an individual with twice as many chromosomes as the parents. Continuation of this process in just a few generations could yield body cells with astronomical numbers of chromosomes.

Meiosis consists of *two* nuclear divisions in which the chromosomes divide only once (Fig. 35-4). The result is that mature gametes (eggs and sperm) have only *one* member of each homologous chromosome pair, or a haploid (n) number of chromosomes. In humans the zygotes and all body cells normally have the diploid number (2n), or 46 chromosomes; the gametes have the haploid number (n), or 23.

Most of the unique features of meiosis occur during the prophase of the first meiotic division (Fig. 35-4). The two members of each pair of homologous chromosomes come into side-by-side contact (**synapsis**) to form a **bivalent.** Each chromosome of the bivalent has already replicated to form two chromatids, each of which will become a new chromosome. The two chromatids are joined at one point, the centromere, so that each bivalent is made up of two pairs of chromatids, or *four* future chromosomes, and is thus called a **tetrad.** The position or location of any gene on a chromosome is the gene **locus** (pl., **loci**), and in synapsis all gene loci on a chromatid normally lie exactly opposite the corresponding loci on the homologous chromatid. Toward the end of prophase, the chromosomes shorten and thicken and are ready to enter into the first meiotic division. In contrast to mitosis, the centromeres holding the chromatids together *do not divide* at the beginning of anaphase. As a result, one of each pair of double-stranded chromosomes (**dyads**) is pulled toward each pole by the microtubules of the division spindle. Therefore, at the end of the first meiotic division, the daughter cells contain *one* of *each* of the homologous chromosomes, so the total chromosome number has been reduced to the haploid. However, because the chromatids are still joined by the centromeres, each cell contains the 2n amount of DNA.

The second meiotic division more closely resembles the events in mitosis. The dyads are split at the beginning of anaphase by division of the centromeres, and single-stranded chromosomes move toward each pole. Thus, by the end of the second meiotic division, the cells have the haploid number of chromosomes and n amount of DNA. Each chromatid of the original tetrad exists in a separate nucleus. Four cells (gametes) are formed, each containing one complete haploid set of chromosomes and only one allele of each gene.

Prophase I

Each chromosome replicates and yields two chromatids; homologous chromosomes pair (synapsis) to form bivalents

Prophase I

Bivalents showing chiasmata

Anaphase I

Homologous chromosomes separate to opposite poles so that each daughter nucleus has only haploid number of chromosomes but diploid amount of DNA

Meiosis I

Meiosis II

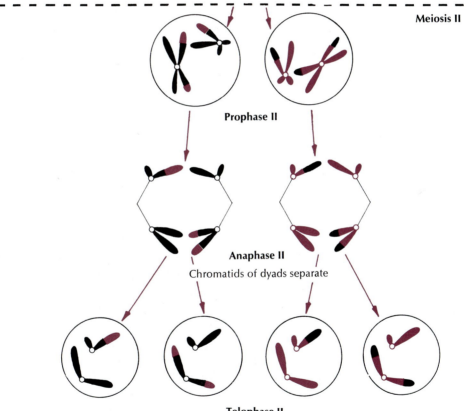

Prophase II

Anaphase II

Chromatids of dyads separate

Telophase II

Four haploid cells (gametes) formed, each with haploid amount of DNA

Figure 35-4

Meiosis in a sex cell with two pairs of chromosomes.

Crossing over

An important event often occurs when the chromatids of a bivalent exchange parts with the adjacent homologous (nonsister) chromatid. This phenomenon, called **crossing over,** is clearly shown in Fig. 35-4. Crossing over is important because the hereditary material is redistributed between homologous chromatids in one bivalent. The chromosomes exchange equivalent sections bearing allelic genes for the same traits, so that each chromatid contains a full set of genes. But the genes are in new combinations.

While the chromosomes are in synapsis, a strand of one chromatid becomes joined with the homologous chromatid. As prophase continues, the homologues begin to move apart, revealing **chiasmata,** the connection points where crossing over has occurred. There may be one or more chiasmata present in each bivalent, depending on the number of times the adjacent homologues have joined. When the chiasmata pull apart, the exchange is complete. The resulting four gametes at the end of meiosis are all genetically different (Fig. 35-4).

___ Gametogenesis

The series of transformations that results in the formation of mature gametes (germ cells) is called gametogenesis. Although the same essential processes are involved in the maturation of both sperm and eggs, there are some important differences. Gametogenesis in the testis is called **spermatogenesis,** and in the ovary it is called **oogenesis.**

Figure 35-5

Mammalian seminiferous tubule. The large primary spermatocyte will give rise to four spermatids by meiosis. Each spermatid will differentiate into a mature spermatozoon. Sertoli cells provide support and protection and probably nutrition for the developing germ cells. (×1100.)

Light micrograph courtesy A. Wayne Vogl.

Spermatogenesis

The walls of the seminiferous tubules contain the differentiating sex cells arranged in a stratified layer five to eight cells deep (electron micrograph on p. 841). The outermost layers contain **spermatogonia** (Fig. 35-2), which have increased in number by ordinary mitosis. Each spermatogonium increases in size and becomes a **primary spermatocyte.** Each primary spermatocyte then undergoes the first meiotic division, as described previously, to become two **secondary spermatocytes.**

Each secondary spermatocyte enters the second meiotic division without the intervention of a resting period. The resulting cells are called **spermatids** (Fig. 35-5), and each contains the haploid number (23 in humans) of chromosomes. A spermatid may have all maternal, all paternal, or both maternal and paternal chromosomes in varying proportions. Without further divisions the spermatids are transformed into mature sperm by losing a great deal of cytoplasm, condensing the nucleus into a head, and forming a whiplike, flagellar tail (Fig. 35-6).

From following the divisions of meiosis, it can be seen that each primary spermatocyte gives rise to four functional sperm, each with the haploid number of chromosomes (Fig. 35-7).

Oogenesis

The early germ cells in the ovary, called **oogonia,** increase in number by ordinary mitosis (Fig. 35-7). Each oogonium contains the diploid number of chromosomes. In females after puberty, one of these oogonia typically develops each menstrual month into a functional egg. After the oogonia cease to increase in number, they grow in size and become **primary oocytes.** Before the first meiotic division, the chromosomes in each primary oocyte meet in pairs, paternal and maternal homologues, just as in spermatogenesis. When the first maturation (reduction) division

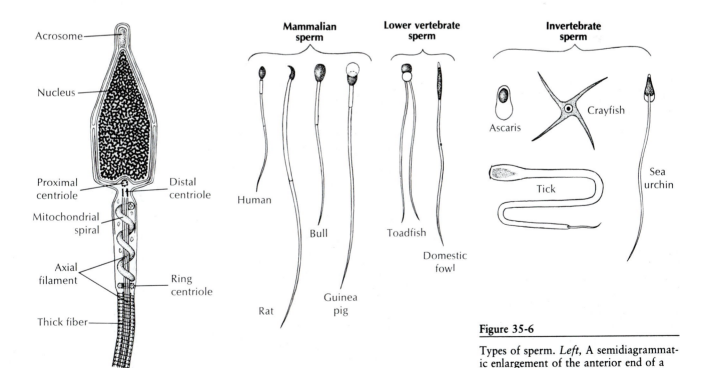

Figure 35-6

Types of sperm. *Left,* A semidiagrammatic enlargement of the anterior end of a human spermatozoon.

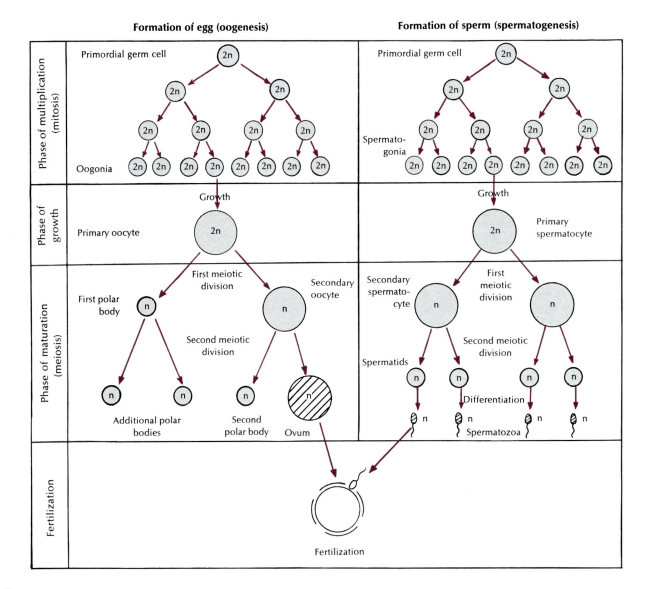

Figure 35-7

Gametogenesis compared in eggs and sperm. *n*, Haploid chromosome number.

occurs, the cytoplasm is divided unequally. One of the two daughter cells, the **secondary oocyte,** is large and receives most of the cytoplasm; the other is very small and is called the **first polar body** (Fig. 35-7). Each of these daughter cells, however, has received half the nuclear material or chromosomes.

In the second meiotic division, the secondary oocyte divides into a large **ootid** and a small polar body. If the first polar body also divides in this division, which sometimes happens, there are three polar bodies and one ootid. The ootid grows into a functional **ovum;** the polar bodies are nonfunctional and disintegrate. The formation of the nonfunctional polar bodies is necessary to enable the egg to get rid of excess chromosomes, and the unequal cytoplasmic division makes possible a large cell with sufficient yolk for the development of the young. Thus, the mature ovum has the haploid number of chromosomes, the same as the sperm. However, each primary oocyte gives rise to only *one* functional gamete instead of four as in spermatogenesis.

——— Gametes and Their Specializations

Eggs

During **oogenesis** the egg becomes a highly specialized, very large cell containing condensed food reserves for subsequent growth. It is of interest that the prolonged growth and enormous accumulation of food reserves in the oocyte occur **before** the meiotic, or maturation, divisions begin. (This contrasts with spermatogenesis, in which differentiation of the mature sperm occurs only **after** the meiotic divisions.) When the maturation divisions do occur, once the growth phase of the oocyte is complete, they are, as already described, highly unequal: the two meiotic divisions produce one very large mature ovum and two or three polar bodies.

In most vertebrates the egg does not actually complete all the meiotic divisions before fertilization occurs. The general rule is that the egg completes the first meiotic division and proceeds to the metaphase stage of the second meiotic division, at which point progress stops. The second meiotic division is completed and the second polar body extruded only if the egg is activated by fertilization.

The most obvious feature of egg maturation is the deposition of yolk. Yolk, usually stored as granules or more organized platelets, is not a definite chemical substance but may be lipid or protein or both. In insects and vertebrates, all having more or less yolky eggs, the yolk may be synthesized within the egg from raw materials supplied by the surrounding follicle cells, or preformed lipid or protein yolk may be transferred by pinocytosis from follicle cells to the oocyte.

The result of the enormous accumulation of yolk granules and other nutrients (glycogen and lipid droplets) is that an egg grows well beyond the normal limits that force ordinary body (somatic) cells to divide. A young frog oocyte 50 μm in diameter, for example, grows to 1500 μm in diameter when mature after 3 years of growth in the ovary, and the volume has increased by a factor of 27,000. Bird eggs attain even greater absolute size; a hen egg will increase 200 times in volume in only the last 6 to 14 days of rapid growth preceding ovulation.

Thus, eggs are remarkable exceptions to the otherwise universal rule that organisms are composed of relatively minute cellular units. This creates a surface area–to–cell volume ratio problem, since everything that enters and leaves the ovum (nutrients, respiratory gases, wastes, and so on) must pass through the cell membrane. As the egg becomes larger, the available surface per unit of cytoplasmic volume (mass) becomes smaller. As we would anticipate, the metabolic rate of the egg gradually diminishes until, when mature, the ovum is in a sort of suspended animation awaiting fertilization. However, large size is not the only factor leading to quiescence. There is increasing evidence that enzyme and nucleic acid inhibitors, which directly repress metabolic and synthetic activity in the egg, appear toward the end of maturation.

Spermatozoa

Sperm in animals show a greater diversity of form than do ova. A typical spermatozoon is made up of a head, a middle piece, and an elongated tail for locomotion (Fig. 35-6). The head consists of the nucleus containing the chromosomes for heredity and an **acrosome** believed to contain an enzyme that assists in egg penetration. The total length of the human sperm is 50 to 70 μm. Some toads have sperm that exceed 2 mm (2000 μm) in length. Most sperm, however, are microscopic in size.

The acrosome is a distinctive feature of nearly all the metazoa (exceptions are the teleost fishes and certain invertebrates). In many species, both invertebrate and vertebrate, the acrosome contains egg-membrane lysins that serve to clear an entrance path through the membranes that form a barrier around the egg. In mammals at least, the lysin is the enzyme hyaluronidase. A striking feature of many invertebrate spermatozoa is the acrosome filament, an extension of varying length in different species that projects suddenly from the sperm head when the latter first contacts the egg membrane. Its penetration of the egg cytoplasm is the initial event of fertilization.

In all sexually reproducing animals the number of sperm in males is far greater than the number of eggs in corresponding females. The number of eggs produced is related to the chances of the young to hatch and reach maturity. This explains the enormous number of eggs produced by certain fishes, as compared with the small number produced by mammals.

HORMONES OF REPRODUCTION

The male and female gonads are endocrine glands as well as gamete-forming glands. Reproduction is a complex process requiring the coordinated action of many hormones, especially in the female. Although the principal features of reproductive endocrinology are understood, the recent search for effective and safe birth control devices has revealed some disturbing gaps in our knowledge. To cite a single but telling example, no one fully understands how the popular birth control pill works.

The female reproductive activities of almost all animals are cyclic. Usually breeding cycles are seasonal and coordinated so that the young are born at a time of year when conditions for growth are most favorable. Mammals have two major reproductive patterns: the **estrous cycle** (characteristic of most mammals) and the **menstrual cycle** (characteristic of primates only). These two cyclic patterns differ in two ways. First, in the estrous cycle, but not in the menstrual cycle, the female is receptive to the male (that is, she is in "heat") only at restricted periods of the year. Second, the menstrual cycle, but not the estrous cycle, ends with the collapse and sloughing of the uterine lining (endometrium). In the estrous animal each cycle ends with the uterine lining simply reverting to its original state, without the bleeding characteristic of the menstrual cycle. (The bleeding that occurs in dogs and cattle when they are in heat is not caused by sloughing of the uterine lining but by red blood cells passing through the wall of the vagina.)

But these differences are really minor variations on a basic theme. The hor-

Figure 35-8

These three sex hormones all show the basic four-ring steroid structure. The female sex hormone estradiol-17β (an estrogen) is a C_{18} (18-carbon) steroid with an aromatic A ring (*first ring to left*). The male sex hormone testosterone is a C_{19} steroid with a carbonyl group (C=O) on the A ring. The female pregnancy hormone progesterone is a C_{21} steroid, also bearing a carbonyl group on the A ring.

Testosterone   Progesterone   Estradiol-17β

monal regulation of the reproductive cycles is so much alike for all mammals that a great deal of what we know about the human reproductive hormones has come from laboratory studies of the ubiquitous white rat, a rodent having an estrous cycle. Differences become more apparent when we study the lower vertebrates, but even fishes share most of the reproductive hormones found in humans. Since our discussion of this vast area must be brief, we will restrict our consideration to humans.

The ovaries produce two kinds of steroid **sex hormones: estrogens** and **progesterone** (Fig. 35-8). Estrogens (principally estradiol) are responsible for the development of the female accessory sex structures (uterus, oviducts, and vagina) and secondary sex characters, such as breast development and the characteristic bone growth, fat deposition, and hair distribution of the female. Progesterone is responsible for preparing the uterus to receive the developing embryo. These hormones are controlled by the pituitary **gonadotropins,** follicle-stimulating hormone (FSH) and luteinizing hormone (LH) (Fig. 35-9).

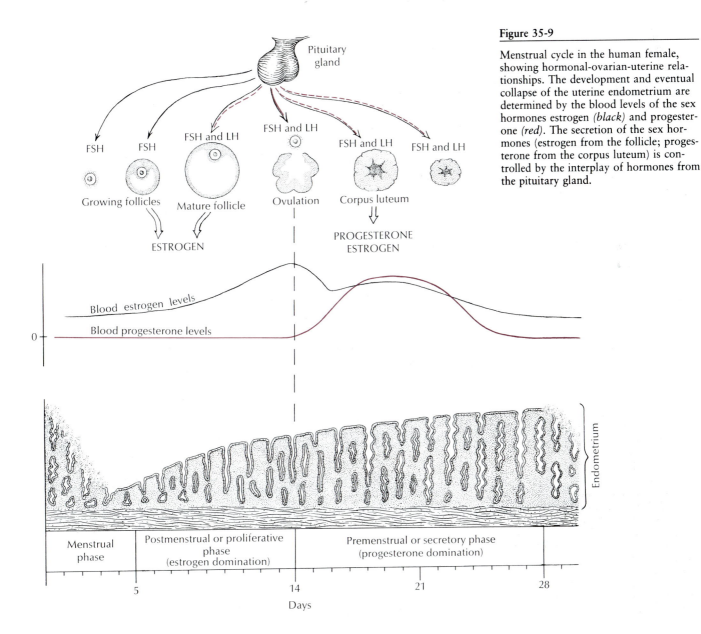

Figure 35-9

Menstrual cycle in the human female, showing hormonal-ovarian-uterine relationships. The development and eventual collapse of the uterine endometrium are determined by the blood levels of the sex hormones estrogen *(black)* and progesterone *(red).* The secretion of the sex hormones (estrogen from the follicle; progesterone from the corpus luteum) is controlled by the interplay of hormones from the pituitary gland.

The menstrual cycle begins with the release into the bloodstream of FSH from the anterior pituitary (Fig. 35-9). Reaching the ovaries, it stimulates the growth of one of the several thousand follicles present in each ovary. As the egg matures, the follicle swells until it bursts, releasing the egg onto the surface of the ovary. This event, called **ovulation,** normally occurs on about the fourteenth day of the cycle.

Now follows the most critical period of the cycle, for unless the mature egg is fertilized within a few hours it will die. During this period the egg is swept into an oviduct (fallopian tube) and begins its journey toward the uterus, pushed along by the numerous cilia that line the oviduct walls. If intercourse occurs at this time, the sperm will traverse the uterus and find their way into the oviducts, where one may meet and fertilize the egg. The developing embryo continues down the oviduct, enters the uterine cavity, where it dwells for a day or two, and then implants in the prepared uterine endometrium. This is the beginning of pregnancy.

Let us now examine the intricate series of events that occurs both before and after the beginning of pregnancy. We have seen that the pituitary hormone FSH begins the reproductive cycle by stimulating the growth of at least one of the ovarian follicles. As the follicle enlarges, it releases estrogens that prepare the uterine lining (endometrium) for reception of the embryo.

The rise in blood estrogen is sensed by the pituitary, which responds by stopping the production of FSH. Estrogen also encourages the production of the second pituitary hormone, LH. Ovulation now occurs. LH causes the cells lining the ruptured follicles to proliferate rapidly, filling the cavity with a characteristic spongy, yellowish body called a **corpus luteum** (Fig. 35-10). The corpus luteum, responding to the continued stimulation of LH, manufactures **progesterone** in addition to estradiol. Progesterone, as its name suggests, stimulates the uterus to undergo the final maturational changes that prepare it for gestation.

The uterus is thus fully ready to house and nourish the embryo by the time the latter settles out onto the uterine surface, usually about 7 days after ovulation. If fertilization has *not* occurred, the corpus luteum disappears, and its hormones are no longer secreted. Since the uterine lining (endometrium) depends on progesterone and estrogen for its maintenance, their disappearance causes the endome-

The widely heralded first "test-tube baby," born in England in July 1978, was a medical and technological triumph, the result of years of collaborative research by R.G. Edwards and P. Steptoe. More properly termed external human fertilization (EHF), the procedure is used to overcome infertility caused usually by a malfunction or malformation of the oviduct that prevents fertilization. First, an egg must be collected from the ovary during the final stages of maturation just before ovulation occurs. A special instrument that combines a fiberoptic light and syringe is introduced through a small incision in the abdominal wall, and the egg is sucked out of the ovarian follicle. The egg is placed in a specially compounded solution in a laboratory dish and fertilized with the husband's sperm. The egg is allowed to develop to the eight-cell stage (about 2 days) until the uterus has reached a receptive condition. The embryo is then introduced into the uterus via a tube passed through the cervix and is allowed to implant. The results of this technically simple step are unpredictable, and only about 20% of replanted embryos develop to advanced stages of gestation. Despite the low rate of success, more than a dozen babies conceived by EHF were born by the end of 1981. This, together with recent improvements in the technique, is encouraging news to childless couples who are able to produce normal eggs and sperm.

Figure 35-10

Section of cat ovary showing corpus luteum *(large body in lower half of photograph)* and primordial follicles containing oogonia *(above).*
Courtesy J.W. Bamberger.

trial lining to dehydrate and slough off, producing the menstrual discharge. However, if the egg has been fertilized and has implanted, the corpus luteum continues to supply the essential sex hormones needed to maintain the mature uterine endometrium. During the first few weeks of pregnancy the developing placenta itself begins to produce the sex hormones progesterone and estrogen and soon replaces the corpus luteum in this function.

As pregnancy advances, progesterone and estrogen prepare the breasts for milk production. The actual secretion and release of milk after birth (lactation) are the result of two other hormones, **prolactin** and **oxytocin**. Milk is not secreted during pregnancy because the placental sex hormones inhibit the release of prolactin by the pituitary. The placenta, like the corpus luteum that preceded it, thus becomes a special endocrine gland of pregnancy. After delivery, many mammals eat the placenta (afterbirth), a behavior that serves to remove telltale evidence of a birth from potential predators.

The male sex hormone **testosterone** (Fig. 35-8) is manufactured by the **interstitial cells** of the testes. Testosterone is necessary for the growth and development of the male accessory sex structures (penis, sperm ducts, glands), for development of secondary male sex characters (hair distribution, voice quality, bone and muscle growth), and for male sexual behavior. The same pituitary hormones that regulate the female reproductive cycle, FSH and LH, are also produced in the male, where they guide the growth of the testes and its testosterone secretion.

DIVERSITY OF REPRODUCTIVE PATTERNS

Animals may be divided into three classes on the basis of the methods they employ to nourish their young. Animals that lay their eggs outside the body for development are called **oviparous** (L., *ovum*, egg, + *parere*, to bring forth). In such cases the eggs may be fertilized inside or outside the body. Some animals retain their eggs in the body (in the oviduct) while they develop, but the embryo derives its sole nourishment from the egg and not from the mother. These are called **ovoviviparous** (L., *ovum*, egg, + *vivere*, to live, + *parere*, to bring forth). In the third type the egg develops in the uterus, but the embryo early in its development forms an intimate relationship with the walls of the uterus and derives its nourishment directly from food furnished by the mother. Such a type is called **viviparous** (L., *vivus*, alive, + *parere*, to bring forth). In both of the last two types the young are born alive. Examples of oviparity are found among many invertebrates and vertebrates. All birds are of this type. Ovoviviparity is common among certain fishes, lizards, and a few of the snakes. Viviparity is confined mostly to the mammals and some elasmobranchs. These patterns in fishes are described in more detail on p. 552.

The structural, physiological, and behavioral aspects of sexual reproduction show an incredible diversity, exceeding that of any other system. The diversity is expressed in the methods for fertilization, kinds of habitats, structure of the reproductive systems, prenatal care of the young, and seasonal and physiological changes in animals. Many examples of this diversity of reproductive adaptations are described in Part Two of this book. The most imaginative evolutionary adaptations seem to have occurred in the area of sexuality. The literature on the subject is fascinating; some suggested readings are included in the references for this chapter.

Is mother's milk superior to artificial formulas? The question is important because only about one baby in three is breast fed, even to 1 month of age, although the trend among new mothers is to breast feed. (By comparison, in 1900 50% of all mothers breast fed their babies until *at least* 12 months of age.) Human milk is different from cow's milk and more complex than a listing of its macronutrient composition (protein, carbohydrate, lipid) suggests. Milk contains several factors known to play vital roles in growth and development, although the function of others remains to be understood. For example, antibodies in human milk help the newborn resist infections. Among the several hormones present in milk is a recently identified class of hormones known as growth factors. The most intensively studied of these is the epidermal growth factor (EGF), which accelerates differentiation of the gastrointestinal tract, stimulates production of digestive enzymes, accelerates maturation of lung tissue (especially important for premature babies), and hastens epidermal growth throughout the body. The numerous effects of EGF are only now being catalogued by researchers, but it seems abundantly clear that no commercial formula can duplicate mother's milk.

White-tailed deer nursing her two juveniles.

Photograph by N. Bolen.

____ Summary

Reproduction is a universal property of all living organisms. Asexual reproduction, characteristic of simple life forms, is a rapid and direct process by which a single organism produces genetically identical copies of itself. It may occur by fission, budding, fragmentation, or sporulation. Sexual reproduction involves the production of sex cells (gametes), usually by two parents, which combine by fertilization to form a zygote that develops into a new individual. The sex cells are formed by meiosis, reducing the number of chromosomes to haploid, and the diploid chromosome number is restored at fertilization. Sexual reproduction recombines parental characters and thus reshuffles and amplifies genetic diversity; this is important for evolution. Two alternatives to typical biparental reproduction are parthenogenesis, the development of an unfertilized egg, and hermaphroditism, the presence of both male and female organs in the same individual.

Sexual reproduction exacts heavy costs in time and energy, requires cooperative investments in mating, and means the 50% loss of genetic representation of each parent in the offspring. Sex probably evolved because it produces variable offspring with superior fitness for environmental change.

The male reproductive system of humans includes the testes, composed of seminiferous tubules in which millions of sperm develop, a duct system (vasa efferentia and vas deferens) that joins the urethra, glands (seminal vesicles, prostate, Cowper's), and the penis. The human female system includes the ovaries, containing thousands of eggs within follicles; egg-carrying oviducts; uterus; and vagina.

In vertebrates the primordial germ cells arise in the yolk sac endoderm, then migrate to the gonad. In mammals the gonad will become a testis in response to masculinizing signals from the Y chromosome of the male, and an ovary in the absence of such signals in the female.

In bisexual animals the genetic material is distributed to the offspring in the gametes (eggs and sperm), produced in the process of meiosis. Each somatic cell in an organism has two chromosomes of each kind (homologous chromosomes) and is thus diploid. Meiosis separates the homologous chromosomes, so that each gamete has half the somatic chromosome number (haploid). In the first meiotic division the centromeres do not divide, and each daughter cell receives one of each of the replicated homologous chromosomes with the chromatids still attached to the centromere. At the beginning of the first meiotic division, the replicated homologous chromosomes come to lie alongside each other (synapsis), forming a bivalent. The gene loci on one set of chromatids lie opposite the corresponding loci on the homologous chromatids. Portions of the adjacent chromatids can exchange with the nonsister chromatids (crossing over) to produce new genetic combinations. At the second meiotic division, the centromeres divide, completing the reduction in chromosome number and amount of DNA. The diploid number is restored when the male and female gametes fuse to form the zygote.

Germ cells mature in the gonads by a process called gametogenesis (spermatogenesis in the male and oogenesis in the female), involving both mitosis and meiosis. In spermatogenesis, each primary spermatocyte gives rise by meiosis and growth to four motile sperm, each bearing the haploid number of chromosomes. In oogenesis, each primary oocyte gives rise to only one mature, nonmotile, haploid ovum. The remaining nuclear material is disposed of as polar bodies. During oogenesis the egg accumulates large food reserves, and DNA and RNA synthesis is intense.

Reproductive cycles are physiologically controlled by hormones to optimize conditions for development of the young. The menstrual cycle of primates and the estrous cycle of all other mammals are orchestrated by pituitary hormones, follicle-stimulating hormone (FSH) and luteinizing hormone (LH), that control the production of steroid sex hormones by the gonads. Estrogens in the female and testosterone in the male control the growth of the accessory sex structures and the secondary sex characteristics.

Selected references

Asdell, S.A. 1964. Patterns of mammalian reproduction, ed. 2. Ithaca, Cornell University Press. *Authoritative compilation of reproductive habits of mammals. Reference work.*

Austin, C.R., and R.V. Short (eds.). 1972-1980. Reproduction in mammals, 8 vols. Cambridge, Eng., Cambridge University Press. *Highly readable and well-illustrated series dealing with germ cells, fertilization, embryonic and fetal development, reproductive hormones and patterns, the artificial control of reproduction, and evolution of reproduction. Paperback.*

Bell, G. 1982. The masterpiece of nature: the evolution and genetics of sexuality. Berkeley, University of California Press. *Scholarly synthesis of ideas on the meaning of sex. Advanced treatment.*

Daly, M., and M. Wilson, 1978. Sex, evolution, and behavior: adaptations for reproduction. Belmont, Calif., Wadsworth Publishing Co., Inc. *Wide-ranging, well-argued account of sexual strategies.*

Djerassi, C. 1981. The politics of contraception. San Francisco, W.H. Freeman & Co. Publishers. *An important book, full of insights. The best of several books on contraception.*

Grobstein, C. 1981. From chance to purpose: an appraisal of external human fertilization. Reading, Mass., Addison-Wesley Publishing Co. *Technique and implications of in vitro human fertilization; for the general reader.*

Hapgood, F. 1979. Why males exist: an inquiry into the evolution of sex. New York, William Morrow & Co., Inc. *Accurate, informative, and witty.*

John, B., and K.R. Lewis. 1973. The meiotic mechanism. Oxford Biology Reader No. 65. London, Oxford University Press. *Well-illustrated and comprehensive overview.*

Johnson, M.H., and B.J. Everitt. 1980. Essential reproduction. Oxford, Eng., Blackwell Scientific Publications. *Detailed but clearly presented mammalian reproductive physiology.*

Maynard Smith, J. 1978. The evolution of sex. Cambridge, Eng., Cambridge University Press. *Important treatment of the origins of sex. Advanced and theoretical.*

Sadleir, R.M. 1973. The reproduction of vertebrates. New York, Academic Press, Inc. *Comparative treatment of reproductive patterns.*

Swanson, H.D. 1974. Human reproduction: biology and social change. New York, Oxford University Press. *Well-written college text dealing with the biological, psychological, sociological, and ethical aspects of the subject.*

Symons, D. 1979. The evolution of human sexuality. New York, Oxford University Press. *Sociobiological approach to differing reproductive interests of men and women.*

Williams, G.C. 1975. Sex and evolution. Princeton, N.J., Princeton University Press. *An important essay on evolutionary biology.*

Selected *Scientific American* articles

Beaconsfield, P., G. Birdwood, and R. Beaconsfield. 1980. The placenta. 243:94-102 (Aug.). *Function of this remarkable organ and how it is used in experimental studies.*

Csapo, A. 1958. Progesterone. 198:40-46 (Apr.). *The role of progesterone in pregnancy.*

Edwards, R.G., and R.E. Fowler. 1970. Human embryos in the laboratory. 223:44-54 (Dec.). *This article describes successes in culturing human and other mammalian eggs and embryos for observation.*

Fuchs, F. 1980. Genetic amniocentesis. 242:47-53 (June). *The amniotic fluid surrounding the fetus can be examined for genetic disorders.*

Grobstein, C. 1979. External human fertilization. 240:57-67 (June). *The procedure and the issues it raises are examined.*

Jaffe, F.S. 1973. Public policy on fertility control. 229:17-23 (July). *Official policy and public attitude toward contraception have undergone substantial changes in the last few years.*

Tietze, C., and S. Lewit. 1977. Legal abortion. 236:21-27 (Jan.). *This age-old and controversial method of fertility control has now been adopted in many countries.*

PRINCIPLES

OF DEVELOPMENT

The dramatic moment of fertilization of a sea urchin egg. This scanning electron micrograph shows the sperm head attached to the egg surface. A fertilization cone, shown lifting from the surface (×29,000), and the rapidly elongating microvilli soon engulf the sperm.

Courtesy Gerald Schatten, Florida State University.

Growth and differentiation are fundamental characteristics of life (see Principles 21 and 22, p. 17). In Chapter 6 a brief survey of early embryonic development was given: types of eggs, fertilization and formation of the zygote, cleavage, and early morphogenesis. In this chapter we will first consider another dimension of development: the coordinating and regulating processes that guide the destiny of a growing embryo. The latter part of the chapter is devoted to the embryology of amniotes, especially humans, and the special adaptations that support development.

The phenomenon of development is a remarkable, and in many ways awesome, process. How is it possible that a tiny, spherical fertilized human egg, scarcely visible to the naked eye, can unfold into a fully formed, unique person, consisting of thousands of billions of cells, each cell performing a predestined functional or structural role? How is this marvelous unfolding controlled? Obviously all the information needed is contained within the egg, principally in the genes of the egg's nucleus. Thus, all development originates from the structure of the nuclear DNA molecules and in the egg cytoplasm surrounding the nucleus. But knowing where the blueprint for development resides is very different from understanding how this control system guides the conversion of a fertilized egg into a fully differentiated animal. This remains a major—many consider it *the* major—unsolved problem of biology. It has stimulated a vast amount of research on the processes and phenomena involved; some early, and in many cases tentative, answers have emerged.

EARLY CONCEPTS: PREFORMATION VERSUS EPIGENESIS

Early scientists and lay people alike speculated at length about the mystery of development long before the process was submitted to modern techniques of biochemistry, molecular biology, tissue culture, and electron microscopy. An early and persistent idea was that the young animal was preformed in the egg and that development was simply a matter of unfolding what was already there. Some claimed they could actually see a miniature of the adult in the egg or the sperm. Even the more cautious argued that all the parts of the embryo were in the egg, needing only to unfold, but so small and transparent they could not be seen. The concept of **preformation** was strongly advocated by most seventeenth- and eighteenth-century naturalist-philosophers.

William Harvey, the great physiologist of blood circulation fame, published a book on embryology in his old age (1651) that contained the conclusion "Omne vivum ex ova" ("Every living thing from the egg"). Harvey could not accept the naive doctrine of preformation but was unable to offer experimental evidence to refute it.

The preformation concept received its death blow in 1759 when the German embryologist Kaspar Friedrich Wolff clearly showed that in the earliest developmental stages of the chick, there was no embryo, only an undifferentiated granular material that became arranged into layers. These continued to thicken in some areas, to become thinner in others, to fold, and to segment, until the body of the embryo appeared. Wolff called this **epigenesis** ("origin upon or after"), an idea that the fertilized egg contains building material only, somehow assembled by an unknown directing force.

Remarkable pictures published at the time depicted a tiny human figure crouched inside a sperm, sometimes shown wearing a nightcap on its head!

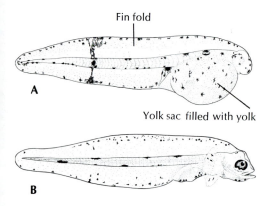

Fin fold

A

Yolk sac filled with yolk

B

Figure 36-1

Fish embryos showing yolk sac. **A,** The 1-day-old larva of a marine flounder has a large yolk sac. **B,** By the time the 10-day-old larva has developed a mouth and primitive digestive tract, its yolk supply has been exhausted. It must now catch its own food to survive and continue growing.

From Hickman, C.P., Jr.: Washington State Fisheries Research Papers 2:38-47, 1959.

Current ideas of development are essentially epigenetic in concept, although we know far more about what directs growth and differentiation. Development is not simply an unfolding of tissues and organs but is the progressive appearance, in stages, of structures not present at an earlier stage. At each stage of development new structures arise from conditions created in preceding stages. But once a particular structure embarks on a course of final differentiation, it becomes irrevocably committed to self-differentiation. It no longer depends on the stages that preceded it, nor does it have the option of forming anything different. Once a structure acquires the power of self-differentiation, it is said to be **determined.** Thus, differentiation is **progressive,** it is **irreversible,** and the final differentiated tissue is relatively **stable.**

DIRECT AND INDIRECT DEVELOPMENT

Even before fertilization, the egg is programmed to follow a special developmental course. The eggs of most marine invertebrates and those of many freshwater vertebrates typically develop into feeding larval forms that look and behave in a totally different manner from the mature adult. In such **indirect** development, the larva represents an adaptive detour in development that enables the animal to exploit microplankton or other food supplies and thus enhance its chances for a successful **metamorphosis** to the juvenile-adult body form. The eggs of animals having indirect development usually contain rather limited food reserves and are programmed for rapid differentiation into tiny, free-swimming larvae that must find their own food to sustain further growth (Fig. 36-1).

The eggs of mammals, birds, and reptiles show **direct** development; that is, the egg develops directly into a juvenile without passing through a highly specialized larval phase. In direct development, either the egg contains a large amount of stored food, as do the huge, yolky bird and reptile eggs, or the early embryo develops a nourishing, parasitic relationship with the maternal body, as do the small, nearly yolkless eggs of mammals. Direct development is more leisurely than indirect. The eggs are programmed to develop first into extensive sheets of unspecialized cells and then to differentiate into tissues and organs of a juvenile.

FERTILIZATION

Fertilization is the union of male and female gametes to form a **zygote.** This process accomplishes two things: it activates development, and it provides for the recombination of paternal and maternal genes. Thus, it restores the original diploid number of chromosomes characteristic of the species.

For a species to survive, it must ensure that fertilization will occur and that enough progeny will survive to continue the population. Many marine fishes simply set their eggs and sperm adrift in the ocean and rely on the random swimming movements of sperm to make chance encounters with eggs. Even though an egg is a large target for a sperm, the enormous dispersing effect of the ocean, the short life span of the gametes (usually just a few minutes for fish gametes), and the limited range of the tiny sperm all conspire against an egg and a sperm coming together. Accordingly, each male releases countless millions of sperm at spawning. The odds against fertilization are further reduced by coordinating the time and place of spawning of both parents.

Ensuring that some eggs are fertilized, however, is not enough. The ocean is a perilous environment for a developing fish, and most never make it to maturity. Most marine fishes are strong r-strategists (p. 1039), with high reproductive rates and high mortality. Thus, the females produce huge numbers of eggs. The common gray cod of the North American east coast regularly spawns 4 to 6 million eggs, of which only two or three eggs on the average will reach maturity. Fishes and other vertebrates that provide more protection to their young produce fewer eggs than do most marine fishes. The chance of the eggs and sperm meeting is also increased by courtship and mating procedures and the simultaneous shedding of the gametes in a nest or closely circumscribed area.

Internal fertilization, characteristic of the sharks and rays as well as reptiles, birds, and mammals, avoids dispersion of the gametes and protects them. However, even with internal fertilization, vast numbers of sperm must be released by the male into the female tract. Furthermore, the events of ovulation and insemination must be closely synchronized, and the gametes must remain viable for several hours to accomplish fertilization. Sperm may have to travel a considerable distance to reach the egg in the female genital tract, many parts of which may be hostile to sperm. Experiments with rabbits have shown that of the approximately 10 million sperm released into the female vagina, only about 100 reach the site of fertilization.

Oocyte Maturation

During oogenesis, described in the preceding chapter, the egg accumulates yolk reserves in preparation for future growth. The nucleus also grows rapidly in size during egg maturation, although not as much as the cell as a whole. It becomes bloated with nuclear sap and so changed in appearance that it was often given another name in older literature: the **germinal vesicle.**

Large amounts of both DNA and RNA accumulate during oogenesis. Early in the oogenesis of large amphibian eggs, the chromosomes become vastly expanded by thin loops thrown out laterally from the chromosomal axis; because of their fuzzy appearance, the chromosomes at this time are called **lampbrush chromosomes** (Fig. 37-20, p. 921). Ribosomal RNA is rapidly synthesized on DNA templates as each chromomere puffs out in lampbrush loops, exposing the double helix of DNA. Messenger RNA is also undergoing intense synthesis by the nucleolus during oocyte growth. The messenger RNA subsequently controls the synthesis of protein in the oocyte. In addition, a considerable quantity of DNA appears in the cytoplasm where it becomes bound to mitochondria and yolk platelets. Its function is unknown. Toward the end of oocyte maturation, this intense nucleic acid and protein synthesis gradually winds down. The lampbrush chromosomes contract and migrate to just beneath the egg surface, in preparation for the maturation divisions. The ribosomal RNA and proteins mix with the egg cytoplasm.

The oocyte is now poised for the maturation (meiotic) divisions, which rid it of excess chromosomal material (in the polar bodies, described in Chapter 35) (p. 854) and ready it for fertilization. A vast amount of synthetic activity has preceded this stage, all of which has packed the egg with reserve materials required for subsequent development.

In many vertebrates the primary oocyte proceeds with the maturation divisions only after it has approached its ultimate size. Even then, however, the divisions typically are interrupted by one or two periods of arrested development before maturation is completed. Human eggs, for example, begin their first meiotic divisions in the ovaries of the prenatal fetus. At birth, all the eggs of the human female infant are developmentally arrested in the diplotene stage of first meiotic prophase. This has been referred to as the "dictyate" stage; the egg is still a primary oocyte, and thus it remains until it is ovulated, a delay of perhaps 12 to 45 years! The first meiotic division is finally completed just before ovulation, and the second meiotic division occurs after the egg is fertilized.

Fertilization and activation

We began this section with the statement that fertilization accomplishes two ends: (1) activation of the quiescent egg to restore metabolic activity and start cleavage, and (2) insertion of a male haploid nucleus into the cytoplasm. However, we have already seen that the eggs of many species can be artificially induced to develop without sperm fertilization and that some species exhibit natural parthenogenesis (such as rotifers, aphids, bees, and wasps [p. 844]). Obviously the paternal genome is not essential for activation, although, in the majority of species, artificial parthenogenesis can seldom be taken past the last cleavage or blastula stage. The artificially activated egg may begin what appears to be normal development, but cleavage soon becomes abnormal and further growth ceases.

One reason that induced parthenogenesis is seldom successful is that the sperm normally contributes the **centriole** needed to form a normal mitotic spindle. For some reason the egg centriole disappears, or at least ceases to function, during the maturation divisions. If either natural or artificial parthenogenesis is to succeed, the egg centriole must be rendered capable of division. This is why in most artificial parthenogenesis experiments a so-called second factor of biological origin (such as blood or tissue fraction) is introduced into the egg cytoplasm. Exactly what this second factor contributes and whether it produces a new self-replicating centriole are not known.

Activation is a dramatic event. In sea urchin eggs, the contact of the spermatozoon with the egg surface sets off almost instantaneous changes in the egg cortex. At the point of contact a **fertilization cone** appears into which the sperm head is later drawn. From this point a visible change travels like a wave across the egg surface, causing immediate elevation of a **fertilization membrane** (Fig. 36-2). The immediate effect of the fertilization membrane is to prevent **polyspermy,** the abnormal entrance of more than one sperm. This is essential for normal development and is especially important for marine invertebrate eggs on which many hundreds of sperm may bind to the surface almost simultaneously (Fig. 36-3). In mammals relatively few sperm even reach the egg, and a rapid block to polyspermy is not important and seems not to occur.

Once the successful sperm binds to the egg surface, **cortical granules,** which form a layer beneath the plasma membrane, rupture and release materials that

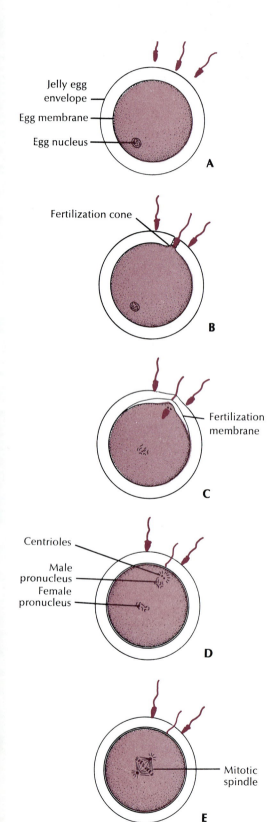

Figure 36-2

Fertilization of an egg. **A,** Many sperm swim to the egg. **B,** The first sperm to penetrate the protective jelly envelope and contact the egg membrane causes the fertilization cone to rise and engulf the sperm head. **C,** The fertilization membrane begins to form at the site of penetration and spreads around the entire egg, preventing the entrance of additional sperm. **D,** Male and female pronuclei approach one another, lose their nuclear membranes, swell, and fuse. **E,** The mitotic spindle forms, signaling creation of a zygote and heralding the first cleavage of a new embryo.

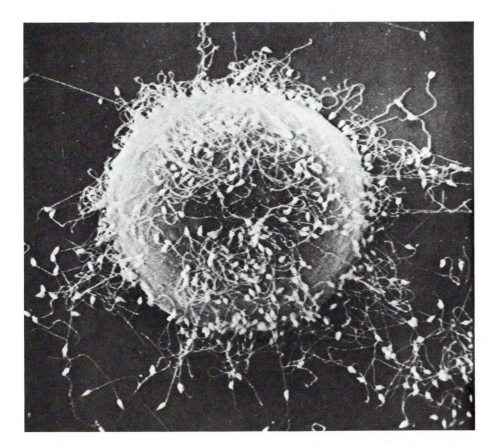

Figure 36-3

Binding of sperm to the surface of a sea urchin egg. Only one sperm penetrates the egg surface, the others being blocked from entrance by the rapid elevation of a fertilization membrane. Unsuccessful sperm soon fall away from the egg. (×1425.)

Courtesy Gerald Schatten, Florida State University.

fuse together to build up a new egg surface, the **hyaline layer.** It lies between the inner plasma membrane and the outer fertilization membrane. Additional sperm continue to bind to the egg for a few seconds, but as the hyaline layer forms, all but the successful sperm detach.

The **cortical reaction,** as these changes are called, is a crucial event in development. It seems to produce a complete molecular reorganization of the egg cortex. It also serves to remove one or more inhibitors that have blocked the energy-yielding systems and protein synthesis in the egg and have kept the egg in its quiescent, suspended-animation state. Almost immediately after the cortical reaction, polyribosomes form from the enormous supply of monoribosomes stored in the cytoplasm and begin producing protein. Normal metabolic activity is restored. The reduction divisions, if not completed, are brought to completion. The male and female pronuclei then fuse, and the zygote enters into cleavage.

___CLEAVAGE AND EARLY DEVELOPMENT

During cleavage the zygote divides repeatedly to convert the large, unwieldy cytoplasmic mass into a large number of small, maneuverable cells (called **blastomeres**) clustered together like a mass of soap bubbles. There is no growth during this period, only subdivision of mass, which continues until normal cell size and nucleocytoplasmic ratios are attained. At the end of cleavage the zygote has been divided into many hundreds of thousands of cells (about 1000 in polychaete worms, 9000 in amphioxus, and 700,000 in frogs). There is a rapid increase in DNA content during cleavage as the number of nuclei and the amount of DNA are doubled with each division. Apart from this, there is little change in chemical composition or displacement of constituent parts of the egg cytoplasm during cleavage. **Polarity**, that is, a polar axis, is present in the egg, and this establishes the direction of cleavage and subsequent differentiation of the embryo. Usually cleavage is very regular although enormously affected by the quantity of yolk present and whether cleavage is radial or spiral, as described previously (p. 129).

____ Regulative and Mosaic Development

In many species belonging to the Deuterostomia division of the animal kingdom (for example, echinoderms and vertebrates), the blastomeres of the early embryo are capable of regulating, or adjusting, their development to imposed damage. If, for example, a sea urchin embryo at the four-cell stage is placed in calcium-free seawater and gently shaken, the blastomeres will separate. Replaced in normal seawater, each separated blastomere will develop into a complete, although small, larva (Fig. 36-4, *A*). Early blastomeres of frog and rabbit embryos also can be separated and yield complete embryos. Such embryos are classified as **regulative** because separated blastomeres can regulate themselves into well-proportioned embryos. One can even fuse two sea urchin embryos together to produce one giant, but otherwise normal, larva. This is another form of regulation, because each of the original embryos is now contributing to only one-half the fused embryo.

The eggs of many invertebrates having spiral cleavage lack this early versatility. If the early blastomeres of a mollusc, annelid, flatworm, or ascidian are separated, each will continue to develop for a period as though it were still part of the whole; each forms a defective, partial embryo (Fig. 36-4, *B*). Such eggs are classified as **mosaic** and are said to have **mosaic development**.

The explanation behind these two types of development seems to lie in the extent to which distinctive regions of the cytoplasm destined for particular organs in the adult become localized during early cleavage. In mosaic eggs, localization of organ-forming regions of the cytoplasm occurs early, even before the first cleavage division. With such mosaic eggs it is often possible to map out the fates of specific areas on the uncleaved egg surface that are known to be presumptive for specific structures (Fig. 36-5). In regulative eggs, localization happens later in cleavage. Once localization is established in either type of egg, blastomeres cannot be damaged or removed from the embryo without corresponding defects in development.

____ Significance of the Cortex

Early cleavage proceeds independent of nuclear genetic information, guided instead by information deposited in the egg during its maturation. It was once believed that the visible particulate material in the cytoplasm had determinative properties. However, it was soon discovered that if the egg is strongly centrifuged so that everything inside—nucleus, mitochondria, lipid droplets, yolk, and other inclusions—is thoroughly displaced, the embryo still develops perfectly. If sea urchin eggs are examined by electron microscopy after being centrifuged for 5 minutes at several thousand times the force of gravity, the only thing not affected is the plasma membrane and a gel-like layer just beneath the plasma membrane (**plasmagel layer**). Yet development proceeds normally.

This and similar experiments show conclusively that the plasmagel (or cor-

Mammalian eggs are highly regulative. Human identical twins are monozygotic because they develop from a single zygote. Since most monozygotic twins share the same placenta, the separation of the embryos must have occurred after implantation when the inner cell mass, from which the embryo will form, consists of dozens of cells. It is possible to fuse two mammalian embryos together to form one giant embryo that develops normally. Recently, mice have been reared from three fused embryos representing six parents!

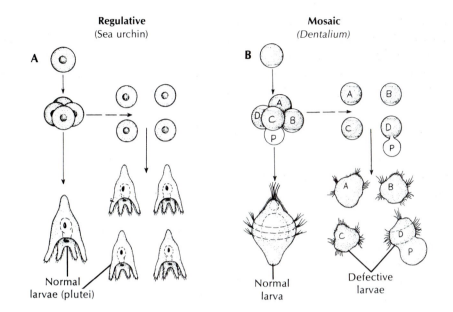

Figure 36-4

Regulative and mosaic cleavage. **A,** Indeterminate cleavage. Each of the early blastomeres (such as that of the sea urchin) when separated from the others develops into a small pluteus larva. **B,** Determinate (mosaic) cleavage. In the mollusc (such as *Dentalium*), when the blastomeres are separated, each gives rise to only a part of an embryo. The larger size of one of the defective larvae is the result of the formation of a polar lobe *(P)* composed of clear cytoplasm of the vegetal pole, which this blastomere alone receives.

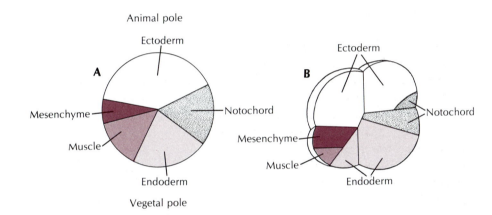

Figure 36-5

Segregation of organ-forming regions in, **A,** an ascidian (tunicate) egg and, **B,** an eight-cell embryo. This is a mosaic egg. Mapping of prospective regions in this way would be impossible in a highly regulative mammalian egg.

tical) layer of the egg contains an invisible but dynamic organization that determines the pattern of cleavage. Cortical organization is at first labile (especially so in regulative eggs) but soon becomes regionally fixed and irreversible. Thus, as cleavage progresses, the cortex and the cytoplasm enclosed become segregated into territories having specific determinative properties. This explains why different blastomeres bear different cytodifferentiation properties.

___ Delayed Nucleation Experiments

Another kind of experiment that demonstrates the importance of specific cortical regions of the egg was first carried out in 1938 by Hans Spemann, a German embryologist. Spemann put ligatures of human hair around newt eggs (amphibian eggs similar to frog eggs) just as they were about to divide, constricting them until they were almost, but not quite, separated into two halves (Fig. 36-6). The nucleus lay in one half of the partially divided egg; the other side was anucleate, containing only cytoplasm. The egg then completed its first cleavage division on the side containing the nucleus; the anucleate side remained undivided. Eventually, when

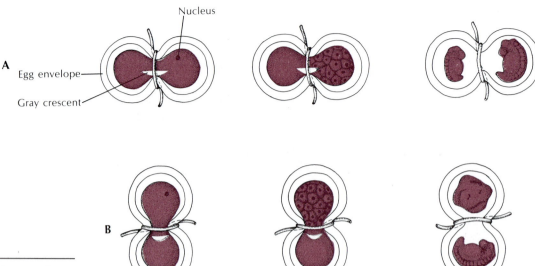

Figure 36-6

Spemann's delayed nucleation experiments. Two kinds of experiments were performed. **A,** Hair ligature was used to partly divide an uncleaved fertilized newt egg. Both sides contained part of the gray crescent. The nucleated side alone cleaved until a descendant nucleus crossed over the cytoplasmic bridge. Then both sides completed cleavage and formed two complete embryos. **B,** Hair ligature was placed so that the nucleus and gray crescent were completely separated. The side lacking the gray crescent became an unorganized piece of belly tissue; the other side developed normally.

the nucleated side had divided into about 16 cells, one of the cleavage nuclei would wander across the narrow cytoplasmic bridge to the anucleate side. Immediately this side began to divide.

With both halves of the embryo containing nuclei, Spemann drew the ligature tight, separating the two halves of the embryo. He then watched their development. Usually two complete embryos resulted. Although the one embryo possessed only one-sixteenth the original nuclear material, and the other contained fifteen sixteenths, they both developed normally. The one-sixteenth embryo was initially smaller, but it caught up in size in about 140 days. This showed that every nucleus of the 16-cell embryo contained a complete set of genes; all were equivalent.

Sometimes, however, Spemann observed that the nucleated half of the embryo developed only into an abnormal ball of "belly" tissue, although the half that received the delayed nucleus developed normally. Why should the more generously endowed fifteen-sixteenths embryo fail to develop and the small one-sixteenth embryo live? The explanation, Spemann discovered, depended on the position of the **gray crescent,** a pigment-free area on the egg surface. In amphibian eggs the gray crescent forms at the moment of fertilization and determines the plane of bilateral symmetry of the future animal. If one half of the constricted embryo lacked any part of the gray crescent, it would not develop.

Obviously, then, there must be cytoplasmic inequalities involved. The egg cortex in the area of the gray crescent contains substances that are essential for normal development. Since all the nuclei of the 16-cell embryo are equivalent, each capable of supporting full development, it is clear that the cytoplasmic environment is crucial to nuclear expression. The nuclei are all alike, but the cytoplasm (or cortex) throughout the embryo is not all alike. In some way chemically different regions of the egg, created during the early growth of the egg (oogenesis), are segregated out into specific cells during early cleavage. Thus, although all nuclei have the same information content, cytoplasmic substances surrounding the nucleus determine what part of the genome will be expressed and when (see Principle 24, p. 18).

___ PROBLEM OF DIFFERENTIATION

The egg cortex contains the primary guiding force for early development (cleavage and blastula formation), and synthetic activities during this period are supported by nucleic acids and reserves laid down in the egg cytoplasm *before* fertilization. However, continued differentiation past cleavage or the blastula stage requires the action of genetic information in the nuclear chromosomes. There is considerable evidence to show that this is so. If the maternal nucleus is removed from an activated but unfertilized frog egg, the anucleate egg will cleave more or less normally but arrest at the outset of gastrulation, when nuclear information is required.

Hybridization experiments have also been carried out in which the maternal nucleus is removed from the egg by microsurgery, just after the egg has been fertilized, but before the pronuclei have time to fuse. Such a zygote, called an **andromerogone,** contains *maternal* cytoplasm and a *paternal* (sperm) nucleus. The egg will cleave to the blastula stage normally; whether it will gastrulate depends on the compatibility of the sperm with the maternal cytoplasm. (Blastula and gastrula formation are described in Chapter 6, pp. 129-131.) If the egg was fertilized with a sperm of the same species, it develops into a haploid (but otherwise normal) tadpole. If it was fertilized with a sperm of a closely related species, it may develop to the neurula stage before development stops. If fertilized with a distantly related species, its development will arrest in the blastula or early gastrula stage. These differences are explained as varying degrees of immunological incompatibilities that appear when the paternal (sperm) genes begin coding for proteins in the embryo. The more foreign the sperm, the greater the incompatibility and the earlier the stage of arrest.

Finally, the most direct evidence that nuclear genes become active at or shortly before gastrulation is that the production of messenger RNA increases sharply at this time, followed by the production of transfer and ribosomal RNA. This has been demonstrated with the use of radioactively labeled RNA precursors.

___ Gene Expression

Gastrulation is a critical time of orderly and integrated cell movements. By folding processes (invagination and evagination) that segregate single epithelial layers and by splitting processes (delamination) that segregate multiple layers, the three prospective germ layers—ectoderm, mesoderm, and endoderm—are formed. This is followed by the rapid differentiation of germ layers into rudimentary, and later functional, tissues and organs.

As cells differentiate, they obviously use only a part of the instructions their nuclei contain. Cells that are differentiating into a thyroid gland are not concerned with that part of the genome that codes for a striated muscle, for example. The unneeded genes are in some way switched off. They are not destroyed, however, because a nucleus from a cell at an advanced stage of development transplanted into an activated egg whose nucleus has been removed can support development of a complete organism (see marginal note).

The basic problem is **gene expression.** What determines that a particular blastomere of, say, a 100-cell embryo will differentiate into muscle or skin or thyroid gland? Presumably the set of genes responsible for the development of a

Two Oxford scientists, J.B. Gurdon and R. Laskey, were able to grow a normal, reproductive adult frog from an unfertilized egg containing the nucleus of a differentiated intestinal cell of a frog tadpole. The technique they used had been developed by R. Briggs and T.J. King at Indiana University in 1952. Using minute glass needles, they were able to pluck out the nucleus from an egg and replace it with a nucleus from a fully differentiated cell. These experiments are of great significance because they demonstrate that a cell, or actually the nucleus from a cell, can be forced backward from its specialized state and once again make available all of its genetic information.

thyroid gland will be set in motion by the chemical environment found *only* in the region of the future thyroid gland. But how can such a unique chemical environment be created unless some *previous* genic action made the thyroid region different from the rest of the body? And even this earlier gene action must have been expressed in a unique chemical environment, or else thyroid glands would grow all over the body.

This kind of argument quickly takes one back to the fertilized egg itself. If genes are the same in all nuclei of the early embryo, the only way differences can develop is through interaction between these nuclei and the surrounding cytoplasm. We have already seen that the basic polarity of the egg and the organizing qualities of the egg cortex provide an early opportunity for such interactions.

Let us briefly summarize what is now known of the transmission of genetic information. Genetic information is coded in the sequence of nucleotides in DNA molecules (see Principle 18, p. 16). DNA serves as a template for the synthesis of messenger RNA in the nucleus. Messenger RNA then migrates out through nuclear pores into the cytoplasm, where it attaches to a ribosome. Here the messenger RNA serves as a template for the synthesis of specific proteins (see Principle 19, p. 16). In this way cytoplasmic proteins are formed that may be specific for that cell.

Evidence to date suggests that at the beginning of development most nuclear genes are inactive. Only small amounts of messenger RNA are being produced on the DNA templates. As development proceeds, new cytoplasmic proteins appear, indicating that more genic DNA is producing messenger RNA. Evidently different genes are activated (or "derepressed") in different parts of the young embryo, and this differential gene activity is responsible for embryonic differentiation.

What is the mechanism by which genes are repressed and then derepressed at specific times during development? We do not know at present. Whatever the mechanism is, it seems certain that the kinds of cytoplasm present in different cells determine what genes come into action. Nucleocytoplasmic interactions form the basis of the organized differentiation of tissues that characterizes animal development.

Embryonic Inductors and Organizers

Embryonic induction is a widespread phenomenon in development. It is the capacity of one tissue to evoke a specific developmental response in another. The classic experiments were reported in 1924 by Hans Spemann and Hilde Mangold. When a piece of dorsal blastopore lip from a salamander gastrula is transplanted into a ventral or lateral position of another salamander gastrula, it invaginates and develops a notochord and muscle somites. It also induces the *host* ectoderm to form a neural tube. Eventually a whole system of organs develops where the graft was placed, and this grows into a nearly complete secondary embryo (Fig. 36-7). This creature is composed partly of grafted tissue and partly of induced host tissue.

It was soon found that *only* grafts from the dorsal lip of the blastopore were capable of inducing the formation of a complete or nearly complete secondary embryo. This area corresponds to the presumptive areas of notochord, muscle somites, and prechordal plate. It was also found that only ectoderm of the host would develop a nervous system in the graft and that the reactive ability is greatest at the early gastrula stage and declines as the recipient embryo gets older.

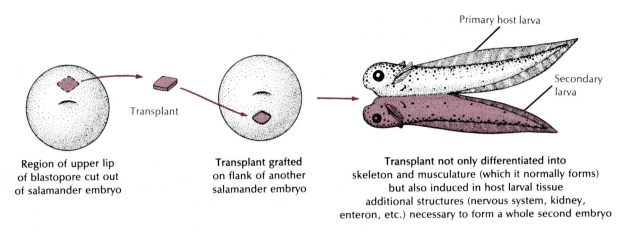

Region of upper lip
of blastopore cut out
of salamander embryo

Transplant

Transplant grafted
on flank of another
salamander embryo

Primary host larva

Secondary
larva

Transplant not only differentiated into
skeleton and musculature (which it normally forms)
but also induced in host larval tissue
additional structures (nervous system, kidney,
enteron, etc.) necessary to form a whole second embryo

Figure 36-7

Spemann's famous organizer experiment.

Spemann called the dorsal lip area the **primary organizer** because it was the only region capable of inducing the development of a complete embryo in the host. This region can be traced back to the gray crescent of the undivided fertilized egg, a cortical area that, as we have already seen, is crucial in directing early development of amphibian embryos (Fig. 36-6). Many other examples of embryonic induction have been discovered, both in amphibians, a favorite for study, and in other vertebrate and invertebrate species.

Efforts to discover the chemical nature of the inductor have met with much less success. Embryologists were dismayed to find that a great variety of denatured animal materials could cause inductive responses. Obviously the dorsal lip graft did not "organize" a particular differentiation; rather it evoked a response that was already part of the induced tissue's total developmental capacity and repertoire. The inductor appears to play a permissive rather than an instructive role by providing a favorable environment in which the stimulated tissue releases a pre-programmed response.

In normal development, induction operates by cell-to-cell contact. However, it may not always require cell-to-cell contact because, when small pieces of inductors and responding tissues are cultured together but separated from one another by a porous nitrocellulose filter, induction still occurs. The inducing substance must be a chemical signal that diffuses through the pores of the filter to reach the responding tissue.

Usually a tissue that has differentiated acts as an inductor for an adjacent undifferentiated tissue. Timing is important. Once a primary inductor sets in motion a specific developmental pattern in one tissue, numerous secondary inductions follow. What emerges is a sequential pattern of development involving not only inductors but cell movement, changes in adhesive properties of cells, and cell proliferation. This is why developmental patterns are so difficult to unravel. There is no master control panel that directs development, but rather a sequence of local patterns in which one step in development is a subunit of another.

The chemical nature of inductors is still unknown. Despite the enormous research effort that has been devoted to induction, the phenomenon has remained so resistant to experimental unveiling that embryologists find themselves with little more insight into the question than they had half a century ago. Nevertheless, in showing that one step in development is a necessary requisite for the next, Hans Spemann's induction experiments were among the most significant events in experimental embryology.

AMNIOTES AND THE AMNIOTIC EGG

Reptiles, birds, and mammals form a natural grouping of vertebrates distinguished by having an amniotic egg. They are called **amniotes,** meaning that they develop an amnion, one of the extraembryonic membranes that make the development of these forms unique among animals.

As rapidly growing living organisms, embryos have the same basic animal requirements as adults—nutrients, fuels, oxygen, and disposal of wastes. For the embryos of the many invertebrates that develop in the external environment, gas exchange is a simple matter of direct diffusion. The egg may contain only enough yolk to sustain the embryo through hatching, when it must begin to feed itself. Beyond hatching, the embryo (now called a free-swimming **larva**) is on its own.

Yolk enclosed in a membranous **yolk sac** is a conspicuous feature of all fish embryos (Fig. 36-1). The yolk is gradually used up as the embryo grows; the yolk sac shrinks and finally is enclosed within the body of the embryo. The mass of yolk is an **extraembryonic** structure, since it is not really a part of the embryo proper, and the yolk sac is an **extraembryonic membrane.** Bird and reptile eggs are also provided with large amounts of yolk to support early development. In birds (direct development), the yolk reaches relatively massive proportions, since it must nourish a baby bird to a much more advanced stage of development at hatching than a larval fish.

In abandoning an aquatic life for a land existence, the first terrestrial animals had to evolve a sophisticated egg containing a complete life-support system. Thus appeared the **amniotic egg,** equipped to protect and support the growth of embryos on dry land. In addition to the **yolk sac** containing the nourishing yolk are three other membranous sacs: **amnion, chorion,** and **allantois.** All are referred to as extraembryonic membranes because, again, they are accessory structures that develop beyond the embryonic body and are discarded when the embryo hatches. (We should note that since the amnion is only one of four extraembryonic membranes, the "amniotic" egg could just as well be called a "chorionic" or an "allantoic" egg.)

The **amnion** is a fluid-filled bag that encloses the embryo and provides a private aquarium for development (Fig. 36-8). Floating freely in this aquatic environment, the embryo is fully protected from shocks and adhesions. The evolution of this structure, from which the amniotic egg takes its name, was crucial to the successful habitation of land.

The **allantois,** another component in the support system for embryos of land animals, is a bag that grows out of the hindgut of the embryo (Fig. 36-8). It collects the wastes of metabolism (mostly uric acid). At hatching, the young animal breaks its connection with the allantois and leaves it and its refuse behind in the shell.

The **chorion** (also called **serosa**) is an outermost extraembryonic membrane that completely encloses the rest of the embryonic system. It lies just beneath the shell (Fig. 36-8). As the embryo grows and its need for oxygen increases, the allantois and chorion fuse to form a **chorioallantoic membrane.** This double membrane is provided with a rich vascular network, connected to the embryonic circulation. Lying just beneath the porous shell, the vascular chorioallantoic membrane serves as a provisional lung across which oxygen and carbon dioxide can freely exchange. Although nature did not plan for it, the chorioallantoic mem-

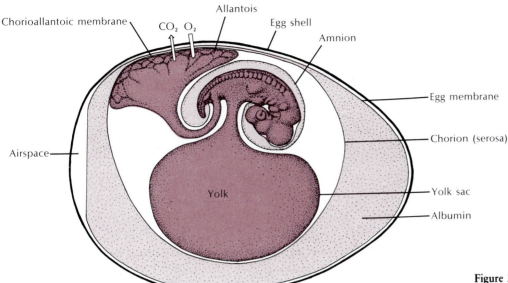

Chorioallantoic membrane

CO₂ O₂

Allantois

Egg shell

Amnion

Egg membrane

Chorion (serosa)

Airspace

Yolk

Yolk sac

Albumin

Figure 36-8

Amniotic egg at early stage of development showing a chick embryo and its extraembryonic membranes. Porous shell allows gaseous exchange of oxygen and carbon dioxide. Circulatory channels from embryo's body to allantois and yolk sac are not shown.

brane of the chicken egg has been used extensively by generations of experimental embryologists as a place to culture chick and mammalian tissues.

The great importance of the amniotic egg to the establishment of a land existence cannot be overemphasized. Amphibians must return to water to lay their eggs. But the reptiles, even before they took to land, developed the amniotic egg with its self-contained aquatic environment enclosed by a tough outer shell. Protected from drying out and provided with yolk for nourishment, such eggs could be laid on dry land, far from water. Reptiles were thus freed from aquatic life and could become the first true terrestrial tetrapods.

Incidentally, the sexual act itself comes from the requirement that the egg be fertilized *before* the eggshell is wrapped around it, if it is to develop. Thus, the male must introduce the sperm into the female tract so that the sperm can reach the egg before it passes to that part of the oviduct where the shell is secreted. Hence, as one biologist put it, it is the eggshell, and not the devil, that deserves the blame for the happy event we know as sex.

HUMAN DEVELOPMENT

The amniotic egg, for all its virtues, has one basic flaw: placed neatly in a nest, it makes fine food for other animals. It was left for the mammals to evolve the best solution for early development: allow the embryo to grow within the protective confines of the mother's body. This has resulted in important modifications in the development of mammals as compared with other vertebrates. The earliest mammals, descended from early reptiles, were egg layers. Even today the most primitive mammals, the monotremes (for example, duck-billed platypus, spiny anteater), lay large yolky eggs that closely resemble bird eggs. In the marsupials (pouched mammals such as the opossum and kangaroo), the embryos develop for a time within the mother's uterus. But the embryo does not "take root" in the uterine wall, as do the embryos of the more advanced **placental mammals,** and consequently it receives little nourishment within the mother. The young of mar-

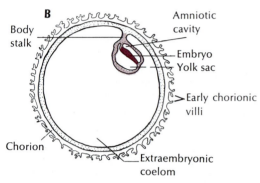

Figure 36-9

Early development of human embryo. **A,** Blastocyst at about 7 days. The trophoblast gives rise to the chorion, which later becomes part of the placenta; the inner cell mass becomes the embryo. **B,** Blastocyst at about 15 days. Note the amniotic cavity and yolk sac; primary villi are developing from the chorion to begin establishment of the placenta.

supials are therefore born immature and are sheltered and nourished in a pouch of the abdominal wall.

All other mammals, the placentalians, nourish their young in the uterus by means of a **placenta**.

Early Development of the Human Embryo

The eggs of all placental mammals, although relatively enormous on a cellular scale, are small by egg standards. The human egg is approximately 0.1 mm in diameter and barely visible to the unaided eye. It contains very little yolk. After fertilization in the oviduct, the dividing egg begins a 5-day journey down the oviduct toward the uterus, propelled by a combination of ciliary action and muscular peristalsis. Cleavage is very slow: 24 hours for the first cleavage and 10 to 12 hours for each subsequent cleavage. By comparison, frog eggs cleave once every hour. Cleavage produces a small ball of 20 to 30 cells (called the morula) within which appears a fluid-filled cavity, the **segmentation** cavity (Fig. 36-9). This is comparable to the blastocoele of a frog's egg (Fig. 6-6, p. 130). The embryo is now called a **blastocyst.**

At this point, development of the mammalian embryo departs radically from that of lower vertebrates. A mass of cells, called the **inner cell mass,** develops on one side of the peripheral cell, or **trophoblast,** layer (Fig. 36-9). The inner cell mass forms the embryo, whereas the surrounding trophoblast forms the placenta. When the blastocyst is approximately 6 days old and composed of approximately 100 cells, it contacts and implants into the uterine endometrium (Fig. 36-10). Very little is known of the forces involved in implantation, or why, incidentally, the intrauterine birth control devices (coil and loop) are so effective in preventing successful implantation. On contact, the trophoblast cells proliferate rapidly and produce enzymes that break down the epithelium of the uterine endometrium. This allows the blastocyst to sink into the endometrium. By the eleventh or twelfth day the blastocyst, totally buried, has eroded through the walls of capillaries and small arterioles; this releases a pool of blood that bathes the embryo. At first the minute embryo derives what nourishment it requires by direct diffusion from the surrounding blood. But very soon a remarkable fetal-maternal structure, the **placenta,** develops to assume these exchange tasks.

Placenta

The placenta is a marvel of biological engineering. Serving as a provisional lung, intestine, and kidney for the embryo, it performs elaborate selective activities without ever allowing the maternal and fetal blood to intermix (very small amounts of fetal blood may regularly escape into the maternal system without causing harm). The placenta permits the entry of foodstuffs, hormones, vitamins, and oxygen and the exit of carbon dioxide and metabolic wastes. Its action is highly selective; it allows some materials to enter that are chemically quite similar to others that are rejected.

The two circulations are physically separated at the placenta by an exceedingly thin membrane (in places only 2 µm thick), across which materials are transferred by diffusive interchange. The transfer occurs across thousands of tiny, fingerlike projections, called **chorionic villi,** which develop from the original chorion membrane (Figs. 36-9 and 36-10). These projections sink like roots into the

12 days   4 weeks   5 weeks

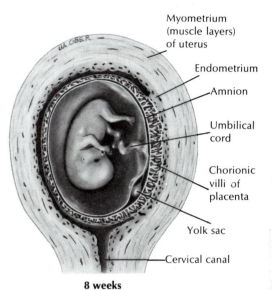

Figure 36-10

Development of a human embryo from 12 days to 12 weeks. The 8-week-old embryo and uterus are drawn to actual size. As the embryo grows, the placenta develops into a disclike structure attached to one side of the uterus. Note the vestigial yolk sac.

8 weeks

12 weeks
(fetus)

uterine endometrium after the embryo implants. As development proceeds and embryonic demands for food and gas exchange increase, the great proliferation of villi in the placenta vastly increases its total surface area. Although the human placenta at term measures only 18 cm (7 inches) across, its total absorbing surface is approximately 13 square meters—50 times the surface area of the skin of the newborn infant.

Since the mammalian embryo is protected and nourished by the placenta, what becomes of the various embryonic membranes of the amniotic egg whose functions are no longer required? Surprisingly perhaps, all of these special membranes are still present, although they may be serving a new function. The yolk sac is retained, and during early development it is the source of lymphocytes that later migrate to the spleen and liver (later still they migrate again to the bone marrow) to originate the body's immune system. The amnion remains unchanged, a protective water jacket in which the embryo floats. The remaining two extraembryonic membranes, the allantois and chorion, have been totally redesigned. The allantois is no longer needed as a urinary bladder. Instead it becomes the stalk, or **umbilical cord,** that links the embryo physically and functionally with the placenta. The chorion, the outermost membrane, forms most of the placenta itself.

One of the most intriguing questions the placenta presents is why it is not rejected by the mother's tissues. The placenta is a uniquely successful foreign transplant, or **allograft.** It (as well as the embryo) is genetically foreign in the sense that it consists of tissue derived not only from the mother but also from the father. We should expect it to be rejected by the uterine tissues, just as a piece of a child's skin is rejected by the child's mother when a surgeon attempts a grafting transplant (p. 708). The placenta in some way circumvents the normal rejection phenomenon, a matter of greatest interest to immunologists seeking ways to transplant tissues and organs successfully.

Development of Systems and Organs

Pregnancy may be divided into four phases: the first phase, lasting 6 or 7 days, is the period of cleavage and blastocyst formation and ends when the blastocyst implants in the uterus. The second phase, about 2 weeks, is the period of gastrulation and formation of the neural plate. The third phase, called the **embryonic period,** is a crucial and sensitive period of primary organ system differentiation. This phase ends at about the eighth week of pregnancy. The last phase, known as the **fetal period,** is characterized by rapid growth, proportional changes in body parts, and final preparation for birth.

During gastrulation the three germ layers are formed. These differentiate, as we have seen, first into primordial cell masses and then into specific organs and tissues. During this process, cells become increasingly committed to specific directions of differentiation.

Derivatives of ectoderm: nervous system and nerve growth

The brain, spinal cord, and nearly all the outer epithelial structures of the body develop from the primitive ectoderm. They are among the earliest organs to appear. Just above the notochord, the **ectoderm** thickens to form a **neural plate** (Fig. 36-11). The edges of this plate rise up, fold, and join together at the top to create an elongated, hollow **neural tube.** The neural tube gives rise to most of the nervous system: anteriorly it enlarges and differentiates into the brain, cranial nerves, and eyes; posteriorly it forms the spinal cord and spinal motor nerves. Sensory nerves arise from special **neural crest** cells pinched off from the neural tube before it closes.

How are the billions of nerve axons in the body formed? What directs their growth? Biologists were intrigued with these questions that seemed to have no easy solutions. Since a single nerve axon may be more than a meter in length (for example, motor nerves running from the spinal cord to the toes), it seemed impossible that a single cell could spin out so far. It was suggested that a nerve fiber grew from a series of preformed protoplasmic bridges along its route. The answer had to await the development of one of the most powerful tools available to biologists, the cell culture technique.

In 1907 embryologist Ross G. Harrison discovered that he could culture living neuroblasts (embryonic nerve cells) for weeks outside the body by placing them in a drop of frog lymph hung from the underside of a cover slip. Watching nerves grow for periods of days, he saw that each nerve fiber was the outgrowth of a single cell. As the fibers extended outward, materials for growth flowed down the axon center to the growing tip where they were incorporated into new protoplasm.

The second question—what directs nerve growth—has taken longer to unravel. An idea held well into the 1940s was that nerve growth is a random, diffuse process. It was believed that the nervous system developed as an equipotential network, or blank slate, that later would be shaped by usage into a functional system. The nervous system just seemed too incredibly complex for us to imagine that nerve fibers could find their way selectively to so many predetermined destinations. Yet it appears that this is exactly what they do! Recent work indicates that each of the billions of nerve cell axons acquires a chemical identification tag that in some way directs it along a correct path. Many years ago Harrison observed that a growing nerve axon terminated in a "growth cone," from which extend numerous tiny threadlike processes (Fig. 36-12). These are constantly reaching out and testing the environment in all directions to guide the nerve chemically to its proper destination. This chemical guidepost system, which must, of course, be genetically directed, is just one example of the amazing precision that characterizes the entire process of differentiation.

Derivatives of endoderm: digestive tube and survival of gill arches

In the frog embryo the primitive gut makes its appearance during gastrulation with the formation of an internal cavity, the **archenteron.** From this simple endodermal cavity develop the lining of the digestive tract, the lining of the pharynx

The tissue culture technique developed by Ross G. Harrison is now used extensively by scientists in all fields of active biomedical research, not just by embryologists. The great impact of the technique has been felt only in recent years. Harrison was twice considered for the Nobel Prize (1917 and 1933), but he failed ever to receive the award because, ironically, the tissue culture method was then believed to be "of rather limited value."

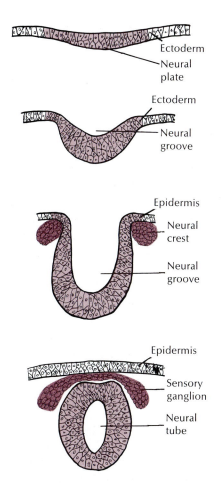

Ectoderm
Neural plate

Ectoderm
Neural groove

Epidermis
Neural crest
Neural groove

Epidermis
Sensory ganglion
Neural tube

Figure 36-11

Development of neural tube and neural crest from neural plate ectoderm (cross section).

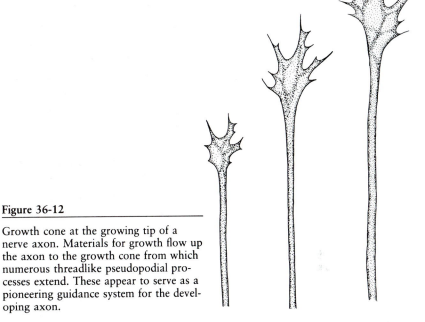

Figure 36-12

Growth cone at the growing tip of a nerve axon. Materials for growth flow up the axon to the growth cone from which numerous threadlike pseudopodial processes extend. These appear to serve as a pioneering guidance system for the developing axon.

and lungs, most of the liver and pancreas, the thyroid and parathyroid glands, and the thymus.

The **alimentary canal** develops from the primitive gut and is folded off from the yolk sac by the growth and folding of the body wall (Fig. 36-13). The ends of the tube open to the exterior and are lined with ectoderm, whereas the rest of the tube is lined with endoderm. The **lungs, liver,** and **pancreas** arise from the foregut.

Among the most intriguing derivatives of the digestive tract are the pharyngeal (gill) arches and pouches, which make their appearance in the early embryonic stages of all vertebrates (Fig. 36-14). In fishes, the gill arches develop into gills and supportive structures and serve as respiratory organs. When the early vertebrates moved onto land, gills were unsuitable for aerial respiration and were replaced by lungs.

Why then do gill arches persist in the embryos of terrestrial vertebrates? Certainly not for the convenience of biologists who use these and other embryonic structures to reconstruct lines of vertebrate descent. Even though the gill arches serve no respiratory function in either the embryos or adults of terrestrial vertebrates, they remain as necessary primordia for a great variety of other structures. For example, the first arch and its endoderm-lined pouch (the space between adjacent arches) form the upper and lower jaws and inner ear of higher vertebrates. The second, third, and fourth gill pouches contribute to the tonsils, parathyroid gland, and thymus. We can understand then why gill arches and other fishlike structures appear in early mammalian embryos. Their original function

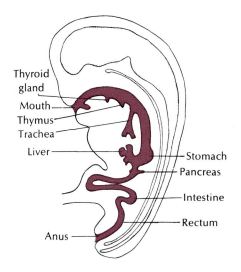

Thyroid gland
Mouth
Thymus
Trachea
Liver
Stomach
Pancreas
Intestine
Rectum
Anus

Figure 36-13

Derivatives of the alimentary canal of a human embryo.

Figure 36-14

Comparison of gill arches of different vertebrate embryos at equivalent stages of development.

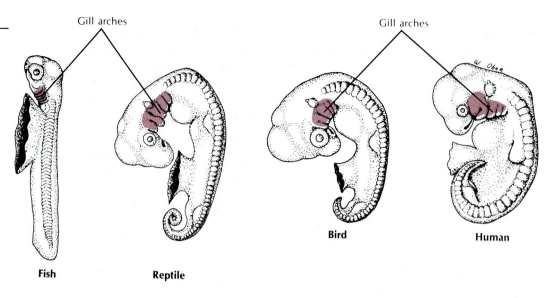

Gill arches

Gill arches

Fish

Reptile

Bird

Human

Figure 36-15

Human embryo showing muscle somites.

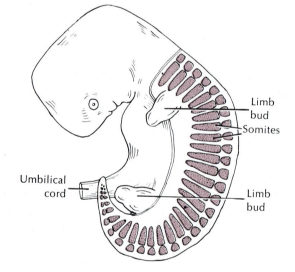

Limb bud
Somites

Umbilical cord

Limb bud

has been abandoned, but the structures are retained for new purposes. It is the great conservatism of early embryonic development that has so conveniently provided us with a telescoped evolutionary history.

Derivatives of mesoderm: support, movement, and beating heart

The intermediate germ layer, the mesoderm, forms the vertebrate skeletal, muscular, and circulatory structures and the kidney. As vertebrates have increased in size and complexity, the mesodermally derived supportive, movement, and transport structures make up an ever greater proportion of the body bulk.

Most **muscles** arise from the mesoderm along each side of the spinal cord (Fig. 36-15). This mesoderm divides into a linear series of somites (38 in humans), which by splitting, fusion, and migration become the muscles of the body and axial parts of the skeleton. The **limbs** begin as buds from the side of the body. Projections of the limb buds develop into fingers and toes.

Although the primitive mesoderm appears after the ectoderm and endoderm, it gives rise to the first functional organ, the embryonic heart. Guided by the underlying endoderm, clusters of precardiac mesodermal cells move ameba-like into a central position between the underlying primitive gut and the overlying neural tube. Here the heart is established, first as a single, thin tube.

Even while the cells group together, the first twitchings are evident. In the chick embryo, a favorite and nearly ideal animal for experimental embryology studies, the primitive heart begins to beat on the second day of the 21-day incubation period; it begins beating before any true blood vessels have formed and before there is any blood to pump. As the ventricle primordium develops, the spontaneous cellular twitchings become coordinated into a feeble but rhythmical beat. Then, as the atrium develops behind the ventricle, followed by the development of the sinus venosus behind the atrium, the heart rate quickens. Each new heart chamber has an intrinsic beat that is faster than its predecessor.

Finally a specialized area of heart muscle called the **sinoatrial** node develops in the sinus venosus and takes command of the entire heartbeat. This becomes the heart's **pacemaker.** As the heart builds up a strong and efficient beat, vascular channels open within the embryo and across the yolk. Within the vessels are the first primitive blood cells suspended in plasma.

The early development of the heart and circulation is crucial to continued embryonic development because without a circulation the embryo could not obtain materials for growth. Food is absorbed from the yolk and carried to the embryonic body; oxygen is delivered to all the tissues, and carbon dioxide and other wastes are carried away. The embryo is totally dependent on these extraembryonic support systems, and the circulation is the vital link between them.

Fetal Circulation

The fetal circulation is another engineering marvel. During fetal development the placenta must function for the lungs, since these of course are nonfunctional in the fetus, which has no access to air. Thus, the blood must be diverted to the placenta from the fetal lungs, and done so in such a way that instantaneous conversion to the adult pattern of circulation is allowed when the newborn infant takes its first breath. There are several parts of the solution, as explained in the following paragraphs and illustrated in Fig. 36-16.

The interchange of nutrients and respiratory gases occurs via the **umbilical cord,** which is composed of one umbilical vein and two umbilical arteries. The umbilical vein, which carries oxygenated blood from the placenta, passes through the umbilical cord and then to the liver, through which the blood passes via a special embryonic vessel, the **ductus venosus.** This vessel joins the inferior vena cava, which enters the right atrium. At this point in the normal adult pattern, the venous blood would be pumped into the right ventricle and from there to the pulmonary artery and lungs. However, the collapsed fetal lungs cannot possibly accept the total volume of blood entering the right side of the heart. A partial solution to this problem is the provision of a large connection, the **ductus arteriosus,** between the pulmonary artery and the aorta into which the blood is diverted. Not all the venous blood follows this route, however, because a second diversionary passage, a hole in the interatrial septum called the **foramen ovale,** allows about half the blood to pass directly from the right to the left atrium. Thus, both ventricles receive approximately equal amounts of blood to pump, as they do in the postnatal condition, even though their usual connection, the pulmonary circuit, is not yet operating. The fetal circuit is completed by two umbilical arteries from the iliac arteries that return blood to the placenta.

Figure 36-16

Fetal circulation. Blood carrying food
and oxygen from the placenta is brought
by the umbilical vein to the liver, is
shunted through the ductus venosus to
the vena cava where it mixes with deoxygenated blood returning from fetal tissues, and then is carried to the right atrium. Two fetal shortcuts bypass the non-
functioning lungs. Some blood goes directly from the right atrium to the left
atrium by an opening, the foramen ovale,
and so enters the systemic circulation.
Some blood passes from the pulmonary
trunk into the aorta by a temporary duct,
the ductus arteriosus. At birth, placental
exchange ceases; the ductus venosus, foramen ovale, umbilical arteries, and ductus arteriosus all close; and regular postnatal pulmonary and systemic circuits
take over.

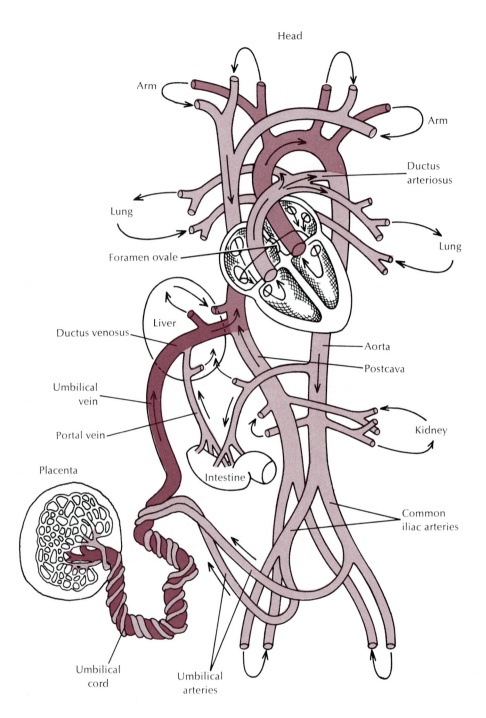

At birth, the placental bloodstream is cut off, and the pulmonary circulation
opens as the infant draws the first lung-expanding breath. The system is ingeniously prepared for this sudden event. The muscular walls of the ductus arteriosus are particularly sensitive to the blood-oxygen tension. As soon as the blood
oxygen rises with the onset of breathing, the ductus arteriosus closes. The other
diversionary opening, the foramen ovale, is provided with a flap valve that shuts
automatically at birth as the blood pressure in the more powerful left side of the
heart rises above that of the right side. In time, all traces of the foramen ovale are
obliterated, and the ductus arteriosus and the umbilical vessels become reduced to
fibrous cords.

___ Birth (Parturition)

Hormonal changes preceding birth

During pregnancy the placenta gradually takes over most of the functions of regulating growth and development of the uterus and the fetus. As an endocrine gland, it secretes estradiol and progesterone, hormones that are secreted by the ovaries and corpus luteum in the early periods of pregnancy (p. 858). The placenta also produces **chorionic gonadotropin,** a hormone that now assumes the role of the LH and FSH pituitary hormones. These cease their secretions at about the second month of pregnancy. Chorionic gonadotropin maintains the corpus luteum so that the latter may continue secreting progesterone and estradiol necessary for the integrity of the placenta. In the later stages of pregnancy the placenta becomes a totally independent endocrine organ, not requiring support from either the corpus luteum or the pituitary gland.

What stimulates birth? Why does pregnancy not continue indefinitely? What factors produce the onset of labor (the rhythmical contractions of the uterus)? Thus far we have only tentative answers to these questions. It has long been known that estrogens stimulate uterine contractions, whereas progesterone, which is also secreted by the placenta, inhibits uterine activity. Just before birth there is a very sharp increase in the plasma level of estrogens and a decrease in progesterone. This appears to remove the "progesterone block" that keeps the uterus in a quiescent state throughout pregnancy. Thus, labor contractions can proceed.

Recently much more information on the control of birth has emerged, involving **prostaglandins,** a group of hormonelike long-chain fatty acids. Prostaglandins have complex actions on virtually all body tissues and organs. They are especially powerful in stimulating contractions and, when used pharmacologically, are very effective in inducing labor or abortion. There is increasing evidence from studies on sheep (which, like human females, have an endocrine placenta during pregnancy) that the fetus itself controls the onset of labor. In some way not yet understood, the fetus, when it reaches normal term weight, releases an endocrine signal that stimulates the placenta to produce prostaglandins and thus initiates labor.

Stages in childbirth

The first major signal that birth is imminent is the so-called labor pains, caused by the rhythmical contractions of the uterine musculature. These are usually slight at first and occur at intervals of 15 to 30 minutes. They gradually become more intense, longer in duration, and more frequent. Some women compare the contractions to menstrual cramps. To some they are painful; to others they are not. Labor contractions may last anywhere from 4 to 24 hours, usually longer with the first child. The squeezing action of these contractions changes the position of the baby, usually so that the head presses against the cervix.

Childbirth occurs in three stages. In the first stage the neck (cervix), or opening of the uterus into the vagina, is enlarged by the pressure of the baby in its bag of amniotic fluid, which may be ruptured at this time. In the second stage the baby is forced out of the uterus and through the vagina to the outside (Fig. 36-17). In the third stage the placenta, or afterbirth, is expelled from the mother's body, usually within 10 minutes after the baby is born.

Figure 36-17

Birth of a baby.
Courtesy American Museum of Natural History.

Multiple births

Many mammals give birth to more than one offspring at a time or to a litter, each member of which has come from a separate egg. Most higher mammals, however, have only one offspring at a time, although occasionally they may have plural young. The armadillo *(Dasypus)* is almost unique among mammals in giving birth to four young at one time—all of the same sex, either male or female, and all derived from one zygote.

Human twins may come from one zygote (identical twins) or two zygotes (nonidentical, or fraternal, twins). Triplets, quadruplets, and quintuplets may include a pair of identical twins. The other babies in such multiple births usually come from separate zygotes. Fraternal twins do not resemble each other more than other children born separately in the same family, but identical twins are, of course, strikingly alike and always of the same sex. Embryologically, each member of fraternal twins has its own placenta, chorion, and amnion. Usually (but not always) identical twins share the same chorion and the same placenta, but each has its own amnion. Sometimes identical twins fail to separate completely and form Siamese twins, in which the organs of one may be a mirror image of the organs of the other. The frequency of twin births in comparison to single births is approximately 1 in 86, that of triplets approximately 1 in 86^2, and that of quadruplets approximately 1 in 86^3.

——LONGEVITY, AGING, AND DEATH

We will end our consideration of development with one aspect that some might wish to ignore: the inevitability of death. Each animal has a characteristic life span. The allotted lifetime of a human being would appear to be the biblical 3 score and 10 years. Even today, despite the achievements of modern medicine, the average life span is still about 70 years. Life spans among other animals vary enormously, and it is a common understanding that large animals live longer than small ones. The Indian elephant may reach 70 years; a hippopotamus or rhinoceros, 50 years; a horse, 45 years; a black bear or gorilla, 25 years; a beaver, 20 years; dogs and cats, 15 years; a gray squirrel, 10 years; a chipmunk, 5 years; a house mouse, 2 years; and a shrew, 1 year. Among birds, some parrots and owls may exceed 60 years (the record appears to be a 68-year-old eagle owl). Cranes and ostriches may live 40 years. However, most of our familiar songbirds are fortunate to reach 10 years, even under the benign conditions of captivity.

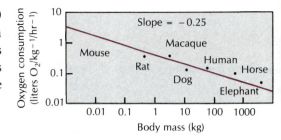

Figure 36-18

Rate of oxygen consumption ($\log_{10}$) of various mammals plotted against body weight ($\log_{10}$). Points tend to fall along a straight line on logarithmic coordinates, with a slope of -0.25.

___ Why Do Humans Live So Long?

Reptiles are noted for longevity, and centenarians are common among giant Galápagos tortoises. However, they are probably the only animals than can routinely outlive people. We live far longer—perhaps three times longer—than other mammals of our body size. Our exceptional longevity has been attributed to **neoteny**: retention of larval or juvenile characteristics in the adult form. "The life course of man runs slowly," wrote Louis Bolk, Dutch advocate of this hypothesis. Compared with the development of any other primate, ours is severely retarded. We are born as helpless embryos and have a protracted infancy, childhood, and juvenility. Nearly 30% of our life span is devoted to growing. Our bones ossify late. At birth, the brain is still growing at fetal rates and continues to grow rapidly for the first year after birth. It is thought that gestation is shortened (it "should" be 21 months) because the extension of rapid early embryonic growth rates produces a large birth weight in only 9 months. Birth occurs when the brain is just one-fourth its ultimate size. To prolong gestation even to 1 year would require radical redesign of the birth canal (Gould, 1977).

The nineteenth-century physiologist Max Rubner had a hypothesis of aging that has recently received renewed support. He concluded that all mammals in their lifetimes use up about the same number of calories per unit of body weight. A mouse that lives for 2 years lives its life far more intensively than an elephant that lives for 70 years. This relationship is explained by **scaling theory,** an interpretation of the structural and functional consequences of a change in size (or in scale) among similar groups of animals. For example, the rate of oxygen consumption decreases consistently with increasing body size. This means that among mammals—the group that reveals scaling relationships most clearly—small mammals consume more oxygen and generate more heat in proportion to their body weight than do large mammals. When we plot the logarithm of body weight against the logarithm of oxygen consumption (Fig. 36-18), we obtain a straight line with a negative slope of -0.25. Thus, the rate of oxygen consumption of a 10 kg animal is only three-fourths that of a 1 kg animal. Certain physiological properties such as heart rate and breathing rate are scaled, like oxygen consumption, to body weight. In other words, heart rates and breathing rates slow down as animals increase in size. Significantly, lifetimes scale approximately at a three-quarter power of body weight: a 10 kg mammal should live about 7.5 times as long as a 1 kg mammal. Combining lifetimes with heart rate, we arrive at the amazing conclusion that the hearts of all mammals, regardless of size, beat about the same number of times—800 million—in their allotted life spans. Because the breathing rate is about one-fourth the heart rate, a mammal will breathe about 200 million times. Lifetime is scaled to life's pace, and all mammals, should they live out their "natural" lives, will survive about the same length of *biological* time. But we humans deviate dramatically from our mammalian kin: our hearts beat three times as often, and we take three times as many breaths, as any other mammal of comparable body size.

___ The Aging Process

The outward signs of aging are obvious, but the basic process remains obscure. Until recently, aging was attributed to progressively defective cellular function that followed an orderly program of senescence encoded in the cell's genes. However, rather than animals having "suicide instructions" built into their genetic repertoire, the weight of evidence supports the general hypothesis that aging is a mixed variety of side effects from genes that confer reproductive advantages early in life. Since consideration of all contemporary hypotheses of cellular aging is well beyond the scope of this book, we will mention only certain well-documented observations.

In one approach to the study of aging, structural cells called fibroblasts are removed from a piece of tissue, transferred to a culture dish containing a nutrient medium, and allowed to divide. After a few divisions a small number of cells are subcultured in a new dish. After several subculturings, a point is reached when the cells fail to divide, and they die. The number of divisions is accepted as a measure of the life span of the cell type. Human fibroblasts taken from embryonic tissue will undergo approximately 50 population doublings before they die; those taken from a young adult are capable of about 30 doublings; and those taken from older individuals will divide about 20 times (Hayflick, 1968). The declining potential for cell division has been taken as evidence of progressive cellular deterioration with increasing age of the cell donor.

Cells from short-lived species have less potential for cell division than do those from a long-lived animal. Fibroblasts from the Galápagos tortoise have been observed to undergo as many as 114 doublings and live far longer in culture than human fibroblasts, a not unexpected finding in view of this creature's life span, which may exceed 150 years.

Current hypotheses view aging as the result of random accumulation of molecular damage. Errors in somatic cell DNA gradually accumulate as animals age. Cells have mechanisms for mending DNA damage, but these repair mechanisms become less effective in old animals. There is much more visible damage in chromosomal structure in cells from aged animals than from young animals. As cells age, defective proteins, especially inactive enzymes, begin to accumulate in the cells. It is possible, too, that the hormonal control systems that regulate enzyme activity may deteriorate with senescence, leading to a breakdown in intercellular communication.

There is ample evidence that degenerative molecular cross-linking between side groups of several kinds of macromolecules occurs with aging. Cross-linked "age pigment" appears in aging cells, and even nuclear chromatin becomes progressively cross-linked with aging. The extracellular fibrous protein **collagen,** which accounts for 40% of all body protein, has long been known to undergo cross-linking as it ages. Because collagen is a major component of tendons, ligaments, bone, and the lining of blood vessels, its deteriorative hardening causes senescent alterations in these structures.

Why do animals age at all? Although the cause of senescence is poorly understood, its value as a deteriorative process that inevitably leads to death is obvious: it prevents disastrous overpopulation. All organisms have impressive reproductive potential. For example, a pair of houseflies in a single summer could produce 19×10^{19} offspring and descendants, if all reproduce and live at least until autumn. Under these circumstances the earth would disappear beneath a thick blanket of flies. Another, more fundamental reason is that death is essential to natural selection. Natural selection is equated with reproductive success (see p. 10). But individuals cannot remain as reproductive or postreproductive adults indefinitely because they would compete with their own offspring for limited resources. No offspring could survive in such a world. The species would cease to adapt to environmental change (and consequently would cease to evolve) because selection for favorable variations would end. Consequently there has been a selection for life spans that terminate in postreproductive years. Senescence is only one of several agencies that lead to death—disease, starvation, predation, and adverse climate all take their toll—and few animals, other than most humans, live out their full potential life span.

Parenthetically, we must admit that unicellular organisms may have what is in one sense "eternal life": the parent cell does not die; it divides to produce two or more progeny and continues to do so as long as conditions compatible with its survival persist. Nevertheless, unicellular organisms are as subject to natural selection as are multicellular ones. As environmental conditions change, only organisms within the range of variation in the population that have the characteristics allowing survival will transmit those characteristics to their progeny.

___ Summary

Developmental biology is concerned with the emergence of order and complexity during the development of a new individual from a fertilized egg, and with the control of this process. The early preformation concept of development gave way in the eighteenth century to the theory of epigenesis, which holds that development is the progressive appearance of new structures that arise as the products of antecedent development.

Development of reptiles, birds, and mammals is direct, proceeding by a more or less prolonged period of growth toward the adult body form. Fish, amphibians, and many members of all major invertebrate groups develop indirectly, with one or more larval stages interposed in the life cycle.

When the egg and sperm combine at fertilization, metabolic activity of the previously quiescent egg is suddenly renewed, and important changes occur in the egg cortex that prepare the egg for cleavage. During cleavage the zygote divides repeatedly, producing numerous small cells (blastomeres).

The eggs of most invertebrate groups develop during cleavage as rigid mosaics of blastomeres having predestined developmental fates. Echinoderm and vertebrate eggs show varying degrees of regulative development, in which the blastomeres do not at first have readily identifiable developmental fates.

Despite the different developmental fates of embryonic cells, all cells have the same number and kinds of genes, as has been demonstrated by nuclear transplantation experiments. During development, certain parts of each cell's genome are expressed while the remainder are switched off (repressed) but not destroyed. Differential gene expression in embryonic cells is controlled by cytoplasmic substances that are unequally distributed in the egg during egg maturation. Early development depends on information supplied by nucleic acids and reserves deposited in the egg cytoplasm before fertilization; with the approach of gastrulation, a process of cellular reorganization when germ layers (ectoderm, mesoderm, and endoderm) are formed, nuclear genes become active.

The harmonious differentiation of tissues depends in large part on induction, the ability of one tissue to react to the developmental response of another.

Induction guides a sequence of permissive events along a specific developmental pathway. Inductors are chemical signals produced by responding cells. Their chemical nature is still unknown.

Reptiles, birds, and mammals are amniotes: terrestrial animals that develop extraembryonic membranes during embryonic life. The four membranes are the amnion, allantois, chorion, and yolk sac, each serving a specific life-support function for the embryo that develops within a self-contained egg (reptiles and birds) or within the maternal uterus (mammals).

The mammalian embryo is nourished by the placenta, a complex fetal-maternal structure that develops in the uterine wall. During pregnancy the placenta becomes an independent nutritive, endocrine, and regulatory organ for the embryo.

The germ layers formed at gastrulation differentiate into tissues and organs. The ectoderm gives rise to the skin and nervous system; the endoderm gives rise to the alimentary canal, pharynx, lungs, and certain glands; and the mesoderm forms the muscular, skeletal, circulatory, and excretory systems.

Before birth the human baby is nourished from the placenta by a special fetal circulation. At birth the umbilical blood supply is suddenly interrupted, and the circulatory shunts that exist during fetal development are closed; the pulmonary circuit opens and the infant's circulation becomes independent.

Childbirth is initiated by strong uterine contractions (labor), followed by expulsion of the baby into the birth canal. After delivery the placenta detaches from the uterine wall and is expelled.

The life span of animals has been correlated with the metabolic pace of life, as predicted by scaling theory. Among mammals, small species have more intense respiratory rates and faster heart rates than large species and age more rapidly. Humans, however, live much longer than any other mammal. Our exceptional longevity has been attributed to neoteny, the retention of juvenile characteristics in the adult, and to protracted growth extending nearly one-third the life expectancy.

Aging and death are inevitable for all multicellular animals. Aging results from the gradual accumulation of molecular damage, although the specific causes remain obscure.

Selected references

Austin, C.R., and R.V. Short (eds.). 1972-1980. Reproduction in mammals, 8 vols. Cambridge, Eng., Cambridge University Press. *Highly readable and well-illustrated series dealing with germ cells, fertilization, embryonic and fetal development, reproductive hormones and patterns, the artificial control of reproduction, and evolution of reproduction.*

Brachet, J. 1974. Introduction to molecular embryology. London, The English Universities Press Ltd. *Molecular approach.*

Calow, P. 1978. Life cycles: an evolutionary approach to the physiology of reproduction, development and aging. London, Chapman & Hall, Ltd. *An evolutionary and ecological approach that considers events throughout the life cycle.*

Comfort, A. 1979. The biology of senescence, ed. 3. New York, Elsevier North Holland, Inc. *Comprehensive treatment.*

Dryden, R. 1978. Before birth. London, Heinemann Educational Books, Ltd. *Descriptive human development.*

Gould, S.J. 1977. Ontogeny and phylogeny. Cambridge, Mass., Harvard University Press. *This important book is an argument for the evolutionary importance of heterochrony, the change in timing of appearance of ancestral characters.*

Gurdon, J.B. 1978. Gene expression during cell differentiation. Carolina Biology Reader No. 25. Burlington, N.C., Carolina Biological Supply Co. *Nature and mechanisms of gene-controlling substances.*

Ham, R.G., and M.J. Veomett. 1980. Mechanisms of development. St. Louis, The C.V. Mosby Co. *Emphasis on molecular and cellular mechanisms.*

Hopper, A.F., and N.H. Hart. 1980. Foundations of animal development. New York, Oxford University Press. *Well-written introductory text, combining classical and experimental embryology.*

Karp, G., and N.J. Berrill. 1981. Development, ed. 2. New York, McGraw-Hill Book Co. *Balanced developmental biology text, emphasizing mechanisms.*

Nelsen, O.E. 1953. Comparative embryology of the vertebrates. New York, McGraw-Hill Book Co. *This treatise is a comprehensive study of the comparative developmental morphology of the vertebrates and protochordates. Contains a wealth of comparative information difficult to find in other texts.*

Roe, S.A. 1981. Matter, life, and generation: eighteenth-century embryology and the Haller-Wolff debate. Cambridge, Eng., Cambridge University Press. *Historical development of embryological thought.*

Sacher, G.A. 1978. Longevity and aging in vertebrate evolution. Bioscience 28(8):497-501. *Argues against the idea that "senescence genes" are responsible for aging.*

Saunders, J.W., Jr. 1982. Developmental biology: patterns, problems, principles. New York, Macmillan, Inc. Textbook emphasizing mechanisms of development. *Excellent comprehensive chapter summaries.*

Spemann, H. 1938. Embryonic development and induction. New Haven, Conn., Yale University Press. *An authoritative and classic work by a pioneer in this aspect of embryology.*

Timiras, P.S. 1978. Biological perspectives on aging. Am. Sci. 66:605-613. *Theorizes that a brain "pacemaker" center controls growth, aging, and death.*

Wolpert, L. 1977. The development of pattern and form in animals. Carolina Biology Reader No. 51. Burlington, N.C., Carolina Biological Supply Co. *How embryonic cells and tissues take up positions. Also deals with induction and regeneration.*

Selected *Scientific American* articles

Bryant, P.J., S.V. Bryant, and V. French. 1977. Biological regeneration and pattern formation. 237:66-81 (July). *Studies of regeneration reveal much about basic principles of development.*

DeRobertis, E.M., and J.B. Gurdon. 1979. Gene transplantation and the analysis of development. 241:74-82 (Dec.). *Purified genes injected into a frog oocyte are transcribed.*

Ebert, J.D. 1959. The first heartbeats. 201:87-96 (Mar.). *The formation and early function of the heart are studied with chick embryos.*

Epel, D. 1977. The program of fertilization. 237:128-138 (Nov.). *Describes the fusion of egg and sperm and the initial events of development.*

Fischberg, M., and A.W. Blackler. 1961. How cells specialize. 205:124-140 (Sept.). *Early steps in differentiation of the embryo are programmed into the egg before fertilization.*

Gray, G.W. 1957. "The organizer." 197:79-88 (Nov.). *The history of embryological studies on the organizing qualities of the blastopore lip of amphibian embryos. The famous experiments of Spemann and others are recounted.*

Gurdon, J.B. 1968. Transplanted nuclei and cell differentiation. 219:24-35 (Dec.).

Hayflick, L. 1968. Human cells and aging. 218:32-37 (Mar.).

Jacobson, M., and R.K. Hunt. 1973. The origins of nerve-cell specificity. 228:26-35 (Feb.). *How nerves find direction during growth.*

Levi-Montalcini, R., and P. Calissano. 1979. The nerve-growth factor. 240:68-77 (June). *The biological effects of this protein are examined.*

Moscona, A.A. 1961. How cells associate. 205:142-162 (Sept.). *Describes the forces that promote cellular aggregation and binding.*

Patterson, P.H., D.D. Potter, and E.J. Furshpan. 1978. The chemical differentiation of nerve cells. 239:50-59 (July).

Reynolds, S.R.M. 1952. The umbilical cord. 187:70-74 (July). *Some facts about its performance.*

Singer, M. 1958. The regeneration of body parts. 199:79-88 (Oct.). *Studies on the remarkable ability of amphibians to regrow lost limbs.*

Stent, G.S., and D.A. Weisblat. 1982. The development of a simple nervous system. 246:136-146 (Jan.). *Development of nerve cells in leeches.*

Wessells, N.K. 1971. How living cells change shape. 225:76-82 (Oct.). *How microtubules and microfilaments make cell movement possible, so important in development.*

Wessells, N.K., and W.J. Rutter. 1969. Phases in cell differentiation. 220:36-44 (Mar.). *Cultivation of embryonic pancreas tissues reveals stages of specialization.*

CHAPTER 37

PRINCIPLES
OF INHERITANCE

Human chromosome isolated during interphase. (×34,000.)

Electron micrograph by G.F. Bahr, Armed Forces Institute of pathology.

Heredity establishes the continuity of life forms. Although offspring and parents in a particular generation may look different, there is nonetheless a basic sameness that runs from generation to generation for any species of plant or animal. In other words, "like begets like." Yet children are not precise replicas of their parents. Some of their characteristics show resemblances to one or both parents, but they also demonstrate many traits not found in either parent. What is actually inherited by an offspring from its parents is a certain type of germinal organization (**genes**) that, under the influence of environmental factors, guides the orderly sequence of differentiation of the fertilized egg into a human being, bearing the unique physical characteristics as we see them. Each generation hands on to the next the instructions required for maintaining continuity of life (see Principle 13, p. 14).

The gene is the unit entity of inheritance, the germinal basis for every characteristic that appears in an organism (see Principle 14, p. 14). In a sense the primary function of an organism is to reproduce genes. The organism is a device, a vehicle for the transfer of genes from one generation to its descendants. It is a repository in which a portion of the gene "pool" of the population has been temporarily entrusted.

The study of what genes are and how they work is the science of genetics. It is a science that deals with the underlying causes of *resemblance,* as seen in the remarkable fidelity of reproduction, and of *variation,* which is the working material for organic evolution. Genetics has shown that all living forms use the same information storage, transfer, and translation system, and thus it has provided an explanation for both the stability of all life and its probable descent from a common ancestral form. This is one of the most important unifying concepts of biology.

We will approach the subject in a historical sequence, since this leads us from the general to the specific and enables us to comprehend certain principles that govern inheritance. This places us in a better position to understand the mechanisms of inheritance and the molecular organization of the genetic material, topics that are taken up in later sections of this chapter.

MENDEL'S INVESTIGATIONS

The first man to formulate the cardinal principles of heredity was Gregor Johann Mendel (1822-1884) (Fig. 37-1), who lived with the Augustinian monks at Brünn (Brno), Moravia. At that time Brünn was a part of Austria, but now it is in the central part of Czechoslovakia. While conducting breeding experiments in a small monastery garden from 1856 to 1864, Mendel examined with great care the progeny of many thousands of plants. He worked out in elegant simplicity the laws governing the transmission of characters from parent to offspring. His discoveries, published in 1866, were of great potential significance, coming just after Darwin's publication of *The Origin of Species.* Yet these discoveries remained unappreciated and forgotten until 1900—some 35 years after the completion of the work and 16 years after Mendel's death.

Mendel's classic observations were based on the garden pea because it had been produced in pure strains by gardeners over a long period of time by careful selection. For example, some varieties were definitely dwarf and others were tall. A second reason for selecting peas was that they were self-fertilizing but also capable of cross-fertilization. To simplify his problem Mendel chose single characters and characters that were sharply contrasted. He carefully avoided mere

In not reporting conflicting findings, which must surely have arisen as they do in any original research, Mendel has been accused of "cooking" his results. The chances are, however, that he carefully avoided ambiguous material to strengthen his central message, which we still regard as an exemplary achievement in experimental analysis.

quantitative and intermediate characters. He selected pairs of contrasting characters, such as tall plants, dwarf plants, smooth seeds, and wrinkled seeds (Fig. 37-1).

Mendel crossed plants having one of these characters with others having the contrasting character. He did this by removing the stamens from a flower to prevent self-fertilization and then placing, on the stigma of this flower, pollen from the flower of the plant that had the contrasting character. He also prevented the experimental flowers from being pollinated from other sources such as wind and insects. When the cross-fertilized flower bore seeds, he noted the kind of plants (hybrids) that were produced from the planted seeds. Subsequently he crossed these hybrids among themselves to see what would happen.

Round-wrinkled seeds
F_1 all round
F_2 5474 round
1850 wrinkled
Ratio 2.96:1

Colored-white flowers
F_1 all colored
F_2 705 colored
224 white
Ratio 3.15:1

Yellow-green cotyledons
F_1 all yellow
F_2 6022 yellow
2001 green
Ratio 3.01:1

Green-yellow pods
F_1 all green
F_2 428 green
152 yellow
Ratio 2.82:1

Inflated-constricted pods
F_1 all inflated
F_2 882 inflated
299 constricted
Ratio 2.95:1

Long-short stems
F_1 all long
F_2 787 long
277 short
Ratio 2.84:1

Axial-terminal flowers
F_1 all axial
F_2 651 axial
207 terminal
Ratio 3.14:1

Figure 37-1

Seven experiments on which Gregor Mendel based his postulates. These are the results of monohybrid crosses for first and second generations.

Photograph courtesy American Museum of Natural History.

MENDELIAN LAWS OF INHERITANCE
Mendel's First Law

In one of Mendel's original experiments, he pollinated pure-line tall plants with the pollen of pure-line dwarf plants. He found that all the progeny, the first generation (F_1), were tall, just as tall as the tall parents of the cross. The reciprocal cross—dwarf plants pollinated with tall plants—gave the same result. This always happened no matter which way the cross was made. Obviously, this kind of inheritance was not a blending of two characteristics, since none of the progeny was of intermediate size.

Next Mendel selfed (self-fertilized) the tall F_1 plants and raised several hundred progeny, the second (F_2) generation. This time, *both* tall and dwarf plants appeared. Again, there was no blending (no plants of intermediate size), but the appearance of dwarf plants from all tall parental plants was surprising. The dwarf characteristic, present in the grandparents but not in the parents, had reappeared. When he counted the actual number of tall and dwarf plants in the F_2 generation, he discovered that there were almost exactly three times more tall plants than dwarf ones.

Mendel then repeated this experiment for the six other contrasting characters that he had chosen, and in every case he obtained ratios very close to 3:1 (Fig. 37-1). At this point it must have been clear to Mendel that he was dealing with hereditary determinants for the contrasting characters that did not blend when brought together. Even though the dwarf characteristic disappeared in the F_1 generation, it reappeared fully expressed in the F_2 generation. He realized that the F_1 generation plants carried determinants (which he called "factors") of both tall and dwarf parents, even though only the tall characteristic was expressed in the F_1 generation.

Mendel called the tall factor **dominant** and the short **recessive**. Similarly, the other pairs of characters that he studied showed dominance and recessiveness. Whenever a dominant factor (gene) is present, the recessive one cannot produce an effect. The recessive factor will show up *only* when both factors are recessive, or in other words, in a pure condition.

In representing his crosses, Mendel used letters as symbols; dominant characters were represented by capital letters, and for recessive characters he used the corresponding lowercase letters. Modern geneticists still follow this custom. Thus, the factors for pure tall plants might be represented by T/T, the pure recessive by t/t, and the mix, or hybrid, of the two plants by T/t. The slash mark is to indicate that the genes are on different chromosomes. When the gametes unite in any fertilization, a zygote is formed. The zygote bears the complete genetic constitution of the organism. All the gametes produced by T/T must necessarily be T, whereas those produced by t/t must be t. Therefore a zygote produced by union of the two must be T/t, or a **heterozygote**. On the other hand, the pure tall plants (T/T) and pure dwarf plants (t/t) are **homozygotes**, meaning that the factors (genes) are alike on the homologous chromosomes. A cross involving only one pair of contrasting characters is called a monohybrid cross.

In the cross between tall and dwarf plants there are two types of *visible* characters: tall and dwarf. These are called **phenotypes**. On the basis of genetic formulas there are three *hereditary* types: T/T, T/t, and t/t. These are called **genotypes**. A genotype is a gene combination (T/T, T/t, or t/t), and the phenotype is the appearance of the organism (tall or dwarf).

In diagram form, one of Mendel's original crosses (tall plant and dwarf plant) could be represented as follows:

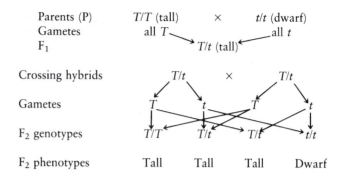

In other words, all possible combinations of F$_1$ gametes in the F$_2$ zygotes will yield a 3:1 phenotype ratio and a 1:2:1 genotype ratio. It is convenient in such crosses to use the checkerboard method devised by Punnett for representing the various combinations resulting from a cross. In the F$_2$ cross the following scheme would apply:

Sperm \ Eggs	½ T	½ t
½ T	¼ T/T (homozygous tall)	¼ T/t (hybrid tall)
½ t	¼ T/t (hybrid tall)	¼ t/t (homozygous dwarf)

Ratio: 3 tall to 1 dwarf.

The next step was an important one because it enabled Mendel to test his hypothesis that every plant contained nonblending factors from both parents. He self-fertilized the plants in the F$_2$ generation; that is, the stigma of a flower was fertilized by the pollen of the same flower. The results showed that self-pollinated F$_2$ dwarf plants produced only dwarf plants, whereas one third of the F$_2$ tall plants produced tall and the other two thirds produced both tall and dwarf in the ratio of 3:1, just as the F$_1$ plants had done. Genotypes and phenotypes were as follows:

F$_2$ plants: Tall $\begin{cases} ¼\ T/T & \xrightarrow{\text{Selfed}} & \text{all } T/T \text{ (homozygous tall)} \\ ½\ T/t & \xrightarrow{\text{Selfed}} & 1\ T/T : 2\ T/t : 1\ t/t\ (3 \text{ tall} : 1 \text{ dwarf}) \end{cases}$

Dwarf ¼ t/t $\xrightarrow{\text{Selfed}}$ all t/t (homozygous dwarf)

This experiment showed that the dwarf plants were pure because they at all times gave rise to short plants when self-pollinated; the tall plants contained both pure tall and hybrid tall. It also demonstrated that, although the dwarf character disappeared in the F$_1$ plants, which were all tall, the character for dwarfness appeared in the F$_2$ plants.

Mendel reasoned that the factors for tallness and dwarfness were units that did not blend when they were together. The F$_1$ generation (the first generation of hybrids, or first filial generation) contained both of these units or factors, but when these plants formed their germ cells, the factors separated so that each germ cell had only one factor. In a pure plant both factors were alike; in a hybrid they were different. He concluded that individual germ cells were always pure with respect to a pair of contrasting factors, even though the germ cells were formed from hybrids in which the contrasting characters were mixed.

This idea formed the basis for his first principle, the **law of segregation,** which states that whenever two factors are brought together in a hybrid, they segregate into separate gametes that are produced by the hybrid. Either one of the pair of genes of the parent passes with equal frequency to the gametes. We now understand that the factors segregate because there are two alleles for the trait, one on each chromosome of a homologous pair, but the gametes receive only one of each in meiosis. (Alleles are alternative forms of genes for the same trait; Chapter 35, p. 850.)

Mendel's great contribution was his quantitative approach to inheritance. This really marks the birth of genetics, since, before Mendel, people believed that traits were blended like mixing together two colors of paint, a notion that unfortunately still lingers in the minds of many. If this were true, variability would be lost in hybridization between individuals. With particulate inheritance, on the other hand, different variations are retained and can be shuffled about and resorted like blocks.

Testcross

When one of the alleles is dominant, the offspring of a cross are all of the same phenotypes whether they are homozygous or heterozygous. For instance, in Mendel's experiment of tall and dwarf characters, it is impossible to determine the genetic constitution of the tall plants of the F_2 generation by mere inspection of the tall plants. Three fourths of this generation are tall, but which of them are heterozygotes?

As Mendel reasoned, the test is to cross the questionable individuals with pure recessives. If the tall plant is homozygous, all the plants in such a testcross are tall, thus:

Parents	T/T(tall) $\times$ t/t (dwarf)
Offspring	T/t (hybrid tall)

If, on the other hand, the tall plant is heterozygous, half of the offspring are tall and half dwarf, thus:

Parents	$T/t \times t/t$
Offspring	T/t (tall) or t/t (dwarf)

The testcross is often used in modern genetics for the analysis of the genetic constitution of the offspring, as well as for a quick way to make desirable homozygous stocks of animals and plants.

Intermediate inheritance

In some cases neither allele is completely dominant over the other, and the heterozygote phenotype shows characteristics intermediate between or even quite distinct from those of the parents. In the four-o'clock flower *(Mirabilis)* (Fig. 37-2), homozygotes are red or white flowered, but heterozygotes have pink flowers. In a certain strain of chickens, a cross between black and splashed white produces offspring that are not gray, but a distinctive color called blue Andalusian. In each case, if the F_1s are crossed, the F_2s have a ratio of 1:2:1 in colors, or

Figure 37-2

Cross between red and white four-o'clock flowers. Red and white are homozygous; pink is heterozygous.

1 red : 2 pink : 1 white and 1 black : 2 blue : 1 white, respectively. This can be illustrated for the four-o'clocks as follows:

	(red flower)		(white flower)	
Parents	R/R	×	R'/R'	
Gametes	all R		all R'	
F_1		R/R'		
		(all pink)		
Crossing hybrids		R/R'	×	R/R'
Gametes		R,R'		R,R'
F_2 genotypes	R/R	R/R'	R/R'	R'/R'
F_2 phenotypes	Red	Pink	Pink	White

In this kind of a cross, the heterozygote is indeed a blending of both red and white characters. It is easy to see how observations of this type would encourage the notion of the blending theory of inheritance. However, in the cross of red and white four-o'clock flowers, *only* the hybrid is a phenotypic blend; the homozygous strains breed true to the parental phenotypes (red or white).

When neither of the alleles is recessive, it is customary to represent both by capital letters and to distinguish them by the addition of a "prime" sign (R') or by superscript letters, for example, R^r (equals red flowers) and R^w (equals white flowers).

——Mendel's Second Law

Thus far we have considered crosses involving alleles of a single gene (monohybrid cross). Mendel also carried out experiments on peas that differed from each other by two or more genes, that is, experiments involving two or more phenotypic characters.

Mendel had already established that tall plants were dominant to dwarf. He also noted that crosses between plants bearing yellow cotyledons and plants bearing green cotyledons produced plants with yellow cotyledons in the F_1 generation; therefore yellow was dominant to green. The next step was to make a cross between plants differing in these two characteristics. When a tall plant with yellow cotyledons $(A/A \ B/B)$ was crossed with a dwarf plant with green cotyledons $(a/a \ b/b)$, the F_1 plants were tall and yellow as expected $(A/a \ B/b)$.

Parents	$A/A \ B/B$	×	$a/a \ b/b$
	(tall, yellow)		(dwarf, green)
Gametes	all AB		all ab
F_1		$A/a \ B/b$	
		(tall, yellow)	

When the F_1 hybrids were crossed with each other, the result was the following four different phenotypes of plants in a ratio of 9:3:3:1:

> 9 tall with yellow cotyledons
> 3 tall with green cotyledons
> 3 dwarf with yellow cotyledons
> 1 dwarf with green cotyledons

Mendel already knew that a cross between two plants bearing a single pair of alleles of the genotype A/a would yield a 3:1 ratio. Similarly, a cross between two plants with the genotypes B/b would yield the same 3:1 ratio. If we examine *only* the tall and dwarf phenotypes in the outcome of the dihybrid experiment, they total up to 12 tall and 4 dwarf, giving a ratio of 3:1. Likewise, a total of 12 plants have yellow cotyledons and 4 plants have green—again a 3:1 ratio. Thus, the monohybrid ratio prevails for both traits when they are considered independently. The 9:3:3:1 ratio is nothing more than two 3:1 ratios combined.

$$3:1 \times 3:1 = 9:3:3:1$$

The F$_2$ genotypes and phenotypes are as follows:

1 *A/A B/B*			
2 *A/a B/B*			
2 *A/A B/b*	9 *A/— B/—*	9 tall yellow	
4 *A/a B/b*			
1 *A/A b/b*	3 *A/— b/b*	3 tall green	
2 *A/a B/b*			
1 *a/a B/B*	3 *a/a B/—*	3 dwarf yellow	
2 *a/a B/b*			
1 *a/a b/b*	1 *a/a b/b*	1 dwarf green	

When one of the alleles is unknown, it can be designated by a dash *(A/—)*. This designation can also be used when it is immaterial whether the genotype is heterozygote or homozygote, as when we total all of a certain phenotype. The dash could be either *A* or *a*.

The results of this experiment show that the segregation of alleles for plant height is entirely independent of the segregation of alleles for cotyledon color. Neither has any influence on the other. This is the basis of Mendel's second law, the **law of independent assortment,** which states: whenever two or more pairs of contrasting characters are brought together in a hybrid, the alleles of different pairs segregate independently of one another. The reason is that during meiosis the member of any pair of homologous chromosomes received by a gamete is independent of the other chromosomes it receives. Of course, independent assortment assumes that the genes are on different chromosomes. If they were on the same chromosome, they would assort together unless crossing over occurred (p. 908).

The dihybrid experiment is shown in the Punnett square below:

Parents	*A/A B/B* (tall yellow)	×	*a/a b/b* (dwarf green)
Gametes	all *AB*		all *ab*
F$_1$		*A/a B/b* (hybrid tall, hybrid yellow)	
Crossing hybrids	*A/a B/b*	×	*A/a B/b*
Gametes	*AB, Ab, aB, ab*		*AB, Ab, aB, ab*
F$_2$		(see checkerboard)	

	AB	Ab	aB	ab
AB	*A/A B/B* Pure tall Pure yellow	*A/A B/b* Pure tall Hybrid yellow	*A/a B/B* Hybrid tall Pure yellow	*A/a B/b* Hybrid tall Hybrid yellow
Ab	*A/A B/b* Pure tall Hybrid yellow	*A/A b/b* Pure tall Pure green	*A/a B/b* Hybrid tall Hybrid yellow	*A/a b/b* Hybrid tall Pure green
aB	*A/a B/B* Hybrid tall Pure yellow	*A/a B/b* Hybrid tall Hybrid yellow	*a/a B/B* Pure dwarf Pure yellow	*a/a B/b* Pure dwarf Hybrid yellow
ab	*A/a B/b* Hybrid tall Hybrid yellow	*A/a b/b* Hybrid tall Pure green	*a/a B/b* Pure dwarf Hybrid yellow	*a/a b/b* Pure dwarf Pure green

Ratio: 9 tall yellow to 3 tall green; 3 dwarf yellow to 1 dwarf green.

One way to estimate numbers of progeny from a cross with a given genotype or phenotype is to construct a Punnett square and count them up. With a mono-hybrid cross, this is very easy; with a dihybrid cross, a Punnett square is rather laborious; and with a trihybrid cross, it is very tedious. We can make such estimates much more easily by taking advantage of simple probability calculations. The basic assumption is that all the genotypes of gametes of one sex have an equal chance of uniting with all the genotypes of gametes of the other sex, in proportion to the numbers of each present. This is generally true when the sample size is large enough, and the actual numbers observed come close to those predicted by the laws of probability.

We may define probability as follows:

$$\text{Probability (p)} = \frac{\text{Number of times an event happens}}{\text{Total number of trials or possibilities for the event to happen}}$$

For example, the probability (p) of a coin falling heads when tossed is ½ because the coin has two sides. The probability of rolling a three on a die is ⅙ because the die has six sides.

The probability of independent events occurring together (ordered events) involves the **product rule,** which is simply the product of their individual probabilities. When two coins are tossed together, the probability of getting two heads is ½ × ½ = ¼, or 1 chance in 4. The probability of rolling two threes simultaneously with two dice is as follows:

$$\text{Probability of two threes} = \frac{1}{6} \times \frac{1}{6} = \frac{1}{36}$$

Note, however, that a small sample size may give a result quite different from that predicted. Thus, if we tossed the coin three times and it fell heads each time, we would not be much surprised. But, if we tossed the coin 1000 times, and the number of times it fell heads diverged very much from 500, we would strongly suspect that there was something wrong with the coin or with the way we were tossing it.

We can use the product rule to predict the ratios of inheritance in monohybrid or dihybrid (or larger) crosses if the genes sort independently in the gametes (as they did in all of Mendel's experiments). In other words, the mechanism of placing A into a gamete is independent of the mechanism of putting a into a gamete. Therefore in a monohybrid cross the probability that a sperm carries the dominant is ½, and the same applies to an egg. In a dihybrid cross involving A/a and B/b, the same thing applies; the probability of any gene appearing in a gamete is ½. Now we can apply the product rule to an F_1 plant A/a B/b to determine the frequency of each kind of gamete:

Probability of gamete being *AB* = ½ × ½ = ¼
Probability of gamete being *Ab* = ½ × ½ = ¼
Probability of gamete being *aB* = ½ × ½ = ¼
Probability of gamete being *ab* = ½ × ½ = ¼

From this point the probabilities for the genotype in each box of the Punnett square on p. 897 can be easily derived as follows:

Probability of plant being *A/A B/B* = ¼ × ¼ = 1/16
Probability of plant being *A/A B/b* = ¼ × ¼ = 1/16

and so on for all 16 boxes.

Collecting all similar phenotypes together we get:

Tall, yellow cotyledon	9/16 = 9
Tall, green cotyledon	3/16 = 3
Dwarf, yellow cotyledon	3/16 = 3
Dwarf, green cotyledon	1/16 = 1

Thus, we have the $9:3:3:1$ ratio, derived by the product rule. In fact, one quickly learns by experience how to determine the ratios of phenotypes without using either the Punnett squares or the product rule. In a dihybrid ($9:3:3:1$ ratio), for instance, those phenotypes that make up the dominants of each gene are $9/16$ of the whole F_2 generation; each of the $3/16$ phenotypes consists of one dominant and one recessive; and the $1/16$ phenotype consists of two recessives.

The F_2 ratios in any cross involving more than one pair of contrasting pairs can be found by combining the ratios in the cross of one pair of alleles. Thus, the number of genotypes is $(3)^n$ and the proportion of phenotypes $(3:1)^n$ when one allele is dominant and the other recessive. For example, let us suppose that in a cross of two pairs of alleles the phenotypes are in the ratio of $(3:1)^2$, or $9:3:3:1$. The genotypes in such a cross are $(3)^2$, or 9. If three pairs of characters are involved (trihybrid cross), the proportions, or ratios, of the phenotypes are then $(3:1)^3$, or $27:9:9:9:3:3:3:1$. The genotypes are $(3)^3$, or 27. Obviously, as the number of gene pairs increases, the number of phenotypes and genotypes rises steeply.

Multiple Alleles

Previously we defined alleles as the alternate forms of a gene. Many dissimilar alleles may occupy the same gene locus on a chromosome but not of course all at one time. Thus, more than two alternative genes may affect the same character. An example is the set of multiple alleles that affects coat color in rabbits. The different alleles are C (normal color), c^{ch} (chinchilla color), c^h (Himalayan color), and c (albino). The four alleles fall into a dominance series with C dominant over everything. The dominant allele is always written to the left and the recessive to the right:

$$C/c^h = \text{Normal color}$$
$$c^{ch}/c^h = \text{Chinchilla color}$$
$$c^h/c = \text{Himalayan color}$$

Multiple alleles arise through mutations at the gene locus over long periods of time. Any gene may mutate in many different places (p. 929) if given time and thus can give rise to slightly different genes or alleles at the same locus. Examples of multiple alleles in humans are the ABO blood types and Rh factors (Chapter 29, p. 708).

Gene Interaction

The types of crosses previously described are simple in that the characters involved result from the action of a single gene, but many cases are known in which the characters are the result of two or more genes. Mendel probably did not appreciate the real significance of the genotype, as contrasted with the visible character—the phenotype. We now know that many different genotypes may be expressed as a single phenotype.

Also, many genes have more than a single effect. A gene for eye color, for instance, may be the ultimate cause for eye color, yet at the same time it may be responsible for influencing the development of other characters as well. Some of these special forms of inheritance are described in the following discussions of supplementary factors, epistasis, and polygenic inheritance.

The description in Chapter 29 assumed that inheritance of the Rh factor was as a single dominant gene. Actually, the genetics of the Rh factor are much more complicated than was believed when the factor was discovered. Some authorities believe that three genes located close together on the same chromosome are involved, whereas others think the system is one gene with many alleles. In 1968 a revision of the single-gene concept listed 37 alleles necessary to account for the phenotypes then known. Furthermore, the frequency of the various alleles varies greatly between whites, Orientals, and blacks.

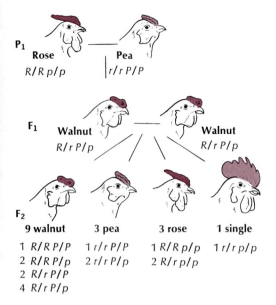

Figure 37-3

Heredity of comb forms in chickens.

Supplementary factors

The variety of comb forms found in chickens illustrates the interaction of supplementary genes (Fig. 37-3). The common forms of comb are rose, pea, walnut, and single. Of these, the pea comb and the rose comb are dominant to the single comb. For example, when a pea comb is crossed with a single comb, all the F_1 offspring have pea combs and the F_2 offspring show a ratio of 3 pea combs to 1 single. When the two dominant combs, pea and rose, are crossed with each other, an entirely new kind of comb, walnut, is found in the F_1 generation. Each of these genes supplements the other in the production of a kind of comb different from each of the dominants. In the F_2 generation the ratio is 9 walnut to 3 rose to 3 pea to 1 single. The walnut comb cannot thus be considered a unit character but is merely the phenotype's expression of pea and rose combs when they act together.

Inspection of the ratio reveals that two genes are involved. If P represents the gene for the pea comb and p represents its recessive allele, and if R represents the gene for the rose comb and r its recessive allele, then the pea comb formula would be $r/r\ P/P$; the formula for rose comb would be $R/R\ p/p$. Any individual having both dominant alleles has a walnut comb. When no dominant allele is present, the comb is single. The cross may be diagrammed as follows:

Parents	$r/r\ P/P$	$\times$	$R/R\ p/p$
	(pea comb)		(rose comb)
Gametes	all rP		all Rp
F_1	$R/r\ P/p$	$\times$	$R/r\ P/p$
	(walnut)		(walnut)
Gametes	RP, rP, Rp, rp		RP, rP, Rp, rp

By the checkerboard method, the F_2 generation shows 9 walnut, 3 pea, 3 rose, and 1 single. Genotypes with the combinations of $R/—\ P/—$ give walnut phenotypes; those with $r/r\ P/—$, pea; those with $R/—\ p/p$, rose; and those lacking in both P and R, single.

Epistasis

When a gene at one locus masks or prevents the expression of a gene at another locus acting on the same trait, the first is said to be epistatic to the second. In rabbits the gene for pigment (of any kind) is epistatic to that for agouti, a barred pigment pattern of the fur. The gene for pigment has two alleles, A and a. If the allele A is present, the rabbit is pigmented and the color depends on other genes. If the individual is homozygous recessive, a/a, the rabbit is albino, no matter what other genes for pigment may be present.

The expression of the second gene, B for agouti, depends on the presence or absence of the A gene. This interaction can be summarized as follows:

Parents	$A/A\ B/B$	$\times$	$a/a\ b/b$
	(agouti)		(albino)
Gametes	All AB		All ab
F_1	$A/a\ B/b$	$\times$	$A/a\ B/b$
	(agouti)		(agouti)
Gametes	AB, Ab, aB, ab		AB, Ab, aB, ab

The F_2 genotypes and phenotypes are as follows:

$$\left.\begin{array}{l} 1\ A/A\ B/B \\ 2\ A/a\ B/B \\ 2\ A/A\ B/b \\ 4\ A/a\ B/b \end{array}\right\}\quad 9\ A/-\ B/- \qquad 9\ \text{agouti}$$

$$\left.\begin{array}{l} 1\ A/A\ b/b \\ 2\ A/a\ b/b \end{array}\right\}\quad 3\ A/-\ b/b \qquad 3\ \text{black}$$

$$\left.\begin{array}{l} 1\ a/a\ B/B \\ 2\ a/a\ B/b \end{array}\right\}\quad 3\ a/a\ B/- \qquad \left.\begin{array}{l} \\ \\ \end{array}\right\}$$

$$1\ a/a\ b/b \qquad\qquad 1\ a/a\ b/b \qquad\qquad 4\ \text{albino}$$

The F$_2$ phenotypic ratio if 9:3:4. This happens because the last two phenotypic classes are both albino and are combined. The dominant allele A must be present for any color to appear. Also, if only the recessive gene for agouti is present (homozygous b/b), the animal's color becomes black, an intermediate between agouti and albino.

Epistasis is not the same as dominance, with which it might be confused. Dominance is the phenotypic expression of one member of a pair of alleles of a **single** gene. In epistasis the alleles of **two** genes on separate loci are involved, with one gene affecting the phenotypic expression of the other gene.

Polygenic inheritance

Whenever several sets of alleles produce a cumulative effect on the same character, they are called **multiple genes,** or **polygenic** factors. Several characteristics in humans are influenced by multiple genes. In such cases the characters, instead of being sharply marked, show continuous variation between two extremes. This is sometimes called **blending,** or **quantitative inheritance.** In this kind of inheritance the children are often more or less intermediate between the two parents.

One illustration of such a type is the degree of pigmentation in crosses between the black and white human races. The cumulative genes in such crosses have a quantitative expression. Many genes are believed to be involved in skin pigmentation, but we will simplify our explanation by assuming that there are only two pairs of independently assorting genes. Thus, a person with very dark pigment has two genes for pigmentation on separate chromosomes $(A/A\ B/B)$. Each dominant allele contributes one unit of pigment. A person with very light pigment has alleles $(a/a\ b/b)$ that contribute no color. (Freckles that commonly appear in the skin of very light people represent pigment contributed by entirely separate genes.) The offspring of very dark and very light parents would have an intermediate skin color $(A/a\ B/b)$.

The children of parents having intermediate skin color show a range of skin color, depending on the number of genes for pigmentation they inherit. Their skin color ranges from very dark $(A/A\ B/B)$, to dark $(A/A\ B/b$ or $A/a\ B/B)$, intermediate $(A/A\ b/b$ or $A/a\ B/b$ or $a/a\ B/B)$, light $(A/a\ b/b$ or $a/a\ B/b)$, to very light $(a/a\ b/b)$. It is thus possible for parents heterozygous for skin color to produce children with darker or lighter colors than themselves.

The relationships can be seen in the following diagram:

Parents	$A/A\ B/B$	$\times$	$a/a\ b/b$
	(very dark)		(very light)
Gametes	AB		ab
F$_1$	$A/a\ B/b$	$\times$	$A/a\ B/b$
	(intermediate)		(intermediate)
Gametes	$AB,\ Ab,\ aB,\ ab$		$AB,\ Ab,\ aB,\ ab$

The F₂ generation shows this ratio:

1 *A/A B/B*	Very dark
2 *A/a B/B*	Dark
2 *A/A B/b*	Dark
4 *A/a B/b*	Intermediate
1 *A/A b/b*	Intermediate
2 *A/a b/b*	Light
1 *a/a B/B*	Intermediate
2 *a/a B/b*	Light
1 *a/a b/b*	Very light

Collecting the phenotypes, the ratio becomes: 1 very dark: 4 dark: 6 intermediate: 4 light: 1 very light.

When there are many genes involved in the production of traits, this situation may be represented in graphs as distribution curves, usually bell shaped. A graph of frequency distribution for height indicates that the height of most people is near the average, indicated by the high point of such a bell-shaped curve, and that few people are much shorter or taller than average. If one locus is much more important than others, the alleles at this locus might split the graph into two or three bell-shaped curves represented different genotypes. Because we never find this kind of graph for the height of human populations, we know that humans do not have a principle for tall and dwarf lines like that of garden peas.

___ Penetrance and Expressivity

Penetrance refers to the percentage frequency with which a gene manifests a phenotypic effect. If a dominant gene or a recessive gene in a homozygous state always produces a detectable effect, it is said to have **complete penetrance.** If dominant or homozygous recessive genes fail to show phenotypic expression in every case, it is called **incomplete** or **reduced penetrance.** Environmental factors may be responsible for the degree of penetrance in some cases because some genes may be more sensitive to such influences than others. The genotype responsible for diabetes mellitus, for instance, may be present, but because of reduced penetrance, the disease does not always occur. Usually we do not know the reason for incomplete penetrance in particular cases, although incomplete penetrance sometimes depends on epistasis, as in the example of rabbit fur pigment, discussed previously. All of Mendel's experiments apparently had 100% penetrance.

The phenotypic variation in the expression of a gene is known as **expressivity.** For instance, a heritable allergy may cause more severe symptoms in one person than in another. Environmental factors may cause different degrees in the appearance of a phenotype. Temperature affects the expression of the genes for dark-colored fur in Siamese cats and Himalayan rabbits. Normally the tail, feet, ears, and nose—the areas that have a cooler body temperature—are dark, but under warm conditions there may be less than normal darkening, whereas in colder environmental temperatures there may be some darkening of the entire animal. Other genes in the hereditary constitution may also modify the expression of a trait. What is inherited is a certain genotype, but how it is expressed phenotypically is determined by the environment and other factors.

Genes that have more than one effect are called **pleiotropic.** Most genes may have multiple effects. Even those genes that produce visible effects probably have numerous physiological effects not detected by the geneticist. The recessive gene in fruit flies that produces (in a homozygous condition) vestigial wings also affects other traits such as the halteres (balancers), bristles, reproductive organs, and length of life.

Lethal Genes

A **lethal gene** is one whose effects result in conditions incompatible with continued life. Lethal genes may be dominant or recessive, and they may cause death at various stages of the life cycle, from the early embryo through adulthood. Some cases of spontaneous abortion in humans are believed caused by lethal genes operating during embryogenesis. Another example is the gene for yellow coat color in mice, which is lethal in the homozygote. It has been known for a long time that the yellow strain of the house mouse *(Mus musculus)* is heterozygous, with the allele for yellow coat dominant to the allele for wild-type gray coat. When two yellow mice are bred together, some of the progeny are yellow and some are gray, always in a ratio of 2:1. This is a marked departure from the expected Mendelian 3:1 ratio consisting of 1 pure yellow *(Y/Y)*, 2 hybrid yellow *(Y/y)*, and 1 pure gray *(y/y)*. The explanation is that the homozygous yellow always dies as an embryo because the *Y/Y* genotype is lethal. The peculiar feature of this inheritance is that the *Y* allele is *dominant* in its effect on coat color (the *Y/y* hybrid is always yellow, never gray) but is *recessive* in its lethality because it must be homozygous *(Y/Y)* to express its lethal effect. This is a good example of a pleiotropic effect, since the gene affects the phenotype of the mouse in two different ways.

Sex Determination and Sex-Linked Inheritance

Genes for some traits are inherited on the chromosomes that also determine sex; therefore expression of those traits depends on the sex of the individual and the sex chromosomes present. However, before discussing how these traits are inherited, we must explain the chromosomal basis of sex determination.

Before the importance of the chromosomes in heredity was realized in the early 1900s, how gender was determined was totally unknown. The first really scientific clue to the determination of sex came in 1902 when C. McClung observed that bugs (Hemiptera) produced two kinds of sperm in approximately equal numbers. One kind contained among its regular set of chromosomes a so-called accessory chromosome that was lacking in the other kind of sperm. Since all the eggs of these species had the same number of haploid chromosomes, half the sperm would have the same number of chromosomes as the eggs, and half of them would have one chromosome less. When an egg was fertilized by a spermatozoon carrying the accessory (sex) chromosome, the resulting offspring was a female; when fertilized by the spermatozoon without an accessory chromosome, the offspring was a male. There are therefore two kinds of chromosomes: X chromosomes, which determine sex (and sex-linked traits), and **autosomes,** which determine the other body traits. The particular type of sex determination just described is often called the XX-XO type, which indicates that the females have two X chromosomes and the males only one X chromosome (the O indicates absence of the chromosome). The XX-XO method of sex determination is depicted in Fig. 37-4.

Later, other types of sex determination were discovered. In humans and many other forms each sex has the same number of chromosomes; however, the sex chromosomes (XX) are alike in the female but unlike (XY) in the male. Hence the human egg contains 22 autosomes + 1 X chromosome; the sperm are of two

Speculation on how sex was determined in animals produced several incredible beliefs, for example, that the two testicles of the male contain different types of semen, one begetting males, the other females. It is not difficult to imagine the abuse and mutilation of domestic animals that occurred when attempts were made to alter the sex ratios of herds. Another idea asserted that sex of the offspring was determined by the more heavily sexed parent. An especially masculine father should produce sons, an effeminate father only daughters. Such ideas were not testable and have lingered until recently.

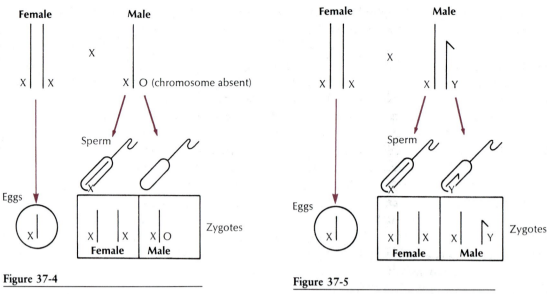

Figure 37-4

XX-XO sex determination.

Figure 37-5

XX-XY sex determination.

kinds; half carry 22 autosomes + 1 X and half bear 22 autosomes + 1 Y. The Y chromosome is much smaller than the X. At fertilization, when two X chromosomes come together, the offspring are female; when X and Y chromosomes come together, the offspring are male. The XX-XY kind of determination is shown in Fig. 37-5.

A third type of sex determination is found in birds, moths, and butterflies in which the male has two X (or sometimes called ZZ) chromosomes and the female an X and a Y (or ZW).

We should note that, in the case of X and Y chromosomes, the homologous chromosomes are unlike in size and shape. Therefore they do not both carry the same genes. The genes of the Y chromosome are not alleles of those on the X chromosome. This fact is very important in sex-linked inheritance, which we shall discuss later.

The Y chromosome is small and apparently carries no sex-linked genes. It consists of repetitious DNA base sequences of no known functional significance. The Y appears to contain just one important gene, the male-determining gene, located on the short arm of the chromosome.

Since the X chromosome carries several genes that are essential for normal cellular function and the Y chromosome carries none, every individual must have *at least* one X chromosome. And of course the XX-XY system ensures that they will: the female has two, the male one. To keep the balance between X-chromosome genes and autosome genes the same in the female as in the male, one of the female's X chromosomes is always inactivated. This happens very early in development when the embryo consists of only a few cells, according to the widely accepted Lyon hypothesis (after Mary Lyon, who discovered this and other aspects of human sex determination). At this time it is strictly a matter of chance whether the maternal or paternal X chromosome is the one inactivated in each cell. All descendants of that cell, however, retain the same inactivated chromosome. Consequently, tissues of adult females are a patchwork of cells (mosaic) expressing the genes of one or the other X chromosome, never both. Interestingly, the inactivated X chromosome condenses in the interphase nucleus of most somat-

Normally this odd feature is of no consequence in human females, but it has a dramatic effect in cats. Tortoise-shell (calico, tabby) cats, which are spotted black and yellow, are *always* females; the males are either all black or all yellow. This happens because the genes for fur color are located on the X chromosome; that is, they are sex linked. A male, having only one X chromosome, will be either black or yellow. But a female has two X chromosomes and, if she is heterozygous for fur color, her fur will be a mosaic of yellow and black patches. Each patch represents the descendants of an early embryonic skin cell having one operating and one inactive X chromosome.

ic cells into a tiny, darkly staining object called a Barr body (Fig. 37-6). This furnishes a simple method for determining whether an individual is a genetic male or female, as has been done, for example, in examination of entrants in women's athletic events.

Genetic sex is just one aspect of sex determination. Having an XX or an XY genetic constitution does not in itself produce a female or male. The embryo is at first totally indifferent sexually, despite its genetic sex. Even the gonad is sexually indifferent and bipotential, since it can differentiate into either a testis or an ovary. Gonad differentiation was discussed in Chapter 35 (p. 849), and we pointed out there that the primordial gonad has an inherent tendency to become an ovary, and the rest of the body to become female, *unless* the male-determining gene on the Y chromosomes redirects gonadal differentiation into a testis. As the presumptive gonad differentiates into an ovary or testis, it begins to secrete sex hormones (androgens by the testes, estrogens by the ovaries). These hormones influence the other developing organs to become male or female.

Sex-linked inheritance

It has long been known that the inheritance of some characters depends on the sex of the parent carrying the gene and the sex of the offspring. One of the best-known sex-linked traits of humans is hemophilia (Chapter 29, p. 702). Another example is red-green color blindness in which red and green colors are indistinguishable to varying degrees. Color-blind men greatly outnumber color-blind women. When color blindness does appear in women, their fathers are color blind. Furthermore, if a woman with normal vision who is a carrier of color blindness bears sons, half of them are likely to be color blind, regardless of whether the father had normal or affected vision. How are these observations explained?

The color-blindness and hemophilia defects are recessive traits carried on the X chromosome that are visibly expressed either when both genes are defective in the female or when only one defective gene is present in the male. The inheritance pattern of these defects is shown for color-blindness in Fig. 37-7. When the mother is a carrier and the father is normal, half of the sons but none of the daughters are color blind. However, if the father is color blind and the mother is a carrier, half of the sons *and* half of the daughters are color blind (on the average and in a large sample). It is easy to understand then why such defects are much more prevalent in males: a single sex-linked recessive gene in the male has a visible effect. What would be the outcome of a mating between a homozygous normal woman and a color-blind man?

Another example of a sex-linked character was discovered by Thomas Hunt Morgan (1910) in *Drosophila*. The normal eye color of this fly is red, but mutations for white eyes do occur. The genes for eye color are known to be carried in the X chromosome. If a white-eyed male and a red-eyed female are crossed, all the F_1 offspring are red eyed because this trait is dominant (Fig. 37-8). If these F_1 offspring are interbred, all the females of F_2 have red eyes, half the males have red eyes, and the other half have white eyes. No white-eyed females are found in this generation; only the males have the recessive character (white eyes). The gene for being white eyed is recessive and should appear in a homozygous condition. However, since the male has only one X chromosome (the Y does not carry a gene for eye color), white eyes appear whenever the X chromosome carries the gene for this trait. If the reciprocal cross is made in which the females are white eyed and the males red eyed, all the F_1 females are red eyed and all the males are white eyed

Figure 37-6

Nuclei from three epithelial cells taken from the mouth of a normal human female. The darkly staining Barr bodies *(arrows)* are the heterochromatinized (inactive) X chromosome.
Courtesy M.L. Barr.

We might wonder how these observations on sex-linked defects are reconciled with the inactivation of one X chromosome in females. If the normal X chromosome was the one inactivated in cells of heterozygous females, would the person not show the recessive trait because the active chromosome was the one with the gene? The answer is that which X chromosome is inactivated is entirely random in cells of the embryo, and there are almost always enough cells with normal X chromosomes that the recessive trait is not expressed.

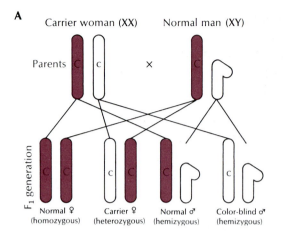

Figure 37-7

Sex-linked inheritance of red-green color blindness in humans. **A,** Carrier mother and normal father produce color blindness in one half of their sons but in none of their daughters. **B,** Half of both sons and daughters of carrier mother and color-blind father are color blind.

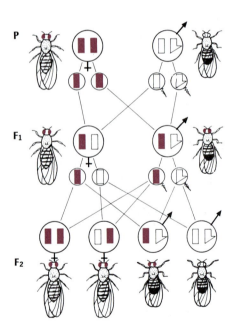

Figure 37-8

Sex-linked inheritance of eye color in fruit fly *Drosophila*. Genes for eye color are carried on X chromosome; Y carries no genes for eye color. Normal red is dominant to white. Homozygous red-eyed female mated with white-eyed male gives all red-eyed in F_1. F_2 ratios from F_1 cross are one homozygous red-eyed female and one heterozygous red-eyed female to one red-eyed male and one white-eyed male.

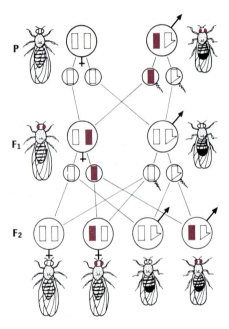

Figure 37-9

Reciprocal cross of Fig. 37-8 (homozygous white-eyed female with red-eyed male) gives white-eyed males and red-eyed females in F_1. F_2 shows equal numbers of red-eyed and white-eyed females and red-eyed and white-eyed males.

(Fig. 37-9). If these F_1 offspring are interbred, the F_2 generation shows equal numbers of red-eyed and white-eyed males and females.

If the allele for red eyes is represented by W, white eyes by w, the female sex chromosome by X, and the male sex chromosome lacking a gene for eye color by Y, the following diagrams show the inheritance of this eye color:

Parents	X^W/X^W (red ♀)		×	X^w/Y (white ♂)	
F_1	X^W/X^w (red ♀)		×	X^W/Y (red ♂)	
Gametes	X^W, X^w			X^W, Y	
F_2 genotypes	X^W/X^W	X^W/Y		X^w/Y	X^w/X^W
F_2 phenotypes	Red ♀	Red ♂		White ♂	Red ♀

Reciprocal cross

Parents	X^w/X^w (white ♀)		×	X^W/Y (red ♂)	
F_1	X^w/X^W (red ♀)		×	X^w/Y (white ♂)	
Gametes	X^w, X^W			X^w, Y	
F_2 genotypes	X^w/X^w	X^w/Y		X^W/X^w	X^W/Y
F_2 phenotypes	White ♀	White ♂		Red ♀	Red ♂

___ Autosomal Linkage and Crossing Over
Linkage

Since Mendel's laws were rediscovered in 1900, it has become apparent that, contrary to Mendel's second law, not all factors segregate independently. Indeed, many traits are inherited together. Since the number of chromosomes in any organism is relatively small compared to the number of traits, each chromosome must contain many genes. All genes present on a chromosome are said to be **linked.** Linkage simply means that the genes are on the same chromosome, and all genes present on homologous chromosomes belong to the same linkage groups. Therefore there should be as many linkage groups as there are chromosome pairs.

In *Drosophila,* in which this principle has been worked out most extensively, there are four linkage groups that correspond to the four pairs of chromosomes found in these fruit flies. Usually, small chromosomes have small linkage groups, and large chromosomes have large groups. More than 500 genes have been mapped in the fruit fly, and they all are distributed among the four pairs of chromosomes.

Let us see how the Mendelian ratios can be altered by linkage, as illustrated by one of Morgan's experiments on *Drosophila.* In fruit fly genetics, the normal allele of any gene is called the **wild type,** since that allele is the most widespread in the wild state. It is usually dominant over its sister alleles, which are considered mutations of the normal wild allele. Morgan made a cross between wild-type fruit flies with normal bodies and wings and flies bearing two recessive mutant characters of black bodies and vestigial wings.

As expected, the F_1 generation of this cross was phenotypically the wild type, confirming that the alleles for black bodies and vestigial wings were recessive.

Morgan then made a testcross to learn more about the genotype of the F_1 generation. This was done by breeding back the F_1 hybrid generation *(AB/ab)* to the double-recessive flies of the parental generation *(ab/ab).* With independent

Geneticists commonly use the word "linkage" in two somewhat different senses. Sex linkage refers to inheritance of a trait on the sex chromosomes, and thus its phenotypic expression depends on the sex of the organism and the factors already discussed. Autosomal linkage, or simply, linkage, refers to inheritance of the genes on a given autosomal chromosome. Letters used to represent such genes are normally written without a slash mark between them, indicating that they are on the same chromosome. For example, *AB/ab* shows that genes *A* and *B* are on the same chromosome, and *a* and *b* are on the homologous chromosome. Interestingly, Mendel studied seven characteristics of garden peas, which assorted independently because they were on seven different chromosomes. If he had studied eight characteristics, he would not have found independent assortment in two of the traits because garden peas have only seven pairs of homologous chromosomes.

Figure 37-10

Crossing over during meiosis. Nonsister chromatids exchange portions, so that none of the resulting gametes is genetically the same as any other. Gene A is farther from gene B than B is from C; therefore gene A is more frequently separated from B in crossing over than B is from C.

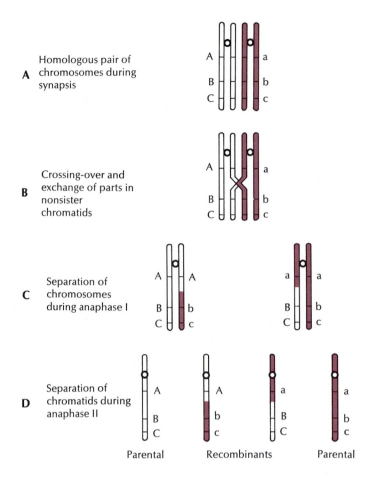

A Homologous pair of chromosomes during synapsis

B Crossing-over and exchange of parts in nonsister chromatids

C Separation of chromosomes during anaphase I

D Separation of chromatids during anaphase II

Parental   Recombinants   Parental

assortment we should expect four different phenotypes in approximately equal numbers:

Phenotype	Expected ratio	Numbers obtained
Wild type	1	586 (46%)
Normal body, vestigial wing	1	106 (8%)
Black body, normal wing	1	111 (9%)
Black body, vestigial wing	1	465 (37%)

Instead Morgan obtained an excess of **parental** types (wild type and double-recessive type) and a deficiency of the two gene recombinations (called **recombinant** types). In a testcross such as this, linkage is indicated if the proportion of parental types exceeds 50%. This cross yielded 83% parental types and 17% recombinant types. Morgan concluded that the wild type and black-vestigial type had entered the dihybrid cross together and stayed together, or were linked.

Crossing over

Linkage, however, is usually not complete. In the experiment just described, the parental forms totaled 83% rather than 100% as expected if linkage were complete. The fact that some recombinant types appear means that the linked genes have indeed separated, in this experiment 17% of the time. Separation of genes located on the same chromosome occurs because of **crossing over.**

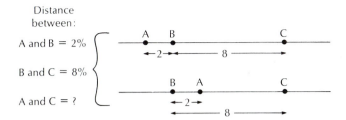

Distance between:

A and B = 2%

B and C = 8%

A and C = ?

Figure 37-11

Tentative arrangement of three genes on a chromosome. Distances are given in linkage map units with each unit defined as equal to 1% frequency of recombination. The third cross, *A* and *C*, is necessary to resolve which of the two possible arrangements proposed by the first two crosses is correct.

As described in Chapter 35 (p. 850), during the protracted prophase of the first meiotic division, homologous chromosomes break and exchange equivalent portions; genes "cross over" from one chromosome to its homologue, and vice versa (Fig. 37-10). Each chromosome consists of two sister chromatids held together by means of a synaptonemal complex. Breaks and exchanges occur at corresponding points on nonsister chromatids. (Breaks and exchanges also occur between sister chromatids but usually have no genetic significance because sister chromatids are identical.) Crossing over is a means for exchanging genes between homologous chromosomes and as such greatly increases the amount of genetic recombination. The frequency of crossing over varies depending on the species, but usually at least one and often several crossovers occur each time chromosomes pair.

Gene mapping

Crossing over makes possible the construction of chromosome maps and provides proof that the genes lie in a linear order on the chromosomes. Crossing over does not occur randomly throughout the length of the chromosome. The greater the distance between genes, the greater the probability that a crossover may occur between them. Two genes located at opposite ends of the chromosome are separated almost every time a break occurs; if they are located close together, they are separated only when the chromosome chances to break between them. Therefore the *frequency of recombination* is proportional to the distance between gene loci on a chromosome.

In our example of the cross between wild-type and black-vestigial-type flies, the frequency of recombination (percentage of offspring that are recombinants) is 17%. By itself, this value does not indicate the location of the two genes involved. But, if a third gene is added, their arrangement can be determined by making three crosses. Let us take a hypothetical example of three genes *(A, B, C)* on the same chromosome (Fig. 37-11).

In the determination of their comparative linear position on the chromosome, we first need to find the crossing-over value between any two of these genes. If *A* and *B* have a crossing-over rate of 2% and *B* and *C* of 8%, then the crossing-over percentage between *A* and *C* should be either the sum (2 + 8) or the difference (8 − 2). If it is 10%, *B* lies between *A* and *C*; if 6%, *A* is between *B* and *C*. By laborious genetic experiments for many years, the famed chromosome maps in *Drosophila* were worked out in this manner (Fig. 37-12). More recent cytological investigations on the giant chromosomes present in the salivary glands of fruit fly larvae tend to prove the correctness of the linear order, although they have not shown the actual position of the genes on the chromosomes.

Figure 37-12

Linkage map of the four chromosomes of the fruit fly *Drosophila melanogaster*. Figures refer to distances from upper end of chromosome.

From Sinnott, E.W., L.C. Dunn, and T. Dobzhansky. 1958. Principles of genetics. New York, McGraw-Hill Book Co. Used with permission of McGraw-Hill Book Co.

____ Chromosomal Aberrations

Structural and numerical deviations from the norm that affect many genes at once are called chromosomal aberrations. They are sometimes called chromosomal mutations, but most cytogeneticists prefer to use the term "mutation" to refer to qualitative changes within a gene; gene mutations will be discussed on p. 929.

Despite the incredible precision of meiosis, chromosomal aberrations do occur, and they are more common than one might think. They have great economic benefit in agriculture. Unfortunately, they are also responsible for many human genetic malformations. It is estimated that five out of every 1000 humans are born with *serious* genetic defects attributable to chromosomal anomalies. An even greater number of embryos with chromosomal defects are aborted spontaneously, far more than ever reach term.

Changes in chromosome numbers are called **euploidy** when there is the addition or deletion of whole chromosome sets and **aneuploidy** when a single chromosome is added to or subtracted from a diploid set. The most common kind of euploidy is **polyploidy,** the carrying of one or more additional sets of chromosomes. Such aberrations are much more common in plants than in animals. Animals are much less tolerant of chromosomal aberrations because sex determination requires a delicate balance between the numbers of sex chromosomes and autosomes. Many domestic plant species are polyploid (cotton, wheat, apples, oats, tobacco, and others), and perhaps 40% of flowering plants are believed to have originated in this manner. Horticulturists favor polyploids and often try to develop them because they have more intensely colored flowers and more vigorous vegetative growth.

Aneuploidy is usually caused by nondisjunctional separation of chromosomes during meiosis. If a pair of chromosomes fails to separate during the first or second meiotic divisions, both members go to one pole and none to the other. This results in one gamete having n − 1 number of chromosomes and another having n + 1 number of chromosomes. If the n − 1 gamete is fertilized by a normal n gamete, the result is a **monosomic** animal. Survival is rare because the lack of one chromosome gives an uneven balance of genetic instructions. **Trisomy,** the result of the fusion of a normal n gamete and an n + 1 gamete, is much more common, and several kinds of trisomic conditions are known in humans. Perhaps the most familiar is **trisomy 21,** or **Down's syndrome.** As the name indicates, it involves an extra chromosome 21 combined with the chromosome pair 21, and it is caused by nondisjunction of that pair during meiosis. It occurs spontaneously, and there is seldom any family history of the abnormality. However, the risk of its appearance rises dramatically with increasing age of the mother; it occurs 40 times as often in women over 40 years old as among women between the ages of 20 and 30.

Structural aberrations involve whole sets of genes within a chromosome. A portion of a chromosome may be reversed, placing the linear arrangement of genes in reverse order (inversion); nonhomologous chromosomes may exchange sections (translocation); entire blocks of genes may be lost (deletion); or an extra section of chromosome may attach to a normal chromosome (duplication). These are all structural changes that usually do not produce phenotypic changes. Duplications, although rare, are important for evolution because they supply additional genetic information that may enable new functions.

PHYSICAL STRUCTURE OF GENETIC MATERIAL

Genetic transmission depends on the replication of molecules of deoxyribonucleic acid (DNA) (see principle 17, p. 16). The student should review the structure of DNA (pp. 47 to 50) before proceeding with the remainder of this chapter.

Prokaryotes, Plasmids, and Viruses

Prokaryotes (bacteria and cyanobacteria, p. 67) have a single, circular chromosome comprised of a helical, double strand of DNA. It has little protein associated with it and is not enclosed in a nucleus. Although it is visible with the electron microscope, the bacterial chromosome never condenses into the bodies we identify as chromosomes during eukaryotic mitosis and meiosis. Virtually all bacterial species and most individual cells carry an additional source of genetic informa-

A syndrome is a group of symptoms associated with a particular disease or abnormality, although not every symptom is necessarily shown by every patient with the condition. In 1866 an English physician, John Langdon Down, described the syndrome that we know is caused by trisomy 21. Because of Down's belief that the facial features of affected individuals were mongoloid in appearance, the condition has been known as mongolism. The resemblances are superficial, however, and the currently accepted names are trisomy 21 and Down's syndrome. Among the numerous characteristics of the condition, the most disabling is severe mental retardation. This, as well as other conditions caused by chromosomal aberrations and several other birth defects, can be diagnosed *prenatally* by a procedure involving amniocentesis. The physician inserts a hypodermic needle through the abdominal wall of the mother and into the fluids surrounding the fetus (*not into the fetus*) and withdraws some of the fluid, which contains some fetal cells. The cells are grown in culture, their chromosomes are examined, and other tests are done. If a severe birth defect is found, the mother has the option of having an abortion performed. As an extra "bonus," the sex of the fetus is learned after amniocentesis. How?

It was originally believed that the asexual prokaryotes could only stamp out carbon copies of the parental cells, genetic change occurring solely when a mutation intervened. However, several processes of genetic recombination are now known in bacteria. For example, when certain viruses infect bacterial cells, the viruses may pick up a fragment of the bacterial DNA and transfer it to new cells during the course of subsequent infection (transduction). Sometimes DNA in the environment (released by cell death or other processes) can somehow penetrate the cell wall and membrane of the bacteria and be incorporated into their genetic complement (transformation). Under certain circumstances, bacteria of differing "mating types" can actually form cytoplasmic bridges between each other and transfer segments of DNA (conjugation). During conjugation, plasmids are exchanged.

tion: the **plasmid.** Plasmids are not part of the bacterial chromosome, although in some instances they may be incorporated into it. They are normally present as small circles of double-stranded DNA, comprising from a fraction of 1% to 3% of the cell's genome. Nevertheless, they may carry important genetic information, such as ability to withstand a variety of toxic agents, including antibiotics; virulence in many disease-causing bacteria of plants and animals; and information for conjugation. Plasmids are regarded by some workers as separate organisms, even simpler than viruses, which live as endosymbionts in bacteria. Among the reasons for considering plasmids organisms is that they can be exchanged by conjugation between bacteria of different species and even genera. They cannot, however, replicate outside a host cell. Plasmids have been an important tool in recombinant DNA technology, described later in this chapter. Although best known in bacteria, plasmids also occur in yeast, and there is some evidence that they are present in vertebrate cells.

Another genetic system unable to replicate by itself is the **virus.** Viruses are essentially molecules of nucleic acid (DNA or RNA) encased in a protein coat. After penetrating the host cells, which may be prokaryotes or eukaryotes, they induce the host to replicate viral nucleic acid and protein, thus manufacturing more virus particles. For RNA viruses, the RNA must first be copied into DNA by an enzyme called **reverse transcriptase.**

___ Eukaryotes

Mitochondria and plastids

Plastids in plant cells (for example, chloroplasts) and mitochondria, found in most eukaryotic cells, are self-replicating and have their own complement of DNA. The DNA is in the form of small circles with little protein, reminiscent of plasmids. Although mitochondrial and plastid DNA carries genetic information for some of their proteins and their ribosomes, some of the proteins of these organelles are specified by nuclear genes.

Chromosomes

The eukaryotic nuclear chromosome carries much more DNA than any of the foregoing, and its organization and regulation are much more complex. The nucleus of a typical human somatic cell contains 2000 times as much DNA as a typical bacterial cell. If the DNA were pulled out of the nucleus as a continuous string, it would measure 2 m, compared to a 1.5 mm length of DNA from one bacterial cell. Clearly, eukaryote chromosomes must be exquisitely organized to direct the synthesis of proteins, be capable of exact duplication before each cell division, and avoid becoming hopelessly entangled during cell division.

During interphase the chromosomes are not condensed into bodies as in mitosis and meiosis but are present in a state referred to as **chromatin,** whose structure cannot be distinguished with the light microscope. In special preparations, the chromatin can be extracted from nuclei and visualized under the electron microscope (Fig. 37-13). Its appearance is that of beads on a string. The "beads" are called **nucleosomes,** and it is believed that they are the structural quantum in chromosomes. They are formed by a molecule of DNA winding around molecules of proteins. The currently accepted model of nucleosomes is shown in Fig. 37-14. The proteins, called **histones,** have long been known to comprise a large proportion of the protein associated with eukaryotic DNA. There

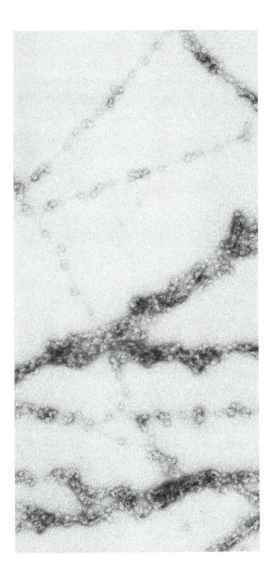

Figure 37-13

Chromatin prepared from chicken red
blood cells. Some strands are stretched
and demonstrate individual nucleosomes.
(Original magnification ×100,000.)
Electron micrograph courtesy C.L.F. Woodcock.

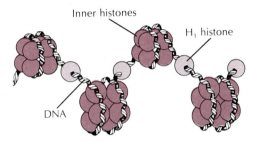

Figure 37-14

Current model of chromatin showing nucleosome organization. The DNA molecule winds one and three fourths turns
around a group of eight histone molecules, two each of four different kinds. A
fifth class of histones (H_1) is found in the
spacer region.

are five kinds of histones. The "inner histones," around which the DNA winds,
are in the form of octomers: two molecules each of four different histone types.
The fifth type is found on the DNA in the "spacer" regions between the nucleosomes. The histones are highly basic; 25% of the amino acids in the inner
histones and 37% of those in the spacer histone consist of lysine, arginine, and
histidine. This property is important in holding them in close association with the
acidic DNA. The nature of higher-order packaging (coiling, folding, and so on) of
chromatin is still unclear, but the spacer histones apparently are very important
factors. Nonhistone proteins may also be important. Whatever the structure, it
must be modified to permit genetic expression. Part of the thread must be unrav-
eled and the nucleosome structure altered as RNA is synthesized.

   Finally, the threads of chromatin must be condensed into the rodlike mitotic
chromosome at each cell division (see Fig. 4-21, p. 92). Evidence indicates that this
compactness is achieved by assembly of the chromatin into a large series of radial
loops (Fig. 37-15), probably on a scaffold of nonhistone protein. Stabilization of
the scaffold involves either calcium or copper ions. There is some evidence that a
scaffold exists during interphase, and its reorganization may bring about the condensation of the mitotic chromosome.

Figure 37-15

Probable arrangement of chromatin in
condensed chromosome. The loops extend radially from a central scaffolding of
nonhistone protein.

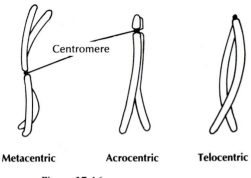

Centromere

Metacentric   Acrocentric   Telocentric

Figure 37-16

Diagram showing positions of centromere on different metaphase chromosomes.

By prophase in mitosis, the chromosomes have already replicated (during interphase); therefore the chromatids can be seen, joined together by their **centromere** (point of spindle fiber attachment). The position of the centromere is characteristic for a particular chromosome and can be used to help identify it. Centromere positions may be described as **metacentric** (arms of the chromatids equal on each side), **acrocentric** (centromere closer to one end), and **telocentric** (centromere at the very end) (Fig. 37-16). The staining reactions of different parts of the chromosomes vary. Some parts stain densely (**heterochromatin**), and some parts take up little stain (**euchromatin**). It is believed that heterochromatic regions of the chromosomes represent areas where the genes are inactive. The Barr body (p. 905) is an entire chromosome of heterochromatin. The particular regions of euchromatin and heterochromatin change during development as different sets of genes become active or inactive. Some authors use these terms to designate active and inactive (dispersed and condensed) interphase chromatin; genetic expression does not occur from condensed chromatin.

Giant chromosomes

Normally manifestations of gene activity on chromosomes, that is, transcription of DNA into RNA, cannot be seen with the light microscope. However, in a few instances they can. In the salivary glands of *Drosophila* and some other insects, the chromatin strands replicate repeatedly without undergoing mitosis and are known as **polytene chromosomes** (Fig. 37-17). These giant chromosomes are easily distinguishable with the light microscope. The chromatin strands are too close for efficient synthesis of RNA along them, but as genes in a particular region become active, they separate to form an observable "puff" (Fig. 37-18). Another example is the **lampbrush chromosomes** found in the oocytes of vertebrates at the first meiotic prophase. They are so called because of their resemblance to brushes used to clean kerosene lamps. Large amounts of RNA and protein are needed during the development of the ovum, and the parts of the chromosome with the appropriate genes are looped out laterally from the central chromosomal axis. Parts of the chromosome with inactive genes are tightly compact.

Figure 37-17

Chromosomes from a salivary gland cell of larval fruit fly *Drosophila*. These are among the largest chromosomes found in animal cells. Such chromosomes are called polytene because they are made up of many replicated chromatin strands. These chromosomes are not confined to salivary glands but are also known to occur in other organs, such as gut and malpighian tubules of most dipteran insects. The technique for their study is simply to crush salivary glands in a drop of aceto-carmine, between a cover glass and a slide, so that the chromosomes are set free from the nuclei and are spread out as shown in the photograph.

Courtesy General Biological Supply House, Inc., Chicago.

GENE THEORY
Gene Concept

The term "gene" (Gr., *genos*, descent) was coined by W. Johannsen in 1909 to refer to the hereditary factors of Mendel (1865). Both cytological and genetic studies showed that genes, although of unknown chemical nature, were the fundamental units of inheritance. They were regarded as indivisible units of the chromosomes on which they were located. Studies with multiple mutant alleles demonstrated that alleles are in fact divisible by recombination; that is, *portions* of a gene are separable, and they have a fine structure. Furthermore, parts of many genes in eukaryotes are separated by sections of DNA that do not specify a part of the finished product (introns).

As a result of new insights into gene structure and function, developed after 1950, the gene emerged as a **unit of function,** called a **cistron.** A cistron is by no means the smallest divisible unit of a gene because mutations may occur within a cistron, but it is the smallest *functional* region on a chromosome. In general, the term "gene" is synonymous with "cistron," although a classical Mendelian gene may consist of more than one cistron. The reader may already detect a semantic problem here and may wonder if introducing the synonym "cistron" for gene is helpful. To the geneticist it is helpful because it replaces the unitary concept of the physical gene with the concept of an operational gene composed of one or more functional components, each of which embraces an array of mutant sites. Out of this, the concept of a gene as a unit that behaves in a Mendelian fashion emerges more or less intact.

As the chief functional unit of genetic material, genes determine the basic architecture of every cell, the nature and life of the cell, the specific protein syntheses, the enzyme formation, the self-reproduction of the cell, and, directly or indirectly, the entire metabolic function of the cell. Because of their ability to mutate, to be assorted and shuffled around in different combinations, genes have become the basis for our modern interpretation of evolution. Genes are molecular patterns that can maintain their identities for many generations, can be self-duplicated in each generation, and can control cell processes by allowing their specificities to be copied.

One Gene–One Enzyme Hypothesis

Since genes act to produce different phenotypes, we may infer that their action follows the scheme: gene → gene product → phenotypic expression. Furthermore, we may suspect that the gene product is usually a protein, because proteins, acting as enzymes, antibodies, hormones, and structural elements throughout the body, are the single most important group of biomolecules.

The first clear, well-documented study to link genes and enzymes was carried out on the common bread mold *Neurospora* by Beadle and Tatum in the early 1940s. This organism was ideally suited to a study of gene function for several reasons: these molds are much simpler to handle than fruit flies, they grow readily in well-defined chemical media, and they are haploid organisms that are consequently unencumbered with dominance relationships. Furthermore, mutations were readily induced by irradiation with ultraviolet light. Ultraviolet light–induced mutants, grown and tested in specific nutrient media, were found to have single-gene mutations that were inherited in accord with Mendelian principles of segregation. Each mutant strain was shown to be defective in one enzyme, which

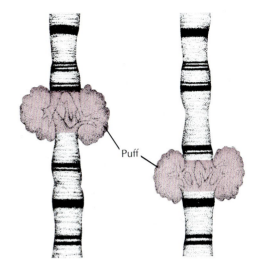

Figure 37-18

Puffing in one of the bands of a salivary gland chromosome of a midge larva *Chironomus.* Swelling, or puff, indicates activity in a region where RNA (and perhaps some DNA) is being produced, and it may include single bands or a group of adjacent ones. Puffs always include the same bands that occur in a definite sequence during development of the larva.

prevented that strain from synthesizing one or more complex molecules. Putting it another way, the ability to synthesize a particular molecule was controlled by a single gene.

From these experiments Beadle and Tatum set forth an important and exciting formulation: **one gene produces one enzyme** (see Principle 20, p. 17). For this work they were awarded the Nobel Prize in 1958. The new hypothesis was soon validated by the research of others who studied other biosynthetic pathways. Hundreds of inherited disorders, including dozens of human hereditary diseases, are caused by single mutant genes that result in the loss of a specific essential enzyme. We now know that a particular protein may be made of several chains of amino acids (polypeptides), each of which may be specified by a different gene. Thus, the Beadle-Tatum hypothesis is expressed as **one gene–one polypeptide.** This hypothesis has proved to be of enormous value as a stimulus to a biochemical approach to gene function. Today we recognize that while most genes direct the synthesis of polypeptides and proteins of enzymes, others code for antibodies, hormones, and various kinds of RNA.

STORAGE AND TRANSFER OF GENETIC INFORMATION
Nucleic Acids: Molecular Basis of Inheritance

It has been known for many years that genes and chromosomes are made up chiefly of nucleoproteins; that is, they are macromolecules composed of nucleic acids, histones, and nonhistone proteins. To review briefly, nucleic acids are polymers of nucleotides, which are in turn composed of a purine or pyrimidine base, a sugar (ribose or deoxyribose), and a phosphate group.

On the basis of the kind of sugar, the nucleic acids are divided into two main groups: **deoxyribonucleic acid (DNA)** and **ribonucleic acid (RNA).** DNA occurs in the nucleus, in mitochondria, and in plastids, where it is the major structural component of genes (see Principle 17, p. 16); RNA is found throughout the cell, being especially abundant in nucleoli and in the cytoplasm. Thus, a nucleic acid molecule is made up of many nucleotides joined to form long chains (Fig. 2-33, p. 49). The purine units are adenine and guanine; the pyrimidines are cytosine, thymine, and uracil. Small amounts of other bases occur, such as 5-methyl cytosine. The kinds of nucleotides differ on the basis of these purines and pyrimidines: (1) adenine-sugar-phosphate, (2) guanine-sugar-phosphate, (3) cytosine-sugar-phosphate, (4) thymine-sugar-phosphate, and (5) uracil-sugar-phosphate. The DNA molecule is composed chiefly of the first four of these nucleotides (Fig. 2-35, p. 50); RNA has the first three and the last one. Although the phosphate-sugar part of the long chain of nucleotides is regular, the purine or pyrimidine base attached to the sugar is not always the same. The order of these bases varies from one section of the nucleic acid molecule to another. Depending on the sequence of the nucleotides, there is an almost unlimited variety of nucleic acids.

The positive identification of the nucleic acids as the repository of genetic information came in the early 1950s after many decades of research. Although DNA was first isolated by Miescher (who called it nuclein) in 1869, just 4 years after Mendel published his findings, it was not until 1944 that O.T. Avery and his associates suggested that DNA is the genetic material in bacteria. However, many geneticists were reluctant to accept these conclusions, arguing that Avery's findings were a special case having little relevance to inheritance in other organisms. Then, in 1952, Hershey and Chase established beyond all reasonable doubt that DNA is the heritable material. This launched intensive activity in laboratories all over the world, culminating in the momentous discovery of the structure of DNA by James Watson and Francis Crick at Cambridge University in 1953. A lively and absorbing personal account of the discovery is given in Watson's book *The Double Helix*.

Double helix

The Watson-Crick model of DNA structure had to suggest plausible answers to such problems as (1) how specific directions are transmitted from one generation to another, (2) how DNA could control protein synthesis, and (3) how the DNA molecule could duplicate itself. Classical genetics and cytology had shown how a cell divides to form two cells and how each cell receives a set of chromosomes with their genes identical in structure to the preexisting set. But nothing was known about how a chemical substance could carry out the specifications required by the genetic substance of a gene. The elegance of the Watson-Crick hypothesis lies in the perfect manner in which it fits the data and in the way that it can be tested.

Maurice Wilkins succeeded in getting sharp x-ray diffraction patterns that revealed three major periodic spacings in crystalline DNA. These periodicities of 0.34, 2, and 3.4 nm were interpreted by Watson and Crick as the space distance between successive nucleotides in the DNA chains, the width of the chain, and the distance between successive turns of the helix, respectively. The x-ray diffraction photograph, with certain limitations, also gave indications of the spatial arrangement of some of the atoms within the large molecule. Watson and Crick came up with the idea that the molecule is bipartite, with an overall helical configuration. Accordingly, their model showed that the DNA molecule looks like two interlocked coils. Each "coil" consists of a sugar-phosphate backbone held together by phosphodiester bonds. The two interlocked coils are held together by hydrogen bonds between the purine and pyrimidine bases that form the core of the double helix (Fig. 2-35, p. 50).

Base pairing

The two DNA strands run in opposite directions, that is, they are **antiparallel**. This is evident from an examination of Fig. 2-35 (p. 50). The two strands are also **complementary**—the sequence of bases along one strand specifies the sequence of bases along the other strand. Each strand could thus serve as a **template** for the production of its complement.

From examination of their original wire model of DNA, Watson and Crick proposed a base-pairing rule. Adenine at one point on a strand must bond with thymine at the corresponding point on the other strand. Similarly, guanine must bond with cytosine. This happens because only these pairs are of proper size and arrangement of hydrogens and acceptor atoms for efficient bonding.

The purine bases adenine and guanine (A and G) are large, whereas the pyrimidine bases thymine and cytosine (T and C) are small. To fit into the structure of the DNA molecule, each pair must consist of one large and one small base; thus, the small bases T and C, T and T, or C and C could not bond in pairs because they would not meet in the middle. The big bases (A and G) could not bond in any combination because they would produce a bulge in the helix. Neither can A and

Figure 37-19

Replication of DNA. The parent strands of DNA part, and DNA polymerase synthesizes daughter strands using the base sequence of parent strands as a template.

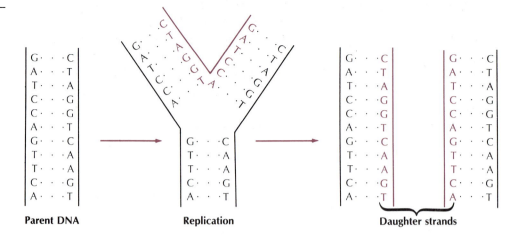

Parent DNA   Replication   Daughter strands

C nor G and T (although in these pairs one is large and one is small) form bond mates because their hydrogen bonds would not pair off properly. Thus, there is only one correct way for the bases to bond: A with T and G with C. This is shown in the circled cross sections to the right of the DNA molecule in Fig. 2-35 (p. 50).

Although all DNA molecules have the same general pattern, each one is unique because of the varying sequence of bases. This sequence spells out the genetic instructions that determine the sequence of amino acids in a protein organized by the gene (see Principle 17, p. 16). This genetic message, or "code," is written in a language of only four symbols (adenine, guanine, thymine, and cytosine) and is translated into protein amino acid sequences (see Principle 18, p. 16). The coding will be discussed subsequently.

___ DNA Replication

Every time the cell divides, the structure of the nuclear DNA must be precisely copied in the daughter cells. The wonder of the DNA double helix model was that its structure suggested how it could be replicated: each existing strand of the DNA molecule serves as a template for the synthesis of a new strand. This is the essential requirement of a genetic molecule, which was not satisfied by other models (such as single or triple helix) proposed before the Watson-Crick model. The two strands of the helix could unwind to expose the nucleotide bases. The double helix then separates, perhaps like a zipper, and new nucleotides are incorporated to synthesize new strands. Each of the four kinds of nucleotides consists of one of the DNA bases, one sugar unit, and three phosphate groups. Only one of the three phosphate groups is used in making the backbone of the new strand; the other two are necessary to provide energy for synthesis.

Because of the strict complementarity (base-pairing) rule, each exposed base will pair only with its complementary base. Thus, each of the two strands will form a double helix identical with the parental molecule. Note that each daughter molecule will contain one parental strand and one new strand (Fig. 37-19).

An enzyme, **DNA polymerase,** is essential for replication. The enzyme does not determine which of the four bases will be added to the new chain (base selection is determined by complementation with the base sequence in the parent strand), but it does hold the reacting molecules in position and vastly accelerates the reaction.

If replication proceeds as predicted, a replication "fork" should be visible where the double helix is "unzipping" during replication. Forks have in fact been seen in the circular bacterial chromosomes and plasmids. How the fork is formed is still unclear. Nor is it yet known how the two intertwined strands of DNA untwist during replication. They may rotate during the process, but it is inconceivable that the entire chromosomal DNA molecule, millions of base pairs in length, flips about within the chromosome. When the hydrogen bonds holding base pairs together are broken during replication, the two strands move apart from one another, even though in the double helical form they appear to be interlocked.

DNA coding by base sequence

Since DNA is the genetic material and is composed of a linear sequence of base pairs, an obvious extension of the Watson-Crick model is that the sequence of base pairs in DNA codes for, and is colinear with, the sequence of amino acids in a protein (see Principle 18, p. 16). The coding hypothesis had to account for the way a string of four different bases—a four-letter alphabet—could dictate the sequence of 20 different amino acids.

In the coding procedure, obviously there cannot be a 1:1 correlation between four bases and 20 amino acids. If the coding unit (often called a word, or **codon**) consists of two bases, only 16 words (4^2) can be formed, which cannot account for 20 amino acids. Therefore the protein code must consist of at least three bases or three letters because 64 possible words (4^3) can be formed by four bases when taken as triplets. This means that there could be a considerable redundancy of triplets (codons), since DNA codes for just 20 amino acids. Later work by Crick confirmed that nearly all of the amino acids are specified by more than one code triplet (Table 37-1).

DNA shows a surprising stability, both in prokaryotes and in eukaryotes. Interestingly, it is very susceptible to damage by harmful chemicals in the environment and radiation. Such damage is usually not permanent because cells have an efficient repair system. Various types of damage and repair are known, one of which is called **excision repair.** Ultraviolet irradiation often causes adjacent pyrimidines to link together by covalent bonds (dimerize), preventing transcription and replication. A series of several enzymes "recognizes" the area of the damaged strand and excises the pair of dimerized pyrimidines and several bases following them. DNA polymerase then synthesizes the missing strand along the remaining one, according to the base-pairing rules, and the enzyme **DNA ligase** joins the end of the new strand to the old one.

_____ Transcription and the Role of Messenger RNA

Information is coded in DNA, but DNA does not participate directly in protein synthesis. It is obvious that an intermediary is required. This intermediary is another nucleic acid called **messenger RNA (mRNA)** (see Principle 19, p. 16). Recall from Chapter 2 (p. 49) that RNA differs from DNA in three important ways: (1) it is _single_ stranded and not a double helix, (2) it has ribose sugar in its nucleotides instead of deoxyribose, and (3) it has the pyrimidine uracil (U) instead of thymine (T). Despite these differences, RNA is constructed very much like a single strand of DNA.

Ribosomal, transfer, and messenger RNAs are **transcribed** directly from

Table 37-1 Genetic Code: Codons (Code Triplets) between Messenger RNA and Specific Amino Acids

Codons	Amino acid
GCU, GCC, GCA, GCG	Alanine
CGU, CGC, CGA, CGG, AGA	Arginine
AAU, AAC	Asparagine
GAU, GAC	Aspartic acid
UGU, UGC	Cysteine
GAA, GAG	Glutamic acid
CAA, CAG	Glutamine
GGU, GGC, GGA, GGG	Glycine
CAU, CAC	Histidine
AUU, AUC, AUA	Isoleucine
CUU, CUC, CUA, CUG, UUA, UUG	Leucine
AAA, AAG	Lysine
AUG	Methionine; initiation of message
UUU, UUC	Phenylalanine
CCU, CCC, CCA, CCG	Proline
AGU, AGC, UCU, UCC, UCA, UCG	Serine
ACU, ACC, ACA, ACG	Threonine
UGG	Tryptophan
UAU, UAC	Tyrosine
GUU, GUC, GUA, GUG	Valine
UAA, UAG, UGA	Termination of message of one gene

DNA (Fig. 37-20), with each of the many mRNAs being determined by a gene or particular segments of DNA. In this process of making a complementary copy of one strand or gene of DNA in the formation of mRNA, an enzyme, **RNA polymerase,** is needed. (In fact, each type of RNA [ribosomal, transfer, and messenger] is transcribed by a specific type of RNA polymerase.) The mRNA contains a sequence of bases that complements the bases in one of the two DNA strands just as the DNA strands complement each other. Thus, A in the coding DNA strand is replaced by U in mRNA; C is replaced by G; G is replaced by C; and T is replaced by A. Only one of the two chains is used as the template for RNA synthesis because only one bears the AUG codon that initiates a message (Table 37-1). The reason why only one strand of the double-stranded DNA is a "coding strand" is that mRNA otherwise would always be formed in complementary pairs, and enzymes also would be synthesized in complementary pairs. In other words, two different enzymes would be produced for every DNA coding sequence instead of one. This would certainly lead to metabolic chaos.

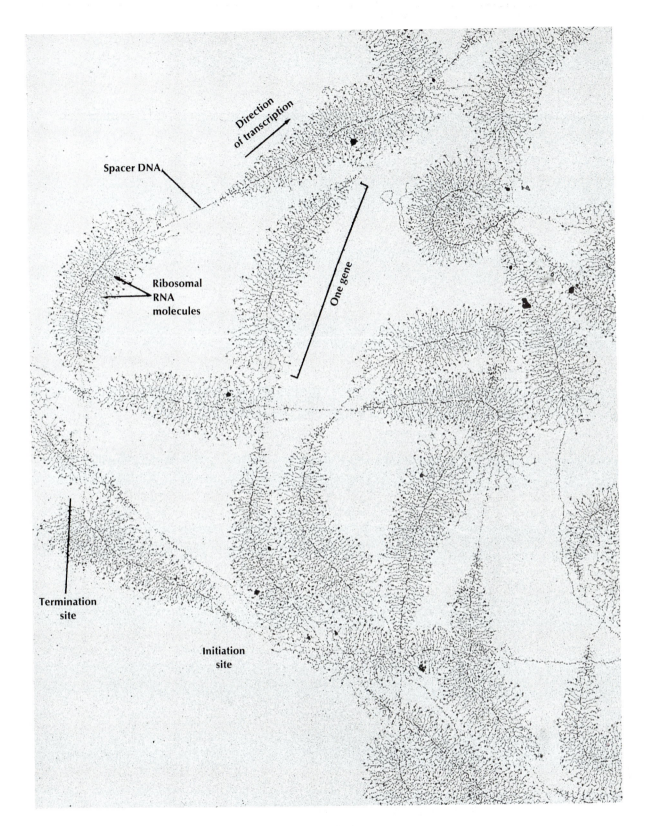

Figure 37-20

Genes in action. This remarkable electron micrograph shows DNA transcribing ribosomal RNA molecules in the oocyte nucleoli of the spotted newt *Diemictylus viridescens*. These are tandemly repeated genes separated by spacer (nontranscribing) segments of DNA. The newest and shortest ribosomal RNA transcripts are close to the initiation site on the gene. When completed molecules reach the termination site, they are freed to move out of the nucleus into the cytoplasm, where they form ribosomes. Enormous quantities of ribosomes are synthesized in maturing amphibian eggs. (×25,000.)

From Miller, O.L., Jr., and D.L. Beatty. Science **164** (cover). 1969. Copyright 1969 by the American Association for the Advancement of Science.

Figure 37-21

Transcription and maturation of ovalbumin gene of chicken. The entire gene of 7700 base pairs is transcribed to form the primary mRNA, then the cap of methyl guanine and the polyadenylate tail are added. After the introns are spliced out, the mature mRNA is transferred to the cytoplasm.
Redrawn from Chambon, P. 1981. Sci. Am. **244:**60-71 (May).

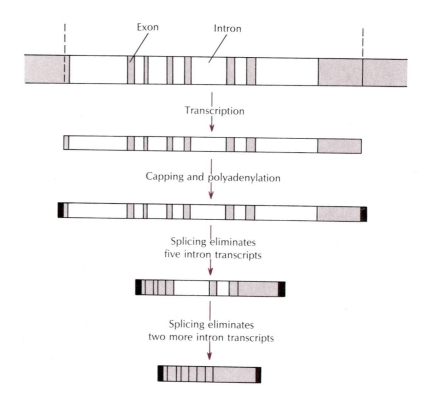

Genes on the DNA of prokaryotes are coded on a continuous stretch of DNA, which is transcribed into mRNA and then translated (see the following section). It was assumed that this was also the case for eukaryote genes until the surprising discovery a few years ago that stretches of DNA are transcribed in the nucleus into mRNA that does not encode the finished product. In other words, the mRNA that is translated into protein in the cytoplasm is not the same mRNA that is transcribed in the nucleus; pieces of the nuclear mRNA have been spliced out (Fig. 37-21). It was thus discovered that many genes are split, interrupted by sequences of bases that do not code for the final product, and the mRNA transcribed from them must be edited or "matured" before translation in the cytoplasm. The intervening segments of DNA are now known as **introns,** while those that code for part of the mature RNA and are translated into gene product are called **exons.** Before the mRNA leaves the nucleus, the introns are spliced out and a methylated guanine "cap" is added at one end, while a tail of adenine nucleotides (poly-*A*) is added at the other (Fig. 37-21). The cap and the poly-*A* tail are characteristic of mRNA molecules.

It has now been found that the genes coding for many (but not all) proteins are split; in mammals the genes coding for the histones and for interferon are on continuous stretches of DNA. In lymphocyte differentiation the parts of the split genes coding for immunoglobulins are actually *rearranged* during development, so that different proteins result from subsequent transcription and translation. This partially accounts for the enormous diversity of antibodies manufactured by the descendants of the lymphocytes (p. 706).

Even more recently it was found that the belief that introns are noncoding regions is not necessarily true. At least in some mitochondrial mRNAs, the introns may code for proteins, and in one case for a ribosomal component. In most of those studied so far, the proteins coded by the introns are "maturases," enzymes that control the splicing of the introns from which they came or introns from

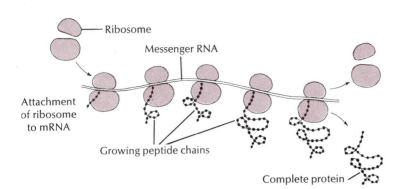

Figure 37-22

How the protein chain is formed. As ribosomes move along messenger RNA, the amino acids are added stepwise to form the polypeptide chain.

different genes. Finally, base sequences in some introns have been found that are complementary to other base sequences in the intron, suggesting that the intron could fold so that the complementary sequences would pair. This may be necessary to control proper alignment of intron boundaries before splicing.

Translation: Final Stage in Information Transfer

The **translation** process takes place on **ribosomes**, granular structures composed of protein and **ribosomal RNA (rRNA)** (see Principle 18, p. 16). The mRNA molecules fix themselves to the ribosomes to form a messenger RNA–ribosome complex. Since only a short section of an mRNA molecule is in contact with a single ribosome, the mRNA usually fixes itself to several ribosomes at once. The entire complex, called a **polyribosome** or **polysome,** allows several proteins of the same kind to be synthesized at once, one on each ribosome of the polyribosome (Fig. 37-22).

The assembly of proteins on the mRNA–ribosome complex requires the action of another kind of RNA called **transfer RNA (tRNA).** The tRNA molecules collect the free amino acids from the cytoplasm and deliver them to the polysome, where they are assembled into a protein. There is a special tRNA molecule for every amino acid. Furthermore each tRNA is accompanied by a special **activating enzyme.** These enzymes are necessary to sort out and attach the correct amino acid to each tRNA by a process called **loading.**

The tRNAs are surprisingly large molecules that are folded in a complicated way in the form of a cloverleaf (Fig. 37-23). On this cloverleaf a special sequence of three bases (the **anticodon**) is exposed in just the right way to form base pairs with complementary bases (the codon) in the mRNA. The anticodon of the tRNA is the key to the correct sequencing of amino acids in the protein being assembled.

For example, alanine is assembled into a protein when it is signaled by the codon GCG in an mRNA. This translation is accomplished by alanine tRNA in which the anticodon is CGC. The alanine tRNA is first loaded with alanine by its activating enzyme. The loaded alanine tRNA enters the polysome where it fits precisely into the right place on the mRNA strand. Then the next loaded tRNA specified by the mRNA code (glycine tRNA, for example) enters the polysome and attaches itself beside the alanine tRNA. The two animo acids are united with a peptide bond (with the energy from a molecule of guanosine triphosphate), and the alanine tRNA falls off. The process continues stepwise as the protein chain is built (Fig. 37-22). A protein of 500 amino acids can be assembled in less than 30 seconds.

Figure 37-23

Formation of polypeptide chain on messenger RNA. As ribosome moves down messenger RNA molecule, transfer RNA molecules with attached amino acids enter ribosome *(left)*. Amino acids are joined together into polypeptide chain, and transfer RNA molecules leave ribosome *(right)*.

Regulation of Gene Function

In the preceding chapter we saw how the orderly differentiation of an organism from fertilized egg to adult requires the involvement of genetic material at every stage of development. Developmental biologists have provided convincing evidence that every cell in a developing embryo is genetically equivalent (see Principle 24, p. 18). This was first demonstrated by Spemann's delayed nucleation experiments (p. 869) and more recently confirmed with the elegant nuclear transplantation experiments of Gurdon and his associates in England (p. 871). Thus, it is clear that as tissues differentiate, they use only a part of the genetic instruction present in every cell (unless chromatin diminution occurs [p. 926]). Certain genes express themselves only at certain times and not at other times. Indeed, there is reason to believe that in a particular cell or tissue, most of the genes are inactive at any given moment. The problem in development is to explain how, if every cell has a full gene complement, certain genes are "turned on" and produce proteins that are required for a particular developmental stage while the other genes remain silent.

Actually, although the developmental process brings the question of gene activation clearly into focus, gene regulation is necessary throughout an organism's existence. The cellular enzyme systems that control all functional processes obviously require genetic regulation because enzymes have powerful effects even in minute amounts. Enzyme synthesis must be responsive to the influences of supply and demand.

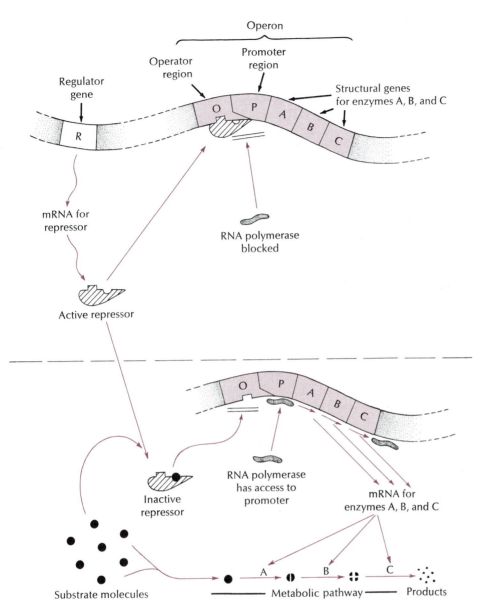

Figure 37-24

One method of genetic regulation found in bacteria. In this case, the presence of substrate molecules prevents the repressor protein from binding to the operator, thus allowing the enzyme, RNA polymerase, to start at the promoter and synthesize the messenger RNA necessary for the synthesis of enzymes A, B, and C. In the absence of substrate, the repressor blocks the promoter, and no enzymes A, B, and C are produced. This is an *inducible* system because the presence of the substrate induces synthesis of enzymes necessary to metabolize it. An alternative system would be one in which products of the metabolic pathway are bound with the repressor to activate it, thus cutting off synthesis of the enzymes and shutting down the pathway.

Operon model for gene regulation

Our understanding of how genetic material is used to regulate the synthesis of proteins has advanced greatly since the discoveries of two French scientists, J. Monod and F. Jacob, using bacteria (Fig. 37-24). The basic unit carrying the genetic code for synthesis of a protein is the **structural gene,** whose actions are regulated in a complex way. Adjacent to the structural gene is a special segment of DNA called the **operator.** Together, the structural gene and operator comprise a genetic unit called the **operon.** The operon may contain a single structural gene or several structural genes of related function. Close to, and perhaps overlapping, the operator is a region called the **promoter,** where mRNA transcription begins. If access to the promoter is blocked, the mRNA cannot be synthesized, and so the enzyme is not produced. Still another gene, called a **regulator** gene, which may be at some distance from the operator, directs synthesis of a protein **repressor.** The

Figure 37-25

Some genes in eukaryotes are apparently turned off by the methylation of some cytosine residues in the chain. **A,** Structure of 5-methyl cytosine. **B,** Cytosine residues next to guanine are those that are methylated in a strand, thus allowing both strands to be symmetrically methylated.

repressor may bind with the operator, thus blocking access to the promoter and preventing the synthesis of mRNA. What determines whether the repressor will bind with the operator? The repressor is affected by other substances in the cell, which may activate or inactivate it. If, for example, a particular substrate is present, and certain enzymes are needed to metabolize that substrate, it may bind with and *inactivate* the repressor, preventing the repressor from binding with the operator. When this happens, mRNA molecules are formed on the structural genes and the needed enzymes are produced. Alternatively, after a buildup of the end product of a metabolic pathway, the end product may *activate* the repressor, which then binds the operator, blocks access of the RNA polymerase to the promoter, and turns off the synthesis of the enzymes in that metabolic pathway.

Gene regulation in eukaryotes

Since the work of Jacob and Monod, it has been realized that the operon concept has little if any applicability to gene regulation in eukaryotes. Genes in eukaryotes are not arranged as operons. We now know of a number of different phenomena in eukaryotic cells that could serve as control points. Brown (1981) has categorized possible genetic mechanisms for control as those in which the genes are altered (diminution, amplification, rearrangement, and modification), those in which gene expression is modulated (transcriptional, postranscriptional, and translational control), and control of expression of multigene families. Thorough discussion of all of these is beyond the scope of this book, but we will give a few examples.

Chromatin diminution

During differentiation of somatic cells or nuclei of some nematodes, protozoa, crustaceans, and insects, some chromatin or even entire chromosomes are discarded, so that only the germ cells (or micronuclei in protozoa) retain the entire genetic complement. Clearly, the products coded by the lost genes cannot be expressed by the cells. How widely applicable this mechanism may be has yet to be determined.

Gene amplification

Polytenization of the chromosomes in some insects has already been mentioned. This is an example of a case in which large amounts of a particular product, for example, rRNA, may be required at a given stage. The macronucleus of ciliates may contain multiple copies of some genes (amplification), while other genes are lost (diminution), and the micronucleus retains the full genetic complement.

Gene rearrangement

The rearrangement of genes for immunoglobulins during differentiation of lymphocytes was mentioned previously. Such rearrangement may also be responsible for a switch in mating types in yeast.

DNA modification

An important mechanism for turning genes off appears to be methylation of cytosine residues in the 5′ position, that is, adding a methyl group (CH₃-) to the carbon in the 5′ position in the cytosine ring (Fig. 37-25, *A*). This usually happens when the cytosine is next to a guanine residue; thus, the bases in the complementary DNA strand would also be a cytosine and a guanine (Fig. 37-25, *B*). When the

DNA is replicated, an enzyme recognizes the CG sequence and quickly methylates the daughter strand, maintaining the gene in an inactive state. In a recent report the gene for fetal hemoglobin was turned on in an adult by treatment with a drug that causes demethylation of DNA. Because the fetal hemoglobin is functionally adequate, treatment with the drug results in a dramatic improvement in the clinical condition of persons with sickle cell anemia and β-thalassemia, which are caused by a defect in the gene for one of the adult hemoglobin chains.

Transcriptional control

Some hormones act by entering the cell and affecting gene transcription directly. Progesterone, for example, enters the cells of the chicken oviduct and binds with a receptor protein, and this complex binds with the chromatin in the nucleus. The effect is to turn on genes that code for specific cellular products; that is, molecules of mRNA are produced that result in synthesis of egg albumin and other substances.

___ Methods in Molecular Genetics

Progress in our understanding of genetic mechanisms on the molecular level, as discussed in the last few pages, has been almost breathtaking in the last few years. We can expect many more discoveries in the near future. This progress has been due largely to the effectiveness of many biochemical techniques now used in molecular biology. We have space to describe only a few briefly.

One of the most important tools in this technology is a series of enzymes called **restriction endonucleases.** Each of these enzymes, derived from bacteria, cleaves double-stranded DNA at particular sites determined by the particular base sequences at that point. Many of these endonucleases cut the DNA strands so that one has several bases projecting farther than the other strand (Fig. 37-26), leaving what are called "sticky ends." When these DNA fragments are mixed with others that have been cleaved by the same endonuclease, and in the presence of DNA ligase, they tend to anneal (join) by the rules of complementary base pairing.

If the DNA annealed after cleavage by the endonuclease is from two different sources, for example, a plasmid and a mammal, the product is **recombinant DNA.** To make use of the recombinant DNA, the modified plasmid must be cloned in bacteria. The bacteria are treated with dilute calcium chloride to make them more susceptible to taking up the recombinant DNA, but the plasmids do not enter most of the cells present. The bacterial cells that have taken up the recombinant DNA can be identified if the plasmid has a marker, for example, resistance to an antibiotic. Then, only the bacteria that will grow in the presence of the antibiotic are those that have absorbed the recombinant DNA. Some viruses have also been used as carriers for recombinant DNA. The plasmids and viruses retain the ability to replicate in the bacterial cells; therefore the mammalian gene is amplified.

Clearly, for this technique to be useful, the cloned bacteria must manufacture (and the mammalian gene in the recombinant DNA must code for) a product of some interest, such as a hormone. To find and isolate that gene from the entire mammalian genome is a formidable task, particularly when the DNA contains numerous introns. One way is to determine the amino acid sequence in the protein, deduce the sequence of DNA codons responsible for that amino acid sequence, and then synthesize DNA of the proper sequence, one base at a time.

This last step is very difficult, and the method is only practical for short

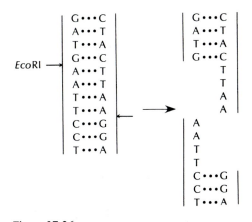

Figure 37-26

Action of restriction endonuclease, *Eco*RI. Such enzymes recognize specific base sequences that are palindromic (a palindrome is a word spelled the same backward and forward). *Eco*RI leaves "sticky ends," which are easily matched to other DNA fragments cleaved by the same enzyme and linked by DNA ligase.

Figure 37-27

Steps in preparing DNA for a mammalian gene for cloning in bacteria and for determining that the gene has been cloned.

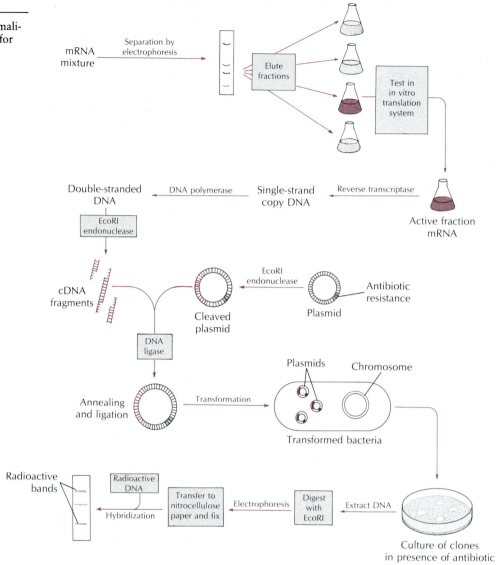

polypeptides. It is easier to synthesize a copy DNA (cDNA) from mRNA. In this procedure, RNA must be extracted from the cells, and the mRNA must be separated from the much more plentiful rRNA by some method such as affinity chromatography, taking advantage of the poly-*A* tail on the mature mRNA. In some instances the desired mRNA is present in great abundance and can be purified. The mixture of mRNAs is fractionated according to size (molecular weight) by a technique called gel electrophoresis, the fractions are recovered, and activity is tested in a cell-free translation system. The cDNA is then prepared from the mRNA that mediates synthesis of the desired protein by the action of reverse transcriptase (Fig. 37-27). The second strand of DNA is synthesized by DNA polymerase using the first cDNA strand as a template. Thus, a molecule of DNA is prepared for insertion into a plasmid and cloning in bacteria.

In many cases, however, the desired mRNA is present in small quantities, and the cDNA prepared from the partially purified RNA is very impure. A mixture of DNA fragments containing many different genes is "shotgunned" into bacteria, and their colonies are screened for the desired product by one of several methods, such as antibody binding.

When colonies of bacterial clones have been identified, their DNA can be extracted, cleaved by the endonuclease, and fractionated by gel electrophoresis, and the cDNA is used as a probe to confirm whether the mammalian gene was being replicated in the bacteria. In this assay the DNA fractions on the electrophoresis plate are heated to separate them into single strands (denaturation), then transferred and fixed to a nitrocellulose filter paper by a kind of blotting technique. A solution containing radioactive cDNA is spread over the plates, and they are washed. Wherever radioactive spots remain on the plates, cDNA has hybridized with the denatured DNA and reformed the double strands according to the rules of base pairing, indicating the identity of the two (Fig. 37-27).

To obtain a useful product from the bacterial colonies containing the mammalian genes, the mammalian genes must be transcribed and translated by the bacteria. This can be accomplished by inserting the proper messages into the plasmid DNA, causing the little chemical factories of the bacterial colonies to turn out large quantities of important substances, such as human insulin and interferon.

The genetic complement of mammalian cells has also been artificially manipulated. Techniques include somatic cell hybridization (to produce monoclonal antibodies [see marginal note on p. 706]) and microinjection of genes into the nuclei of cells in culture.

SOURCES OF PHENOTYPIC VARIATION

We will conclude this chapter by considering the creative force of evolution: biological variation. Without variability among individuals, there could be no continued adaptation to a changing environment and no evolution.

There are actually several sources of variability, some of which we have already described. The independent assortment of chromosomes during meiosis is a random process that creates new chromosomal recombinations in the gametes. In addition, chromosomal crossing over during meiosis allows recombination of linked genes between homologous chromosomes, further increasing variability. The random fusion of gametes from both parents produces still another source of variation.

Thus, sexual reproduction multiplies variation and provides the diversity and plasticity necessary for a species to survive environmental change. Sexual reproduction with its sequence of gene segregation and recombination, generation after generation, is, as the geneticist T. Dobzhansky has said, the "master adaptation which makes all other evolutionary adaptations more readily accessible."

Although sexual reproduction reshuffles and amplifies whatever genetic diversity exists in the population, there must be ways to generate *new* genetic material. This happens through gene mutations and, sometimes, through chromosomal aberrations.

There is a story that George Bernard Shaw once received a letter from a famous actress who suggested that they conceive a perfect child who would combine her beauty and his brains. He declined the offer, pointing out that the child could just as well inherit her brains and his beauty. Shaw was correct; the fusion of parental gametes is not only random, it is unpredictable.

Gene Mutations

Gene mutations are chemicophysical changes in genes resulting in an alteration of the original character. Although the actual mutation cannot be visually detected under the microscope, all gene mutations are believed to be changes of nucleotides in chromosomal DNA. A mutation may involve a codon substitution, the deletion of one or more bases from a codon, or the insertion of additional bases into the DNA chain. Most mutations are "point" mutations involving a single base pair (p. 49).

Mutations are random because they are unpredictable and unrelated to the needs of the organism. Once a gene is mutated, it faithfully reproduces its new self just as it did before it was mutated. *Many, perhaps nearly all, mutant genes are actually harmful because they replace adaptive genes that have evolved and served the organism through its long evolution.* Sometimes, however, mutations are advantageous. These are of great significance to evolution because they furnish new possibilities on which natural selection works. Natural selection determines which new genes merit survival; the environment imposes a screening process that passes the fit and eliminates the unfit.

When an allele of a gene is mutated to the new allele, it tends to be recessive and its effects are normally masked by its partner allele. Only in the homozygous condition can such mutant genes be expressed. Thus, a population carries a reservoir of mutant recessive genes, some of which are lethal but seldom expressed. Inbreeding encourages the formation of homozygotes and increases the probability of recessive mutants appearing.

Most mutations are destined for a brief existence. There are cases, however, in which mutations may be harmful or neutral under one set of environmental conditions and helpful under a different set. Should the environment change, there could be a new adaptation beneficial to the species. The earth's changing environment has provided numerous opportunities for new gene combinations and mutations, as evidenced by the great diversity of animal life today.

Frequency of mutations

Although whether or not a mutation occurs is random, different mutation rates prevail at different loci. Some *kinds* of mutations are more likely to occur than others, and individual genes differ considerably in length. A long gene (more base pairs) is more likely to have a mutation than a short gene. Nevertheless, it is possible to estimate average spontaneous rates for different organisms and traits.

Relatively speaking, genes are extremely stable. In the well-studied fruit fly *Drosophila* there is approximately one detectable mutation per 10,000 loci (rate of 0.01% per locus per generation). The rate for humans is one per 10,000 to one per 100,000 loci per generation. If we accept the latter, more conservative figure, then a single normal allele is expected to go through 100,000 generations before it is mutated. However, since human chromosomes contain 100,000 loci, every person carries approximately one new mutation. Similarly, each spermatozoon produced contains, on the average, one mutant allele.

Since most mutations are deleterious, these statistics are anything but cheerful. Fortunately, most genes are recessive and are not detected by natural selection until by chance they have increased enough in frequency for homozygotes to be produced. At that point most are eliminated, since the zygote or individual carrying the mutants does not reproduce.

All animals carry large numbers of lethal and semilethal alleles in their gene pools. In human populations this has been called the "genetic load," or load of hidden mutations. By genetic recombination these continue to surface to produce mutant individuals less "fit" (in the Darwinian sense) than the "wild-type" genotype.

____ Summary

Genes are the unit entities that determine all the characteristics of an organism and are inherited by offspring from their parents. Genes may be dominant, recessive, or intermediate; the recessive gene in the heterozygous genotype will not be expressed in the phenotype but requires the homozygous condition for overt expression. In a monohybrid cross involving a dominant gene and its recessive allele (both parents homozygous), the F_1 generation will all be heterozygous, whereas the F_2 genotypes will occur in a $1:2:1$ ratio, and the phenotypes in a $3:1$ ratio. This demonstrates Mendel's law of segregation. Heterozygotes in intermediate inheritance show phenotypes intermediate between the homozygous phenotypes, or sometimes they show a different phenotype altogether, with corresponding alterations in the phenotypic ratios. Dihybrid crosses (in which the alleles for the two traits are carried on separate pairs of homologous chromosomes) demonstrate Mendel's law of independent assortment, and the phenotypic ratios will be $9:3:3:1$ with dominant and recessive characters. The ratios for monohybrid and dihybrid crosses can be determined by construction of a Punnett square, but the laws of probability allow calculation of the ratios in crosses of two or more characters much more easily.

Genes can have more than two alleles, and different combinations of alleles can produce different phenotypic effects. Nonallelic genes can interact, as in supplementary genes, epistasis, and polygenic inheritance, in which one gene affects the expression of another gene. Some genes may not always produce a phenotypic effect, even though they are dominant or present in the homozygous recessive genes (incomplete penetrance). Some genes may vary in the degree of effect produced (expressivity), and many genes have more than one effect (pleiotropic). Lethal genes cause death, either of the embryo or of the organism later in its life.

Gender is determined in most animals by the sex chromosomes; in humans, fruit flies, and many other animals, females have two X chromosomes, and males have an X and a Y. A gene on the X chromosome shows sex-linked inheritance and will produce an effect in the male, even if it is recessive, because the Y chromosome does not carry a corresponding allele. All genes on a given autosomal chromosome are linked and do not assort independently unless crossing over occurs. Crossing over increases the amount of genetic recombination in a population. Since the frequency of crossing over between two genes increases with the distance between the loci of the genes on the chromosome, gene maps of each chromosome can be constructed.

Occasionally, nondisjunction of one of the chromosomes in meiosis occurs, and one of the gametes ends up with one chromosome too many and the other with $n - 1$ chromosomes. Resulting zygotes usually do not survive; humans with $2n + 1$ chromosomes may live, but they are born with serious defects, such as Down's syndrome.

The genetic material in prokaryotes is carried in the DNA of their single, circular chromosome, which never condenses into the rodlike bodies we see in mitosis of eukaryotes. Most bacteria also have plasmids, which are small circles of DNA carrying relatively few, but often important, parts of the bacterial genome. Viruses also carry genetic information in DNA and sometimes in RNA. Neither viruses nor plasmids can replicate outside the host cell.

Genetic information in eukaryotes is found in the DNA of their mitochondria, plastids, and nuclear chromosomes. The chromosomes carry far more DNA than bacterial chromosomes or the other organelles mentioned. During interphase the eukaryotic chromosomes are dispersed into long strands of chromatin. The chromatin is comprised of DNA molecules organized with basic proteins called histones in repeating units known as nucleosomes. During mitosis the chromosomes are tightly contracted into rodlike bodies that avoid entanglement of the genetic material during its division between two daughter cells.

The position of the centromere is characteristic of a given chromosome. The locations of heterochromatin and euchromatin indicate regions where genes are inactive and active, respectively. Evidence of gene activity can be observed with the light microscope in the puffs of the polytene chromosomes of insects and the lampbrush chromosomes in the oocytes of vertebrates.

The unit of genetic function is the cistron. One gene most commonly controls the production of one protein or polypeptide (one gene–one polypeptide hypothesis), but the various types of RNA are also encoded on the genes.

The nucleic acids in the cell are DNA and RNA, which are large polymers of nucleotides composed of a nitrogenous base, pentose sugar, and phosphate group. The nitrogenous bases in DNA are adenine (A), guanine (G), thymine (T), and cytosine (C), and those in RNA are the same except that uracil (U) is substituted for thymine. DNA is a double-stranded, helical molecule in which the bases extend toward each other from the sugar-phosphate backbone: A always paired with T and G with C. Thus, the strands are antiparallel and complementary, being held in place by hydrogen bonds between the paired bases. In DNA replication the strands part, and the enzyme DNA polymerase synthesizes a new strand along each parent strand, using the parent strand as a template.

The sequence of the bases in DNA is a code for the amino acid sequence in the ultimate product protein. Each three bases (triplet) make up a codon specifying a particular amino acid. Cells have considerable ability to repair damaged DNA strands.

Proteins are synthesized by transcription of the information coded into DNA into the base sequence of a molecule of messenger RNA (mRNA), which functions in concert with ribosomes (containing ribosomal RNA [rRNA] and protein) and transfer RNA (tRNA). Ribosomes attach to the strand of mRNA and move along it, assembling the amino acid sequence of the protein. Each amino acid is brought into position for assembly by a molecule of tRNA, which itself bears a base sequence (anticodon) complementary to the respective codons of the mRNA. In eukaryotes the sequences of bases in DNA coding for amino acids in a protein (exons) are interrupted by intervening sequences (introns). The introns are spliced out of the primary mRNA before it leaves the nucleus, and the protein is synthesized in the cytoplasm.

On a molecular level, a gene is a portion of DNA bearing the information necessary to synthesize a functional product, whether mRNA (and therefore ultimately a protein), rRNA, or tRNA. Genes, and the synthesis of the products for which they are responsible, must be regulated: turned on or off in response to varying environmental conditions or cell differentiation. One important mode of gene regulation in prokaryotes is the interaction of a repressor protein with the operator portion of an operon (the operator plus one or more structural genes). The repressor is coded for by a regulator gene, and the repressor may be inactivated by a substrate for a metabolic reaction or activated by the end product of a reaction. Gene regulation in eukaryotes is more complex, and a number of possible mechanisms are known. One inactivation mechanism is the methylation of cytosine residues that lie next to guanine residues in the DNA strand, thus preventing transcription. In some cells genes are activated by the direct action of a hormone in the nucleus.

Modern methods in molecular genetics have made spectacular advances possible. Restriction endonucleases cleave DNA at specific base sequences, and such cleaved DNA from different sources can be rejoined to form recombinant DNA. Combining mammalian with plasmid or viral DNA, a mammalian gene can be introduced into bacterial cells, which then multiply and express the mammalian gene, for example, the gene for synthesis of insulin or interferon.

A mutation is a physicochemical alteration in the bases of the DNA that changes the effect of the gene. Although rare and usually detrimental to the survival and reproduction of the organism, mutations are occasionally beneficial and provide new genetic material on which natural selection can work.

Selected references

Abelson, J. 1980. A revolution in biology. Science **209**:1319-1321. *This is the lead-off article in an entire issue of* Science *devoted to recombinant DNA. Highly recommended, much information.*

Brown, D.D. 1981. Gene expression in eukaryotes. Science **211**:667-674. *A review of current knowledge concerning gene regulation in eukaryotes.*

Check, W. 1982. Plasmids: more than genetic debris. Mosaic **13**:27-32. *Role of plasmids in bacterial genetics. They may be present in vertebrate cells.*

Dunn, L.C. 1965. A short history of genetics. New York, McGraw-Hill Book Co. *Engaging account of the development of the science of genetics.*

Ehrlich, M., and R.Y.-H. Wang. 1981. 5-Methylcytosine in eukaryotic DNA. Science **212**:1350-1357. *Review of the possible functions of the small proportion of cytosine residues in eukaryotic DNA that is methylated.*

Goodenough, U. 1978. Genetics, ed. 2. New York, Holt, Rinehart & Winston.

Gould, S.J. 1980. Dr. Down's syndrome. Natural History **89**:142-148. *The term "mongolism," often used to describe Down's syndrome, originated in an involved and defamatory attempt to erect a racist social system.*

Hexter, W., and H.T. Yost, Jr. 1976. The science of genetics. Englewood Cliffs, N.J., Prentice-Hall, Inc. *Introductory text.*

Jenkins, J.B. 1979. Genetics, ed. 2. Boston, Houghton Mifflin Co. *Comprehensive introductory text.*

Kolata, G. 1982. Fetal hemoglobin genes turned on in adults. Science **218**:1295-1296. *Administration of a leukemia drug, 5-azacytidine, which causes undermethylation of newly synthesized DNA, produced dramatic clinical improvement in patients with sickle cell anemia and thalassemia. Apparently it turned on the gene for fetal hemoglobin.*

Kornberg, W. (ed.). 1980. The structures that make DNA work. Mosaic **11**:2-9. *Structure and function of nucleosomes.*

Lewin, R. 1982. A baroque turn for intron processing. Science **218**:1293-1295. *Higher-order structure is probably important in the splicing of mitochondrial and perhaps nuclear introns.*

Lewis, C.D., and U.K. Laemmli. 1982. Higher order metaphase chromosome structure: evidence for metalloprotein interactions. Cell **29**:171-181. *The scaffolding that organizes the chromatin in condensed chromosomes may be stabilized by copper or calcium ions.*

Mange, A.P., and E.J. Mange. 1980. Genetics: human aspects. Philadelphia, Saunders College. *A readable, introductory text concentrating on the genetics of the animal species of greatest concern to most of us.*

Marx, J.L. 1982. Is RNA copied into DNA by mammalian cells? Science **216**:969-970. *Some mammalian intronless genes have structures that suggest that they were copied from mature mRNA and then reinserted into chromosomes. The mechanisms involved are still a mystery.*

Marx, J.L. 1982. Building bigger mice through gene transfer. Science **218**:1298. *Genes for rat growth hormone were inserted into newly fertilized mouse eggs, which were then surgically implanted in uteri of foster mothers. Some of the mice that developed carried the rat gene and weighed 70% to 80% more than controls at 74 days after birth.*

Mayr, E. 1970. Population, species, and evolution. Cambridge, Mass., Harvard University Press. *This excellent reference is an abridgement of the author's* Animal Species and Evolution.

McKnight, S.L., and R. Kingsbury. 1982. Transcriptional control signals of a eukaryotic protein-coding gene. Science **217**:316-324. *Three distinct transcriptional control signals have been identified within 105 nucleotide residues immediately "upstream" from where transcription begins.*

Motulsky, A.G. 1983. Impact of genetic manipulation on society and medicine. Science **219**:135-140. *A summary of ethical considerations raised by genetic engineering. We must improve biological education for everyone so that we can make informed decisions.*

Olins, D.E., and A.L. Olins. 1978. Nucleosomes: the structural quantum in chromosomes. Am. Sci. **66**:704-711. *Structure and higher-order packaging of chromatin.*

Razin, A., and A.D. Riggs. 1980. DNA methylation and gene function. Science **210**:604-610.

Methylation of cytosine residues is a key element in the control mechanisms of vertebrate genes.

Suzuki, D.T., and A.J.F. Griffiths. 1981. An introduction to genetic analysis, ed. 2. San Francisco, W.H. Freeman & Co. Publishers. *Concepts and experimental basis of genetics presented in a historical sequence.*

Watson, J.D. 1969. The double helix. New York, Atheneum Publishers. *An enlightening and entertaining history of events leading to an understanding of the genetic code.*

Watson, J.D. 1976. Molecular biology of the gene, ed. 3. New York, The Benjamin Co., Inc. *Concise, well-illustrated popular text.*

Yelton, D.E., and M.D. Scharff. 1980. Monoclonal antibodies. Am. Sci. 68:510-516. *Principles and problems in monoclonal antibody production.*

Selected *Scientific American* articles

Anderson, W.F., and E.G. Diacumakos. 1981. Genetic engineering in mammalian cells. 245:106-121 (July). *Thymidine kinase deficiency in cultured cells was corrected by cloning the thymidine kinase gene with plasmids in bacteria, recovering the plasmids, and microinjecting the DNA into the deficient cells.*

Bauer, W.R., F.H.C. Crick, and J.H. White. 1980. Supercoiled DNA. 243:118-133 (July). *In many of the smaller genomes known (such as plasmids, mitochondrial DNA, and some viruses), the double helix of DNA itself forms a helix. The biological consequences are important.*

Chambon, P. 1981. Split genes. 244:60-71 (May). *Noncoding sequences (introns) in the DNA of higher organisms are transcribed and then spliced out of the mRNA.*

Cohen, S.N. 1975. The manipulation of genes. 233:24-33 (July). *It is now possible to transfer the DNA of one species into an unrelated species.*

Cohen, S.N., and J.A. Shapiro. 1980. Transposable genetic elements. 242:40-49 (Feb.). *A new source of genetic variability has been found: DNA sequences that can join together unrelated segments of DNA, transferring groups of genes among bacterial plasmids, viruses, and perhaps animal and plant chromosomes.*

Crow, J.F. 1979. Genes that violate Mendel's rules. 240:134-146 (Feb.). *Certain genes have been discovered that somehow violate the law of segregation, favoring their own survival and impairing the survival of the gamete bearing their allele.*

De Robertis, E.M., and J.B. Gurdon. 1979. Gene transplantation and the analysis of development. 241:74-82 (Dec.). *Cloned genes can be microinjected into nuclei of amphibian oocytes and are then transcribed and expressed in the oocyte.*

Fuchs, F. 1980. Genetic amniocentesis. 242:47-53 (June). *A good description of amniocentesis and the variety of genetic abnormalities that can be detected by its use.*

Gilbert, W., and L. Villa-Komaroff. 1980. Useful proteins from recombinant bacteria. 242:74-94 (Apr.). *Recombinant DNA methods are explained, including how bacteria are induced to synthesize such useful molecules as interferon and insulin. An important and timely topic!*

Howard-Flanders, P. 1981. Inducible repair of DNA. 245:72-80 (Nov.). *Several systems by which cells repair damaged DNA have been discovered.*

Leder, P. 1982. The genetics of antibody diversity. 246:102-115. *Rearrangement of parts of genes plus mutations in somatic cells may account for the enormous diversity of antibodies that can be synthesized by vertebrates.*

Miller, O.L. 1973. The visualization of genes in action. 228:34-42 (Mar.). *Remarkable electron micrographs of the transcription and translation processes in the cell.*

Novick, R.P. 1980. Plasmids. 243:103-127 (Dec.). *The author contends that plasmids are symbiotic organisms.*

Rich, A., and S.H. Kim. 1978. The three-dimensional structure of transfer RNA. 238:52-62 (Jan.).

Stein, G.S., J.S. Stein, and L.J. Kleinsmith. 1975. Chromosomal proteins and gene regulation. 232:46-57 (Feb.). *The possible role of histone and nonhistone proteins in turning genes off and on is explained.*

Wang, J.C. 1982. DNA topoisomerases. 247:94-109 (July). *These enzymes control the topological form of DNA molecules; one can supercoil the DNA helix, and another can uncoil it. Such enzymes may be important in control of transcription and translation.*

C H A P T E R   3 8

ORGANIC EVOLUTION

Workers in a quarry at Dinosaur National Park removing dinosaur bones
from sedimentary rock. Although imperfect, the fossil record provides
a glimpse of ancient life on earth and is crucial to the interpretation
of animal phylogeny.

Photograph by J.N.A. Lott, McMaster University/BPS.

A

B

Figure 38-1

Founders of theory of natural selection. **A,** Charles Robert Darwin (1809-1882), as he appeared in 1881, the year before his death. **B,** Alfred Russel Wallace (1823-1913) in 1895. Darwin and Wallace independently arrived at the same conclusion. A letter and essay from Wallace written to Darwin in 1858 spurred Darwin to write *The Origin of Species,* published in 1859.

The singularity of the earth is not that it harbors life, since life must surely exist elsewhere in the universe. It is that life on earth is so enormously diverse and pervasive. Even from space the ubiquity of life is evident in the kaleidoscopic patterns of grasslands, forests, lakes, and croplands stretching across the earth's surface, their colors changing with the seasons.

Each ecosystem is biologically and physically distinct. Each is occupied by a great variety of organisms, living interdependently and manifesting every conceivable kind of adaptation to their surroundings. Nutrients are withdrawn and again released; energy captured by plants flows through the system bringing order out of disorder in apparent defiance of the second law of thermodynamics; organisms die and are replaced by offspring, a renewal that threads its descent faithfully through generations of ancestors. It is a drama of incalculable complexity that has been and is now unfolding before our eyes.

Yet despite the apparent permanence of the natural world, change characterizes all things on earth and in the universe. Countless kinds of animals and plants have flourished and disappeared, leaving behind an imperfect fossil record of their existence.

The earth itself bears its own record of change, transformed as it is by processes that have occurred over a vast span of time and still are at work today. These changes are irreversible, and for life at least they appear in the broad sense to be directional and progressive, as primitive organisms of the young earth have yielded to the advanced, complex creatures of the present. We call this historical change in the set of instructions for building an organism **organic evolution.** Because every feature of life as we know it today is a product of the evolutionary process, biologists consider organic evolution to be the keystone of all biological knowledge.

The great contribution of Charles Robert Darwin and Alfred Russel Wallace (Fig. 38-1) was that they simultaneously provided the first credible explanation for evolutionary change, the **principle of natural selection.** The principal alternative explanation to account for the diversity of life on earth is that of special creation, which holds that all life forms were divinely created much as we find them today. However, special creation rests on premises that are not verifiable and thus must be accepted on faith. The study of biology, on the other hand, must account for the physical evidence that life has evolved and changed over time. Students should be aware that the extensive evidence for evolution and acceptance of the fact that evolution has occurred are not necessarily incompatible with religious concepts of creation. Indeed, evolution can be viewed as a creative process operating over long periods of time. How matter and life may have appeared in our universe is not at issue in evolutionary theory. It is regrettable, therefore, that the recent reemergence of rigid antievolutionary views, in the guise of "creation science," should portray creation by a supernatural being and evolution as irreconcilable.

In our treatment of the principle of organic evolution in this chapter, we consider Darwin's theory of natural selection and the evidence for evolution, the concept of species and how they change with time, and the question of how new species arise. Before reading this chapter, you may find it helpful to reread the summary of the evolutionary concept and the mechanism of natural selection (pp. 9 and 10).

DEVELOPMENT OF THE IDEA OF ORGANIC EVOLUTION

Evolution is no longer a subject for debate among biologists; as a process it is known and accepted, even though the forces that determine the course of evolution are not fully understood. Yet, before the eighteenth century, much of the speculation on the origin of species rested on myth and superstition rather than on observation. Nevertheless, long before this time, there were those who were thinking about and attempting to interpret the order of nature.

Some of the early Greek philosophers, notably Xenophanes, Empedocles, and Aristotle, developed the germ of the idea of change and natural selection within the restrictions of belief in spontaneous generation. They recognized fossils as evidence of a former life that they believed had been destroyed by some natural catastrophe. Despite their spirit of intellectual inquiry, the Greeks failed to establish an evolutionary concept, probably because of their limited experience with the natural world.

With the gradual decline of ancient science, beginning well before the rise of Christianity, debate on evolution nearly ended. The opportunity for fresh thinking became even more restricted as the biblical account of the earth's creation became accepted as a tenet of faith. The year 4004 BC was fixed by Archbishop James Ussher (mid-seventeenth century) as the time of true creation of life. In this atmosphere evolutionary views were considered rebellious and heretical.

Still, some speculation continued. The French naturalist Buffon (1707-1788) stressed the influence of environment on the modifications of animal type. He also extended the age of earth to 70,000 years from 6000 years.

Figure 38-2

Jean Baptiste de Lamarck (1744-1829), French naturalist who developed the first reasoned account of evolution. The scientific establishment of his time was contemptuous of his "use-and-disuse" theory of evolution. Yet, in France today, where Darwinism has never been fully accepted, Lamarck is regarded as the father of evolution. This engraving was made in 1821. Courtesy British Museum (Natural History), London.

Lamarckism: the First Scientific Theory of Evolution

The first complete theory of evolution was authored by Jean Baptiste de Lamarck (1744-1829) (Fig. 38-2), a pioneering French biologist. Lamarck, who published his theory in 1809, the year of Darwin's birth, was the first biologist to make a convincing case for the idea that fossils were the remains of extinct animals and not, as some argued, stones molded in chance imitations of life. Lamarck's theory of **inheritance of acquired characteristics** was engagingly simple: organisms, by striving to adapt to their environment, acquire adaptations during their lives that are passed on by heredity to their offspring. The giraffe, according to Lamarck, developed its long neck by constantly stretching for food. Genetic variation then arose preferentially in this direction, and the trait of long necks became common in the population. Snakes lost their legs, Lamarck believed, because legs were a handicap in moving through dense vegetation. A man who developed his muscles by exercise was supposed to pass his strength on to his sons. Lamarck's attitude toward adaptation was straightforward: an organism could get any adaptation it needed. Despite the uncluttered appeal and efficiency of Lamarck's theory, it was effectively disproved in this century by geneticists who could find no mechanism that would make such a process possible. The unveiling of the genetic code showed that DNA transcription and translation are a one-way process with no known way for the environment to feed information back into the cell's DNA.

Lamarckian inheritance enjoyed a brief rehabilitation in 1981 when two researchers claimed that mice that developed tolerance to foreign skin grafts could pass the trait on to their offspring. However, other scientists who repeated the experiments failed to reproduce the results.

Figure 38-3

Sir Charles Lyell (1797-1875), English
geologist and friend of Darwin. His book
Principles of Geology greatly influenced
Darwin during Darwin's formative period. The photograph was made about
1856.

Courtesy British Museum (Natural History), London.

Charles Lyell and the Doctrine of Uniformitarianism

While eighteenth- and early nineteenth-century zoologists wrestled with conflicting concepts of organic evolution, geologists were marshaling sound evidence for
the physical evolution of the earth's crust. The geologist Sir Charles Lyell (1797-
1875) (Fig. 38-3) in his *Principles of Geology* (1830-1833) stated that the changes
in the earth's surface were the result of ongoing natural forces operating with
uniformity over great periods of time. The idea that processes occurring now are
the same as those in the past came to be called the doctrine of uniformitarianism.
As one writer of the time stated, "no vestige of a beginning—no prospect of an
end."

Lyell was able to show that such forces, acting over long periods of time,
could account for all observed changes, including the formation of fossil-bearing
rocks. His familiarity with fossils, with the natural history of contemporary
marine and freshwater animals, and with sedimentary rocks led him to conclude
that the earth's age must be reckoned in millions of years rather than in thousands.

Charles Darwin (1809-1882) was thus not the first to propose the idea of
evolution nor even to suggest a mechanism for its action. His predecessors had
already established an intellectual climate that made a hypothesis of evolutionary
mechanism possible, if not inevitable. Darwin himself later acknowledged that the
theory of natural selection had been suggested by others before him. But so forcefully did Darwin present his ideas and his array of carefully collected scientific
data that no one since has been able to challenge his preeminence in this field.
Today the fact of organic evolution can be denied only by abandoning reason. As
the noted English biologist Sir Julian Huxley wrote, "Charles Darwin effected the
greatest of all revolutions in human thought, greater than Einstein's or Freud's or
even Newton's, by simultaneously establishing the fact and discovering the mechanism of organic evolution."*

DARWIN'S GREAT VOYAGE OF DISCOVERY

"After having been twice driven back by heavy south-western gales, Her Majesty's
ship *Beagle*, a ten-gun brig, under the command of Captain Fitz Roy, R.N., sailed
from Devonport on the 27th of December, 1831." Thus began Charles Darwin's
account of the historic 5-year voyage of the *Beagle* around the world (Fig. 38-4).
Darwin, not quite 23 years old, had been invited to serve as naturalist without pay
on the *Beagle*, a small vessel only 90 feet in length, which was about to depart on a
second extensive surveying voyage to South America and the Pacific. It was the
beginning of one of the most important voyages of the nineteenth century.

During the voyage (1831-1836) (Fig. 38-5), Darwin endured almost constant seasickness and the erratic companionship of the authoritarian Captain Fitz
Roy. But his youthful physical strength and early training as a naturalist equipped
him for his work. The *Beagle* made many stops along the harbors and coasts of
South America and adjacent regions. Darwin made extensive collections and
observations on the fauna and flora of these regions. He unearthed numerous

*Huxley, J. In Bowman, R.I. 1966. The Galápagos. Berkeley, University of California Press.

Figure 38-4

Voyage of the *Beagle*.

Modified from Moorhead, A. 1969. Darwin and the *Beagle*. New York, Harper & Row, Publishers, Inc.

A   B

Figure 38-5

Charles Darwin and H.M.S. *Beagle*. **A,** Darwin in 1840, 4 years after the *Beagle* returned to England. **B,** H.M.S. *Beagle* in the Straits of Magellan.

A, From a watercolor by George Richmond; B, courtesy American Museum of Natural History.

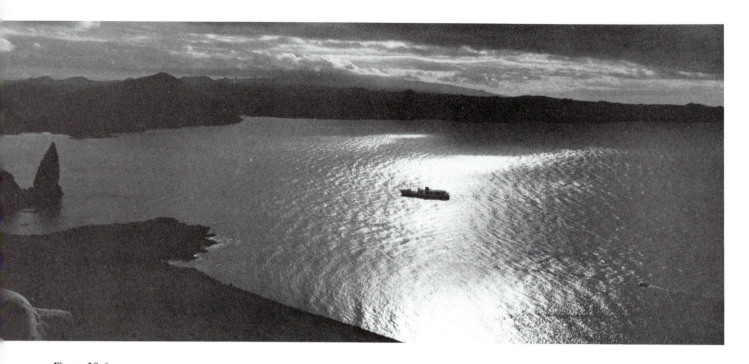

Figure 38-6

The Galápagos Islands.
Photograph by C.P. Hickman, Jr.

fossils of animals long since extinct and noted the resemblance between fossils of the South American pampas and the known fossils of North America. In the Andes he encountered seashells embedded in rocks at 13,000 feet. He experienced a severe earthquake and watched the mountain torrents that relentlessly wore away the earth—observations that strengthened his conviction that natural forces were responsible for the geological features of the earth. Finally, he realized that he was witnessing the results of evolution.

In mid-September of 1835, the *Beagle* arrived at the Galápagos Islands, a volcanic archipelago straddling the equator 600 miles west of the coast of Ecuador (Fig. 38-6). The fame of the islands stems from their infinite strangeness. They are unlike any other islands on earth. Some visitors today are struck with awe and wonder; others with a sense of depression and dejection. Circled by capricious currents, surrounded by shores of twisted lava, bearing skeletal brushwood baked by the equatorial sun, almost devoid of vegetation, inhabited by strange reptiles and by convicts stranded by the Ecuadorian government, the islands indeed had few admirers among mariners. By the middle of the seventeenth century, the islands were already known to the Spaniards as "Las Islas Galápagos"—the tortoise islands. The giant tortoises, used for food first by buccaneers and later by American and British whalers, sealers, and ships of war, were the islands' principal attraction. At the time of Darwin's visit, the tortoises were already being heavily exploited.

During the *Beagle's* 5-week visit to the Galápagos, Darwin began to develop his views of the evolution of life on earth. His original observations of the giant tortoises, marine iguanas that feed on seaweed, and drab ground finches, a family that had evolved into several species, each with distinct beak and feeding adaptations, all contributed to the turning point in Darwin's thinking.

Darwin was struck by the fact that, although the Galápagos Islands and the Cape Verde Islands (visited earlier in this voyage of the *Beagle*) were similar in climate and topography, their fauna and flora were altogether different. He recognized that Galápagos plants and animals were related to those of the South

1

American mainland, yet differed from them sometimes in curious ways. Each island often contained a unique species of a particular group of animals that was nonetheless related to forms on other islands. In short, Galápagos life must have originated in continental South America and then undergone modification in the various environmental conditions of the separate islands. He concluded that living forms were neither divinely created nor immutable; they were, in fact, the products of evolution. Although Darwin devoted only a few pages to Galápagos animals and plants in his monumental *Origin of Species,* published more than two decades after visiting the islands, his observations on the unique character of the animals and plants were, in his own words, the "origin of all my views."

On October 2, 1836, the *Beagle* landed in England. Most of Darwin's extensive collections had long since preceded him to England, as had most of his notebooks and diaries kept during the cruise. Three years after the *Beagle*'s return to England, Darwin's journal was published. It was an instant success and required two additional printings within the first year. In later versions, Darwin made extensive changes and abbreviated the original ponderous title typical of nineteenth-century books to simply *The Voyage of the Beagle.* The fascinating account of his observations written in a simple, appealing style has made the book one of the most lasting and popular travel books of all time.

Curiously, the main product of Darwin's voyage, his theory of evolution, did not appear in print for more than 20 years after the *Beagle*'s return. In 1838 he "happened to read for amusement" an essay on populations by T.R. Malthus (1766-1834), who stated that animal and plant populations, including human populations, tend to increase beyond the capacity of the environment to support them. Darwin had already been gathering information on the artificial selection of animals under domestication by humans. After reading Malthus's article, Darwin realized that a process of selection in nature, a "struggle for existence" because of overpopulation, could be a powerful force for evolution of wild species.

He allowed the idea to develop in his own mind until it was presented in an essay in 1844—still unpublished. Finally in 1856 he began to pull together his voluminous data into a work on the origin of species. He expected to write four volumes, a "very big" book, "as perfect as I can make it." However, his plans were to take an unexpected turn.

In 1858, he received a manuscript from Alfred Russel Wallace (1823-1913), an English naturalist in Malaya with whom he had been corresponding. Darwin was stunned to find that in a few pages, Wallace summarized the main points of the natural selection theory that Darwin had been working on for two decades. Rather than withhold his own work in favor of Wallace as he was inclined to do, Darwin was persuaded by two close friends, the geologist Lyell and the botanist Hooker, to publish his views in a brief statement that would appear together with Wallace's paper in the *Journal of the Linnaean Society.* Portions of both papers were read before an unimpressed audience on July 1, 1858.

For the next year, Darwin worked urgently to prepare an "abstract" of the planned four-volume work. This was published in November 1859, with the title *On the Origin of Species by Means of Natural Selection, or the Preservation of Favoured Races in the Struggle for Life.* The 1250 copies of the first printing were sold the first day! The book instantly generated a storm that has never completely abated. Darwin's views were to have extraordinary consequences on scientific and religious beliefs and remain among the greatest intellectual achievements of all time.

Once Darwin's excessive caution had been swept away by the publication of

Why was Darwin so successful? Although a famous scientist in his time, Darwin remained a mysterious figure to all but his family and a close circle of friends. From these sources emerges the portrait of a man possessing many abilities. He was a patient thinker with the capacity to weave together a theoretical structure from a mountain of empirical data. He kept meticulous records, enjoyed experimentation, and maintained a set and ordered routine in his life. Certainly he possessed a streak of competitiveness and the desire to excel. Perhaps most important of all, his intellectual development was strongly influenced by his scientific friends and, especially, his devoted family, an unfailing wellspring of love, respect, and support.

Figure 38-7

Reconstruction of the appearance of *Corythosaurus*, a dinosaur from the upper Cretaceous of North America, approximately 90 million years ago. **A,** Portion of skeleton as discovered and partially worked out of rocks in New Mexico quarry. **B,** Skeleton, 30 feet in length on slab. **C,** Drawing prepared from skeleton. **D,** Artist's reconstruction of living animal.

A and **B,** Courtesy American Museum of Natural History; **C** and **D,** from Colbert, E.H. 1969. Evolution of the vertebrates, ed. 2. New York. Copyright © 1969. Reprinted by permission of John Wiley & Sons, Inc.

A

B

C

Corythosaurus

D

The Origin of Species, he entered an incredibly productive period of evolutionary thinking for the next 23 years, producing book after book. He died April 19, 1882, and was buried in Westminster Abbey. The little *Beagle* had already disappeared, having been retired in 1870 and presumably broken up for scrap.

EVIDENCES FOR EVOLUTION
Reconstructing the Past
Fossils and their formation

The strongest and most direct evidence for evolution, and the evidence that first persuaded Darwin to think seriously about evolution, is the fossil record of the past, even though fossils and the sediments containing them provide dim and imperfect views of an ancient life (Fig. 38-7). The complete record of the past is always beyond our reach, since so many organisms left no fossils. Yet, incomplete as the record is, biologists rely on the discoveries of new fossils and the continued study of existing fossils to interpret phylogeny and relationships of both plant and animal life. It would be difficult indeed to make sense out of the evolutionary patterns or classification of organisms without the support of the fossil record. The documentary evidence of evolution as a general process, progressive changes in life from one geological era to another, past distribution of lands and seas, and environmental conditions of the past (paleoecology) all depend on what fossils teach us.

A fossil may be defined as the remains of past life uncovered from the crust of the earth. It refers not only to complete remains (mammoths and amber insects), actual hard parts (teeth and bones), and petrified skeletal parts that are infiltrated with silica or other minerals by water seepage (ostracoderms and molluscs), but also to molds, casts, impressions, and fossil excrement (coprolites).

The fossil record is biased because preservation is selective. Vertebrate skeletal parts and invertebrates with shells and other hard structures have left the best record (Fig. 38-8). It is unlikely that jellyfish, worms, caterpillars, and such fossilize, but now and then a rare chance discovery such as the Burgess shale deposits of British Columbia or the Precambrian fossil bed of south Australia reveals an enormous amount of information about soft-bodied organisms. Certain regions have apparently provided ideal conditions for fossil formation—for example, the tar pits of Rancho La Brea in Hancock Park, Los Angeles; the great dinosaur beds of Alberta, Canada, and Jensen, Utah; and the Olduvai Gorge of South Africa.

A common method of fossil formation is the quick burial of animals under waterborne sediments. Rapid burial is usually important because it slows or prevents decomposition by oxidation, solution, and bacterial action.

Most fossils are laid down in deposits that become stratified. If left undis-

Fossil remains may on rare occasions include soft tissues preserved so well that recognizable cell organelles can be viewed with the electron microscope! Insects are frequently found entombed in amber, the fossilized resin of trees. One study of a fly entombed in 40 million year old amber revealed structures corresponding to muscle fibers, nuclei, ribosomes, lipid droplets, endoplasmic reticulum, and mitochondria (Fig. 38-9). This extreme case of mummification probably occurred because chemicals in the plant sap diffused into the embalmed insect's tissues.

Figure 38-8

This bit of Green River shale from Farson, Wyoming, bears the impression of a "double-armored herring" *(Knightia)*, approximately 4 inches long, which swam there during the Eocene epoch, approximately 55 million years ago.

turbed, which is rare, the older strata are the deeper ones; however, the layers are usually tilted or folded or show faults (cracks). Often old deposits exposed by erosion are later covered with new deposits in a different plane. Sedimentary rock such as limestone may be exposed to tremendous pressures or heat during mountain building and may be metamorphosed into rocks such as crystalline quartzite, slate, or marble. Fossils are often destroyed during these processes.

Since various fossils are correlated with certain strata, they often serve as a means of identifying the strata of different regions. Certain widespread marine invertebrate fossils such as various foraminiferans and echinoderms are such good indicators of specific geological periods that they are called "index," or "guide," fossils.

Geological time

Long before the age of the earth was known, geologists began dividing its history into a table of succeeding events, using as a basis the accessible deposits and correlations from sedimentary rock. Time was divided into eons, eras, periods, and epochs. These are shown on the endpaper inside the back cover of this book. Time during the last eon (Phanerozoic) is expressed in eras (for example, Cenozoic), periods (for example, Tertiary), epochs (for example, Paleocene), and sometimes smaller divisions of an epoch.

As far as the fossil record is concerned, the recorded history of life begins near the base of the Cambrian period of the Paleozoic era approximately 600 million years BP. The period before the Cambrian is called the Precambrian era. Although the Precambrian era occupies 85% of all geological time, it is a puzzling era because of the lack of macrofossils. It has received much less attention than later eras, partly because of the absence of fossils and partly because oil, which provides the commercial incentive for much geological work, seldom exists in Precambrian formations. There are, however, evidences for life in the Precambrian era: well-preserved bacteria and algae, as well as casts of jellyfish, sponge spicules, soft corals, segmented flatworms, and worm trails. Most, but not all, are microfossils.

Figure 38-9

Electron micrograph of tissue from a 40 million year old fossilized fly. Membranous arrays characteristic of endoplasmic reticulum cisternae are visible. The scale bar is 1 μm.

Courtesy G.O. Poinar, Jr., University of California, Berkeley.

1 μm

Then, a few million years before the Cambrian period, nearly all major invertebrate groups suddenly appear in the fossil record—the **Cambrian "explosion."** Although the Cambrian explosion was once considered illusory, an artifact of poor fossil preservation in Precambrian rocks, almost all paleontologists now agree that an extraordinary diversification of animal life occurred at the beginning of the Cambrian. There is little agreement on what may have triggered the Cambrian explosion, but there can be no dispute about its consequences. Virtually all basic multicellular animal designs evolved at this time, and the earth's oceans became stocked with them.

We might expect animal evolution to have now proceeded apace in unencumbered radiation. In fact, the subsequent history is punctuated by periodic and dramatic extinctions followed by radiations of the survivors. The most cataclysmic of these extinction episodes happened about 225 million years ago, when at least half of the families of shallow-water marine invertebrates, and fully 90% of marine invertebrate species, disappeared within a few million years. This was the **Permian extinction.**

Another great extinction, marking the end of the dinosaurs as well as numerous marine invertebrates, occurred at the end of the Cretaceous period, about 65 million years ago. Other great extinctions are used by geologists to mark the end of the earth's geological periods: Cambrian, Ordovician, Silurian, and so on. Each time a major disruption in the equilibrium of the earth's life forms occurred.

There are various explanations for these extinctions. The Permian, for example, coincides with the formation of Pangaea, a huge supercontinent formed from the joining together of all the continents. The area of shallow seas was greatly reduced and there may have been a drastic lowering of the sea level, reducing the available habitat. Furthermore, populations of organisms that previously were separated were brought together into competition. Another explanation attributes at least one or more of the great extinctions to the impact on earth of a giant asteroid or comet (marginal note on p. 582).

Dating of fossils and geological formations

Only relatively recently have paleontologists developed accurate methods for dating the layers in which fossils are embedded. Before about 1950, scientists applied the "law of stratigraphy," a relative dating method that relied on the sequence of layers of rock: the oldest at the bottom and the youngest at the top. Paleontologists knew that dinosaurs and ichthyosaurs were animals of the Mesozoic era, that amphibians originated in the Devonian period, and that saber-toothed tigers and mastodons roamed the forests of the Pleistocene epoch. At the end of the nineteenth century, the earth was thought to be 100 million years old, and the geological time scale was adjusted accordingly. But with no measure of the absolute passage of time, figures of 1 billion or 10 billion years could just as well have been accepted.

In the late 1940s, radiometric dating methods were developed for determining the absolute age in years of rock formations. At least five independent methods are now used for dating geological formations, all based on the radioactive decay of naturally occurring elements into other elements. These "radioactive clocks" proceed independent of pressure and temperature changes and therefore are not affected by often violent earth-building activities.

One method, potassium-argon dating, depends on the decay of potassium-40 (^{40}K) to argon-40 (^{40}A) (12%) and calcium-40 (^{40}Ca) (88%).

The half-life of potassium-40 is 1.3 billion years. This means that half the original atoms will decay in 1.3 billion years, and half the remaining atoms will be gone at the end of the next 1.3 billion years. This continues until all the radioactive potassium-40 atoms are gone. To measure the age of the rock, one calculates the ratio of remaining potassium-40 atoms to the amount of potassium-40 originally there (the remaining potassium-40 atoms plus the argon-40 into which they have decayed).

Perhaps the best radioactive clock depends on the decay of uranium into lead. When granitic magma solidifies, uranium usually forms and the radioactive clock starts. As time passes, uranium-238 decays to lead-206, and uranium-235 decays to lead-207. Under favorable conditions both isotopes of lead remain locked in the rock and, after isolation in the laboratory, can be accurately measured by mass spectrometry. Rocks over 2 billion years old can be dated with a probable error of less than 1%.

There are many uncertainties in radioactive dating, and the techniques require sophisticated instrumentation and great care in methodology. Not all rocks or fossils can be dated. But if two or more different methods provide concordant answers, the age can be accepted as reliable, since it is most improbable that different isotopes would leach out of the sample at the same rate. In fact, in many thousands of analyses, rocks have been dated by three or more independent clocks and the ages determined have been in close agreement.

Classification and Homology

Biologists long before Darwin discovered that, despite the great diversity of life, it was possible to arrange living things into a logical system of classification. The "natural system of classification" that originated with Aristotle and later was formalized by Linnaeus (p. 147) is based on the degree of similarity of morphological characters.

For example, the domestic cat is clearly related to the wild cats and jungle cats of the Old World, and all are included in the same genus, *Felis*. This genus shares an obvious relationship with the "big cats" (lions, tigers, leopards, and jaguars of the genus *Panthera*), as well as lynxes and bobcats (genus *Lynx*), so all are grouped into a set of higher rank, the family Felidae. All members of this family share a number of traits that set them apart from all other families, such as a round head, 30 teeth, and digitigrade feet with retractile claws. At the same time, the cat family is clearly related as a group to a number of other families (for example, the dog, bear, raccoon, weasel and otter, and hyena families). All of these bear a distinctive anatomy and way of life that characterize them as flesh eaters; they are grouped together in the order Carnivora.

Thus, animals can be grouped with respect to certain combinations of traits. Linnaeus had introduced his classification system partly as a means for cataloging nature and partly to reveal the Creator's purpose, since he believed that each group carried a set of similar features that corresponded to God's plan. Darwin, however, recognized an alternative explanation: the marvelous similarities that allowed plants and animals to be classified into neat hierarchies existed because of

The well-known carbon-14 (^{14}C) dating method is of little help in estimating the age of geological formations because the short half-life of ^{14}C restricts its use to quite recent events (less than about 40,000 years). It is especially useful, however, for archeological studies. This method is based on the production of radioactive ^{14}C (half-life of approximately 5570 years) in the upper atmosphere by bombardment of nitrogen-14 (^{14}N) with cosmic radiation. The radioactive ^{14}C enters the tissue of living animals and plants, and an equilibrium is established between atmospheric ^{14}C and ^{14}N in the organism. At death, ^{14}C exchange with the atmosphere stops. In 5570 years only half of the original ^{14}C remains in the preserved fossil. Its age is found by comparing the ^{14}C content of the fossil with that of living organisms.

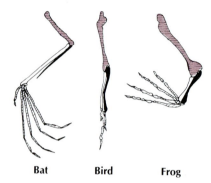

Figure 38-10

Forelimbs of five vertebrates, showing skeletal homologies. *Red,* humerus; *white,* radius; *black,* ulna; *white striated,* wrist and phalanges. The most generalized or primitive limb is that of humans—the feature that has been a primary factor in human evolution because of its wide adaptability. Various types of limbs have been structurally modified for adaptations to particular functions.

a "blood" relationship, caused by descent and divergence from a common ancestor. This became one of the strongest arguments for his theory.

One of the most important tools used by Linnaeus and his successors to search out natural relationships was the concept of homology, discussed in Chapter 6 (p. 143). Homology is the term used to describe structures that, because of common ancestry, share a fundamental structure and relative position. The classic example we cited on p. 143 was the vertebrate pentadactyl limb. The human arm, front leg of a frog, wing of a bat or bird, and flipper of a whale are homologous because they are built of the same bones, even though they look different and function differently (Fig. 38-10). Each forelimb has about the same number of bones arranged in a similar way. Common structures, constructed of the same building blocks, must reflect common descent from an ancestor having these structures.

Embryological homologies remind us of our kinship with distant vertebrate ancestors. Gill slits, which in fish develop into respiratory organs, appear in the embryos of all vertebrates (Fig. 36-14, p. 880). In the adults of terrestrial vertebrates the gill arches disappear altogether or become modified beyond recognition. Such persistence of history in our embryonic development occurs because early embryonic sequences are not easily modified. Embryological similarities, like anatomical homologies, attest to evolution.

As the evolutionary theory gained acceptance, the unveiling of homologies received new impetus because it was seen as a key to understanding the course of evolution. The example of the pentadactyl limb tells us that all these vertebrates are related by common ancestry and should be grouped together as four-footed, five-toed vertebrates. But, if we want to know if bats are more closely related to frogs or humans, the pentadactyl limb cannot help us because all three forms in question have it. We would discover, however, that bats and humans are warm blooded, have hair, suckle their young, and possess other homologous features that relate them, whereas the frog has none of these things. The frog, on the other hand, possesses its own set of characteristics that relate it to salamanders and other amphibians. Working in this way, looking for more and more restricted homologies, we can characterize groups and subgroups, arriving at a classification that represents natural and true ancestry.

Biochemical homologies

Common ancestry and homology can now be demonstrated even more forcefully for proteins than for anatomical structures, mainly because protein chains have many more recognizable units (100 or more amino acids) than do anatomical structures, which seldom contain more than a dozen or so parts. By comparing amino acid chains of homologous proteins (hemoglobin, for example) from different animals, we can derive a molecular genealogical tree in much the same way that phylogenetic trees are constructed from fossils.

It has been possible to trace the evolution of at least one protein, cytochrome c, to the origin of eukaryotic cells more than 1 billion years ago. Cytochrome c is a small enzyme composed of 104 amino acid units. As different mutations accumulated, the amino acid sequences of the molecule in descendant species became different. Just how much any two species differ corresponds with the distance that they are separated on the phylogenetic tree. Elaborate family trees constructed entirely from sequence diversion agree remarkably well with those obtained by classical morphology and embryology. Such studies are of great importance because they carry evolutionary study much closer to the understanding of the genetic variation that underlies all evolutionary adaptation.

NATURAL SELECTION
Darwin's Theory of Natural Selection

The concept of natural selection, often expressed in the phrase "survival of the fittest," was the centerpiece of Darwin's theory of evolution. It was the first plausible alternative to Lamarck's theory of evolution by inheritance of acquired characteristics. Darwin's theory of natural selection was nearly as simple as Lamarck's (although less obvious) but was based on observable facts and supported by an abundance of evidence.

1. **All organisms show variation.** No two individuals are exactly alike. They differ in size, color, physiology, behavior, and other ways. Darwin realized that much of this variation is inherited even though he did not understand how. The mechanism of genetic mutation was to be discovered many years later. Darwin pointed out that humans have taken advantage of inherited variation to produce useful new breeds and races of livestock and plants. He believed that, if selection is possible under human control, it can also be produced by agencies operating in nature. He reasoned that *natural* selection can have the same effect as *artificial* selection.

2. **In nature all organisms produce more offspring than can survive.** In every generation the young are more numerous than the parents. Darwin calculated that, even in a slow-breeding species such as the elephant, a single pair breeding from age 30 to 90 and having only six young in this span could give rise to 19 million elephants in 750 years. Why, he asked, are there not more elephants?

3. **Accordingly, there is a struggle for survival.** If more individuals are born than can possibly survive, there must be a severe struggle for existence among them. Darwin wrote in *The Origin of Species* that "it is the doctrine of Malthus applied with manifold force to the whole animal and vegetable kingdoms." Competition for food, shelter, and space becomes increasingly severe as overpopulation develops.

4. **Some individuals of a species have a better chance for survival than others.** Because individuals of a species differ, some are favored in the struggle for survival; others are handicapped and eliminated.

5. **The result is natural selection.** Out of the struggle for existence results the survival of the fittest. Under natural selection, individuals bearing favorable variations survive and have a chance to breed and transmit their characteristics to their offspring. The less fit die without reproducing. Natural selection is simply the differential survival or reproduction of favored variants. The process continues with succeeding generations so that organisms gradually become better adapted to their environment. Should the environment change, there must also be a change in the characters that have survival value, or the species is eliminated. Reproduction is what really counts in natural selection.

6. **Through natural selection new species originate.** The differential reproduction of variants can gradually transform species and result in the long-term "improvement" of types. According to Darwin, when different parts of an animal or plant population are confronted with slightly different environments, each

The use of the word "theory" to describe evolutionary science has caused many people to believe that the principle carries little more weight than an idea or a conjecture, since we often use the word in common speech (for example, "I have a theory about what really happened there"). When creationists charge that evolution is "just a theory," this may be what they have in mind. Scientists, on the other hand, use "theory" to refer to a body of generalizations and principles developed within a field of inquiry, such as mathematics or physics or biology (p. 8). Thus, we have the theory of numbers, theory of gravitation, and theory of evolution. Such theories are built from sets of facts, not conjectures and speculations. It is also important to emphasize that evolution as a process is a fact, and the only argument among scientists today is with the details of how it operates, not whether it operates.

The popular phrase "survival of the fittest" was not originated by Darwin but was coined a few years earlier by the British philosopher Herbert Spencer, who anticipated some of Darwin's principles of evolution. Unfortunately the phrase later came to be coupled with unbridled aggression and violence in a bloody, competitive world. In fact, natural selection operates through many other characteristics of living things. The fittest animal may be the most helpful, the most caring, or the most loving. Fighting prowess is only one of several means toward successful reproductive advantage.

diverges from the other. In time they differ enough from each other to form separate species. In this way two or more species may arise from a single ancestral species. Through adaptation to a changed environment, a group of animals may also diverge enough from their ancestors to become a different species.

____ Appraisal of Darwin's Theory

Darwin supported his theory of evolution by an overwhelming amount of evidence that had never before been accumulated. He convincingly demonstrated evolution and then provided a logical explanation for it. Through the well-chosen body of evidence so lucidly expounded in *The Origin of Species*, he made evolution understandable. Nevertheless, despite its elegance, it is hardly surprising that parts of his theory have been modernized because of more recent biological knowledge. When Darwin wrote *The Origin of Species*, nothing was known about the inheritance of variation. It was not even known that sexual reproduction involved the combination of a single sperm with a single egg. One always marvels that Darwin's deductions and conclusions were so sound in view of the scientific ignorance that prevailed at the time.

The most serious weakness in Darwin's theory was his failure to identify correctly the mechanism of inheritance. Darwin saw heredity as a blending phenomenon; in other words, the characteristics of the parents melded together in the offspring. In the 1860s Darwin proposed the hypothesis of **pangenesis,** an idea that little particles were given off by various cells in the body; these circulated about, eventually collecting in the sex organs to combine into sex cells. Darwin thought that the particles could be altered by external conditions and that these acquired characteristics could be passed on to the next generation—an explanation for Lamarckism! (Although Darwin wrongly believed that the effects of use and disuse could be inherited, he did not regard Lamarckian inheritance of acquired characteristics as essential to his theory.) We now know that many of the kinds of variations that Darwin thought were inheritable are not. Darwin himself was not very enthusiastic about his pangenesis hypothesis (he did not incorporate it into later revisions of *The Origin of Species*), and it received a decidedly cool reception during his lifetime.

Eventually, Mendelian genetics provided the particulate kind of inheritance that Darwin's theory of natural selection required. Only variations arising from changes in the genes (mutations) are inherited and furnish the material on which natural selection can act. Gregor Mendel published his theories on inheritance in 1868, 14 years before Darwin died. Darwin presumably never read the work (although it was found in his extensive library after his death), and, if there were others who knew of it, they failed to bring it to his attention. Had Mendel written Darwin about his results, it is possible that Darwin would have modified his theory. However, it is also possible that Darwin would not have seen the relationship of the hereditary mechanisms to gradual changes and continuous variations that represent the hub of Darwinian evolution. It took other scientists years to establish the relationship of genetics to Darwin's natural selection theory.

The first step in modernizing Darwin's theory was the demonstration that the operative units in inheritance are self-reproducing, nonblending genes. Next was the discovery of chromosomes in which genes were found to be precisely located in linkage groups. Biologists could then understand how the ultimate source of variation—mutations—could be inherited in the usual Mendelian fashion.

"If I lived twenty more years and was able to work, how I should have to modify the Origin, and how much the views on all points will have to be modified! Well it is a beginning and that is something . . ."
Charles Darwin, in a letter to Joseph Hooker, 1869

Ironically, when Mendel's work was rediscovered in 1900, it was viewed as antagonistic to Darwin's theory of natural selection. During the early part of this century, the popularity of Darwin's theory continued to ebb. When mutations were discovered, most geneticists accepted the idea that "mutation pressure"—continuously recurring mutations—was the basis of evolutionary change. Natural selection was relegated to the role of executioner, a negative force that merely eliminated the obviously unfit.

___ Emergence of Modern Darwinism: the Synthetic Theory

In the 1930s a new breed of geneticists began to reevaluate Darwin's theory from a different perspective. These were population geneticists, scientists who studied variation in natural populations of animals and plants and who had a sound knowledge of statistics and mathematics, disciplines that earlier geneticists woefully lacked. Gradually, a new comprehensive theory emerged that brought together population genetics, paleontology, biogeography, embryology, systematics, and, later, animal behavior.

Population genetics, which combines Darwinian natural selection with modern principles of heredity, shows that evolution is a change in the genetic composition of populations. Such changes occur when the population is exposed to an environmental challenge—some change in the physical or biotic environment. Interactions between population and environment have become the dominant theme of the modern synthetic theory of evolution.

We can recognize three ways in which populations respond to an environmental challenge. First, they may become extinct. This is the fate suffered by most species that have been confronted with a drastic environmental change.

Following a second course, a population may somehow successfully meet all environmental challenges to which they are exposed, undergoing only minor changes in their genetic makeup and persisting through time relatively unaltered. Examples include the tuatara of New Zealand (p. 597), the modern lungfishes, and the modern oysters—all forms that closely resemble their ancestors of millions of years ago. Internal changes that we cannot detect may take place, but for the most part the stability of these populations is real.

The third response to environmental challenge is the evolution of adaptations in a population that enable it to invade a new ecological habitat. Populations with this response are the winners in an evolutionary sense, since they generate new species and enrich the earth's biota with the great diversity we find today.

We should not leave the impression that all debate ended once the modern synthetic theory (often called neo-Darwinism) emerged. Some of the major areas of controversy today will be discussed in the pages that follow.

Figure 38-11

Thomas Henry Huxley (1825-1895), one of England's greatest zoologists, on first reading the convincing evidence for natural selection in Darwin's *Origin of Species,* is said to have exclaimed, "How extremely stupid not to have thought of that!" He became Darwin's foremost advocate and engaged in often bitter debates with Darwin's critics. Darwin, who disliked publicly defending his own work, was glad to leave such encounters to his "bulldog," as Huxley called himself.
Courtesy British Museum (Natural History), London.

___ MICROEVOLUTION: GENETIC CHANGE WITHIN POPULATIONS AND SPECIES

Microevolution is the change of gene frequencies within single, natural populations. These are the small evolutionary events that are going on all the time. The evolutionary process is much too slow to be observable in a single lifetime. Nevertheless, within individual populations it is often possible to observe shifts in gene frequencies that produce new adaptive traits. Occasionally we can witness the emergence of new species. We have stressed that evolution is the result of interaction between populations and their environments. How these interactions cause evolution is the subject of this section.

Genetic Variation within Species

Biological variation exists within all natural populations. We can verify this fact simply by measuring a single character is several dozen specimens selected from a local population: tail length in mice, length of a leg segment in grasshoppers, number of gill rakers in sunfish, number of peas in pods, and height of adult males of the human species. When the values are graphed with respect to frequency distribution, they tend to approximate a normal, or bell-shaped, probability curve. Most individuals fall near the mean, fewer fall above or below the mean, and the extremes make up the "tails" of the frequency curve with increasing rarity. The larger the population sample, the closer the frequencies resemble a normal curve. Sometimes significant deviations from normality are discovered in populations, and such instances may reveal important facts about variations within the population.

As pointed out in Chapter 37, the ultimate source of all genetic variation is the mutation of genes. The *immediate* source of genetic variation, however, is not mutations because a mutation is a rare event. Rather it is the recombination of existing alleles by sexual reproduction.

All of the alleles of all genes possessed by members of a population are referred to collectively as the **gene pool.** The interbreeding population is the visible manifestation of the gene pool, which thus has continuity through successive generations. The gene pool of large populations must be enormous, because at observed mutation rates many mutant alleles can be expected at all gene loci. Let us suppose that two alleles are present at a chromosomal locus: A and a. Two kinds of sex cells would be produced, and among individuals in the population there are three possible genotypes: A/A, A/a, and a/a. When two pairs of alleles are involved, 2^2 or four kinds of sex cells can be produced (see the Punnett square on p. 897), and within the population there are nine possible genotypes. With larger numbers of loci and pairs of alleles, the potential number of different kinds of sex cells rises rapidly, that is, 2^3, 2^4, 2^5, and so on.

Most animals have thousands of gene loci. If the number of gene loci in an individual were 10,000 (about average for many mammal species), and 10% (1000) of these loci were heterozygous, the individual could produce a staggering 2^{1000} genetically different kinds of sex cells, a number larger than all the atoms in the universe! So, with just two alleles existing for 10% of the genome, there is obviously copious material on which natural selection can act. Even if no new mutations occurred, the shuffling of existing genes would provide enough variation to fuel natural selection for a long time.

Variation and natural selection

What does variation signify for evolution? As already stated, genetic variation produced in whatever manner furnishes the material on which natural selection works to produce evolution. Natural selection does this by favoring beneficial variations and eliminating those harmful to the organism. Selective advantages of

In fact, the amount of potential variation is even greater than our example suggests. After protein electrophoresis (a method used to distinguish different forms of the same enzyme [allozymes]) was introduced in the 1960s, geneticists were surprised to discover that at least 30% of the roughly 10,000 loci in *Drosophila* are polymorphic, with two to six alleles at each locus. These alleles appear at such high frequencies that the average fly is likely to be heterozygous at about 12% of its loci. But this is not the whole story because genes exert different influences in the presence of other genes. Gene A may act differently in the presence of gene B from what it does in the presence of gene C (epistasis, p. 900). The diversity produced by this interaction and the addition of new mutations now and then add to the complexity of population genetics.

this type represent a very slow process, but on a geological time scale they can bring about striking evolutionary changes represented by the various taxonomic units (species, genera, and so on), adaptive radiation groups, and the various kinds of adaptations.

The fact must be stressed, however, that natural selection works on the whole animal and not on a single hereditary characteristic. The organism that possesses the most beneficial combination of characteristics is going to be selected over one not so favored. This concept may help to explain some of those puzzling instances in which an animal may have certain characteristics, or a "hand of cards," that have no advantage or are actually harmful, but in the overall picture has a winning combination. Thus, in a population, pools of variations are created on which natural selection can work to produce evolutionary change.

Genetic Equilibrium

In the human population, brown eyes are dominant to blue, curly hair is dominant to straight, and a Roman nose is dominant to a straight nose. Why has the dominant gene not gradually supplanted the recessive one in each instance so that we are all brown eyed, curly haired, and Roman nosed? It is a common belief that a character dependent on a dominant gene increases in proportion because of its dominance. This is not the case because there is a tendency in *large* populations for genes to remain in equilibrium generation after generation. A dominant gene does not change in frequency with respect to its recessive allele(s).

This principle is based on a basic law of population genetics called the **Hardy-Weinberg equilibrium.** According to this law, gene frequencies and genotype ratios in large biparental populations reach an equilibrium in one generation and remain constant thereafter unless disturbed by new mutations, natural selection, or genetic drift (chance).

A rare gene, according to this principle, does not disappear merely because it is rare. That is why certain rare traits, such as albinism and cystic fibrosis, persist for endless generations. Variation is retained even though evolutionary processes are not in active operation. Whatever changes occur in a population—gene flow from other populations, mutations, natural selection, and migration—involve the establishment of a new equilibrium with respect to the gene pool, and this new balance is maintained until upset by disturbing factors.

The Hardy-Weinberg law is a logical consequence of Mendel's first law of segregation and expresses the tendency toward equilibrium inherent in Mendelian heredity.

Let us select for our example a population having a single locus bearing just two alleles, T and t. The phenotypic expression of this gene might be, for example, the ability to taste a chemical compound called phenylthiocarbamide. Individuals in the population will be of three genotypes for this locus: T/T, T/t (both tasters), and t/t (nontasters). In a sample of 100 individuals, let us suppose we have determined that there are 20 of T/T genotype, 40 of T/t genotype, and 40 of t/t genotype. We could then set up a table showing the allelic frequencies as follows (remember that every individual has two loci for the gene and thus two alleles):

Genotype	Number of individuals	Number of T alleles	Number of t alleles
T/T	20	40	
T/t	40	40	40
t/t	40		80
TOTAL	100	80	120

Of the 200 alleles, the proportion of the T allele is 80/200 = 0.4 (40%), and the proportion of the t allele is 120/200 = 0.6 (60%). It is customary in presenting this equilibrium to use p and q to represent the two allele frequencies. The dominant gene is represented by p, the recessive by q. Thus:

$$p = \text{Frequency of } T = 0.4$$
$$q = \text{Frequency of } t = 0.6$$
$$\text{Therefore} \quad p + q = 1$$

Having calculated allele frequencies in the sample, let us determine whether these frequencies will change spontaneously in a new generation of a population. Assuming the mating is random (and this is important; all mating combinations of genotypes must be equally probable), each individual will contribute an equal number of gametes to the "common pool" from which the next generation is formed. This being the case, the frequencies of gametes in the "pool" will be proportional to the allele frequencies in the sample. That is, 40% of the gametes will be T, and 60% will be t (ratio of 0.4:0.6). Both eggs and sperm will, of course, show the same frequencies. The next generation is formed as follows:

Sperm \ Eggs	Probability of $T = 0.4$	Probability of $t = 0.6$
Probabilty of $T = 0.4$	Probability of T/T individual = $0.4 \times 0.4 = 0.16$	Probability of T/t individual = $0.4 \times 0.6 = 0.24$
Probability of $t = 0.6$	Probability of T/t individual = $0.4 \times 0.6 = 0.24$	Probability of t/t individual = $0.6 \times 0.6 = 0.36$

Collecting the genotypes, we have:

$$\text{Frequency of } T/T = 0.16$$
$$\text{Frequency of } T/t = 0.48$$
$$\text{Frequency of } t/t = 0.36$$

Next, we determine the values of p and q from the randomly mated population:

$$T\ (p) = \frac{0.16 + \frac{1}{2}\ (0.48)}{1} = 0.4$$

$$t\ (q) = \frac{0.36 + \frac{1}{2}\ (0.48)}{1} = 0.6$$

The new generation bears exactly the same genotype frequencies as the parent population! There has been no increase in the frequency of the dominant gene T. Thus, *in a freely interbreeding, sexually reproducing population, the frequency of each allele remains constant generation after generation.* The more mathematically minded reader will recognize that the genotype frequencies T/T, T/t, and t/t are actually a binomial expansion of $(p + q)^2$:

$$(p + q)^2 = p^2 + 2\ pq + q^2 = 1$$

This algebraic approach is a convenient way to calculate the frequency of genotypes in a population. For example, albinism in humans is caused by a recessive allele a. Only one person in 20,000 is an albino, and this individual must be homozygous (a/a) for the recessive allele. Obviously there are many carriers in the population with normal pigmentation, that is, people who are heterozygous *(A/a)* for albinism. What is their frequency? Assuming again that mating is random (a questionable assumption for albinos, but one that we will accept for our example), genotype distribution will be $p^2 = A/A$, $2\ pq = A/a$, and $q^2 = a/a$. Only the frequency of genotype *a/a* is known with certainty, 1/20,000; therefore:

$$q^2 = 1/20,000$$

$$q = \sqrt{1/20,000} = \frac{1}{141}$$

$$p = 1 - q \qquad = \frac{140}{141}$$

The frequency of carriers is as follows:

$$A/a = 2\ pq = 2 \times \frac{140}{141} \times \frac{1}{141} = \frac{1}{70}$$

One person in every 70 is a carrier! Even though a recessive trait may be rare, it is amazing how common a recessive allele may be in a population. There is a message here for anyone proposing a eugenics program designed to free a population of a "bad" gene. It is practically impossible. Since only the homozygous recessives reveal the phenotype to be artificially selected against (by sterilization, for example), the gene continues to surface from the heterozygous carriers. For a recessive allele present in two of every 100 persons (but homozygous in only one in 10,000 persons), it would require 50 generations of complete selection against the homozygotes just to reduce its frequency to one in 100 persons.

_____ Processes of Evolution: How Genetic Equilibrium Is Upset

The Hardy-Weinberg law shows that populations do not change—and thus do not evolve—as long as certain conditions are met: (1) very large population, (2) random mating, (3) no mutations, (4) no selection, and (5) no migration. We already know that these conditions cannot all prevail indefinitely and that the Hardy-Weinberg equilibrium can be disturbed by mutations, genetic drift, natural selection, and migration. Earlier (p. 929) we discussed mutations, the ultimate source of variability in all populations. We will now look at other factors that cause gene frequencies to change and thus lead to evolution.

Genetic drift and neutral mutations

Genetic drift refers to changes in gene frequency resulting from purely random sampling fluctuations. By such means a new mutant gene may be able to spread through a small population until it becomes homozygous in all the organisms of a population (random fixation), or it may be lost altogether from a population (random extinction). Such a condition naturally would upset the gene frequency equilibrium.

How does the principle apply? Let us suppose that a few individuals at random become isolated from a large general population. This could happen by some freakish accident of physical conditions, such as a flood carrying a small group of field mice to a remote habitat or a disease epidemic wiping out most of a population. In the general population individuals would be represented by both

Figure 38-12

Frequencies of the blood-type allele B among humans in Europe. The allele is common in the east and rare in the west. The allele may have arisen as a new mutant gene in a small population of people in Asia that were, or became, isolated from their parent population eastward where the allele did not exist. By random genetic drift, the new allele may have spread through the founding population. The spread of the allele westward began when the founding population lost its isolation and intermixed with people in the west.

Modified from Mourant, A.E. 1954. The distribution of human blood. Toronto, Ryerson Press.

homozygotes, T/T, for example, and heterozygotes, T/t. It would be possible for the small isolated group to be made up only of T/T individuals and the t gene would be lost altogether. Also, when only a small number of offspring are produced, certain genes may by chance be included in the germ cells, and others may not be represented. It is possible in this way for heterozygous genes to become homozygous. The new group may in time have gene pools different from those of the ancestral population.

During the 1960s, genetic drift was deemphasized as a factor of much importance in evolution because it could operate only in small populations. However, evolutionists now realize that most breeding populations of animals *are* small. A natural barrier such as a stream, or a ravine between two hilltops, may effectively separate a breeding population into two separate and independent units of selection.

Small populations of colonizers are especially subject to genetic drift. The smaller the colonies, the greater are random changes in gene frequencies that can lead to new species. It is no surprise, therefore, that speciation occurs often and rapidly on islands.

Neutral mutations are those that do not confer differences in fitness and are therefore not affected by natural selection. If a mutation is truly neutral, that is, is neither beneficial nor harmful, it will remain in the population at some frequency determined largely by accidents of genetic drift. The mutation may by chance be lost or may increase in frequency (again purely by chance) and become fixed in the gene pool.

Over the last 10 years or so, geneticists have discovered far more variation in protein structure—mostly enzymes—than could ever have been predicted. The presence of different forms of the same protein in a population is called **protein polymorphism.** Most of these protein variants are neutral because they are unaffected by Darwinian selection.

The discovery of neutral mutations has given rise to the "neutralist school," which maintains that most if not all biochemical variation in gene pools is neutral with respect to adaptation and natural selection. If the advocates of the neutralist school are correct, molecular evolution (for example, protein structure) occurs by genetic drift. This has led to a lively debate between "selectionists," who believe that natural selection is the dominant force in evolution, and "neutralists," who maintain that most evolution is determined by drift and is therefore "non-Darwinian."

Much biochemical variation appears to be trivial and neutral with respect to adaptation. For example, there have been many attempts to discover adaptive properties in the ABO blood group system of humans. The blood groups of this system are distributed unevenly among human populations in different parts of the world (Fig. 38-12). Some correlation has been found between the frequency of certain blood groups and the incidence of particular diseases, but most geneticists now believe that the blood groups are neutral in humans. Genetic drift appears to be responsible for differences in frequencies of the blood groups among different human populations.

Nevertheless, not all "invisible" protein polymorphism is neutral. Experiments have shown that many enzymatic differences are adaptive. For example, animals living in cold climates have enzymes that are more active at lower temperatures, whereas populations of the same species living in warmer climates possess enzymes that are more active at higher temperatures. Discoveries of this kind suggest to selectionists that much protein polymorphism is adaptive in ways not yet understood. Thus, the debate between selectionists and neutralists continues, and at this time there is not enough evidence to know which school is correct.

Natural selection

We have already stated that natural selection is the principal guiding force in evolution, and we have alluded to its mechanism. We will now more firmly define what it does. *Natural selection guides evolution by sorting out new adaptive combinations from a population gene pool derived from mutations, recombination, and other sources of genetic variation acting over many generations.*

Let us examine this definition. Sexually reproducing populations are composed of many individuals, and each individual has a different genotype. These differences have arisen by mutations, genetic recombinations, and perhaps genetic drift, nonrandom mating, or migration. Suppose that one of these genotypes is better than any of the others; that is, the animal bearing it is *better adapted* to the environment than are other animals having different genotypes. What basis have we for concluding that a particular genotype is better, that is, has greater **adaptive value** than others? The basis is reproductive success. Most organisms contribute progeny to the next generation. The genotype that contributes the most progeny, and therefore the most genotypes to the next generation, has the greatest adaptive value and chance of success. If this differential reproduction continues systematically generation after generation, the genotype will increase in frequency while others decline in frequency. Natural selection, then, produces differences in gene pools from one generation to the next.

We have stressed, and will stress once more, that natural selection works on the whole organism—the entire phenotype—and not on individual genes. The winning genotype may well contain genes that have detrimental effects on the individual but are preserved because other genes are strongly beneficial.

Natural selection at work

Despite the current debate over the importance of neutral mutations, natural selection remains the centerpiece of evolutionary biology. Differential survival and reproduction of different genotypes change the genetic composition of populations. Changing gene frequency therefore is the whole basis of evolution.

There are many examples that show how natural selection alters populations in nature. Sometimes selection can proceed very rapidly as, for example, in the development of high resistance to insecticides by insects, especially flies and mosquitoes. Doses that at first killed almost all pests later were ineffective in controlling them. As a result of selection, mutations bestowing high resistance, but previously rare in the population, increased in frequency.

Perhaps the most famous instance of rapid selection is that of **industrial melanism** (dark pigmentation) in the peppered moth of England (Fig. 38-13). Before 1850 the peppered moth was always white with black speckling in the wings and body. In 1849 a mutant black form of the species appeared. It became increasingly common, reaching frequencies of 98% in Manchester and other heavily industrialized areas by 1900. The peppered moth, like most moths, is active at night. It rests during the day in exposed places, depending on its cryptic coloration for protection. The mottled pattern of the normal white form blends perfectly with the lichen-covered tree trunks. With increasing industrialization, the soot and grime from thousands of chimneys killed the lichens and darkened the bark of trees for miles around centers such as Manchester. (This part of England was known as the "Black Country.") Against a dark background the white moth is conspicuous to predatory birds, whereas the mutant black form is camouflaged. The result was rapid natural selection: the easier-to-see white form was preferentially selected by birds, whereas the melanic form was subject to far less predation. Selection pressure thus tended to eliminate the white form while favoring the genes that contributed to black wings and body.

Another way to describe the selective quality of the genes that determine color is in terms of their **fitness**. Fitness, or adaptive value, describes the way individuals differ in their reproductive success because of differences in the genes they carry. In this case the single dominant mutation for the black form of the peppered moth increased its fitness in England's "Black Country." This same trait, however, confers low fitness in nonpolluted countryside areas. On the other hand, genes for the white form confer high fitness in nonpolluted countryside areas but low fitness near industrial centers.

Of special interest is the rapidity of the change. Rather than requiring thou-

Figure 38-13

Light and melanic forms of the peppered moth *Biston betularia* on, **A,** a lichen-covered tree in unpolluted countryside and, **B,** a soot-covered oak near industrial Birmingham, England. The dark melanic coloration that appeared in 1850 is controlled by a dominant allele.
Photographs by H.B.D. Kettlewell.

sands of years, the change occurred in only about 50 years. White moths still survived in nonpolluted areas of England, and with the recent institution of pollution-control programs the white forms are reappearing in the woods around cities. Industrial melanism is a dramatic example of rapid directional selection caused by a changing environment and leading to shifting gene frequencies.

EVOLUTION OF NEW SPECIES

We have described how populations change over periods of time because of genetic variation. Mutations are the fundamental source of genetic variation, further enhanced by sexual interchange and recombination. Natural selection acting on these variations is the force that produces evolutionary change and maintains the adaptive well-being of populations. In this discussion we consider how new species arise. The process of species multiplication, that is, the division of a parent species into several daughter species, is called **speciation.**

Species Concept

Although a definition of species is needed before we can theorize about species formation, biologists do not agree on a single rigid definition that applies in all cases. The traditional concept of species is as static and immutable units subject only to minor and unimportant variations. According to this view, a species is a group within which the individuals closely resemble one another but are clearly distinguishable from those of any other group. The flaw in this definition is the fact of biological variation. Many species are made up of individuals that can be arranged into completely intergrading series. Sometimes the gaps between species can be detected only with the greatest difficulty, and it becomes almost impossible to decide where two species are to be separated. Yet species are realities in nature. We observe and collect them, study them, sample their populations, and describe their behavior.

The difficulty with the traditional system is that classification is based on appearance alone (size, color, length of various parts, and so on). Other criteria can be used: behavioral differences, reproductive characteristics, genetic composition, and ecological niche. The single property that maintains the integrity of a species more than any other property, especially among biparental organisms, is *interbreeding.* The members of a species can interbreed freely with each other, produce fertile offspring, and share a common gene pool. Interbreeding of different species usually is either physically or behaviorally impossible, or it produces sterile offspring. There are of course exceptions, but they are rare. Species are thus usually considered genetically closed systems, whereas **races** within a species are open systems and can exchange genes. A species therefore may be defined as *a group of organisms of interbreeding natural populations that is reproductively isolated from other such groups and that shares a common gene pool* (Dobzhansky, 1951; Mayr, 1970).

How Species Become Reproductively Isolated

The definition of a species states that gene pools of different species are **reproductively isolated** from each other. With the exception of occasional hybridization, gene flow between species does not occur. Reproductive isolation, then, ensures the independence of a new species. No new species could maintain its integrity if it freely interbred with other species. If it did interbreed with another species, and the offspring from these matings were just as viable and fertile as those of matings within the species, the two species would simply amalgamate. Reproductive isolation, then, is the *result* of successful speciation. How does it happen?

New species do not arise easily. The origin of a new animal species is probably never accomplished by a single large mutation that would bestow instant reproductive isolation, as geneticists once thought. Speciation in animals could be instantaneous only if a new mutation would prevent its bearer from exchanging genes with the rest of the population. But how could the new mutant find a mate? The chance that two members of the opposite sex would mutate at the same locus, in the same way, and at the same time is infinitely remote. Instantaneous speciation does occur, however, by allopolyploidy in plants, as we will explain later.

There appears to be only one certain way for barriers to be built between animal species: **geographical isolation.** Unless some individuals of a population can be segregated for many generations from the parent population, new adaptive variations that may arise may become lost through interbreeding with the parent population. Geographical isolation permits a unique sample of the population gene pool to be "pinched off," or segregated, so that diversification can occur.

____ Allopatric Speciation

Allopatric ("in another land") populations of a species are those that occupy different geographical areas and do not interbreed. Speciation that occurs as a result of geographical isolation is known as allopatric speciation.

Let us imagine a single interbreeding population of mammals that is split into two isolated populations by some geographical change—the uplifting of a mountain barrier, the sinking and flooding of a geological fault, or a climatic change that creates a hostile ecological barrier such as a desert. Gene flow between the two isolated populations is no longer possible. The populations are almost certainly different from each other even when first isolated, since just by chance alone one population contains alleles not present in the other.

With the passage of time, genetic recombination accentuates the difference, especially if the populations are small. Mutations that appear in the separated populations are certain to be different. Furthermore, the climatic conditions of the separated regions are usually different; one may be warm and moist, the other cool and dry. Natural selection acting on the isolated gene pools favors those mutations and recombinations that best adapt the populations to their respective environments, unique food supplies, and new predator-prey relationships.

The two populations continue to diverge morphologically, physiologically, and behaviorally until distinct geographical races are formed. After some indefinite time span, perhaps only a few thousand years, but possibly a much longer period of time, evolutionary diversification progresses until the two races are reproductively isolated. If the barrier separating them fails (erosion of mountains, shifting of river flow, reestablishment of a hospitable ecological bridge), the two populations again intermix. However, they may no longer interbreed because fertility between them is impaired by their accumulated gene differences. They are now distinct species.

Speciation under these conditions is by no means inevitable. It happens only under the most ideal conditions: small population (and gene pool) size, fortunate

Geographical isolation is not the same thing as reproductive isolation. Geographical isolation refers to the spatial separation of two populations. It prevents gene exchange and is a precondition for speciation. Reproductive isolation is the result of speciation, and refers to the various physical, physiological, ecological, and behavioral barriers that prevent interbreeding with any other species.

mutations, and the right combination of selection pressures. The chances are good, in fact, that one or both populations isolated in this way will become extinct. But over the vast span of time that organic evolution has had to work, the special conditions required for speciation have been repeated numerous times, indeed millions of times.

Adaptive radiation on islands

Many times in the earth's history, a single parental population has given rise not just to one or two new species, but to an entire family of species. The rapid multiplication of related species, each with its unique specializations that fit it for a particular ecological niche, is called **adaptive radiation.**

Young islands are especially ideal habitats for rapid evolution. If they are formed by volcanoes that rose from a platform on the ocean floor, as were the Galápagos Islands, they are at first devoid of life. In time they are colonized by plants and animals from the continent or from other islands. These newcomers encounter an especially productive situation for evolution because of the abundance of new opportunities.

On the crowded mainland almost every ecological niche is already occupied. (An ecological niche is an animal's unique way of life in an environment; see Chapter 41.) Every animal is specialized and adapted for a particular way of life, and all food sources are exploited by one species or another. Although variations continue to appear within a population, those offspring in each generation most like their parents are most likely to survive, because they are best suited for that particular set of environmental conditions. Competition between different species is too keen on the mainland, where evolution has been proceeding for a very long time, for many new evolutionary experiments to succeed.

On a young island, however, new arrivals find new ecological opportunities and no competitors. Those surviving the sea or air voyage and the landfall may be able to become established, multiply, and spread out. They are in a new land that in all probability differs ecologically from their original home. New variations may serve some of the descendants of the colonizers in establishing themselves in new niches. Offspring that differ slightly from their parents may find that these differences enable them to exploit alternate food sources as yet unused by other animals. They thus flourish and produce offspring, some of which bear similar characteristics. With each passing generation these animals become increasingly successful at this alternative way of life, at the same time becoming increasingly different from their ancestors. The outcome is a new genetic blueprint, in short, a new species. Equally well, immigrants to an island may fail to become established if the limited variety that is provided by a small group of colonizers does not happen to fit the new environment.

On archipelagoes, such as the Galápagos Islands, isolation plays an extremely important evolutionary role. Not only is the entire archipelago isolated from the continent, but each island is geographically isolated from the others by the sea, the most inhospitable environment for land animals. Moreover, each island is different from every other to a greater or lesser extent in its physical, climatic, and biotic characteristics. As colonizing animals find their way to the different islands, they are presented with an environmental challenge that is unique for each island. Moreover, each new arrival carries with it only a small fraction, a biased sample, of the population's gene pool. This further stimulates diversification, already encouraged by isolation, new ecological opportunities, and lack of competition.

Figure 38-14

Adaptive radiation in Darwin's finches of the Galápagos Islands.

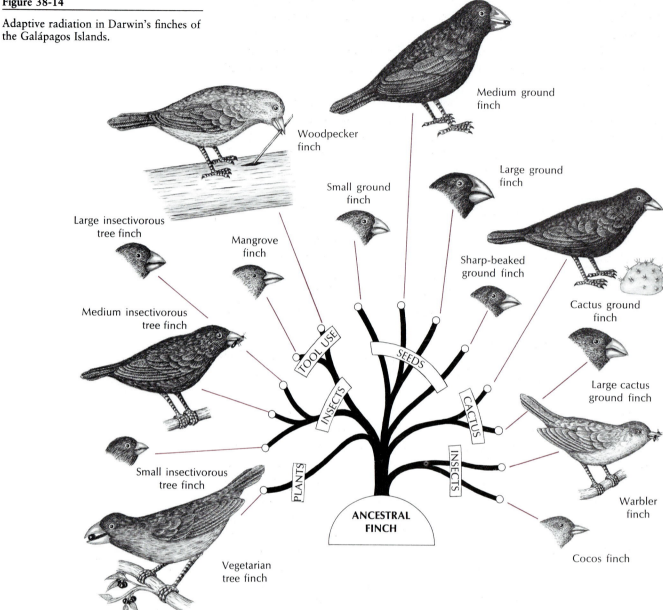

Archipelagoes, more than any other place on the earth's surface, offer the raw materials and opportunities for rapid evolutionary changes of great magnitude.

Darwin's finches

Let us consider the evolution of the family of 13 famous Galápagos finch species (Fig. 38-14). Their fame rests not on their beauty—they are, in fact, inconspicuous, dull colored, and rather unmusical in song—but on the enormous impact they had in molding Darwin's theory of natural selection. Darwin noticed that the Galápagos finches (the name "Darwin's finches" was popularized in the 1940s by the British ornithologist David Lack) are clearly related to each other, but that each species differs from the others in several respects, especially in size and shape of the beak and in feeding habits. Darwin reasoned that, if the finches were specially created, it would require the strangest kind of coincidence for 13 similar finches to be created on the Galápagos Islands and nowhere else.

Darwin's finches are an excellent example of how new forms may originate from a single colonizing ancestor. Lacking competition from other land birds, they underwent adaptive radiation, evolving along various lines to occupy available niches that on the mainland would have been denied to them. They thus assumed the characteristics of mainland families as diverse and unfinchlike as warblers and woodpeckers.

A fourteenth Darwin's finch is found on isolated Cocos Island, far to the north of the Galápagos archipelago. It is similar in appearance to the Galápagos finches and almost certainly has descended from the same ancestral stock. Since Cocos Island is a single small island with no opportunities for isolation of finch populations, there has been no species multiplication.

Sympatric Speciation

The Cocos Island example emphasizes the fundamental requirement for geographical isolation in speciation. In its absence, there is no other reasonable way for gene pools of animals to become separated long enough for genomic differences to accumulate. Is there any mechanism for sympatric ("in the same land") speciation in animals to occur? Most biologists think not, while acknowledging that it may occur under special circumstances and as an isolated event.

Examples of sympatric speciation are found among polyploid species of plants. Polyploidy refers to an increase in the haploid number of chromosomes of an organism by some multiple above the normal diploid level: tripling (triploidy), quadrupling (tetraploidy), and so on.

One clear case of sympatric speciation is the artificial creation of new species by hybridization. In 1924 Karpechenko crossed the radish *(Raphanus sativus)* with the cabbage *(Brassica oleracea)*, each having 18 chromosomes. The 18 chromosome hybrids (nine chromosomes from each parent) were sterile, as hybrids usually are, but by chance some of the hybrids doubled their chromosome number, becoming tetraploid. This event is called spontaneous allopolyploidy.

The tetraploid plant with 36 chromosomes, bearing characteristics of both the radish and the cabbage, proved to be fertile. A new sympatric "instant species" was formed called *Raphanobrassica*. It could not be crossed with either of the parents and was reproductively isolated. Unfortunately the new species is of no practical use because it has roots like a cabbage and leaves like a radish.

Spontaneous allopolyploidy has probably occurred as a natural event for the production of some of our food plants such as the bread wheats, potatoes, and raspberries. Although it may be a significant factor in plant evolution, it is probably a rare process in animal evolution. There is some evidence that sympatric speciation might occur (although it is impossible to prove) in certain insects and in animal parasites.

MACROEVOLUTION: MAJOR EVOLUTIONARY EVENTS

We have seen that the gradual accumulation of small changes in gene frequency within a population, leading to the formation of new species by classical Darwinian natural selection, is called microevolution. **Macroevolution** is the term used to describe large-scale events in organic evolution operating over millions of years.

Time

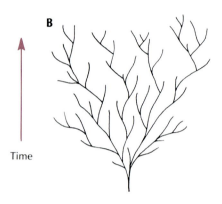

Time

Figure 38-15

Punctuation and gradualism compared.
A, The punctuation model sees evolutionary change as being concentrated in relatively rapid bursts *(straight lateral lines)* followed by prolonged periods of little or no change *(straight vertical lines).* **B,** The gradualistic (Darwinian) model views evolution as proceeding more or less steadily through time.

The appearance of major groups (for example, molluscs, land vertebrates, and birds) represents completely new designs for living. Can historical trends of this magnitude be explained by shifting gene frequencies within populations (that is, by microevolution) operating over vast time scales? The orthodox answer is yes, and the supporting evidence comes especially from molecular and physiological studies showing that organisms share homologies at many levels (DNA, RNA, blood proteins, cellular organization, metabolic pathways, and so on).

Nevertheless, many evolutionists are troubled by the idea that evolution has always progressed at a stately pace, with new lineages appearing gradually over vast periods of time. More often than not, the fossil record suggests that evolution moves in leaps. Many species remain virtually unchanged for millions of years, then suddenly disappear to be replaced by a quite different, but related, form. Moreover, most major groups of animals appear abruptly in the fossil record, fully formed, and with no fossils yet discovered that form a transition from their parent groups. Thus, it has seldom been possible to piece together ancestor-dependent sequences from the fossil record that show gradual, smooth transitions between species.

There are two principal explanations for the absence of transitional forms in the fossil record. The traditional explanation is that evolution has always progressed at the same steady pace, and that "gaps" in the record are imperfections because transitions occur by microevolution in restricted localities and in small populations, under circumstances not favorable to fossil formation. In this view, fossils appear in the record only after a major group has become widely established by migration. The alternative view, which appears to be gaining favor among paleontologists, is that the abruptness of the fossil record is a true record of macroevolutionary "spurts."

One emerging explanation for rapid speciation events is that of **punctuated equilibria** (Eldredge and Gould, 1972). In this view, new species emerge rather suddenly, then remain mostly unchanged until they become extinct. In other words, long periods of equilibrium are abruptly "punctuated" by the extinction of a species, and its replacement by a new descendant species. It has been observed that most species survive for 5 to 10 million years before becoming extinct, and during this time they apparently change very little. A speciation event that occurs in a small, isolated population over perhaps 50,000 years represents 1% or less of the species' life span. Fifty thousand years is a "geological instant" in the earth's history but represents thousands of generations in the evolving species. We know that gradual Darwinian selection can accomplish dramatic genetic changes much more rapidly than this. Thus, punctuated equilibrium does not require a new explanation for speciation because 50,000 to 100,000 years is sufficient time for a new species to evolve by Darwinian selection. Eldredge and Gould have repeatedly emphasized that the long periods of stasis following the rapid transition are the more interesting phenomenon. Fig. 38-15 compares the punctuated equilibrium model with the conventional Darwinian (gradualistic) model of evolution.

Evolutionists who have long bewailed the imperfect state of the fossil record were treated in 1981 to the opening of an uncensored page of fossil history in Africa. Peter Williamson, a British paleontologist working in fossil beds 400 m deep near Lake Turkana, was able to document a remarkably clear record of speciation events in freshwater molluscs. The geology of the Lake Turkana basin reveals a history of instability. Earthquakes, volcanic eruptions, and climatic changes caused the waters of the lake to rise and fall periodically, sometimes by hundreds of feet. The 13 lineages of snails collected by Williamson show long periods of stability interrupted at intervals by relatively brief periods of rapid change in shell shape when the waters of the lake receded, isolating the snail populations from each other. Then the newly evolved species remained unchanged through thick deposits before becoming extinct and being replaced by new fossils resembling (but clearly distinct from) the ancestral form. The transitions took place within 5000 to 50,000 years. In the few meters of sediment where the speciation event had occurred, all the transition forms were visible.

Williamson's study is a remarkably fine-grained record of evolution at work. It conforms well to the punctuated equilibrium model of Eldredge and Gould.

Evolution of the Horse

The fossil record of horse evolution (Fig. 38-16) provides us with an excellent example of the changing tempo of evolution. The evolution of this form extends back to the Eocene epoch some 60 million years ago, and much of it took place in North America. This record would at first seem to indicate a straight-line evolution, but actually the history of the horse family is made up of many lineages, that is, descent of many lines. The phylogeny of the horse is extensively branched, with most of the branches now extinct. There were millions of years when little change occurred; there were other epochs when changes took place relatively rapidly.

No real change in the feet occurred during the Eocene epoch, but at least three types of feet developed later and were found in different groups during the late Cenozoic era. Only one of these three types is found today.

There was extensive adaptive radiation throughout the horse's evolutionary history. In the evolution of the horse the morphological changes of the limbs and teeth were of primary importance, along with a progressive increase in size of most of the types in the direct line of descent.

The earliest member of the horse phylogeny is considered to be *Hyracotherium,* also known as *Eohippus,* the dawn horse (Fig. 38-16). It was rodentlike in appearance and about the size of a small dog. Its forefeet had four digits, and the hindlegs had three. Most of the weight was borne on pads, making the feet well adapted for travel on the soft earth of tropical North America. The teeth had short crowns and long roots and were specialized for browsing on shrubs.

As the tropical conditions of central North America later gave way to open, grassy plains, the horse gradually developed feet better suited for rapid travel on dry land and grinding teeth for grazing. This transition began with *Mesohippus,* which flourished in the Oligocene epoch some 40 million years ago. *Mesohippus,* although still a browser, was larger than *Eohippus* and had three toes on each foot. *Mesohippus* gave rise to several lineages, one of which, *Merychippus,* was the direct ancestor of modern horses. *Merychippus* lived during the Miocene epoch, some 25 million years ago, when grassy prairies were becoming widespread all over the earth under the influence of an increasingly cooler and drier climate. Its teeth were high crowned, with complex crests and ridges for grinding; this development made possible the complete switch to a grazing diet. It was still three toed, but the lateral toes were high above the ground so that the weight of the body was thrown on the middle toe.

Pliohippus, a descendant of *Merychippus,* persisted into the Pleistocene epoch, some 2 million years ago. *Pliohippus* lost the side toes (although splint

Figure 38-16

Evolution of the horse family, showing the transition
from browsing to grazing and evolution of the front leg.
Only a few of the many lines of horse evolution are
shown. See text for further explanation.

bones remained to attest to their former existence) and became a single-toed horse. It gave rise to *Equus,* the modern horse, of which there are some 60 domesticated breeds, and to zebras and asses. During the Pleistocene Ice Age, the *Equus* genus spread from North America into Eurasia, Africa, and South America.

The origin of the modern horse from its diminutive ancestor *Hyracotherium* is often incorrectly portrayed as a single line of gradual transformation—a ladder of progress. In fact, the history of the horse is more like a bush than a ladder. *Equus* is not the inevitable product of a trend but a tip of one of many branches that have diverged sharply from the trunk.

The development of this remarkable animal, which has had an enormous influence on the course of human history, was closely associated with the climatic and ecological changes of its habitat. As the habitat changed, so did the horse. It became a grazer instead of a browser and developed the body size and foot structure conducive for fleetness over a firm, prairie surface. It is an extraordinary example of evolutionary adaptation to changing ecological opportunity (Principle 5, p. 12).

The sequel to the horse evolution story is strange. Having pursued a remarkable evolution on the North American continent for 60 million years, the horse became extinct in both Americas toward the end of the Pleistocene epoch. The cause of its demise is unknown, but excessive hunting by early Indians, infectious disease, predation, or some climatic catastrophe may have been responsible. It is certain that no horses were present when white people first came to the Americas. However, horses still existed in Europe and Asia and were reintroduced into America from Europe by the early Spanish colonists.

___ Summary

Organic evolution explains the diversity of living organisms, their characteristics, and their distribution as the historical outcomes of gradual, continuous change from previously existing forms. Evolutionary theory is strongly identified with Charles Robert Darwin who, with Alfred Russel Wallace, presented the first credible explanation for evolutionary change, the principle of natural selection. An alternative nineteenth-century scientific theory of evolution, Jean Baptiste de Lamarck's concept of inheritance of acquired characteristics, was disproved early in this century by geneticists. Darwin derived most of the material later used to construct his theory when, as a young man, he made a 5-year voyage around the world on the H.M.S. *Beagle.*

Evidences of organic evolution come from several sources. Fossils, the preserved remains of long-dead organisms, form an incomplete record of the progression of ancient life through geological time. Following the Cambrian explosion some 600 million years ago, when most multicellular animal phyla originated, animal evolution has been punctuated by periodic mass extinctions followed by rapid radiations of the survivors.

The age of fossils can be reliably estimated because the geological formations in which they lie can be dated by measuring the radioactive decay of naturally occurring elements.

The similarities that allow organisms, both living and extinct, to be classified into neat hierarchies is also evidence of evolution because of the presence of homologies. Homologies are structures that, because of common ancestry, share a fundamental structural plan and relative position. Common ancestry is also revealed by molecular evolution, which involves comparing homologous proteins and other molecules in different species.

Natural selection is the guiding force of evolution. The principle is founded on the observed facts that no two organisms are exactly alike, that at least some variations are inheritable, that all species tend to overproduce their kind, and that more individuals are produced than can survive. Therefore, survival and reproduction of some variants are favored over others; that is, organisms possessing those adaptations making them better adapted to the environment will survive and produce more offspring than those with less favorable variations. Thus, their inheritable characteristics will appear in greater proportion in the next generation. The essence of natural selection is reproductive success.

Darwin's theory of natural selection was gradually modified in this century when the mechanisms of heredity were established by geneticists. The modern synthesis, a new view of evolution that emerged in the 1930s, emphasized natural selection by gradual shifting of gene frequencies within populations. This is also known, especially today, as microevolution.

Mutations are the ultimate source of all new variation. However, sexual reproduction, in which the genotypes of two parents are mixed in the offspring, is the immediate source of variation among individuals in a population.

In very large, interbreeding populations, gene frequencies tend to remain stable as predicted by the Hardy-Weinberg equilibrium. Such populations will not evolve unless disturbed by mutations, genetic drift, natural selection, or migration.

Genetic drift is the change in gene frequencies in small populations as a result of chance alone, in the absence of natural selection. Once considered to be an unimportant force in evolution, genetic drift has received new attention from advocates of the neutralist school of evolution, who argue that most evolutionary changes represent the fixation of neutral mutations by random drift.

Natural selection, on the other hand, works on the products of the genetic code, and it guides evolution by sorting out better-adapted organisms from a population composed of individuals with different genotypes. The spread of the mutant melanic form of the peppered moth in industrial England is an example of natural selection in action.

A species is defined as a natural, interbreeding population of organisms sharing a common gene pool that is reproductively isolated from other groups. The evolution of new species (speciation) may occur when some individuals become geographically isolated from the parent population. This is called allopatric speciation. Young islands, with their new ecological opportunities and absence of competitors for colonizing forms, are ideal habitats for adaptive radiation: multiplication of related species. The 13 finch species of the Galápagos Islands illustrate the crucial importance of isolation in speciation.

Sympatric speciation, the origin of new species in the absence of geographical isolation, sometimes occurs in plants but has never been convincingly demonstrated in animals.

Large-scale events in life's history and the origin of new evolutionary trends are called macroevolution. Some scientists believe macroevolution can be explained by long-term extrapolation of microevolutionary mechanisms, that is, gradual changes in gene frequencies. This is the traditional view. Others more recently have viewed evolution as making sudden leaps, with new designs arising rapidly. The punctuated equilibrium hypothesis asserts that new species arise almost instantaneously in geological time, then remain almost unchanged during their subsequent history on earth. The fossil record appears to support this view.

The evolution of the horse is an excellent example of adaptive radiation and the changing tempo of evolution.

Galápagos tortoise.
Photograph by C.P. Hickman, Jr.

Selected references

Attenborough, D. 1979. Life on earth: a natural history. Boston, Little, Brown & Co. *Nontechnical account of the course of animal evolution, developed from the superb television series of the same name.*

Ayala, F.J., and J.W. Valentine. 1979. Evolving: the theory and processes of organic evolution. Menlo Park, Calif., The Benjamin-Cummings Publishing Co. *Well-written textbook.*

Boag, P.T., and P.R. Grant. 1981. Intense natural selection in a population of Darwin's finches (Geospizinae) in the Galápagos. Science **214:**82-85. *Beautiful example of natural selection at work.*

Darlington, P.J., Jr. 1980. Evolution for naturalists: the simple principles and complex reality. New York, John Wiley & Sons, Inc. *A delightfully written view of evolution by a scientist with a deep understanding of the natural world.*

Darwin, C. 1839. The voyage of the Beagle. New York, Doubleday Publishing Co. (1962). *This Natural History Library edition contains an excellent introduction by Leonard Engel.*

Darwin, C. 1859. On the origin of species by means of natural selection, or the preservation of favoured races in the struggle for life. London, John Murray. *There were five subsequent editions by the author. The Mentor Book edition (1958) is introduced by Sir Julian Huxley.*

Dobzhansky, T. 1951. Genetics and the origin of species, ed. 3. New York, Columbia University Press. *Important although advanced treatise.*

Dobzhansky, T., F.J. Ayala, G.L. Stebbins, and J.W. Valentine. 1977. Evolution. San Francisco, W.H. Freeman & Co. Publishers. *Comprehensive but somewhat uneven treatment.*

Eldredge, N., and S.J. Gould. 1972. Punctuated equilibria: an alternative to phyletic gradualism. In T.J.M. Schopf (ed.). Models in paleobiology, San Francisco, Freeman, Cooper & Co.

Futuyma, D.J. 1979. Evolutionary biology. Sunderland, Mass., Sinauer Associates, Inc. *Textbook of evolutionary theory, emphasizing mechanisms.*

Gillespie, N.C. 1979. Charles Darwin and the problem of creation. Chicago, University of Chicago Press. *Theological issues were important for Darwin and greatly influenced his thinking.*

Gould, S.J. 1982. The meaning of punctuated equilibrium and its role in validating a hierarchical approach to macroevolution. In R. Milkman (ed.). Perspectives on evolution. Sunderland, Mass., Sinauer Associates, Inc. *Punctuation explained and defended.*

Hanson, E.D. 1981. Understanding evolution. New York, Oxford University Press. *Textbook of evolution, with up-to-date treatment of a broad range of topics.*

Harris, C.L. 1981. Evolution: genesis and revelations, with readings from Empedocles to Wilson. Albany, State University of New York Press. *Opinionated but original, humorous, and thoughtful history of evolutionary ideas.*

Irvine, W. 1955. Apes, angels, and Victorians: the story of Darwin, Huxley, and evolution. New York, McGraw-Hill Book Co. *Masterly description of two central figures in the nineteenth century Darwinian revolution, told with skill and wit.*

Jukes, T.H. 1980. Silent nucleotide substitutions and the molecular evolutionary clock. Science **210:**973-978. *Shows that perhaps half the nucleotide substitutions in DNA during evolution are "silent" (neutral) changes and argues that genetic drift plays a leading role in evolution.*

Kitcher, P. 1982. Abusing science: the case against creationism. Cambridge, Mass., The M.I.T. Press. *One of the best scientific and philosophical analyses of creationism.*

Lack, D. 1947. Darwin's finches: an essay on the general biological theory of evolution. New York, Cambridge University Press. *A classic study of adaptive radiation in the famous Galápagos finches.*

Mayr, E. 1970. Population, species and evolution. Cambridge, Mass., Harvard University Press. *This excellent reference is an abridgement of the author's* Animal Species and Evolution.

Mayr, E. 1976. Evolution and the diversity of life: selected essays. Cambridge, Mass., Harvard University Press. *Collection of writings covering the full range of thought of one of the great evolutionary biologists of this century.*

Mayr, E. 1982. The growth of biological thought: diversity, evolution, and inheritance. Cambridge, Mass., Harvard University Press. *An important monograph of almost epic proportions, chronicling and interpreting the development of ideas in systematics, evolutionary theory, and genetics.*

Miller, J., and B. Van Loon. 1982. Darwin for beginners. New York, Pantheon Books, Inc. *Delightful presentation of the major concepts of natural selection, modern genetics, and isolating mechanisms, told with humor.*

Ospaovat, D. 1981. The development of Darwin's theory: natural history, natural theology, and natural selection, 1838-1859. Cambridge, Eng., Cambridge University Press. *In this scholarly work, the author argues that Darwin's theory underwent a radical change between its first formulation in the late 1830s and its publication in* The Origin of Species *in 1859.*

Patterson, C. 1978. Evolution. London, Routledge & Kegan Paul Ltd. *Lucid explanation of evolutionary theory. Highly recommended.*

Ruse, M. 1979. The Darwinian revolution: science red in tooth and claw. Chicago, University of Chicago Press. *A highly readable account of Darwin's role in converting the nineteenth-century British scientific community to a belief in evolution.*

Ruse, M. 1982. Darwinism defended: a guide to the evolution controversies. Reading, Mass., Addison-Wesley Publishing Co., Inc. *A personal view of evolutionary theory, ending with a critique of "scientific creationism."*

Simpson, G.G. 1980. Splendid isolation: the curious history of South American mammals. New Haven, Conn., Yale University Press. *Excellent documentation of how the South American mammals developed in a "closed system" during the age of mammals, written by a dean of American paleontologists.*

Stanley, S.M. 1979. Macroevolution. San Francisco,

W.H. Freeman & Co. Publishers. *Exploration of macroevolution from the paleontologist's viewpoint.*

Stanley, S.M. 1981. The new evolutionary timetable: fossils, genes, and the origin of species. New York, Basic Books, Inc., Publishers. *Readable and simplified account of the emergence of the punctuational view of evolution.*

Stebbins, G.L. 1982. Darwin to DNA, molecules to humanity. San Francisco, W.H. Freeman & Co. Publishers. *Insightful, well-written treatment of the evolutionary process.*

Stebbins, G.L., and F.J. Ayala. 1981. Is a new evolutionary synthesis necessary? Science 213:967-971. *Argument that macroevolution cannot be explained by microevolutionary principles.*

Stone, I. 1980. The origin: a biographical novel of Charles Darwin. Garden City, N.Y., Doubleday & Co., Inc. *Delightfully written, meticulously researched historical novel of Darwin's life, a must for Darwin aficionados.*

Selected *Scientific American* articles

In addition to the articles listed, the September 1978 issue is devoted exclusively to organic evolution, with articles by Ernst Mayr, F.J. Ayala, J.W. Schopf, J. Maynard Smith, and others.

Barghoorn, E.S. 1971. The oldest fossils. **244**:30-42 (May).

Bishop, J.A., and L.M. Cook. 1975. Moths, melanism and clean air. **232**:90-99 (Jan.). *The evolution of industrial melanism in moths is described.*

Cavalli-Sforza, L.L. 1969. "Genetic drift" in an Italian population. **221**:30-37 (Aug.).

Clarke, B. 1975. The causes of biological diversity. **233**:50-60 (Aug.). *Argues that diversity is maintained by, as well as is the basis of, natural selection.*

Cole, F.C. 1959. A witness at the Scopes trial. **200**:120-130 (Jan.).

Darlington, C.D. 1959. The origins of Darwinism. **200**:60-66 (May).

Dickerson, R.E. 1980. Cytochrome c and the evolution of energy metabolism. **242**:136-153 (Mar.). *Molecular pedigree of an ancient protein.*

Eiseley, L.C. 1959. Alfred Russel Wallace. **200**:70-84 (Feb.).

Gilbert, L.E. 1982. The coevolution of a butterfly and a vine. **247**:110-121 (Aug.). Heliconius *butterflies lay their eggs on* Passiflora *vines, which in defense have evolved fake eggs.*

Kettlewell, H.B.D. 1959. Darwin's missing evidence. **200**:48-53 (Mar.).

Kimura, M. 1979. The neutral theory of molecular evolution. **241**:98-126 (Nov.). *This theory holds that at the molecular level most evolutionary change results from random drift of selectively equivalent genes, rather than from natural selection.*

Kurten, B. 1969. Continental drift and evolution. **220**:54-64 (Mar.).

Lack, K. 1953. Darwin's finches. **188**:66-72 (Apr.).

Newell, N.D. 1972. The evolution of reefs. **226**:54-65 (June). *Major events in the earth's history are reflected in changes in tropical reef communities.*

Russell, D.A. 1982. The mass extinctions of the late Mesozoic. **246**:58-65 (Jan.). *They may have been caused by a falling asteroid.*

Wilson, E.O. (ed.). 1974. Ecology, evolution, and population biology. San Francisco, W.H. Freeman & Co. Publishers. *Collection of* Scientific American *articles with introductions by E.O. Wilson.*

CHAPTER 39

HUMAN EVOLUTION

Reconstructed fossil skull of the hominid *Australopithecus afarensis,* a near human believed to represent a direct ancestor of modern humans.

Courtesy The Cleveland Museum of Natural History.

While the question of human origins has preoccupied human thoughts for centuries and has formed the basis of many of the world's religions, the case for human antiquity is rooted in Darwin's 1859 publication of *The Origin of Species*. Darwin did not include the human species among the evidences used to support his theory of natural selection, but few missed the implication: humans have evolved slowly from lower forms of life. It was an idea repugnant to the Victorian world, which reacted with predictable outrage to the suggestion that humans might be descended from chimpanzees or orangutans. Actually, neither Charles Darwin nor Thomas H. Huxley, who vigorously supported and defended Darwin's theory (Fig. 38-11, p. 949), argued that humans were descended *directly* from apes, but rather that apes are the closest relatives of humans. However, to the British, being related to an ape even distantly was degrading and quite unacceptable. After all, the Bible stated that God had created man on the sixth day and said nothing about kinship to orangutans, chimpanzees, or any other ape.

Today, this storm of controversy seems quaint if not ridiculous to most people, but we should remember that the Victorian era was a turning point in the history of human knowledge, especially in our attitudes toward *Homo sapiens* as an animal species and toward our place in nature. Furthermore, there was at that time virtually no fossil evidence linking humans with apelike creatures. Darwin and Huxley rested their case mostly on cogent anatomical comparisons between humans and apes. The close resemblance of many features of human anatomy to those of apes could be explained only by assuming a common origin. Most differences in anatomy were related to the upright human posture.

The search for fossils, especially for a "missing link" that would prove a connection between apes and people, began slowly but was spurred by the unearthing of two excellent skeletons of the Neanderthal man in the 1880s and then by the discovery of the famous Java man *(Homo erectus)* by Eugene Dubois in 1891. The most spectacular discoveries, however, have been made in the last three decades in Africa, especially in the period 1967 to 1977, which American paleoanthropologist Donald C. Johanson refers to as the "golden decade."

There is great excitement now among paleontologists and anthropologists, although it is not yet possible to reconstruct fully the descent of genus *Homo* from the existing fossil evidence (which is still disappointingly meager compared with that of many nonprimate mammals).

We are no longer searching for a mythical "missing link" between living apes and humans. Both descended from a common primate ancestor in the past and, although closely related much as cousin is to cousin, they have evolved along independent lineages. Today's refined methods of investigation and modern dating techniques have established beyond reasonable doubt the authenticity and antiquity of the fossil evidence. Misunderstandings, disputes, and contradictions have been cleared up; elaborate hoaxes exposed; and doubt and ridicule gradually reduced. Nevertheless, old ideas die hard, and some people are still reluctant to accept the fact that humans are mutable creatures like other animals.

We will begin our story by looking beyond apes and monkeys to a more distant past when mammalian forms bearing primate characteristics emerged; then we will investigate the hominid evolutionary record leading to modern humans.

Figure 39-1

Common tree shrew *Tupaia glis* of tropical rain forests and montane forests of Southeast Asia.
Photograph by Ron Garrison, San Diego Zoo.

OUR CLOSEST RELATIVES—PRIMATES

Humans are primates, a fact that even the nonevolutionist Linnaeus recognized. (The classification of order Primates, the most advanced of mammalian orders, is found on p. 662.) Order Primates is divided into two suborders: Prosimii and Anthropoidea. The prosimians include the more primitive primates, such as the lemurs, lorises, and tarsiers (Figs. 39-2 and 39-3). The more advanced anthropoids are separated into three superfamilies: (1) Ceboidea, or New World monkeys (Fig. 39-4), with prehensile tail and nonopposable thumb; (2) Cercopithecoidea, or Old World monkeys (Fig. 39-5), with opposable thumb and nonprehensile tail; and (3) Hominoidea, the great apes and humans. The hominoids are in turn divided into two families: Pongidae and Hominidae. The pongids (great apes) include the gibbons (three species), gorilla (one species), orangutan (one species), and chimpanzees (two species) (Fig. 39-7). The hominids include one living species, *Homo sapiens*.

The reader should beware of the potential confusion between the term hominoid, which encompasses the great apes and humans, and the term hominid, which refers only to humanlike types, both living and extinct.

Earliest Primates

What were the basic adaptive features that guided the evolution of the primates, eventually giving rise to humans? To answer this question, we must explore the evolution of our primate ancestors. Primates share a number of important characteristics, such as grasping fingers on all four limbs, flat fingernails instead of claws, and forward-pointing eyes with binocular vision and excellent depth perception. Some have large brains and high intelligence, although the brains of most primates are no larger, in relation to body size, than the brains of other mammals.

The fossil record of the early primates is sketchy, but we know that it began in the Cretaceous period (late Mesozoic era), about 80 million years BP. Many authorities believe that the earliest primate was a nocturnal animal about the size of a **tree shrew** (Fig. 39-1), which took to living in trees. Tree shrews were formerly considered to be the most primitive of the primates, but most zoologists today place the tree shrews in the order Insectivora, a primitive group of mammals that includes several more familiar species such as moles and shrews. Whatever their correct classification may be, the tree shrews give us an idea of what a transition form between the insectivores and the primates might have looked like.

The small, nimble tree shrews gave rise in the Paleocene epoch to **lemurs** (Fig. 39-2), which have toenails instead of claws, a longer tail for balance, and a larger brain. The first digit can be opposed to the others, giving that digit greater independence of movement and facilitating the ability to grasp objects. The brain is relatively large, with a well-developed visual cortex, an adaptation for life in the trees.

Do these adaptations for an arboreal life presage the kind of existence ultimately adopted by the modern primates? We have reason to believe that they do, and furthermore, that an arboreal life was important in guiding the evolution of increased intelligence. Flexible limbs are essential for active animals moving through trees. Grasping hands and feet, in contrast to the clawed feet of squirrels and rodents, enable the primates to grip limbs, hang from branches, seize food and manipulate it, and, most significantly, use tools. Highly developed sense organs, especially good vision, and proper coordination of limb and finger muscles are essential for an active arboreal life and were selected for. Of course, sense organs

Figure 39-2

Black lemur *Lemur macaco* of Madagascar and Comoro islands.
Photograph by Ron Garrison, San Diego Zoo.

Figure 39-3

Mindanao tarsier *Tarsius syrichta carbonarius* of Mindanao island in the Philippines.
Courtesy San Diego Zoo.

are no better than the brain that processes sensory information. Precise timing, judgment of distance, and alertness were necessary concomitants of an arboreal life and required a large cerebral cortex. The early primates had enemies, such as snakes and owls, and those that survived and produced the most young were those with the best-developed senses and agility.

Tarsiers appeared in the Eocene epoch. They were aboreal, nocturnal forms as are their descendants today (Fig. 39-3). Their large eyes have shifted to a forward position to give them a stereoscopic view of the world.

Thus, as the prosimians evolved in their arboreal habitat, the pressures of stalking their insect prey along slender branches gradually molded the two main primate characteristics: grasping hands with flat nails instead of claws, and forward-facing eyes with binocular vision. Many other mammalian predators have binocular vision, but only the primates have both grasping hands and binocular vision.

Evolution of Monkeys and Apes

With the appearance of the anthropoids, a revolution in life-style occurred. For some reason these primates became day active rather than nocturnal. This change had far-reaching effects on anatomy and behavior. Smell, so important to nocturnal animals for finding food and detecting enemies in the dark, gave way as the dominant sense to vision, which is much more important than smell in daylight. Stereoscopic vision, inherited from the prosimians, greatly enhanced the ability to judge distance, recognize predators, locate food, and scamper about the trees, leaping from branch to branch. Cones appeared in the retina, enriching vision with color. The brain case became rounded and more vaulted as the improved senses became governed by an expanded brain. The long tail of lemurs that aided them in balance was reduced as more reliance was placed on improved limb coordination. Later, the tail virtually disappeared in Old World monkeys and apes, but in the New World the tail was put to a new use as a prehensile, clinging organ.

The earliest fossils of monkeys and apes appeared in late Eocene and early Oligocene deposits, 40 million years BP. By far the most important source of these early fossils is the Fayum Depression—a hot, dry desert about 60 miles southwest of Cairo, Egypt. In the Oligocene epoch, however, Fayum was a tropical rain forest, laced with rivers, on the edge of the Mediterranean, which extended much farther inland than it does today. Here a relatively abundant fossil record indicates that several genera of both monkeys and apes, all very small but clearly monkey-like and not prosimian like, scampered among the trees along the swamp-lined rivers. Thus, no later than the Oligocene epoch, both monkeys and apes arose independently from prosimian stocks.

Some of these monkeys migrated, perhaps by rafting on felled trees or masses of vegetation, to South America, where their isolated descendants gave rise to the New World monkeys. Although it seems impossible that any primate could survive the journey from Africa to South America today, the two continents were much closer together 40 million years ago (see maps of continental drift on p. 1016). The New World monkeys (superfamily Ceboidea) are more primitive and are usually smaller than Old World monkeys, although they are similar in appearance. Their nostrils are far apart, and they have long prehensile tails (Fig. 39-4).

A   B

Figure 39-4

Representative New World monkeys. **A,** Red howler *Alouatta seniculus* of tropical rain forests and deciduous forests throughout South America. **B,** Squirrel monkey *Saimiri sciureus* of the tropical rain forests of central and northern South America. Note the round, widely separated nostrils, the flat appearance of the faces, and the prehensile tails. New World monkeys are completely arboreal, exhibit little sexual dimorphism, and lack the ischial callosities (sitting pads) of Old World monkeys.

Courtesy San Diego Zoo; **A,** photograph by Ron Garrison.

The thumb is only slightly opposable to the other fingers. Because the New World monkeys split off early from the prosimians and are not closely related to Old World monkeys despite many anatomical and behavioral resemblances, they are not important to human evolution.

The Old World monkeys have their nostrils close together, and they do not use their tails as prehensile organs (Fig. 39-5). Like the New World monkeys, they are four footed in terrestrial locomotion, walking on their palms and soles. Most are arboreal, but the short-tailed baboons show a tendency for ground dwelling.

The Old World monkeys cannot be considered ancestral to the anthropoid apes or humans. The primitive, hominoid apes evolved independently from prosimian ancestors. Many fossils of these small, monkey-sized animals have been found in Miocene and Pliocene deposits. Although apelike, they lack certain specializations of modern apes. One early form of particular interest, because it may represent an early lineage that founded both ape and human lines of descent, is *Aegyptopithecus* (Fig. 39-6), the "dawn ape." This spaniel-sized form is known from several late Oligocene (30 million years BP) fossil remains, including a nearly complete skull with cranium, upper and lower jaws, and virtually all teeth. The dentition is distinctly apelike, but the skull is monkeylike. This fact, together with limb bones discovered at Fayum in 1977, suggests that the animal was a quadruped. Many paleontologists believe that *Aegyptopithecus* is a transition form leading to the hominids.

Figure 39-5

Representative Old World monkeys. **A,** Mandrill *Mandrillus sphinx* of high forested regions of central Africa. **B,** Kikuyu colobus *Colobus polykomos kikuyuensis* and baby of rain and montane forests of central Africa. **C,** Hamadryas (sacred) baboon *Papio hamadryas* of extreme east-central Africa. **D,** Olive baboon *Papio anubis* and baby of central Africa. Note the comma-shaped, thinly separated nostrils, downward-pointing noses, and absence of prehensile tails. Old World monkeys are of robust form, may be either arboreal or ground dwelling, exhibit distinct sexual dimorphism, and possess ischial callosities.

A, B, and C, Courtesy San Diego Zoo; A and C, photographs by Ron Garrison; D, photograph by L.L. Rue, III.

ANCESTORS OF APES AND HUMANS
Dryopithecines

In the Miocene epoch, beginning about 25 million years BP, several new and significant characters enter the story. Lines of descent become clearer (although by no means complete) because the fossils are more abundant and not so old. The earth was becoming cooler, and this trend continued into the Pliocene epoch, at which time polar ice caps were beginning to form. Winters were longer and summers were shorter in many parts of the world. Tropical and subtropical forests gave way to grasslands over vast areas of North America, Europe, and Asia. In this setting the anthropoid apes (pongids) began an adaptive radiation that lasted well into the Pliocene epoch. Of the numerous pongid fossils from the Miocene and Pliocene epochs, one in particular revealed an intriguing blend of monkey, ape, and human traits. This was *Dryopithecus* (Gr., *drys*, tree, + *pithecus*, ape), a diverse genus that embraces several African, European, and Indian species (Fig. 39-6). One species, *D. africanus*, resembled chimpanzees and is believed to be in a direct line of descent leading to modern chimpanzees. Another much larger species (*D. major*) was probably a predecessor of the gorilla. Still another form having obvious affinities to the chimpanzee was Proconsul, discovered at Lake Victoria in Africa in 1930. Proconsul's position in ape evolution has been long disputed, but most authorities now agree that Proconsul was not a distinct genus, but an African member of the widespread genus *Dryopithecus*. *Dryopithecus* appeared in the late Oligocene, some 30 million years BP, and flourished until about 10 million years BP.

The confusingly diverse Miocene apes have now been collected as a subfamily of pongids called the **dryopithecines**. They clearly are ancestral to the pongids and probably to the hominids as well, although the exact lineages remain to be worked out. As a group they were essentially arboreal fruit-eaters of woodland savannas. They were probably good brachiators (swinging by the arms), with arms and legs of about the same length. On the ground they were quadrupedal, but most of them walked using their front leg knuckles, much as chimpanzees do today. Their large size (one was as large as the modern gorilla) and intelligence enabled them to exploit both arboreal and terrestrial environments in relative safety.

The pongids today (gibbons, orangutan, chimpanzees, and gorilla) (Fig. 39-7) have longer arms than legs, a long trunk compared with lower limbs, curved legs with the knees turned outward, large canines, a laterally compressed (not rounded) dental arch, a long protruding face, and a brain about one third as large as ours. Some modern apes have largely abandoned the arboreal way of life. Chimpanzees and gorillas are quite at home on the ground. A more or less erect posture is characteristic of many of them, although they may use their long arms for support while walking. More abundant food on the ground may have induced them to come down out of the trees and enter the savanna as pioneers.

Genetic similarity of apes and humans

Despite the large gap that separates humans from apes, there is abundant evidence for common ancestry that becomes ever more convincing. By using a variety of new biochemical techniques to estimate the "genetic distance" between humans and chimpanzees, we find that their macromolecules are almost all alike. Humans and apes are in fact genetically more alike than are different species of fruit flies of

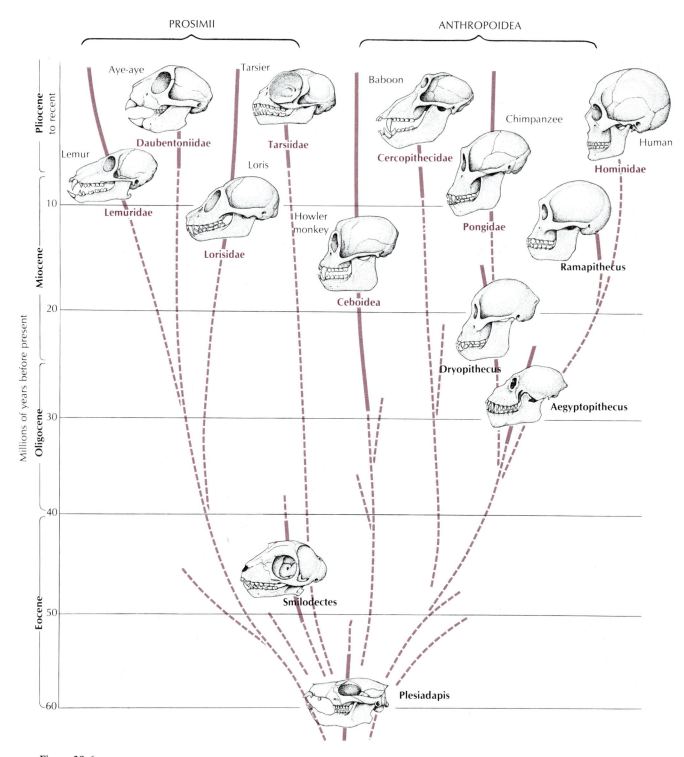

PROSIMII   ANTHROPOIDEA

Aye-aye   Tarsier   Baboon   Chimpanzee   Human

Daubentoniidae   **Tarsiidae**   **Cercopithecidae**   **Hominidae**

Lemur   Loris

Lemuridae   Howler   **Pongidae**

monkey   Ramapithecus

Lorisidae

Ceboidea   Dryopithecus

Aegyptopithecus

Smilodectes

Plesiadapis

Millions of years before present

Pliocene to recent — Miocene — Oligocene — Eocene

10 — 20 — 30 — 40 — 50 — 60

Figure 39-6

Phylogeny of the primates, showing evolutionary relationships. Extinct forms are indicated by their generic names. Extant groups are indicated by the family name (superfamily in the case of Ceboidea) and common name of the example. Skulls are not drawn to the same scale.

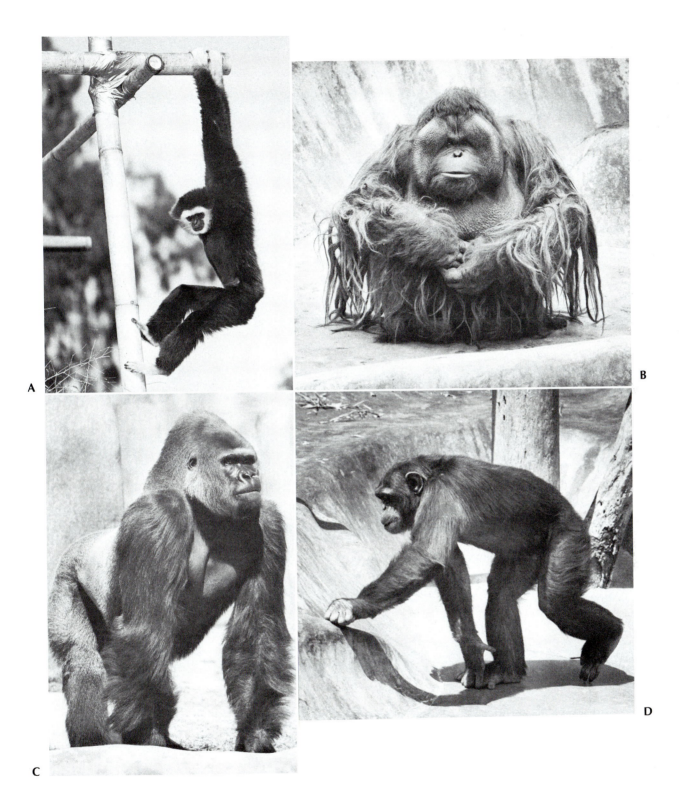

Figure 39-7

Anthropoid apes (pongids). **A,** White-handed gibbon *Hylobates lar* of rain forests, semideciduous forests, and montane forests of Southeast Asia. **B,** Bornean orangutan *Pongo pygmaeus* of the rain forests of Borneo. **C,** Lowland gorilla *Gorilla gorilla gorilla* of rain forests of equatorial Africa. **D,** Chimpanzee *Pan troglodytes* of western Africa.

Courtesy San Diego Zoo; A and D, photographs by Ron Garrison.

the genus *Drosophila!* The two kinds of polypeptide chains (alpha and beta) comprising the protein globin of the blood pigment hemoglobin are identical in primary structure in humans and chimpanzees. The gorilla's globin differs from ours by only a single amino acid in each chain. All three genera share biochemically identical molecules of cytochrome c, an enzyme of the electron transport chain. Even the genes of apes and humans are nearly alike. Humans and gibbons differ from each other in only 5.1% of the nucleotide sequences of DNA. Humans and chimpanzees are even more alike; they differ in only 2.5% of their genes. By comparison, sheep and cows differ in 11.2% of their genes, and rats and mice in 30%.

Yet chimpanzees are obviously very different biologically from people, and, given their genetic similarity, we would like to know the reason why. First, the 2.5% genetic difference adds up to a respectable 2500 gene pairs—certainly enough to account for the anatomical and mental differences between chimpanzees and humans. Second, by affecting the *expression* of other genes, even a single gene mutation can profoundly influence embryonic timing and development and lead to significant phenotypic change. It has been suggested that such **regulatory mutations** that alter timing and patterns of expression of several genes simultaneously—macromutations—were responsible for the rapid evolution of primates in general and the remarkable speciation of humans in particular.

First Hominids

At some point the hominids separated from the apes and underwent a radiation of their own. Giving up an arboreal life was a necessary prelude to their amazing evolution. The climatic changes during the Miocene and Pliocene epochs that greatly reduced the forests also provided an impetus to an existence on the open savannas. The upright carriage of the human body, of no advantage for tree dwelling, can be advantageous in open country. Because there are more dangerous predators on the ground than in trees, selection pressures would have fostered longer and stronger hindlegs for faster upright running. Standing upright offers other benefits. It provides a better view over tall grasses and bushes. It reduces the solar heat load at noon on the hot savanna and increases warming in the morning when the air is cool and the sun is low in the sky. Perhaps most important, it frees the hands for using tools, gathering food, and carrying babies.

Thus, during the Miocene and Pliocene epochs, emerging hominids slowly evolved toward an upright posture. This important transition was really an enormous leap because it required extensive redesigning of the skeleton and muscle attachments. Unfortunately we have only a glimpse of how it may have proceeded.

A late Miocene fossil fragment discovered in 1932 by G.E. Lewis, and long ignored by paleontologists, was *Ramapithecus brevirostris,* dated at about 12 to 14 million years BP (Fig. 39-6). Since *Ramapithecus* was found in the Siwalik Hills of India, Lewis named his discovery after the Hindu epic hero Rama. Interest in this form was rekindled when in 1961 the husband-and-wife team of Louis and Mary Leakey discovered more fragments of *Ramapithecus* in South Africa. Other discoveries followed, and by 1977 some two dozen separate jaw and tooth fossils of the baboon-sized *Ramapithecus* had been described. The dental arch is conspicuously hominid in form. The cheek teeth are larger and flatter and the front teeth smaller than those of apes, suggesting that *Ramapithecus* had to deal with tougher, less nutritious food such as roots, instead of the soft shoots and fruits

"Rapid" speciation, as in horses and primates, represents about one speciation event every 50 to 200 thousand years. The average speciation rate for most other vertebrates is closer to one event every 2 to 3 million years.

eaten by forest apes. This indicates that *Ramapithecus* lived at least part of the time on the ground in open woodlands, away from the dense, protective forests.

Ramapithecus, with its big molars bearing heavy enamel and its small canines, clearly foreshadows the hominid line. But is *Ramapithecus* the earliest known hominid? Until recently it was thought so, but Harvard paleontologist David Pilbeam disputes this. Other important fossil finds strengthen his position. In 1982 Pilbeam announced the discovery and painstaking reconstruction of a partial skull of *Sivapithecus*, an apelike hominoid that lived between 8 and 12 million years ago. Pilbeam believes that *Sivapithecus* is closely related to the orangutans and may be their ancestor. Because *Ramapithecus* closely resembles *Sivapithecus*, it can no longer be considered to be in the direct line leading to humans. With the ramapithecines, as the group may be called, now out of the running as human ancestors, no fossil has yet been discovered that can be considered the common ancestor of African apes and hominids.

___ Australopithecines—Near Humans

After the ramapithecines, there is an early Pliocene gap from 8 million to 4 million years BP, for which virtually no hominid fossils, other than a few tantalizing fragments, have been discovered. Yet the early Pliocene epoch was an eventful one in which the hominid line began to branch into different routes. One in particular gave rise to the first certain bipedal genus *Australopithecus*. The fossil skull of an immature anthropoid was discovered in 1924 at Tuang, South Africa, by Raymond Dart, an anatomy professor at Johannesburg University. He named his find

Figure 39-8

Skull and cranial endocast of the southern African hominid *Australopithecus africanus*.

From Dillon, L.S. 1978. Evolution, ed. 2. St. Louis, The C.V. Mosby Co.

Australopithecus (L., *auster,* south, + Gr., *pithecus,* ape) *africanus,* "the southern African ape," and he was certain from the beginning that it was in the direct lineage to humans. The skull was beautifully preserved but mostly enclosed in a rock-hard mixture of sand, soil, and pebbles (breccia). Dart picked away at his find for several months, at last fully revealing the gracile skull of a juvenile, aged 5 or 6 years, containing the endocast of a brain and a fully developed set of milk teeth (Fig. 39-8).

Dart's discovery of *A. africanus* opened a new era in the search for human ancestors. In 1938, another fossil turned up in South Africa. This was a stockier ape man and consequently was named *A. robustus.* Still, firm dating was lacking for either *A. africanus* or *A. robustus.*

The focus now shifts to Olduvai Gorge in Tanzania (Fig. 39-9) where, over four decades, Louis and Mary Leakey, later joined by their son Richard, recorded the geological, animal, and human history of the region. Olduvai is one of the most important sources on earth of information about human ancestors. The stratigraphy of Olduvai is clear, so that absolute dating is possible. There is an abundance of both animal fossils and primitive human tools.

Perhaps the most exciting find at Olduvai was Mary Leakey's discovery (1959) of a nearly intact skull, lacking the jaw, of *Australopithecus boisei.* It was originally described as *Zinjanthropus boisei,* the Olduvai Gorge man. This young male, even more solidly built than *A. robustus,* has been dated as 1.7 million years old, but more recent finds by Richard Leakey at Koobi Fora in Kenya (Figs. 39-9 and 39-10) have pushed the age of *A. boisei* back to nearly 3 million years BP.

The super-robust *A. bosei,* which is thought to have split off from *A. robustus,* inhabited eastern and southern Africa for perhaps a million years before becoming extinct in the mid-Pleistocene epoch, about 1 million years BP.

Although Africa seems to be the basic home of this group, similar fossils have been found as far away as Java. The volume of their brain casts varied from

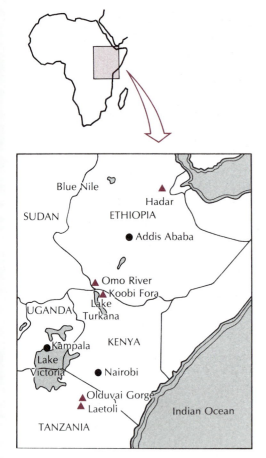

Figure 39-9

Some of the important fossil-bearing sites in eastern Africa.

Figure 39-10

Intact cranium of *Australopithecus boisei* discovered by Richard Leakey and his wife Meave at Koobi Fora (Lake Turkana) in 1969. Ten years earlier Mary Leakey had discovered the original cranium of this species, which became known as the Olduvai Gorge man.

Photograph by Peter Kain. © Richard Leakey.

about 450 to 600 cc and overlapped the range of the chimpanzee and gorilla. Certain bones, such as those in the pelvis, were hominid rather than pongid. The australopithecines walked in an erect or semierect position, as attested by the shape of the leg and foot bones. Their dentition was more human than apelike. They may be regarded as the earliest known type with distinctly humanlike characteristics.

Discovery of Lucy and the "First Family"

Hadar is a remote wasteland of rock, gravel, and sand in the center of the Afar Desert of Ethiopia (Fig. 39-9). The site is the bed of an ancient lake, long since disappeared, that is cut with gullies from infrequent but heavy rainfalls. At this site in 1974, Donald Johanson and expedition colleagues made the stunning discovery of the most complete, best-preserved skeleton of a hominid ever found (Fig. 39-11). Nicknamed Lucy, the skeleton was 40% complete. It was potassium-argon dated at 3.3 to 3.4 million years old but a recent (1983) redating indicated that it may be just 2.9 million years old. The shape of the pelvis indicated that Lucy was a female, and the leg bones showed that she walked upright (Fig. 39-12). The next year, Johanson discovered a concentration of several hundred bones that represented at least 13 and possibly more individuals. This find was named the First Family. The story of these extraordinarily important finds and the fierce rivalries that surround recent hominid discoveries is vividly recounted in Johanson's book *Lucy: the Beginnings of Humankind* (1981).

The new fossils, eventually named *Australopithecus afarensis* after the Afar region where they were found, represented a short but powerful, bipedal hominid with a head more ape shaped than human shaped (p. 969). The face resembled that of a chimpanzee, and the brain was chimpanzee sized (about 400 cc). There is no evidence that *A. afarensis* used stone tools.

Figure 39-11

Lucy *(Australopithecus afarensis)*, the most complete skeleton of an early hominid ever found, was discovered by Don Johanson in 1974 in Ethiopia. Lucy has recently been redated at 2.9 million years old.

Courtesy The Cleveland Museum of Natural History.

Figure 39-12

Lucy *(Australopithecus afarensis)* beside a modern human being *(Homo sapiens)*. Lucy was only 1.07 m (3½ feet) tall and probably weighed about 27 kg (60 pounds). She was about 25 years old when she died.

Figure 39-13

Donald C. Johanson *(left)* with colleague
Timothy White. Their announcement in
1979 of a new hominid species, *Australopithecus afarensis,* and the suggestion
that it is ancestral to all later hominids,
stimulated controversy among paleoan-
thropologists.

Courtesy The Cleveland Museum of Natural History.

Figure 39-14

Alternative phylogenies of the hominids.
Three schemes are shown, representing
some of the current hypotheses. Other
schemes have been proposed. The second
scheme shown is favored by D. Johanson,
discoverer of Lucy, and the scheme at top
is favored by R. Leakey.

More recent finds at Hadar, announced in 1982, have pushed the age of *A. afarensis* back to at least 4 million years BP. Perhaps the most significant aspect of the Hadar finds is that they prove that our ancestors began to walk upright before they developed large brains.

Where should *A. afarensis* be placed on the hominid family tree? Johanson and his colleague Timothy White (Fig. 39-13) are convinced that *A. afarensis* was ancestral to all other hominids (Fig. 39-14). Others disagree. Richard Leakey believes that the Hadar finds, as well as some hominid fossils discovered recently by Mary Leakey at Laetoli (and which Johanson includes in the *afarensis* taxon), represent two separate species, one larger than the other. The smaller, according to Leakey, is an unknown australopithecine, and the larger is an early *Homo*. Johanson, on the other hand, believes the large individuals to be males, and the smaller, females, of the same *afarensis* species. The Leakeys therefore see the *Homo* line as emerging 3, 4, or even 5 million years ago. At this writing, there are partisans for both sides of the debate, which is unlikely to be settled until more fossils are found.

Let us turn now to *Homo habilis*, the earliest hominid that has gained membership in the "true human" club.

EMERGENCE OF HOMO, THE TRUE HUMAN
Homo habilis—the "Handy Man"

In the early 1960s a series of hominid fossils, together with stone tools, was found at Olduvai close to the site where Mary Leakey had discovered *A. boisei*. The Leakeys, at Raymond Dart's suggestion, gave their find the binomen *Homo habilis,* meaning "handy man," because of their conviction that this hominid was the first user of primitive stone tools. Although the fossils were badly crushed, a laborious reconstruction of the pieces enabled the Leakeys to estimate that the cranial capacity was about 640 cc. This is minute by modern human standards (average 1350 cc), but it is significantly larger than the australopithecine range of 400 to 530 cc. There were many dissenters who argued that it was premature to award human status to these new finds, preferring instead to consider them australopithecines. However, in 1972 Richard Leakey (Fig. 39-15) discovered a virtually complete skull at Lake Turkana so clearly *Homo* that, in time, all but the most stubborn critics were silenced.

Leakey's dramatic find, known simply by its registration number as skull 1470—"1470 man"—is at least 1.6 million years old (Fig. 39-16). Skull 1470 had a firmly established cranial capacity of 775 cc and resembled the skull of *Homo erectus* (see the following discussion) in several significant ways, yet was clearly distinct from the latter. *Homo habilis* is now fully accepted as a valid taxon. Of the many fossils now assigned to *Homo habilis*, the oldest are dated at 1.76 million years. The discovery and acceptance of *Homo habilis* proved that it was a contemporary of *Australopithecus;* that is, the two species coexisted as the Leakeys had claimed for some time. The Leakeys contended that *Homo* and *Australopithecus* broke off from a common ancestral line some 4 million years ago BP. *Homo* coexisted with *Australopithecus* for 3 million years, but unlike the latter, which was probably a vegetarian, *Homo* used tools made from stones and bones to kill animals for food. *Homo* was, of course, fully erect and bipedal.

Figure 39-15

Richard Leakey, son of Louis and Mary Leakey, and discoverer of the famous 1470 skull.

Photograph by Peter Kain. © Richard Leakey.

Figure 39-16

Skull 1470 *(Homo habilis)* was discovered by a member of Richard Leakey's team at Koobi Fora in 1972. It was originally dated at close to 3 million years BP but has since been dated more firmly at 1.6 to 1.8 million years BP.

Photograph by Peter Kain. © Richard Leakey.

Figure 39-17

Peking man *(Homo erectus)*. Pictured is a cast of the best preserved of 14 skulls discovered at a site near Peking, China.

From Dillon, L.S. 1978. Evolution, ed. 2. St. Louis, The C.V. Mosby Co.

Homo erectus—Pleistocene Hominids

Unlike *Homo habilis,* whose qualifications for full membership in the "true human" club are in dispute, *Homo erectus* was uncontestably a true human. The story of the discovery and eventual respectability of *Homo erectus* begins with Dutch anatomist Eugene Dubois's famous fossil find in eastern Java in 1891. Dubois named his find *Pithecanthropus erectus* ("erect ape man"). Dubois's ape man, consisting of only a skull cap and thigh bone, was so much older than anything else humanlike discovered up to that time that no one knew how to interpret it. Dubois himself vacillated over its relationship to apes and hominids, and finally, piqued by publicized suspicion of their authenticity, he secreted his specimens under the floorboards of his dining room and for 30 years refused to let anyone see them.

In 1927 Davidson Black, a Canadian anatomist teaching in a Peking university, announced the discovery near Peking of a skull that closely resembled the Java man (Fig. 39-17). Continued excavation at the site after Black's death in 1933 eventually revealed 14 skulls, some in excellent state of preservation, together with several lower jaws and other skeletal parts. Several crudely worked tools were also found and, most important, ash heaps indicating the use of fire. Black's Peking man and Dubois's Java man are now recognized as separate races of the same species *Homo erectus* ("erect-walking man").

Homo erectus was a large hominid standing 150 to 170 cm (5 to 5.5 feet) tall. It had a low but distinct forehead, strong browridges, and no chin (Fig. 39-18). Both jaws were fairly massive and bore large teeth. The cranial capacity averaged about 1000 cc. The pelvic and leg bones indicate that *Homo erectus* had long, straight legs and was an excellent walker.

How old is *Homo erectus?* A 1976 discovery by Richard Leakey of a complete *Homo erectus* skull has been reliably dated at 1.5 million years BP. This is much older than either the Java or Peking hominids are thought to be (about 0.5 to 0.7 million years BP, although neither has been accurately dated). *Homo erectus* lived until about 300,000 years ago, thus spanning a period of about 1.2 million years.

Homo erectus occupied much of the Old World, as indicated by fossil finds in eastern and northern Africa and in Europe, as well as China and Java. *Homo erectus* successfully hunted large animals, butchered them using stone and bone tools, and cooked them at campsites, often in cave chambers. Fire was probably also used for warmth. The site near Peking, China, has yielded the remains of some 60 species of animals used by *Homo erectus* as food: small rodents, bats, bears, horses, deer, and even rhinoceroses and elephants. However, *Homo erectus,* who was really a vegetarian turned meat-eater, also ate many vegetable foods. Some authorities believe that as much as 75% of the diet was vegetarian.

Homo erectus was a social species, living in tribes of 20 to 50 people. The tribes interbred and migrated across the tropical Old World and even into temperate regions where they survived severe winters by wrapping themselves in animal skins and using fire for warmth. They often used caves for shelter, but there are clear indications that they also built crude wooden shelters. Their brain size and brain configuration suggest that they communicated by speech. All in all, *Homo erectus* had a complex culture. At the time of their disappearance about 300,000 years BP, they had become dependent on cooperative social behavior.

Figure 39-18

Artist's conception of the Java man, depicting *Homo erectus* as somewhat more brutish than he probably was.

Courtesy of the artist, Zdeněk Burian. From Dillon, L.S. 1978. Evolution, ed. 2. St. Louis, The C.V. Mosby Co.

___ Homo sapiens—Modern Hominids
Swanscombe and Steinhelm skulls

Between *Homo erectus* and the establishment of the modern polytypic species of *Homo sapiens* ("wise man"), hominid evolution has threaded a complex course. The earliest fossils showing clear-cut *Homo sapiens* features are the Swanscombe hominid from southeastern England and the Steinhelm hominid from near Stuttgart, West Germany. These skulls are 250,000 to 350,000 years old. They had prominent browridges and a brain capacity of 1200 cc (Steinhelm) to 1300 cc (Swanscombe), which places them well within the range of variation of modern humans (1000 to 2000 cc). These skulls are of particular interest because they are intermediate in position between *Homo erectus* and modern *Homo sapiens*. Compared with *Homo erectus*, they have larger brains; decreased face, jaw, and tooth sizes; smaller browridges; and thinner skulls. Indeed, the major evolutionary changes from *Homo erectus* on are confined to the head. *Homo sapiens* was becoming more intelligent, as manifested not only by increasing brain volume but by increasing complexity of social culture, communication, and environmental manipulation.

Neanderthals

The matching of stone tools with fossil evidence shows that a large number of human subcultures developed during the Pleistocene epoch. These became increasingly varied and tangled as the Neanderthals, modern humans' immediate predecessors, emerged about 130,000 years ago. The first Neanderthal find to be described came from a cave in the Neander Valley (Neander Thal in Old German) near Düsseldorf, West Germany, in 1856. New discoveries have been made repeatedly since then, and the Neanderthals are perhaps the best-documented fossil humans. These European fossil finds have been associated with a rich array of tools belonging to a Paleolithic (Mousterian) culture. It is characterized by a particular pattern of flaking in a wide variety of blades, borers, spear points, axes, scrapers, and numerous specialized tools. The Neanderthals used such tools for hunting, killing and butchering, food processing, hide preparation, woodworking, and tool making. Their populations dominated the Old World from Europe to Africa and Asia in late Pleistocene times. The species was not a homogeneous one, but varied from place to place in response to local conditions and the isolation of populations from one another.

The "classical" Neanderthals, who ranged widely in Europe and North Africa, had a large skull, comparable to that of modern Europeans, but the brain was probably less convoluted. The face was relatively massive with forward projecting jaws, heavy browridges, and weakly formed chin (Fig. 39-19). However, in the Middle East the so-called "progressive" Neanderthals were becoming more like modern humans. These modern traits—less massive browridges and a more rounded skull in the back—were first revealed in the Mount Carmel "man" (probably a woman) discovered in Israel in 1931. Then in 1957 several superb skulls, even complete skeletons, were dug out of a cave at Shanidar in northern Iraq (Fig. 39-20). These and other discoveries indicate that the Neanderthals were extremely varied. This resulted from portions of the total gene pool becoming isolated for thousands of years at a time in different areas of the Old World. As a whole, however, the gene pool was slowly drifting toward modern humans.

Figure 39-19

European Neanderthal skull. This "classic" form is the La Ferrassie skull from a site near Burgue, France.
Courtesy Musée de l'Homme; from Dillon, L.S. 1978. Evolution, ed. 2. St. Louis, The C.V. Mosby Co.

Cro-Magnons

During the last interglacial period about 30,000 to 40,000 years ago, the Cro-Magnon race emerged rather suddenly from an unknown source (Fig. 39-21). They may have been descendants of early, generalized Neanderthals of Asia and perhaps were responsible for the eventual extermination of the Neanderthals. Like the Neanderthals, the Cro-Magnons were not homogeneous but rather a mixture of people who showed considerable physical variations in different localities. They had a far superior culture (Perigordian) and left artistic paintings and carvings in their caves. They are considered ancestors of modern humans and represent the modern type of human. They were about 183 cm (6 feet) tall and had a high forehead but no supraorbital ridges, a rather prominent chin, and a brain capacity as large as (or larger than) that of present-day humans. Their physical characteristics are matched today by the Basques in northern Spain and certain Swedes in southern Sweden. Attempts to discern the characteristics of present-day races in early populations of *Homo sapiens* have been unsuccessful. It is not known whether they were white, black, or brown.

The evolutionary course of modern humans in the last 30,000 to 40,000 years has exhibited the same pattern of divergence and extinction demonstrated by our forebears and other organisms. The essential characteristics of human phylogeny, such as a superior brain and wide adaptability, can all be attributed to the strictly quantitative effects of mutations that could have happened at any evolutionary level. In other words, we are the outcome of the basic forces of evolution that have directed the evolution of every organism from the time life first originated. Mutation, isolation, population factors, genetic drift, and natural selection—all general processes of evolutionary progress—have operated in the same way for us as for other animals. Human evolution, however, has been exceptionally rapid.

A

B

Figure 39-20

Shanidar I skull. **A,** The skull still partly enclosed in the rocky matrix in which it was found in the Shanidar cave in northern Iraq. **B,** The skull after restoration. This well-preserved specimen, about 46,000 years old, is from a Neanderthal man, who died at about 40 years of age.
Courtesy R.S. Solecki, Columbia University.

Figure 39-21

Restoration of prehistoric hominids. A Cro-Magnon *(right)* is compared with a Neanderthal *(center)* and a Java man *(left)*.
Courtesy J.M. McGregor.

___OUR UNIQUE POSITION

We are animals and the products of evolution. However, we have what no other animal has: a nongenetic, cultural evolution that involves a constant feedback between past and future experience. Although human evolution has become increasingly cultural as opposed to genetic, we are still subjected to the same biological forces and principles that affect the lives and evolution of other animals. All animals are adapted to their environment, but through culture, we have found ways to surround ourselves with an environment of our own making.

We are a definite species. Our population is commonly divided into races or populations that are genetically distinguished from others. A so-called race has certain genes or gene combinations that may be more or less unique, although races grade into each other and do not have definite boundaries. Pure races are nonexistent, and there is no fixed number of races. Races are adaptations to local conditions. It is believed that, as primitive peoples spread over geographical areas, they became adapted to certain regions, and natural selection stamped on them certain distinguishing features. Races at present are losing their biological significance because human adaptation to environment is becoming largely cultural. Rapid mobility and communication have shrunk the size of our planet so that isolation of races seldom exists. Genes can shift through human populations now with amazing speed, and racial intermixtures are far more common than formerly. Since all races have more or less unique potentialities, hybrid vigor could operate within racial interbreeding just as it does for other animals.

We are the only animal that knows how to make and use tools effectively. Perhaps this capability more than any other has been responsible for our dominant position in the animal kingdom. We are able to expend enormous energy in manipulating the environment to suit ourselves, often resulting in destructive consequences to other living forms and not infrequently to ourselves.

Another unique characteristic is our capacity for conceptual thought. We have a symbolic language of wide and specific expression. With words we can carve concepts out of experience. This has resulted in cumulative experience that can be transmitted from one generation to another. In other animals, transmission never spans more than one generation. We owe much to our arboreal ancestry. This promoted binocular vision, a fine visuotactile discrimination, and manipulative skills in the use of our hands. If a horse (with one toe instead of five fingers) had human intellect and culture, could it accomplish what humans have?

____ Summary

The publication of Charles Darwin's book *The Origin of Species* in 1859 precipitated an intellectual revolution in people's views of human origins. At the time that Darwin's views were first debated, few prehuman fossils had been unearthed, but the current accumulation of fossil evidence has strongly vindicated Darwin's belief that humans descended from primate ancestors.

Humans are primates, a generalized group having an arboreal ancestry and characterized by having grasping fingers and forward-facing eyes capable of stereoscopic vision. Modern primates are divided into the prosimians (lemurs, lorises, bush babies, and tarsiers) and the anthropoids (monkeys, apes, and hominids). The anthropoids are active during the day and have color vision. The ancestors of New World monkeys, which are distinguished by having prehensile tails and divergent nostrils, separated at least 40 million years ago from the ancestors of Old World monkeys, which lack prehensile tails and have close-set nostrils.

At the beginning of the Miocene epoch (about 25 million years BP), the dryopithecines emerged, a hominoid group that moved on all four legs and were fruit-eaters. These were the ancestors of the pongids (great apes) and hominids. About 14 million years BP, a group of hominoids, collectively called ramapithecines, appeared, moved from forests to open woodlands, and may have ventured onto the savanna.

Following a gap in the fossil record from 8 to 4 million years ago, the bipedal genus *Australopithecus* emerged in Africa. The earliest australopithecine, *A. afarensis*, with a brain capacity of 400 cc, lived from 4 to 2.9 million years BP. It was probably ancestral to all later hominids. About 2 million years ago two australopithecines *(A. africanus* and *A. robustus)* coexisted with a more delicate but larger-brained (about 700 cc capacity) hominid, *Homo habilis*. *Homo habilis* was the first user of stone tools. *Homo erectus* appeared 1½ million years ago, probably a descendant of *Homo habilis*. *Homo erectus* was a proficient hunter and had a brain capacity averaging 1000 cc.

The fully modern human with a 1300 cc brain capacity developed gradually. The Neanderthals, who lived from about 130,000 to 100,000 years ago, were proficient tool-users and built shelters for themselves. Cro-Magnons, regarded as modern humans, appeared about 40,000 years ago. Implement crafting improved rapidly, and human culture became enriched by esthetics, artistry, and sophisticated language.

Selected references

Brace, C.L., and J. Metress (eds.). 1973. Man in evolutionary perspective. New York, John Wiley & Sons, Inc. *Readings in physical anthropology with excellent explanatory introductions to each selection.*

Buttner-Janusch, J. 1973. Physical anthropology: a perspective. New York, John Wiley & Sons, Inc. *Lucid presentation of human evolution.*

Cronin, J.E., N.T. Boaz, C.B. Stringer, and Y. Rak. 1981. Tempo and mode in hominid evolution. Nature **292**:113-122. *The authors examine hominid evolution as a model of punctuated equilibrium and conclude that human evolution has been gradual instead.*

Darwin, C. 1871. Descent of man. London, J. Murray. *Darwin's essay on human evolution deals largely with sexual selection.*

Day, M.H. 1977. Guide to fossil man: a handbook of human palaeontology, ed. 3. Chicago, The University of Chicago Press. *A useful catalog of descriptions and photographs of fossil hominids, although lacking important recent finds.*

Edey, M.A. 1972. The emergence of man: the missing link. New York, Time-Life Books. *Survey of the australopithecines.*

Eimerl, S., I. DeVore, and editors of Time-Life Books. 1974. The primates. Life Nature Library. New York, Time-Life Books. *Superbly illustrated natural history of our nearest relatives.*

Howells, W.W. 1973. Evolution of the genus *Homo.* Reading, Mass., Addison-Wesley Publishing Co.

Johanson, D.C., and M.A. Edey. 1981. Lucy: the beginnings of humankind. New York, Simon & Schuster. *Informative, lucid, often spicy account of the Hadar, Ethiopia, discoveries, and the personalities of the scientists involved.*

Jolly, C.J. (ed.). 1978. Early hominids of Africa. New York, St. Martin's Press. *Contributed chapters, advanced.*

Klein, R.G. 1977. The ecology of early man in southern Africa. Science **197**:115-126. *Traces human ecology through 3 million years.*

Leakey, R.E. 1981. The making of mankind. New York, E.P. Dutton. *Beautifully illustrated and clearly written nonpolemical review of paleoanthropology and human and primate prehistory, leading up to the present. Well presented and highly recommended.*

Leakey, R.E., and R. Lewin. 1977. Origins. New York, E.P. Dutton. *Clear discussion of the fossil record and human cultural history and behavior. Enjoyable reading; aimed at the popular audience but scientifically accurate.*

Leakey, R.E., and R. Lewin. 1979. The people of the lake: man, his origins, nature and future. New York, Doubleday. *Readable essay on human origins and the narrow borderline between apes and humans.*

Lovejoy, C.O. 1981. The origin of man. Science **211**:341-350. *An argument that bipedality originated because it enhanced reproductive fitness in evolving hominids.*

Solecki, R.S. 1972. Shanidar: the first flower people. New York, Alfred A. Knopf, Inc. *Describes the exciting discovery and excavation of the Iraq Neanderthals.*

Stebbins, G.L. 1982. Darwin to DNA, molecules to humanity. San Francisco, W.H. Freeman & Co. Publishers. *Written for the nonspecialist, the closing chapters deal in an interesting way with human biological and cultural evolution.*

Szalay, F.S., and E. Delson. 1979. Evolutionary history of the primates. New York, Academic Press, Inc. *Thorough and encyclopedic review of fossil primates.*

Tuller, R.M. 1977. The human species: its nature, evolution, and ecology. New York, McGraw-Hill Book Co. *Clearly presented, well-illustrated treatment.*

Wood, B.A. 1978. Human evolution: outline studies in biology, London, Chapman & Hall. *Useful condensed interpretation of hominid fossil finds up to 1977.*

Yunis, J.J., and O. Prakash. 1982. The origin of man: a chromosomal pictorial legacy. Science **215**:1525-1530. *A high-resolution chromosomal technique reveals that 18 of 23 pairs of human chromosomes are virtually identical to those of the orangutan, gorilla, and chimpanzee.*

Selected *Scientific American* articles

Hay, R.L., and M.D. Leakey. 1982. The fossil footprints of Laetoli. **246**:50-57 (Feb.). *Remarkable footprints of a bipedal hominid discovered in Tanzania are some 3.5 million years old.*

Holloway, R.L. 1974. The casts of fossil hominid brains. **231**:106-115 (July). *Molds made from fossil hominid skulls indicate the human brain began enlargement some 3 million years ago.*

Howells, W.W. 1966. Homo erectus. **215**:46-53 (Nov.).

Issac, G. 1978. The food-sharing behavior of protohuman hominids. **238**:90-108 (Apr.).

MacNeish, R.S. 1971. Early man in the Andes. **224**:36-46 (Apr.). *Humans have lived in Peru for at least 22,000 years.*

Rukang, W., and L. Shenglong. 1983. Peking man. **248**:86-94 (June).

Simons, E.L. 1964. The early relatives of man. **211**:50-62 (July).

Simons, E.L. 1967. The earliest apes. **217**:28-35 (Dec.).

Simons, E.L. 1977. Ramapithecus. **236**:28-35 (May).

Smith, P.E.L. 1976. Stone-age man on the Nile. **235**:30-38 (Aug.). *Hunters and gatherers lived along the Nile for thousands of years before the Pharaohs.*

Trinkaus, E., and W.W. Howells. 1979. The Neanderthals. **241**:118-133 (Dec.).

Walker, A., and R.E.F. Leakey. 1978. The hominids of East Turkana. **239**:54-66 (Aug.).

Washburn, S.L. 1978. The evolution of man. **239**:194-208 (Sept.). *A personal evaluation of human evolution based on recent fossil finds.*

PART FIVE

Reindeer drive in Lapland.

THE ANIMAL AND
ITS ENVIRONMENT

Photograph by C.P. Hickman, Jr.

Life was created and shaped by environmental forces. No organism is for an instant free from the requirements of the surroundings in which it lives. The environment therefore is the totality of all extrinsic factors, both physical and biotic, that in any way affect the life and behavior of an organism.

In the following chapters we deal with the relationships of animals to the world around them and with the special human impact on the creatures that share the biosphere with us.

Chapter 40

THE BIOSPHERE AND ANIMAL
DISTRIBUTION

Chapter 41

ANIMAL ECOLOGY

Chapter 42

ANIMALS IN THE HUMAN
ENVIRONMENT

CHAPTER 40

THE BIOSPHERE AND ANIMAL DISTRIBUTION

Canada geese *Branta canadensis* lift off from a marsh within the grasslands biome, one of the principal biomes within the biosphere.

Photograph by L.L. Rue, III.

BIOSPHERE

All life is confined to a thin veneer of the earth called the **biosphere.** From the first remarkable photographs of earth taken from the Apollo spacecraft, revealing a beautiful blue and white globe lying against the limitless backdrop of space, viewers were struck and perhaps humbled by our isolation and insignificance in the enormity of the universe. The phrase "spaceship earth" became a part of the vocabulary, and the realization evolved that all the resources we will ever have for sustaining life are restricted to a thin layer of land and sea and a narrow veil of atmosphere above it. We could better appreciate just how thin the biosphere is if we could shrink the earth and all of its dimensions to a 1 m sphere. We would no longer perceive vertical dimensions on the earth's surface. The highest mountains would fail to penetrate a thin coat of paint applied to our shrunken earth; a fingernail's scratch on the surface would exceed the depth of the ocean's deepest trenches.

Fitness of the Earth's Environment

Astronomers have estimated conservatively that in the vastness of the universe there are millions of stars, similar to our sun, that have planetary systems. The astronomer Harlow Shapley believes that in our galaxy alone there are *at least* 100,000 planets having conditions suitable for life. If he is correct, we can no longer maintain that only the earth harbors life. Nevertheless, there are so many requirements for life that only a small number of planets can fulfill the special conditions that would permit evolution of life at all similar to that on earth.

First, a planet suitable for life must receive a steady supply of light and heat from its sun for many billions of years. This means that its orbit must be nearly circular.

Second, water must be present on the planet to permit the evolution of complex biochemical systems based on carbon. Earth is indeed a watery planet, with water covering 71% of its surface. Viewed from space, water, not land, is earth's most conspicuous surface feature.

Third, the temperature must be suitable, meaning practically within the range of −50° to +100° C, as it is over most of the earth's surface. Life at temperatures above 100° C is impossible because biopolymers based on carbon and water would be rapidly hydrolyzed. Temperatures much below the freezing point of water prevent growth of organisms by slowing chemical processes.

Fourth, all life requires a suitable array of major and minor elements. Oxygen, carbon, hydrogen, and nitrogen form 95% of living matter and thus dominate the composition of life on earth. These four are supported by seven other major elements (phosphorus, calcium, potassium, sulfur, sodium, chlorine, and magnesium) and a large number of minor or "trace" elements. Perhaps 46 elements in all are found in living matter; many are essential for life, whereas others are present only because they exist in the environment with which the organism interacts. Not all planets possess elements in the same proportions, even in our solar system.

There are many other properties of earth that make it an especially fit environment for life. It is large enough to have a surface density that permits molecules to collect and align properly. Matter in cells is in a colloidal state, an intermediate between conditions too solid to allow change and conditions too fluid or gaseous to permit molecular organization. The earth's gravity is strong enough to hold an extensive gaseous atmosphere but not so strong that more than a trace of free hydrogen remains. Another consideration, especially important for life on earth today, is the oxygen-ozone atmospheric screen that absorbs lethal ultraviolet radiation from the sun. So effective is this absorption that rays with wavelengths shorter than 283 nm (nanometer = 10^{-12} m) fail to reach the earth's surface.

In his classic book *The Fitness of the Environment,* published in 1913, the biochemist L.J. Henderson maintained that earth possesses "the best of all possible environments for life." We may agree; however, we realize that the surface of any body that is the size and age of earth in a similar orbit revolving about a similar sun and having a similar elemental composition should also have an excellent environment for life.

The organism and its environment share a reciprocal relationship. The environment is fit for the organism, and the organism is fitted to the environment and adapts to its changes. As an open system, an animal is forever receiving and giving off materials and energy. The building materials for life are obtained from the physical environment, either directly by producers such as green plants or indirectly by consumers that return inorganic substances to the environment by excretion or by the decay and disintegration of their bodies.

The living form is a transient link that is built up out of environmental materials, which are then returned to the environment to be used again in the re-creation of new life. Life, death, decay, and re-creation have been the cycle of existence since life began.

In this continuous interchange between organism and environment, both are altered in the process, and a favorable relationship is preserved. The environment of earth, with its living and nonliving components, is not a static entity but has undergone an evolution in every way as dramatic as the evolution of the animal kingdom. It is still changing today, more rapidly than ever before, under the heavy-handed influence of humans.

The primitive earth of 3.5 billion years ago, barren, stormy, and volcanic with a reducing atmosphere of ammonia, methane, and water, was wonderfully fit for the prebiotic syntheses that led to life's beginnings. Yet, it was totally unsuited, indeed lethal, for the kinds of living organisms that inhabit the earth today, just as early forms of life could not survive in our present environment. The appearance of free oxygen in the atmosphere, produced largely if not almost entirely by life, is an example of the reciprocity between organism and environment. Although oxygen was at first poisonous to early forms of life, its gradual accumulation over the ages from photosynthesis forced protective biochemical alterations to appear that led eventually to complete dependence on oxygen for life.

Earth's biosphere and the organisms in it have evolved together. Again, as living organisms adapt and evolve, they act on and produce changes in their environment; in so doing they must themselves change.

DISTRIBUTION OF LIFE ON EARTH
Ecosphere and Its Subdivisions

The **ecosphere** includes all life on earth and the physical environments in which it lives and with which it interacts. It is the largest biological system we can recognize. It includes the biosphere, which, as we have already seen, is the blanket of life surrounding the earth. The biosphere is supported by three more subdivisions of the ecosphere: lithosphere, hydrosphere, and atmosphere.

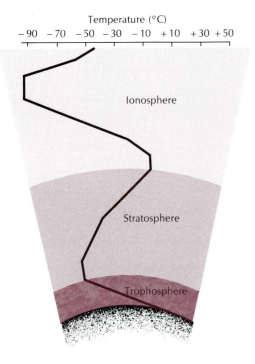

Temperature (°C)

−90 −70 −50 −30 −10 +10 +30 +50

Ionosphere

Stratosphere

Trophosphere

Figure 40-1

Earth's atmosphere, showing three major subdivisions and temperature profile.

The **lithosphere** is the rocky material of the earth's outer shell. It is the substrate of life and the ultimate source of all mineral elements required by living organisms. Life does not extend very far into the lithosphere; soil animals seldom extend beyond a depth of 5 m, although termite burrows have been found as deep as 50 m in the forests of Madagascar. Caves are natural underground extensions of the earth's surface and often support a remarkably varied animal life.

The **hydrosphere** is the body of water on or near the earth's surface. Most of this water is in the oceans, but water also extends into the lithosphere and the atmosphere.

Water is distributed over the earth by a global hydrological cycle that consists of three principal phases: evaporation, precipitation, and runoff. Evaporation occurs from oceans, from land, and from other water surfaces. Some five sixths of the evaporation is from the ocean; the quantity of water that evaporates from its surface is equivalent to a depth of about 1 m annually. One important aspect of the global water balance is that more water is evaporated from the ocean than is returned to it by precipitation. Ocean evaporation therefore provides much of the rainfall that supports land ecosystems.

On land, more water is received via precipitation than is lost by evaporation from the surface and by plant transpiration. The excess is intercepted by living organisms, especially plants, runs off the land surface into streams, or filters into the ground-water system (aquifers).

Runoff from land produces erosion and wears away the surfaces of continents. This leveling process, however, is offset by geological uplift, thus bringing marine sediments above sea level. Living things also carry water through their bodies in addition to what they need themselves and in doing so speed up the return of water to the atmosphere. The metabolism of organisms thus accelerates the cycle of water and may profoundly influence weather conditions, not only locally, but also over extensive areas, such as the vegetation of jungles. For example, South America, with its enormous tropical rain forests, receives twice as much precipitation per unit of area as do other continents, and evaporation and runoff are correspondingly high.

The **atmosphere** is commonly subdivided into three great strata: **troposphere**, **stratosphere**, and **ionosphere** (Fig. 40-1). The troposphere, the layer nearest the earth, extends upward to about 8 km above the poles and 15 km above the equator. All life is confined to this layer, as are haze, dust, clouds, and air currents. Air masses warmed in the tropics rise, those cooled at the poles sink, and all are shifted laterally by the rotation of the earth. These effects produce enormous weather systems that profoundly influence life on the earth's surface.

Above the troposphere is the stratosphere, which extends to about 50 km above the earth's surface. In the lower stratosphere is the oxygen-ozone atmospheric screen layer mentioned previously; it is concentrated mostly between 20 and 25 km. Above the stratosphere is the ionosphere, the outer reaches of which extend some 3500 km from the earth. Air particles in this extremely rarified atmosphere are largely ionized by solar radiation. Temperatures are cold (to −90° C) in the lower ionosphere but rise with increasing altitude and may reach 1650° C in the upper region during periods of high solar activity.

The gases present in the lower atmosphere (troposphere) are (by volume) nitrogen, 78%; oxygen, 21%; argon, 0.93%; carbon dioxide, 0.03%; variable amounts of water vapor; and trace amounts of neon, helium, methane, krypton, ozone, and xenon.

Figure 40-2

"Greenhouse effect." Carbon dioxide and water vapor in the atmosphere are transparent to sunlight but absorb heat energy reradiated from the earth, leading to warming of atmospheric air.

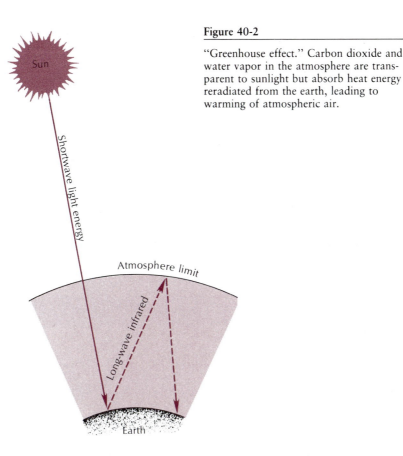

Atmospheric oxygen has originated almost entirely from plant photosynthesis. As discussed in Chapter 3, the primitive earth contained a reducing atmosphere devoid of oxygen. When oxygen-evolving photosynthesis appeared about 3 billion years ago, oxygen gradually began to accumulate in the atmosphere. It is believed that by the mid-Paleozoic era, some 400 million years BP, the oxygen concentration had reached its present level of about 21%. Since then oxygen consumption by animals and plants has approximately equaled oxygen production. The present surplus of free oxygen in the atmosphere resulted from the fossilization of plants before they could decay or be consumed by animals. As these vast stores of fossil fuels are burned by our industrialized civilization, the oxygen surplus that accumulated over the ages could conceivably be depleted. Fortunately, this is unlikely for two reasons: (1) most of the total fossilized carbon is deposited in noncombustible shales and rocks, and (2) the oxygen reserves in the atmosphere and in the oceans are so enormous that the supply could last thousands of years, even if all photosynthetic replenishment suddenly were to cease.

There is concern, however, that the rapid input of carbon dioxide into the atmosphere from the burning of fossil fuels may significantly affect the earth's heat budget. Much of the sun's short-wave light energy absorbed by the earth's surface is reradiated as longer-wave infrared heat energy (Fig. 40-2). Materials in the atmosphere, especially carbon dioxide and water vapor, impede this heat loss and allow the atmosphere to warm up. The accumulation of carbon dioxide could lead to an increase in the temperature of the biosphere as a whole. This is called the "greenhouse effect," since the atmosphere acts to trap reradiated heat from the earth in much the same way the glass of a greenhouse traps the heat absorbed by the plants and soil inside.

The concern over the long-range effects of increasing atmospheric carbon dioxide, primarily from burning of fossil fuel, stems not from mere conjecture. Atmospheric carbon dioxide increased from about 280 parts per million (ppm) before the Industrial Revolution to an average 335 ppm today and is increasing at a rate of 1.3 ppm per year. It is expected to exceed 600 ppm in the next century. In the past century the global temperature has increased 0.4° C, and it will have increased 3° C when the carbon dioxide has doubled in the next century, a warming of unprecedented magnitude. This is expected to shift climatic zones profoundly, creating drought conditions in the American wheatlands and wetter conditions along the coasts. Melting of the earth's ice sheets is another possibility, with flooding of coastal lowlands throughout the world. Whatever the outcome, a fascinating, unplanned global experiment is under way.

Figure 40-3

Some of the major biomes of North America.

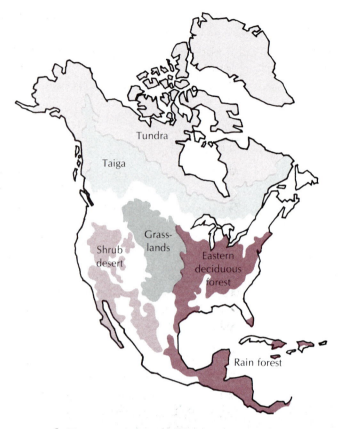

___ Terrestrial Environment: Biomes

A biome is a major biotic unit bearing a characteristic and easily recognized array of plant life. Botanists long ago recognized that the terrestrial environment of the earth could be divided into large units having a distinctive vegetation: forests, prairies, deserts, and so on. Animal distribution has always been more difficult to map, even after naturalists had accumulated the basic information about animal ranges and centers of distribution from around the world. Plant and animal distributions do not coincide. Eventually zoogeographers accepted plant distribution as the basic biotic units and recognized the biomes as distinctive combinations of plants and animals. A biome is therefore identified by its dominant plant formation (Fig. 40-3), but, since animals depend on plants, each biome supports a characteristic fauna.

Each biome is distinctive, but its borders are not. Anyone who has traveled across the United States knows that plant communities grade into one another over broad areas. The moist deciduous forests of the Appalachians give way gradually to the drier oak forests of the upper Mississippi states, and then to oak woodlands with grassy understory. This yields to tall and mixed prairie (now corn and wheatlands), then to desert grasslands, and finally to desert shrublands. The indistinct boundaries where the dominant plants of adjacent biomes are mixed together form an almost continuous gradient called an **ecocline.** The main factors determining an ecocline are temperature and precipitation.

From what we have said, it is obvious that biomes are mainly a convenient way to organize our concepts about different life communities. Nevertheless, anyone can distinguish a grassland, deciduous forest, coniferous forest, or shrub desert by the dominant plants in each. And we can make reasonable assumptions about the kinds of animals that live in each biome.

The principal terrestrial biomes are temperate deciduous forest, temperate coniferous forest, tropical forest, grassland, tundra, and desert. In this brief survey, we will refer especially to the biomes of North America and will consider predominant features of each.

Temperate deciduous forest

The temperate deciduous forest, best developed in eastern North America, encompasses several forest types that change gradually from the northeast to the south. Deciduous, broad-leaved trees such as oak, maple, and beech that shed their leaves in winter predominate. Seasonal aspects are better defined in this biome than in any other. The deciduous habit is an adaptation of dormancy for low energy levels from the sun in winter and freezing winter temperatures. In summer, the relatively dense forests form a closed canopy that creates deep shade below. Consequently there has been a selection for understory plants that grow rapidly in the spring and flower early before the canopy develops. The mean annual precipitation is relatively high (75 to 125 cm, or 30 to 50 inches) and rain falls periodically throughout the year.

The heavy exploitation of the deciduous forests of North America began in the seventeenth century and reached a peak in the nineteenth century. Logging removed nearly all of the once-magnificent stands of temperate hardwoods. With the opening of the prairie for agriculture, many eastern farms were abandoned and allowed to return gradually to deciduous forests.

Animal communities in deciduous forests respond to seasonal change in various ways. Some, such as the insect-eating warblers, migrate. Others, such as the woodchuck, hibernate away the winter months. Others that are unable to escape survive by using the available food (for example, deer) or stored food supplies (for example, squirrels). Hunting and habitat loss have eliminated virtually all the large carnivores that once roamed the eastern forests, such as mountain lions, bobcats, and wolves. Deer, on the other hand, thrive in the second-growth eastern forests under the protection of strict hunting management. Insect and invertebrate communities are abundant in deciduous forests because decaying logs and forest floor litter provide excellent shelter.

Coniferous forest

In North America the coniferous forests form a broad, continuous, continent-wide belt stretching across Canada and Alaska, and south through the Rocky Mountains into Mexico. It is dominated by evergreens—pine, fir, spruce, and cedar—which are adapted to withstand freezing and take full advantage of short summer growing seasons. The conical trees with their flexible branches shed snow loads easily. The northern area is the **boreal** (northern) **forest,** often referred to as **taiga** (a Russian word, pronounced "tie-ga"). The taiga is dominated by white and black spruce, balsam, subalpine fir, larch, and birch. In the central region of North America, the taiga merges into **lake forest,** dominated by white pine, red pine, and eastern hemlock. However, most of this forest was destroyed by logging and is replaced by shrubby wasteland that characterizes much of Michigan, Wisconsin,

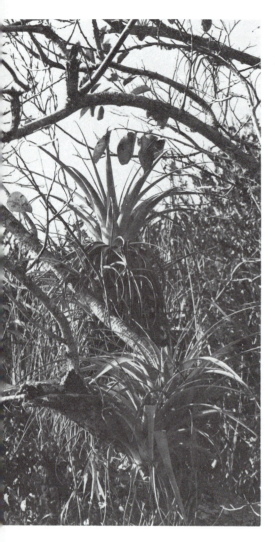

Figure 40-4

Air plants (bromeliads) in a tropical forest. The pineapple-like bromeliads and other epiphytes (plants that live on the surface of other plants) are common in tropical America. They tolerate lack of soil and a precarious water supply. Large bromeliads are often little ecosystems in themselves, supporting a variety of small, interdependent plant and animal life.
Photograph by L.L. Rue, III.

and Minnesota today. The large **southern pine forests** occupy much of the southeastern United States.

Mammals of the boreal and lake coniferous forests are deer, moose, elk, snowshoe hare, several furbearers, and a variety of rodents. They are adapted physiologically or behaviorally for long, cold, snowy winters. Common birds are chickadees, nuthatches, warblers, and jays. One bird, the red crossbill, has a beak specialized for picking seeds from cones. Mosquitoes and flies are pests to both animals and humans in this biome. Southern coniferous forests lack many mammals found in the north, but they have more snakes, lizards, and amphibians.

Tropical forest

The worldwide equatorial belt of tropical forests are areas of high rainfall, high humidity, relatively high and constant temperatures, and little seasonal variation in day length. These conditions have nurtured luxurious, uninterrupted growth that reaches its greatest intensity in the rain forests. In sharp contrast to temperate deciduous forests, dominated as they are by a relatively few tree species, tropical forests contain thousands of species, none of which is dominant. A single hectare typically contains 50 to 70 tree species as compared with 10 to 20 tree species in an equivalent area in the eastern United States. Climbing plants and epiphytes are common among the trunks and limbs (Fig. 40-4). A distinctive feature of tropical forests is the stratification of life into six, and occasionally as many as eight, feeding strata (Fig. 40-5).

Insectivorous birds and bats occupy the air above the canopy; below it birds, fruit bats, and mammals feed on leaves and fruit. In the middle zones are arboreal mammals (such as monkeys and tree sloths), numerous birds, insectivorous bats, insects, and amphibians. A distinct group of animals ranges up and down the trunks, feeding from all strata. On the ground are large mammals lacking climbing ability, such as the large rodents of South America (for example, capabara, paca, and agouti). Finally, a mixed group of small insectivorous, carnivorous, and herbivorous animals searches the litter and lower tree trunks for food. No other biome can match the tropical forest in incredible variety of animal species. Food webs are intricate and notoriously difficult for ecologists to unravel.

The tropical forests, especially the enormous expanse centered in the Amazon Basin, are the most seriously threatened of forest ecosystems. Large areas are being cleared for agriculture by "slash-and-burn" methods, but, because of low fertility, farms are soon abandoned. It may seem paradoxical that a biome as luxuriant as the tropical forest should have poor soil. This occurs because nutrients released by decomposition are rapidly absorbed by plants, leaving no reservoir of humus. Once the plants are removed, the soil rapidly becomes a hard, bricklike crust called laterite. Tropical plants cannot recolonize such areas.

Each month an area of undisturbed tropical forest the size of El Salvador is being converted to other uses. Unlike the forest clearing in the temperate zones, which made possible sustained, productive agriculture, tropical soils quickly become depleted, forcing farmers to move on to clear more forest. Another pressure on tropical forests is multinational timber companies that own and cut large tracts of timber for furniture of developed countries. Cattle ranchers also clear huge forest tracts to raise beef that is later sold to North America's fast-food chains. As one specialist remarked, "Everyone's hand is on the chain saw."

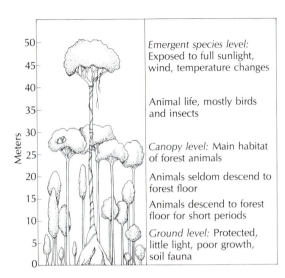

50
45
40
35
30
Meters
25
20
15
10
5
0

Emergent species level: Exposed to full sunlight, wind, temperature changes

Animal life, mostly birds and insects

Canopy level: Main habitat of forest animals

Animals seldom descend to forest floor

Animals descend to forest floor for short periods

Ground level: Protected, little light, poor growth, soil fauna

Figure 40-5

Profile of tropical rain forest, showing stratification of animal life. The animal biomass is small compared with the biomass of the trees.

Grassland

One of the most extensive prairie biomes in the world is in North America. In the early nineteenth century this sea of grass, broken only by occasional woodlands of pine, juniper, and oak, supported vast herds of bison, totaling perhaps 60 million animals. Both the plant and animal components of this biome have been almost completely destroyed by humans. By 1888 fewer than 1000 bison remained (Chapter 42). Virtually all of the major native grasses have been replaced by cultivated grains in croplands and by alien species of grasses in grazing lands. In other grasslands of the world such as the Eurasian steppe, the African veldt, and the South American pampas, some areas of virgin grassland remain. Most, however, have been severely altered by grazing and agricultural activities.

The original North American grasslands were controlled by the climate. Rainfall is too scant to support trees but is sufficient to prevent the formation of deserts. Although the dominant herbivore, the bison, is gone, several typical prairie herbivores remain, for example, jackrabbits, prairie dogs, ground squirrels, and antelope. Mammalian predators include coyotes, ferrets, and badgers, although, of these, only coyotes are common. Wolves that once followed the bison herds have disappeared with their prey.

Tundra

The tundra is characteristic of severe, cold climatic regions, especially the treeless Arctic regions and high mountaintops. Plant life must adapt itself to a short growing season of about 60 days and to a soil that remains frozen for most of the year. Most tundra regions are covered with bogs, marshes, ponds, and a spongy mat of decayed vegetation, although high tundras may be covered only with lichens and grasses. Despite the thin soil and short growing season, the vegetation of dwarf woody plants, grasses, sedges, and lichens may be quite profuse. The plants of the alpine tundra of high mountains, such as the Rockies and Sierra Nevadas, may differ from the Arctic tundra in some respects. Characteristic animals of the Arctic tundra are the lemming, caribou, musk-ox, arctic fox, arctic hare, ptarmigan, and (during the summer) many migratory birds.

Sonoran desert of Arizona and central Mexico has a diversified vegetation. Conspicuous here are giant saguaro cactus, creosote bushes, and bur sage.
Photograph by L.L. Rue, III.

Desert

Deserts are extremely arid regions where rainfall is low (less than 25 cm a year), and water evaporation is high. The largest desert in the world is the huge Sahara-Arabian-Gobi desert, stretching from west Africa to central Asia and occupying 8% of the earth's nonpolar land mass. In large portions of this area, it may rain only every few years. The deserts of western North America and Mexico are often called "near desert" because rainfall is substantially greater than on the great desert of Africa and Asia. Desert plants, such as various shrubs and cacti, have reduced foliage and other adaptations for conserving water (Fig. 40-6). Many large desert animals have developed remarkable anatomical and physiological adaptations for keeping cool and conserving water (p. 649). Most smaller animals avoid the most severe desert conditions by living in burrows. Many are nocturnal. Mammals found there include the white-tailed deer, peccary, cottontail, jackrabbit, kangaroo rat, pocket mouse, ground squirrel, badger, gray fox, skunk, and the like. Birds typical to desert life are the roadrunner, cactus wren, turkey vulture, cactus woodpecker, burrowing owl, Gambel's quail, raven, hummingbird, and flicker. Reptiles are numerous, such as the horned lizard, Gila monster, race runner, collared lizard, chuckwalla, coral snake, rattlesnake, and bull snake. A few species of toads are also common. Arthropods include a great variety of scorpions, spiders, centipedes, and insects.

Inland Waters

Freshwater environments include the running-water, or **lotic,** habitats, and the standing-water, or **lentic,** habitats. Freshwater streams are running-water habitats. Standing-water habitats include ponds and lakes.

A   B

Figure 40-7

A, Running-water habitats such as this brook rapids contain many organisms having adaptations for maintaining their position in the current. **B,** A water penny, larva of the riffle beetle *Psephenus*. This flat larva is 3.5 to 6 mm long and is adapted for clinging to lower surfaces of stones in swift brooks. The adult is a somewhat flattened, blackish beetle, 4 to 6 mm long, that may be found in the water or in bordering vegetation.
Photographs by F.M. Hickman.

Running-water habitats

Freshwater streams are lotic habitats that follow a gradient from mountain brooks to streams and rivers. From its origin at a spring, pond, or mountain lake, a permanent stream flows downward at a rate determined by the vertical face, volume of flow, and stream-bed volume. As the stream enlarges at lower altitudes, the current diminishes, the temperature tends to rise, oxygen content tends to drop, and bottom silting increases. Lotic habitats have a high primary productivity, as much as 30 times that of standing-water habitats, because flowing water continually brings in nutrients and carries away wastes. Oxygen is usually at or near saturation for the existing temperature in the swifter portions of a stream because of the constant contact of moving water with the atmosphere.

All animals that live in streams are adapted for maintaining position in the unremitting current (Fig. 40-7). Many of the forms found in such habitats have organs of attachment, such as suckers and modified appendages, streamlined body shapes for reducing surface resistance, or stages adapted for creeping under stones.

Ponds

Unlike streams, ponds have feeble currents or none at all. Most ponds contain a great deal of vegetation that tends to increase with the age of the pond. Many have very little open water in the center, for the vegetation, both rooted and floating types, has largely taken over. As ponds fill up, the higher plants become progressively more common. The bottoms of ponds vary from sandy and rocky (young ponds) to deep and mucky (old ponds). The water varies in depth from a few centimeters to a meter or two, although some may be deeper. Ponds are too shallow to be stratified, for the force of the wind is usually sufficient to keep the entire mass of water in circulation. Because of this, the gases (oxygen and carbon dioxide) are uniformly distributed through the water, and the temperature is fairly uniform.

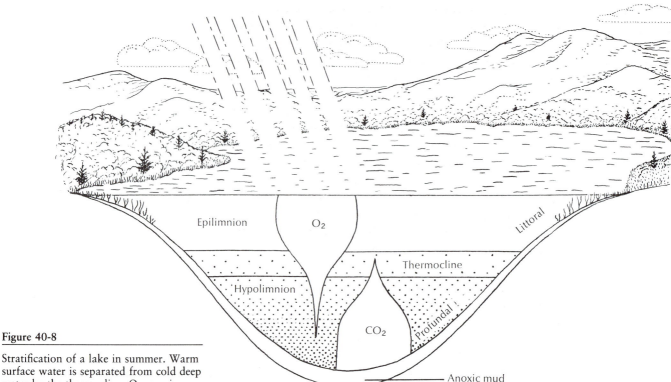

Figure 40-8

Stratification of a lake in summer. Warm surface water is separated from cold deep water by the thermocline. Oxygen is abundant in the well-illuminated, wind-stirred epilimnion, but scanty or absent at the bottom. Carbon dioxide may be abundant at the bottom where respiration and organic decomposition predominate.

Animal communities of ponds are usually similar to those of bays in larger bodies of water (lakes). The large amount of vegetation and plant decomposition products affords an excellent habitat for many forms. Among the common forms found are varieties of snails and mussels, larvae of flies, beetles, caddis flies, dragonflies, many kinds of crustaceans and midges, and many species of frogs. The community of animals that live on the bottom or among the submerged vegetation is called **benthos.** Many swimming forms, called **nekton,** are also found in the larger ponds. Because of the abundance of food, many birds are usually found in and around ponds. These include herons, killdeers, ducks, grebes, and blackbirds. Most ponds also have plankton composed of microscopic plants and animals, such as protozoa, crustaceans, worms, rotifers, diatoms, and algae.

Forms found in ponds ordinarily require less oxygen than those living in streams or rapids.

Lakes

The distinction between lakes and ponds is not sharply defined. Lakes are usually distinguished from ponds by having continuous and permanent water in their centers and by having some sandy shores. The bottoms of lakes depend to a great extent on exposure to winds. Where waves are common, the bottoms are usually sandy, but protected areas may contain a great deal of deposited bottom muck. The surface of water in proportion to the total volume of water is less in a lake than in a pond, for lakes are deeper. In large lakes, such as the Great Lakes of North America, the depth may exceed 500 m; in moderate-sized lakes the depth is much less. Oxygen is scarcer in the deeper regions where there is little circulation. Light penetration depends on the particles suspended in water. Most of the light is absorbed by the first meter of surface water, and little penetrates beyond a few meters.

Waters of many northern, temperate lakes undergo seasonal changes in temperature that cause them to become stratified (Fig. 40-8). After the ice melts in the spring, the sun warms the surface water. When the temperature reaches 4° C, the temperature at which water attains its greatest density, the strong winds of spring mix the water from top to bottom until it is uniformly 4° C. This is the **spring overturn,** an important event that brings nutrients up from the bottom and carries oxygen down from the top. As the surface water continues to warm in early summer, its density decreases. Eventually, the warmer and lighter surface water ceases to mix with the colder and heavier bottom water, even during periods of strong winds. Stratification has occurred, and the warm surface water, the **epilimnion,** remains separated from the deeper water, the **hypolimnion,** for the rest of the summer. The area of separation is a temperature barrier called the **thermocline,** a zone where the temperature drops steeply. Above the thermocline, the surface water continues to warm during the summer. Below the thermocline, the water remains still and cold, often only a degree or two warmer than it was in winter.

The decomposition of organic material at the bottom may deplete the hypolimnion of oxygen during the summer and increase the concentration of carbon dioxide and methane. This summer stagnation period requires special adaptations by the animals living there: some are anaerobic (bacteria), some tolerate extended oxygen debts (worms), some make nightly excursions into the epilimnion to obtain oxygen (certain insect larvae), and some encyst and wait out the stagnation period in a dormant condition (certain crustaceans).

In the autumn, colder weather cools the surface, causing the water to sink. The thermocline begins to disappear, and soon the water temperature is uniformly cold (4° C) from top to bottom. Winds again stir the lake throughout, recharging it with nutrients and oxygen. This is the **fall overturn.** In winter the surface water cools, becomes lighter, and may freeze, while the bottom water remains at 4° to 5° C. If the lake is covered with ice and snow, there may be a winter stagnation period during which the oxygen concentration gradually falls as a result of consumption by animals and decomposition of organic matter.

Several habitats are found in lakes. In the terrigenous bottom habitat where the water is shallow and vegetation is absent, snails and mayfly nymphs might be found. In the cove habitat, which has a great deal of vegetation—submerged, emergent, and floating—one might find bryozoans, small crustaceans, snails, and some insect larvae; in open water one might find plankton and nekton. On the bottom (benthic habitat) are animals that require little light and oxygen, such as a few annelids, bivalves, and midge larvae.

Oceans

By almost any measure, the oceans represent by far the largest portion of the earth's biosphere. They cover 71% of the earth's surface to an average depth of 3.75 km (2.3 miles), with their greatest depths reaching to more than 11.5 km (7.2 miles) below sea level. Life occurs throughout this enormous volume, whereas on land, life is confined to within a few meters above and below the land's surface. The marine world is relatively uniform as compared with land, and in many respects it is less demanding on life forms. However, the evident monotony of the ocean's surface belies the variety of life below. The oceans are the cradle of life, and this is reflected in the variety of organisms living there—more than 200,000 species of plants and animals. The vast majority of these forms, about 98%, live

Acid rain, caused mainly by the industrial emissions of sulfur and nitrogen oxides from the burning of fossil fuels, has led to serious deterioration of water quality in lakes, ponds, and rivers of southern Scandinavia and eastern North America. These emissions interact with atmospheric moisture to yield high concentrations of hydrogen, sulfate, and nitrate ions. Acid rains having a pH below 4 are not uncommon. Most sensitive to acid rain are recently glaciated areas having low buffering capacity. The acidity of Maine's lakes increased eightfold between 1937 and 1974; hundreds of lakes in the Adirondacks are now sterile, or are approaching sterility, and are lost to practical and recreational purposes.

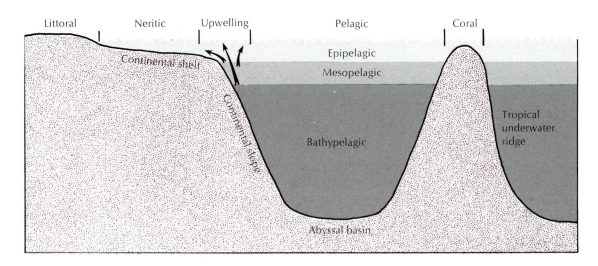

Figure 40-9

Major marine zones.

on the sea bed (**benthic**); only 2% live freely in the open ocean (**pelagic**). Of the benthic forms, most occur in the intertidal zone or shallow depths of the oceans. Less than 1% live in the deep ocean below 2000 m.

The two principal determinants of such uneven distribution of biomass in the ocean are nutrient availability and light penetration into the water. The most productive areas are concentrated along continental margins and a few open areas where the waters are enriched by organic nutrients (principally phosphates and nitrates) and organic debris lifted by upwelling currents into the sunlit, or **photic**, zone. Photosynthetic activity is limited to the depth of the photic zone, usually less than 150 m, although in especially clear waters it may extend to more than 300 m. Below the photic zone, the lack of both nutrients and light prevents the growth of phytoplankton, which forms the base of the food pyramid. In the zone of perpetual darkness all life depends on the "rain" of organic debris from the photic zone above.

In addition to the principal division of the marine habitat into benthic (bottom) and pelagic (open water), we can distinguish several zones based on depth and distance from shore (Fig. 40-9). The **epipelagic** zone is equivalent to the photic zone and reaches down to 100 to 200 m. Below this is the **mesopelagic** zone, extending down to 1000 m. Only shorter (blue) wavelengths of light penetrate this zone, too little to support effective photosynthesis. This is followed by the **bathypelagic** zone (1000 m to the bottom). The total biomass may be in excess of 1000 g/m² in the inshore photic zone. At 200 m the biomass drops to about 50 g/m² and the deeper one goes, the sparser life becomes. At 1000 m the biomass is 1 g/m², and in the abyssal depths of the ocean it is only 0.1 g/m². These figures emphasize the importance of the inshore region, even though it makes up less than 2.5% of the total oceanic area.

An important faunistic boundary is the permanent thermocline in the tropics in which the water temperature drops from the mixed surface temperature to the cold water of the deep ocean. The thermocline occurs between 50 m and 500 m. Below 2000 m the water temperature averages about 3.3° C at the equator. Unlike the seasonal thermocline of freshwater lakes, described previously, the permanent thermocline of the ocean is unaffected by climatic changes on the surface. Nutrients captured by the phytoplankton biomass tend to sink below the thermocline, becoming unavailable to surface productivity unless flushed upward by upwelling.

The life of the ocean is divided into regions, or provinces, each with its own distinctive life forms (Fig. 40-9). Five major regions are the (1) **littoral,** or intertidal, zone, and **sublittoral** zone, where sea and land meet; (2) **neritic,** or shallow-water zone, surrounding the continents and extending out to a depth of about 200 m; (3) **upwelling,** where nutrient-rich water is carried up into the photic zone; (4) **pelagic,** the vast open sea; and (5) **coral reefs,** built by carbonate-secreting organisms where tropical land masses protrude into the photic zone. Coral reefs were described in Chapter 10, so will not be included in the brief survey of the marine environment that follows.

Littoral-sublittoral zones

The littoral zone is biologically one of the richest and, paradoxically, physically the harshest of all marine environments. At its margins it is subjected to pounding surf (as much as 15,000 kg/cm^2), sun, wind, rain, extreme temperature fluctuations, erosion, and sedimentation. These influences have created numerous distinctive habitats, often in proximity to one another, each harboring a specialized fauna. Animals living here must be firmly attached and strongly protected. Barnacles, snails, chitons, limpets, and mussels are shielded by their shells and either grow permanently to the rocky surface or maintain position with powerful suction organs. Some species of sea urchins bore recesses into the rocks to become permanently imprisoned in their stony cups as they grow. On sandy and muddy shores, animals possess adaptations for burrowing and surviving a shifting matrix.

The littoral-sublittoral zone of temperate regions of the earth actually embraces three zones. The upper **spray zone,** moistened by saltwater spray above the high-tide mark, supports a few green algae and lichens on which periwinkle snails (*Littorina* sp.) graze. Small spray-zone barnacles (*Chthamalus* sp.) also survive here. The middle **tidal zone** is typically covered with brown and red algae, especially the common brown alga ("seaweed") with its distinctive floats (*Fucus* sp.). Barnacles (*Balanus* sp.), limpets, chitons, snails, and other herbivores are common in this region. The lower **subtidal zone** (sublittoral), which is always submerged, supports forests of brown algae (*Laminaria* sp.) and a great variety of smaller algae, sea urchins, starfishes, anemones, molluscs, and fishes.

Estuaries may be considered part of the littoral-sublittoral environment. An **estuary** is a semienclosed transition zone where fresh water flows into the sea. Depending on the substrate, currents, climate, and other physical conditions, an estuary may take the form of a mud or sand flat, tidal marsh, or mangrove swamp. Salinity is variable because the amount of fresh water entering the estuary varies throughout the year. Temperature extremes are often severe. Despite their physical harshness, estuaries are typically rich in nutrients and consequently support a diverse fauna. Most estuarine organisms are benthic, either burrowing into or attaching to the bottom. Conspicuous features of estuaries are oyster communities, around which a host of symbiotic organisms associate. Motile inhabitants of estuaries are chiefly fishes and crustaceans. All estuarine animals must tolerate fluctuations in salinity, which is always changing with the ebb and flow of the tide and variable discharge of fresh water from rivers and streams. The different ways animals meet this problem are discussed in Chapter 30.

Neritic zone

The neritic zone overlies the continental shelf, an area usually defined as extending from the subtidal zone out to a depth of 200 m. Although it occupies only 7.5% of the total oceanic area, it ranks high in importance because here are concentrated most of the world's fisheries. The neritic zone is more productive than the open sea because upwelling at the shelf edge together with the greater turbulence of continental shelf waters brings nutrients into all strata of the water. Furthermore, the continental shelf benefits from nutrients washed into the sea by streams and rivers. Sinking nutrients, rather than disappearing into the ocean's depths, fall on the shelf floor where they stimulate a rich growth of seaweed, marine grasses, and other plants. The increased plant growth in turn supports a diverse animal life.

Upwelling

Upwelling supports much of the productivity of the neritic zone as well as a rich fishery of its own. Areas of upwelling, although small in area and restricted to a few regions, are important sources of nutrient renewal for the surface photic zone of the oceans. In such regions deep, low-temperature water in which nutrients have accumulated well up to slowly replace surface water swept away by prevailing winds.

Among the most important upwelling regions is the Peru Current. Until recently, the Peruvian anchovy (or anchoveta) comprised 22% of all the fish caught in the world. The total catch of all the fish in the United States in 1969 was only 20% of the Peruvian anchovy catch! Anchovies are converted into fish meal, which is exported as livestock feed, and fish oil, which is used in margarine, paint, and other products. The base of this food chain is principally photosynthetic colonial diatoms, which convert upwelling inorganic nutrients into energy-rich organic compounds. The diatoms are harvested directly by crustaceans and by the anchovies, which have gill rakers adapted for filter-feeding. Predation on the anchovies is intense. "Guano" birds (principally cormorants and gannets) that feed almost exclusively on anchovies have over the centuries deposited vast accumulations of droppings (guano) along the coastal deserts of Peru. Tuna, sea lions, and squid also feast on the anchovies. In recent years humans have become the greatest predator of all. Following more than a decade of intense commercial fishing, the Peruvian anchovy fishery suffered a collapse in 1972 from which it has not yet recovered. An additional blow was dealt the fishery during years when the upwelling failed. There is concern that this great industry will experience the same fate that befell the California sardine fishery and the Japanese herring fishery, both fisheries of upwelling regions. These intensively harvested fisheries fell below the point of spontaneous recovery and may have disappeared forever.

Open ocean

The open ocean beyond the continental shelves occupies 90% of the total oceanic area. Despite its vastness, it is relatively impoverished biologically because the constant rain of sinking plankton and detritus from the photic zone carries nutrients below the permanent thermocline and into the bathypelagic zone where they are immobilized. Nitrates and phosphates, the most important limiting nutrients, are commonly 100 times more concentrated in the neritic than in the epipelagic zone. Productivity is high only in areas where nutrients are replenished by current convergences (Arctic and Antarctic seas) and upwelling. The polar areas are in fact enormously productive. Phytoplankton, the base of the food chain, is eaten by euphausiid shrimp (krill), which are harvested by blue and fin whales. Before their egregious overexploitation by humans, the whales are estimated to have consumed 77 million tons of Antarctic krill per year, far more than the entire catch of all the fishes, crustaceans, and molluscs taken by all the world's fishing fleets in any one year! Because the baleen whales have been nearly destroyed by hunting, the Antarctic krill now remain mostly unharvested.

Far below the epipelagic zone exists the abyssal habitat, characterized by enormous pressure, perpetual darkness, and a constant temperature near 0° C. It has remained a world unknown to humans until recently, when baited cameras, bathyscaphs, and deep-water trawls have been lowered to view and sample the ocean bottom. Benthic forms of the sea floor survive on that meager portion of the gentle rain of organic debris from above that escapes consumption by organisms in the water column. Despite the unusual properties of the habitat, sea anemones, sea urchins, crustaceans, and polychaete worms—indeed nearly all major invertebrate groups—exist here as well as fishes (Fig. 40-10).

—ANIMAL DISTRIBUTION (ZOOGEOGRAPHY)

The study of zoogeography tries to explain why animals are found where they are, their patterns of dispersal, and the factors responsible for their dispersal. With the exception of the human species, which is able to live nearly anywhere on earth, and creatures such as the house mouse and the cockroach, which share human habitations, the different kinds of animals occupy limited habitats on earth. It is not always easy to explain why animals are distributed as they are, since similar habitats on separate continents may be occupied by quite different kinds of animals. A particular species may be absent from a region that supports similar animals for any of three reasons: (1) there may be barriers that prevent it from getting there; (2) having gotten there, it may be unable to adapt to the new habitat or compete successfully with resident species and may become extinct; or (3) having once arrived and adapted, it has subsequently evolved into a distinct species.

Thus, there are always good reasons why animals are found where they are (or are not found where one thinks they ought to be), and it is the task of the zoogeographer to discover what these reasons are. Usually this means going back into the past. The fossil record plainly shows that animals once flourished in regions from which they are now absent. Extinction has played a major role, but many groups left descendants that migrated to other regions and survived. For example, camels originated in North America, where their fossils are found, but spread to Eurasia by way of Alaska (true camels) and to South America (llamas) during the Pleistocene epoch. Then they became extinct in North America at the close of the Ice Age. Thus, the history of an animal species or its ancestor must be known before one can understand why it is where it is. The earth's surface is undergoing constant change. Many areas that are now land were once covered with seas; fertile plains may be claimed by advancing desert; impassable mountain barriers may arise where none existed before; or inhospitable ice fields may retreat before a warmer climate to be replaced by forests. Geological change has been responsible for much of the alteration in animal (and plant) distribution and has been a powerful influence in shaping organic evolution.

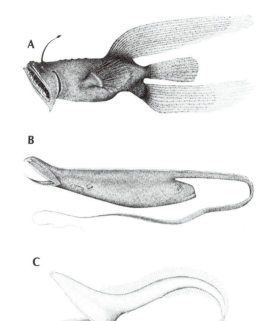

Figure 40-10

Fishes of the abyssal habitat. Because their entire lives are spent in absolute darkness, their eyes are degenerate and often functionless. Huge mouths and capacious stomachs are adaptations for large but very infrequent meals, the organic debris drifting down from above. **A**, *Caulophryne* sp. **B**, *Saccopharynx ampullaceus*. **C**, *Eurypharynx pelecanoides*. Courtesy Smithsonian Institution.

Figure 40-11

The six major faunal realms of the earth.

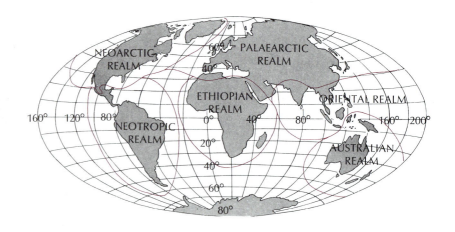

Major Faunal Realms

The nineteenth-century naturalists recognized that it was possible to divide the terrestrial world into several distinct realms of animal distribution, separated from one another by topographical and climatic barriers. Philip L. Sclater (1858) first proposed a region system based on bird families. Later (1876), Alfred Russel Wallace, codiscoverer with Charles Darwin of the principle of natural selection, modified Sclater's pattern and applied it to vertebrates in general. Wallace recognized six land realms based on animal ranges. Although later scientists slightly modified his biogeographical boundaries, the Wallacean regions are the ones we recognize today (Fig. 40-11). Great oceanic barriers serve as longitudinal dividers between the Nearctic and Palaearctic realms in the north and the Neotropic and Australian realms in the south. The great northern land mass is divided by a subtropic, warm temperate dry belt into Palaearctic, Ethiopian, and Oriental realms. These realms are better recognized by the differences between them than by faunal similarities within them. As with the biomes described earlier, the boundaries between realms are transition zones that are often poorly defined, especially if the barrier between them is largely climatic. Or they may be clear and distinct if the separation is a mountain range or salt water; to land animals, even a narrow saltwater strait is an effective barrier.

Distributional Processes

The association of animals in ways that enable zoogeographers to recognize faunal realms suggests that the major realms have been separated from each other for long periods of time. Of particular interest are the numerous instances of **discontinuous, or disjunct, distributions**: the same or closely related organism or group living in widely separated areas of a continent, or even the world (Fig. 40-12). How could an animal group become separated in this way? In some cases they may be **evolutionary relics**, the scattered remnants of a once widespread and successful group that can no longer compete (or can compete only marginally) with modern forms. The three surviving genera of lungfishes—one each in South America, Africa, and Australia—are good examples (Fig. 23-19, p. 535). But this explanation cannot apply to many species of modern animals—mammals, for instance—that compete successfully in their habitats, yet may be widely but unevenly distributed around the world. Nor can it explain the appearance of new animal species, which has occurred millions of times over the history of the earth.

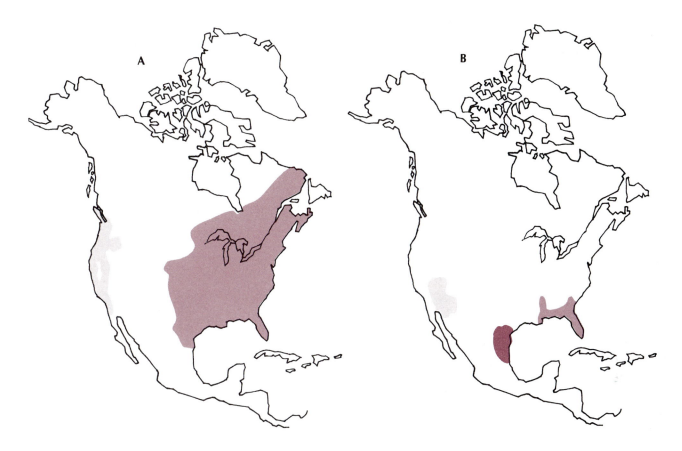

Any convincing explanation of animal distribution must also explain speciation.

There are only two ways for disjunct distributions to arise. Either an organism moves to a new location (**dispersal**), or the location moves, carrying the organism passively with it (**vicariance**).

Distribution by dispersal

By dispersal, animals spread into new localities from their place of origin. Changes in environment may force animals to shift their domiciles, although most great groups have spread to gain favorable conditions, not to avoid unfavorable ones. The reproductive rate of animals is so great that there is continuous pressure on individuals to move into new areas, reducing the competition for food, shelter, and space to live and breed. This **population pressure** expands the range of the species and maintains healthy populations. Survival of the species may depend on successful dispersal to new areas when the old habitat ceases to be habitable because of geographical and ecological changes through time. Dispersal followed by isolation is also a biological prerequisite for the formation of new species because, as we pointed out previously (p. 958), geographical isolation of a founding colony from the parent population permits new adaptive variations to arise.

Dispersal movements involve emigration from one region and immigration into another. Dispersal is a *one-way,* outward movement that must be distinguished from migration, a *periodic* movement back and forth between two localities, such as the seasonal migration of birds. Dispersing animals may move **actively** under their own power, whether they are creepers, climbers, runners, hoppers,

Figure 40-12

Disjunct distributions in North America. **A,** Moles of the family Talpidae probably entered North America during the Tertiary across the Bering land bridge that once joined North America and Asia. Eastern and western populations are now separated by the Rocky Mountains. **B,** Gopher turtles of the genus *Gopherus* are now separated into three fully isolated populations.

A, Redrawn from Burt, W.H.; B, redrawn from Blair, W.F. Both in C.L. Hubbs (ed.). 1958. Zoogeography, Washington, D.C., AAAS Pub. No. 51. Copyright 1958 by AAAS.

Figure 40-13

Centers of origin of, **A,** pheasants of the subfamily Phasianinae and, **B,** crocodiles of the order Crocodilia. The figures indicate numbers of species or genera within each contour. The center of origin is considered to be the area of highest taxon density.

Redrawn from Pielou, E.C. 1979. Biogeography. New York, John Wiley & Sons, Inc.

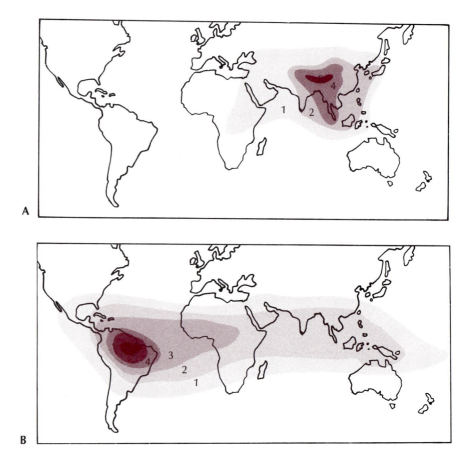

or flyers; or they may be **passively** dispersed by wind and air currents, by floating or rafting on rivers, lakes, or the sea, or by hitching rides on other animals. The chief deterrents to the spread of animals are barriers such as mountain chains, cliffs, canyons, sand dunes, lava flows, rivers, and, most effective of all, oceans. However, what comprises a barrier to one animal may serve as an avenue of dispersal for another. A river may obstruct the dispersal of a gray squirrel but facilitate the movement of a beaver. In addition to the physical barriers listed are climatic barriers, such as deserts, and biotic barriers, such as competition between species, predators, changes in vegetation, and absence of suitable food. Deserts are especially important barriers to most animals because they have an inhospitable climate, too hot and dry for most species, and are lacking in vegetation for cover, in food, and in suitable places to live. Deserts are of course the chosen habitats for a variety of animals bearing appropriate desert adaptations; to these animals, nondesert habitats are barriers to dispersal.

Distribution by vicariance

Disjunct distributions of animals may be created by the splitting of ancestral populations by changing geography—separation of areas that were once joined—rather than by dispersal. The study of fragmentation of biotas in this manner is called **vicariance** (L., *vicarius*, a substitute) **biogeography.** Vicariance distribution can occur when a species is separated by some new barrier, such as a mountain range or a desert, or when landmasses become fragmented, resulting in the separation of their fauna and flora. Many biogeographers use the word "vicariance" as a synonym for "allopatry," which, as we have seen, is simply a way for new species to arise in geographically separated areas. Vicariance biogeography, however, has recently attracted a school of enthusiastic adherents who claim that vicariance is a primary principle of biogeography, to the virtual exclusion of dispersal. In their view, dispersal can only lead to competition, and often to extinction, as species expand into already occupied habitats, whereas vicariance is responsible for the multiplication of species. The vicariance explanation fits in well with the accepted idea of allopatric speciation: biotas must be geographically separated before speciation can occur (p. 958). It does not, however, explain the common observation that many taxonomic groups have centers of origin (Fig. 40-13). The **center of origin,** the place where a group is believed to have originated, can be located by drawing a contour map composed of lines of equal species (or genus) richness. The center of origin is outlined by the contour surrounding the highest species (or genus) density for the group (Fig. 40-13). The problem for the vicariance advocate is to explain how species multiplication can occur within a restricted area, as center-of-origin maps imply, if virtually all speciation occurs allopatrically, that is, by geographical splitting of ancestral populations. Various models have been offered as solutions to this problem, but the explanations are beyond the scope of this book. The reasonable conclusion is that both dispersal and vicariance occur, separately and in combination. It may be true that most speciation happens by vicariance (allopatry), but this places no restriction on dispersal after (or even before) speciation occurs.

Continental drift theory

It is no accident that the current enthusiasm for vicariance biogeography coincides with the recent acceptance of the continental drift theory by geologists. The continental drift theory is not new (it was proposed in 1912 by the German meteorologist Alfred Wegener) but it remained controversial and largely rejected until the newly proposed theory of **plate tectonics** provided a mechanism to account for drifting continents. According to the theory of plate tectonics (tectonics means "deforming movement"), the earth's surface is composed of six to 10 rocky plates, about 100 km thick, that shift about on a more malleable underlying layer. Wegener proposed that the earth's continents had been drifting like rafts following the breakup of a single great landmass called Pangaea ("all land"). According to recent workers who have considerably revised Wegener's dating, this occurred some 200 million years ago. Two great supercontinents were formed: a northern Laurasia and a southern Gondwana, separated from each other by the Tethys Sea (Fig. 40-14). At the end of the Jurassic period, some 135 million years ago, the supercontinents began to fragment and drift apart. Laurasia split into North America, most of Eurasia, and Greenland. Gondwana split into South America, Africa, Madagascar, Arabia, India, Australia, and Antarctica. This theory is supported by the appearance of fit between the continents, by recent airborne paleomagnetic surveys, by seismographic studies, by the presence of midoceanic ridges where the tectonic plates are born, and by a wealth of biological data.

Continental drift explains several otherwise puzzling distributions of animals, such as the similarity of invertebrate fossils in Africa and South America, as well as certain similarities in present-day fauna at the same latitudes on the two continents. However, the continents have been separated for all of the Cenozoic era and probably for much of the Mesozoic era as well, much too long to explain the dispersal of modern organisms such as the placental mammals. Continental

200 million years ago

Figure 40-14

Hypothesized drift of continents over the past 200 million years from an original single land mass to their present positions. The universal land mass Pangaea first separated into two supercontinents (Laurasia and Gondwana). These later broke up into smaller continents. The black arrows indicate vector movements of the continents. The black crescent labeled *A* is a modern geographical reference point representing the Antilles arc in the West Indies.

Modified from Dietz, R.S., and J.C. Holden. 1970. Sci. Am. **223**:30-41 (Oct.).

180 million years ago

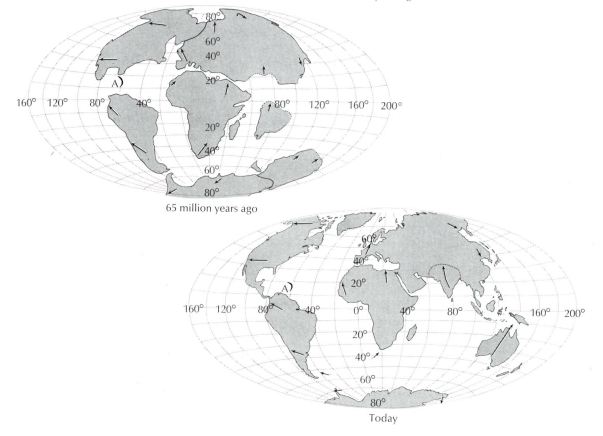

65 million years ago

Today

Old Northerners

Stopped by filter
Shrews
Pocket mice
Pocket gophers
Beavers
Bobcats
Pronghorns
Bison
Sheep

Crossing filter
Rabbits
Squirrels
Field mice
Dogs
Bears
Raccoons
Weasels
Otters
Skunks
Pumas
Deer

*Now stopped in or
south of filter*
Coatis
Kinkajous
Many cats
Tapirs
Peccaries
Camels

Crossing filter
Porcupines
Opossum

Stopped by filter
Most armadillos
Anteaters
Sloths
Guinea pigs
Pacas
Capybaras
Etc.

Old Southerners

Figure 40-15

Central America as a filter zone. The Isthmus of Panama emerged 3 to 4 million years ago, permitting the extensive interchange of many groups of mammals but preventing the passage of others. "Old Northerners" and "Old Southerners" are extant mammals of northern and southern ancestry, respectively.
Modified from Simpson, G.G. 1980. Splendid isolation. New Haven, Conn., Yale University Press.

drift theory is, nevertheless, enormously useful in explaining interconnections between flora and fauna of the past.

The present distribution of the marsupial mammals is an excellent example of the influence of continental breakup. The marsupials appeared in the Middle Cretaceous period, about 100 million years BP, probably in South America. Because South America was at that time connected to Australia through Antarctica (which was then much warmer than it is today), the marsupials spread through all three continents. They also moved into North America, but there they met the placental mammals, which had dispersed to that continent from Asia. The marsupials evidently could not compete with placentals and so became extinct in North America. (North American marsupials today, that is, the opossums, are relatively recent arrivals from South America.) The placentals followed the marsupials into South America, but by that time the marsupials had expanded and were too firmly established to be driven into extinction. In the meantime, about 50 million years BP, Australia drifted apart from Antarctica, barring entrance to the placentals. Australia remained in isolation, allowing the marsupials to diversify into the present rich and varied fauna.

Temporary land bridges have also been important pathways of dispersal. An important and well-established land bridge that no longer exists connected Asia and North America across the Bering Strait. It was across this corridor that the placentals moved from Asia into North America.

Today a land bridge connects North and South America at the Isthmus of Panama, but from the mid-Eocene epoch (50 million years BP) to the end of the Pliocene epoch (3 million years BP), the two continents were completely separated by a water barrier. During this long period, all of the major groups of placental mammals were evolving in distinctive directions on each continent. When the land bridge was reestablished at the end of the Pliocene epoch, a tide of mammals began to flow in both directions. For a period both continents gained in mammal diversity, but direct competition for similar ecological niches soon led to the extinction of large numbers of mammals on both continents. North American invaders such as deer, foxes, bears, raccoons, tapirs, llamas, mastodons, and antelopes displaced many South American residents occupying similar niches, and today nearly half of the South American mammals are descendants of recent North American invaders (Fig. 40-15). Only a few South American invaders survived in North America: porcupines, armadillos, and opossums. Several other South American groups, including the giant ground sloths and the giant armadillos, entered North America but subsequently died out.

____ Summary

The biosphere is the thin blanket of life surrounding the earth. The presence of life on earth is possible because numerous conditions for life are fulfilled on this planet. These include a steady supply of energy from the sun, the presence of water, a suitable range of temperatures, the correct proportion of major and minor elements, and the screening of lethal ultraviolet radiation by atmospheric ozone.

The earth environment and living organisms have evolved together, each deeply marking the other.

The ecosphere is composed of the biosphere, the thin film of life on the earth's surface; the lithosphere, the earth's rocky shell; the hydrosphere, the global distribution of water; and the atmosphere, the blanket of gas surrounding the earth.

The earth's terrestrial environment is composed of biomes that bear a distinctive array of plant life and associated animal life. The eastern deciduous forest is characterized by distinct seasons and autumn leaf fall. North of the deciduous forest is the coniferous forest, which in its northern range is called taiga, an area dominated by needle-leafed trees adapted for heavy snowfall. Animals of the taiga are adapted for long, snowy winters.

The tropical forest is the richest biome, characterized in part by a great diversity of plant species and the vertical stratification of animal habitats. Tropical forest soils rapidly deteriorate when the forest is removed.

The most modified biome is the grassland, or prairie, biome, which has been largely converted to agriculture and grazing. The tundra biome of the far north and the desert biome are both severe environments for animal life, but they are populated nevertheless with organisms that have evolved appropriate adaptations.

Freshwater environments include rivers and streams (lotic habitats) and ponds and lakes (lentic habitats). Ponds are shallow, usually have vegetation across the entire bottom, and do not stratify thermally with changing seasons. Lakes, because of their depth, become thermally stratified, but they turn over in spring and fall, replenishing the oxygen of the hypolimnion and redistributing nutrients.

The oceans occupy 71% of the earth's surface. The photic, or sunlit, zone supports photosynthetic activity by phytoplankton. The rain of nutrients from the photic zone supports the great diversity of life below on the sea bed (benthos). The littoral, or tidal, zone is biologically rich but physically harsh. The neritic, or shallow-water, zone overlying the continental shelf is the locus of the world's great fisheries, which are especially productive in areas of upwelling where nutrients are constantly renewed. The open ocean, or pelagic zone, occupies most of the ocean's area but has low biological productivity.

Zoogeography is the study of animal distribution on earth. Several great faunal realms are recognized by distinctive animal associations. These are the Nearctic, Neotropical, Palearctic, Ethiopian, Oriental, and Australian realms.

Animals have become distributed around the earth by dispersal, the spread of populations from the centers of origin, and by vicariance, the separation of populations by barriers or continental drift. Continental drift, now strongly supported by plate tectonic theory, helps to explain how animal groups become geographically separated so that speciation can occur. It also explains how certain groups, such as the marsupial mammals, can become isolated from competing groups. Temporary land bridges have also served as important pathways for animal dispersal.

Selected references

Andrewartha, H.G., and L.C. Birch. 1954. The distribution and abundance of animals. Chicago, University of Chicago Press. *Classic analysis of animal populations and the factors that influence their abundance and distribution.*

Brown, J.H., and A.C. Gibson. 1983. Biogeography. St. Louis, The C.V. Mosby Co. *Readable current synthesis of the field.*

Cox, C.B., and P.D. Moore. 1980. Biogeography: an ecological and evolutionary approach, ed. 3. New York, John Wiley & Sons, Inc. *Introductory textbook with lucid explanations. Ecological emphasis.*

Darlington, P.J. 1957. Zoogeography: the geographical distribution of animals. New York, John Wiley & Sons, Inc. *Out of date, but still a classic, and better than many recent books on the subject.*

Elton, C.S. 1958. The ecology of invasions by animals and plants. New York, John Wiley & Sons, Inc. *A classic on animal dispersal.*

Engel, L., and the editors of Time-Life Books. 1972. The sea. Life Nature Library. New York, Time-Life Books. *This handsomely illustrated volume provides a popularized yet balanced treatment of the sea and its biota.*

Flessa, K.W. 1980. Biological effects of plate tectonics and continental drift. BioScience 30:518-523. *Clear statement on the impact of plate tectonics on biogeography.*

Hansen, J., D. Johnson, A. Lacis, S. Lebedeff, P. Lee, D. Rind, and G. Russell. 1981. Climate impact of increasing atmospheric carbon dioxide. Science 213:957-966. *Documentation of the increasing load of atmospheric carbon dioxide and its anticipated effects.*

Henderson, L.J. 1913. The fitness of the environment. New York, Macmillan, Inc. *Explains how conditions on our planet made life possible.*

Marshall, L.G., S.D. Webb, J.J. Sepkoski, Jr., and D.M. Raup. 1982. Mammalian evolution and the great American interchange. Science 215:1351-1357. *North American mammalian immigrants to South America over the Panama land bridge were remarkably successful. The reasons are explored.*

McConnaughey, B.H. 1978. Introduction to marine biology, ed. 3. St. Louis, The C.V. Mosby Co. *Unified presentation of the marine environment and its life.*

Müller, P. 1974. Aspects of zoogeography. The Hague, Dr. W. Junk b.v., Publishers. *Descriptive approach.*

Nelson, G., and D.E. Rosen (eds.). 1981. Vicariance biogeography: a critique. New York, Columbia University Press. *Twelve contributed chapters with extensive discussions by symposium contributors. Conflicting views of vicariance theory are aired.*

Pielou, E.C. 1979. Biogeography. New York, John Wiley & Sons, Inc. *A landmark publication in the field with a superb analysis of contemporary thinking in biogeography. Highly recommended.*

Simmons, I. 1982. Biogeographical processes. London, George Allen & Unwin. *Concise introduction to the subject.*

Simpson, G.G. 1953. Evolution and geography. Eugene, Ore., State System of Higher Education. *An excellent appraisal of the main concepts of animal distribution.*

Simpson, G.G. 1980. Splendid isolation: the curious history of South American mammals. New Haven, Conn., Yale University Press. *The "great American interchange," the dispersal of animals between North and South America, is beautifully described.*

Udvardy, M.D.F. 1969. Dynamic zoogeography. New York, Van Nostrand Reinhold Co. *Textbook stressing ecology and mechanisms of dispersal of land animals.*

Williamson, M. 1981. Island populations. Oxford, Eng., Oxford University Press. *Island biogeography with emphasis on ecology and evolution.*

Selected *Scientific American* articles

The biosphere. 1970. **223**:44 (Sept.). *This special issue includes articles on the various cycles—energy, water, oxygen, nitrogen, and mineral—and also on human food and energy and materials production as processes in the biosphere.*

Bullard, E. 1969. The origin of the oceans. **221**:66-75 (Sept.).

Dietz, R.S., and J.C. Holden. 1970. The breakup of Pangaea. **223**:30-41 (Oct.). *The sequence of continental drift since the early Mesozoic era is mapped.*

Fairbridge, R.W. 1960. The changing level of the sea. **202**:70-79 (May).

Gautier, T.N. 1955. The ionosphere. **193**:123-138 (Sept.).

Gregg, M.C. 1973. The microstructure of the ocean. **228**:64-77 (Feb.).

Hallam, A. 1975. Alfred Wegener and the hypothesis of continental drift. **232**:88-97 (Feb.). *Wegener's theory that anticipated the modern concept of continental drift remained unaccepted for some 50 years by the scientific community.*

Idyll, C.P. 1973. The anchovy crisis. **228**:22-29 (June). *The Peruvian anchovy fishery and its recent collapse are described.*

Koehl, M.A.R. 1982. The interaction of moving water and sessile organisms. **247**:124-134 (Dec.). *Describes the adaptations of coastal marine organisms to the forces of waves.*

Kurtén, B. 1969. Continental drift and evolution. **220**:54-64 (Mar.). *The breakup of early supercontinents in the past helps to explain the diversification of mammals.*

Landsberg, H.E. 1953. The origin of the atmosphere. **189**:82-85 (Aug.).

McNeil, M. 1964. Lateritic soils. **211**:97-102 (Nov.). *Soil in much of the tropics is protected by the native vegetation, but when this is cleared, the soil becomes hard and bricklike. This is a grave problem for agriculture in many Third World countries.*

Milne, L.J., and M. Milne. 1978. Insects of the water surface. **238**:134-142 (Apr.). *The surface of ponds creates a special environment for four types of insects.*

Revelle, R. 1982. Carbon dioxide and world climate. **247**:35-43 (Aug.). *Atmospheric carbon dioxide levels are increasing. What will be the effects?*

Welty, C. 1957. The geography of birds. **197**:118-126 (July). *Despite their mobility, most birds are confined to restricted zoogeographical regions.*

CHAPTER 41

ANIMAL ECOLOGY

Lesser flamingoes *Phoeniconaias minor* and other birds on Lake Nakuru, Kenya.
The enormous flamingo population, sometimes approaching 2 million birds, is entirely
supported by a cyanobacterium (blue-green alga) having a primary productivity
exceeding 10 g carbon/m²/day.

Photograph by B. Tallmark.

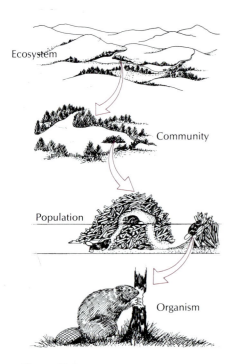

Life is confined largely to the interfaces between land, air, and water. It does not penetrate very far below the land surface, very high into the atmosphere, or very abundantly into the depths of the ocean. In the preceding chapter we defined where life does occur in the biosphere. Living things within the biosphere may be examined at several different levels of organization.

The most inclusive level of organization below the biosphere is the **ecosystem** (Fig. 41-1). An ecosystem is a complex, self-sustaining natural system of which living organisms are a part, together with the nonliving components. All the interactions that bind the living (**biotic**) and nonliving (**abiotic**) components together are included in the ecosystem. A particular ecosystem is usually defined by the investigator studying it, and it may be quite large, such as a grassland, a forest, a lake, or even an ocean, or it may be more restricted, such as a river bank or treehole. Whatever the size or the biological structures it contains, certain characteristics of any ecosystem can usually be described. The sun's energy is fixed by plants and then transferred to consumers and decomposers. Nutrients are cycled and recycled through the various living components of the ecosystem. No ecosystem is ever completely closed, however. There is always some flow of resources and organisms into and out of an ecosystem.

The next level of organization is the **community,** an assemblage of living organisms sharing the same environment and having a certain distinctive unity (Fig. 41-1). Communities comprise the living elements of an ecosystem. Like ecosystems, communities may be large or small, ranging from the coniferous forest community that may span a continent to the inhabitants of a rotting log community or the community of microorganisms living in a human's large intestine. The elements of a community are closely interdependent.

The **population,** the next lower level of organization, is an interbreeding group of organisms of the *same species* sharing a particular space. Every community is composed of several populations, including those of plants, animals, and microorganisms. Energy and nutrients flow through a population. Its size is regulated by its relationships to other populations in the community and by the abiotic characteristics of the ecosystem in which it is found. Because members of a population are interbreeding, they share a **gene pool** and thus are a distinct genetic unit.

The lowest level of organization within the biosphere, in ecological terms, is the **organism** itself. It is the living expression of the species. Each organism responds to its environment. To understand why animals are distributed as they are, ecologists must examine the varied mechanisms that animals use to compensate for environmental stresses and alterations.

Ecologists have, in fact, become increasingly interested in the physiological and behavioral mechanisms of animals. Both are intrinsic to the animal-habitat interrelationship. For example, the success of certain warm-blooded species under extreme temperature conditions such as in the Arctic or in a desert depends on near-perfect balance between heat production and heat loss and between appropriate insulation and special heat exchangers. Other species succeed in these situations by escaping the most extreme conditions by migration, hibernation, or torpidity. Insects, fishes, and other poikilotherms (animals having variable body temperature) compensate for temperature change by altering biochemical and cellular processes involving enzymes, lipid organization, and the neuroendocrine system. Thus, the physiological capacities with which the animal is endowed permit it to live under changing and often adverse environmental conditions. Physiological studies are necessary to answer the "how" questions of ecology.

The animal's behavioral responses are also part of the animal-habitat interaction and of interest to the ecologist. Behavior is involved in obtaining food, finding shelter, escaping enemies and unfavorable environments, finding a mate, courting, and caring for the young. Genetically determined mechanisms such as behavioral repertoires are acted on by natural selection. Those that improve adaptability to the environment assist in survival and the evolution of the species.

The term **ecology**, coined in the last century by the German zoologist Ernst Haeckel, is derived from the Greek *oikos*, meaning "house" or "place to live." Haeckel called ecology the "relation of the animal to its organic as well as inorganic environment." Although we no longer restrict ecology to animals alone, Haeckel's definition is still basically sound.

The term **environment** is frequently used in reference to the organism's immediate surroundings, but it is not always clear whether it is meant to include the living, as well as the nonliving, surroundings. To the ecologist it certainly includes both. Ultimately the environment consists of everything in the universe external to the organism. Since ecology is really biology of the environment, it obviously is a broad and far-flung field of study.

The ecologist may choose to focus on any level of organization within the biosphere. **Ecosystem analysis** is largely interdisciplinary, incorporating physics, chemistry, and other sciences to assist in the comprehension of the role of the environment in determining the distribution and abundance of organisms. **Community ecology** is similar but of more restricted scope; it is possible to focus on the interactions of a few species and to study energy transfers in detail. **Population biology** stresses genetics, evolution, seasonal changes, and other phenomena affecting population dynamics. Some ecologists study the organism itself (**organismic biology**) to see how it responds to the environment, hour by hour, day by day; such studies have become physiological and behavioral. All contribute to ecological understanding. None stands alone.

In the last several years the word "ecology" has come into popular misuse as a synonym for environment, which often makes biologists wince. As people concerned about the environment, we can be environmentalists; a person engaged in the scientific study of the relationship of organisms and their environment is an ecologist. He or she is usually an environmentalist too, but environment is not the same as ecology.

___ECOSYSTEM ECOLOGY

The abiotic component of an ecosystem can be characterized by its physical parameters such as temperature, moisture, light, and altitude and by its chemical features, which include various essential nutrients. These characteristics determine the basic nature of the ecosystem.

The biotic component—the populations of plants, animals, and microorganisms that form the communities of the ecosystem—may be categorized into producers, consumers, and decomposers. The **producers,** mostly green plants, are **autotrophs,** which use the energy of the sun to synthesize sugars from carbon dioxide by photosynthesis. This energy is made available to the **consumers** and **decomposers.** They are **heterotrophs,** which exploit the self-nourishing autotrophs by converting organic compounds of plants into compounds required for their own growth and activity. In this discussion we consider the flow of energy through the ecosystem, which involves the concepts of productivity and the food chain, biogeochemical cycling, and limiting factors within the environment.

Figure 41-2

Narrowing of spectrum of sunlight by atmospheric absorption and by absorption in seawater. The solid red line from top to bottom represents wavelengths of maximum intensity. Broken red lines locate the wavelength boundaries within which 90% of the solar energy is concentrated.

Modified from Wald, G. 1959. Life and light. Sci. Am. 201:92-108.

Solar Radiation and Photosynthesis

Virtually all life depends on the energy of the sun. The sun releases energy produced by the nuclear transmutation of hydrogen to helium. Solar radiation is received at the earth's surface in wavelengths of approximately 280 to 13,500 nm. Ultraviolet radiation with wavelengths of less than 280 nm is cut off sharply by the ozone layer in the upper atmosphere (Fig. 41-2). Radiation with wavelengths greater than 760 nm is long-wave infrared radiation that heats the atmosphere, warms the earth, and produces currents of air and water. The most important part of solar radiation is the wavelengths between 310 and 760 nm; this is the portion that we call **visible light** because of its effect on the human retina. It is also the range that drives all important photobiological processes, including photosynthesis, photochemical effects, phototropism (orientation of plants toward light), and animal vision.

The flow of energy through the ecosystem begins with **photosynthesis.** Energy enters the ecosystem as visible light; plants use it to produce adenosine triphosphate (ATP) and synthesize carbon compounds for themselves and for animals that feed on them. Although certain details of photosynthesis remain unknown, the major events can be outlined.

Light striking a green plant is absorbed by chlorophyll, sending low-energy electrons into a higher energy level. These excited electrons drop back to a ground state in approximately 10^{-7} seconds, but in this brief interval their energy is channeled into a sequence of energy-yielding reactions. Part of the energy is used to synthesize ATP; the remainder causes the reduction of pyridine nucleotides (NADP). Both ATP and reduced NADP are then used to synthesize sugars from

A   B

Figure 41-3

Animal communities near a Galápagos
Rift thermal vent, photographed at 2800
m (about 9000 feet) from the deep sub-
mersible *Alvin*. **A,** "Spaghetti worms"
(acorn worm of the phylum Hemichordata) lie in a tangled web across rocks. **B,**
Giant pogonophoran worms *Riftia pachyptila* grow in dense profusion among
rocks covered with mussels, limpets,
polychaete worms, and crabs. An unknown fish swims by.

A, Photograph by J. Childress, University of California,
Santa Barbara; **B,** photograph by J. Edmond, Massachusetts Institute of Technology.

carbon dioxide and water. Photosynthesis in the individual leaf begins at low light
intensity and increases at first linearly; that is, the rate of photosynthesis increases
as light intensity increases until it reaches a maximum.

The amount of solar energy that reaches the earth's atmosphere is estimated
at 15.3×10^8 gram calories per square meter each year (g cal/m^2/yr). Much of this
energy is dissipated by dust particles or consumed in the evaporation of water.
Only a very small fraction is used in the photosynthetic conversion of carbon
dioxide to carbohydrates. Calculated on an annual or growing season basis, the
photosynthetic efficiency of land area is approximately 0.3% and that of the
ocean approximately 0.13%. These estimates are low because they are based on
the total energy available for the year rather than on the growing season alone.
During brief intervals of very active growth, plants may store a maximum of 19%
of the available light energy.

Life without the Sun

Until recently it was believed that all animals depended directly or indirectly on
primary production from solar energy. Even benthic organisms of the deep sea
(abyssal) that live far below the depth to which light penetrates (200 to 300 m)
depend on the rain of organic debris from the sunlit world above. However, in
1977 and 1979, dense communities of animals were discovered living on the sea
floor adjacent to vents of hot water issuing from rifts (Galápagos Rift and East
Pacific Rise) where tectonic plates on the sea floor are slowly spreading apart.
These communities (Fig. 41-3) included several species of molluscs, some crabs,
polychaete worms, enteropneusts (acorn worms), and giant pogonophoran
worms (see marginal note on p. 444). The seawater above and immediately
around vents is 7° to 23° C where it is heated by basaltic intrusions, whereas the
surrounding normal seawater is 2° C.

It was immediately apparent that these vents must supply nutrients to support such a rich fauna. It was discovered that the producers in the vent communities are chemoautotrophic bacteria that derive energy from the oxidation of the
large amounts of hydrogen sulfide in the vent water and fix carbon dioxide into
organic carbon. Some of the animals in the vent communities, for example, the
bivalve molluscs, are filter feeders that ingest the bacteria. Others, such as the

giant pogonophoran tubeworms, which lack mouths and digestive tracts, harbor colonies of symbiotic bacteria in their tissues and use the organic carbon that these bacteria synthesize.

Thus, the deep-sea vent communities are self-contained, closed systems that depend entirely on energy issuing from the earth's interior. Each is a miniature ecosystem, altogether separate from other known ecosystems, all of which depend on solar energy and photosynthesis.

Production and the Food Chain

The energy accumulated by plants in photosynthesis is called **production.** Because it is the first step in the input of energy into the ecosystem, the *rate* of energy storage (that is, energy storage per unit of time) by plants is known as **primary productivity.** The total rate of energy storage, the **gross productivity,** is not entirely available for growth because plants also use energy for maintenance and reproduction. When this energy consumption, or plant **respiration,** is subtracted from the gross productivity, the **net primary productivity** remains. Plant growth results in the accumulation of plant **biomass.** Biomass is expressed as the *weight* of dry organic matter per unit of area and thus differs from productivity, which is the *rate* at which organic matter is formed by photosynthesis.

The level of productivity of different ecosystems depends on the availability of nutrients and the limitations of temperature levels and moisture availability. Highly productive ecosystems are floodplain forests, swamps and marshes, estuaries, coral reefs, and certain crop ecosystems (for example, rice and sugar cane). In such systems net production can exceed 3000 $g/m^2/yr$ of dry organic matter. Less productive (1000 to 2000 $g/m^2/yr$) ecosystems are most temperate forests, most agricultural crops, lakes and streams, and grasslands. Least productive (70 to 200 $g/m^2/yr$) ecosystems are tundra and alpine regions, deserts, and the open ocean. Extreme desert, rock, and ice regions have virtually zero productivity.

The net productivity of plants is the energy that supports almost all the rest of life on earth. Plants are eaten by consumers, which are themselves consumed by other consumers, and so on in a series of steps called the **food chain.** Food chains are descriptions of the way energy flows through the ecosystem. A diagram of a food chain shows arrows leading from one species to another, meaning that the first species is food for the second. But the first may be food for several other organisms as well. Seldom, in fact, does one organism live exclusively on another. Although some food chains are simple and short, for example, the one in which the whale feeds mainly on plankton, it is more common for several food chains to be interwoven into a complex **food web** (Fig. 41-4).

Despite their complexity, food chains tend to follow a pattern. Green plants, the base of the food chain, are eaten by grazing **herbivores,** which can convert the energy stored in plants into animal tissue. Herbivores may be eaten by small **carnivores** and these by large carnivores. There may be two or three, sometimes even four, levels of carnivores. At the end of the chain are the **top carnivores,** which, lacking predators, die and decompose, replenishing the soil with nutrients for plants that start the chain. At each level, beginning with the plants, are parasites, which qualify as herbivores or carnivores depending on whether they are parasites of plants or animals. They usually deprive their hosts of only insignificant amounts of energy, but other detrimental effects may be significant. Sometimes the parasites have parasites.

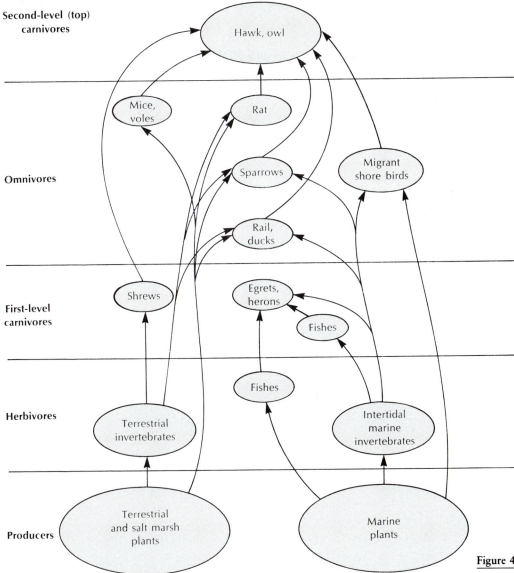

Second-level (top) carnivores

Omnivores

First-level carnivores

Herbivores

Producers

Hawk, owl

Mice, voles

Rat

Sparrows

Migrant shore birds

Rail, ducks

Shrews

Egrets, herons

Fishes

Fishes

Terrestrial invertebrates

Intertidal marine invertebrates

Terrestrial and salt marsh plants

Marine plants

Figure 41-4

A midwinter food web in a *Salicornia* (perennial glasswort) salt marsh of the San Francisco Bay area.

Modified from Smith, R.L. 1980. Ecology and field biology, ed. 3. New York, Harper & Row, Publishers, Inc.; after Johnston, R.F. 1956. Wilson Bull. **68:**91.

There are numerous examples of food chains. In the forest, for instance, many small insects (primary consumers) feed on plants (producers). A smaller number of spiders and carnivorous insects (secondary consumers) prey on small insects; still fewer birds (tertiary consumers) live on the spiders and carnivorous insects; and finally one or two hawks (quaternary or top consumers) prey on the birds.

The decomposers have traditionally been considered the final step in the herbivore-carnivore food chain, since they reduce organic matter into nutrients that become available again to the producers. Ecologists now recognize that the decomposers comprise their own distinct **detritus food chain,** consisting of **detritus feeders,** such as earthworms, mites, millipedes, crabs, aquatic worms, and molluscs, and **microorganisms,** such as bacteria and fungi. Dead organic matter, such as fallen leaves or dead animals, is decomposed and used by fungi, bacteria, and protozoa. Detritus feeders then eat the microorganisms as well as much of the dead organic matter directly. They are in turn eaten by small carnivores; the detritus food chain thus leads up into herbivore-carnivore food chains.

___ Ecological Pyramids

At each transfer within the food chain, 80% to 90% of the available energy is lost as heat. This limits the number of steps in the chain to four or five. Therefore the number of top consumers that can be supported by a given biomass of plants depends on the length of the chain.

"R.F.D.2."

Steve Stinson and Roanoke Times and World-News

Humans, who occupy a position at the end of the chain, may eat the grain that fixes the sun's energy; this very short chain represents an efficient use of the potential energy. Humans also may eat beef from animals that eat grass that fixes the sun's energy; the addition of a step in the chain decreases the available energy by an order of 10. In other words, it requires 10 times as much plant biomass to feed humans as meat eaters as to feed humans as grain eaters. Let us consider the person who eats the bass that eats the sunfish that eats the zooplankton that eats the phytoplankton that fixes the sun's energy. The 10-fold loss of energy occurring at each level in this five-step chain explains why bass do not form a very large part of the human diet. In this food chain, for a person to gain a pound by eating bass, the pond must produce 5 tons of phytoplankton biomass.

These figures must be considered as we look to the sea for food. The productivity of the oceans is very low and limited largely to regions of upwelling where nutrients are brought up and made available to the phytoplankton producers and to estuaries, marshes, and reefs. Such areas occupy only a small part of the ocean. The rest is a watery desert.

Ocean fisheries supply 18% of the world's protein, but most of this is used to supplement livestock and poultry feed. If we remember the rule of 10-to-1 loss in energy with each transfer of material, the use of fish as food for livestock rather than as food for humans is a poor use of a valuable resource in a protein-deficient world. Of the fishes that we do eat, the preference is for species such as flounder, tuna, and halibut, which are three or four steps up the food chain. Every 125 g of tuna requires 1 metric ton of phytoplankton food to produce. If humans are to derive greater benefit from the oceans as a food source in the future, we must eat more of the fishes that are lower in the food chain.

When we examine the food chain in terms of biomass at each level, it is apparent that we can construct **ecological pyramids** of numbers or of biomass. A pyramid of numbers (Fig. 41-5, *A*), also known as an **Eltonian pyramid** (after the British ecologist Charles Elton, who first devised the scheme), depicts the numbers of individual organisms that are transferred between each level in the food chain. Although providing a vivid impression of the great difference in numbers of organisms involved in each step of the chain, a pyramid of numbers does not indicate the actual weight of organisms at each level.

Figure 41-5

Ecological pyramids of numbers, biomass, and energy. Pyramids are generalized, since the area within each level is
not scaled proportionally to quantitative
differences in the units given.
Redrawn from Smith, R.L. 1980. Ecology and field biology, ed. 3. New York, Harper & Row, Publishers, Inc.; and
Odum, E.P. 1971. Fundamentals of ecology, ed. 3. Philadelphia, W.B. Saunders Co.

More instructive are pyramids of biomass (Fig. 41-5, *B*), which depict the
total bulk of organisms. Such pyramids usually slope upward because mass and
energy are lost at each transfer. However, in some aquatic ecosystems in which the
producers are the algae, which have short life spans and rapid turnover rates, the
pyramid is inverted. This happens because the algae can tolerate heavy exploitation by the zooplankton consumers. Therefore the base of the pyramid is smaller
than the biomass it supports.

A third type of pyramid is the pyramid of energy, which shows rate of energy
flow between levels (Fig. 41-5, *C*). An energy pyramid is never inverted because
less energy is transferred from each level than was put into it. A pyramid of energy
gives the best overall picture of community structure because each level reveals its
true importance in the community regardless of its biomass.

Nutrient Cycles

All of the elements essential for life are derived from the environment, where they
are present in the air, soil, rocks, and water. When plants and animals die and
their bodies decay, or when organic substances are burned or oxidized, the elements and inorganic compounds essential for life processes (nutrients) are released
and returned to the environment. Decomposers fulfill an essential role in this
process by feeding on plant and animal remains and on fecal material. The result is
that nutrients flow in a perpetual cycle between the biotic and abiotic components
of the ecosystem.

Nutrient cycles are often called **biogeochemical cycles** because they involve
exchanges between living organisms (bio-) and the rocks, air, and water of the

Figure 41-6

Nutrient cycles and energy flow in a terrestrial ecosystem. Note that nutrients are recycled, whereas energy flow *(red)* is one way.

earth's crust (geo-). Geochemistry is the discipline that deals with the chemical composition of the earth and the exchange of elements therein.

Nutrient and energy cycles are closely interrelated, since both influence the abundance of organisms in an ecosystem. However, unlike nutrients, which recirculate, energy flow follows one direction; it does not follow a cycle because it is lost as heat as it is used. The continuous input of energy from the sun keeps nutrients flowing and the ecosystem functioning. This interrelationship is depicted in Fig. 41-6. Among the most important biogeochemical cycles are those of carbon and nitrogen.

Carbon cycle

Carbon is the basic constituent of organic compounds and living tissue and is required by plants for the fixation of energy by photosynthesis. It is hardly necessary to emphasize the total dependence of life on the availability of this element. Carbon circulates between carbon dioxide (CO_2) gas in the atmosphere and living organisms through assimilation and respiration; it is also withdrawn into long-term reserves of fossil fuel deposits (humus and peat and finally coal and oil) (Fig. 41-7).

The cycling of carbon parallels and is linked to the flow of energy that begins with the fixation of energy during photosynthetic production. Plants synthesize glucose, a 6-carbon compound, from CO_2 that is withdrawn from the atmosphere; they then use this sugar to build higher carbohydrates, especially cellulose, the main structural carbohydrate of plants. Plants require 1.6 kg of CO_2 from the atmosphere for each kilogram of cellulose produced. The concentration of CO_2 in the atmosphere today is only 0.03%, in contrast to the relative abundance of atmospheric oxygen, 21% of air.

Two aspects of the low concentration of CO_2 require emphasis. The first is that CO_2 availability limits energy fixation by plants. Physiologists have shown

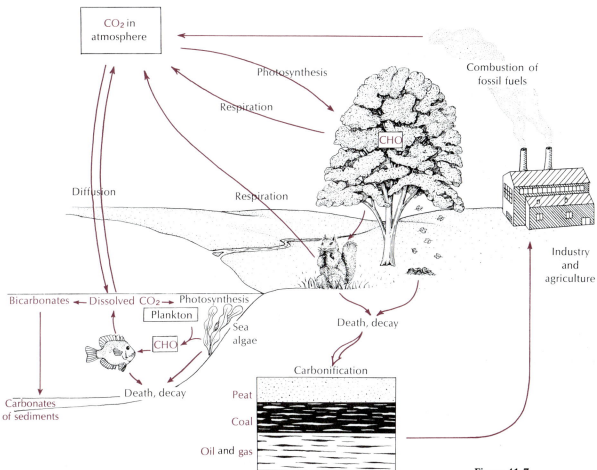

Figure 41-7

Carbon cycle showing circulation of carbon as carbon dioxide gas between living components of environment and long-term storage as fossil fuels.

that, if the atmospheric CO_2 is increased by 10%, plant photosynthesis increases 5% to 8%.

The second point is that there has been a tremendous increase in the consumption of fossil fuels by humans in the last two decades. More than 10 billion tons of CO_2 enters the atmosphere each year from industrial and agricultural activities; of this 75% comes from burning fossil fuels and 25% from the release of CO_2 from soil because of frequent plowing (a surprising and unappreciated effect of agricultural practice). Some authorities argue that the input of CO_2 into the atmosphere by human activities is not really chemical pollution, since the increase is removed by photosynthesis or by precipitation as carbonates in the ocean. There is concern, however, that even small increases in CO_2, which traps radiated heat, may increase the temperature of the earth's biosphere (p. 999).

Nitrogen cycle

Like carbon, nitrogen (N_2) is a basic and essential constituent of living material, particularly in proteins and nucleic acids. Despite the high concentration of N_2 in the atmosphere (78% of air), it is almost totally unavailable to life forms in its gaseous state. The nitrogen cycle converts N_2 into a chemical form that living organisms can use. This conversion is called **nitrogen fixation.** Some atmospheric N_2 is fixed by lightning, which produces ammonia and nitrates that are carried to earth by rain and snow. But at least 10 times as much N_2 is biologically fixed by bacteria and blue-green algae (Fig. 41-8).

Figure 41-8

Nitrogen cycle showing circulation of nitrogen between organisms and through environment *(red)*. Microorganisms responsible for key conversions are indicated in circles and boxes.

Most important in terrestrial systems are bacteria associated with legumes (members of the pea family), whose nitrogenous contribution to soil enrichment is well known. The old agricultural practice of allowing fields to lie fallow (without crops) for a season every few years enabled N_2 fixers to replenish the element in a usable form. Aerobic rhizobia bacteria produce nodules on the roots of legumes in which molecular N_2 is converted to ammonia and nitrates, which plants can use to build protein. Plant proteins are transferred to consumers, which build their own proteins from the amino acids supplied. Plants' and animals' waste products (urea and excreta) and their ultimate decomposition provide for the return of organic nitrogen to the substrate. Then decomposers break down proteins, freeing ammonia, which is used by bacteria in a series of steps as shown in Fig. 41-8. Finally nitrate (NO_3^-) is produced, which may be used once again by plants or may be degraded to inorganic nitrogen by denitrifying bacteria and returned to the atmosphere. Nitrates also are carried by runoff to streams and lakes and eventually to the sea. A cycle similar to this terrestrial cycle occurs in aquatic ecosystems except that there is a steady loss of nitrogen to deep-sea sediments.

The nitrogen cycle is a near-perfect, self-regulating cycle in which losses in one phase are balanced by gains in another. There is little absolute change in nitrogen in the biosphere as a whole. However, human activities have caused steady losses of soil nitrogen by slowing natural addition of organic nitrogen through current agricultural practice and by the harvesting of timber. The latter causes an especially heavy outflow, from both timber removal and soil disturbance.

COMMUNITIES

Communities represent the most tangible concept in ecology. We are all familiar with the differences between forest, grassland, desert, and salt marsh, and we have little trouble picturing, at least in a general way, the kinds of plant and animal communities associated with each of these ecosystems. Communities comprise the *biotic* portion of the ecosystem; each consists of a certain combination of species that forms a functional unit. Although communities are sometimes difficult to define because the assemblages of species within similar communities are not always the same, communities do exist, and they all possess a number of attributes. It is beyond the scope of this book to discuss all the aspects of community form and function. In this discussion we examine two important principles that operate in community organization.

Ecological Dominance

Biological communities are typically dominated by a single species or limited group of species that greatly influences the nature of the local environment. All other species in that community must adapt to conditions created by the dominants. Communities often are named for the dominant organisms, for example, black spruce forest, beech-maple forest, oyster community, and coral reef. It is not always easy to specify just what constitutes a dominant organism. It may be the most numerous, the largest, or the most productive, or it may in some other manner exert the greatest influence on the rest of the community. In a woodland a tree obviously means more to the community than a poison ivy plant (even though a casual visitor may carry away a more lasting impression of the poison ivy).

Dominant species are often so because they occupy space that might otherwise be occupied by other species. When a dominant species is eliminated for some reason, the community changes. The American chestnut once dominated large regions of the eastern United States, where it comprised more than 40% of the overstory trees in climax deciduous forests. After the invasion in 1900 of the chestnut blight (a fungus), which was apparently brought into New York City on nursery stock from Asia, the chestnut was eliminated from its entire range within a few years (Fig. 41-9). The chestnut position was filled by oak, hickory, beech, and red maple, and chestnut-oak forests became oak and oak-hickory forests. Tree squirrel populations that relied on chestnuts as their major food decreased to a small fraction of their former abundance.

The appearance of the forests changed. To the subdominant species, whose specialized environmental requirements were attuned to the particular conditions of a chestnut forest, the change required adjustments that some could not meet. The shift in dominance produced changes throughout the community.

Ecological Niche Concept

An animal's position in the environment is characterized by more than the habitat in which we expect to find it; it also has a "profession," a special role in life that distinguishes it from all other species. This is its **niche,** which Elton defined as the animal's place in the biotic environment, that is, what it does and its relation to its food and its enemies. The niche concept has now been broadened to include an

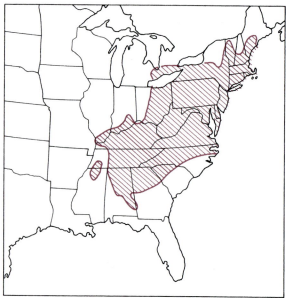

Figure 41-9

American chestnut tree *Castanea dentata* and its original distribution in North America. Photograph taken circa 1900.

Map from Krebs, C.J. 1972. Ecology, New York, Harper & Row, Publishers, Inc.

animal's position in time and space and its relation to all abiotic factors in the environment. The expression "every animal has its niche" conveys the idea well.

It is an accepted rule that no two species can occupy the same niche at the same time and place. If they did, they would be in direct competition for exactly the same food and space. Should this happen, one species would have to diverge into a different niche, move to a different habitat, or face extinction.

Related populations that live in the same geographical area are called **sympatric** (meaning literally "same country") species, as opposed to **allopatric** ("different country") species that occupy different locations. Sympatric species might be expected to have similar niches and be in danger of direct competition. This can be avoided in a number of ways, as the following examples illustrate.

In parts of eastern and southern Africa the two species of rhinoceros, the black and the white, are sympatric: they share the same habitat. However, the black rhinoceros is a browser, feeding on leaves and woody plants, whereas the white rhinoceros is a grazer, eating grasses and herbs. They do not compete for the same food, and consequently they occupy distinct ecological niches.

The three species of boobies of the Galápagos Islands—the white, blue-footed, and red-footed—offer a second example. All three are plunge divers that feed on the same kinds of marine fish frequenting the ocean around the islands. The blue-footed booby, however, always fishes close to the shore; the white booby flies a mile or two from land to fish; and the red-footed booby makes long hunting forays many miles from shore. Again, although sympatric, they do not compete

Figure 41-10

Mutualism (or protocooperation) between African Cape buffalo and cattle egret. Egrets benefit by feeding on parasites embedded in buffaloes' skin and on insects disturbed by buffaloes as they graze. Buffaloes in turn are rid of pests and warned of approaching danger when watchful egrets take to the air in noisy flight.

Photograph by L.L. Rue, III.

for the same food. The three species have divided up the food resources so that a different portion of the sea becomes the undisputed hunting territory of each species. This is an example of **niche diversification.**

The niche concept is a fundamental one to the biologist because it explains how animals avoid endless struggles with other animals. A species and its niche are reflections of the same thing: a unique way of life. A species is master of its own niche and thus is not in direct competition with similar species, even though competition was used to decide the boundaries of the niche in the first place. This concept was discussed in Chapter 38, p. 959.

POPULATIONS

A population is a group of organisms belonging to the same species that shares a particular space. Whether the population is gray squirrels in an eastern woods or bluegill sunfish in a farm fishpond, it bears a number of attributes unique to the group. A population shares a common gene pool; it has a certain density, birth rate, death rate, age ratio, and reproductive potential; and it grows and differentiates much like the individual organisms of which it is composed.

Population Interactions

Populations in a community may affect each other in various ways, although in certain cases there may be no apparent interaction (**neutral** effect). One interaction, **competition,** has already been mentioned. Although it is true that two populations cannot occupy the same niche at the same time and place, some degree of competition often occurs in natural populations. Because natural selection favors decreased competition, this often leads to niche diversification, such as the three species of boobies in the Galápagos Islands. Another adaptation may be that the two populations use the same resource but at different times of the year. One population may be excluded by a superior competitor from a habitat it could otherwise occupy. When two such populations occupy adjacent habitats, competition may be intense along the border between them.

Another interaction is the **predator-prey** relationship, in which individuals of one population kill and feed on individuals in the prey population. Often a population is preyed on by more than one species of predator, and predators commonly have more than one prey species. Predators are large relative to their prey, and they usually consume several to many prey animals in their lifetime. A conceptually related interaction is the **parasite-host** relationship. Both parasites and predators feed at the expense of their host-prey. However, parasites are small relative to their hosts, and parasites have only one host—at least at a given stage in their life cycle. In most cases, parasites do not kill their hosts because, if the host dies, the parasite perishes along with it. Most parasites are **symbiotic;** that is, they live in (**endoparasites**) or on (**ectoparasites**) the body of their host. Organisms such as mosquitoes and biting flies are intermediate between parasites and predators as we have defined them; they are sometimes referred to as **micropredators** or **intermittent parasites.**

Another type of interaction that is sometimes symbiotic is **commensalism,** in which the commensal enjoys some benefit from the relationship but does not harm the host. Some cases of commensalism grade into **mutualism,** an interaction in which both species are benefitted (Fig. 41-10). Mutualism has been recognized in

Most people are aware that lions, tigers, and wolves are predators, but the world of invertebrates also includes predaceous animals. These range from protozoa, jellyfish and their relatives, and various worms to predaceous insects, starfish, and many others. Examples of parasites include many bacteria, protozoa (such as those causing malaria and African sleeping sickness), tapeworms, roundworms, ticks and mites, and insects. Humans have many commensal bacteria, and often protozoa, living in the intestines. There are a large number of other cases of commensalism, especially in marine ecosystems, of which the association of pilot fishes and remoras with sharks is a classic example. These fish get the "crumbs" left over when the host makes its kill, but we now know that some remoras also feed on ectoparasites of the sharks; thus, they grade into mutualism. An often-cited case of mutualism is that of the termite and the protozoa living in its gut. The protozoa can digest the wood eaten by the termite, although the termite cannot, and the termite lives on the waste products of the protozoa metabolism. In return, the protozoa gain a congenial place to live and a food supply. Less obvious examples of mutualism would include flowering plants that are pollinated by insects, which are furnished with a nectar food by the plant, and the association of humans with their domestic animals and plants, although these might be considered protocooperation.

Carrying capacity

Number of individuals

Time ⟶

Figure 41-11

Population growth curve.

The logistic equation for a population growth curve may be written as follows:

$$\frac{dN}{dt} = \frac{rN(K - N)}{K}$$

where N = number of individuals in the population, t = units of time, r = a constant, intrinsic rate of increase of the population, and K = a constant, the carrying capacity of the environment.

Without further explanation of the mathematics of this equation, it is clear that when N exceeds K, r becomes negative, and the numbers in the population will decline. The ultimate result, if the situation continues, is extinction of the population.

recent years as much more prevalent in the animal kingdom than previously believed. Many cases of mutualistic interactions are symbiotic, but many are not. Some investigators prefer to distinguish **protocooperation** from mutualism. Protocooperation describes mutually beneficial interactions that are not physiologically necessary to the survival of the partners.

Population Growth

Living organisms have reproductive potential beyond that required for replacement of their numbers, some far in excess of such requirement. Some female insects lay thousands of eggs, field mice can produce as many as 17 litters of four to seven young each year, and a single female codfish may spawn 6 million eggs per season. It has been calculated that a bacterium dividing three times per hour would produce a colony a foot deep over the entire earth in 1½ days, and the colony would be over our heads 1 hour later. The growth potential of a population, the so-called biotic potential rate, never proceeds unchecked indefinitely because of the limitations of the environment. Most populations reach a certain level and then fluctuate about the level. What keeps populations in check? How is the "balance of nature" explained?

If numbers of individuals are plotted on a graph against units of time, a growth curve of the population may be derived. The growth curve of a population with limited resources will be sigmoid in shape (Fig. 41-11). In the beginning, with ample space and abundant food, the starting population breeds and grows as fast as its reproductive potential allows. As births exceed deaths, and more animals join the reproductive population, the increase is exponential. But, as the environmental resistance increases, commonly because of a depletion of food and space, the growth rate decreases as the upper population limit is approached. The simple sigmoid curve can be demonstrated easily with populations in the laboratory (bacteria, protozoa, and some insects), but the situation in nature is usually more complex. Annual plankton blooms in ponds and lakes, eruptions of insect pests, and growth of weeds in old fields may demonstrate the sigmoid population growth curve.

Construction of mathematical models to describe population dynamics can be valuable, both to predict population behavior over periods of time and the outcome of artificial manipulations of the populations, and to discover heretofore unknown biological principles.

The sigmoid population growth curve can be described by the so-called logistic equation and is an example of a simple mathematical model. The mathematics of the logistic equation are not necessary for our discussion here, but some of its terms are useful for our understanding. The intrinsic rate of increase, r, is the difference between births and deaths. With any positive r, the rate of increase will be exponential. With a negative r (more deaths than births), the population will decrease. The carrying capacity of the environment is referred to as K. When populations first approach K, they may overshoot and crash (mass mortality caused by depletion of resources), or they may decline and then oscillate about the carrying capacity.

For example, when sheep were introduced on the island of Tasmania around 1800, their growth was represented by a sigmoid curve with a small overshoot, followed by mild oscillations around a final population size of 1,700,000 sheep (Fig. 41-12, *A*). A similar pattern but with larger fluctuations was recorded for a

A   **Growth of a sheep population introduced into an island**

Carrying capacity

B   **Growth curve for ring-necked pheasant on an island**

Carrying capacity

C   **World population growth curve**

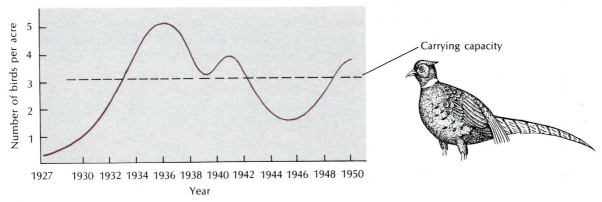

Human population growth

Black death, 1348

1976

Figure 41-12

Growth curves for, **A**, sheep, **B**, ring-necked pheasant, and, **C**, human populations.

population of ring-necked pheasants introduced on an island in Ontario, Canada (Fig. 41-12, *B*).

The growth of the human population was slow for a very long time. For most of their evolutionary history, humans were hunters and gatherers who depended on and were limited by the natural productivity of the environment. With the development of agriculture, the carrying capacity of the environment increased, and the population grew steadily from 5 million around 8000 BC, when agriculture was introduced, to 16 million around 4000 BC. Despite the toll taken by terrible famines, disease, and war, the population reached 500 million by 1650.

With the coming of the Industrial Revolution in Europe and England in the eighteenth century, followed by a medical revolution, discovery of new lands for colonization, and better agriculture practices, the carrying capacity of the earth for humans increased dramatically. The population doubled to 1 billion around 1850. It doubled again to 2 billion by 1930 and to 4 billion in 1976. Thus, the growth has been exponential and remains high (Fig. 41-12, C).

However, recent surveys provide hope that the world population growth is slackening. In just 5 years (1970 to 1975) the annual growth rate decreased from 1.9% to 1.64%. At 1.64%, it will take 42 years for the world population to double rather than 36 years at the higher annual growth rate figure. The decrease is credited to better family planning programs, but increasing deaths from starvation and disease also are contributing factors.

Unlike other animals, which can do little to increase the carrying capacity of their environment, humans have done so repeatedly. Unfortunately, when the carrying capacity is increased, humans respond as would any animal by increasing their population. Because the earth's resources are finite, the time will inevitably come when the carrying capacity can be extended no further. The question is whether humans will be able to anticipate this limit and check population growth in time or whether we will overshoot the resources and experience a crash. Indeed, for millions of Third World people time has already run out. The rapid population growth is not something that thinking people view with equanimity.

—— How Population Growth Is Curbed

What determines the number of animals in a natural population? For a laboratory culture of animals the answer seems fairly clear. They grow until they reach K, at which point growth is suppressed by competition for the limited resources of space and food. Thus, the forces that limit growth arise from within the population; they are **density-dependent** mechanisms caused by crowding. Food and space limitations are commonly observed density-dependent factors, but others, such as disease and predation, may operate as well.

In wild populations, competitive limitations may be due to crowding within the species (**infraspecific**) or competition with another species (**interspecific**) with an overlapping niche. The population growth of both species may be roughly according to the logistic equation, but the K for each is lowered, making necessary the introduction of additional terms in the mathematical model.

Crowding promotes other agents of death that help to regulate populations. Transmission of infectious **disease** may be much higher under crowded conditions, so that much higher mortality resulting from parasitism occurs than would prevail at lower population densities. Epidemics may sweep through crowded populations as did the terrible bubonic plague (black death) through the crowded, dirty cities of Europe in the fourteenth century. **Predation** increases when prey becomes abundant and easy to catch, and larger populations of prey are often followed by an increase in the predator populations. **Shelter** for suitable nest sites and as refuge from bad weather becomes less available with crowding.

The continuous competition for food and space to live brings forth yet another density-dependent force: **stress.** Although the physiology of stress is not thoroughly understood, there is ample evidence that, when certain natural populations become crowded, such as populations of lemmings, voles, and snowshoe hares, a neuroendocrine imbalance involving the pituitary and adrenal glands appears. Growth is suppressed. Reproduction fails, and individuals become irritable and aggressive. Under such conditions snowshoe hares suffer from a lethal "shock disease" that results in a population crash.

Overcrowding may also cause **emigration** away from the birth area. Overcrowded mice increase their locomotor activity and begin to explore new areas. In the case of lemmings, overpopulation produces the famous mass "marches" recorded at intervals in Scandinavia. When songbird populations become overcrowded, the less successful become "vagabond" birds that are forced out into less preferred habitats. Emigration is one major force resulting in the colonization of new habitats. The rapid dispersal of the European starling throughout the United States and southern Canada, following its introduction into New York City in 1890, is an excellent example (p. 628).

Not all of the forces that limit growth are density dependent. Extreme changes in the weather or unusually cold, hot, wet, or dry weather is a **density-independent** hazard of varying severity to animal populations. Local insect populations are sometimes pushed to the point of extinction by a severe winter. Hurricanes and volcanic eruptions may destroy entire populations. Hailstorms have been known to kill most of the young of wading-bird populations. Prairie grass and forest fires kill everything unable to escape.

Ecologists have distinguished between organisms whose populations are controlled more by density-dependent factors and those controlled by density-independent factors. Organisms with a range of adaptations to survive density-dependent control are called K-selected (from the K term in the logistic equation), and those with adaptations for density-independent control are r-selected (from the r term). In natural populations of various species, there is a continuum of highly r-selected to highly K-selected, and the terms are relative; that is, species A may be r-selected with respect to species B and K-selected compared with species C. Nevertheless, certain characteristics of each can be recognized. Organisms that are r-selected generally have very high reproductive rates, high (often catastrophic) mortality, short life, and population sizes variable in time, usually well below the carrying capacity of the environment, whereas K-selected organisms have the opposite characteristics. K-selected populations tend to be comprised of larger, long-lived individuals able to compete in crowded circumstances (N close to K), not making a heavy commitment to reproduction because that would reduce the chance of individual survival. Populations that are r-selected can rapidly exploit an unstable environment before better competitors arrive, producing large numbers of young that disperse quickly and increase the chances that at least a few will find another favorable place to grow. All such characteristics are genetically determined and are the products of relentless natural selection over the millenia.

Thus, population numbers are influenced by factors generated within the population and by forces from without, and usually no single mechanism can account fully for how growth is curbed in a given population. Natural populations are controlled by density-dependent and density-independent forces. Humans are the greatest force of all. By altering animal habitats we change the balances that set the old limits to animal numbers. Our activities can increase or exterminate whole populations of animals.

K-selected species are often known as K-strategists, and r-selected organisms as r-strategists. For many r-strategists the carrying capacity of the environment for the adults is rarely reached because the mortality of the progeny is so high. This is true for many marine organisms that produce enormous numbers of offspring. Many parasites are r-strategists; unless the hosts are crowded, transmission to a new host may be hazardous, and the reproductive capacity of the parasite is high to offset this loss. Examples of r-strategists among plants would include the annual weeds that quickly colonize disturbed ground, reproduce, and disperse their seed before perennial species can mature, shading and crowding out the annuals, thus altering and stabilizing the environment.

Redwood forest.
Photograph by L.L. Rue, III.

Summary

The most inclusive level of environmental organization below the biosphere is the ecosystem, which includes interacting biotic and abiotic components. The biotic components are communities of various species of organisms, each species being comprised of a population, and each population being the sum of the individual organisms that share a gene pool.

Energy flows into the ecosystem as sunlight. Nearly all life depends on the conversion of that energy into organic compounds by the fixation of carbon dioxide in green plants. Recently, however, rich communities of animal life have been discovered to be associated with deep-sea thermal vents. These vent communities, which are supported by chemoautotrophic bacteria, are the only animal communities known to be completely independent of solar energy.

Food chains of producers (plants) and consumers (herbivores and carnivores) may be recognized, but in nature, complex food webs exist. Ecological pyramids can be constructed to show the decrease in numbers of individuals, biomass, and energy at each level of the food chain. Nutrients, such as carbon, nitrogen, and other elements, are cycled and recycled in the ecosystem. Each community is usually dominated by one or a few species that greatly influence the nature of the local environment. Each species has its own niche, or the role it plays in the ecosystem. Populations in the community may have no interaction (neutral), or they may interact as competitors, predators and prey, parasites and hosts, commensals, mutuals, or protocooperators.

Populations introduced into an environment where there is an upper limit to resources usually grow in a manner that can be described by a sigmoid curve; at first, when food and space are not limiting, the growth is exponential, and then the curve levels off as the carrying capacity of the environment is reached. The curve can be expressed mathematically as the logistic equation. This equation takes into account the intrinsic rate of increase of the population (r) and the carrying capacity of the environment (K). Species of organisms can be categorized as to their adaptations to survive their mechanisms of population growth regulation. Species whose populations approach K and are regulated by density-dependent factors are K-selected, and species that generally do not approach K and are regulated by density-independent factors are r-selected. Populations that are r-selected are opportunists, quickly moving into an unstable environment and producing large numbers of progeny before better competitors arrive. Density-dependent mechanisms of population control include competition, disease, and predation; density-independent mechanisms include extreme weather, abrupt environmental change, and hazardous conditions for the progeny with accompanying high mortality.

Selected references

Allee, W.C., A.E. Emerson, O. Park, T. Park, and K.P. Schmidt. 1949. Principles of animal ecology. Philadelphia, W.B. Saunders Co. *A valuable comprehensive text and reference, although dated.*

Andrewartha, H.G. 1970. Introduction to the study of animal populations. Chicago, University of Chicago Press. *A summary of the classic 1954 text by Andrewartha and Birch.*

Bates, M. 1960. The forest and the sea. New York, Random House, Inc. *Several editions available. Excellent general approach to ecology. Highly recommended.*

Colinvaux, P.A. 1973. Introduction to ecology. New York, John Wiley & Sons, Inc. *Highly readable and interesting approach to general ecology. Stresses population ecology.*

Colinvaux, P.A. 1978. Why big fierce animals are rare: an ecologist's perspective. Princeton, N.J., Princeton University Press. *A personal and engagingly written view of ecology.*

Dasmann, R.F. 1981. Wildlife biology, ed. 2. New York, John Wiley & Sons, Inc. *Brief, well-written primer of ecological principles applied to mammals and birds.*

Ehrlich, P.R., A.H. Ehrlich, and J.P. Holdren. 1977. Ecoscience: population, resources, environment. San Francisco, W.H. Freeman & Co. Publishers. *Well-written approach to human ecology.*

Elton, C.S. 1927. Animal ecology. London, Sidgwick & Jackson. *This classic contains many insights and is still worth reading.*

Henderson, L.J. 1913. The fitness of the environment (reprint). Boston, Beacon Press. *A classic that should still be read.*

Hutchinson, G.E. 1978. An introduction to population ecology. New Haven, Conn., Yale University Press. *Population ecology with a minimum of mathematics. Clear examples and numerous historical diversions.*

Ito, Y. 1980. Comparative ecology (translated by J. Kikkawa). Cambridge, Eng., Cambridge University Press. *Population and behavioral ecology.*

Krebs, C.J. 1978. Ecology: experimental analysis of distribution and abundance, ed. 2. New York, Harper & Row, Publishers, Inc. *Important treatment of population ecology.*

Leopold, A. 1949. A Sand County almanac. New York, Oxford University Press, Inc. *Several editions available. A beautiful account by a great conservationist; now a favorite of the environmental movement.*

MacArthur, R.H. 1972. Geographical ecology. New York, Harper & Row, Publishers, Inc. *One of the most important and influential books of recent years.*

Odum, E.P. 1983. Basic ecology. Philadelphia, Saunders College/Holt, Rinehart & Winston. *This is the author's successful* Fundamentals of Ecology *trimmed and updated.*

Remmert, H. 1980. Ecology: a textbook. Berlin, Springer-Verlag. *Clear presentation of basic principles, with good examples.*

Ricklefs, R.E. 1979. Ecology, ed. 2. New York, Chiron Press. *Respected, readable, broad-ranging general ecology text with solid evolutionary approach.*

Smith, R.L. 1980. Ecology and field biology, ed. 3. New York, Harper & Row, Publishers, Inc. *Comprehensive, clearly written, well-illustrated general ecology text. An excellent summary follows each chapter.*

Selected *Scientific American* articles

Beddington, J.R., and R.M. May. 1982. The harvesting of interacting species in a natural ecosystem. 247:62-69 (Nov.). *Heavy harvesting of animals from the southern ocean provides a testing ground for management of a resource.*

Bell, R.H.V. 1971. A grazing ecosystem in the Serengeti. 225:86-93 (July). *The migration of grazers across Tanzania is synchronized with the availability of specific tissues of grasses.*

Bolin, B. 1970. The carbon cycle. 223:124-132 (Sept.).

Bormann, F.H., and G.E. Likens. 1970. The nutrient cycles of an ecosystem. 223:92-101 (Oct.).

Cloud, P., and A. Gibor, 1970. The oxygen cycle. 223:110-123 (Sept.).

Coale, A.J. 1974. The history of the human population. 231:40-51 (Sept.). *The relative stability of the human population was due to the balance of high birth and death rates until about 200 years ago, when death rates began to fall.*

Cole, L.C. 1958. The ecosphere. 198:83-92 (Apr.).

Deevey, E.S., Jr. 1970. Mineral cycles. 223:148-158 (Sept.).

Delwiche, C.C. 1970. The nitrogen cycle. 223:136-146 (Sept.).

Denison, W.C. 1973. Life in tall trees. 228:75-80 (June). *The interesting ecosystem of the high forest canopy, where entire communities of plants and animals live.*

Freedman, R., and B. Berelson. 1974. The human population. 231:30-39 (Sept.). *The present rapid growth in the human population cannot last much longer. Will it level off because of higher death rates or lower birth rates?*

Gates, D.M. 1971. The flow of energy in the biosphere. 224:88-100 (Sept.). *Plants capture only a fraction of the solar energy that falls on the earth, but this fraction maintains all life.*

Janick, J., C.H. Noller, and C.L. Rhykerd. 1976. The cycles of plant and animal nutrition. 235:74-86 (Sept.). *Energy and nutrients of human consumption are processed by chains of organisms.*

Koehl, M.A.R. 1982. The interaction of moving water and sessile organisms. 247:124-134 (Dec.). *Adaptations of animals living in heavy currents.*

Myers, J.H., and C.J. Krebs. 1974. Population cycles in rodents. 230:38-46 (June). *The cyclical rise and fall in rodent populations are associated with genetic changes in the population.*

Wynne-Edwards, V.C. 1964. Population control in animals. 211:68-74 (Aug.).

CHAPTER 42

ANIMALS IN THE HUMAN ENVIRONMENT

The Still Hunt by James Henry Moser. This painting was commissioned for the Smithsonian Institution and was first displayed at the 1888 Cincinnati Exhibition as part of a crusade to save the bison from extinction. Although vast herds like this no longer existed in 1888—the bison was already an endangered species—many who had crossed the prairies in the first half of the nineteenth century attested to the painting's authenticity. Market hunters such as the one portrayed commonly shot more than 100 bison from a single position before moving on.

Courtesy Mammoth Museum, Yellowstone National Park.

In 1846, 23-year-old Francis Parkman, guided by a desire to study American Indians and haunted by images of a western wilderness yet unseen, began a journey westward on the Oregon Trail. Near the Platte River in what is now Nebraska, he described the prairie scene that unfolded before him while he rode back to camp after a furious buffalo chase.*

> The face of the country was dotted far and wide with countless hundreds of buffalo. They trooped along in files and columns, bulls, cows, and calves, on the green faces of the declivities in front. They scrambled away over the hills to the right and left; and far off, the pale swells in the extreme distance were dotted with innumerable specks. Sometimes I surprised shaggy old bulls grazing alone, or sleeping behind the ridges I ascended. They would leap up at my approach, stare stupidly at me through their tangled manes, and then gallop heavily away. The antelope were very numerous, and as they are always bold when in the neighborhood of buffalo, they would approach to look at me, gaze intently with their great round eyes, then suddenly leap aside, and stretch lightly away over the prairie, as swiftly as a race horse. Squalid, ruffian-like wolves sneaked through the hollows and sandy ravines. Several times I passed through villages of prairie dogs, who sat, each at the mouth of his burrow, holding his paws before him in a supplicating attitude, and yelping away most vehemently, whisking his little tail with every squeaking cry he uttered. Prairie dogs are not fastidious in their choice of companions; various long checkered snakes were sunning themselves in the midst of the village, and demure little gray owls, with a large white ring around each eye, were perched side by side with the rightful inhabitants. The prairie teemed with life.

When the first British settlements were founded in Virginia and Massachusetts, there could not have been fewer than 60 million bison, inaccurately called buffalo *(Bison bison)*, roaming the American wilderness. The two recognized subspecies, *B.b. bison*, the plains bison, and the somewhat larger and darker wood bison, *B.b. athabascae*, extended from northwestern Canada to Mexico and from the Rocky Mountains to the Atlantic seaboard from New York to Florida (Fig. 42-1). On the great plains, where their domain was most secure, the bison made enormous annual migrations in vast herds numbering millions of animals. In the spring they moved northward to graze on new grass that had sprung up behind the retreating snow; in autumn they returned southward. Late eighteenth- and early nineteenth-century observers recorded moving herds of bison covering areas of several square miles so densely that nowhere was the ground visible. Because they were nomadic, bison did not overgraze the land despite their incredible numbers. There was also ample herbage to feed the numerous antelopes and prairie dogs observed by Parkman. The bison population easily sustained losses inflicted from predation by their natural enemies—the wolves, grizzly bears, and pumas—and even the hunting pressure by Indians had very little effect on their numbers.

To the Plains Indians the bison were providers of virtually every necessity of life. The high-quality meat was eaten fresh or was dried, pounded, and stored as pemmican for future use. The skins provided homes, clothing, moccasins, and warm robes. The rawhide was turned into saddles, ropes, and quivers, and the sinews became bowstrings. Spoons and other utensils were carved out of the horns; hooves were reduced to glue; and the ribs became scrapers and sled runners.

The bison culture of the Plains Indians reached full flower in the seventeenth and eighteenth centuries after the Indians acquired horses, which had been introduced into North America by the Spaniards at the end of the sixteenth century. With their new mobility, hunting became easier, and the tribes could follow the

*Parkman, F. 1931. The Oregon Trail. New York, Farrar & Rinehart.

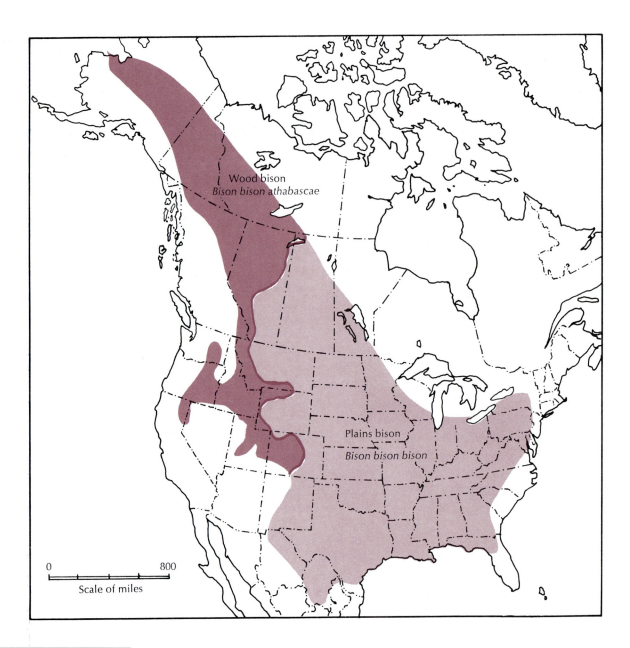

Figure 42-1

Distribution of American bison before the arrival of Europeans in North America.

From Hall, E.R., and K.R. Kelson. 1959. The mammals of North America. New York, The Ronald Press Co.

bison migrations, carrying all their belongings with them. When rifles were introduced to the Indians by white traders along the Missouri, Platte, and Arkansas rivers, hunting pressure increased substantially, but even this made few inroads on the total bison population because the Indian population was low.

In eastern America the rapid westward advance of pioneers was accompanied by decimation of the bison. By 1810 no bison remained east of the Mississippi. Their extinction clearly portended the ultimate fate of the plains bison. In 1846, when Parkman traveled the Oregon Trail, the bison were restricted to the western plains and mountains, although there were still probably 30 million left. The final act in the great bison slaughter began in the mid-nineteenth century. Congress in 1864 authorized the building of the Union Pacific Railroad across the heart of the continent, directly through the bison range. Thousands of hunters moved over the plains, killing bison to feed the huge construction gangs. As the railroad penetrated westward, "buffalo" robes and tongues, the latter considered a delicacy in the East, were collected and shipped east by rail. The carcasses were

Figure 42-2

Huge stacks of skulls and other bones representing approximately 25,000 bison await shipment beside a Saskatchewan railway siding in 1890. For a brief period following the bison slaughter, bones collected from the prairies were shipped east to be ground into fertilizer.

From Hewitt, C.G. 1921. The conservation of wildlife of Canada. New York, The Scribner Book Companies, Inc.

left to rot on the ground. Hunting pressure reached its zenith in the early 1870s when some 4 million bison were killed each year.

Contributing to the slaughter were thousands of soldiers instructed to kill bison in order to starve out the Plains Indians. By 1883 the annihilation was virtually complete, except for a single herd of about 10,000 animals in North Dakota. In September of that year, hunters were sent to North Dakota, and by guarding all available water holes, they destroyed the last free herd of bison (Fig. 42-2).

Those who protested the destruction were ignored by politicians, who believed it to be a justifiable means to deprive the Plains Indians of a way of life. Fortunately, small groups of semidomesticated bison still existed on a few private estates. A census taken in 1889 estimated the total remnant population throughout the United States and Canada at 541 animals. Following the senseless North Dakota slaughter of 1883, strong voices of protest from a few influential individuals aroused public interest in the bison's plight. In Yellowstone National Park, a herd of 20 bison that was constantly threatened by poachers was given full protection in 1890. Some farmers succeeded in building up small breeding herds from remnant groups they had been protecting.

By the turn of the century the bison population was beginning to recover. The American Bison Society, formed in 1905, received both federal government backing and powerful private support in its mission to reestablish the American bison as a viable species secure from extinction. The National Bison Range was established in Montana in 1908, and other reserves in both the United States and Canada followed. Shortly after the turn of the century, a large herd of wood bison was discovered near Lake Athabasca in western Canada. The 17,300-square-mile Wood Buffalo National Park in Alberta and Northwest Territories was established in 1922. By 1967, there were 23,000 bison in North America, including plains bison, wood bison, hybrids of the two subspecies, and zoo captives. Most exist today as wards of humans.

The destruction of the American bison was a tragic episode in American history that becomes only slightly more comprehensible when viewed in the context of the exploitive spirit of the times. Within a few decades 60 million large animals of a single species were destroyed, a holocaust of unprecedented magnitude. The herds were vast, probably the largest aggregation of land animals on

Figure 42-3

"Black blizzards" of the 1930s moved millions of tons of soil off the prairies, darkening the skies to the Atlantic seaboard. Thousands of "dusted out" families streamed westward to California, a migration later portrayed in John Steinbeck's novel *The Grapes of Wrath*. This photograph was taken in 1936 in Gregory County, South Dakota.

Courtesy U.S. Department of Agriculture, Soil Conservation Service, Washington, D.C.

earth, and few people could foresee their fate. The same mentality resulted in the annihilation of the passenger pigeon. Fortunately, unlike the passenger pigeon, the bison were able to flourish in captivity and could recover from remnant populations. It was inevitable that the bison would disappear from the plains, since roaming herds of half-ton animals were incompatible with a West given over to agriculture. We cannot deny that the human species must exploit nature to live, but the destruction of the bison was cataclysmic in scope, senseless in direction, and erosive of human values. Their fate is a sobering commentary on the turbulent relationship between wildlife and advancing human civilization.

It is of interest to compare the great prairies that "teemed with life" when Francis Parkman saw them in 1846 with their appearance at the turn of the century just a few years after the arrival of homesteaders. Bison were replaced by longhorn cattle and sheep, and the ranges were overstocked. Sheep, with their close-cropping teeth, were especially destructive; within a few years the highly palatable prairie grasses, legumes, and forbs disappeared. These species were replaced by wheat grasses, bromegrasses, and annual weeds—rapidly converting the prairie into low-grade pasture. With continued grazing, mesquite appeared, and the topsoil thinned. Boomtime "sodbusting" for growing wheat accelerated soil deterioration. No longer bound by grass roots, the soil was lifted by wind and washed away by rain. The American naturalist and conservationist William Temple Hornaby wrote in 1908 of the Montana prairie, where "the awful sheep herds have gone over it, like swarms of locusts, and now the earth looks scalped and bald and lifeless. Today it is almost as bare of cattle as of buffaloes, and it will be years in recovering from the fatal passage of sheep."

Conditions were ideal for the creation of the Dust Bowl, requiring only an extended drought, which occurred in the 1930s. From Texas to Canada the "black blizzards" swept across an exhausted land, joining economic depression in bringing misery to prairie farmers (Fig. 42-3). A single storm on May 12, 1934,

Figure 42-4

Harvesting wheat near Regina, Saskatch-ewan, in the North American grain belt. Sound soil conservation practices insti-tuted after the Dust Bowl have trans-formed the prairies into the world's most productive cropland. Today, the average North American farmer, using irrigation, fertilizers, machines, and a considerable input of fossil fuel energy, produces enough to feed himself and 70 others.
Photograph by L.L. Rue, III.

lifted an estimated 300 million tons of soil from Texas, Oklahoma, Colorado, and Kansas and deposited it eastward in amounts up to 100 tons per square mile.

Today the American prairie is a changed land. Soil conservation practices introduced in the late 1930s eventually transformed the prairies into the most productive agricultural region of the world, dominated by a monoculture of cereal grains (Fig. 42-4). These grains comprise more than one half of the world's grain exports and are the single most important export factor in the U.S. balance of trade. Except for pests, few animals exist in the uniformly cultivated fields, but certain areas are still important refuges for wildlife. One of these is the broad Platte River valley in Nebraska, through which Francis Parkman traveled in 1846. In south-central Nebraska, where the Platte River curves eastward through an enormous bordering marshy area, migratory birds are attracted in great numbers: hundreds of thousands of ducks, countless songbirds, and most of the mid-con-tinent population of sandhill cranes and white-fronted geese. Over the years, how-ever, the marshy wetlands have been gradually drained for cropland until only 20% of the original area remains for wildlife.

The Platte River itself is seriously threatened by an unremitting demand for water for irrigation and other human needs. The yearly flow today is only 16% of what it was before the Nebraska Territory became a state. If the additional water developments that are planned for the Platte River are all carried out, the river will be dry within 35 years. Attempts by the U.S. Fish and Wildlife Service to set aside a portion of the wetlands as a permanent refuge for wildlife have up to this time been defeated, primarily by suspicious landowners who fear that they will be displaced from their land. Meanwhile, cattle raisers, farmers, and industry vigor-ously compete for the remaining water, a dispute in which the wildlife has no voice.

Little remains of the vast climax grasslands that occupied the heart of North America only 150 years ago. No other ecosystem on this continent has been as thoroughly transformed from its natural state. It emphasizes our capacity as humans to reshape the face of nature and manipulate the environment to suit our own needs. This capacity is both the outcome of our biological success as a species and the origin of our ecological problems.

ENVIRONMENT AND HUMAN EVOLUTION
Humans as Hunters

Hunting is an ancient human activity. For most of the period that true humans (genus *Homo*) have walked the earth, their survival depended on the success of the hunt. Only in the last evolutionary instant of human existence on earth have humans of necessity replaced hunting with work. However, the ancient hunting urge, basically a male pursuit, is abundantly manifested today in big-game hunting, fox hunting, game-bird hunting, angling, and numerous other expressions of sport hunting that have survived cultural suppression.

While humans today stand fully revealed as predators, we have our origins in an apelike lineage called the dryopithecines, which thrived on a diet of fruit rather than meat. Human evolution, treated in Chapter 39, was a sequence of fundamental changes in anatomy, behavior, and intelligence from which humans emerged as hunters. Our early dryopithecine ancestors were creatures of the forest. However, climatic changes in the late Miocene and early Pliocene epochs (about 8 million years BP) produced major environmental transformations in North America and Asia. Tropical and subtropical forests yielded to temperate forests and great expanses of grasslands. The early hominids gradually left the dwindling forests altogether to become creatures of the open terrain. As they did so, they consumed more meat and fewer plant foods because plant foods were much scarcer on the savanna than in the forests. Manual dexterity and excellent eye-hand coordination, together with superior intelligence and upright posture, were advantages that enabled the hominid lineage to surpass the rest of the wildlife. They became increasingly dependent on animal food, ranging from insects, tortoises, lizards, and rodents to carrion abandoned by predators on the savanna.

We can speculate that carrion feeding and the first use of tools—sharpened pebbles used to tear away parts of hoofed animals killed by predators—appeared together. Weapons, too, doubtless were needed, since lions and hyenas could not be expected to relinquish their kills voluntarily. Hominids were now aggressors. Using tools and weapons of their own invention, they became hunters, fully equipped for a predatory existence.

The effectiveness of early tools was demonstrated by the late Louis Leakey, who skinned and butchered an antelope in less than 20 minutes using a pebble tool found at Olduvai Gorge in Tanzania.

Emergence of the family unit

These changes occurred slowly, since some 10 million years separate the first true hominid from *Homo erectus,* the first indisputable big-game hunter. The beginnings of social organization, as well as the use of tools, appeared among the Pleistocene australopithecines that lived in open habitats 2 to 3 million years BP. A new social order, especially the family unit, developed to maximize food-foraging potentials. Division of labor between the sexes was required: men ranged widely to hunt game and collect kills abandoned by lions, while women cared for the young, gathered plant foods, and guarded the home site. Family coherence was strengthened by the length of human childhood and associated necessary parental care. The use of language, which presumably existed in at least rudimentary form some 3 million years ago, also reinforced the family bond and facilitated inter-group communication. With individuals united into families and tribes and clans, cooperative hunting behavior was employed, making early humans far more formidable adversaries of wildlife. The stage was readied for humans to use their intelligence to exploit a new way of life on the open savanna. Gradually, early hominids acquired the biblical dominion "over the fish of the sea, and over the fowl of the air, and over the cattle, and over all the earth, and over every creeping thing that creepeth upon the earth" (Genesis 1).

Impact of human hunting

There is no evidence that the small-brained australopithecines used any but the smallest stone tools. Nor had they discovered the use of fire. The large-brained *Homo erectus*, who shared much of the Pleistocene epoch with the australopithecines, took a much larger step toward environmental conquest. Wooden clubs and spears entered the arsenal of hunting weapons, and there is evidence that bolas were employed about 400,000 years ago to capture antelopes. Even more significant, *Homo erectus* learned the use of fire, perhaps as early as 800,000 years ago. With fire they warmed themselves, smoked animals from caves, lighted the darkness to ward off real and imagined terrors of the night, and cooked and tenderized their meat. There is also evidence that Pleistocene humans set fire to the vegetation to concentrate their prey, perhaps stampeding them over cliffs or into swamps where they would be trapped. They also must have discovered that the new growth that sprang up following grass and forest fires attracted wildlife and eased the task of finding it. Humans were thus beginning to modify the environment for their own needs. They were also conducting cooperative big-game drives that were having an increasing impact on wildlife.

Modern humans' immediate predecessors, the Neanderthals, which appeared about 130,000 years ago, left a relatively rich array of fossils, artifacts, and evidences of cultural activities. Already the world's most formidable predators, they depended entirely on their skill as hunters for their survival. The refinement of mass harvesting techniques coincided with a human population explosion that brought the total world population to perhaps 4 million about 20,000 years ago. Large mammal herds could not sustain their numbers against mass slaughter techniques employed by nomadic peoples who followed the herds wherever they went. Animal populations went into serious decline. Magic hunting rituals and polychrome cave art of primitive hunters are thought to be attempts to restore animals to their former abundance as well as to achieve spiritual dominion over the quarry.

For countless millennia humans had drawn all their sustenance from the animal kingdom. If the hunter outwitted the quarry, the family could eat; if he failed, they starved. Animals that shared the hunter's world occupied his thoughts and plans and were the center of all his activities. Although he killed the animals ruthlessly, he nevertheless respected them, felt a kinship with them, and believed himself closely related to them. But as successful hunters, humans were putting themselves out of the hunting business.

Transition from Hunting to Agriculture

Agriculture, the domestication and cultivation of plants, especially cereal crops, arose independently in the Near East and Central America as the hunter-gatherer economies began to fail. The first cultivated cereals, perhaps wheat and barley,

Mass slaughters of animals by early humans were not uncommon. At one site at the foot of a high rock cliff in southern France were discovered the bones of at least 40,000 wild horses in a deposit up to 245 cm (8 feet) thick. These were presumably stampeded over the cliff by Neanderthal hunters who set grass fires.

were probably selected from natural hybrids of wild species. Sites along the Nile Valley in Egypt provide evidence that milled grain was used for food as early as 15,000 years ago. The domestication of animals soon followed. Sheep were domesticated in Iraq at least 11,000 years ago, and evidence of domesticated goats was discovered in 10,000-year-old Palestinian sites. Cattle (8000 years BP) and pigs (5000 to 6000 years BP) soon followed. Cattle became perhaps the earliest beasts of burden, used for pulling carts, turning waterwheels, and carrying people, as well as providing milk and meat.

The advent of agriculture was nothing less than a revolution. No subsequent human event—not the great plagues nor the Industrial Revolution nor the devastating wars of humankind—has had a greater permanent impact on the course of human history. The hunter-gatherer economy that had persisted for more than 2 million years was brought rapidly to a close, although certain hunting populations persisted, some to the present century (such as Australian aborigines, pygmies of the Congo rain forest, and North American Eskimos). A nomadic economy was replaced by more or less permanent villages and communities centered in agricultural areas. Civilization, defined as a state of social culture that is organized around cities and that practices agriculture, was born. The most important result of the new agricultural technology was a vast increase in the carrying capacity of the human environment. A given area of agricultural land could support hundreds of times more people than it could during the early hunter economy. The human population began to soar. Agricultural production continued to diversity, and more and more land was turned to the production of crops and domesticated animals.

As limits to growth were reached, new lands were conquered and exploited. The human species now emerged as a powerful reshaper of the earth. Forests were cut or burned, irrigation systems were built, hillsides were terraced, and grasslands were converted to barren wastelands by overgrazing. Landscapes have suffered the greatest ravages where civilization has existed the longest. The vegetation of the Mediterranean region was largely destroyed 2500 years ago. Most of the pastureland of Spain, Italy, Greece, and Yugoslavia was severely damaged by erosion, which was caused by grazing of domestic animals, especially goats. Before the birth of Christ large sections of northern Africa and the Middle East were so heavily overcropped that they became deserts or wastelands, largely abandoned by both humans and animals. Great civilizations that once flourished in Mesopotamia (Iraq), Palestine, Greece, Italy, and China fell victim to exploitive overgrazing.

Despite the calamities that had befallen the Mediterranean area, until about 300 years ago most of the earth's biosphere was virtually unmarked by human activity. In the Americas, the forests, lakes, prairies, and rivers lay wild and natural and rich in native fauna and flora. Most of northern Europe and Asia was dominated by virgin forests, and the soil remained untouched. The environments of Australia, New Zealand, the East Indies, and the Pacific islands were yet to feel the violent impact of civilization's arrival. The seas were clean and abounded in marine life undisturbed by humans.

This was the scene that the Swedish zoologist-conservationist K. Curray-Lindahl calls "the last idyll." It was a heritage of incalculable richness for future generations. At that point, 300 years ago, history provided abundant warnings of the bitter harvest to be reaped from unbridled human exploitation of nature. Tragically, they were lessons unheeded. Human population was about to begin an

The human population, estimated to be 5 million at the beginning of the agricultural age 10,000 years ago, reached an estimated 40 million by 3500 BC and 100 million by 2000 BC. It probably stood at nearly 200 million at the time of the birth of Christ.

unprecedented growth. Stimulated by the Industrial Revolution, the discovery of abundant fossil fuels for energy, the colonization of new lands, improved agricultural technology, and medical advances, the human population doubled between the years 1650 and 1850, reaching 1 billion people. It doubled again to 2 billion people by 1930; in 1976 it stood at 4 billion people. Now, with each passing day, the problem of feeding so many people intensifies. The population of the human species has reached plague proportions.

Today very little of the earth's biosphere resembles its original pristine state. Numerous animal species have been destroyed by human activities in the last three centuries, and many others are threatened with extinction. According to the American biologist W.H. Murdy (1975), the present ecological crisis is a "crisis in human evolution." We must, he argues, participate in our own evolution, using our knowledge to ensure our survival and the enhancement of human cultural values in an environment of which all living things are a part. We alone have the enormous responsibility of preserving that which is not yet destroyed by countering the destructive forces within us. Our options are rapidly diminishing.

WILDLIFE AND PEOPLE

Pitting Wildlife against Progress

In June 1978, the U.S. Supreme Court ruled that construction on the $120 million Tellico dam project nearing completion in Tennessee must be stopped to save from certain extinction an endangered species of fish, the snail darter. The snail darter, discovered only in 1973, requires shallow, fast-flowing water for spawning, a critical habitat that could be destroyed by the dam's reservoir.

The ruling did nothing to dissipate polarization of public opinion that had already developed over the issue. Proponents of the dam maintained that it would provide badly needed power, improve downstream flood control, and create hundreds of miles of shoreline for recreation. Tennessee already has 85 to 90 species of darters of interest only to ichthyologists, said proponents, and one species would never be missed. Their viewpoint was summed up by Senator Jake Garn of Utah, who stated, "I do not believe that any animal, no matter how worthless, ought to be allowed to halt any project, no matter how valuable."

Preservationists, rather than defending the snail darter's right to survive, questioned the necessity of the dam itself. They argued that the 16,000 acres of productive cropland to be inundated was of much greater value than the benefits of the dam (the General Accounting Office later confirmed the argument). As with all dams, the life of this one would not exceed a few decades because of silting within the reservoir, whereas the inundated land would be lost forever. Further- more, 200 historic and archeological sites, including the old Cherokee village of Tenasi, from which the state takes its name, would be lost. Finally, opponents pointed out, the flood control benefits would cut the flood crest by only 2 inches at Chattanooga, the nearest city. Their viewpoint was perhaps best expressed by then U.S. Secretary of the Interior Cecil D. Andrus, who said, "Common sense dictates that we shouldn't dam every river, stream, or creek in America. Let me suggest that we may have developed the best hydroelectric sites, that we have built some of the best reclamation projects, and that having done this, the law of diminishing returns requires that we proceed with every caution."

The emotion-charged snail darter—Tellico dam issue brought clearly into focus the continuing confrontation between human beings and their environment—a conflict that has no easy resolution and from which no winners can emerge. It pits wildlife against "progress," intangible, long-term benefits of nature against the tangible, short-term benefits of public works projects, principles against practicality. That a small fish could quite literally bring to a halt an enormously expensive construction project astounded Congress, delighted preservationists, and left the average citizen incredulous.

The cause of the snail darter's sudden rise to fame was the Endangered Species Act, a surprisingly powerful piece of legislation passed by Congress in 1966 and expanded and reinforced in 1973. Congress declared in 1966 that "one of the unfortunate consequences of growth and development . . . has been the extermination of some native fish and wildlife . . . and serious losses in other species of native wild animals." It pledged through the act to conserve and protect native fish and wildlife threatened with extinction. The most significant section of the act prohibits federal agencies from jeopardizing endangered species or habitats that have been designated as critical. This legislation was a landmark in wildlife protection because it was the first time that a U.S. domestic law was not enacted mainly to promote human, rather than wildlife, interests. In the past, wildlife reserves or seasons closed to hunting, trapping, and fishing were usually established to perpetuate animals for sport, future market use, or some other nonaltruistic motive.

The snail darter's reprieve from extinction turned out to be short lived. The Endangered Species Act was amended by Congress in 1978 to create a committee empowered to grant exemptions to the act when the benefits of a project "clearly outweigh" the benefits of species preservation. The committee was soon dubbed the God Committee because its decisions could save a species or send it to extinction. It was becoming apparent that the Tellico dam project was a boondoggle and that even with the dam mostly completed, it would be profitable to abandon construction and leave the valley unflooded for agriculture and recreation. A new study showed that the dam's electricity would actually be produced at an economic loss. The God Committee then ruled in favor of the snail darter. But in 1979 the dam's proponents fashioned an amendment to a large water projects appropriation that exempted the Tellico dam from *all* laws that stood in its way. Congress, disgruntled with the whole matter, passed it without debate and it was signed into law in September 1979. Dam construction immediately resumed, and within a year the reservoir began to fill.

Extinction

The Endangered Species Act grew out of rapidly rising public concern for the destructive effects of civilization on wildlife. One measure of human impact is the extinction rate of animals. Since 1600, when reasonably accurate record-keeping began, approximately 225 species of vertebrate animals are known to have become extinct (the true extinction total is far higher but includes numerous invertebrates and tropical animals unknown to biologists). The rate of extinction increased significantly between 1600 and 1900: 21 extinctions in the seventeenth century, 36 in the eighteenth century, and 84 in the nineteenth century. Toward the end of the nineteenth century the number of extinctions increased alarmingly, and although conservation efforts instituted after 1920 stabilized the rate somewhat, 85 more species had disappeared forever by 1974. Furthermore, numerous animal species are today on the verge of extinction; these are the approximately 185 critically endangered species and subspecies recognized by the U.S. Fish and Wildlife Service and by the International Union for the Conservation of Nature and Natural Resources.

In North America the rapid transition from wilderness to a highly industrialized society has had an especially severe impact on native wildlife. Sixteen mammals, eight birds, and nine fishes are known to have vanished in the continental United States alone. If animals from Hawaii and Puerto Rico are included, the list rises to 62 birds, mammals, and fishes that have become extinct since 1600, most of them in the twentieth century. The victims include, among mammals, the great sea mink (last seen in 1860), Merriam's elk (1906), and six subspecies of North American wolf. Extinct birds include the great auk (1833), the Labrador duck (1875), the passenger pigeon (1914), the Carolina parakeet (1914), and the heath hen (1932).

Extinction is, of course, a natural event in organic evolution, as we have discussed previously (especially in Chapter 38). Sometimes individual species disappear gradually as their populations wane in competition with better-adapted forms. At other times whole taxa become extinct within a relatively brief geological period, as for example the complete demise of the dinosaurs at the end of the Cretaceous period (70 million years BP) or the concurrent extinction of many large mammals and ground-nesting birds at the end of the Pleistocene epoch of the Cenozoic era (11,000 years BP). Extinctions may be associated with global or regional climatic changes that adversely affect vegetation and habitat or with the invasion of exotic animals that are able to outcompete the endemic fauna; in the case of recent extinctions, they may have been the result of human predation.

One theory of the massive Pleistocene extinction that by no means has been discredited proposes that early populations of *Homo sapiens*, using weapons, fire, and ingenious hunting techniques, exterminated vulnerable large mammals and ground-nesting birds. Within a relatively brief period, giant bison, wild horses, long-necked camels, ground sloths, mammoths, and mastodons disappeared from the American plains. In Eurasia, mammoths, wooly rhinoceroses, Irish elk, and cave bears became extinct. It has been possible to trace the path of early human immigrations into Africa and Asia, the Americas, Australia, and New Zealand and to note an associated drastic reduction in certain groups of Pleistocene fauna. Nevertheless, humans were still relatively rare creatures during the Pleistocene epoch. Their weapons were primitive. Many question the capacity of early humans to exterminate big-game animals, when eighteenth- and nineteenth-century American Indians, using horses and firearms, had little noticeable effect on the populations of plains bison.

Although we cannot fully assess the impact of early humans on animal extinction, the spread of civilization across the earth has unmistakably been linked to the demise of many animal species. Historically, waves of extinction have attended the arrival of explorers and colonizers to each new continent, island, or archipelago. At first, most extinctions were caused by direct hunting, usually for food but often for commercial products such as furs and ornamental feathers. The development of the musket was responsible for the sharp rise in bird extinctions during the late eighteenth and early nineteenth centuries. Later, various indirect causes of extinction assumed prominence: habitat destruction, exotic animal introductions, and pest and predator control.

The International Union for the Conservation of Nature and Natural Resources of Lausanne, Switzerland, periodically publishes a *Red Data Book* listing threatened wildlife. The recognized categories are (1) critically endangered species that are in immediate danger of extinction, such as the California condor, the whooping crane, and the blue whale; (2) vulnerable or threatened species that are still abundant but are depleted and are under threat, for example, the grizzly bear, the California bighorn, and the prairie falcon; and (3) rare species, which comprise small populations and, although not threatened, are subject to risk, for example, the Galápagos tortoise and the Komodo dragon. This and other such lists published by federal agencies of different nations are unfortunately replete with statistical confusion arising from differences of opinion as to when species or subspecies should be added or removed from the lists, and to which category each belongs.

Causes of extinction today
Habitat alteration

The destruction of animal habitats is today the major threat to survival of endangered species. When habitats are destroyed—whether by logging, drainage of marshes, damming of rivers, urban development, or agriculture—animals must move and adapt to other habitats or die. Although it has been difficult to educate the public about the importance of habitat preservation—many still believe that conservation is primarily the protection of animals against wanton killing—nearly everyone is aware that the destruction of an ecosystem by strip mining, clean-cut logging, or subdivision development adversely affects animals.

Habitat encroachment by humans often has subtle and far-flung effects that are not so readily apparent. Development and land exploitation more frequently than not cause habitat fragmentation. As patches of habitat become smaller and more isolated from each other, many animals that require large home ranges find themselves restricted to areas too small for their food, shelter, and reproductive requirements. Animals in isolated habitats of restricted size become much more vulnerable to nearby human activities, such as pesticide use, air pollution, noise, and human intrusion. Sometimes the exploitation of a small area has widespread ramifications to wildlife in undisturbed areas. A pond or stream may be the only source of water to wildlife for miles around; if it is destroyed by pollution or diverted for irrigation, large numbers of animals are adversely affected.

Migratory animals are especially vulnerable to habitat alteration. The habitat of ducks, geese, and other migratory waterfowl embraces the northern breeding grounds, southern wintering grounds, and all the areas they visit in between. All portions are necessary for their survival. Migratory fishes, such as salmon and steelhead trout, if barred from their spawning grounds by a dam or polluted stretch of river, will be destroyed just as effectively as if they were decimated by overfishing.

Yet another dimension of habitat alteration is successional changes that follow the clearing or burning of a mature forest. Species requiring stable, mature forest wilderness (such as grizzly bears, wolverines, bighorn sheep, caribou, and ivory-billed woodpeckers) decrease in numbers following a severe forest fire, whereas the luxurious new plant growth that follows a fire, fertilized by nutrients in the ash, encourages successional species such as deer, elk, rabbits, grouse, and quail (Fig. 42-5). Not all forest fires are bad, despite the admonitions of Smokey the Bear. Periodic forest fires stimulate forest diversity, recirculate nutrients, and control diseases that tend to flourish in overmature forest stands. Some species such as Kirtland's warbler depend on fires for their survival. This endangered species requires 8- to 20-year-old jack pines for nesting. Jack pine cones remain tightly sealed by resins, opening only during a fire to release their seeds. Fire suppression in the Kirtland warbler's Michigan habitat resulted in uniform stands of trees too old for the birds' narrow habitat requirement. In 1964, when the cause of the warbler's demise was discovered, the U.S. Forest Service instituted periodic controlled burns to encourage the species' recovery.

The rapid destruction of the tropical forests has alarming implications for both humans and animals. Some 40% of the tropics of the world has been destroyed during the past 150 years, and virtually all the rest may be cleared by the year 2000. Some 400 million people make their living by slash-and-burn techniques, growing crops for a year or two, then moving on. Within 25 years, when the human population is expected to have at least doubled in size, there will be little tropical forest left. Enormous economic disruption and widespread starvation of

Figure 42-5

Regrowth after a forest fire in Oregon (Tillamook Burn) provides excellent habitat for game species such as deer, elk, bear, grouse, and quail. Controlled fires are now considered an important forest management tool for removing diseased trees and opening land to new growth.
Photograph by L.L. Rue, III.

truly frightening proportions seem inevitable. Most tropical countries, beset as they are by overwhelming human problems arising from explosive population growth, have neither the resources nor the motivation to study and protect the natural communities on which they depend. Nevertheless, several Latin American countries have plans to create reserves and parks in large portions of rain forest that still remain intact. Developed countries should be offering every possible encouragement and economic assistance to help these countries implement their plans. Areas already under protection have not fared well in Latin America because of haphazard protection and strong social and economic pressures to use the reserves for other purposes. Reserves in Latin America may slow the loss of natural habitat, but sweeping social changes will be required to prevent its eventual destruction.

Hunting

Until relatively recently, uncontrolled hunting for meat and oil and for commercial animal products (furs, hides, ornamental feathers, horns, and tusks) was the most serious menace to wildlife. Historically, the marine mammals, especially the furbearers (fur seals, harp seals, and sea otters) were subjected to egregious mass slaughters wherever they were discovered around the globe. The sea otter suffered 170 years of unrelenting persecution along northern Pacific coasts until, in 1910, it was considered extinct. Belatedly, the animal was granted international protection, a move that encountered no objections from the fur hunters who found no profit in hunting for any remnant colonies that might still exist. Fortunately, some had survived and were first sighted in 1938 off Bixby Creek on the California coast. Other colonies were soon discovered in Alaska and elsewhere. Slowly, under strict protection, the species is recovering.

The northern fur seal was nearly exterminated by a century and a half of sealing on the Pribilof Islands by Russian, American, Canadian, and British sealers. After the United States purchased Alaska and the Pribilofs from Russia in 1867, it attempted to limit harvesting, but Canadian and British sealers continued indiscriminate and wasteful shooting in the open sea. Finally in 1911, the United States arranged an international treaty that stopped open-sea hunting. From a low of about 125,000 seals, the population is approaching its former size of an estimated 2 to 3 million animals. Some 30,000 fur seals are collected annually by licensed sealers, operating in a rational, well-managed industry. The baby harp seal industry along the coast of Labrador and in the Gulf of St. Lawrence is also well managed, but the bloody method of harvesting has sparked an outcry from animal lovers and protectionists that may well bring an end to the persecution. It must be remembered that seal harvesting is supported by human demand for fur coats, not by the sealers' putative desire for butchery.

The vigorous public denunciation of harp seal hunting stems in part from the "Bambi factor"—our separation of animals into "good" and "bad" based on human illusions of imaginary animal characteristics. Baby harp seals, with their big, dark, liquid eyes, look lovable and innocent; it seems inconceivable that anyone could club them to death by the thousands and skin them for their fur—or, for that matter, any other reason. Yet snakes, coyotes, and weasels, which are just as innocent (although perhaps not so lovable), seldom benefit from public outcries over their persecution. As long as an irrational public is concerned only about furry creatures with warm brown eyes, conservation organizations will use them as a selling point. The conservation movement, however, is firmly committed to the preservation of the entire pyramid of life.

Costa Rica has established enormous areas of unbroken rain forest as national parks and plans to extend the parks until they occupy 10% of the nation's territory—proportionately more than any other Latin American country. Brazil has set aside 175,000 square kilometers (68,000 square miles) of Amazonia as parks and reserves and has ambitious plans to expand this about 10 fold. Peru, Venezuela, and Colombia are also establishing new parks, some of which embrace huge areas of rain forest. Unfortunately, many of these are little more than "paper parks," poorly understood by politicians and subject to constant invasion by people for farming, logging, and other disruptive activities.

Figure 42-6

Starving white-tailed deer. Hunting is necessary to crop deer populations that otherwise quickly proliferate beyond the capacity of the land to support them in winter. Humans have replaced natural predators.

Photograph by L.L. Rue, Ill.

Poaching of African elephants for the illegal ivory trade has reached massive proportions. The price of ivory reached $34 per pound in 1980, up from $2.30 per pound in 1970. It was estimated in 1980 that 50,000 to 150,000 elephants are killed illegally each year from a total African population of 1.3 million elephants.

Perhaps the saddest and least comprehensible slaughter of animal life today is the exploitation of the great whales. It is a true war of extermination, and the two major whaling nations, the Soviet Union and Japan, are fully aware of it. Despite rapidly growing international pressure, which has placed the whaling industry on the defensive, it appears that whaling will cease only when whale populations are driven so low that hunting becomes unprofitable. The whaling fleets will disappear, their crews will disperse, and substitutes will be discovered for the raw materials derived from whales. Then, if it is not too late, the whales may recover to their former magnificence.

Present-day game hunting and angling are, as we mentioned earlier, atavistic displays of an ancient hunting urge. "There is in the passion for hunting," wrote Charles Dickens, "something deeply implanted in the human breast." Sport hunting is a well-managed industry in the United States and Canada, probably the best managed in the world. None of the 74 bird species and 35 mammal species hunted legally in the United States is either threatened or endangered. Nevertheless, much of the urban public associates hunting with the wanton and repugnant killing of beautiful forest creatures. The confrontation between the nation's 21 million hunters and the numerous antihunting organizations is not new, but the polarization of viewpoints is more intense than ever before. However one views hunting emotionally, the morality of killing animals and the arguments about cruelty are side issues to conservation, often obscuring more important issues.

Two inescapable facts are that (1) hunting interests in North America have been a principal force in acquiring land for wildlife refuges and migratory bird sanctuaries and (2) until humans are prepared to reestablish wolves, coyotes, mountain lions, lynxes, and other natural predators in animal habitats, controlled hunting is necessary to manage game populations (Fig. 42-6). It should be added, however, that because hunters killed the carnivores and raptors in the first place to keep them from feeding on the hunters' game, hunters themselves are responsible for the present predator-prey imbalance. It is unlikely that the hunter-nonhunter controversy will disappear. As long as hunters continue to shatter the peacefulness of autumn, endanger hikers, and annoy farmers, the American public's tolerance for hunting will continue to decline.

In other parts of the world, game hunting still is a major threat to numerous species such as Bengal tigers, leopards, cheetahs, rhinoceroses, crocodiles, and elephants (Fig. 42-7). Animal poaching in game preserves is increasingly prevalent as the rising human population of Africa and Asia places enormous strains on available food supplies. How long can national parks and game preserves be protected for the enjoyment of tourists, while natives adjacent to the preserves starve to death? Here, as elsewhere, it is human problems that conflict with wildlife.

Feral domestic and introduced animals

Humans have introduced numerous species into new habitats all over the world, where they affect the indigenous fauna by preying on them (cats, dogs, mongooses) or competing with them for food and habitat (rabbits, rats, mice, cattle, goats, sheep, pigs). Many introductions are deliberate, others are accidental, and both are facilitated by the mobility of humans. In 1929 a noted tropical entomologist, while on a rice ship from Trinidad to Manila, amused himself by listing every kind of animal on board, from cockroaches and fleas to rats and pet animals. He found no less than 41 species, mostly insects. When he opened his luggage in Manila, out walked several beetles.

Of course, not every animal introduced to a new land manages to establish itself, but of those that do, nearly all change the balance of the ecosystem in some way. Many have inflicted an enormous cost to agriculture—the fire ant, the boll weevil, and the gypsy moth are a few latter-day examples in the United States— and are responsible for much, if not most, of the heavy use of pesticides on crops and forests. The demise of both the American elm and the chestnut (p. 1034) was caused by accidental introduction of diseases carried by insect vectors.

The natural balance of island communities is especially vulnerable to damage by introduced animals. In the absence of natural checks that keep their populations regulated on the continent, introduced species often flourish at the expense of the native island fauna, many of which have evolved in the absence of mammalian predators and consequently lack protective avoidance behavior. Flightless birds are highly vulnerable. A classic example is the dodo, a very large flightless member of the pigeon family, which inhabited the island of Mauritius. Its fate was sealed by the first Dutch colonists who arrived in 1644 with pigs and dogs. Both the colonists and the introduced animals preyed on the dodos, annihilating the last of them in 1693. The dodo thus bears the distinction of being the first extinct animal whose demise could be fully documented.

No archipelago has suffered more disfigurement of the native fauna and flora than the Hawaiian Islands, where the whole of the native lowland forest community has been destroyed by introduced plants and animals. Sixteen species of birds became extinct between 1837 and 1945, half of them members of the extraordinary honeycreeper family. Only 14 species of honeycreepers survive, nearly all endangered. Although some of the original forest remains in Hawaii, especially in upland habitats where cultivation is impractical, nearly all is overrun by feral domestic animals, rats, and a host of other introduced vertebrate and invertebrate pests. It is only a matter of time before what remains of the marvelous indigenous fauna and flora of Hawaii has either vanished forever or is disfigured beyond recognition.

Rhinoceros horns (actually the "horn" is a compacted mass of hairs) are in great demand by Indians and Chinese who consider them to be a powerful aphrodisiac (in part because of their phallic shape) and remedy for a variety of ailments. Daggers with intricately carved rhinoceros horn handles are traditional gifts at puberty rites in the Middle East. Carvers in North Yemen prepared more than 2000 horns in 1975 and 1976 alone.

Figure 42-7

Elephant tusks taken from poachers by Kenya conservation authorities. These are only a few from an enormous warehouse in Mombasa containing thousands of huge tusks, representing, of course, the slaughter of thousands of elephants.
Photograph by F.M. Hickman.

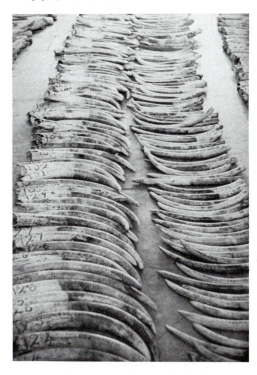

Figure 42-8

Introduced birds and mammals that have established populations in New Zealand, with countries of origin.

From Elton, C.S. 1958. The ecology of invasions by animals and plants. New York, John Wiley & Sons, Inc.; after Wodzicki, K.A. 1950. Bull. D.S.I.R., New Zealand 98:1-255.

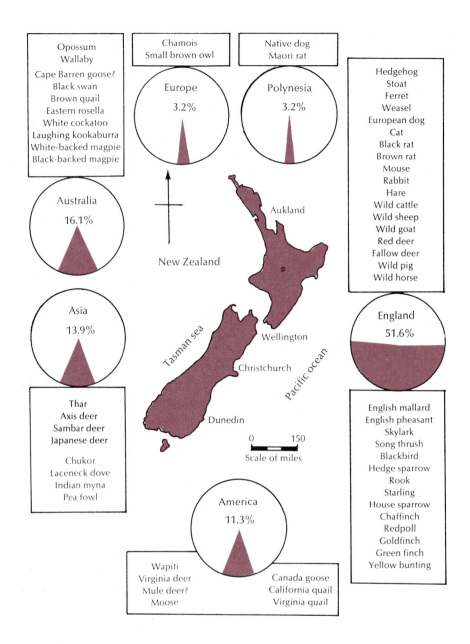

The unique Pleistocene fauna of New Zealand, which still flourished when the Polynesians arrived in the ninth century AD, was dominated by large ratite (flightless) birds (21 species of moas and four species of kiwis) and had a rich representation of other birds, reptiles, and amphibians. The only land mammals were two bats and perhaps a rodent. Today, largely as a result of the depredations of introduced animals, all 21 moa species are extinct. Three kiwi species survive under strict protection. Nearly one third of the original fauna has vanished in a thousand years of human habitation. Approximately 60 species of birds and mammals have been introduced (Fig. 42-8), of which about half have become problem animals. While conservation programs are vigorously supported in New Zealand, it will never be possible to reconstitute the original fauna and flora.

Predator and pest control

Predators and pests that compete with humans for the same food have long been relegated to the category of "bad" living things. Among mammalian predators, wolves, coyotes, bobcats, grizzly bears, and cougars kill livestock and game and in doing so have engendered the wrath of sheepherders and hunters. In the United States and Canada, millions of taxpayer dollars have been spent to shoot, poison, and trap predators to benefit a relatively small but vociferous group. As a result, cougars, grizzly bears, and wolves have virtually disappeared from western grazing lands. The adaptable coyote, however, has been able to maintain a relatively healthy population despite vigorous control programs. Biologists had long argued that elimination of all predators by mass poisoning programs was poor management, since a large part of the coyotes' diet consists of rodents, which compete with sheep for forage. In 1972, yielding finally to citizen protests over mass poisoning programs—stimulated in part by such polemics as Jack Olsen's book *Slaughter the Animals, Poison the Earth*—the U.S. Fish and Wildlife Service banned all poisoning on public lands. Contrary to fears expressed by the sheep industry, the ban neither resulted in a dramatic increase in coyotes nor was responsible for decline in the sheep industry, which was already waning for economic reasons.

Animal traffic

The pet trade is big business in North America, England, and Europe. Between 1967 and 1974, American imports of exotic mammals, birds, and reptiles increased sixfold, reaching nearly 4 million annually in the mid-1970s. More than 100 million fishes, mostly tropical, are imported each year for the 20 million Americans who own aquariums. An astonishing variety of endangered species are sold illegally as pets, especially in the United States. The list includes monkeys of various species, cheetahs, leopards of three species, ocelots, numerous species of endangered and threatened birds, lizards, snakes, and fishes. The result is that the exotic pet trade, a curious phenomenon that seems to be associated with an affluent public's avidity for new kinds of gratification, is rapidly assuming a prominent position among the causes of extinction.

The collection and shipment of animals from Southeast Asia and Central and South America by careless hunters and callous dealers are extraordinarily wasteful—only about one animal in 10 survives the numerous hazards and gross mistreatment that occur between capture and purchase by the ultimate owner. Most collecting is done by indigenous peasant hunters who know little about live-capture techniques. Mortality is high at the time of capture. Many species are collected by shooting the mother to capture the baby; not infrequently several females are killed to secure a single uninjured infant. The rarer the animal, the greater is the price it will fetch, and the more enterprising are its human pursuers. Thus, an animal's rarity often promotes those elements that were responsible for its demise in the first place. Of the wild animals that survive the perilous trip to American homes, most die within a few weeks from improper care. Most of the rest are disposed of as people become bored with them or discover they cannot cope with them.

Some 60% of all wild mammals imported into the United States are destined for biomedical research, and of these, the great majority are primates. They are used for the preparation of vaccines, for physiological and behavioral experiments, and for defense-related research. The global demand for primates for research is of such proportions, estimated at 200,000 animals per year, that many species of both New World and Old World monkeys have been pushed close to extinction. Fifty-four of the 149 species of primates (36%) are severely threatened today. The demand by zoos and circuses for primates, especially for the pongids (chimpanzees, orangutans, gorillas, and gibbons) also contributes to the drain, although in general, zoos are far less damaging to wildlife than the general public imagines. For example, in 1974 zoos imported into the United States only 4% of the wild mammals and 2% of the wild birds; the pet trade and biomedical research consumed the rest. Furthermore, nearly all of the larger zoos breed animals in captivity; zoos trade animals with each other and in some instances have been able to rebuild stocks of severely endangered species.

To relieve the stress that biomedical research places on native primate populations, several American users have begun breeding programs for rhesus monkeys and other primates. Although demand is certain to outpace the production of home-breeding programs for some years to come, biomedical researchers can only welcome any move that will reduce their contribution to the world wildlife crisis.

ENVIRONMENTAL MOVEMENT

In the 1854 Chief Seattle of the Dunwanish tribe in Puget Sound admonished president Franklin Pierce in a moving and visionary letter:

> The great Chief in Washington sends word that he wishes to buy our land. How can you buy or sell the sky—the warmth of the land? The idea is strange to us. Yet we do not own the freshness of the air or the sparkle of the water. How can you buy them from us? Every part of this earth is sacred to my people. Every shiny pine needle, every sandy shore, every mist in the dark woods, every clearing and humming insect is holy in the memory and experience of my people.
>
> We know that the white man does not understand our ways. One portion of the land is the same to him as the next, for he is a stranger who comes in the night and takes from the land whatever he needs. The earth is not his brother but his enemy, and when he has conquered it he moves on. He leaves his father's graves, and his children's birthright is forgotten.

The American Indians, harmoniously and inextricably linked with the creatures around them and in spiritual kinship with nature, could not comprehend the white settlers' reckless and indifferent exploitation of land. The Indians venerated nature; the white settlers abused it. We may never fully understand why the ethics of these two people diverged as far as they did, but it is possible to reconstruct historical events that led to the white settlers' attitude—an attitude that threatens our very survival today.

We have already traced the beginnings of human society. Early humans were merely a part of wildlife's ecological web. People exploited nature for food and shelter as did the animals around them, but as long as people were fundamentally hunters and gatherers, their environmental requirements were small, and they remained in harmony with their surroundings. As civilization developed, people began to draw away from nature, spinning an increasingly artificial world around themselves. To satisfy their needs, new and more effective ways were developed to obtain them from the environment. When this caused habitat destruction and diminishing returns, the change was regarded as an inevitable and acceptable consequence of a chosen way of life. Agriculture, as we have already seen, vastly accelerated both habitat alteration and wildlife extermination, since wild animals now became competitors with humans for their food. Changes often occurred so slowly that people were unaware of how altered their environment had become.

At the time the first settlers came to America, much of the wildlife of England and Europe belonged to the privileged classes. Only the nobility hunted deer and grouse; the peasants hunted rabbits. Such nonegalitarian restraints were in large part responsible for the presence of wild boar and other large mammals in densely settled parts of Europe for hundreds of years.

In America, natural resources and wildlife appeared inexhaustible. From the first, settlers encountered deer, turkey, salmon, and sturgeon in abundance. No aristocracy restricted their right to hunt them; wildlife belonged to everyone. Thus began the "great American experiment," founded on the philosophy that every individual was entitled to any resources that could be gathered through personal initiative. It was an exploitive and destructive ethic, but no one viewed it that way. Living was hard for the settler despite the plenitude of natural resources. It was the pioneer family pitted against trees, wild animals, and hostile Indians—not conditions expected to foster a conservation ethic.

Even before the pioneers had reached the Mississippi River, attitudes were changing along the eastern seaboard. As the wildlife disappeared, eastern colonists began enacting laws to protect game and fish. Poorly enforced and relatively ineffective at first, such laws nevertheless reflected changing public attitudes toward wildlife. Gradually and almost grudgingly, the federal government began to assume leadership in environmental legislation.

The establishment of Yellowstone National Park in 1872 marked the real beginning of the environmental movement in the United States. Environmental wounds were becoming obvious to everyone, and by the turn of the century, an increasing number of determined Americans began to prod a reluctant Congress to act on environmental legislation. Public sentiment for animals in jeopardy had been quickened by the loss of the passenger pigeon and the near miss with the bison, the latter becoming a symbol of vanishing America.

At a time when pollution, energy and economic crises, and burgeoning social problems besiege the nation's conscience, most people are apt to respond indifferently to the passing of a few remote species of animals. If one has never seen a whooping crane or a blue whale—and never expects to see one or any other animal on the endangered species list—of what possible concern is their extinction? And is not the sacrifice of a few insignificant animals and plants necessary for progress? Such myopic views are affirmations of a philosophy at least as old as civilization: that the value of plants and animals is determined by their benefit to humans. This is an anthropocentric position that sees living things merely as instruments to human survival. It ignores the interrelatedness of all living components of the environment while subscribing to the notion that, because humans are the highest animal, they alone can make correct decisions about the exploitation of nature. According to this view, some animals and plants are more valuable to humans than others. Such a narrowly conceived attitude is rejected by modern ecological theory, which reaffirms the value of all living things in nature because all are parts of an interrelated whole.

Extinction therefore is an extremely serious result of environmental abuse because it is irreversible; an extinct animal or plant can never be recreated. Extinction removes a functional part from the web of life, and both diversity and stability of the ecosystem are reduced. Vanishing wildlife is an "early warning signal" of environmental malaise, and when we see the list of endangered animals lengthen year after year, we cannot remain indifferent.

Many people have not remained indifferent. With the establishment of Yellowstone National Park the conservation movement almost at once began to gather momentum. In 1886 Canada created Glacier National Park in British Columbia, followed in 1887 by the magnificent Banff National Park in the Canadian Rockies. Australia and New Zealand followed suit with their own national parks in the next decade; soon national parks were springing up all over the world. Admittedly, during the early decades of the environmental movement, national parks were created to preserve scenic beauty; the preservation of wildlife was incidental. But as the surrounding land became emptied of wildlife, parks acquired status as sanctuaries. And while Americans and Canadians pondered the new idea of establishing parks just for animals, large game preserves were already appearing in Africa. Today, the 386 national wildlife refuges scattered among all but one state in the United States and the hundreds of national parks and game preserves all over the world are manifestations of an environmental movement that has matured far beyond the most fanciful visions of the founders of Yellowstone National Park.

Conservation is much more than trying to fence off beautiful national parks and wildlife sanctuaries from an otherwise deteriorating biosphere. Most of all, it requires a common understanding among all humanity that our fate is inextricably linked to the living world at large. It is a worldwide problem of enormous complexity. In the final analysis, anything we do now or in the future becomes futile unless the growth of the human population can be stemmed. That is the ultimate problem.

Many believe that we are on a threshold of a new awakening, that we will be able to bridle our self-indulgence, our extraordinary propensity to isolate ourselves from nature, and then reaffirm both the meaningfulness of the human experience and our kinship with all living things.

____ Summary

This final chapter concerns one aspect of the humanization of the earth, the human impact on animal extinction. We begin by documenting the great bison slaughter of the nineteenth century, the most cataclysmic known destruction of an animal species by humans. Approximately 60 million large mammals were reduced within a few decades to remnant herds totaling less than 600 animals. The principal domain of the bison, the North American grasslands, was then given over to highly productive croplands.

Humans have always been animal hunters, but the small populations of early hominids could not have had a significant impact on animal numbers or habitat. With the evolution of modern humans (*Homo sapiens*) some 130,000 years ago, more sophisticated hunting techniques appeared. Humans soon proved themselves capable of eliminating species through overhunting and habitat modification with the use of fire.

Habitat disruption increased very rapidly after the introduction of agriculture some 15,000 years ago. Agriculture increased the carrying capacity of the human environment, permitting the human population to increase much more quickly than ever before. Humans soon emerged as powerful reshapers of the earth's natural habitats.

Although extinction is a natural process in organic evolution, the extinction rate of animals has increased measurably, if not alarmingly, with the spread of human civilization. The Endangered Species Act, passed in 1966 by the U.S. Con-

"If I were to name the three most precious resources of life, I should say
books, friends, and nature; and the greatest of these, at least the most constant
and always at hand, is nature. Nature we
have always with us, an inexhaustible
storehouse of that which moves the
heart, appeals to the mind, and fires the
imagination—health to the body, a stimulus to the intellect, and joy to the soul."
John Burroughs,
"Leaf and Tendril," 1908

Photograph by S. Mann.

gress and reinforced in 1973, was the first legislation enacted that was designed to slow the extinction of animals. It is a surprisingly tough and uncompromising law, largely altruistic in purpose, that recognizes the importance of preserving the habitat of an endangered species.

Of the major causes of extinction today, habitat alteration is the greatest threat to species survival because it disrupts or destroys entire communities of organisms on which animals depend. Uncontrolled hunting was until recently a major cause of extinction, but in developed countries hunting and angling today are so closely managed that no legally hunted species is threatened or endangered. In developing countries, however, enormous hunting pressures on endemic animal species continue.

The introduction of nonendemic species into new habitats all over the world has changed natural balances that have evolved in various ecosystems and has led to numerous documented animal extinctions. Predator and pest control on croplands and grazing lands has also endangered several mammalian carnivores. The pet trade has recently emerged as a serious threat to wildlife, largely because of wasteful collecting techniques.

People have become increasingly aware that the endless quest for progress has left deep environmental wounds and forced many species into extinction. Much of the past indifference toward animal extinction stems from the widely held view that animals and plants exist solely as instruments to human survival. This myopic view is rejected by modern ecological theory. Today there are encouraging signs that a new ethic—a conservation strategy—is emerging that cherishes natural systems and recognizes the interdependence of all life forms.

Selected references

The environmental movement has spawned an avalanche of literature, some of which has been given over to emotional condemnation of just about every aspect of human interaction with wildlife, and some of which is concerned principally with pollution. We have not included these kinds of treatment in the following selection.

Allin, C.W. 1982. The politics of wilderness preservation. Westport, Conn., Greenwood Press. *Origin and development of preservation politics in the United States.*

Anglemyer, M., E.R. Seagraves, and C.C. LeMaistre. 1980. A search for environmental ethics: an initial bibliography. Washington, D.C., Smithsonian Institution Press. *Collection of 446 annotated references on environmental ethics.*

Bates, M. 1960. The forest and the sea. New York, Random House, Inc. *A lucid, thoughtful treatment of nature's economy and human intervention.*

Borland, H. 1975. The history of wildlife in America. Washington, D.C., National Wildlife Federation. *Beautifully illustrated overview with an appendix containing a summary of U.S. wildlife habitats.*

Burghardt, G.M., and H.A. Herzog, Jr. 1980. Beyond conspecifics: is Brer Rabbit our brother? BioScience 30:763-768. *Beautiful animals are valued more than ugly ones. How do we develop an acceptable ethic toward our relations with other species?*

Curry-Lindahl, K. 1972. Let them live. New York, William Morrow & Co., Inc. *A continent-by-continent survey of animals threatened with extinction.*

Dubos, R. 1980. The wooing of earth. New York, Charles Scribner's Sons. *The author believes that careful management of nature can create values that transcend those created by natural forces working alone.*

Ehrlich, P., and A. Ehrlich. 1981. Extinction: the causes and consequences of the disappearance of species. New York, Random House, Inc. *Lively and well-documented argument that survival of all species is essential for our own intrinsic good.*

Elton, C.S. 1958. The ecology of invasions by animals and plants. New York, John Wiley & Sons, Inc. *Numerous examples of the often disastrous consequences of purposeful and accidental introductions.*

Emmel, T.C. (ed.). 1977. Global perspective on ecology. Palo Alto, Calif., Mayfield Publishing Co. *Collection of 39 articles on global ecology and environmental problems.*

Fox, M.W. 1980. Returning to Eden: animal rights and human responsibility. New York, The Viking Press. *Explores contemporary human attitudes toward use and abuse of animals.*

Fox, S. 1981. John Muir and his legacy: the American conservation movement. Boston, Little, Brown &

Co. *A biography of John Muir and a chronological history of the conservation movement to 1975.*

Frankel, O.H., and M.E. Soulé. 1981. Conservation and evolution. New York, Cambridge University Press. *The authors examine the processes of extinction from an evolutionary viewpoint and argue that intensive human efforts are required to save threatened species.*

Matthews, L.H. 1975. Man and wildlife. New York, St. Martin's Press, Inc. *Excellent account of human-wildlife conflicts.*

Mitchell, J.G. 1976. Fear and loathing in wolf country. Audubon 78(3):20-39. *Examines conflicting perspectives of wolves by game hunters and preservationists in Minnesota and Alaska.*

Mitchell, L.C. 1981. Witnesses to a vanishing America: the nineteenth-century response. Princeton, N.J., Princeton University Press. *Insightful assessment of the history of the westward conquest in America, which has led Americans to question their culture.*

Murdy, W.H. 1975. Anthropocentrism: a modern version. Science 187:1168-72.

Myers, N. 1979. The sinking ark: a new look at the problem of disappearing species. New York, Pergamon Press. *Outlines broad-scale conservation measures we can take to stop the destruction of species.*

Nietschmann, B. 1977. The Bambi factor. Natural History 86(7):84-87. *Why there are "good" and "bad" animals.*

Nitecki, M.H. (ed.). 1981. Biotic crises in ecological and evolutionary time. New York, Academic Press, Inc. *Collection of symposium papers that explore causes of extinction.*

Odell, R. 1980. Environmental awakening: the new revolution to protect the earth. Cambridge, Mass., Ballinger Publishing Co. *Thoughtful and carefully researched discussion of the key issues in the environmental movement.*

Scheffer, V.B. 1974. A voice for wildlife. New York, Charles Scribner's Sons. *Examines the causes of confrontation between people and wildlife, considers solutions, and takes a look at the future wildlife ethic. A thoughtful and well-developed book.*

Trefethen, J.B. 1975. An American crusade for wildlife. New York, Winchester Press. *Excellent history of the conservation movement in the United States.*

Vogt, B. 1978. Now, the river is dying. National Wildlife 16(4):4-11. *Battle for the water of the Platte River in Nebraska reflects a vastly larger problem throughout the American west.*

Westman, W.E. 1977. How much are nature's services worth? Science 197:960-964. *Measuring social benefits of ecosystem functioning is difficult and controversial but important for public understanding.*

G L O S S A R Y

aboral (ab-o'rəl) (L., *ab*, from, + *os*, mouth). A region opposite the mouth.

acanthor (ə-kan'thor) (Gr., *akantha*, spine or thorn, + *or*). First larval form of acanthocephalans in the intermediate host.

acclimatization (ə-klī'mə-də-zā'shən) (L., *ad*, to, + Gr., *klima*, climate). Gradual physiological adaptation in response to relatively long-lasting environmental changes.

acetabulum (as'ə-tab'ū-lum) (L., a little saucer for vinegar). True sucker, especially in flukes and leeches; the socket in the hip bone that receives the thigh bone.

acinus (as'ə-nəs), pl. **acini** (as'ə-ni) (L., grape). A small lobe of a compound gland or a saclike cavity at the termination of a passage.

acoelomate (a-sēl'ə-māt') (Gr., *a*, not, + *koilōma*, cavity). Without a coelom, as in flatworms and proboscis worms.

acontium (ə-kän'chē-əm), pl. **acontia** (Gr., *akontion*, dart). Threadlike structure bearing nematocysts located on mesentery of sea anemone.

acrocentric (ak'rō-sen'trək) (Gr., *akros*, tip, + *kentron*, center). Chromosome with centromere near the end.

actin (Gr., *aktis*, ray). A protein in the contractile tissue that forms the thin myofilaments of striated muscle.

adaptation (L., *adaptatus*, fitted). An anatomical structure, physiological process, or behavioral trait that improves an animal's fitness for existence.

adaptive value. Degree to which a characteristic helps an organism to survive and reproduce; lends greater fitness in environment; selective advantage.

adductor (ə-duk'tər) (L., *ad*, to, + *ducere*, to lead). A muscle that draws a part toward a median axis, or a muscle that draws the two valves of a mollusc shell together.

adenine (ad'nēn, ad'ə-nēn) (Gr., *adēn*, gland, + *ine*, suffix). A purine base; component of nucleotides and nucleic acids.

adenosine (ə-den'ə-sen) **(di-, tri-) phosphate** (ADP and ATP). A nucleotide composed of adenine, ribose sugar, and two (ADP) or three (ATP) phosphate units; ATP is an energy-rich compound that, with ADP, serves as a phosphate bond—energy transfer system in cells.

adipose (ad'ə-pōs) (L., *adeps*, fat). Fatty tissue; fatty.

adrenaline (ə-dren'ə-lən) (L., *ad*, to, + *renalis*, pertaining to kidneys). A hormone produced by the adrenal, or suprarenal, gland; epinephrine.

adsorption (ad-sorp'shən) (L., *ad*, to, + *sorbere*, to suck in). The adhesion of molecules to solid bodies.

aerobic (a-rō'bik) (Gr., *aēr*, air, + *bios*, life). Oxygen-dependent form of respiration.

afferent (af'ə-rənt) (L., *ad*, to, + *ferre*, to bear). Adjective meaning leading or bearing toward some organ, for example, nerves conducting impulses toward the brain or blood vessels carrying blood toward an organ; opposed to efferent.

aggression (L., *aggredi*, attack). A primary instinct usually associated with emotional states; an offensive behavior action.

agonistic behavior (Gr., *agōnistēs*, combatant). An offensive action or threat directed toward another organism.

alate (ā'lāt) (L., *alatus*, wing). Winged.

allantois (ə-lan'tois) (Gr., *allas*, sausage, + *eidos*, form). One of the extraembryonic membranes of the amniotes that functions in respiration and excretion in birds and reptiles and plays an important role in the development of the placenta in most mammals.

allele (ə-lēl') (Gr., *allēlōn*, of one another). Alternative forms of genes coding for the same trait; situated at the same locus in homologous chromosomes.

allograft (a'lō-graft) (Gr., *allos*, other, + graft). A piece of tissue or an organ transferred from one individual to another individual of the same species, not identical twins; homograft.

allometry (ə-lom'ə-trē) (Gr., *allos*, other, + *metry*, measure). Relative growth of a part in relation to the whole organism.

allopatric (Gr., *allos*, other, + *patra*, native land). In separate and mutually exclusive geographical regions.

alpha helix (Gr., *alpha*, first, + L., *helix*, spiral). Literally the first spiral arrangement of the genetic DNA molecule; regular coiled arrangement of polypeptide chain in proteins; secondary structure of proteins.

altricial (al-tri'shəl) (L., *altrices*, nourishers). Referring to young animals (especially birds) having the young hatched in an immature, dependent condition.

alula (al'yə-lə) (L., dim. of *ala*, wing). The first digit or thumb of a bird's wing, much reduced in size.

alveolus (al-vē'ə-ləs) (L., dim. of *alveus*, cavity, hollow). A small cavity or pit, such as a microscopic air sac of the lungs, terminal part of an alveolar gland, or bony socket of a tooth.

ambulacra (am'byə-lak'rə) (L., *ambulare*, to walk). In echinoderms, radiating grooves where podia of water-vascular system characteristically project to outside.

amebocyte (ə-mē'bə-sīt) (Gr., *amoibē*, change, + *kytos*, hollow vessel). Any free body cell capable of movement by pseudopodia; certain types of blood cells and tissue cells.

ameboid (ə-mē'boid) (Gr., *amoibē*, change, + *oid*, like). Ameba-like in putting forth pseudopodia.

amictic (ə-mik'tic) (Gr., *a*, without, + *miktos*, mixed or blended). Pertaining to female rotifers, which produce only diploid eggs that cannot be fertilized, or to the eggs produced by such females.

amino acid (ə-mē'nō) (amine, an organic compound). An organic acid with an amino group (—NH₂). Makes up the structure of proteins.

amitosis (ā'mī-tō'səs) (Gr., *a*, not, + *mitos*, thread). A form of cell division in which mitotic nuclear changes do not occur; cleavage without separation of daughter chromosomes.

amniocentesis (am'nē-ō-sin-te'səs) (Gr., *amnion*, membrane around the fetus, + *centes*, puncture). Procedure for withdrawing a sample of fluid around the developing embryo for examination of chromosomes in the embryonic cells and other tests.

amnion (am'nē-än) (Gr., *amnion*, membrane around the fetus). The innermost of the extraembryonic membranes forming a fluid-filled sac around the embryo in amniotes.

amniote (am'nē-ōt). Having an amnion; as a noun, an animal that develops an amnion in embryonic life, that is, reptiles, birds, and mammals.

amphiblastula (am'fə-blas'chə-lə) (Gr., *amphi*, on both sides, + *blastos*, germ, + L., *ula*, small). Free-swimming larval stage of certain marine sponges; blastula-like, but with only the cells of the animal pole flagellated; those of the vegetal pole unflagellated.

amphid (am'fəd) (Gr., *amphidea*, anything that is bound around). One of a pair of anterior sense organs in certain nematodes.

amphipathic (am-fi-pa'thək) (Gr., *amphi*, on both sides, + *pathos*, suffering, passion). Adjective to describe a molecule with one part soluble in water (polar) and another part insoluble in water (nonpolar).

amplexus (am-plek′səs) (L., embrace). The copulatory embrace of frogs or toads.

ampulla (am-pūl′ə) (L., flask). Membranous vesicle; dilation at one end of each semicircular canal containing sensory epithelium; muscular vesicle above tube foot in water-vascular system of echinoderms.

amylase (am′ə-lās′) (L., *amylum*, starch, + *ase*, suffix meaning enzyme). An enzyme that breaks down starch into smaller units.

anadromous (an-ad′rə-məs) (Gr., *anadromos*, running upward). Refers to fishes that migrate up streams from the sea to spawn.

anaerobic (an′ə-rō′bik) (Gr., *an*, not, + *aēr*, air, + *bios*, life). Not dependent on oxygen for respiration.

analogy (L., *analogus*, ratio). Similarity of function but not of origin.

anamorphic (a′nə-mor′fik) (Gr., *ana*, again, + *morphē*, form). Gradually changing form to one of greater complexity. In arthropods, involves the acquisition of additional body segments during development.

anastomosis (ə-nas′tə-mō′səs) (Gr., *ana*, again, + *stoma*, mouth). A union of two or more blood vessels, fibers, or other structures to form a branching network.

androgen (an′drə-jən) (Gr., *anēr, andros*, man, + *genēs*, born). Any of a group of vertebrate male sex hormones. Compare estrogen.

androgenic gland (an′drō-jen′ək) (Gr., *anēr*, male, + *gennaein*, to produce). Gland in Crustacea that causes development of male characteristics.

aneuploidy (an′ū-ploid′ē) (Gr., *an*, without, not, + *eu*, good, well, + *ploid*, multiple of). Loss or gain of a chromosome, cells of the organism have one fewer than normal chromosome number, or one extra chromosome, for example, trisomy 21 (Down's syndrome).

angiotensin (an′jē-o-ten′sən) (Gr., *anggeion*, vessel, + L., *tensio*, to stretch). Blood protein formed from the interaction of renin and a liver protein, causing increased blood pressure and stimulating release of aldosterone and ADH.

Angstrom (after Ångström, Swedish physicist). A unit of one ten millionth of a millimeter (one ten thousandth of a micrometer); it is represented by the symbol Å.

anhydrase (an-hī′drās) (Gr., *an*, not, + *hydōr*, water, + *ase*, enzyme suffix). An enzyme involved in the removal of water from a compound. Carbonic anhydrase promotes the conversion of carbonic acid into water and carbon dioxide.

anisogametes (an′īs-ō-gam′ēts) (Gr., *anisos*, unequal, + *gametēs*, spouse). Gametes of a species that differ in form or size.

anlage (än′lä-gə) (Ger., laying out, foundation). Rudimentary form; primordium.

annulus (an′yəl-əs) (L., ring). Any ringlike structure, such as superficial rings on leeches.

antenna (L., sail yard). A sensory appendage on the head of arthropods, or the second pair of the two such pairs of structures in crustaceans.

antennal gland. Excretory gland of Crustacea located in the antennal metamere.

anterior (L., comparative of *ante*, before). The head end of an organism, or (as an adjective) toward that end.

antibody (an′tē-bod′ē). A protein, usually circulating and dissolved in the blood, that is capable of combining with the antigen that stimulated its production.

anticodon (an′tī-kō′don). A sequence of three nucleotides in transfer RNA that is complementary to a codon in messenger RNA.

antigen (an′-ti-jən). Any substance capable of stimulating an immune response, most often a protein.

aperture (ap′ər-chər) (L., *apertura* from *aperire*, to uncover). An opening; the opening into the first whorl of a gastropod shell.

apical (ā′pə-kl) (L., *apex*, tip). Pertaining to the tip or apex.

apical complex. A certain combination of organelles found in the protozoan phylum Apicomplexa.

apopyle (ap′-ə-pīl) (Gr., *apo*, away from, + *pylē*, gate). In sponges, opening of the radial canal into the spongocoel.

appendicular (L., *ad*, to, + *pendere*, to hang). Pertaining to appendages; pertaining to vermiform appendix.

arboreal (är-bōr′ē-al) (L., *arbor*, tree). Living in trees.

archenteron (ärk-en′tə-rän) (Gr., *archē*, beginning, + *enteron*, gut). The main cavity of an embryo in the gastrula stage; it is lined with endoderm and represents the future digestive cavity.

archeocytes (ärk′ē-ō-sites) (Gr., *archaios*, beginning, + *kytos*, hollow vessel). Ameboid cells of varied function in sponges.

areolar (a-rē′ə-ler) (L., *areola*, small space). A small area, such as spaces between fibers of connective tissue.

arginine phosphate. Phosphate storage compound (phosphagen) found in many invertebrates and used to regenerate stores of ATP.

Aristotle's lantern. Masticating apparatus of some sea urchins.

artiodactyl (är′ti-o-dak′təl) (Gr., *artios*, even, + *daktylos*, toe). One of an order or suborder of mammals with two or four digits on each foot.

asconoid (Gr., *askos*, bladder). Simplest form of sponges, with canals leading directly from the outside to the interior.

asexual. Without distinct sexual organs; not involving formation of gametes.

assimilation (L., *assimilatio*, bringing into conformity). Absorption and building up of digested nutriments into complex organic protoplasmic materials.

atoke (ā′-tōk) (Gr., *a*, without, + *tokos*, offspring). Anterior, nonreproductive part of a marine polychaete, as distinct from the posterior, reproductive part (epitoke) during the breeding season.

ATP. Adenosine triphosphate. In biochemistry, an ester of adenosine and triphosphoric acid.

atrium (ā′trē-əm) (L., *atrium*, vestibule). One of the chambers of the heart; also, the tympanic cavity of the ear; also, the large cavity containing the pharynx in tunicates and cephalochordates.

auricle (aw′ri-kl) (L., *auricula*, dim. of *auris*, ear). One of the less muscular chambers of the heart; atrium; the external ear, or pinna; any earlike lobe or process.

auricularia (ə-rik′u-lar′e-ə) (L., *auricula*, a small ear). A type of larva found in Holothuroidea.

autogamy (aw-täg′ə-me) (Gr., *autos*, self, + *gamos*, marriage). Condition in which the gametic nuclei produced by meiosis fuse within the same organism that produced them to restore the diploid number.

autosome (aw′-tō-sōm) (Gr., *autos*, self, + *sōma*, body). Any chromosome that is not a sex chromosome.

autotomy (aw-täd′ə-me) (Gr., *autos*, self, + *tomos*, a cutting). The breaking off of a part of the body by the organism itself.

autotroph (aw′tō-trōf) (Gr., *autos*, self, + *trophos*, feeder). An organism that makes its organic nutrients from inorganic raw materials.

autotrophic nutrition (Gr., *autos*, self, + *trophia*, denoting nutrition). Nutrition characterized by the ability to use simple inorganic substances for the synthesis of more complex organic compounds, as in green plants and some bacteria.

avicularium (L., *avicula*, small bird, + *aria*, like or connected with). Modified zooid that is attached to the surface of the major zooid in Ectoprocta and resembles a bird's beak.

axial (L., *axis*, axle). Relating to the axis, or stem; on or along the axis.

axolotl (ak′sə-lot′l) (Nahuatl, *atl*, water, + *xolotl*, doll, servant, spirit). Larval stage of any of several species of the genus *Ambystoma* (such as *Ambystoma tigrinum*) exhibiting neotenic reproduction.

axoneme (aks′ə-nēm) (L., *axis*, axle, + Gr., *nēma*, thread). The microtubules in a cilium or flagellum, usually arranged as a circlet of nine pairs enclosing one central pair; also, the microtubules of an axopodium.

axopodium (ak′sə-pō′di-um) (Gr., *axon*, an axis, + *podion*, small foot). Long, slender, more or less permanent pseudopodium found in certain sarcodine protozoa. (Also **axopod.**)

B cell. A type of lymphocyte that is most important in the humoral immune response.

basal body. Also known as kinetosome and blepharoplast, a cylinder of nine triplets of microtubules found basal to a flagellum or cilium; same structure as a centriole.

basis, basipodite (bā′səs, bā-si′pə-dīt) (Gr., *basis*, base, + *pous, podos*, foot). The distal or second joint of the protopod of a crustacean appendage.

bathypelagic (bath'ə-pe-laj'ik) (Gr., *bathys*, deep + *pelagos*, open sea). Relating to or inhabiting the deep sea.

benthos (ben'thäs) (Gr., depth of the sea). Organisms that live along the bottom of seas and lakes; adj., **benthic**. Also, the bottom itself.

biogenesis (bī'ō-jen'ə-səs) (Gr., *bios*, life, + *genesis*, birth). The doctrine that life originates only from preexisting life.

bioluminescence. Method of light production by living organisms in which usually certain proteins (luciferins), in the presence of oxygen and an enzyme (luciferase), are converted to oxyluciferins with the liberation of light.

biomass (Gr., *bios*, life, + *maza*, lump or mass). The weight of total living organisms or of a species population per unit of area.

biome (bī'ōm) (Gr., *bios*, life, + *ōma*, abstract group suffix). Complex of plant and animal communities characterized by climatic and soil conditions; the largest ecological unit.

biosphere (Gr., *bios*, life, + *sphaira*, globe). That part of earth containing living organisms.

bipinnaria (L., *bi*, double, + *pinna*, wing, + *aria*, like or connected with). Free-swimming, ciliated, bilateral larva of the asteroid echinoderms; develops into the brachiolaria larva.

biramous (bī-rām'əs) (L., *bi*, double, + *ramus*, a branch). Adjective describing appendages with two distinct branches, contrasted with uniramous, unbranched.

bivalent (bī-vāl'ənt) (L., *bi*, double + *valen*, strength, worth). The pairs of homologous chromosomes at synapsis in the first meiotic division, a tetrad.

blastocoel (blas'tō-sēl) (Gr., *blastos*, germ, + *koilos*, hollow). Cavity of the blastula.

blastomere (Gr., *blastos*, germ, + *meros*, part). An early cleavage cell.

blastopore (Gr., *blastos*, germ, + *poros*, passage, pore). External opening of the archenteron in the gastrula.

blastula (Gr., *blastos*, germ, + L., *ula*, dim.). Early embryological stage of many animals; consists of a hollow mass of cells.

blepharoplast (blə-fā'rə-plast) (Gr., *blepharon*, eyelid, + *plastos*, formed). See basal body.

blood type. Characteristic of human blood given by the particular antigens on the membranes of the erythrocytes, genetically determined, causing agglutination when incompatible groups are mixed; the blood types are designated A, B, O, AB, Rh negative, Rh positive, and others.

Bohr effect. A characteristic of hemoglobin that causes it to dissociate from oxygen in greater degree at higher concentrations of carbon dioxide.

BP. Before the present.

brachial ((brak'ē-əl) (L., *brachium*, forearm). Referring to the arm.

brachiolaria (brak'ē-ō-lār'ē-ə) (L., *brachiola*, little arm, + *aria*, pertaining to). This asteroid larva develops from the bipinnaria larva and has three preoral holdfast processes.

branchial (brank'ē-əl) (Gr., *branchia*, gills). Referring to gills.

brown fat. Mitochondria-rich, heat-generating adipose tissue of endothermic vertebrates.

buccal (buk'əl) (L., *bucca*, cheek). Referring to the mouth cavity.

buffer. Any substance or chemical compound that tends to keep pH levels constant when acids or bases are added.

calorie (kal'ō-ry) (L., *calere*, to be warm). Unit of heat defined as the amount of heat required to heat 1 g of water from 14.5 to 15.5 C; 1 cal = 4.184 joules in the International System of Units.

capitulum (ka-pi'tə-ləm) (L., small head). Term applied to small, headlike structures of various organisms, including projection from body of ticks and mites carrying mouthparts.

carapace (kar'ə-pās) (F., from Sp., *carapacho*, shell). Shieldlike plate covering the cephalothorax of certain crustaceans; dorsal part of the shell of a turtle.

carbohydrate (L., *carbo*, charcoal, + Gr., *hydōr*, water). Compounds of carbon, hydrogen, and oxygen having the generalized formula $(CH_2O)_n$; aldehyde or ketone derivatives of polyhydric alcohols, with hydrogen and oxygen atoms attached in a 2:1 ratio.

carboxyl (kär-bäk'səl) (carbon + oxygen + yl, chemical radical suffix). The acid group of organic molecules —COOH.

carinate (kar'ə-nāt) (L., *carina*, keel) Having a keel, in particular the flying birds with a keeled sternum for the insertion of flight muscles.

carnivore (kar'nə-vōr') (L., *carnivorus*, flesh eating). One of the flesh-eating mammals of the order Carnivora. Also, any organism that eats animals. Adj., **carnivorous**.

carotene (kär'ə-tēn) (L., *carota*, carrot, + *ene*, unsaturated straight-chain hydrocarbons). A red, orange, or yellow pigment belonging to the group of carotenoids; precursor of vitamin A.

cartilage (L., *cartilago*; akin to L., *cratis*, wickerwork). A translucent elastic tissue that makes up most of the skeleton of embryos, very young vertebrates, and adult cartilaginous fishes, such as sharks and rays; in higher forms much of it is converted into bone.

caste (kast) (L., *castus*, pure, separated). One of the polymorphic forms within an insect society, each caste having its specific duties, as queen, worker, soldier, and so on.

catadromous (kə-tad'rə-məs) (Gr., *kata*, down, + *dromos*, a running). Refers to fishes that migrate from fresh water to the ocean to spawn.

catalyst (kad'ə-ləst) (Gr., *kata*, down, + *lysis*, a loosening). A substance that accelerates a chemical reaction but does not become a part of the end product.

cecum, caecum (sē'kəm) (L., *caecus*, blind). A blind pouch at the beginning of the large intestine; any similar pouch.

cellulose (sel'ū-lōs) (L., *cella*, small room). Chief polysaccharide constituent of the cell wall of green plants and some fungi; an insol-

uble carbohydrate $(C_6H_{10}O_5)_n$ that is converted into glucose by hydrolysis.

centriole (sen'trē-ol) (Gr., *kentron*, center of a circle, + L., *ola*, small). A minute cytoplasmic organelle usually found in the centrosome and considered to be the active division center of the animal cell; organizes spindle fibers during mitosis and meiosis. Same structure as basal body or kinetosome.

centrolecithal (sen'tro-les'ə-thəl) (Gr., *kentron*, center, + *lekithos*, yolk, + Eng., *al*, adjective). Pertaining to an insect egg with the yolk concentrated in the center.

centromere (sen'trə-mir) (Gr., *kentron*, center, + *meros*, part). A small body or constriction on the chromosome to which a spindle fiber attaches during mitosis or meiosis.

centrosome (sen'trə-sōm) (Gr., *kentron*, center, + *sōma*, body). Minute body in cytoplasm of many plant and animal cells that contains one or two centrioles and is the center of dynamic activity in mitosis.

cephalization (sef'ə-li-zā-shən) (Gr., *kephale*, head). The process by which specialization, particularly of the sensory organs and appendages, became localized in the head end of animals.

cephalothorax (sef'ə-lä-thō'raks) (Gr., *kephale*, head, + thorax). A body division found in many Arachnida and higher Crustacea, in which the head is fused with some or all of the thoracic segments.

cercaria (ser-kār'ē-ə) (Gr., *kerkͻs*, tail, + L., *aria*, like or connected with). Tadpolelike larva of trematodes (flukes).

chelicera (kə-lis'ə-rə), pl. **chelicerae** (Gr., *chēlē*, claw, + *keras*, horn). One of a pair of the most anterior head appendages on the members of the subphylum Chelicerata.

chelipeds (kēl'ə-peds) (Gr., *chēlē*, claw, + L., *pes*, foot). Pincerlike first pair of legs in most decapod crustaceans; specialized for seizing and crushing.

chiasma (kī-az'mə), pl. **chiasmata** (Gr., cross). An intersection or crossing, as of nerves; a connection point between homologous chromatids where crossing over has occurred at synapsis.

chitin (kī'tən) (Fr., *chitine*, from Gr., *chitōn*, tunic). A horny substance that forms part of the cuticle of arthropods and is found sparingly in certain other invertebrates; a nitrogenous polysaccharide insoluble in water, alcohol, dilute acids, and digestive juices of most animals.

chloragogue cells (klōr'ə-gog) (Gr., *chloros*, light green, + *agōgos*, a leading, a guide). Modified peritoneal cells, greenish or brownish, clustered around the digestive tract of certain annelids; apparently they aid in elimination of nitrogenous wastes and in food transport.

chlorocruorin (klō'rō-kroo'ə-rən) (Gr., *chloros*, light green, + L., *cruor*, blood). A greenish iron-containing respiratory pigment dissolved in the blood plasma of certain marine polychaetes.

chlorophyll (klō'rō-fil) (Gr., *chloros*, light green, + *phyllon*, leaf). Green pigment found in plants and in some animals; necessary for photosynthesis.

chloroplast (klō'rō-plast) (Gr., *chloros*, light green, + *plastos*, molded). A plastid containing chlorophyll and usually other pigments, found in cytoplasm of plant cells.

choanocyte (kō-an'ō-sīt) (Gr., *choanē*, funnel, + *kytos*, hollow vessel). One of the flagellate collar cells that line cavities and canals of sponges.

cholinergic (kōl'-i-nər'jik) (Gr., *chōle*, bile, + *ergon*, work). Type of nerve fiber that releases acetylcholine from axon terminal.

chorion (kō'rē-on) (Gr., *chorion*, skin). The outer of the double membrane that surrounds the embryo of reptiles, birds, and mammals; in mammals it contributes to the placenta.

choroid plexus (kōr'oid plek'sus) (Gr., *chorion*, skin, + *eidos*, form; L., *plexus*, interwoven). Vascular network in the brain ventricles that regulates secretion and absorption of cerebrospinal fluid.

chromatid (krō'mə-tid) (Gr., *chromato*, from *chrōma*, color, + L., *id*, feminine stem for particle of specified kind). A replicated chromosome joined to its sister chromatid by the centromere; separates and becomes daughter chromosome at anaphase of mitosis or anaphase of the second meiotic division.

chromatin (krō'mə-tin) (Gr., *chrōma*, color). The nucleoprotein material of a chromosome; the hereditary material containing DNA.

chromatophore (krō-mat'ə-fōr) (Gr., *chrōma*, color, + *pherein*, to bear). Pigment cell, usually in the dermis, in which usually the pigment can be dispersed or concentrated.

chromomere (krō'mō-mir) (Gr., *chrōma*, color, + *meros*, part). One of the chromatin granules of characteristic size on the chromosome; may be identical with a gene or a cluster of genes.

chromonema (krō-mə-nē'mə) (Gr., *chrōma*, color, + *nēma*, thread). A convoluted thread in prophase of mitosis or the central thread in a chromosome.

chromoplast (krō'mō-plast) (Gr., *chrōma*, color, + *plastos*, molded). A plastid containing pigment.

chromosome (krō'mə-sōm) (Gr., *chrōma*, color, + *sōma*, body. A complex body, spherical or rod shaped, that arises from the nuclear network during mitosis, splits longitudinally, and carries a part of the organism's genetic information as genes composed of DNA.

chrysalis (kris'ə-lis) (L., from Gr., *chrysos*, gold). The pupal stage of a butterfly.

cilium (sil'i-əm), pl. **cilia** (L., eyelid). A hairlike, vibratile organelle process found on many animal cells. Cilia may be used in moving particles along the cell surface or, in ciliate protozoans, for locomotion.

cinclides (sing'klid-əs), sing. **cinclis** (sing'kləs) (Gr., *kinklis*, latticed gate or partition). Small pores in the external body wall of sea anemones for extrusion of acontia.

circadian (sər'kə-dē'-ən) (L., *circa*, around, + *dies*, day). Occurring at a period of approximately 24 hours.

cirrus (sir'əs) (L., curl). A hairlike tuft on an insect appendage; locomotor organelle of fused cilia; male copulatory organ of some invertebrates.

cisternae (sis-ter'nē) (L., *cista*, box). Space between membranes of the endoplasmic reticulum within cells.

cistron (sis'trən) (L., *cista*, box). A series of codons in DNA that code for an entire polypeptide chain.

cladistics (klad-is'-təks) (Gr., *cladus*, branch, sprout). A system of arranging taxa by analysis of primitive and derived characteristics so that the arrangement will reflect phylogenetic relationships.

cleavage (O.E., *cleofan*, to cut). Process of nuclear and cell division in animal zygote.

climax (klī'maks) (Gr., *klimax*, ladder). Stage of relative stability attained by a community of organisms, often the culminating development of a natural succession. Also, orgasm.

cline (klīn) (Gr., *klinein*, slope, bend). A pattern of gradual genetic change in a population according to its geographical range.

clitellum (klī-tel'əm) (L., *clitellae*, packsaddle). Thickened saddlelike portion of certain midbody segments of many oligochaetes and leeches.

cloaca (klō-ā'kə) (L., sewer). Posterior chamber of digestive tract in many vertebrates, receiving feces and urogenital products. In certain invertebrates, a terminal portion of digestive tract that serves also as respiratory, excretory, or reproductive duct.

clone (klōn) (Gr., *klōn*, twig). All descendants derived by asexual reproduction from a single individual.

cnidocil (nī'dō-sil) (Gr., *knidē*, nettle, + L., *cilium*, hair). Triggerlike spine on nematocyst.

cnidocyte (nī'dō-sīt) (Gr., *knidē*, nettle, + *kytos*, hollow vessel). Modified interstitial cell that holds the nematocyst; during development of the nematocyst, the cnidocyte is a cnidoblast.

coacervate (kō'ə-sər'vət) (L., *coacervatus*, to heap up). An aggregate of colloidal droplets held together by electrostatic forces.

cochlea (kōk'lēə) (L., snail, from Gr., *kochlos*, a shellfish). A tubular cavity of the inner ear containing the essential organs of hearing; occurs in crocodiles, birds, and mammals; spirally coiled in mammals.

cocoon (kə-kun') (Fr., *cocon*, shell). Protective covering of a resting or developmental stage, sometimes used to refer to both the covering and its contents; for example, the cocoon of a moth or the protective covering for the developing embryos in some annelids.

codon (kō'dän) (L., code, + on). A sequence of three adjacent nucleotides that code for one amino acid.

coelenteron (sē-len'tər-on) (Gr., *koilos*, hollow, + *enteron*, intestine). Internal cavity of a cnidarian; gastrovascular cavity; archenteron.

coelom (sē'lōm) (Gr., *koilōma*, cavity). The body cavity in triploblastic animals, lined with mesodermal peritoneum.

coelomocyte (sē'lō'mə-sīt) (Gr., *koilōma*, cavity, + *kytos*, hollow vessel). Another name for amebocyte; primitive or undifferentiated cell of the coelom and the water-vascular system.

coelomoduct (sē-lō'mə-dukt) (Gr., *koilos*, hollow, + L., *ductus*, a leading). A duct that carries gametes or excretory products (or both) from the coelom to the exterior.

coenecium, coenoecium (sə-nēs[h]'ē-um) (Gr., *koinos*, common, + *oikion*, house). The common secreted investment of an ectoproct colony; may be chitinous, gelatinous, or calcareous.

coenocytic (sē'nə-sit'ik) (Gr., *koinos*, common, + *kytos*, hollow vessel). A tissue in which the nuclei are not separated by cell membranes; syncytial.

coenzyme (kō-en'zīm) (L., prefix, *co*, with, + Gr., *enzymos*, leavened, from *en*, in, + *zymē*, leaven). A required substance in the activation of an enzyme; a prosthetic or nonprotein constituent of an enzyme.

collagen (käl'ə-jən) (Gr., *kolla*, glue, + *genos*, descent). A tough, fibrous protein occurring in vertebrates as the chief constituent of collagenous connective tissue; also occurs in invertebrates, for example, the cuticle of nematodes.

collenchyme (käl'ən-kīm) (Gr., *kolla*, glue, + *enchyma*, infusion). A gelatinous mesenchyme containing undifferentiated cells; found in cnidarians and ctenophores.

collencyte (käl'lən-sīt) (Gr., *kolla*, glue, + *en*, in, + *kytos*, hollow vessel). A type of cell in sponges that is star shaped and apparently contractile.

colloblast (käl'ə-blast) (Gr., *kolla*, glue, + *blastos*, germ). A glue-secreting cell on the tentacles of ctenophores.

colloid (kä'loid) (Gr., *kolla*, glue, + *eidos*, form). A two-phase system in which particles of one phase are suspended in the second phase.

columella (kä'lə-mel'ə) (L., small column). Central pillar in gastropod shells.

comb plate. One of the plates of fused cilia that are arranged in rows for ctenophore locomotion.

commensalism (kə-men'səl-iz'əm) (L., *cum*, together with, + *mensa*, table). A relationship in which one individual lives close to or on another and benefits, and the host is unaffected; often symbiotic.

community (L., *communitas*, community, fellowship). An assemblage of organisms that are associated in a common environment and interact with each other in a self-sustaining and self-regulating relation.

competition. Some degree of overlap in ecological niches of two populations in the same community, such that they both depend on the same food source, shelter, or other resources.

complement. Collective name for a series of enzymes and activators in the blood, some of which may bind to antibody and may lead to rupture of a foreign cell.

conjugation (kon′jū-gā′shən) (L., *conjugare*, to yoke together). Temporary union of two ciliate protozoa while they are exchanging chromatin material and undergoing nuclear phenomena resulting in binary fission. Also, formation of cytoplasmic bridges between bacteria for transfer of plasmids.

conspecific (L., *com*, together, + *species*). A member of the same species.

contractile vacuole. A clear fluid-filled cell vacuole in protozoa and a few lower metazoa; takes up water and releases it to the outside in a cyclical manner, for osmoregulation and some excretion.

copulation (Fr., from L., *copulare*, to couple). Sexual union to facilitate the reception of sperm by the female.

copy DNA (cDNA). DNA "copied" from an mRNA molecule using the viral enzyme reverse transcriptase.

corium (kō′re-um) (L., *corium*, leather). The deep layer of the skin; dermis.

cornea (kor′nē-ə) (L., *corneus*, horny). The outer transparent coat of the eye.

corneum (kor′nē-əm) (L., *corneus*, horny). Epithelial layer of dead, keratinized cells. Stratum corneum.

cornified (kor′nə-fīd) (L., *corneus*, horny). Adjective for conversion of epithelial cells into nonliving, keratinized cells.

corona (kə-rō′nə) (L., crown). Head or upper portion of a structure; ciliated disc on anterior end of rotifers.

corpora allata (kor′pə-rə əl-la′tə) (L., *corpus*, body + *allatum*, aided). Endocrine glands in insects that produce juvenile hormone.

cortex (kor′teks) (L., bark). The outer layer of a structure.

coxa, coxopodite (kox′ə, kəx-ä′pə-dīt) (L., *coxa*, hip, + Gr., *pous*, *podos*, foot). The proximal joint of an insect or arachnid leg; in crustaceans, the proximal joint of the protopod.

creatine phosphate. High-energy phosphate compound found in the muscle of vertebrates and some invertebrates, used to regenerate stores of ATP.

crista (kris′tə), pl. **cristae** (L., *crista*, crest). A crest or ridge on a body organ or organelle; a platelike projection formed by the inner membrane of mitochondrion.

crossing over. Exchange of parts of nonsister chromatids at synapsis in the first meiotic division.

cryptobiotic (Gr., *kryptos*, hidden, + *bioticus*, pertaining to life). Living in concealment; refers to insects and other animals that live in secluded situations, such as underground or in wood; also tardigrades and some nematodes, rotifers, and others that survive harsh environmental conditions by assuming for a time a state of very low metabolism.

ctenoid scales (ten′oid) (Gr., *kteis*, *ktenos*, comb). Thin, overlapping dermal scales of the more advanced fishes; exposed posterior margins have fine, toothlike spines.

cuticle (kū′ti-kəl) (L., *cutis*, skin). A protective, noncellular, organic layer secreted by the external epithelium (hypodermis) of many invertebrates. In higher animals the term refers to the epidermis or outer skin.

cyanobacteria (sī-an-ō-bak-ter′ē-ə) (Gr., *kyanos*, a dark-blue substance, + *bakterion*, dim. of *baktron*, a staff). Photosynthetic prokaryotes, also called blue-green algae, cyanophytes.

cyanophyte (sī-an′ō-fīt) (Gr., *kyanos*, a dark-blue substance, + *phyton*, plant). A cyanobacterium, blue-green alga.

cycloid scales (sī′-kloid) (Gr., *kyklos*, circle). Thin, overlapping dermal scales of the more primitive fishes; posterior margins are smooth.

cydippid larva (sī-dip′pid) (Gr., *kydippe*, mythological Athenian maiden). Free-swimming larva of most ctenophores; superficially similar to the adult.

cyrtocyte (ser′tō-sīt) (Gr., *kyrtē*, a fish basket, cage, + *kytos*, hollow vessel). A protonephridial cell with a single flagellum enclosed in a cylinder of cytoplasmic rods.

cysticercoid (sis′tə-ser′coəd) (Gr., *kystis*, bladder, + *kerkos*, tail, + *eidos*, form). A type of juvenile tapeworm comprised of a solid-bodied cyst containing an invaginated scolex; contrast with cysticercus.

cysticercus (sis′tə-ser′kəs) (Gr., *kystis*, bladder, + *kerkos*, tail). A type of juvenile tapeworm in which an invaginated and introverted scolex is contained in a fluid-filled bladder; contrast with cysticercoid.

cystid (sis′tid) (Gr., *kystis*, bladder). In an ectoproct, the dead secreted outer parts plus the adherent underlying living layers.

cytochrome (sī′tə-krōm) (Gr., *kytos*, hollow vessel, + *chrōma*, color). Several iron-containing pigments that serve as electron carriers in aerobic respiration.

cytokinesis (sī′tə-kin-ē′sis) (Gr., *kytos*, hollow vessel, + *kinesis*, movement). Division of the cytoplasm of a cell.

cytopharynx (Gr., *kytos*, hollow vessel, + *pharynx*, throat). Short tubular gullet in ciliate protozoa.

cytoplasm (sī′tə-plasm) (Gr., *kytos*, hollow vessel, + *plasma*, mold). The living matter of the cell, excluding the nucleus.

cytoproct (sī′tə-prokt) (Gr., *kytos*, hollow vessel, + *prōktos*, anus). Site on a protozoan where undigestible matter is expelled.

cytosol (sī′tə-sol) (Gr., *kytos*, hollow vessel, + L., *sol*, from *solutus*, to loosen). Unstructured portion of the cytoplasm in which the organelles are bathed.

cytosome (sī′tə-sōm) (Gr., *kytos*, hollow vessel, + *sōma*, body). The cell body inside the plasma membrane.

cytostome (sī′tə-stōm) (Gr., *kytos*, hollow vessel, + *stoma*, mouth). The cell mouth in many protozoa.

Darwinism. Theory of evolution by natural selection.

definitive host. The host in which sexual reproduction of a symbiont takes place; if no sexual reproduction, then the host in which the symbiont becomes mature and reproduces; contrast intermediate host.

deme (dēm) (Gr., populace). A local population of closely related animals.

demography (də-mäg′grə-fē) (Gr., *demos*, people, + *graphy*). The properties of the rate of growth and the age structure of populations.

deoxyribonucleic acid (DNA). The genetic material of all organisms, characteristically organized into linear sequences of genes.

deoxyribose (dē-ok′sē-rī′bōs) (L., *deoxy*, loss of oxygen, + ribose, a pentose sugar). A 5-carbon sugar having 1 oxygen atom less than ribose; a component of deoxyribonucleic acid (DNA).

dermal (Gr., *derma*, skin). Pertaining to the skin; cutaneous.

dermis. The inner, sensitive mesodermal layer of skin; corium.

desmosome (dez′mə-sōm) (Gr., *desmos*, bond, + *sōma*, body). Buttonlike plaque serving as an intercellular connection.

determinate cleavage. The type of cleavage, usually spiral, in which the fate of the blastomeres is determined very early in development; mosaic cleavage.

detritus (də-trī′tus) (L., that which is rubbed or worn away). Any fine particulate debris of organic or inorganic origin.

Deuterostomia (dū′də-rō-stō′mē-ə) (Gr., *deuteros*, second, secondary, + *stoma*, mouth). A group of higher phyla in which cleavage is indeterminate and primitively radial. The endomesoderm is entercoelous, and the mouth is derived away from the blastopore. Includes Echinodermata, Chordata, and a number of minor phyla. Compare with Protostomia.

dextral (dex′trəl) (L., *dexter*, right-handed). Pertaining to the right; in gastropods, shell is dextral if opening is to right of columella when held with spire up and facing observer.

diapause (dī′ə-pawz) (Gr., *diapausis*, pause). A period of arrested development in the life cycle of insects and certain other animals in which physiological activity is very low and the animal is highly resistant to unfavorable external conditions.

diffusion (L., *diffusus*, dispersion). The movement of particles or molecules from area of high concentration of the particles or molecules to area of lower concentration.

digitigrade (dij′ə-də-grād) (L., *digitus*, finger, toe, + *gradus*, step, degree). Walking on the digits with the posterior part of the foot raised; compare plantigrade.

dihybrid (dī-hī′brəd) (Gr., *dis*, twice, + L., *hibrida*, mixed offspring). A hybrid whose parents differ in two distinct characters; an offspring having different alleles at two different loci, for example, A/a B/b.

dimorphism (dī-mor′fizm) (Gr., *di*, two, + *morphē*, form). Existence within a species of two distinct forms according to color, sex, size, organ structure, and so on. Occurrence of two kinds of zooids in a colonial organism.

dioecious (dī-ē′shəs) (Gr., *di*, two, + *oikos*, house). Having male and female organs in separate individuals.

diphycercal (dif′i-ser′kəl) (Gr., *diphyēs*, twofold, + *kerkos*, tail). A tail that tapers to a point, as in lungfishes; vertical column extends to tip without upturning.

diphyodont (di'fi-ə-dänt) (Gr., *diphyēs*, two-fold, + *odous*, tooth). Having deciduous and permanent sets of teeth successively.

dipleurula (dī-ploor'ū-lə) (Gr., *di*, two, + *pleura*, rib, side, + L., *ula*, small). A hypothetical, simple ancestral form of echinoderms; elongated and bilaterally symmetrical, with three pairs of coelomic sacs.

diploblastic (di'plə-blas'tək) (Gr., *diploos*, double, + *blastos*, bud). Organism with two germ layers, endoderm and ectoderm.

diploid (dip'loid) (Gr., *diploos*, double, + *eidos*, form). Having the somatic (double, or 2n) number of chromosomes or twice the number characteristic of a gamete of a given species.

DNA. See deoxyribonucleic acid.

dominance hierarchy. A social ranking, formed through agonistic behavior, in which individuals are associated with each other so that some have greater access to resources than do others.

dorsal (dor'səl) (L., *dorsum*, back). Toward the back, or upper surface, of an animal.

Down's syndrome. A congenital syndrome including mental retardation, caused by the cells in a person's body having an extra chromosome 21; also called trisomy 21.

drive. A state of activity directed toward satisfying a specific need.

dyad (dī'əd) (Gr., *dyas*, two). One of the groups of two chromosomes formed by the division of a tetrad during the first meiotic division.

ecdysis (ek'də-sis) (Gr., *ekdysis*, to strip off, escape). Shedding of outer cuticular layer; molting, as in insects or crustaceans.

ecdysone (ek-dī'sōn) (Gr., *ekdysis*, to strip off). Molting hormone of arthropods, stimulates growth and ecdysis, produced by prothoracic glands in insects and Y organs in crustaceans.

ecology (Gr., *oikos*, house, + *logos*, discourse). Part of biology that deals with the relationship between organisms and their environment.

ecosystem (ek'ō-sis-təm) (eco[logy]) from Gr., *oikos*, house, + system). An ecological unit consisting of both the biotic communities and the nonliving (abiotic) environment, which interact to produce a stable system.

ecotone (ek'ō-tōn) (eco[logy] from Gr., *oikos*, home, + *tonos*, stress). The transition zone between two adjacent communities.

ectoderm (ek'tō-derm) (Gr., *ektos*, outside, + *derma*, skin). Outer layer of cells of an early embryo (gastrula stage); one of the germ layers, also sometimes used to include tissues derived from ectoderm.

ectolecithal (ek'tō-les'ə-thəl) (Gr., *ektos*, outside, + *lekithos*, yolk). Yolk for nutrition of the embryo contributed by cells that are sep-

arate from the egg cell and are combined with the zygote by envelopment within the eggshell.

ectoplasm (ec'tō-plazm) (Gr., *ektos*, outside, + *plasma*, form). The cortex of a cell or that part of cytoplasm just under the cell surface; contrasts with endoplasm.

ectothermic (ek'tō-therm'ic) (Gr., *ektos*, outside, + *thermē*, heat). Having a variable body temperature derived from heat acquired from the environment; contrasts with **endothermic.**

effector (L., *efficere*, bring to pass). An organ, tissue, or cell that becomes active in response to stimulation.

efferent (ef'ə-rənt) (L., *ex*, out, + *ferre*, to bear). Leading or conveying away from some organ, for example, nerve impulses conducted away from the brain, or blood conveyed away from an organ; contrasts with **afferent.**

eleocyte (el'ē-ə-sīt) (Gr., *elaion*, oil, + *kytos*, hollow vessel). Fat-containing cells in annelids that originate from the chlorogogue tissue.

elephantiasis (el-ə-fən-tī'ə-səs). Disfiguring condition caused by chronic infection with filarial worms *Wuchereria bancrofti* and *Brugia malayi*.

embryogenesis (em'brē-ō-jen'ə-səs) (Gr., *embryon*, embryo, + *genesis*, origin). The origin and development of the embryo; embryogeny.

emigrate (L., *emigrare*, to move out). To move *from* one area to another to take up residence; contrasts with immigrate.

emulsion (ə-məl'shən) (L., *emulsus*, milked out). A colloidal system in which both phases are liquids.

endemic (en-dem'ik) (Gr., *en*, in, + *demos*, populace). Peculiar to a certain region or country; native to a restricted area; not introduced.

endergonic (en-dər-gän'ik) (Gr., *endon*, within, + *ergon*, work). Used in reference to a chemical reaction that requires energy; energy absorbing.

endite (en'dīt) (Gr., *endon*, within). Medial process on an arthropod limb.

endocrine (en'də-krən) (Gr., *endon*, within, + *krinein*, to separate). Refers to a gland that is without a duct and that releases its product directly into the blood or lymph.

endocytosis (en'dō-sī-tō'sis) (Gr., *endon*, within, + *kytos*, hollow vessel). The engulfment of matter by phagocytosis and of macromolecules by pinocytosis.

endoderm (en'də-dərm) (Gr., *endon*, within, + *derma*, skin). Innermost germ layer of an embryo, forming the primitive gut; also may refer to tissues derived from endoderm.

endolecithal (en'də-les'ə-thəl) (Gr., *endon*, within, + *lekithos*, yolk). Yolk for nutrition of the embryo incorporated into the egg cell itself.

endolymph (en'do-limf) (Gr., *endon*, within, + *lympha*, water). Fluid that fills most of the membranous labyrinth of the vertebrate ear.

endometrium (en'də-mē'trē-əm) (Gr., *endon*, within, + *mētra*, womb). The mucous membrane lining the uterus.

endoplasm (en'də-pla-zm) (Gr., *endon*, within, + *plasma*, mold or form). The portion of cytoplasm that immediately surrounds the nucleus.

endoplasmic reticulum. A complex of membranes within a cell; may bear ribosomes (rough) or not (smooth).

endopod, endopodite (en'də-päd, en-dop'ə-dīt) (Gr., *endon*, within, + *pous, podos,* foot). Medial branch of a biramous crustacean appendage.

endopterygote (en'dəp-ter'i-gōt) (Gr., *endon*, within, + *pteron*, feather, wing). Insect in which the wing buds develop internally; has holometabolous metamorphosis.

endorphin (en-dor'fin) (contraction of endogenous morphine). Group of opiate-like brain neuropeptides that modulate pain perception and are implicated in many other functions.

endoskeleton (Gr., *endon*, within, + *skeletos*, hard). A skeleton or supporting framework within the living tissues of an organism; contrasts with **exoskeleton.**

endosome (en'də-sōm) (Gr., *endon*, within, + *sōma*, body). Nucleolus in nucleus of some protozoa that retains its identity through mitosis.

endostyle (en'də-stīl) (Gr., *endon*, within, + *stylos*, a pillar). Ciliated groove(s) in the floor of the pharynx of tunicates, cephalochordates, and larval cyclostomes, useful for accumulating and moving food particles to the stomach.

endothermic (en'də-therm'ic) (Gr., *endon*, within, + *thermē*, heat). Having a body temperature determined by heat derived from the animal's own oxidative metabolism; contrasts with **ectothermic.**

enkephalin (en-kef'lin) (Gr., *endon*, within, + *kephale*, head). Group of small brain neuropeptides with opiate-like qualities.

enterocoel (en'tər-ō-sēl') (Gr., *enteron*, gut, + *koilos*, hollow). A type of coelom formed by the outpouching of a mesodermal sac from the endoderm of the primitive gut.

enterocoelic mesoderm formation. Embryonic formation of mesoderm by a pouchlike outfolding from the archenteron, which then expands and obliterates the blastocoel, thus forming a large cavity, the coelom, lined with mesoderm.

enterocoelomate (en'ter-ō-sēl'ō-māte) (Gr., *enteron*, gut, + *koilōma*, cavity, + Eng., *ate*, state of). An animal having an enterocoel, such as an echinoderm or a vertebrate.

enteron (en'tə-rän) (Gr., intestine). The digestive cavity.

entozoic (en-tə-zō'ic) (Gr., *entos*, within, + *zōon*, animal). Living within another animal; internally parasitic (chiefly parasitic worms).

entropy (en'trə-pē) (Gr., *en*, in, on, + *tropos*, turn, change in manner). A quantity that is the measure of energy in a system not available for doing work.

enzyme (en'zīm) (Gr., *enzymos*, leavened, from *en*, in, + *zyme*, leaven). A protein substance, produced by living cells, that is capable of speeding up specific chemical transformations, such as hydrolysis, oxidation, or reduction, but is unaltered itself in the process; a biological catalyst.

ephyra (ef´ə-rə) (Gr., *Ephyra*, Greek city). Refers to castlelike appearance. Medusa bud from a scyphozoan polyp.

epidermis (ep´ə-dər´məs) (Gr., *epi*, on, upon, + *derma*, skin). The outer, nonvascular layer of skin of ectodermal origin; in invertebrates, a single layer of ectodermal epithelium.

epididymis (ep´ə-did´ə-məs) (Gr., *epi*, on, upon, + *didymos*, testicle). Part of the sperm duct that is coiled and lying near the testis.

epigenesis (ep´ə-jen´ə-sis) (Gr., *epi*, on, upon, + *genesis*, birth). The embryological (and generally accepted) view that an embryo is a new creation that develops and differentiates step by step from an initial stage; the progressive production of new parts that were nonexistent as such in the original zygote.

epigenetics (ep´ə-jə-net´iks) (Gr., *epi*, on, upon, + *genesis*, birth). Study of mechanisms by which the genes produce phenotypic effects.

epilimnion (ep-ə-lim´ne-än) (Gr., *epi*, on, upon, + *limnē*, lake). Upper water that overlies the thermocline of a lake or sea.

epimorphic (ep´ə-mor´fik) (Gr., *epi*, on, upon, + *morphē*, form). Having the same form in successive stages of growth; pertains especially to insects and crustaceans in which the juvenile hatching from the egg is morphologically similar to the adult.

epipod, epipodite (ep´ē-päd, e-pip´ə-dīt) (Gr., *epi*, on, upon, + *pous, podos*, foot). A lateral process on the protopod of a crustacean appendage, often modified as a gill.

epistasis (ə-pis´tə-səs) (Gr., *epi*, on, upon, + *stasis*, a standing still). Masking or prevention of the expression of one gene by another gene at another locus.

epithelium (ep´i-thē´lē-um) (Gr., *epi*, on, upon, + *thele*, nipple). A cellular tissue covering a free surface or lining a tube or cavity.

epitoke (ep´i-tōk) (Gr., *epitokos*, fruitful). Posterior part of a marine polychaete when swollen with developing gonads during the breeding season; contrast with **atoke**.

erythroblastosis fetalis (ə-rith´-rō-blas-tō´səs fə-tal´əs) (Gr., *erythros*, red, + *blastos*, germ, + *osis*, a disease; L., *fetalis*, relating to a fetus). A disease of newborn infants caused when Rh-negative mothers develop antibodies against the Rh-positive blood of the fetus. See **blood type**.

erythrocyte (ə-rith´rō-sīt) (Gr., *erythros*, red, + *kytos*, hollow vessel). Red blood cell; has hemoglobin to carry oxygen from lungs or gills to tissues; during formation in mammals, erythrocytes lose their nuclei, those of other vertebrates retain the nuclei.

estrus (es´trəs) (L., *oestrus*, gadfly, frenzy). The period of heat, or rut, especially of the female during ovulation of the egg. Associated with maximum sexual receptivity.

estuary (es´chə-we´rē) (L., *aestuarium*, estuary). An arm of the sea where the tide meets the current of a freshwater stream.

ethology (e-thäl´-ə-jē) (Gr., *ethos*, character, + *logos*, discourse). The study of animal behavior in natural environments.

euchromatin (ū´krō-mə-tən) (Gr., *eu*, good, well, + *chrōma*, color). Part of the chromatin that takes up stain less than heterochromatin, contains active genes.

eukaryotic, eucaryotic (ū´ka-rē-ot´ik) (Gr., *eu*, good, true, + *karyon*, nut, kernel). Organisms whose cells characteristically contain a membrane-bound nucleus or nuclei; contrasts with **prokaryotic.**

euploidy (ū´ploid´ē) (Gr., *eu*, good, well, + *ploid*, multiple of). Change in chromosome number from one generation to the next in which there is an addition or deletion of a complete set of chromosomes in the progeny; the most common type is polyploidy.

euryhaline (ū´-rə-hā´līn) (Gr., *eurys*, broad, + *hals*, salt). Able to tolerate wide ranges of saltwater concentrations.

euryphagous (yə-rif´ə-gəs) (Gr., *eurys*, broad, + *phagein*, to eat). Eating a large variety of foods.

eurytopic (ū-rə-täp´ik) (Gr., *eurys*, broad, + *topos*, place). Refers to an organism with a wide distribution range.

eutely (u´te-lē) (Gr., *euteia*, thrift). Condition of a body composed of a constant number of cells or nuclei in all adult members of a species, as in rotifers, acanthocephalans, and nematodes.

evagination (ē-vaj´ə-nā´shən) (L., *e*, out, + *vagina*, sheath). An outpocketing from a hollow structure.

evolution (L., *evolvere*, to unfold). Organic evolution is any genetic change in organisms, or more strictly a change in gene frequency from generation to generation.

excision repair. Means by which cells are able to repair certain kinds of damage (dimerized pyrimidines) in their DNA.

exergonic (ek´sər-gän´ik) (Gr., *exō*, outside of, + *ergon*, work). An energy-yielding reaction.

exite (ex´īt) (Gr., *exō*, outside). Process from lateral side of an arthropod limb.

exocrine (ek´sə-krən) (Gr., *exō*, outside, + *krinein*, to separate). A type of gland that releases its secretion through a duct; contrasts with **endocrine.**

exon (ex´ən) (Gr., *exō*, outside). Part of the mRNA as transcribed from the DNA that contains a portion of the information necessary for final gene product.

exopod, exopodite (ex´ə-päd, ex-äp´ə-dīt) (Gr., *exō*, outside, + *pous, podos*, foot). Lateral branch of a biramous crustacean appendage.

exopterygote (ek´səp-ter´i-gōt) (Gr., *exō*, without, + *pteron*, feather, wing). Insect in which the wing buds develop externally during nymphal instars; has hemimetabolous metamorphosis.

exoskeleton (ek´sō-skel´ə-tən) (Gr., *exō*, outside, + *skeletos*, hard). A supporting structure secreted by ectoderm or epidermis; external, not enveloped by living tissue, as opposed to endoskeleton.

expressivity. The magnitude of a phenotypic effect as produced by a gene, as opposed to the frequency of the phenotypic effect in a population (penetrance).

exteroceptor (ek´stər-ō-sep´tər) (L., *exter*, outward, + *capere*, to take). A sense organ excited by stimuli from the external world.

facilitated transport. Mediated transport of a substance into a cell in the direction of a concentration gradient, contrast with active transport.

FAD. Abbreviation for flavine adenine dinucleotide, an electron acceptor in the respiratory chain.

fatty acid. Any of a series of saturated organic acids having the general formula $C_nH_{2n}O_2$, occurs in natural fats of animals and plants.

fermentation (L., *fermentum*, ferment). Enzymatic transformation, without oxygen, of organic substrates, especially carbohydrates, yielding products such as alcohols, acids, and carbon dioxide.

fiber, fibril (L., *fibra*, thread). These two terms are often confused. Fiber is a fiberlike cell or a strand of protoplasmic material produced or secreted by a cell and lying outside the cell. Fibril is a strand of protoplasm produced by a cell and lying within the cell.

filipodium (fi´li-pō´de-əm) (L., *filum*, thread, + Gr., *pous, podos*, a foot). A type of pseudopodium that is very slender and may branch but does not rejoin to form a mesh.

filter feeding. Any feeding process by which particulate food is filtered from water in which it is suspended.

fission (L., *fissio*, a splitting). Asexual reproduction by a division of the body into two or more parts.

fitness. Degree of adjustment and suitability for a particular environment. Genetic fitness is relative contribution of one genetically distinct organism to the next generation; organisms with high genetic fitness are naturally selected and become prevalent in a population.

flagellum (flə-jel´əm)(L., a whip). Whiplike organelle of locomotion.

flame bulb. Specialized hollow excretory or osmoregulatory structure of one or several small cells containing a tuft of cilia (the "flame") and situated at the end of a minute tubule; connected tubules ultimately open to the outside. See **solenocyte, protonephridium.**

fluke (O.E., *flōc*, flatfish). A member of class Trematoda or class Monogenea. Also, certain of the flatfishes (order Pleuronectiformes).

FMN. Abbreviation for flavin mononucleotide, the prosthetic group of a protein (flavoprotein) and a carrier in the electron transport chain in respiration.

food vacuole. A digestive organelle in the cell.

fouling. Contamination of feeding or respiratory areas of an organism by excrement, sediment, or other matter. Also, accumulation of sessile marine organisms on the hull of a boat or ship so as to impede its progress through the water.

fovea (fō´vē-ə) (L., a small pit). A small pit or depression; especially the fovea centralis, a small rodless pit in the retina of some vertebrates, a point of acute vision.

free energy. The energy available for doing work in a chemical system.

gamete (ga´mēt, gə-mēt´) (Gr., *gamos*, marriage). A mature haploid sex cell; usually, male and female gametes can be distinguished. An egg or a sperm.

gametic meiosis. Meiosis that occurs during formation of the gametes, as in humans and other higher animals.

gametocyte (gə-mēt′ə-sīt) (Gr., *gametēs*, spouse, + *kytos*, hollow vessel). The mother cell of a gamete, that is, immature gamete.

ganoid scales (ga′noid) (Gr., *ganos*, brightness). Thick, bony, rhombic scales of some primitive bony fishes; not overlapping.

gap junction. An area of tiny canals communicating the cytoplasm between two cells.

gastrodermis (gas′tro-dər′mis) (Gr., *gaster*, stomach, + *derma*, skin). Lining of the digestive cavity of cnidarians.

gastrovascular cavity (Gr., *gaster*, stomach, + L., *vasculum*, small vessel). Body cavity in certain lower invertebrates that functions in both digestion and circulation and has a single opening serving as both mouth and anus.

gastrula (gas′tro-lə) (Gr., *gaster*, stomach, + L., *ula*, dim.). Embryonic stage, usually cap or sac shaped, with walls of two layers of cells surrounding a cavity (archenteron) with one opening (blastopore).

gastrulation (gas′tro-lā′shən) (Gr., *gaster*, stomach). Process by which an early metazoan embryo becomes a gastrula, acquiring first two and then three layers of cells.

gel (jel) (from gelatin, from L., *gelare*, to freeze). That state of a colloidal system in which the solid particles form the continuous phase and the fluid medium the discontinuous phase.

gemmule (je′mūl) (L., *gemma*, bud, + *ula*, dim.). Asexual, cystlike reproductive unit in freshwater sponges; formed in summer or autumn and capable of overwintering.

gene (Gr., *genos*, descent). The part of a chromosome that is the hereditary determiner and is transmitted from one generation to another. It is a section of DNA that occupies a characteristic chromosomal locus and can best be defined only in a physiological or operational sense.

gene pool. A collection of all of the alleles of all of the genes in a population.

genetic drift. Change in gene frequencies by chance processes in the evolutionary process of animals. In small populations, one allele may drift to fixation, becoming the only representative of that gene locus.

genome (jē′nōm) (Gr., *genos*, offspring, + L., *ōma*, abstract group). All the genes in a haploid set of chromosomes.

genotype (jēn′ō-tīp) (Gr., *genos*, offspring, + *typos*, form). The genetic constitution, expressed and latent, of an organism; the total set of genes present in the cells of an organism; contrasts with **phenotype.**

genus (jē-nus), pl. **genera** (L., race). A group of related species with taxonomic rank between family and species.

germ layer. In the animal embryo, one of three basic layers (ectoderm, endoderm, mesoderm)

from which the various organs and tissues arise in the multicellular animal.

germ plasm. The germ cells of an organism, as distinct from the somatoplasm; the hereditary material (genes) of the germ cells.

gestation (je-stā′shən) (L., *gestare*, to bear). The period in which offspring are carried in the uterus.

glochidium (glō-kid′e-əm) (Gr., *glochis*, point, + *idion*, dim.). Bivalved larval stage of freshwater mussels.

glomerulus (glä-mer′u-ləs) (L., *glomus*, ball). A tuft of capillaries projecting into a renal corpuscle in a kidney. Also, a small spongy mass of tissue in the proboscis of hemichordates, presumed to have an excretory function. Also, a concentration of nerve fibers situated in the olfactory bulb.

glycogen (glī′kə-jən) (Gr., *glykys*, sweet, + *genēs*, produced). A polysaccharide constituting the principal form in which carbohydrate is stored in animals; animal starch.

glycolysis (glī-kol′i-sis) (Gr., *glykys*, sweet, + *lyein*, to loosen). Enzymatic breakdown of glucose (especially) or glycogen into phosphate derivatives with release of energy.

gnathobase (nāth′ə-bās′) (Gr., *gnathos*, jaw, + base). A median basic process on certain appendages in some arthropods, usually for biting or crushing food.

Golgi complex (gōl′jē) (after Golgi, Italian histologist). An organelle in cells that serves as a collecting and packaging center for secretory products.

gonad (gō′nad) (N.L., *gonas*, a primary sex organ). An organ that produces gametes (ovary in the female and testis in the male).

gonangium (gō-nan′jē-əm) (N.L., *gonas*, primary sex organ + *angeion*, dim. of vessel). Reproductive zooid of hydroid colony (Cnidaria).

gonoduct (Gr., *gonos*, seed, progeny, + duct). Duct leading from a gonad to the exterior.

gonopore (gän′ə-pōr) (Gr., *gonos*, seed, progeny, + *poros*, an opening). A genital pore found in many invertebrates.

green gland. Excretory gland of certain Crustacea; the antennal gland.

gregarious (L., *grex*, herd). Living in groups or flocks.

guanine (gwä′nēn) (Sp., from Quechura, *huanu*, dung). A white crystalline purine base, $C_5H_5N_5O$, occurring in various animal tissues and in guano and other animal excrements.

gynandromorph (ji-nan′dra-mawrf) (Gr., *gyn*, female, + *andr*, male + *morphē*, form). A bisexual form with the characteristics of both sexes; bisexual mosaic.

gynocophoric canal (gī′nə-kə-fōr′ik) (Gr., *gynē*, woman, + *pherein*, to carry). Groove in male schistosomes (certain trematodes) that carries the female.

habitat (L., *habitare*, to dwell). The place where an organism normally lives or where individuals of a population live.

habituation. A kind of learning in which continued exposure to the same stimulus produces diminishing responses.

halter (hal′tər), pl. **halteres** (hal-ti′rēz) (Gr., leap). In Diptera, small club-shaped structure on each side of the metathorax representing

the hindwings; believed to be sense organs for balancing; also called balancer.

haploid (Gr., *haploos*, single). The reduced, or n, number of chromosomes, typical of gametes, as opposed to the diploid, or 2n, number found in somatic cells. In certain lower phyla, some mature animals have a haploid number of chromosomes.

hectocotylus (hek-tə-kät′ə-ləs) (Gr., *hekaton*, hundred, + *kotylē*, cup). Specialized, and sometimes autonomous, arm that serves as a male copulatory organ in cephalopods.

hemal system (hē′məl) (Gr., *haima*, blood). System of small vessels in echinoderms; function unknown.

hemerythrin (hē′mə-rith′rin) (Gr., *haima*, blood, + *erythros*, red). A red, iron-containing respiratory pigment found in the blood of some polychaetes, sipunculids, priapulids, and brachiopods.

hemimetabolous (he′mi-mə-ta′bə-ləs) (Gr., *hēmi*, half, + *metabolē*, change). Refers to gradual metamorphosis during development of insects, without a pupal stage.

hemoglobin (Gr., *haima*, blood, + L., *globulus*, globule). An iron-containing respiratory pigment occurring in vertebrate red blood cells and in blood plasma of many invertebrates; a compound of an iron porphyrin heme and a protein globin.

hemolymph (hē′mə-limf) (Gr., *haima*, blood, + L., *lympha*, water). Fluid in the coelom or hemocoel of some invertebrates that represents the blood and lymph of higher forms.

hemozoin (hē-mə-zo′ən) (Gr., *haima*, blood, + *zōon*, an animal). Insoluble digestion product of malaria parasites produced from hemoglobin.

hepatic (hə-pat′ic) (Gr., *hēpatikos*, of the liver). Pertaining to the liver.

herbivore ([h]ərb′ə-vōr′) (L., *herba*, green crop, + *vorare*, to devour). Any organism subsisting on plants. Adj., **herbivorous.**

hermaphrodite (hə[r]-maf′rə-dīt) (Gr., *hermaphroditos*, containing both sexes; from Greek mythology, Hermaphroditos, son of Hermes and Aphrodite). An organism with both male and female functional reproductive organs. **Hermaphroditism** may refer to an aberration in unisexual animals; **monoecism** implies that this is the normal condition for the species.

hermatypic (hər-mə-ti′pik) (Gr., *herma*, reef, + *typos*, pattern). Relating to reef-forming corals.

heterocercal (het′ər-o-sər′kəl) (Gr., *heteros*, different, + *kerkos*, tail). In some fishes, a tail with the upper lobe larger than the lower, and the end of the vertebral column somewhat upturned in the upper lobe, as in sharks.

heterochromatin (he′tə-rō-krōm′ə-tən) (Gr., *heteros*, different, + *chrōma*, color). Chromatin that stains intensely and appears to represent inactive genetic areas.

heterochrony (hed′ə-rō-krōn-y) (Gr., *heteros*, different, + *chronos*, time). Change in the relative time of appearance and rate of development of characters already present in ancestors.

heterodont (hed′ə-ro-dänt) (Gr., *heteros*, different, + *odous*, tooth). Having teeth differentiated into incisors, canines, and molars for different purposes.

heterotroph (hət′ə-rō-träf) (Gr., *heteros*, different, + *trophos*, feeder). An organism that obtains both organic and inorganic raw materials from the environment in order to live; includes most animals and those plants that do not carry on photosynthesis.

heterozygote (het′ə-rō-zī′gōt) (Gr., *heteros*, different, + *zygotos*, yoked). An organism in which the pair of alleles for a trait is composed of different genes (usually dominant and recessive); derived from a zygote formed by the union of gametes of dissimilar genetic constitution.

hexamerous (hek-sam′ər-əs) (Gr., *hex*, six, + *meros*, part). Six parts, specifically, symmetry based on six or multiples thereof.

hibernation (L., *hibernus*, wintry). Condition, especially of mammals, of passing the winter in a torpid state in which the body temperature drops nearly to freezing and the metabolism drops close to zero.

histogenesis (his-tō-jen′ə-sis) (Gr., *histos*, tissue, + *genesis*, descent). Formation and development of tissue.

histone (hi′stōn) (Gr., *histos*, tissue). Any of several simple proteins found in cell nuclei and complexed at one time or another with DNA. Histones yield a high proportion of basic amino acids on hydrolysis; characteristic of eukaryotes.

holoblastic cleavage (Gr., *holo*, whole, + *blastos*, germ). Complete and approximately equal division of cells in early embryo. Found in mammals, amphioxus, and many aquatic invertebrates that have eggs with a small amount of yolk.

holometabolous (hō′lō-mə-ta′bə-ləs) (Gr., *holo*, complete, + *metabolē*, change). Complete metamorphosis during development.

holophytic nutrition (hōl′ō-fit′ik) (Gr., *holo*, whole, + *phyt*, plant). Occurs in green plants and certain protozoa and involves synthesis of carbohydrates from carbon dioxide and water in the presence of light, chlorophyll, and certain enzymes.

holozoic nutrition (hōl′ō-zō′ik) (Gr., *holo*, whole, + *zoikos*, of animals). Type of nutrition involving ingestion of liquid or solid organic food particles.

home range. The area over which an animal ranges in its activities. Unlike territories, home ranges are not defended.

homeostasis (hō′mē-ō-stā′sis) (Gr., *homeo*, similar, + *stasis*, state or standing). Maintenance of an internal steady state by means of self-regulation.

homeothermic (hō′mē-ō-thər′mik) (Gr., *homeo*, alike, + *thermē*, heat). Having a nearly uniform body temperature, regulated independent of the environmental temperature; "warm blooded."

hominid (häm′ə-nid) (L., *homo, hominis,* man). A member of the family Hominidae, now represented by one living species, *Homo sapiens.*

hominoid (häm′ə-noid). Relating to the Hominoidea, a superfamily of primates to which the great apes and humans are assigned.

homocercal (hō′mə-ser′kal) (Gr., *homos*, same, common, + *kerkos*, tail). A tail with the upper and lower lobes symmetrical and the vertebral column ending near the middle of the base, as in most teleost fishes.

homodont (hō′mō-dänt) (Gr., *homos*, same, + *odous*, tooth). Having all teeth similar in form.

homograft. See **allograft.**

homology (hō-mäl′ə-jē) (Gr., *homologos*, agreeing). Similarity of parts or organs of different organisms caused by similar embryonic origin and evolutionary development from a corresponding part in some remote ancestor. Also, correspondence in structure of different parts of the same individual. May also refer to a matching pair of chromosomes. Adj., **homologous.**

homozygote (hō-mə-zī′gōt) (Gr., *homos*, same, + *zygotos*, yoked). An organism in which the pair of alleles for a trait is composed of the same genes (either dominant or recessive but not both). Adj., **homozygous.**

humoral (hū′mər-əl) (L., *humor*, a fluid). Pertaining to an endocrine secretion.

hyaline (hī′ə-lən) (Gr., *hyalos*, glass). Adj., glassy, translucent. Noun, a clear, glassy, structureless material occurring, for example, in cartilage, vitreous body, mucin, and glycogen.

hybridoma (hī-brid-ō′mah) (contraction of hybrid + myeloma). Fused product of a normal and a myeloma (cancer) cell, which has some of the characteristics of the normal cell.

hydatid cyst (hī-da′təd) (Gr., *hydatis*, watery vesicle). A type of cyst formed by juveniles of certain tapeworms (*Echinococcus*) in their vertebrate hosts.

hydranth (hī′dranth) (Gr., *hydōr*, water, + *anthos*, flower). Nutritive zooid of hydroid colony.

hydroid. The polyp form of a cnidarian as distinguished from the medusa form. Any cnidarian of the class Hydrozoa, order Hydroida.

hydrolysis (Gr., *hydōr*, water, + *lysis*, a loosening). The decomposition of a chemical compound by the addition of water; the splitting of a molecule into its groupings so that the split products acquire hydrogen and hydroxyl groups.

hydrosphere (Gr., *hydōr*, water, + *sphaira*, ball, sphere). Aqueous envelope of the earth.

hydrostatic skeleton. A mass of fluid or plastic parenchyma enclosed within a muscular wall to provide the support necessary for antagonistic muscle action; for example, parenchyma in acoelomates and perivisceral fluids in pseudocoelomates serve as hydrostatic skeletons.

hydroxyl (hydrogen + oxygen, + yl). Containing an OH^- group, a negatively charged ion formed by alkalies in water.

hyperosmotic (Gr., *hyper*, over, + *osmos*, impulse). Refers to a solution whose osmotic pressure is greater than that of another solution with which it is compared; contains a greater concentration of dissolved particles and gains water through a semipermeable

membrane from a solution containing fewer particles; contrasts with **hypoosmotic.**

hyperparasitism (hī′pər-par′ə-sid-iz-əm) (Gr., *hyper*, over, + *para*, beside, + *sitos*, food). Parasitism of a parasite by another parasite.

hypertrophy (hī-pər′trə-fē) (Gr., *hyper*, over, + *trophē*, nourishment). Abnormal increase in size of a part or organ.

hypodermis (hī′pə-dər′mis) (Gr., *hypo*, under, + L., *dermis*, skin). The cellular layer lying beneath and secreting the cuticle of annelids, arthropods, and certain other invertebrates.

hypolimnion (hī-pō-lim′nē-än) (Gr., *hypo*, under, + *limnē*, lake). The water below the thermocline of a lake.

hypoosmotic (Gr., *hypo*, under, + *osmos*, impulse). Refers to a solution whose osmotic pressure is less than that of another solution with which it is compared or taken as standard; contains a lesser concentration of dissolved particles and loses water during osmosis; contrasts with **hyperosmotic.**

hypophysis (hī-pof′ə-sis) (Gr., *hypo*, under, + *physis*, growth). Pituitary body.

hypostome (hī′pə-stōm) (Gr., *hypo*, under, + *stoma*, mouth). Name applied to structure in various invertebrates (such as mites and ticks), located at posterior or ventral area of mouth.

hypothalamus (hī-pō-thal′ə-mis) (Gr., *hypo*, under, + *thalamos*, inner chamber). A ventral part of the forebrain beneath the thalamus; one of the centers of the autonomic nervous system.

imago (ə-mā′gō). The adult and sexually mature insect.

immunoglobulin (im′yə-nə-glä′byə-lən) (L., *immunis*, free, + *globus*, globe). Any of a group of plasma proteins, produced by plasma cells, that participates in the immune response by combining with the antigen that stimulated its production. Antibody.

imprinting (im′print-ing) (L., *imprimere*, to impress, imprint). Rapid and usually stable learning pattern appearing early in the life of a member of a social species and involving recognition of its own species; may involve attraction to the first moving object seen.

indeterminate cleavage. A type of embryonic development in which the fate of the blastomeres is not determined very early as to tissues or organs, for example, in echinoderms and vertebrates.

indigenous (ən-dij′ə-nəs) (L., *indigena*, native). Pertains to organisms that are native to a particular region; not introduced.

inductor (in-duk′ter) (L., *inducere*, to introduce, lead in). In embryology, a tissue or organ that causes the differentiation of another tissue or organ.

inflammation (in′fləm-mā′shən) (L., *inflammare*, from *flamma*, flame). The complicated physiological process in mobilization of body defenses against foreign substances and infectious agents and repair of damage from such agents.

infraciliature (in-frə-sil′e-ə-tər) (L., *infra*, below, + *cilia*, eyelashes). The organelles just below the cilia in ciliate protozoa.

infundibulum (in′fun-dib′u-ləm) (L., funnel). Stalk of the neurohypophysis linking the pituitary to the diencephalon.

innate (i-nāt′) (L., *innatus*, inborn). A characteristic based partly or wholly on gene differences.

instar (inz′tär) (L., form). Stage in the life of an insect or other arthropod between molts.

instinct (L., *instinctus*, impelled). Stereotyped, predictable, genetically programmed behavior. Learning may or may not be involved.

integument (ən-teg′ū-mənt) (L., *integumentum*, covering). An external covering or enveloping layer.

intermediary meiosis. Meiosis that occurs neither during gamete formation nor immediately after zygote formation, resulting in both haploid and diploid generations, such as in foraminiferan protozoa.

intermediate host. A host in which some development of a symbiont occurs, but in which maturation and sexual reproduction do not take place (contrasts with **definitive host**).

interstitial (in-tər-sti′shəl) (L., *inter*, among, + *sistere*, to stand). Situated in the interstices or spaces between structures such as cells, organs, or grains of sand.

intron (in′trän) (L., *intra*, within). Portion of mRNA as transcribed from DNA that will not form part of mature mRNA, that is, that does not include part of message for gene product.

introvert (L., *intro*, inward, + *vertere*, to turn). The anterior narrow portion that can be withdrawn (introverted) into the trunk of a sipunculid worm.

invagination (in-vaj′ə-nā′shən) (L., *in*, in, + *vagina*, sheath). An infolding of a layer of tissue to form a saclike structure.

inversion (L., *invertere*, to turn upside down). A turning inward or inside out, as in embryogenesis of sponges; also, reversal in order of genes or reversal of a chromosome segment.

irritability (L., *irritare*, to provoke). A general property of all organisms involving the ability to respond to stimuli or changes in the environment.

isogametes (īs′o-gam′ēts) (Gr., *isos*, equal, + *gametēs*, spouse). Gametes of a species in which both sexes are alike in size and appearance.

isolecithal (ī′sə-les′ə-thəl) (Gr., *isos*, equal, + *lekithos*, yolk, + *al*). Pertaining to a zygote (or ovum) with yolk evenly distributed. Homolecithal.

isotonic (Gr., *isos*, equal, + *tonikos*, tension). Said of solutions having the same or equal osmotic pressure; isosmotic.

isotope (Gr., *isos*, equal, + *topos*, place). One of several different forms (species) of a chemical element, differing from each other in atomic mass but not in atomic number.

juvenile hormone. Hormone produced by the corpora allata of insects; among its effects are maintenance of larval or nymphal characteristics during development.

juxtaglomerular apparatus (jək′stə-glä-mer′yə-lər) (L., *juxta*, close to, + *glomus*, ball). Complex of sensory cells located in the afferent arteriole adjacent to the glomerulus and a loop of the distal tubule, which produces the enzyme renin.

keratin (ker′ə-tən) (Gr., *kera*, horn, + *in*, suffix of proteins). A scleroprotein found in epidermal tissues and modified into hard structures such as horns, hair, and nails.

kinesis. (kə-nē′səs) (Gr., *kinēsis*, movement). Movements by an organism in random directions in response to a stimulus.

kinetodesma (kə-nē′tə-dez′mə), pl. **kinetodesmata** (Gr., *kinein*, to move, + *desma*, bond). Fibril arising from the kinetosome of a cilium in a ciliate protozoan, and passing along the kinetosomes of cilia in that same row.

kinetosome (kin-et′ə-sōm) (Gr., *kinētos*, moving, + *sōma*, body). The self-duplicating granule at the base of the flagellum or cilium; similar to centriole, also called basal body or blepharoplast.

kinety (kə-nē′tē) (Gr., *kinein*, to move). All the kinetosomes and kinetodesmata of a row of cilia.

kinin (kī′nin) (Gr., *kinein*, to move, + *in*, suffix of hormones). A type of local hormone that is released near its site of origin; also called parahormone or tissue hormone.

K-selection (from the K term in the logistic equation). Natural selection under conditions that favor survival when populations are controlled primarily by density-dependent factors.

kwashiorkor (kwash-ē-or′kər) (from Ghana). Malnutrition caused by diet high in carbohydrate and extremely low in protein.

labium (lā′bē-əm) (L., a lip). The lower lip of the insect formed by fusion of the second pair of maxillae.

labrum (lā′brəm) (L., a lip). The upper lip of insects and crustaceans situated above or in front of the mandibles; also refers to the outer lip of a gastropod shell.

labyrinthodont (lab′ə-rin′thə-dänt) (Gr., *labyrinthos*, labyrinth, + *odous, odontos*, tooth). A group of fossil-stem amphibians from which most amphibians later arose. They date from the late Paleozoic era.

lacteal (lak′te-əl) (L., *lacteus*, of milk). Noun, one of the lymph vessels in the villus of the intestine. Adj., relating to milk.

lacuna (lə-kū′nə), pl. **lacunae** (L., pit, cavity). A sinus; a space between cells; a cavity in cartilage or bone.

lagena (lə-jē′nə) (L., large flask). Portion of the primitive ear in which sound is translated into nerve impulses; evolutionary beginning of cochlea.

Lamarckism. Hypothesis, as expounded by Jean Baptiste de Lamarck, of evolution by the acquisition during an organism's lifetime of characteristics that are transmitted directly to offspring.

lamella (lə-mel′ə) (L., dim. of *lamina*, plate). One of the two plates forming a gill in a bivalve mollusc. One of the thin layers of bone laid concentrically around an osteon (Haversian) canal. Any thin, platelike structure.

larva (lar′və), pl. **larvae** (L., a ghost). An immature stage that is quite different from the adult.

lek (lek) (Sw., play, game). An area where animals assemble for communal courtship display and mating.

lemniscus (lem-nis′kəs) (L., ribbon). One of a pair of internal projections of the epidermis from the neck region of Acanthocephala, which functions in fluid control in the protrusion and invagination of the proboscis.

lentic (len′tik) (L., *lentus*, slow). Of or relating to standing water such as swamp, pond, or lake.

leukemism (lū′kə-mi-zəm) (Gr., *leukos*, white, + *ismos*, condition of). Presence of white pelage or plumage in animals with normally pigmented eyes and skin.

leukocyte (lū′kə-sīt) (Gr., *leukos*, white, + *kytos*, hollow vessel). A blood cell with a nucleus and ameboid properties; a white blood cell. Has no hemoglobin.

limax form (lī′məx) (L., *limax*, slug). Form of pseudopodial movement in which entire organism moves without extending a discrete pseudopodium.

lipase (lī′pās) (Gr., *lipos*, fat, + *ase*, enzyme suffix). An enzyme that accelerates the hydrolysis or synthesis of fats.

lipid, lipoid (li′pid) (Gr., *lipos*, fat). Certain fatlike substances, often containing other groups such as phosphoric acid; lipids combine with proteins and carbohydrates to form principal structured components of cells.

lithosphere (lith′ə-sfir) (Gr., *lithos*, rock, + *sphaira*, ball). The rocky component of the earth's surface layers.

littoral (lit′ə-rəl) (L., *litoralis*, seashore). Adj., pertaining to the shore. Noun, that portion of the sea floor between the extent of high and low tides, intertidal; in lakes, the shallow part from the shore to the lakeward limit of aquatic plants.

lobopodium (lō′bə-pō′de-əm) (Gr., *lobos*, lobe, + *pous, podos*, foot). Blunt, lobelike pseudopodium.

locus (lō′kəs), pl. **loci** (lō′sī) (L., place). Position of a gene in a chromosome.

logistic equation. A mathematical expression describing an idealized sigmoid curve of population growth.

lophocyte (lō′fə-sīt) (Gr., *lophos*, crest, + *kytos*, hollow vessel). Type of sponge amebocyte that secretes bundles of fibrils.

lophophore (lōf′ə-fōr) (Gr., *lophos*, crest, + *phoros*, bearing). Tentacle-bearing ridge or arm within which is an extension of the coelomic cavity in lophophorate animals (ectoprocts, brachiopods, and phoronids).

lorica (lo′rə-kə) (L., corselet). Protective external case found in some protozoa, rotifers, and others.

lotic (lō′tik) (L., *lotus*, action of washing or bathing). Of or pertaining to running water, such as a brook or river.

lumen (lū′mən) (L., light). The cavity of a tube or organ.

lymphocyte (lim′fō-sīt) (L., *lympha*, water, goddess of water, + Gr., *kytos*, hollow vessel). Cell in blood and lymph that has central role in immune responses. See **T cells** and **B cells**.

lysosome (lī′sə-sōm) (Gr., *lysis*, loosing, + *sōma*, body). Intracellular organelle consisting of a membrane enclosing several digestive enzymes that are released when the lysosome ruptures.

macromolecule. A very large molecule, such as a protein, polysaccharide, or nucleic acid.

macronucleus (ma′krō-nū′klē-əs) (Gr., *makros*, long, large, + *nucleus*, kernel). The larger of the two kinds of nuclei in ciliate protozoa; controls all cell functions except reproduction.

madreporite (ma′drə-pōr′īt) (Fr., *madrépore*, reef-building coral, + *ite*, suffix for some body parts). Sievelike structure that is the intake for the water-vascular system of echinoderms.

malacostracan (mal′ə-käs′trə-kən) (Gr., *malako*, soft, + *ostracon*, shell). Any member of the crustacean subclass Malacostraca, which includes both aquatic and terrestrial forms of crabs, lobsters, shrimps, pill bugs, sand fleas, and others.

Malpighian tubules (mal-pig′ē-ən) (Marcello Malpighi, Italian anatomist, 1628-1694). Blind tubules opening into the hindgut of nearly all insects and some myriapods and arachnids, and functioning primarily as excretory organs.

mantle. Soft extension of the body wall in certain invertebrates, for example, brachiopods and molluscs, which usually secretes a shell; thin body wall of tunicates.

marasmus (mə-raz′məs) (Gr., *marasmos*, to waste away). Malnutrition, especially of infants, caused by a diet deficient in both calories and protein.

marsupial (mär-sū′pē-əl) (Gr., *marsypion*, little pouch). One of the pouched mammals of the subclass Metatheria.

mastax (mas′təx) (Gr., jaws). Pharyngeal mill of rotifers.

matrix (mā′triks) (L., *mater*, mother). The intercellular substance of a tissue, or that part of a tissue into which an organ or process is set.

maturation (L., *maturus*, ripe). The process of ripening; the final stages in the preparation of gametes for fertilization.

maxilla (mak-sil′ə) (L., dim. of *mala*, jaw). One of the upper jawbones in vertebrates; one of the head appendages in arthropods.

maxilliped (mak-sil′ə-ped) (L., *maxilla*, jaw, + *pes*, foot). One of the pairs of head appendages located just posterior to the maxilla in crustaceans, a thoracic appendage that has become incorporated into the feeding mouthparts.

mediated transport. Transport of a substance across a cell membrane mediated by a carrier molecule in the membrane.

medulla (mə-dul′ə) (L., marrow). The inner portion of an organ in contrast to the cortex or outer portion. Also, hindbrain.

medusa (mə-dū′sə) (Gr. mythology, female monster with snake-entwined hair). A jellyfish, or the free-swimming stage in the life cycle of cnidarians.

Mehlis' gland (me′ləs). Glands of uncertain function surrounding the ootype of trematodes and cestodes.

meiofauna (mī′ō-faa-nə) (Gr., *meion*, smaller, + L., *faunus*, god of the woods). Small invertebrates found in the interstices between sand grains.

meiosis (mī-ō′səs) (Gr. from *meioun*, to make small). The nuclear changes by means of which the chromosomes are reduced from the diploid to the haploid number; in animals, usually occurs in the last two divisions in the formation of the mature egg or sperm.

melanin (mel′ə-nin) (Gr., *melas*, black). Black or dark-brown pigment found in plant or animal structures.

menopause (men′ō-pawz) (Gr., *men*, month, + *pauein*, to cease). In the human female, that time of life when ovulation ceases; cessation of the menstrual cycle.

menstruation (men′stroo-ā′shən) (L., *menstrua*, the menses, from *mensis*, month). The discharge of blood and uterine tissue from the vagina at the end of a menstrual cycle.

meroblastic (mer-ə-blas′tik) (Gr., *meros*, part, + *blastos*, germ). Partial cleavage occurring in zygotes having a large amount of yolk at the vegetal pole; cleavage restricted to a small area on the surface of the egg.

merozoite (me′rə-zō′īt) (Gr., *meros*, part, + *zōon*, animal). A very small trophozoite at the stage just after cytokinesis has been completed in multiple fission of a protozoan.

mesenchyme (me′zn-kīm) (Gr., *mesos*, middle, + *enchyma*, infusion). Embryonic connective tissue; irregular or amebocytic cells often embedded in gelatinous matrix.

mesocoel (mez′ō-sēl) (Gr., *mesos*, middle, + *koilos*, hollow). Middle body coelomic compartment in some deuterostomes, anterior in lophophorates, corresponds to hydrocoel in echinoderms.

mesoderm (me′zə-dərm) (Gr., *mesos*, middle, + *derma*, skin). The third germ layer, formed in the gastrula between the ectoderm and endoderm; gives rise to connective tissues, muscle, urogenital and vascular systems, and the peritoneum.

mesoglea (mez′ō-glē′ə) (Gr., *mesos*, middle, + *glia*, glue). The layer of jellylike or cement material between the epidermis and gastrodermis in cnidarians and ctenophores; also may refer to jellylike matrix between epithelial layers in sponges.

mesohyl (me′sə-hil) (Gr., *mesos*, middle, + *hylē*, wood). Gelatinous matrix surrounding sponge cells; mesoglea, mesenchyme.

mesonephros (me-zō-nef′rōs) (Gr., *mesos*, middle, + *nephros*, kidney). The middle of three pairs of embryonic renal organs in vertebrates. Functional kidney of fishes and amphibians; its collecting duct is a wolffian duct. Adj., **mesonephric.**

messenger RNA (mRNA). A form of ribonucleic acid that carries genetic information from the gene to the ribosome, where it determines the order of amino acids as a polypeptide is formed.

metabolism (Gr., *metabolē*, change). A group of processes that includes digestion, production of energy (respiration), and synthesis of molecules and structures by organisms; the sum of the constructive (anabolic) and destructive (catabolic) processes.

metacentric (me′tə-sen′trək) (Gr., *meta*, among, + *kentron*, center). Chromosome with centromere at or near the middle.

metacercaria (me′tə-sər-ka′rē-ə) (Gr., *meta*, after, + *kerkos*, tail, + L., *aria*, connected with). Fluke larva (cercaria) that has lost its tail and has become encysted.

metacoel (met′ə-sēl) (Gr., *meta*, after, + *koilos*, hollow). Posterior coelomic compartment in some deuterostomes and lophophorates; corresponds to somatocoel in echinoderms.

metamere (met′ə-mēr) (Gr., *meta*, after, + *meros*, part). A repeated body unit along the longitudinal axis of an animal; a somite, or segment.

metamerism (mə-ta′mə-ri′zəm) (Gr., *meta*, between, after, + *meros*, part). Condition of being made up serially repeated parts (metameres); serial segmentation.

metamorphosis (Gr., *meta*, after, + *morphē*, form, + *osis*, state of). Sharp change in form during postembryonic development, for example, tadpole to frog or larval insect to adult.

metanephridium (me′tə-nə-fri′di-əm) (Gr., *meta*, after, + *nephros*, kidney). A type of tubular nephridium with the inner open end draining the coelom and the outer open end discharging to the exterior.

metanephros (me′tə-ne′fräs) (Gr., *meta*, between, after, + *nephros*, kidney). Embryonic renal organs of vertebrates arising behind the mesonephros; the functional kidney of reptiles, birds, and mammals. It is drained from a ureter.

microfilament (mī′krō-fil′ə-mənt) (Gr., *mikros*, small, + L., *filum*, a thread). A thin, linear structure in cells; of actin in muscle cells and others.

micron (μ) (mī′krän) (Gr., neuter of *mikros*, small). One one thousandth of a millimeter; about 1/25,000 of an inch. Now largely replaced by micrometer (μm).

microneme (mī′krə-nēm) (Gr., *mikros*, small, + *nēma*, thread). One of the types of structures comprising the apical complex in the phylum Apicomplexa, slender and elongate, leading to the anterior and thought to function in host cell penetration.

micronucleus. A small nucleus found in ciliate protozoa; controls the reproductive functions of these organisms.

microthrix (mī′krə-thrix), pl. **microtriches** (Gr., *mikros*, small, + *thrix*, hair). A small microvillus-like structure on the surface of a tapeworm's tegument.

microtubule (Gr., *mikros*, small, + L., *tubule*, pipe). A long, tubular cytoskeletal element with an outside diameter of 20 to 27 μm.

Microtubules influence cell shape and play important roles during cell division.

microvillus (Gr., *mikros*, small, + L., *villus*, shaggy hair). Narrow, cylindrical cytoplasmic projection from epithelial cells; microvilli form the brush border of several types of epithelial cells.

mictic (mik′tik) (Gr., *miktos*, mixed or blended). Pertaining to haploid egg of rotifers or the females that lay such eggs.

miracidium (mīr′ə-sid′ē-əm) (Gr., *meirakidion*, youthful person). A minute ciliated larval stage in the life of flukes.

mitochondrion (mīd′ə-kän′drē-ən) (Gr., *mitos*, a thread, + *chondrion*, dim. of *chondros*, corn, grain). An organelle in the cell in which aerobic metabolism takes place.

mitosis (mī-tō′səs) (Gr., *mitos*, thread, + *osis*, state of). Nuclear division in which there is an equal qualitative and quantitative division of the chromosomal material between the two resulting nuclei; ordinary cell division (indirect).

monocyte (mon′ə-sīt) (Gr., *monos*, single, + *kytos*, hollow vessel). A type of leukocyte that becomes a phagocytic cell (macrophage) after moving into tissues.

monoecious (mə-nē′shəs) (Gr., *monos*, single, + *oikos*, house). Having both male and female gonads in the same organism; hermaphroditic.

monohybrid (Gr., *monos*, single + L., *hybrida*, mongrel). A hybrid offspring of parents different in one specified character.

monomer (mä′nə-mər) (Gr., *monos*, single, + *meros*, part). A molecule of simple structure, but capable of linking with others to form polymers.

monophyletic (mä′nə-phī-le′tik) (Gr., *monos*, single, + *phyletikos*, pertaining to a phylum). Referring to a taxon whose units all evolved from a single parent stock; contrasts with **polyphyletic.**

monosaccharide (mä′nə-sa′kə-rīd) (Gr., *monos*, one, + *sakcharon*, sugar, from Sanskrit *sarkarā*, gravel, sugar). A simple sugar that cannot be decomposed into smaller sugar molecules; the most common are pentoses (such as ribose) and hexoses (such as glucose).

monozoic (mo′nə-zō′ik) (Gr., *monos*, single, + *zōon*, animal). Tapeworms with a single proglottid, do not undergo strobilation to form chain of proglottids.

morphogenesis (mor′fə-je′nə-səs) (Gr., *morphē*, form, + *genesis*, origin). Development of the architectural features of organisms; formation and differentiation of tissues and organs.

morphology (Gr., *morphē*, form, + L., *logia*, study, from Gr., *logos*, work). The science of structure. Includes cytology, the study of cell structure: histology, the study of tissue structure; and anatomy, the study of gross structure.

bat / āpe / ärmadillo/ herring / fēmale / finch / līce / crocodile / crōw / duck / ūnicorn / ə indicates unaccented vowel sound "uh" as in mammal, fishes, cardinal, heron, vulture / stress as in bi-ol′o-gy, bi′o-log′i-cal

morula (mär′u-lə) (L., *morum*, mulberry, + *ula*, dim.). Solid ball of cells in early stage of embryonic development.

mosaic cleavage. Type characterized by independent differentiation of each part of the embryo; determinate cleavage.

Müller's larva. Free-swimming ciliated larva that resembles a modified ctenophore, characteristic of certain marine polyclad turbellarians.

mutation (mū-tā′shən) (L., *mutare*, to change). A stable and abrupt change of a gene; the heritable modification of a character.

mutualism (mū′chə-wə-li′zəm) (L., *mutuus*, lent, borrowed, reciprocal). A type of interaction in which two different species derive benefit from the association and in which the association is necessary to both; often symbiotic.

myofibril (Gr., *mys*, muscle, + L., dim. of *fibra*, fiber). A contractile filament within muscle or muscle fiber.

myogenic (mī′o-jen′ik) (Gr., *mys*, muscle, + N.L., *genic*, giving rise to). Originating in muscle, such as heart beat arising in vertebrate cardiac muscle because of inherent rhythmical properties of muscle rather than because of neural stimuli.

myoneme (mī′ə-nēm′) (Gr., *mys*, muscle, + *nēma*, thread). Long contractile fibril in certain protozoa.

myosin (mī′ə-sin) (Gr., *mys*, muscle, + *in*, suffix, belonging to). A large protein of contractile tissue that forms the thick myofilaments of striated muscle. During contraction it combines with actin to form actomyosin.

myotome (mī′ə-tōm′) (Gr., *mys*, muscle + *tomos*, cutting). A voluntary muscle segment in cephalochordates and vertebrates: that part of a somite destined to form muscles; the muscle group innervated by a single spinal nerve.

nacre (nā′kər) (F., mother-of-pearl). Innermost lustrous layer of mollusc shell, secreted by mantle epithelium. Adj., **nacreous.**

NAD. Abbreviation of nicotinamide adenine dinucleotide, an electron acceptor or donor in many metabolic reactions.

naiad (nā′əd) (Gr., *naias*, a water nymph). An aquatic, gill-breathing immature insect (nymph).

nares (na′rēz), sing. **naris** (L., nostrils). Openings into the nasal cavity, both internally and externally, in the head of a vertebrate.

natural selection. A nonrandom reproduction of genotypes that results in the survival of those best adapted to their environment and elimination of those less well adapted; leads to evolutionary change.

nauplius (naw′plē-əs) (L., a kind of shellfish). A free-swimming microscopic larval stage of certain crustaceans, with three pairs of appendages (antennules, antennae, and mandibles) and median eye. Characteristic of ostracods, copepods, barnacles, and some others.

nekton (nek′tən) (Gr., neuter of *nēktos*, swimming). Term for actively swimming organisms, essentially independent of wave and current action. Compare with plankton.

nematocyst (ne-mad′ə-sist′) (Gr., *nēma*, thread, + *kystis*, bladder). Stinging organoid of cnidarians.

neoteny (nē′ə-tē′nē, nē-ot′ə-nē) (Gr., *neos*, new, + *teinein*, to extend). The attainment of sexual maturity in the larval condition. Also, the retention of larval characters into adulthood.

nephridium (nə-frid′ē-əm) (Gr., *nephridios*, of the kidney). One of the segmentally arranged, paired excretory tubules of many invertebrates, notably the annelids. In a broad sense, any tubule specialized for excretion and/or osmoregulation; with an external opening and with or without an internal opening.

nephron (ne′frän) (Gr., *nephros*, kidney). Functional unit of kidney structure of vertebrates, consisting of a Bowman's capsule, an enclosed glomerulus, and the attached uriniferous tubule.

neritic (nə-rid′ik) (Gr., *nērites*, a mussel). Portion of the sea overlying the continental shelf, specifically from the subtidal zone to a depth of 200 m.

neurogenic (nū-rä-jen′ik) (Gr., *neuron*, nerve, + N.L., *genic*, give rise to). Originating in nervous tissue, as does the rhythmical beat of some arthropod hearts.

neuroglia (nū-räg′le-ə) (Gr., *neuron*, nerve, + *glia*, glue). Tissue supporting and filling the spaces between the nerve cells of the central nervous system.

neurolemma (nū-rə-lem′ə) (Gr., *neuron*, nerve, + *lemma*, skin). Delicate nucleated outer sheath of a nerve cell; sheath of Schwann.

neuron (Gr., nerve). A nerve cell.

neuropodium (nū′rə-pō′de-əm) (Gr., *neuron*, nerve, + *pous, podos*, foot). Lobe of parapodium nearer the ventral side in polychaete annelids.

neurosecretory cell (nu′rō-sə-krēd′ə-rē). Any cell (neuron) of the nervous system that produces a hormone.

niche. The role of an organism in an ecological community; its unique way of life and its relationship to other biotic and abiotic factors.

nitrogen fixation (Gr., *nitron*, soda, + *gen*, producing). Reduction of molecular nitrogen to ammonia by some bacteria and cyanobacteria, often followed by **nitrification,** the oxidation of ammonia to nitrites and nitrates by other bacteria.

notochord (nōd′ə-kord′) (Gr., *nōtos*, back + *chorda*, cord). An elongated cellular cord, enclosed in a sheath, which forms the primitive axial skeleton of chordate embryos and adult cephalochordates.

notopodium (nō′tə-pō′de-əm) (Gr., *nōtos*, back, + *pous, podos*, foot). Lobe of parapodium nearer the dorsal side in polychaete annelids.

nucleic acid (nu′klē′ik) (L., *nucleus*, kernel). One of a class of molecules composed of joined nucleotides; chief types are deoxyribonucleic acid (DNA), found in cell nuclei (chromosomes and mitochondria), and ribonucleic acid (RNA), found both in cell nuclei (chromosomes and nucleoli) and in cytoplasmic ribosomes.

nucleoid (nu′klē-oid) (L., *nucleus*, kernel, + *oid*, like). The region in a prokaryotic cell where the chromosome is found.

nucleolus (nu-klē′ə-ləs) (dim. of L., *nucleus*, kernel). A deeply staining body within the nucleus of a cell and containing RNA; nucleoli are specialized portions of certain chromosomes that carry multiple copies of the information to synthesize ribosomal RNA.

nucleoplasm (nu′klē-ə-plazm′) (L., *nucleus*, kernel, + Gr., *plasma*, mold). Protoplasm of nucleus, as distinguished from cytoplasm.

nucleoprotein. A molecule composed of nucleic acid and protein; occurs in the nucleus and cytoplasm of all cells.

nucleosome (nu′klē-ə-som) (L., *nucleus*, kernel, + *sōma*, body). A repeating subunit of chromatin in which one and three quarters turns of the double-helical DNA are wound around eight molecules of histones.

nucleotide (nu′klē-ə-tīd). A molecule consisting of phosphate, 5-carbon sugar (ribose or deoxyribose), and a purine or a pyrimidine; the purines are adenine and guanine, and the pyrimidines are cytosine, thymine, and uracil.

nuptial flight (nup′shəl). The mating flight of insects, especially that of the queen with male or males.

nymph (L., *nympha*, nymph, bride). An immature stage (following hatching) of a hemimetabolous insect that lacks a pupal stage.

ocellus (ō-sel′əs) (L., dim. of *oculus*, eye). A simple eye or eyespot in many types of invertebrates.

octomerous (ok-tom′ər-əs) (Gr., *oct*, eight, + *meros*, part). Eight parts, specifically, symmetry based on eight.

ommatidium (ä′mə-tid′ē-əm) (Gr., *omma*, eye, + *idium*, small). One of the optical units of the compound eye of arthropods and molluscs.

oncomiracidium (än′kō-mīr′ə-sid′ē-əm) (Gr., *onkos*, barb, hook, + *meirakidion*, youthful person). A ciliated larva of a monogenetic trematode.

ontogeny (än-tä′jə-nē) (Gr., *ontos*, being, + *geneia*, act of being born, from *genēs*, born). The course of development of an individual from egg to senescence.

oocyst (ō′ə-sist) (Gr., *ōion*, egg, + *kystis*, bladder). Cyst formed around zygote of malaria and related organisms.

ooecium (ō-ēs′ē-əm) (Gr., *ōion*, egg, + *oikos*, house, + L., *ium*, from Ger. ion, dim.). Brood pouch; compartment for developing embryos in ectoprocts.

oogonium (ō′ə-gōn′ē-əm) (Gr., *ōion*, egg, + *gonos*, offspring). A cell that, by continued division, gives rise to oocytes; an ovum in a primary follicle immediately before the beginning of maturation.

ookinete (ō-ə-kī′nēt) (Gr., *ōion*, egg, + *kinein*, to move). The motile zygote of malaria organisms.

ootype (ō′ə-tīp) (Gr., *ōion*, egg, + *typos*, mold). Part of oviduct in flatworms that receives ducts from vitelline glands and Mehlis' gland.

operator. A section of DNA near a structural gene, which helps control transcription of the gene into messenger RNA.

operculum (ō-per′kū-ləm) (L., cover). The gill cover in bony fishes; horny plate in some snails.

operon (äp′ə-rän). A genetic unit consisting of a cluster of genes that are under the control of an operator and a repressor, found in prokaryotes.

ophthalmic (äf-thal′mik) (Gr., *ophthalmos*, an eye). Pertaining to the eye.

opisthaptor (ä′pəs-thap′tər) (Gr., *opisthen*, behind, + *haptein*, to fasten). Posterior attachment organ of a monogenetic trematode.

opisthosoma (ō-pis′thə-sō′mə) (Gr., *opisthe*, behind, + *sōma*, body). Posterior body region in arachnids and pogonophorans.

opsonization (op′sən-i-zā′shən) (Gr., *opsonein*, to buy victuals, to cater). The facilitation of phagocytosis of foreign particles by phagocytes in the blood or tissues, mediated by antibody bound to the particles.

organelle (Gr., *organon*, tool, organ, + L., *ella*, dim.). Specialized part of a cell; literally, a small organ that performs functions analogous to organs of multicellular animals.

organizer (or′gan-ī-zer) (Gr., *organos*, fashioning). Area of an embryo that directs subsequent development of other parts.

osmole. Molecular weight of a solute, in grams, divided by the number of ions or particles into which it dissociates in solution. Adj., **osmolar.**

osmoregulation. Maintenance of proper internal salt and water concentrations in a cell or in the body of a living organism, active regulation of internal osmotic pressure.

osmosis (oz-mō′sis) (Gr., *ōsmos*, act of pushing, impulse). The flow of solvent (usually water) through a semipermeable membrane.

osmotic potential Osmotic pressure.

osphradium (äs-frā′dē-əm) (Gr., *osphradion*, small bouquet, dim. of *osphra*, smell). A sense organ in aquatic snails and bivalves that tests incoming water.

ossicles (L., *ossiculum*, small bone). Small separate pieces of echinoderm endoskeleton. Also, tiny bones of the middle ear of vertebrates.

osteoblast (os′tē-ō-blast) (Gr., *osteon*, bone, + *blastos*, bud). A bone-forming cell.

osteoclast (os′tē-ō-clast) (Gr., *osteon*, bone, + *klan*, to break). A large, multinucleate cell that functions in bone dissolution.

osteon (äs′tē-än) (Gr., bone). Unit of bone structure; Haversian system.

ostium (L., door). Opening.

otolith (ōd′əl-ith′) (Gr., *ous*, *otos*, ear, + *lithos*, stone). Calcareous concretions in the membranous labyrinth of the inner ear of lower vertebrates, or in the auditory organ of certain invertebrates.

oviger (ō′vi-jər) (L., *ovum*, egg, + *gerere*, to bear). Leg that carries eggs in pycnogonids.

oviparity (ō′və-pa′rəd-ē) (L., *ovum*, egg, + *parere*, to bring forth). Reproduction in which eggs are released by the female; development of offspring occurs outside the maternal body. Adj., **oviparous** (ō-vip′ə-rəs).

ovipositor (ō′və-päz′əd-ər) (L., *ovum*, egg, + *positor*, builder, placer, + *or*, suffix denoting agent or doer). In many female insects a structure at the posterior end of the abdomen for laying eggs.

ovoviviparity (ō′vo-vī-və-par′ə-dē) (L., *ovum*, egg, + *vivere*, to live, + *parere*, to bring forth). Reproduction in which eggs develop within the maternal body without additional nourishment from the parent and hatch within the parent or immediately after laying. Adj., **ovoviviparous** (ō′vo-vī-vip′ə-rəs).

oxidation (äk′sə-dā′shən) (Fr., *oxider*, to oxidize, from Gr., *oxys*, sharp, + *ation*). The loss of an electron by an atom or molecule; sometimes addition of oxygen chemically to a substance. Opposite of reduction, in which an electron is accepted by an atom or molecule.

oxidative phosphorylation (äk′sə-dād′iv fäs′fər-i-lā′shən). The conversion of inorganic phosphate to energy-rich phosphate of ATP, involving electron transport through a respiratory chain to molecular oxygen.

paedogenesis (pē-dō-jen′ə-sis) (Gr., *pais*, child, + *genēs*, born). Reproduction by immature or larval animals caused by acceleration of maturation. Progenesis.

paedomorphosis (pē-dō-mor′fə-səs) (Gr., *pais*, child, + *morphē*, form). Displacement of ancestral juvenile features to later stages of the ontogeny of descendants.

pair bond. An affiliation between an adult male and an adult female for reproduction. Characteristic of monogamous species.

pallium (pal′e-əm) (L., mantle). Mantle of a mollusc or brachiopod.

pangenesis (pan-jen′ə-sis) (Gr., *pan*, all, + *genesis*, descent). Darwin's hypothesis that hereditary characteristics are carried by individual body cells that produce particles that collect in the germ cells.

papilla (pə-pil′ə) (L., nipple). A small nipplelike projection. A vascular process that nourishes the root of a hair, feather, or developing tooth.

papula (pa′pū-lə) (L., pimple). Respiratory processes on skin of sea stars; also, pustules on skin.

parabiosis (pa′rə-bī′sis) (Gr., *para*, beside, + *biosis*, mode of life). The fusion of two individuals, resulting in mutual physiological intimacy.

parapodium (pa′rə-pō′dē-əm) (Gr., *para*, beside, + *pous*, *podos*, foot). One of the paired lateral processes on each side of most segments in polychaete annelids; variously modified for locomotion, respiration, or feeding.

parasitism (par′ə-sīd′izəm) (Gr., *parasitos*, from *para*, beside, + *sitos*, food). The condition of an organism living in or on another organism (host) at whose expense the parasite is maintained; destructive symbiosis.

parasympathetic (par′ə-sim-pə-thed′ik) (Gr., *para*, beside, + *sympathes*, sympathetic, from *syn*, with, + *pathos*, feeling). One of the subdivisions of the autonomic nervous system, whose fibers originate in the brain and in anterior and posterior parts of the spinal cord.

parenchyma (pə-ren′kə-mə) (Gr., anything poured in beside). In lower animals, a spongy mass of vacuolated mesenchyme cells filling spaces between viscera, muscles, or epithelia; in some, the cells are cell bodies of muscle cells. Also, the specialized tissue of an organ as distinguished from the supporting connective tissue.

parenchymula (pa′rən-kī′mū-lə) (Gr., *para*, beside, + *enchyma*, infusion). Flagellated, solid-bodied larva of some sponges.

parthenogenesis (pär′thə-nō-gen′ə-sis) (Gr., *parthenos*, virgin, + L., from Gr., *genesis*, origin). Unisexual reproduction involving the production of young by females not fertilized by males; common in rotifers, cladocerans, aphids, bees, ants, and wasps. A parthenogenetic egg may be diploid or haploid.

pathogenic (path′ə-jen′ik) (Gr., *pathos*, disease, + N.L., *genic*, giving rise to). Producing or capable of producing disease.

peck order. A hierarchy of social privilege in a flock of birds.

pecten (L., comb). Any of several types of comblike structures on various organisms, for example, a pigmented, vascular, and comblike process that projects into the vitreous humor from the retina at a point of entrance of the optic nerve in the eyes of all birds and many reptiles.

pectines (pek′tīnz) (L., comb, pl. of *pecten*). Sensory appendage on abdomen of scorpions.

pectoral (pek′tə-rəl) (L., *pectoralis*, from *pectus*, the breast). Of or pertaining to the breast or chest; to the pectoral girdle; or to a pair of horny shields of the plastron of certain turtles.

pedal laceration. Asexual reproduction found in sea anemones, a form of fission.

pedicel (ped′ə-sel) (L., *pediculus*, little foot). A small or short stalk or stem. In insects, the second segment of an antenna or the waist of an ant.

pedicellaria (ped′ə-sə-lar′ē-ə) (L., *pediculus*, little foot, + *aria*, like or connected with). One of many minute pincerlike organs on the surface of certain echinoderms.

pedipalps (ped′ə-palps′) (L., *pes, pedis*, foot, + *palpus*, stroking, caress). Second pair of appendages of arachnids.

pedogenesis. See paedogenesis.

peduncle (pē′dun-kəl) (L., *pedunculus*, dim. of *pes*, foot). A stalk. Also, a band of white matter joining different parts of the brain.

pelage (pel′ij) (Fr., fur). Hairy covering of mammals.

pelagic (pə-laj′ik) (Gr., *pelagos*, the open sea). Pertaining to the open ocean.

pellicle (pel′ə-kəl) (L., *pellicula*, dim. of *pellis*, skin). Thin, translucent, secreted envelope covering many protozoa.

penetrance. The frequency in a population with which a dominant gene or a recessive gene in the homozygous condition produces a phenotypic effect.

pentadactyl (pen-tə-dak′təl) (Gr., *pente*, five, + *daktylos*, finger). With five digits, or five fingerlike parts, to the hand or foot.

peptidase (pep′tə-dās) (Gr., *peptein*, to digest, + *ase*, enzyme suffix). An enzyme that breaks down simple peptides, releasing amino acids.

peptide bond. A bond that binds amino acids together into a polypeptide chain, formed by removing an OH from the carboxy group of one amino acid and an H from the amino group of another to form an amide group — CO—NH—.

periostracum (pe-rē-äs′trə-kəm) (Gr., *peri*, around, + *ostrakon*, shell). Outer horny layer of a mollusc shell.

periproct (per′ə-präkt) (Gr., *peri*, around, + *prōktos*, anus). Region of aboral plates around the anus of echinoids.

perisarc (per′ə-särk) (Gr., *peri*, around, + *sarx*, flesh). Sheath covering the stalk and branches of a hydroid.

perissodactyl (pə-ris′ə-dak′təl) (Gr., *perissos*, odd, + *daktylos*, finger, toe). Pertaining to an order of ungulate mammals with an odd number of digits.

peristalsis (per′ə-stal′səs) (Gr., *peristaltikos*, compressing around). The series of alternate relaxations and contractions that serve to force food through the alimentary canal.

peristomium (per′ə-stō′mē-əm) (Gr., *peri*, around, + *stoma*, mouth). Foremost true segment of an annelid; it bears the mouth.

peritoneum (per′ə-tə-nē′əm) (Gr., *peritonaios*, stretched around). The membrane that lines the coelom and covers the coelomic viscera.

petaloids (pe′tə-loids) (Gr., *petalon*, leaf, + *eidos*, form). Describes flowerlike arrangement of respiratory podia in irregular sea urchins.

pH (potential of *h*ydrogen). A symbol referring to the relative concentration of hydrogen ions in a solution; pH values are from 0 to 14, and the lower the value, the more acid or hydrogen ions in the solution. Equal to the negative logarithm of the hydrogen ion concentration.

phagocyte (fag′ə-sīt) (Gr., *phagein*, to eat, + *kytos*, hollow vessel). Any cell that engulfs and devours microorganisms or other particles.

phagocytosis (fag′ə-sī-tō-səs) (Gr., *phagein*, to eat, + *kytos*, hollow vessel). The engulfment of a particle by a phagocyte or a protozoan.

phagosome (fa′gə-sōm) (Gr., *phagein*, to eat, + *sōma*, body). Membrane-bound vesicle in cytoplasm containing food material engulfed by phagocytosis.

pharynx (far′inks), pl. **pharynges** (Gr., *pharynx*, gullet). The part of the digestive tract between the mouth cavity and the esophagus that, in vertebrates, is common to both digestive and respiratory tracts. In cephalochordates the gill slits open from it.

phasmid (faz′mid) (Gr., *phasma*, apparition, phantom, + *id*). One of a pair of glands or

sensory structures found in the posterior end of certain nematodes.

phenetics (fen-et′iks) (Gr., *phainein*, to show). A system of arranging taxonomic groupings according to the statistically highest number of similarities without regard to phylogenetic significance.

phenotype (fē′nə-tīp) (Gr., *phainein*, to show). The visible or expressed characters of an organism, controlled by the genotype, but not all genes in the genotype are expressed.

pheromone (fer′ə-mōn) (Gr., *pherein*, to carry, + *hormōn*, exciting, stirring up). Chemical substance released by one organism that influences the behavior or physiological processes of another organism.

phosphagen (fäs′fə-jən) (phosphate + gen). A term for creatine phosphate and arginine phosphate, which store and may be sources of high-energy phosphate bonds.

phosphatide (fäs′fə-tīd′) (phosphate + ide). A lipid with phosphorus, such as lecithin. A complex phosphoric ester lipid, such a lecithin, found in all cells. Phospholipid.

phosphorylation (fäs′fə-rə-lā′shən). The addition of a phosphate group, such as H_2PO_3, to a compound.

photosynthesis (fōd′ō-sin′thə-sis) (Gr., *phōs*, light, + *synthesis*, action or putting together). The synthesis of carbohydrates from carbon dioxide and water in chlorophyll-containing cells exposed to light.

phototaxis (fō-to-tak′sis) (Gr., *phōs*, light, + *taxis*, arranging, order). A taxis in which light is the orienting stimulus. An involuntary tendency for an organism to turn toward (positive) or away from (negative) light.

phyllopodium (fī′lə-pō′dē-əm) (Gr., *phyllon*, leaf, + *pous, podos*, foot). Leaflike swimming appendage of branchiopod crustaceans.

phylogeny (fī-läj′ə-nē) (Gr., *phylon*, tribe, race, + *geneia*, origin). The origin and development of any taxon, or the evolutionary history of its development.

phylum (fī′ləm), pl. **phyla** (N.L. from Gr., *phylon*, race, tribe). A chief category, between kingdom and class, of taxonomic classifications into which are grouped organisms of common descent that share a fundamental pattern of organization.

pilidium (pī-lid′ē-əm) (Gr., *pilidion*, dim. of *pilos*, felt cap). Free-swimming, hat-shaped larva of nemertine worms.

pinacocyte (pin′ə-kō-sīt′) (Gr., *pinax*, tablet, + *kytos*, hollow vessel). Flattened cells comprising dermal epithelium in sponges.

pinna (pin′ə) (L., feather, sharp point). The external ear. Also a feather, wing, or fin or similar part.

pinocytosis (pin′o-sī-tō′sis, pīn′o-sī-to′sis) (Gr., *pinein*, to drink, + *kytos*, hollow vessel, + *osis*, condition). Taking up of fluid by endocytosis; cell drinking.

placenta (plə-sen′tə) (L., flat cake). The vascular structure, embryonic and maternal, through which the embryo and fetus are nourished while in the uterus.

placoid scale (pla′koid) (Gr., *plax, plakos*, tablet, plate). Type of scale found in cartilaginous fishes, with basal plate of dentin embedded in the skin and a backward-pointing spine tipped with enamel.

plankton (plank′tən) (Gr., neuter of *planktos*, wandering). The passively floating animal and plant life of a body of water; compares with **nekton**.

plantigrade (plan′tə-grād′) (L., *planta*, sole, + *gradus*, step, degree). Pertaining to animals that walk on the whole surface of the foot (for example, humans and bears); compares with **digitigrade**.

planula (plan′yə-lə) (N.L., dim. from L., *planus*, flat). Free-swimming, ciliated larval type of cnidarians; usually flattened and ovoid, with an outer layer of ectodermal cells and an inner mass of endodermal cells.

planuloid ancestor (plan′yə-loid) (L., *planus*, flat, + Gr., *eidos*, form). Hypothetical form representing ancestor of Cnidaria and Platyhelminthes.

plasma cell (plaz′mə) (Gr., *plasma*, a form, mold). A descendant cell of a B cell, functions to secrete antibodies.

plasma membrane (plaz′mə) (Gr., *plasma*, a form, mold). A living, external, limiting, protoplasmic structure that functions to regulate exchange of nutrients across the cell surface.

plasmid (plaz′məd) (Gr., *plasma*, a form, mold). A small circle of DNA carried by a bacterium in addition to its large chromosome.

plasmodium (plaz-mō′dē-əm) (Gr., *plasma*, a form, mold, + *eidos*, form). Multinucleate ameboid mass, syncytial.

plastid (plas′təd) (Gr., *plast*, formed, molded, + L., *id*, feminine stem for particle of specified kind). A membranous organelle in plant cells functioning in photosynthesis and/or nutrient storage, for example, chloroplast.

platelet (plāt′lət) (Gr., dim. of *plattus*, flat). A tiny, incomplete cell in the blood that releases substances initiating blood clotting.

pleiotropic (plī-ə-trō′pic) (Gr., *pleiōn*, more, + *tropos*, to turn). Pertaining to a gene producing more than one effect; affecting multiple phenotypic characteristics.

pleopod (plē′ə-päd) (Gr., *plein*, to sail, + *pous*, *podos*, foot). One of the swimming appendages on the abdomen of a crustacean.

pleura (plu′rə) (Gr., side, rib). The membrane that lines each half of the thorax and covers the lungs.

plexus (plek′səs) (L., network, braid). A network, especially of nerves or blood vessels.

pluteus (plü′dē-əs), pl. **plutei** (L., *pluteus*, movable shed, reading desk). Echinoid or ophiuroid larva with elongated processes like the supports of a desk; originally called "painter's easel larva."

podium (pō′dē-əm) (Gr., *pous*, *podos*, foot). A footlike structure, for example, the tube foot of echinoderms.

poikilothermic (poi-ki′lə-thər′mik) (Gr., *poikilos*, variable, + thermal). Pertaining to animals whose body temperature is variable and fluctuates with that of the environment; cold blooded; compares with **ectothermic**.

polarization (L., *polaris*, polar, + Gr., *iz*, make). The arrangement of positive electrical charges on one side of a surface membrane and negative electrical charges on the other side (in nerves and muscles).

Polian vesicles (pō′le-ən) (from G.S. Poli, Italian naturalist). Vesicles opening into ring canal in most asteroids and holothuroids.

polyandry (pol′y-an′drē) (Gr., *polys*, many, + *anēr*, man). Condition of having more than one male mate at one time.

polygamy (pə-lig′ə-mē) (Gr., *polys*, many, + *gamos*, marriage). Condition of having more than one mate at one time.

polygyny (pə-lij′ə-nē) (Gr., *polys*, many, + *gynē*, woman) Condition of having more than one female mate at one time.

polymer (pä′lə-mər) (Gr., *polys*, many, + *meros*, part). A chemical compound composed of repeated structural units called monomers.

polymerization (pə-lim′ər-ə-zā′shən). The process of forming a polymer or polymeric compound.

polymorphism (pä′lē-mor′fī-zəm) (Gr., *polys*, many, + *morphē*, form). The presence in a species of more than one structural type of individual.

polynucleotide (poly + nucleotide). A nucleotide of many mononucleotides combined.

polyp (päl′əp) (Fr., *polype*, octopus, from L., *polypus*, many footed). The sessile stage in the life cycle of cnidarians.

polypeptide (pä-lē-pep′tīd) (Gr., *polys*, many, + *peptein*, to digest). A molecule consisting of many joined amino acids, not as complex as a protein.

polyphyletic (pä′lē-fī-led′ik) (Gr., *polys*, many, + *phylon*, tribe). Derived from more than one ancestral source; opposed to monophyletic.

polyphyodont (pä′lē-fī′ə-dänt) (Gr., *polyphyes*, manifold, + *odous*, tooth). Having several sets of teeth in succession.

polypide (pä′li-pīd) (L., *polypus*, polyp). An individual or zooid in a colony, specifically in ectoprocts, which has a lophophore, digestive tract, muscles, and nerve centers.

polyploid (pä′lə-ploid′) (Gr., *polys*, many, + *ploidy*, number of chromosomes). Characterized by a chromosome number that is greater than two full sets of homologous chromosomes.

polysaccharide (pä′lē-sak′ə-rid, -rīd) (Gr., *polys*, many, + *sakcharon*, sugar, from Sanskrit *sarkarā*, gravel, sugar). A carbohydrate composed of many monosaccharide units, for example, glycogen, starch, and cellulose.

polysome (polyribosome) (Gr., *polys*, many, + *sōma*, body). Two or more ribosomes connected by a molecule of messenger RNA.

polytene chromosomes (pä′li-tēn) (Gr., *polys*, many + *tainia*, band). Chromosomes in the somatic cells of some insects in which the chromatin replicates repeatedly without undergoing mitosis.

polyzoic (pä′lē-zō′ik) (Gr., *polys*, many, + *zōon*, animal). A tapeworm forming a strobila of several to many proglottids; also, a colony of many zooids.

pongid (pän′jəd) (L., *Pongo*, type genus of orangutan). Of or relating to the primate family Pongidae, comprising the anthropoid apes (gorillas, chimpanzees, gibbons, orangutans).

population (L., *populus*, people). A group of organisms of the same species inhabiting a specified geographical locality.

portal system (L., *porta*, gate). System of large veins beginning and ending with a bed of capillaries; for example, hepatic portal and renal portal systems in vertebrates.

preadaptation. The possession of a condition that is selected for in an ancestral environment and that coincidentally predisposes an organism for survival in some other environment.

prebiotic synthesis. The chemical synthesis that occurred before the emergence of life.

precocial (prē-kō′shəl) (L., *praecoquere*, to ripen beforehand). Referring (especially) to birds whose young are covered with down and are able to run about when newly hatched.

predaceous, predacious (prē-dā′shəs) (L., *praeda*, prey). Living by killing and consuming other animals; predatory.

predator (pred′ə-tər) (L., *praeda*, prey). An organism that preys on other organisms for its food.

prehensile (prē-hen′səl) (L., *prehendere*, to seize). Adapted for grasping.

primate (prī′māt) (L., *primus*, first). Any mammal of the order Primates, which includes the tarsiers, lemurs, marmosets, monkeys, apes, and humans.

primitive (L., *primus*, first). Primordial; ancient; little evolved; said of species closely approximating their early ancestral types.

proboscis (prō-bäs′əs) (Gr., *pro*, before, + *boskein*, feed). A snout or trunk. Also, tubular sucking or feeding organ with the mouth at the end as in planarians, leeches, and insects. Also, the sensory and defensive organ at the anterior end of certain invertebrates.

producers (L., *producere*, to bring forth). Organisms, such as plants, able to produce their own food from inorganic substances.

progesterone (prō-jes′tə-rōn′) (L., *pro*, before, + *gestare*, to carry). Hormone secreted by the corpus luteum and the placenta; prepares the uterus for the fertilized egg and maintains the capacity of the uterus to hold the embryo and fetus.

proglottid (prō-gläd′əd) (Gr., *proglōttis*, tongue tip, from *pro*, before, + *glōtta*, tongue, + *id*, suffix). Portion of a tapeworm containing a set of reproductive organs; usually corresponds to a segment.

prokaryotic, procaryotic (pro-kar′ē-ät′ik) (Gr., *pro*, before, + *karyon*, kernel, nut). Not having a membrane-bound nucleus or nuclei. Prokaryotic cells are more primitive than eukaryotic cells and persist today in the bacteria and blue-green algae.

promoter. A region of DNA to which the RNA polymerase must have access for transcription of a structural gene to begin.

pronephros (prō-nef′rəs) (Gr., *pro*, before, + *nephros*, kidney). Most anterior of three pairs of embryonic renal organs of vertebrates;

functional only in adult hagfishes and larval fishes and amphibians; vestigial in mammalian embryos. Adj., **pronephric.**

proprioceptor (prō′prē-ə-sep′tər) (L., *proprius,* own, particular, + receptor). Sensory receptor located deep within the tissues, especially muscles, tendons, and joints, that is responsive to changes in muscle stretch, body position, and movement.

prosimian (prō-sim′ē-ən) (Gr., *pro,* before, + L., *simia,* ape). Any member of a group of primitive, arboreal primates: lemurs, tarsiers, lorises, and so on.

prosoma (prō-sōm′ə) (Gr., *pro,* before, + *sōma,* body). Anterior part of an invertebrate in which primitive segmentation is not visible; fused head and thorax of arthropod; cephalothorax.

prosopyle (präs′ə-pīl) (Gr., *prosō,* forward, + *pylē,* gate). Connections between the incurrent and radial canals in some sponges.

prostaglandins (präs′tə-glan′dəns). A family of fatty acid tissue hormones, originally discovered in semen, known to have powerful effects on smooth muscle, nerves, circulation, and reproductive organs.

prostomium (prō-stō′mē-əm) (Gr., *pro,* before, + *stoma,* mouth). In most annelids and some molluscs, that part of the head located in front of the mouth.

protease (prō′tē-ās) (Gr., *protein,* + *ase,* enzyme). An enzyme that digests proteins; includes proteinases and peptidases.

protein (prō′tēn, prō′tē-ən) (Gr., *protein,* from *proteios,* primary). A macromolecule of carbon, hydrogen, oxygen, and nitrogen and sometimes sulfur and phosphorus; composed of chains of amino acids joined by peptide bonds; present in all cells.

prothoracic glands. Glands in the prothorax of insects that secrete the hormone ecdysone.

prothoracicotropic hormone. Hormone secreted in brain of insects that stimulates the prothoracic glands to secrete ecdysone.

prothrombin (pro-thräm′bən) (Gr., *pro,* before, + *thrombos,* clot). A constituent of blood plasma that is changed to thrombin by a catalytic sequence that includes thromboplastin, calcium, and plasma globulins; involved in blood clotting.

protist (prō′tist) (Gr., *protos,* first). A member of the kingdom Protista, generally considered to include the unicellular eukaryotic organisms (protozoa and eukaryotic algae).

protocoel (prō′tə-sēl) (Gr., *protos,* first, + *koilos,* hollow). The anterior coelomic compartment in some deuterostomes, corresponds to the axocoel in echinoderms.

protocooperation. A mutually beneficial interaction between organisms in which the interaction is not physiologically necessary to the survival of either.

protonephridium (prō′tō-nə-frid′ē-əm) (Gr., *protos,* first, + *nephros,* kidney). Primitive osmoregulatory or excretory organ consisting of a tubule terminating internally with flame bulb or solenocyte; the unit of a flame bulb system.

protoplasm (prō′tə-plazm) (Gr., *protos,* first, + *plasma,* form). Organized living substance; cytoplasm and nucleoplasm of the cell.

protopod, protopodite (prō′tə-päd, prō-top′ə-dīt) (Gr., *protos,* first, + *pous, podos,* foot). Basal portion of crustacean appendage, containing coxa and basis.

Protostomia (prō′də-stō′mē-ə) (Gr., *protos,* first, + *stoma,* mouth). A group of phyla in which cleavage is determinate, the coelom (in coelomate forms) is formed by proliferation of mesodermal bands (schizocoelic formation), the mesoderm is formed from a particular blastomere (called 4d), and the mouth is derived from or near the blastopore. Includes the Annelida, Arthropoda, Mollusca, and a number of minor phyla. Compares with **Deuterostomia.**

proventriculus (pro′ven-trik′ū-ləs) (L., *pro,* before, + *ventriculum,* ventricle). In birds, the glandular stomach between the crop and gizzard. In insects, a muscular dilation of foregut armed internally with chitinous teeth.

proximal (L., *proximus,* nearest). Situated toward or near the point of attachment; opposite of distal, distant.

pseudocoel (sū′do-sēl) (Gr., *pseudēs,* false, + *koilōma,* cavity). A body cavity not lined with peritoneum and not a part of the blood or digestive systems, embryonically derived from the blastocoel.

pseudopodium (sū′də-pō′dē-əm) (Gr., *pseudēs,* false, + *podion,* small foot, + *eidos,* form). A temporary cytoplasmic protrusion extended out from a protozoan or ameboid cell, and serving for locomotion or for taking up food.

puff. Strands of DNA spread apart at certain locations on giant chromosomes of some flies where that DNA is being transcribed.

pupa (pū′pə) (L., girl, doll, puppet). Inactive quiescent stage of the holometabolous insects. It follows the larval stages and precedes the adult stage.

purine (pū′rēn) (L., *purus,* pure, + *urina,* urine). Organic base with carbon and nitrogen atoms in two interlocking rings. The parent substance of adenine, guanine, and other naturally occurring bases.

pyrimidine (pī-rim′ə-dēn) (alter. of pyridine, from Gr., *pyr,* fire, + *id,* adj. suffix, + *ine*). An organic base composed of a single ring of carbon and nitrogen atoms; parent substance of several bases found in nucleic acids.

queen. In entomology, the single fully developed female in a colony of social insects such as bees, ants, and termites, distinguished from workers, nonreproductive females, and soldiers.

radial cleavage. Type in which early cleavage planes are symmetrical to the polar axis, each blastomere of one tier lying directly above the corresponding blastomere of the next layer; indeterminate cleavage.

radial symmetry. A morphological condition in which the parts of an animal are arranged concentrically around an oral-aboral axis, and more than one imaginary plane through this axis yields halves that are mirror images of each other.

radula (ra′jə-lə) (L., scraper). Rasping tongue found in most molluscs.

ratite (ra′tīt) (L., *ratis,* raft) Having an unkeeled sternum; compares with **carinate.**

recapitulation Summing up or repeating; hypothesis that an individual repeats its phylogenetic history in its development.

recombinant DNA. DNA from two different species, such as a virus and a mammal, combined into a single molecule.

redia (rē′dē-ə), pl. **rediae** (rē′dē-ē) (from Redi, Italian biologist). A larval stage in the life cycle of flukes; it is produced by a sporocyst larva, and in turn gives rise to many cercariae.

regulative development. Progressive determination and restriction of initially totipotent embryonic material.

regulator gene. A gene with the information to synthesize a molecule that can block transcription of a structural gene, thus precluding synthesis of the product coded for on the structural gene.

releaser (L., *relaxare,* to unloose). Simple stimulus that elicits an innate behavior pattern.

renin (rē′nin) (L., *ren,* kidney) An enzyme produced by the kidney juxtaglomerular apparatus that initiates changes leading to increased blood pressure and increased sodium reabsorption.

replication (L., *replicatio,* a folding back). In genetics, the duplication of one or more DNA molecules from the preexisting molecule.

respiration (L., *respiratio,* breathing). Gaseous interchange between an organism and its surrounding medium. In the cell, the release of energy by the oxidation of food molecules.

restriction endonuclease. An enzyme that cleaves a DNA molecule at a particular base sequence.

rete mirabile (rē′tē mə-rab′ə-lē) (L., wonderful net). A network of small blood vessels so arranged that the incoming blood runs countercurrent to the outgoing blood and thus makes possible efficient exchange between the two bloodstreams. Such a mechanism serves to maintain the high concentration of gases in the fish swim bladder.

reticular (rə-tīk′ū-lər) (L., *reticulum,* small net). Resembling a net in appearance or structure.

reticuloendothelial system (rə-tic′ū-lō-en-dō-thēl′i-əl) (L., *reticulum,* dim. of net, + Gr., *endon,* within, + *thele,* nipple). The fixed phagocytic cells in the tissues, especially the liver, lymph nodes, spleen, and others; also called RE system.

rhabdite (rab′dīt) (Gr., *rhabdos,* rod). Rodlike structures in the cells of the epidermis or underlying parenchyma in certain turbellarians. They are discharged in mucous secretions.

rheoreceptor (rē′ə-rē-cep′tər) (Gr., *rheos,* a flowing, + receptor). A sensory organ of

bat / āpe / ärmadillo/ herring / fēmale / finch / līce / crocodile / crōw / duck / ūnicorn / ə indicates unaccented vowel sound "uh" as in mammal, fishes, cardinal, heron, vulture / stress as in bi-ol′o-gy, bi′o-log′i-cal aquatic animals that responds to water current.

rhopalium (rō-pā′lē-əm) (N.L. from Gr., *rhopalon*, a club). One of the marginal, club-shaped sense organs of certain jellyfishes; tentaculocyst.

rhoptries (rōp′trēz) (Gr., *rhopalon*, club, + *tryō*, to rub, wear out). Club-shaped bodies in Apicomplexa comprising one of the structures of the apical complex; open at anterior and apparently functioning in penetration of host cell.

rhynchocoel (ring′kō-sēl) (Gr., *rhynchos*, snout, + *koilos*, hollow). In nemertines, the dorsal tubular cavity that contains the inverted proboscis. It has no opening to the outside.

ribosome (rī′bə-sōm). A small organelle composed of protein and ribonucleic acid. May be free in the cytoplasm or attached to the membranes of the endoplasmic reticulum; functions in protein synthesis.

ritualization. In ethology, the evolutionary modification, usually intensification, of a behavior pattern to serve communication.

RNA. Ribonucleic acid, of which there are several different kinds, such as messenger RNA, ribosomal RNA, and transfer RNA (mRNA, rRNA, tRNA).

rostellum (räs-tel′ləm) (L., small beak). Projecting structure on scolex of tapeworm, often with hooks.

rostrum (räs′trəm) (L., ship's beak). A snoutlike projection on the head.

r-selection (from the r term in the logistic equation). Natural selection under conditions that favor survival when populations are controlled primarily by density-independent factors; contrast with **K-selection.**

saccule (sa′kūl) (L., *sacculus*, small bag). Small chamber of the membranous labyrinth of the inner ear.

sagittal (saj′ə-dəl) (L., *sagitta*, arrow). Pertaining to the median anteroposterior plane that divides a bilaterally symmetrical organism into right and left halves.

saprophagous (sə-präf′ə-gəs) (Gr., *sapros*, rotten, + *phagos*, from *phagein*, to eat). Feeding on decaying matter; saprobic; saprozoic.

saprophyte (sap′rə-fīt) (Gr., *sapros*, rotten, + *phyton*, plant). A plant living on dead or decaying organic matter.

saprozoic nutrition (sap-rə-zō′ik) (Gr., *sapros*, rotten, + *zōon*, animal). Animal nutrition by absorption of dissolved salts and simple organic nutrients from surrounding medium; also refers to feeding on decaying matter.

sarcolemma (sär′kə-lem′ə) (Gr., *sarx*, flesh + *lemma*, rind). The thin, noncellular sheath that encloses a striated muscle fiber.

sarcomere (sär′kə-mir) (Gr., *sarx*, flesh, + *meros*, part) Transverse segment of striated muscle believed to be the fundamental contractile unit.

sarcoplasm (sär′kə-plaz′-əm) (Gr., *sarx*, flesh, + *plasma*, mold). Clear, semifluid substance between fibrils of muscle tissue.

schizocoel (skiz′ə-sēl) (Gr., *schizo*, from *schizein*, to split, + *koilōma*, cavity). A coelom formed by the splitting of embryonic meso-

derm. Noun, **schizocoelomate,** an animal with a schizocoel, such as an arthropod or mollusc. Adj., **schizocoelous.**

schizocoelous mesoderm formation (skiz′ō-sēl-ləs). Embryonic formation of the mesoderm as cords of cells between ectoderm and endoderm; splitting of these cords results in the coelomic space.

schizogony (skə-zä′gə-nē) (Gr., *schizein*, to split, + *gonos*, seed). Multiple asexual fission.

sclerite (skle′rit) (Gr., *sklēros*, hard). A hard chitinous or calcareous plate or spicule; one of the plates making up the exoskeleton of arthropods, especially insects.

scleroblast (skler′ə-blast) (Gr., *sklēros*, hard, + *blastos*, germ). An amebocyte specialized to secrete a spicule, found in sponges.

sclerotic (skle-räd′ik) (Gr., *sklēros*, hard). Pertaining to the tough outer coat of the eyeball.

sclerotization (skle′rə-tə-zā′shən). Process of hardening of the cuticle of arthropods by the formation of stabilizing cross linkages between peptide chains of adjacent protein molecules.

scolex (skō′leks) (Gr., *skōlēx*, worm, grub). The holdfast, or so-called head, of a tapeworm; bears suckers and, in some, hooks, and posterior to it new proglottids are differentiated.

scrotum (skrō′təm) (L., bag). The pouch that contains the testes in most mammals.

scyphistoma (sī-fis′tə-mə) (Gr., *skyphos*, cup, + *stoma*, mouth). A stage in the development of scyphozoan jellyfish just after the larva becomes attached, the polyp form of a scyphozoan.

sedentary (sed′ən-ter-ē). Stationary, sitting, inactive; staying in one place.

seminiferous (sem-ə-nif′rəs) (L., *semen*, semen, + *ferre*, to bear). Pertains to the tubules that produce or carry semen in the testes.

semipermeable (L., *semi*, half, + *permeabilis*, capable of being passed through). Permeable to small particles, such as water and certain inorganic ions, but not to larger molecules.

septum, pl. **septa** (L., fence). A wall between two cavities.

serosa (sə-rō′sə) (N.L. from L., *serum*, serum). The outer embryonic membrane of birds and reptiles; chorion. Also, the peritoneal lining of the body cavity.

serotonin (sir′ə-tōn′ən) (L., *serum*, serum). A phenolic amine, found in the serum of clotted blood and in many other tissues, that possesses several poorly understood metabolic, vascular, and neural functions; 5-hydroxytryptamine.

serum (sir′əm) (L., whey, serum). The liquid that separates from the blood after coagulation; blood plasma from which fibrinogen has been removed. Also, the clear portion of a biological fluid separated from its particulate elements.

sessile (ses′əl) (L., *sessilis*, low, dwarf). Attached at the base; fixed to one spot, not able to move about.

seta (sīd′ə), pl. **setae** (sē′tē) (L., bristle). A needlelike chitinous structure of the integument of annelids, arthropods, and others.

siliceous (sə-li′shəs) (L., *silex*, flint). Containing silica.

simian (sim′ē-ən) (L., *simia*, ape). Pertaining to monkeys or apes.

sinistral (si′nə-strəl, sə-ni′stral) (L., *sinister*, left). Pertaining to the left; in gastropods, shell is sinistral if opening is to left of columella when held with spire up and facing observer.

sinus (sī′nəs) (L., curve). A cavity or space in tissues or in bone.

siphonoglyph (sī-fän′ə-glif′) (Gr., *siphōn*, reed, tube, siphon, + *glyphē*, carving). Ciliated furrow in the gullet of sea anemones.

siphuncle (sī′fun-kl) (L., *siphunculus*, small tube). Cord of tissue running through shell of nautiloid, connecting all chambers with body of animal.

solenocyte (sō-len′ə-sīt) (Gr., *solēn*, pipe, + *kytos*, hollow vessel). Special type of flame bulb in which the bulb bears a flagellum instead of a tuft of cilia. See **flame bulb, protonephridium.**

soma (sō′mə) (Gr., body). The whole of an organism except the germ cells (germ plasm).

somatic (sō-mat′ik) (Gr., *sōma*, body). Refers to the body, for example, somatic cells in contrast germ cells.

somatocoel (sə-ma′tə-sel) (Gr., *sōma*, body, + *koilos*, hollow). One of the pair of sacs that form the main body coelom of echinoderms.

somatoplasm (sō′mə-də-pla′zm) (Gr., *sōma*, body, + *plasma*, anything formed). The living matter that makes up the mass of the body as distinguished from germ plasm, which makes up the reproductive cells. The protoplasm of body cells.

somite (sō′mīt) (Gr., *sōma*, body). One of the blocklike masses of mesoderm arranged segmentally (metamerically) in a longitudinal series beside the neural tube of the embryo; metamere.

speciation (spē′sē-ā′shən) (L., *species*, kind). The evolutionary process by which new species arise; the process by which variations become fixed.

species (spē′shez, spē′sēz) sing. and pl. (L., particular kind). A group of interbreeding individuals of common ancestry that are reproductively isolated from all other such groups; a taxonomic unit ranking below a genus and designated by a binomen consisting of its genus and the species name.

spermatheca (spər′mə-thē′kə) (Gr., *sperma*, seed, + *thēkē*, case). A sac in the female reproductive organs for the reception and storage of sperm.

spermatogonium (spər′mad-ə-gō′nē-əm) (Gr., *sperma*, seed, + *gonē*, offspring). Precursor of mature male reproductive cell; gives rise directly to a spermatocyte.

spermatophore (spər-mad′ə-fōr′) (Gr., *sperma*, *spermatos*, seed, + *pherein*, to bear). Capsule or packet enclosing sperm, produced by males of several invertebrate groups and a few vertebrates.

sphincter (sfingk′tər) (Gr., *sphinkter*, band, sphincter, from *sphingein*, to bind tight). A ring-shaped muscle capable of closing a tubular opening by constriction.

spicule (spi′kyul) (L., dim. of *spica*, point). One of the minute calcareous or siliceous skeletal bodies found in sponges, radiolarians, soft corals, and sea cucumbers.

spiracle (spi′rə-kəl) (L., *spiraculum*, from *spirare*, to breathe). External opening of a trachea in arthropods. One of a pair of openings on the head of elasmobranchs for passage of water. Exhalent aperture of tadpole gill chamber.

spiral cleavage. A type of early embryonic cleavage in which cleavage planes are diagonal to the polar axis and unequal cells are produced by the alternate clockwise and counterclockwise cleavage around the axis of polarity; determinate cleavage.

spongin (spun′jin) (L., *spongia*, sponge). Fibrous, scleroprotein material making up the skeletal network of horny sponges.

spongioblast (spun′jeo-blast) (Gr., *spongos*, sponge, + *blastos*, bud). Cell in a sponge that secretes spongin, a protein.

spongocoel (spun′jō-sēl) (Gr., *spongos*, sponge, + *koilos*, hollow). Central cavity in sponges.

sporocyst (spō′rə-sist) (Gr., *sporos*, seed, + *kystis*, pouch). A larval stage in the life cycle of flukes; it originates from a miracidium.

sporogony (spor-äg′ə-ne) (Gr., *sporos*, seed, + *gonos*, birth). Multiple fission to produce sporozoites after zygote formation.

sporozoite (spō′rə-zō′īt) (Gr., *sporos*, seed, + *zōon*, animal, + *ite*, suffix for body part). A stage in the life history of many sporozoan protozoa; released from oocysts.

statoblast (stad′ə-blast) (Gr., *statos*, standing, fixed, + *blastos*, germ). Biconvex capsule containing germinative cells and produced by most freshwater ectoprocts by asexual budding. Under favorable conditions it germinates to give rise to new zooid.

statocyst (Gr., *statos*, standing, + *kystis*, bladder). Sense organ of equilibrium; a fluid-filled cellular cyst containing one or more granules (statoliths) used to sense direction of gravity.

statolith (Gr., *statos*, standing, + *lithos*, stone). Small calcareous body resting on tufts of cilia in the statocyst.

stenohaline (sten-ə-hā′lĭn, -lən) (Gr., *stenos*, narrow, + *hals*, salt). Pertaining to aquatic organisms that have restricted tolerance to changes in environmental saltwater concentration.

stenophagous (stə-näf′ə-gəs) (Gr., *stenos*, narrow, + *phagein*, to eat). Eating few kinds of foods.

stenotopic (sten-ə-tä′pik) (Gr., *stenos*, narrow, + *topos*, place). Refers to an organism with a narrow range of adaptability to environmental change; having a restricted geographical distribution.

stereogastrula (ste′rē-ə-gas′trə-lə) (Gr., *stereos*, solid, + *gastēr*, stomach, + L., *ula*, dim.). A solid type of gastrula, such as the planula of cnidarians.

sternum (ster′nəm) (L., breastbone). Ventral plate of an arthropod body segment; breastbone of vertebrates.

sterol (ste′rōl), **steroid** (ste′roid) (Gr., *stereos*, solid, + L., *ol*, [from *oleum*, oil]). One of a class of organic compounds containing a molecular skeleton of four fused carbon rings; it includes cholesterol, sex hormones, adrenocortical hormones, and vitamin D.

stigma (Gr., *stigma*, mark, tattoo mark). Eyespot in certain protozoa. Spiracle of certain terrestrial arthropods.

stolon (stō′lən) (L., *stolō, stolonis*, a shoot, or sucker of a plant). A rootlike extension of the body wall that gives rise to buds that may develop into new zooids, thus forming a compound animal in which the zooids remain united by the stolon. Found in some colonial anthozoans, hydrozoans, ectoprocts, and ascidians.

stoma (stō′mə) (Gr., mouth). A mouthlike opening.

stomochord (stō′mə-kord) (Gr., *stoma*, mouth, + *chordē*, cord). Anterior evagination of the dorsal wall of the buccal cavity into the proboscis of hemichordates; the buccal diverticulum.

strobila (strō′bə-lə) (Gr., *strobilē*, lint plug like a pine cone [*strobilos*]). A stage in the development of the scyphozoan jellyfish. Also, the chain of proglottids of a tapeworm.

stroma (strō′mə) (Gr., *strōma*, bedding). Supporting connective tissue framework of an animal organ; filmy framework of red blood corpuscles and certain cells.

structural gene. A gene carrying the information to construct a protein.

sycon (sī′kon) (Gr., *sykon*, fig). A type of canal system in certain sponges. Sometimes called syconoid.

symbiosis (sim′bī-ōs′əs, sim′bē-ōs′əs) (Gr., *syn*, with, + *bios*, life). The living together of two different species in an intimate relationship. Symbiont always benefits; host may benefit, may be unaffected, or may be harmed (mutualism, commensalism, and parasitism).

sympatric (sim′pa′-trik) (Gr., *syn*, with, + *patra*, native land). Having the same or overlapping regions of distribution. Noun, **sympatry.**

synapomorphy (si-nap′ō-mor-fē) (Gr., *synapsis*, contact, union, + *morphē*, form). A derived characteristic shared by two or more taxonomic groups; the more synapomorphies shared, the more closely related the groups. See **cladistics.**

synapse (si′naps, si-naps′) (Gr., *synapsis*, contact, union). The place at which a nerve impulse passes between neuron processes, typically from an axon of one nerve cell to a dendrite of another nerve cell.

synapsis (si-nap′səs) (Gr., *synapsis*, contact, union). The time when the pairs of homologous chromosomes lie alongside each other in the first meiotic division.

syncytium (sin-sish′e-əm) (Gr., *syn*, with, + *kytos*, hollow vessel). A mass of protoplasm containing many nuclei and not divided into cells.

syndrome (sin′drōm) (Gr., *syn*, with + *dramein*, to run). A group of symptoms characteristic of a particular disease or abnormality.

syngamy (sin′gə-mē) (Gr., *syn*, with, + *gamos*, marriage). Fertilization of one gamete with another individual gamete to form a zygote, found in most animals with sexual reproduction.

syrinx (sir′inks) (Gr., shepherd's pipe). The vocal organ of birds located at the base of the trachea.

systematics (sis-tə-mad′iks). Science of classification and evolutionary biology.

T cell. A type of lymphocyte most important in cellular immune response.

tactile (tak′til) (L., *tactilis*, able to be touched, from *tangere*, to touch). Pertaining to touch.

tagma, pl. **tagmata** (Gr., *tagma*, arrangement, order, row). A compound body section of an arthropod resulting from embryonic fusion of two or more segments; for example, head, thorax, abdomen.

tagmatization, tagmosis. Organization of the arthropod body into tagmata.

taiga (tī′gä) (Russ.). Habitat zone characterized by large tracts of coniferous forests, long, cold winters, and short summers; most typical in Canada and Siberia.

taxis (tak′sis), pl. **taxes** (Gr., *taxis*, arrangement). An orientation movement by a (usually) simple organism in response to an environmental stimulus.

taxon (tak′son), pl. **taxa** (Gr., *taxis*, arrangement). Any taxonomic group or entity.

taxonomy (tak-sän′ə-mi) (Gr., *taxis*, arrangement, + *nomos*, law). Study of the principles of scientific classification; systematic ordering and naming of organisms.

tectum (tek′təm) (L., roof). A rooflike structure, for example, dorsal part of capitulum in ticks and mites.

tegument (teg′ū-ment) (L., *tegumentum*, from *tegere*, to cover). An integument: specifically external covering in cestodes and trematodes, formerly believed to be a cuticle.

telencephalon (tel′en-sef′ə-lon) (Gr., *telos*, end, + *encephalon*, brain). The most anterior vesicle of the brain; the anterior-most subdivision of the prosencephalon that becomes the cerebrum and associated structures.

teleology (tel′ē-äl′ə-jē) (Gr., *telos*, end, + L., *logia*, study of, from Gr., *logos*, word). The philosophical view that natural events are goal directed and are preordained, as opposed to the scientific view of mechanical determinism.

telocentric (tē′lō-sen′trək) (Gr., *telos*, end, + *kentron*, center). Chromosome with centromere at the end.

telolecithal (te-lō-les′ə-thəl) (Gr., *telos*, end, + *lekithos*, yolk, + *al*). Having the yolk concentrated at one end of an egg.

telson (tel′sən) (Gr., *telson*, extremity). Posterior projection of the last body segment in many crustaceans.

bat / āpe / ärmadillo/ herring / fēmale / finch / līce / crocodile / crōw / duck / ūnicorn / ə indicates unaccented vowel sound "uh" as in mammal, fishes, cardinal, heron, vulture / stress as in bi-ol′o-gy, bi′o-log′i-cal

template (tem′plət). A pattern or mold guiding the formation of a duplicate; often used with reference to gene duplication.

tentaculocyst (ten-tak′u-lō-sist) (L., *tentaculum*, feeler, + Gr., *kystis*, pouch). One of the sense organs along the margin of medusae; a rhopalium.

tergum (ter′gəm) (L., back). Dorsal part of an arthropod body segment.

territory (L., *territorium*, from *terra*, earth). A restricted area preempted by an animal or pair of animals, usually for breeding purposes, and guarded from other individuals of the same species.

test (L., *testa*, shell). A shell or hardened outer covering.

tetrad (te′trad) (Gr., *tetras*, four). Group of two pairs of chromatids at synapsis and resulting from the replication of paired homologous chromosomes; the bivalent.

tetrapods (te′trə-päds) (Gr., *tetras*, four + *pous, podos*, foot). Four-footed vertebrates; the group includes amphibians, reptiles, birds, and mammals.

therapsid (thə-rap′sid) (Gr., *theraps*, an attendant). Extinct Mesozoic mammal-like reptile from which true mammals evolved.

thermocline (thər′mō-klīn) (Gr., *thermē*, heat, + *klinein*, to swerve). Layer of water separating upper warmer and lighter water from lower colder and heavier water in a lake or sea; a stratum of abrupt change in water temperature.

Tiedemann's bodies (tēd′ə-mənz) (from F. Tiedemann, German anatomist). Four or five pairs of pouchlike bodies attached to the ring canal of sea stars, apparently functioning in production of coelomocytes.

tight junction. Region of actual fusion of cell membranes between two adjacent cells.

tornaria (tor-na′rē-ə) (L., *tornare*, to turn). A free-swimming larva of enteropneusts that rotates as it swims; resembles somewhat the bipinnaria larva of echinoderms.

torsion (L., *torquere*, to twist). A twisting phenomenon in gastropod development that alters the position of the visceral and pallial organs by 180 degrees.

toxicyst (tox′i-sist) (Gr., *toxikon*, poison, + *kystis*, bladder). Structures possessed by predatory ciliate protozoa, which on stimulation expel a poison to subdue the prey.

trachea (trā′kē-ə) (M.L., windpipe). The windpipe. Also, any of the air tubes of insects.

transcription. Formation of messenger RNA from the coded DNA.

transduction. Condition in which bacterial DNA (and the genetic characteristics it bears) is transferred from one bacterium to another by the agent of viral infection.

transfer RNA (tRNA). A form of RNA of about seven nucleotides, which are adapter molecules in the synthesis of proteins. A specific amino acid molecule is carried by transfer RNA to a ribosome–messenger RNA complex for incorporation into a polypeptide.

transformation. Condition in which DNA in the environment of bacteria somehow penetrates them and is incorporated into their genetic complement, so that their progeny inherit the genetic characters so acquired.

translation (L., a transferring). The process in which the genetic information present in messenger RNA is used to direct the order of specific amino acids during protein synthesis.

trichinosis (trik-ən-o′səs). Disease caused by infection with the nematode *Trichinella spiralis.*

trichocyst (trik′ə-sist) (Gr., *thrix*, hair, + *kystis*, bladder). Saclike protrusible organelle in the ectoplasm of ciliates, which discharges as a threadlike weapon of defense.

triglyceride (trī-glis′ə-rīd) (Gr., *tria*, three, + *glykys*, sweet, + *ide*, suffix denoting compound). A triester of glycerol with one, two, or three acids.

triploblastic (trip′lō-blas′tik) (Gr., *triploos*, triple, + *blastos*, germ). Pertaining to metazoa in which the embryo has three primary germ layers—ectoderm, mesoderm, and endoderm.

trisomy 21. See **Down's syndrome.**

trochophore (trōk′ə-fōr) (Gr., *trochos*, wheel, + *pherein*, to bear). A free-swimming ciliated marine larva characteristic of most molluscs and certain ectoprocts, brachiopods, and marine worms; an ovoid or pyriform body with preoral circlet of cilia and sometimes a secondary circlet behind the mouth.

trophallaxis (trof′ə-lak′səs) (Gr., *trophē*, food, + *allaxis*, barter, exchange). Exchange of food between young and adults, especially certain social insects.

trophoblast (trof′ə-blast) (Gr., *trephein*, to nourish, + *blastos*, germ). Outer ectodermal nutritive layer of blastodermic vesicle; in mammals it is part of the chorion and attaches to the uterine wall.

trophozoite (trof′ə-zō′īt) (Gr., *trophē*, food, + *zōon*, animal). Adult stage in the life cycle of a protozoan in which it is actively absorbing nourishment.

tropomyosin (trōp′ə-mī′ə-sən) (Gr., *tropos*, turn, + *mys*, muscle). Low–molecular weight protein surrounding the actin filaments of striated muscle.

troponin (trə-pōn′in). Complex of globular proteins positioned at intervals along the actin filament of skeletal muscle; thought to serve as a calcium-dependent switch in muscle contraction.

tube feet (**podia**). Numerous small, muscular, fluid-filled tubes projecting from body of echinoderms; part of water-vascular system; used in locomotion, clinging, food handling, and respiration.

tubulin (tū′bū-lən) (L., *tubulus*, small tube, + *in*, belonging to). Globular protein forming the hollow cylinder of microtubules.

tundra (tun′drə) (Russ. from Lapp, *tundar*, hill). Terrestrial habitat zone, located between taiga and polar regions; characterized by absence of trees, short growing season, and mostly frozen soil during much of the year.

tunic (L., *tunica*, tunic, coat). In tunicates, a cuticular, cellulose-containing covering of the body secreted by the underlying body wall.

turbellarian (tər′bə-lar′ə-an) (L., *turbellae*, a stir or tumult). Flatworm of phylum Platyhelminthes, class Turbellaria.

typhlosole (tif′lə-sōl′) (Gr., *typhlos*, blind, + *sōlēn*, channel, pipe). A longitudinal fold projecting into the intestine in certain invertebrates such as the earthworm.

umbilical (L., *umbilicus*, navel). Refers to the navel, or umbilical cord.

umbo (um′bō), pl. **umbones** (əm-bō′nēz) (L., boss of a shield). One of the prominences on either side of the hinge region in a bivalve mollusc shell. Also, the "beak" of a brachiopod shell.

ungulate (un′gū-lət) (L., *ungula*, hoof). Hoofed. Noun, any hoofed mammal.

urethra (ū-rē′thrə) (Gr., *ourethra*, urethra). The tube from the urinary bladder to the exterior in both sexes.

utricle (ū′trə-kəl) (L., *utriculus*, little bag). That part of the inner ear containing the receptors for dynamic body balance; the semicircular canals lead from and to the utricle.

vacuole (vak′yə-wōl) (L., *vacuus*, empty, + Fr., *ole*, dim.). A membrane-bounded, fluid-filled space in a cell.

valence (vā′ləns) (L., *valere*, to have power). Degree of combining power of an element as expressed by the number of atoms of hydrogen (or its equivalent) that that element can hold (if negative) or displace in a reaction (if positive). The oxidation state of an element in a compound. The number of electrons gained, shared, or lost by an atom when forming a bond with one or more other atoms.

valve (L., *valva*, leaf of a double door). One of the two shells of a typical bivalve mollusc or brachiopod.

vector (L., a bearer, carrier, from *vehere, vectum*, to carry). Any agent that carries and transmits pathogenic microorganisms from one host to another host.

veliger (vēl′ə-jər, vel-) (L., *velum*, veil, covering). Larval form of certain molluscs; develops from the trochophore and has the beginning of a foot, mantle, shell, and so on.

velum (vē′ləm) (L., veil, covering). A membrane on the subumbrella surface of jellyfish of class Hydrozoa. Also, a ciliated swimming organ of the veliger larva.

vestige (ves′tij) (L., *vestigium*, footprint). A rudimentary organ that may have been well developed in some ancestor or in the embryo.

vicariance (vī-kar′ē-ənts) (L., *vicarius*, a substitute). Geographical separation of ancestral populations; allopatry.

villus (vil′əs), pl. **villi** (L., tuft of hair). A small fingerlike, vascular process on the wall of the small intestine. Also one of the branching, vascular processes on the embryonic portion of the placenta.

virus (vī′rəs) (L., slimy liquid, poison). A submicroscopic noncellular particle composed of a nucleoprotein core and a protein shell; parasitic; will grow and reproduce in a host cell.

viscera (vis′ər-ə) (L., pl. of *viscus*, internal organ). Internal organs in the body cavity.

vitalism (L., *vita*, life). The view that natural processes are controlled by supernatural forces and cannot be explained through the laws of physics and chemistry alone, as opposed to mechanism.

vitamin (L., *vita,* life, + *amine,* from former supposed chemical origin). An organic substance required in small amounts for normal metabolic function; must be supplied in the diet or by intestinal flora because the organism cannot synthesize it.

vitellaria (vi′təl-lar′e-ə) (L., *vitellus,* yolk of an egg). Structures in many flatworms that produce vitelline cells, that is, cells that provide eggshell material and nutrient for the embryo.

vitelline membrane (və-tel′ən, vī′təl-ən) (L., *vitellus,* yolk of an egg). The noncellular membrane that encloses the egg cell.

bat / āpe / ärmadillo/ herring / fēmale / finch / līce / crocodile / crōw / duck / ūnicorn / ə indicates unaccented vowel sound "uh" as in mammal, fishes, cardinal, heron, vulture / stress as in bi-ol′o-gy, bi′o-log′i-cal

viviparity (vī′və-par′ə-dē) (L., *vivus,* alive, + *parere,* to bring forth). Reproduction in which eggs develop within the female body, with nutritional aid of maternal parent as in therian mammals, many reptiles, and some fishes; offspring are born as juveniles. Adj., **viviparous** (vī-vip′ə-rəs).

water-vascular system. System of fluid-filled closed tubes and ducts peculiar to echinoderms; used to move tentacles and tube feet that serve variously for clinging, food handling, locomotion, and respiration.

X-organ. Neurosecretory organ in eyestalk of crustaceans that secretes molt-inhibiting hormone.

Y-organ. Gland in the antennal or maxillary segment of some crustaceans that secretes molting hormone.

zoecium, zooecium (zō-ē′shē-əm) (Gr., *zōon,* animal, + *oikos,* house). Cuticular sheath or shell of Ectoprocta.

zoochlorella (zō′ə-klōr-el′ə) (Gr., *zōon,* life, + *Chlorella*). Any of various minute green algae (usually *Chlorella*) that live symbiotically within the cytoplasm of some protozoa and other invertebrates.

zooid (zō-oid) (Gr., *zōon,* life). An individual member of a colony of animals, such as colonial cnidarians and ectoprocts.

zygote (Gr., *zygōtos,* yoked). The fertilized egg.

zygotic meiosis. Meiosis that takes place within the first few divisions after zygote formation; thus, all stages in the life cycle other than the zygote are haploid.

APPENDIX

DEVELOPMENT OF ZOOLOGY

Certain key discoveries have greatly influenced progress in the study of zoology. This appendix presents some of the major landmarks in the development of biology and the individuals whose names are commonly associated with them. It is very difficult to appraise the historical development of any field of study. One investigator often gets the credit for an important discovery when many others should share in the prestige. No one individual has a monopoly on ideas; advances in science are built on the results of many causes and the work of many minds. Especially in recent years, important discoveries have been due to the efforts of teams of investigators. Furthermore, because knowledge of a topic accrues over a period of time, it is often difficult to decide in which year the "discovery" occurred.

In this brief outline the student may be able to see some of the relationships that exist between one discovery and another. The discoveries are not completely isolated as they may sometimes appear. One may note also that fundamental discoveries in a particular branch of biology tend to be grouped fairly close together chronologically because that particular interest may have dominated the thought of biological investigators at that time.

The reader may wish to locate important discoveries in a given area without reading the entire list. Such an effort may be made easier by use of the following list of key symbols. Any such system of classification suffers some limitations, however. Many basic discoveries are not easily categorized because they have implications in wide areas. The list of categories must be short, or it becomes too cumbersome. Nevertheless, we hope that the classification will be useful.

□ Taxonomy, systematics, and environmental fields (behavior, ecology, and the like)
○ Tissue- and organ-level anatomy and physiology
△ Cell biology
✳ Developmental biology
‡ Genetics
✕ Evolution and paleontology
† Of *particular* medical significance

ORIGINS OF BASIC CONCEPTS AND KEY DISCOVERIES IN ZOOLOGY

384-322 BC: *Aristotle. The foundation of zoology as a science.*

Although this great pioneer zoologist and philosopher cannot be appraised by modern standards, there is scarcely a major subdivision of zoology to which he did not make some contribution. He was a true scientist, for he emphasized observational and experimental methods. Despite his lack of scientific background, he was one of the greatest scientists of all time.

○ **130-200 AD:** *Galen. Development of anatomy and physiology.*

This Roman investigator has been praised for his clear concept of scientific methods and blamed for passing down to others certain glaring errors that persisted for centuries. His influence was so great that for centuries after his period students considered him the final authority on anatomical and physiological subjects.

1347: *William of Occam. Occam's razor.*

This principle of science has received its name from the fact that it is supposed to cut out unnecessary and irrelevant hypotheses in the explanation of phenomena. The gist of the principle is that, of several possible explanations, the one that is simplest, has the fewest assumptions, and is most consistent with the data at hand is the most probable.

○ **1543:** *Vesalius, Andreas. First modern interpretation of anatomical structures.*

With his insight into fundamental structure, Vesalius ushered in the dawn of modern biological investigation. Many aspects of his interpretation of anatomy are just now beginning to be appreciated.

○ **1616-1628:** *Harvey, William. First accurate description of blood circulation.*

Harvey's classic demonstration of blood circulation was the key experiment that laid the foundation of modern physiology. He explained bodily processes in physical terms, cleared away much of the mental rubbish of mystical interpretation, and gave an auspicious start to experimental physiology.

○ **1627:** *Aselli, G. First demonstration of lacteal vessels.*

This discovery, coming at the same time as Harvey's great work, supplemented the discovery of circulation.

○ **1649:** *Descartes, René. Early concept of reflex action.*

Descartes postulated that impulses originating at the receptors of the body were carried to the central nervous system where they activated muscles and glands by what he called "reflection."

✳ **1651:** *Harvey, William. Aphorism of Harvey:* Omne vivum ex ovo *(all life from the egg).*

Although Harvey's work as an embryologist is overshadowed by his demonstration of blood circulation, his *De Generatione Animalium*, published in 1651, contains many sound observations on embryological processes.

○ **1652:** *Bartholin, Thomas. Discovery of lymphatic system.*

The significance of the thoracic duct in its relation to the circulation was determined in this investigation.

○ **1658:** *Swammerdam, Jan. Description of red blood corpuscles.*

This discovery, together with Swammerdam's observations on the valves of the lymphatics and the alterations in shape of muscles during contraction, represented early advancements in the microscopical study of bodily structures.

○ **1660:** *Malpighi, Marcello. Demonstration of capillary circulation.*

By demonstrating the capillaries in the lung of a frog, Malpighi was able to complete the scheme of blood circulation. Harvey never saw capillaries and thus never included them in his description.

△ **1665:** *Hooke, Robert. Discovery of the cell.*

Hooke's investigations were made with cork, and the term "cell" fits cork much better than it does animal cells, but by tradition the misnomer has stuck.

△ **1672:** *de Graaf, R. Description of ovarian follicles.*

De Graaf's name is given to the mature ovarian follicle, but he believed that the follicles were the actual ova, an error later corrected by von Baer.

△□ **1675-1680:** *van Leeuwenhoek, Anthony. Discovery of protozoa.*

The discoveries of this eccentric Dutch microscopist revealed a whole new world of biology.

□ **1693:** *Ray, J. Concept of species.*

Although Ray's work on classification was later overshadowed by that of Linnaeus, Ray was really the first to apply the species concept to a particular kind of organism and to point out the variations that exist among the members of a species.

○ **1733:** *Hales, Stephen. First measurement of blood pressure.*

This was further proof that the bodily processes could be measured quantitatively—more than a century after Harvey's momentous demonstration.

✳ **1745:** *Bonnet, Charles. Discovery of natural parthenogenesis.*

Although somewhat unusual in nature, this phenomenon has yielded much information about meiosis and other cytological problems.

□ **1758:** *Linnaeus, Carolus. Development of binomial nomenclature system of taxonomy.*

So important is this work in taxonomy that 1758 is regarded as the starting point in the determination of the generic and specific names of animals. Besides the value of his binomial system, Linnaeus gave taxonomists a valuable working model of conciseness and clearness that has never been surpassed.

✳ **1759:** *Wolff, Kaspar F. Embryological theory of epigenesis.*

This embryologist, the greatest before von Baer, did much to overthrow the preformation theory then in vogue and, despite many shortcomings, laid the basis for the modern interpretation of embryology.

○ **1760:** *Hunter, John. Development of comparative investigations of animal structure.*

This vigorous eighteenth-century anatomist gave a powerful impetus not only to anatomical observations but also to the establishment of natural history museums.

□ **1763:** *Adanson, M. Concept of empirical taxonomy.*

This botanist proposed a scheme of classification that grouped individuals into taxa according to shared characters. A species would have the maximum number of shared characters according to this scheme. The concept has been revived recently by exponents of numerical taxonomy. It lacks the evaluation of the evolutionary concept and has been criticized on this account.

‡ **1763:** *Kölreuter, J.G. Discovery of quantitative inheritance (multiple genes).*

Kölreuter, a pioneer in plant hybridization, found that certain plant hybrids had characters more or less intermediate between the parents in the F_1 generation, but in the F_2 there were many gradations from one extreme to the other. An explanation was not forthcoming until after Mendel's laws were discovered.

□ **1768-1779:** *Cook, James. Influence of geographical exploration on development of biology.*

This famous sea captain made possible a greater range of biological knowledge because of the able naturalists whom he took on his voyages of discovery.

△ 1772: *Priestley, J., and J. Ingenhousz. Concept of photosynthesis.*

These investigators first pointed out some of the major aspects of this important phenomenon, such as the use of light energy for converting carbon dioxide and water into released oxygen and retained carbon.

△ 1774: *Priestley, J. Discovery of oxygen.*

The discovery of this element is of great biological interest because it helped in determining the nature of oxidation and the exact role of respiration in organisms.

△ 1778: *Lavoisier, Antoine L. Nature of animal respiration demonstrated.*

A basis for the chemical interpretation of the life process was given a great impetus by the careful quantitative studies of the changes during breathing made by this great investigator. His work also meant the final overthrow of the mystical phlogiston hypothesis that had held sway for so long.

□ 1781: *Abildgaard, P. First experimental life cycle of a tapeworm.*

Life cycles of parasites may be very complicated, involving several hosts. That a parasitic worm could require more than one host was a revolutionary concept in Abildgaard's day and was widely disbelieved until the work of Küchenmeister over 60 years later.

× 1791: *Smith, William. Correlation between fossils and geological strata.*

By observing that certain types of fossils were peculiar to particular strata, Smith was able to work out a method for estimating geological age. He laid the basis of stratigraphic geology.

○ 1792: *Galvani, L. Animal electricity.*

The lively controversy between Galvani and Volta over the twitching of frog legs led to extensive investigation of precise methods of measuring the various electrical phenomena of animals.

× 1796: *Cuvier, Georges. Development of vertebrate paleontology.*

Cuvier compared the structure of fossil forms with that of living ones and concluded that there had been a succession of organisms that had become extinct and were succeeded by the creation of new ones. To account for this extinction, Cuvier held to the theory of catastrophism, or the simultaneous extinction of animal populations by natural cataclysms.

× 1801: *de Lamarck, J.B. Evolutionary concept of use and disuse.*

De Lamarck gave the first clear-cut expression of a hypothesis to account for organic evolution. His assumption was that acquired characters were inherited; modern evolutionists have refuted this part of the hypothesis.

○ 1802: *Young, T. Hypothesis of trichromatic color vision.*

Young's hypothesis suggested that the retina contained three kinds of light-sensitive substances, each having a maximum sensitivity in a different region of the spectrum and each being transmitted separately to the brain. The three substances combined produced the colors of the environment. The three pigments responsible are located in three kinds of cones. Young's explanation has been modified in certain details by other investigators.

○ 1811: *Bell, C., and F. Magendie. Discovery of the functions of dorsal and ventral roots of spinal nerves.*

This demonstration was a starting point for an anatomical and functional investigation of the most complex system in the body.

∗ 1817: *Pander, C.H. First description of three germ layers.*

The description of the three germ layers was first made on the chick, and later the concept was extended by von Baer to include all vertebrates.

∗ 1827: *von Baer, Karl. Discovery of mammalian ovum.*

The very tiny ova of mammals escaped de Graaf's eyes, but von Baer brought mammalian reproduction into line with that of other animals by detecting the ova and their true relation to the follicles.

△ 1828: *Brown, Robert. Brownian movement first described.*

This interesting phenomenon is characteristic of living matter and sheds some light on the structure of cells.

□ 1828: *Thompson, J.V. Nature of plankton.*

Thompson's collections of these small forms with a tow net, together with his published descriptions, are the first records of the vast community of planktonic animals. He was also the first to work out the true nature of barnacles.

△ 1828: *Wöhler, F. First to synthesize an organic compound.*

Wöhler succeeded in making urea (a compound formed in the body) from the inorganic substance ammonium cyanate; thus, $NH_4OCN \rightarrow NH_2CONH_2$. This success in producing an organic substance synthetically was the stimulus that resulted in the preparation of thousands of compounds by others.

∗× 1830: *von Baer, Karl. Biogenetic law formulated.*

Von Baer's conception of this law was conservative and sounder in its implication than has been the case with many other biologists (Haeckel, for instance). Von Baer stated that embryos of higher and lower forms resemble each other more the earlier they are compared in their development, and *not* that the embryos of higher forms resemble the adults of lower organisms.

× 1830: *Lyell, C. Modern concept of geology.*

The influence of this concept not only did away with the catastrophic theory but also gave a logical interpretation of fossil life and the correlation between the formation of rock strata and the animal life that existed at the time these formations were laid down.

△ 1831: *Brown, Robert. First description of cell nucleus.*

Others had seen nuclei, but Brown was the first to name the structure and to regard the nucleus as a general phenomenon. This description was an important preliminary to the formulation of the cell theory a few years later, for Schleiden acknowledged the importance of the nucleus in the development of the cell concept.

○ 1833: *Hall, Marshall. Concept of reflex action.*

Hall described the method by which a stimulus can produce a response independently of sensation or volition and coined the term "reflex action." It remained for the outstanding work of the great Sir Charles Sherrington in the twentieth century to explain much of the complex nature of reflexes.

†○ 1835: *Bassi, Agostino. First demonstration of a microorganism as an infective agent.*

Bassi's discovery that a certain disease of silkworms was caused by a small fungus represents the beginning of the germ theory of disease that was to prove so fruitful in the hands of Pasteur and other able investigators.

△ 1835: *Dujardin, Felix. Description of living matter (protoplasm).*

Dujardin associated the jellylike substance that he found in protozoa and that he called "sarcode" with the life process. This substance was later called "protoplasm," and the sarcode idea may be considered a significant landmark in the development of the protoplasm concept.

†○ 1835: *Owen, Richard. Discovery of Trichinella.*

This versatile investigator is chiefly remembered for his researches in anatomy, but his discovery of this very common parasite in humans is an important landmark in the history of parasitology.

△○ 1838: *von Liebig, Justus. Foundation of biochemistry.*

The idea that vital activity could be explained by chemicophysical factors was an important concept for biological investigators studying the nature of life.

△ 1838-1839: *Schleiden, M.J., and T. Schwann. Formulation of the cell theory.*

The cell doctrine, with its basic idea that

all plants and animals were made up of similar units, represents one of the truly great landmarks in biological progress. Many biologists believe the work of Schleiden and Schwann has been rated much higher than it deserves in the light of what others had done to develop the cell concept. R. Dutrochet (1824) and H. von Mohl (1831) described all tissues as being composed of cells.

△ **1838:** *Mulder, G.J. Concept of the nature of proteins.*

Mulder proposed the name "protéine," later "protein," for the basic constituents of protoplasmic materials.

△ **1839-1846:** *Purkinje, J.E., and Hugo von Mohl. Concept of protoplasm established.*

Purkinje proposed the name "protoplasm" for living matter, and von Mohl did extensive work on its nature, but it remained for Max Schultze (1861) to give a clear-cut concept of the relations of protoplasm to cells and its essential unity in all organisms.

□ **1839:** *Verhulst, P.F. Logistical theory of population growth.*

According to this theory, animal populations have a slow initial growth rate that gradually speeds up until it reaches a maximum and then slows down to a state of equilibrium. By plotting the logarithm of the total number of individuals against time, an **S**-shaped curve results that is somewhat similar for all populations.

□○ **1840:** *von Liebig, J., and F.F. Blackman. The law of minimum requirements.*

Von Liebig interpreted plant growth as being dependent on essential requirements that are present in minimum quantity; some substances, even in minute quantities, were needed for normal growth. Later Blackman discovered that the rate of photosynthesis is restricted by the factor that operates at a limiting intensity (for example, light or temperature). The concept has been modified in various ways since it was formulated. We now know that a factor interaction other than the minimum ones plays a part.

○ **1840:** *Müller, J. Theory of specific nerve energies.*

This theory states that the kind of sensation experienced depends on the nature of the sense organ with which the stimulated nerve is connected. The optic nerve, for instance, conveys the impression of vision however it is stimulated.

○ **1842:** *Bowman, William. Histological structure of the nephron (kidney unit).*

Bowman's accurate description of the nephron afforded physiologists an opportunity to attack the problem of how the kidney separates waste from the blood, a problem not yet fully solved.

✳ **1842:** *Steenstrup, Johann J.S. Alternation of generations described.*

Metagenesis, or alternation of sexual and asexual reproduction in the life cycle, exists in many animals and plants. The concept had been introduced before this time by L.A. de Chamisso (1819).

✕ **1843:** *Owen, Richard. Concepts of homology and analogy.*

Homology, as commonly understood, refers to similarity in embryonic origin and development, whereas analogy is the likeness between two organs in their functioning. Owen's concept of homology was merely that of the same organ in different animals under all varieties of form and function.

○ **1844:** *Ludwig, C. Filtration theory of renal excretion.*

About the same time that Bowman described the malpighian corpuscle, Ludwig showed that the corpuscle functions as a passive filter and that the filtrate that passes through it from the blood carries into the urinary tubules the waste products that are concentrated by the resorption of water as the filtrate moves down the tubules. Other investigators, Cushny, Starling, and Richards, have confirmed and extended his observations.

○△ **1845:** *von Helmholtz, H., and J.R. von Mayer. The formulation of the law of conservation of energy.*

This landmark in human thinking showed that in any system, living or nonliving, the power to perform mechanical work always tends to decrease unless energy is added from without. Physiological investigation could now advance on the hypothesis that the living organism is an energy machine and obeys the laws of energetics.

‡ **1848:** *Hofmeister, W. Discovery of chromosomes.*

This investigator made sketches of bodies, later known to be chromosomes, in the nuclei of pollen mother cells (*Tradescantia*). Schneider further described these elements in 1873, and Waldeyer named them in 1888.

□ **1848:** *von Siebold, Carl T.E. Establishment of the status of protozoa.*

Von Siebold emphasized the unicellular nature of protozoa, fitted them into the recently developed cell theory, and established them as the basic phylum of the animal kingdom.

○ **1851:** *Bernard, Claude. Discovery of the vasomotor system.*

Bernard showed how the amount of blood distributed to the various tissues by the small arterioles was regulated by vasomotor nerves of the sympathetic nervous system, as he demonstrated in the ear of a white rabbit.

✳ **1851:** *Waller, A.V. Importance of the nucleus in regeneration.*

When nerve fibers are cut, the parts of the fibers peripheral to the cut degenerate in a characteristic fashion. This wallerian degeneration enables one to trace the course of fibers through the nervous system. In the regeneration process the nerve cell body (with its nucleus) is necessary for the downgrowth of the fiber from the proximal segment.

○ **1852:** *von Helmholtz, Herman. Determination of rate of nervous impulse.*

This landmark in nerve physiology showed that the difficult phenomena of nervous activity could be expressed numerically.

○△ **1852:** *von Kölliker, Albrecht. Establishment of histology as a science.*

Many histological structures were described with marvelous insight by this great investigator, starting with the publication of the first text in histology (*Handbuch der Gewebelehre*).

○ **1852:** *Stannius, H.F. Stannius's experiment on the heart.*

By tying a ligature as a constriction between the sinus venosus and the atrium in the frog and also one around the atrioventricular groove, Stannius was able to demonstrate that the muscle tissues of the atria and ventricles have independent and spontaneous rhythms. His observations also indicated that the sinus is the pacemaker of the heartbeat.

†□ **1852:** *Küchenmeister, G.F.H. Relationship of "bladder worms" to adult tapeworms.*

This was the first demonstration that "bladder worms" (cysticerci) were the juveniles of taeniid tapeworms. It was followed rapidly by numerous other lifecycle studies of cestodes.

✳ **1854:** *Newport, G. Discovery of the entrance of spermatozoon into a frog's egg.*

This was a significant step in cellular embryology, although its real meaning was not revealed until the concept of fertilization as the union of two pronuclei was formulated about 20 years later (Hertwig, 1875).

†○ **1855:** *Addison, T. Discovery of adrenal disease.*

The importance of the adrenals in maintaining normal body functions was shown when Addison described a syndrome of general disorders associated with the pathology of this gland.

✕ **1856:** *Discovery of Neanderthal fossil hominid (Homo sapiens).*

Many specimens of this type of fossil hominid have been discovered (Europe, Asia, Africa) since the first one was found near Düsseldorf, Germany. Their culture was Mousterian (100,000 to 40,000 years BP), and although they were of short stature, their cranial capacity was as large as or larger than that of modern humans.

○ 1857: *Bernard, Claude. Discovery of formation of glycogen by the liver.*

Bernard's demonstration that the liver forms glycogen from substances brought to it by the blood showed that the body can build up complex substances as well as tear them down.

□ 1858: *Sclater, P.L. Distribution of animals on basis of zoological regions.*

This was the first serious attempt to study the geographical distribution of organisms, a study that eventually led to the present science of zoogeography. A.R. Wallace worked along similar lines.

✱△ 1858: *Virchow, Rudolf. Aphorism of Virchow: Omnis cellula e cellula (every cell from a cell).*

△ 1858: *Virchow, Rudolf. Formulation of the concept of disease from the viewpoint of cell structure.*

He laid the basis of modern pathology by stressing the role of the cell in diseased tissue.

✕ 1859: *Darwin, Charles. The concept of natural selection as a factor in evolution.*

Although Darwin did not originate the concept of organic evolution, no one has been more influential in the development of evolutionary thought. The publication of *The Origin of Species* represents the greatest single landmark in the history of biology.

○ 1860: *Bernard, Claude. Concept of the constancy of the internal environment (homeostasis).*

Bernard's realization that there are mechanisms in living organisms that tend to maintain internal conditions within relatively narrow limits, despite external change, is one of the most valuable generalizations in physiology.

✱ 1860: *Pasteur, Louis. Aphorism of Pasteur: Omne vivum e vivo (every living thing from the living).*

✱ 1860: *Pasteur, Louis. Refutation of spontaneous generation.*

Pasteur's experiment with the open S-shaped flask proved conclusively that fermentation or putrefaction resulted from microbes, thus ending the long-standing controversy regarding spontaneous generation.

□ 1860: *Wallace, A.R. The Wallace line of faunal delimitation.*

As originally proposed by Wallace, there was a sharp boundary between the Australian and Oriental faunal regions so that a geographical line drawn between certain islands of the Malay Archipelago, through the Makassar Strait between Borneo and Celebes, and between the Philippines and the Sanghir Islands separated two distinct and contrasting zoological regions. On one side Australian forms predominated; on the other, Oriental ones. The validity of this division has been questioned by zoogeographers in the light of more extensive knowledge of the faunas of the two regions.

△ 1861: *Graham, Thomas. Colloidal states of matter.*

This work on colloidal solutions has resulted in one of the most fruitful concepts regarding protoplasmic systems.

□ 1862: *Bates, H.W. Concept of mimicry.*

Mimicry refers to the advantageous resemblance of one species to another for protection against predators. It involves palatable or edible species that imitate dangerous or inedible species that enjoy immunity because of warning coloration against potential enemies.

□ 1864: *Haeckel, Ernst. Modern zoological classification.*

The broad features of zoological classification as we know it today were outlined by Haeckel and others, especially R.R. Lankester, in the third quarter of the nineteenth century. B. Hatschek is another zoologist who deserves much credit for the modern scheme, which is constantly undergoing revision. Other schemes of classification in the early nineteenth century did much to resolve the difficult problem of classification, such as those of Cuvier, de Lamarck, Leuckart, Ehrenberg, Vogt, Gegenbauer, and Schimkevitch.

△ 1864: *Schultze, Max. Protoplasmic bridges between cells.*

The connection of one cell to another by means of protoplasmic bridges has been demonstrated in both plants and animals. Modern techniques, including electron microscopy, have shown that many cells communicate by gap junctions, which have channels capable of passing molecules of up to 1000 daltons in molecular weight.

‡ 1866: *Haeckel, Ernst. Nuclear control of inheritance.*

At the time the hypothesis was formed, the view that the nucleus transmitted the inheritance of an animal had no evidence to substantiate it.

□ 1866: *Kovalevski, A. Taxonomic position of tunicates.*

The great Russian embryologist showed in the early stages of development the similarity between amphioxus and the tunicates and how the latter could be considered a branch of the phylum Chordata.

‡ 1866: *Mendel, Gregor. Formulation of the first two laws of heredity.*

These first clear-cut statements of inheritance made possible an analysis of hereditary patterns with mathematical precision. Rediscovered in 1900, his paper confirmed the experimental data geneticists had found at that time. Since that time Mendelian genetics has been considered the chief cornerstone of hereditary investigation.

○ 1866: *Schultze, Max. Histological analysis of the retina.*

Schultze's fundamental discovery that the retina contained two types of visual cells—rods and cones—helped to explain the differences in physiological vision of high and low intensities of light.

✕✱ 1867: *Kovalevski, A. Germ layers of invertebrates.*

The concept of the primary germ layers laid down by Pander and von Baer was extended to invertebrates by this investigator. He found that the same three germ layers arose in the same fashion as those in vertebrates. Thus, an important embryological unity was established for the animal kingdom.

○ 1869: *Langerhans, P. Discovery of islet cells in pancreas.*

These islets were first found in the rabbit, and since their discovery they have been one of the most investigated tissues in animals. The hypothesis that they have come from the transformation of pancreatic acinus cells has now given way to the belief that they originated from the embryonic tubules of the pancreatic duct.

△ 1869: *Miescher, F. Isolation of nucleoprotein.*

From pus cells, a pathological product, Miescher was able to demonstrate in the nuclei certain phosphorus-rich substances, nucleic acids, which are bound to proteins to form nucleoproteins. In recent years these complex molecules have been the focal point of significant biochemical investigations on the chemical properties of genes, with the wider implications of a better understanding of growth, heredity, and evolution.

1871: *Quetelet, Lambert A. Foundations of biometry.*

The applications of statistics to biological problems is called biometry. By working out the distribution curve of the height of soldiers, Quetelet showed biologists how the systematic study of the relationships of numerical data could become a powerful tool for analyzing data in evolution, genetics, and other biological fields.

□ 1872-1876: Challenger *expedition.*

Not only did this expedition establish the science of oceanography, but a vast amount of material was collected that greatly extended the knowledge of the variety and range of animal life.

□ 1872: *Dohrn, Anton. Establishment of Naples Biological Station.*

The establishment of this famous station marked the first of the great biological stations, and it rapidly attained international importance as a center of biological investigation.

○ 1872: *Ludwig, C., and E.F.W. Pflüger. Gas exchange of the blood.*

By means of the mercurial blood pump, these investigators separated the gases from the blood and thereby threw much light on the nature of gas exchange and the place where oxidation occurs (in the tissues).

×☐ *1874: Haeckel, Ernst H. Taxonomic position of phylum Chordata.*

The great German evolutionist based many of his conclusions on the work of the Russian embryologist Kovalevski, who in 1866 showed that the tunicates as well as amphioxus had vertebrate affinities.

× *1874: Haeckel, Ernst H. Gastrea hypothesis of metazoan ancestry.*

According to this hypothesis, the hypothetical ancestor of all the Metazoa consisted of two layers (ectoderm and endoderm) similar to the gastrula stage in embryonic development, and the endoderm arose as an invagination of the blastula. Thus, the diploblastic stage of ontogeny was to be considered as the repetition of this ancestral form. This concept in modified form has had wide acceptance.

‡✲ *1875: Hertwig, Oskar. Concept of fertilization as the conjugation of two sex cells.*

The fusion of the pronuclei of the two gametes in the process of fertilization paved the way for the concept that the nuclei contained the hereditary factors and that both maternal and paternal factors are brought together in the zygote.

△ *1875: Strasburger, Eduard. Description of "indirect" (mitotic) cell division.*

The accurate description of the processes of cell division that Strasburger made in plants represents a great pioneer work in the rapid development of cytology during the last quarter of the nineteenth century.

△ *1876: Pasteur, Louis. The Pasteur effect.*

In his studies of fermentation processes in wine making, Pasteur discovered that cells consumed much more glucose and produced much more lactic acid in the absence of oxygen than in its presence. It is now known that the effect occurs in many different kinds of cells and is a consequence of the lower energy yield of glycolysis compared with oxidative phosphorylation.

○ *1877: Pfeffer, Wilhelm. Concept of osmosis and osmotic pressure.*

Pfeffer's experiments on osmotic pressure and the determination of the pressure in different concentrations laid the foundation for an understanding of a general phenomenon in all organisms.

○ *1878: Balfour, Francis M. Relationship of the adrenal medulla to the sympathetic nervous system.*

By showing that the adrenal medulla has the same origin as the sympathetic nervous system, Balfour really laid the foundation for the interesting concept of the similarity in the action of epinephrine and sympathetic nervous mediation.

○△ *1878: Kühne, Willy. Nature of enzymes.*

The study of the action of chemical catalysts has steadily increased with biological advancement and now represents one of the most fundamental aspects of biochemistry.

△ *1879: Flemming, Walther. Chromatin described and named.*

Flemming shares with a few others (especially Strasburger, 1875) the description of the details of mitotic cell division. The part of the nucleus that stains deeply he called **chromatin** (colored), which gives rise to the chromosomes.

✲ *1879: Fol, Hermann. Penetration of ovum by a spermatozoon described.*

Fol was the first to describe a thin cone-like body extending outward from the egg to meet the sperm. Compare Dan's acrosome reaction (1954).

△ *1879: Kossel, Albrecht. Isolation of nucleoprotein.*

Nucleoproteins were isolated in the heads of fish sperm; they make up the major part of chromatin. They are combinations of proteins with nucleic acids, and this study was one of the first of the investigations of a topic that interests biochemists at the present time.

Nobel Laureate (1910).

† *1880: Laveran, C.L.A. Protozoa as pathogenic agents.*

This French investigator first demonstrated that the causative organism for malaria is a protozoan. This discovery led to other investigations that revealed the role the protozoa play in causing diseases such as sleeping sickness and kala-azar. It remained for Sir Ronald Ross to discover the role of mosquitoes in spreading malaria.

Nobel Laureate (1907).

○ *1880: Ringer, S. Influence of blood ions on heart contraction.*

The pioneer work of this investigator determined the inorganic ions necessary for contraction of frog hearts and made possible an evaluation of heart metabolism and the replacement of body fluids.

△ *1882: Flemming, Walther. First accurate counts of nuclear filaments (chromosomes) made.*

△ *1882: Flemming, W. Mitosis and spireme named.*

†△ *1882: Metchnikoff, Élie. Role of phagocytosis in immunity.*

The theory that microbes are ingested and destroyed by certain white corpuscles (phagocytes) shares with the theory of chemical bodies (antibodies) the chief explanation for the body's natural immu-

nity. Metchnikoff first studied phagocytosis in the cells of starfish and water fleas (*Daphnia*).

Nobel Laureate (1908).

△ *1882: Strasburger, Eduard. Cytoplasm and nucleoplasm named.*

☐ *1882-1924: The Albatross of the Fish Commission.*

The *Albatross*, under the direction of the U.S. Fish Commission, was second only to the famed *Challenger* in advancing scientific knowledge about oceanography.

○△ *1883: Golgi, Camillo, and R. Cajal. Silver nitrate technique for nervous elements.*

The development and refinement of this technique gave a completely new picture of the intricate relationships of neurons. Modifications of this method have given valuable information concerning the cellular element—the Golgi apparatus.

Nobel Laureates (1906).

✲ *1883: Hertwig, Oskar. Origin of term "mesenchyme."*

This important tissue may arise embryonically from all three germ layers but arises chiefly from the mesoderm. It is a protoplasmic network whose meshes are filled with a fluid intercellular substance. Mesenchyme gives rise to a great variety of tissues, and both its cells and intercellular substance may be variously modified; its most common derivative is connective tissue.

†☐ *1883: Leuckart, Rudolph, and A.P. Thomas. Life history of sheep liver flukes.*

This discovery represents the first time a complete life cycle was worked out for a digenetic trematode. Working independently, these investigators found that the trematode used a snail intermediate host.

‡ *1883: Roux, Wilhelm. Allocation of hereditary functions to chromosomes.*

This hypothesis could not have been much more than a guess when Roux made it, but how fruitful was the idea in the light of the enormous amount of evidence since accumulated!

△ *1884: Flemming, W., E. Strasburger, and E. van Beneden. Demonstration that nuclear filaments (chromosomes) double in number by longitudinal division.*

This concept represented a further step in understanding the precise process in indirect cell division.

○ *1884: Rubner, Max. Quantitative determinations of the energy value of foods.*

Although Liebig and others had estimated calorie values of foods, the investigations of Rubner put their determinations on a sound basis. His work made possible a scientific explanation for metabolism and a basis for the study of comparative nutrition.

‡ **1885:** *Hertwig, Oskar, and E. Strasburger. Concept of the nucleus as the basis of heredity.*

The development of this idea occurred before Mendel's laws of heredity were rediscovered in 1900, but it anticipated the important role the nucleus with its chromosomes was to assume in hereditary transmission.

‡ **1885:** *Rabl, Karl. Concept of the individuality of the chromosomes.*

The view that the chromosomes retain their individuality through all stages of the cell cycle is accepted by all cytologists, and much evidence has accumulated in support of the hypothesis. However, it has been virtually impossible to demonstrate the chromosome's individuality through all stages.

✳ **1885:** *Roux, Wilhelm. Mosaic theory of development.*

In the early development of the frog's egg, Roux showed that the determinants for differentiation were segregated in the early cleavage stages and that each cell or groups of cells would form only certain parts of the developing embryo (mosaic or determinate development). Later, other investigators showed that in many forms blastomeres, separated early, would give rise to whole embryos (indeterminate development).

✳‡ **1885:** *Weismann, August. Formulation of germ plasm theory.*

Weismann's great theory of the germ plasm stresses the idea that there are two types of protoplasm—germ plasm, which gives rise to the reproductive cells or gametes, and somatoplasm, which furnishes all the other cells. Germ plasm, according to the theory, is continuous from generation to generation, whereas the somatoplasm dies with each generation and does not influence the germ plasm.

1886: *Establishment of Woods Hole Biological Station in Massachusetts.*

This station is by all odds the greatest center of its kind in the world. Many of the biologists in America have studied there, and the station has increasingly attracted investigators from many other countries as well. The influence ot Woods Hole on the progress of biology cannot be overestimated.

△ **1887:** *Fischer, Emil. Structural patterns of proteins.*

The importance of proteins in biological systems has made their study the central theme of much modern biochemical work.

Nobel Laureate (1902).

✳ **1887:** *Haeckel, Ernst H. Concept of organic form and symmetry.*

Symmetry refers to the spatial relations and arrangements of parts in such a way as to form geometrical designs. Although many others before Haeckel's time had studied and described types of animal form, Haeckel gave us our present concepts of organic symmetry, as revealed in his monograph on radiolarians collected on the *Challenger* expedition.

‡ **1889:** *Hertwig, R., and E. Maupas. True nature of conjugation in paramecium.*

The process of conjugation was described (even by van Leeuwenhoek) many times and its sexual significance interpreted, but these two investigators independently showed the details of the divisions before conjugation and the mutual exchange of the micronuclei during the process.

†○ **1889:** *von Mering, J., and O. Minkowski. Effect of pancreatectomy.*

The classic experiment of removing the pancreas stimulated research that led to the isolation of the pancreatic hormone insulin by Banting (1922).

† **1890:** *Smith, Theobald. Role of an arthropod in disease transmission.*

The transmission of the sporozoan *Babesia*, which is the active agent in causing Texas cattle fever, by the tick *Boophilus*, represented the first demonstration of the role of an arthropod as a vector of disease.

✳ **1891:** *Driesch, Hans. Discovery of totipotent cleavage.*

The discovery that each of the first several blastomeres, if separated from each other in the early cleavage of the sea urchin embryo, would develop into a complete embryo stimulated investigation on totipotent and other types of development.

× **1890-1891:** *Dubois, Eugene. Discovery of the fossil human* Pithecanthropus erectus *(now* Homo erectus*).*

Although not the first fossil human to be found, the Java man represents one of the first significant primitive humans that have been discovered.

× **1893:** *Dollo, I. Concept of the irreversibility of evolution.*

In general, the overall evolutionary process is one-way and irreversible insofar as a whole complex genetic system is concerned, although back mutations and restricted variations may occur over and over.

○ **1893:** *His, Wilhelm. Anatomy and physiology of the atrioventricular node and bundle.*

The specialized conducting tissue of the heart has given rise to many investigations, not the least of which were those of His, whose name was given to the intricate system of branches that are reflected over the inner surface of the ventricles.

✳ **1894:** *Driesch, Hans. Constancy of nuclear potentiality.*

Driesch's view was that all nuclei of an organism were equipotential but that the activity of nuclei varied as tissues differentiated. More recent studies have emphasized the crucial importance of the cytoplasm of the embryo in determining expression of the nuclear genome.

□ **1894:** *Merriam, C.H. Concept of life zones in North America.*

This scheme is based on temperature criteria and the importance of temperature in the distribution of plants and animals. According to this concept, animals and plants are restricted in their northward distribution by the total quantity of heat during the season of growth and reproduction, and their southward distribution is restricted by the mean temperature during the hottest part of the year.

†□ **1895:** *Bruce, D. Life cycle of protozoan blood parasite* (Trypanosoma).

The relation of this parasite to the tsetse fly and to wild and domestic animal infection in Africa is an early demonstration of the role of arthropods as vectors of disease.

†○ **1895:** *Roentgen, W. Discovery of x-rays.*

This great discovery was quickly followed by its application in the interpretation of bodily structures and processes and represents one of the greatest tools in biological research.

Nobel Laureate (1901).

× **1896:** *Baldwin, J.M. Baldwin evolutionary effect.*

It is the belief that genetic selection of genotypes will be channeled or canalized in the same direction as the adaptive modifications that were formerly nonhereditary. It is now understood that the *capacity* to respond to environmental conditions is itself hereditary.

× **1896:** *Russian Hydrographic Survey. Biology of Lake Baikal.*

This lake in Siberia is more than 800 km long and 80 km wide and has an extreme depth of more than a mile (the deepest lake in the world). Its unique fauna is a striking example of evolutionary results from long-continued isolation. Up to 100% of the species in certain groups are endemic (found nowhere else). This remarkable fauna represents the survival of ancient freshwater animals that have become extinct in surrounding areas.

○ **1897:** *Abel, J.J., and A.C. Crawford. Isolation of the first hormone (epinephrine).*

The purification and isolation of one of the active principles of the suprarenal medulla led to discovery of its chemical nature and naming by J. Takamine (1901) and its synthesis by F. Stolz (1904).

△○ **1897:** *Buchner, E. Discovery of zymase.*

Buchner's discovery that an enzyme (a nonliving substance) manufactured by yeast cells was responsible for fermentation resolved many problems that had baffled Pasteur and other investigators. Zymase is now known to consist of a number of enzymes.

Nobel Laureate (1907).

× **1897:** *Canadian Geological Survey. Dinosaur fauna of Alberta, Canada.*

The discovery and exploration of the Upper Cretaceous fossil beds along the Red Deer River in Alberta revealed one of the richest dinosaur faunal finds known.

†○ **1897:** *Eijkman, Christian. Discovery of the cause of a dietary deficiency disease.*

Eijkman's pioneer work on the causes of beriberi led to the isolation of the antineuritic vitamin (thiamine). This work may be called the key discovery that resulted in the development of the important vitamin concept.

Nobel Laureate (1929).

†□ **1897:** *Ross, Ronald. Life history of malarial parasite* (Plasmodium).

This notable achievement represents a great landmark in the field of parasitology and the climax of the work of many investigators on the problem.

Nobel Laureate (1902).

△○ **1897:** *Sherrington, C.S. Concept of the synapse in the nervous system.*

If the nervous system is composed of discrete units, or neurons, functional connections must exist between these units. Sherrington showed how individual nerve cells could exert integrative influences on other nerve cells by graded excitatory or inhibitory synaptic actions. The electron microscope has in recent years added much to our knowledge of synaptic structure.

Nobel Laureate (1932).

△ **1898:** *Benda, C., and C. Golgi. Discovery of mitochondria and the Golgi apparatus.*

These interesting cytoplasmic inclusions were actually seen by various observers before this date, but they were both named in 1898, and the real study of them began at this time. W. Flemming and R. Altmann first demonstrated mitochondria. The Golgi apparatus was demonstrated by V. St. George (1867) and G. Platner (1855), but Camillo Golgi, with his silver nitrate impregnation method, gave the first clear description of the apparatus in nerve cells. Mitochondria are now known to play an important role in cell respiration and energy production.

× **1898:** *Osborn, Henry F. Concept of adaptive radiation in evolution.*

This concept states that, starting from a common ancestral type, many different forms of evolutionary adaptations may occur. In this way evolutionary divergence can take place, and the occupation of a variety of ecological niches is made possible, according to the adaptive nature of the invading species.

× **1900:** *Chamberlain, T.C. Hypothesis of the freshwater origin of vertebrates.*

The evidence for this hypothesis as first proposed was based mainly on the discovery of early vertebrate fossils in sediments thought to be of freshwater origin, such as Old Red Sandstone. The fossil evidence has been reevaluated by recent investigators, who interpret it to support a marine origin of the vertebrates.

‡ **1900:** *Correns, Karl E., Erick Tschermak von Seysenegg, and Hugo De Vries. Rediscovery of Mendel's laws of heredity.*

In their genetic experiments on plants these three investigators independently obtained results similar to Mendel's, and in their survey of the literature they found that Mendel had published his now-famous laws in 1866. A few years later, W. Bateson and others found that the same laws applied to animals.

× **1900:** *Andrews, C.F. Discovery of fossil beds in the Fayum Depression region of Egypt.*

Here Andrews and others discovered numerous Eocene and Oligocene fossils of protomonkeys believed to be ancestral to Old World monkeys and thus in the lineage leading to hominids.

†○ **1900:** *Landsteiner, Karl. Discovery of blood groups.*

This fundamental discovery made possible successful blood transfusions and initiated intense work on the biochemistry of blood.

Nobel Laureate (1930).

✳ **1900:** *Loeb, Jacques. Discovery of artificial parthenogenesis.*

The possibility of getting eggs that normally undergo fertilization to develop by chemical and mechanical methods has been accomplished in a number of different animals, from sea urchin and frog eggs (Loeb, 1900) to the rabbit egg (Pincus, 1936). The phenomenon has been a useful tool in studying the biology of fertilization.

‡ **1901:** *Montgomery, T.H. Homologous pairing of maternal and paternal chromosomes in the zygote.*

Montgomery showed that in synapsis before reduction division, each pair is made up of a maternal and a paternal chromosome. This phenomenon, verified a year later by W.S. Sutton, is of fundamental importance in the segregation of hereditary factors (genes).

×‡ **1901:** *De Vries, Hugo. Mutation theory of evolution.*

De Vries concluded from his study of the evening primrose *Oenothera lamarckiana* that new characters appear suddenly and are inheritable. Although the variations in *Oenothera* were probably not mutations at all, since many of them represented hybrid combinations, the evidence that mutations are the ultimate source of all new variation has steadily mounted.

‡ **1902:** *McClung, Clarence E. Discovery of sex chromosomes.*

The discovery in the grasshopper that a certain chromosome (X) had a synaptic mate (Y) different in appearance or else lacked a mate altogether gave rise to the theory that certain chromosomes determined sex. H. Henking actually discovered the X chromosome in 1891.

○ **1903:** *Bayliss, William M., and Ernest H. Starling. Action of the hormone secretin.*

The demonstration of the action of secretin, a hormone released from the mucosa of the stomach, marked the real birth of the science of endocrinology. It was the first unequivocal proof that physiological functions could be chemically integrated without participation of the nervous system.

‡ **1903:** *Boveri, Theodor, and W.S. Sutton. Parallelism between chromosome behavior and Mendelian segregation.*

This concept states that synaptic mates in meiosis correspond to the Mendelian alternative characters and that the formula of character inheritance of Mendel could be explained by the behavior of the chromosomes during maturation. This is therefore a cytological demonstration of Mendelian genetics.

‡ **1903:** *Sutton, W.S. Constitution of the diploid group of chromosomes.*

Sutton related Mendelian transmission of inherited characters to cytology by showing that the diploid group of chromosomes is made up of two chromosomes of each recognizable size, one member of which is paternal and the other maternal in origin.

○ **1904:** *Cannon, Walter B. Mechanics of digestion observed by means of x-ray films.*

The clever application of x-rays to a study of the movements and other aspects of the digestive system has revealed an enormous amount of information on the physiology of the alimentary canal. Cannon first used this technique in 1898.

○ **1904:** *Carlson, Anton J. Pacemaking activity of neurogenic hearts.*

Heartbeats may originate in muscle (myogenic hearts) or in ganglion cells (neurogenic hearts). Carlson showed that in the arthropod *Limulus* the pacemaker was located in certain ganglia on the dorsal surface of the heart and that experimental alterations of these ganglia by temperature or other means altered the heart rate. Neurogenic hearts are restricted to certain invertebrates.

□ **1904:** *Jennings, Herbert S. Behavior patterns in protozoa.*

The careful investigations of this lifelong student of the behavior of these lower organisms led to concepts such as the trial-and-error behavior and many of our important beliefs about the various forms of tropisms and taxes.

□ **1904:** *Nuttall, George H.F. Serological relationships of animals.*

This method of determining animal relationships is striking evidence of evolution. It has been used in recent years to help establish the taxonomic position of animals.

○ **1905:** *Haldane, John B.S., and John G. Priestley. Role of carbon dioxide in the regulation of breathing.*

By their clever technique of obtaining samples of air from the lung alveoli, these investigators showed how the constancy of carbon dioxide concentration in the alveoli and its relation to the concentration in the blood were the chief regulators of the mechanism of respiration.

‡ **1906:** *Bateson, William, and Reginald C. Punnett. Discovery of linkage of hereditary units.*

Although Bateson and Punnett first discovered linkage in sweet peas, it was Morgan and associates who correctly interpreted this great genetic concept. All seven pairs of Mendel's alternative characters were on separate chromosomes, which simplified the problem.

○ **1906:** *Einthoven, W. Mechanism of the electrocardiogram.*

The invention of the string galvanometer (1903) by Einthoven supplied a precise tool for measuring the bioelectrical activity of the heart and quickly led to the electrocardiogram, which gives accurate information about disturbances of the heart's rhythm.

Nobel Laureate (1924).

○ **1906:** *Hopkins, Frederick G. Analysis of dietary deficiency.*

Hopkins tried to explain dietary deficiency by a biochemical investigation of the lack of essential amino acids in the diet, an approach that has led to many important investigations in nutritional requirements.

Nobel Laureate (1929).

△ **1906:** *Tswett, M. Principle of chromatography.*

This is the separation of chemical components in a mixture by differential migration of materials according to structural

properties within a special porous sorptive medium. It was refined and became a widely used method 30 or 40 years later (Martin and Synge, 1941). The technique was first used by Tswett to separate pigments of plants.

† **1906-1913:** *Gorgas, William C. Control of malaria and yellow fever.*

By intelligent and industrious application of the knowledge that mosquitoes carry malaria and yellow fever, Gorgas saved 71,000 lives and made possible the construction of the Panama Canal.

✳ **1907:** *Boveri, Theodor. Qualitative differences of chromosomes.*

Boveri showed in his classic experiment with sea urchin eggs that chromosomes have qualitatively different effects on development. He found that only those cells that had one of each kind of chromosome developed into larvae; those cells that did not have representatives of each kind of chromosome failed to develop.

○△ **1907:** *Harrison, Ross. Tissue culture technique.*

The culturing of living tissues in vitro, that is, outside the body, has given biologists an important tool for studying tissue structure and growth. Harrison overcame great technical difficulties to successfully culture living tissues in suitable media.

✕ **1907:** *Discovery of the Heidelberg fossil human* (Homo heidelbergensis *now* H. erectus heidelbergensis).

This fossil consisted of a lower jaw with all its teeth. The jaw shows many simian characteristics, but the teeth show patterns of primitive humans. This type is supposed to have existed during mid-Pleistocene times and is more or less intermediate between Java man and modern humans.

○ **1907:** *Hopkins, Frederick G. Relationship of lactic acid to muscular contraction.*

Hopkins showed that, after being formed in muscular contraction, a part of the lactic acid is oxidized to furnish energy for the resynthesis of the remaining lactic acid into glycogen. This discovery did much to clarify part of the metabolic reactions involved in the complicated process of muscular contraction.

Nobel Laureate (1929).

✳ **1907:** *Wilson, H.V. Reorganization of sponge cells.*

In this classic experiment, Wilson showed that the disaggregation of sponges, by squeezing them through fine silk bolting cloth so that they are separated into minute cell clumps, resulted in the surviving cells coming together and organizing themselves into small sponges when they were in seawater.

‡ **1908:** *Garrod, A.E. Discovery that gene products are proteins.*

Certain hereditary disorders are caused by enzyme deficiencies wherein the mutations of a single gene may be responsible for controlling the specificity of a particular enzyme in certain disorders. Garrod's work was largely ignored until 1940.

✕‡ **1908:** *Hardy, Godfrey H., and W. Weinberg. Hardy-Weinberg population formula.*

This important theorem states that, in the absence of factors (such as mutation and selection) causing change in gene frequency, the frequency of a particular gene in any large population will reach an equilibrium in one generation and thereafter will remain stable regardless of whether the genes are dominant or recessive. Its mathematical expression forms the basis for the calculations of population genetics.

○△ **1909:** *Arrhenius, S., and S.P.L. Sörensen. Dissociation theory.*

The sensitivity of most biological systems to acid and alkaline conditions has made pH values of the utmost importance in biological research.

Arrhenius, Nobel Laureate (1903).

‡ **1909:** *Castle, William E., and J.C. Philips. The inviolability of germ cells to somatic cell influences.*

That germ cells are relatively free from somatic cell influences was shown by the substitution of a black guinea pig ovary in a white guinea pig, which gave rise to black offspring when mated with a black male.

✕ **1909:** *Johannsen, W.L. Limitations of natural selection on pure lines.*

This investigator found that when a hereditary group of characters becomes genetically homogeneous, natural selection cannot change the genetic constitution with regard to these characters. He showed that selection could not itself create new genotypes but was effective only in isolating genotypes already present in the group; it therefore could not effect evolutionary changes directly.

†□ **1909:** *Nicolle, Charles J.H. Body louse as vector of typhus fever.*

The demonstration that typhus fever was transmitted from patient to patient by the bite of the body louse paved the way for the control of this dreaded epidemic disorder by using DDT to delouse populations.

Nobel Laureate (1928).

○ **1910:** *Dale, Henry H. Nature of histamine.*

Dale and colleagues found that an extract from ergot had the properties of histamine (β-imidazolyl ethylamine), which can be produced synthetically by splitting off carbon dioxide from the amino acid histidine. It is also a constituent of all tissue cells, from which it may be released by injuries or other causes. The pronounced effect of histamine in dilating small blood vessels, contracting smooth muscle, and stimulating glands has caused it to be associated with many physiological phenomena, such as anaphylaxis, shock, and allergies.

Nobel Laureate (1936).

† 1910: *Ehrlich, Paul. Chemotherapy in the treatment of disease.*

The discovery of salvarsan as a cure for syphilis represents the first great discovery in this field. Another was the dye sulfanilamide, discovered by Domagk in 1935.

Nobel Laureate (1908).

□ 1910: *Heinroth, O. Concept of imprinting as a type of behavior.*

This is a special type of learning that is demonstrated by birds (and possibly other animals). It is based on the fact that in many species of birds the hatchlings are attracted to the first large object they see and thereafter will follow that object to the exclusion of all others.

‡ 1910: *Morgan, Thomas H. Discovery of sex linkage.*

Morgan and colleagues discovered that the results of a cross between a white-eyed male and a red-eyed female in *Drosophila* were different from those obtained from the reciprocal cross of a red-eyed male with a white-eyed female. This was a crucial experiment because it showed for the first time that how a trait behaved in heredity depended on the sex of the parent, in contrast to most Mendelian characters, which behave genetically the same way whether introduced by a male or female parent.

‡ 1910-1920: *Morgan, Thomas H. Establishment of the theory of the gene.*

The extensive work of Morgan and associates on the localization of hereditary factors (by genetic experiments) on the chromosomes of the fruit fly *(Drosophila)* represents some of the most significant work ever performed in the field of heredity.

Nobel Laureate (1933).

□ 1910: *Murray, J., and J. Hjort. Deep-sea expedition of the* Michael Sars.

Of the many expeditions for exploring the depths of the oceans, the *Michael Sars* expedition, made in the North Atlantic regions, must rank among the foremost. The expedition yielded an immense amount of information about deep-sea animals, as well as important data regarding the ecological pattern of animal distribution in the sea.

□ 1910: *Pavlov, Ivan P. Concept of the conditioned reflex.*

The idea that acquired reflexes play an important role in the nervous reaction patterns of animals has greatly influenced the development of modern psychology.

Nobel Laureate (1904).

✳ 1911: *Child, Charles M. Axial gradient hypothesis.*

This hypothesis attempts to explain the pattern of metabolism from the standpoint of localized regional differences along the axes of organisms. The differences in the metabolic rate of different areas have made possible an understanding of certain aspects of regeneration, development, and growth.

✕ 1911: *Cuénot, L. The preadaptation concept.*

Preadaptation refers to a morphological or physiological character that has been selected for (arisen) in one environment, but that is coincidentally adaptive in a new environment. This favorable conjunction of characters and suitable environment is considered to be an important factor in progressive evolution (opportunistic evolution).

† 1911: *Funk, Casimer. Vitamin hypothesis.*

Vitamin deficiency diseases are those in which effects can be definitely traced to the lack of some essential constituent of the diet. Thus, beriberi is caused by an insufficient amount of thiamine, scurvy by a lack of vitamin C, and so on.

✳ 1911: *Harvey, E.B. Cortical changes in the egg during fertilization.*

In the mature egg, cortical granules gather at the surface of the egg, but on activation of the egg these granules, beginning at the point of sperm contact, disappear in a wavelike manner around the egg. These granules are supposed to release material during their breakdown that helps form the ensuing fertilization membrane.

△ 1911: *Rutherford, Ernest. Concept of the atomic nucleus.*

This cornerstone of modern physics must be of equal interest to the biologist in the light of the rapid advances of molecular biology. Rutherford also discovered (1920) the proton, one of the charged particles in the atomic nucleus.

Nobel Laureate (1908).

✕ 1911: *Walcott, Charles D. Discovery of Burgess shale fossils.*

The discovery of a great assemblage of beautifully preserved invertebrates in the Burgess shale of British Columbia and their careful study by an American paleontologist represent a landmark in the fossil record of invertebrates. These fossils date from the middle Cambrian age and include the striking *Aysheaia*, which has a resemblance to the extant *Peripatus*.

○✳ 1912: *Gudernatsch, J.F. Role of the thyroid gland in the metamorphosis of frogs.*

This investigator found that the removal of the thyroid gland of tadpoles pre-

vented metamorphosis into frogs, and also that the feeding of thyroid extracts to tadpoles induced precocious metamorphosis. In 1919 W.W. Swingle showed that the presence and absence of inorganic iodine would produce the same results.

□ 1912: *Wegener, Alfred L. Concept of continental drift.*

This theory postulates that the continents were originally joined together in one or two large masses that gradually broke up during geological time, and the fragments drifted apart to form the current landmasses. The theory has been revived recently on the basis of surveys of paleomagnetism, seismographic studies, tectonic plate studies, and a wealth of biological evidence, for example, the finding of an amphibian fossil in Antarctic regions.

△ 1913: *Michaelis, L., and M. Menton. Enzyme-substrate complex.*

On theoretical and mathematical grounds these investigators showed that an enzyme forms an intermediate compound with its substrate (the enzyme-substrate complex) that subsequently decomposes to release the free enzyme and the reaction products. D. Keilin of Cambridge University and B. Chance of the University of Pennsylvania later demonstrated the presence of such a complex by color changes and measurements of its rate of formation and breakdown that agree with theoretical predictions.

✕ 1913: *Reck, H. Discovery of Olduvai Gorge fossil deposits.*

This region in East Africa has yielded an immense number of early mammalian fossils as well as the tools of Stone Age humans, such as stone axes. Among the interesting fossils discovered were elephants with lower jaw tusks, horses with three toes, the odd ungulate (chalicothere) with claws on the toes, and, more recently, several hominid fossils (see Leakey, Mary D., 1959).

□ 1913: *Shelford, Victor E. Law of ecological tolerance.*

This law states that the potential success of an organism in a specific environment depends on how it can adjust within the range of its toleration to the various factors to which the organism is exposed.

‡ 1913: *Sturtevant, A.H. Formation of first chromosome map.*

By the method of crossover percentages, it has been possible to locate the genes in their relative positions on chromosomes—one of the most fruitful discoveries in genetics, for it led to the extensive mapping of the chromosomes in *Drosophila*.

○ 1913: *Tashiro, Shiro. Metabolic activity of propagated nerve impulse.*

The detection of slight increases in carbon dioxide production in stimulated nerves, as compared with inactive ones, was evidence that conduction in nerves is a chemical change. Later (1926), A.V. Hill was able to measure the heat given off during the passage of an impulse. Increased oxygen consumption and other metabolic changes have also been measured in excited nerves.

○ **1914:** *Kendall, Edward C. Isolation of thyroxine.*

The isolation of thyroxine in crystalline form was a landmark in endocrinology. It was artificially synthesized by Harington in 1927.

✳ **1914:** *Lillie, Frank R. Role of fertilizin in fertilization.*

According to this theory, the jelly coat of eggs contains a substance, fertilizin, now known to be an acid mucopolysaccharide, which combines with the antifertilizin on the surface of sperm and causes the sperm to clump together.

‡ **1914:** *Shull, George H. Concept of heterosis.*

When two standardized strains or races are crossed, the resulting hybrid generation may be noticeably superior to both parents as shown by greater vigor, vitality, and resistance to unfavorable environmental conditions. First worked out in corn (maize), such hybrid vigor may also be manifested by other kinds of hybrids. Although its exact nature is still obscure, the phenomenon may be caused by the bringing together in the hybrid of many dominant genes of growth and vigor that were scattered among the two inbred parents, or it may be caused by the complementary reinforcing action of genes when brought together.

‡ **1916:** *Bridges, Calvin B. Discovery of nondisjunction.*

Bridges explained an aberrant genetic result by a suggested formula that later he was able to confirm by cytological examination. A pair of chromosomes failed to disjoin at the reduction division so that both chromosomes passed into the same cell. It was definite proof that genes are located on the chromosomes.

☐ **1917:** *Grinnell, Joseph. Concept of the ecological niche.*

The niche is the role of an animal in relation to all of the resources in its environment, both physical and biological. C. Elton has done much to develop the concept.

○ **1918:** *Krogh, August. Regulation of the motor mechanism of capillaries.*

The mechanism of the differential distribution of blood to the various tissues has posed many problems from the days of Harvey and Malpighi, but Krogh showed that capillaries were not merely passive in this distribution but that they had the power to contract or dilate actively, according to the needs of the tissues. Both nervous and chemical controls are involved.

Nobel Laureate (1920).

☐ **1918:** *Loeb, Jacques. Forced movements, tropisms, and animal conduct.*

Regarded as the founder of a mechanist "school," Loeb opposed the generally anthropomorphic and teleological interpretations of animal behavior. While Loeb carried his mechanistic doctrine to an extreme, he did inspire more rigorous, experimental approaches in animal behavior studies.

○ **1918:** *Starling, Ernest H. The law of the heart.*

Within physiological limits, the more the ventricles are filled with incoming blood, the greater is the force of their contraction at systolé. This is an adaptive mechanism for supplying more blood to tissues when it is needed. It is now recognized that only the hearts of lower vertebrates obey Starling's law; the intact heart of mammals is regulated principally by nervous and hormonal controls.

1919: *Aston, Francis W. Discovery of isotopes.*

Radioactive isotopes have proved of the utmost value in biological research because of the possibility of tracing the course of various elements in living organisms.

Nobel Laureate (1922).

△ **1920:** *Herzog, R.O., and W. Jancke. Development of x-ray diffractometry.*

When a parallel beam of x-rays is passed through crystallized biological material, the rays are spread and an image of the diffracted pattern is recorded (by rings, spots, and the like). By measurements and mathematical calculations information about structure can be obtained.

△ **1921:** *Hopkins, Frederick G. Isolation of glutathione.*

The discovery of this sulfur-containing compound gave a great impetus to the study of the complicated nature of cellular oxidation and metabolism.

Nobel Laureate (1929).

○ **1921:** *Langley, John N. Concept of the functional autonomic nervous system.*

Langley's concept of the functional aspects of the autonomic system dealt mainly with the mammalian type, but the fundamental principles of the system have been applied with modification to other groups as well. Two divisions—sympathetic and parasympathetic—are recognized in the functional interpretation of excitation and inhibition in the antagonistic nature of the two divisions.

○ **1921:** *Loewi, Otto, and H.H. Dale. Isolation of acetylcholine.*

This key demonstration led to the neurohumoral concept of the transmission of nerve impulses to muscles.

Nobel Laureates (1936).

○ **1921:** *Richards, A.N. Collection and analysis of glomerular filtrate of the kidney.*

This experiment was direct evidence of the role of the glomeruli as mechanical filters of cell-free and protein-free fluid from the blood and was striking confirmation of the Ludwig-Cushny theory of kidney excretion.

✳ **1921:** *Spemann, Hans. Organizer concept in embryology.*

Certain parts of the developing embryo known as organizers induce specific developmental patterns in responding tissue. While many aspects of induction remain obscure, Spemann's work was important in showing that development is a sequence of programmed stages and that each stage is necessary for the next.

Nobel Laureate (1935).

†○ **1921, 1922:** *Banting, Frederick, C.H. Best, and J.J.R. Macleod. Extraction of insulin.*

The great success of this hormone in relieving a distressful disease, diabetes mellitus, and the dramatic way in which active extracts were obtained have made the isolation of this hormone the best known in the field of endocrinology.

Banting and Macleod, Nobel Laureates (1923).

○ **1922:** *Erlanger, Joseph, and H.S. Gasser. Differential conduction of nerve impulses.*

By using the cathode-ray oscillograph, these investigators found that there were several different types of mammalian nerve fibers that could be distinguished structurally and that had different rates of conducting nervous impulses according to the thickness of the nerve sheaths (most rapid in the thicker ones).

Nobel Laureates (1944).

○ **1922:** *Kopeč, S. Concept of neurosecretory systems.*

This concept has emerged from the work of many investigators. R. Cajalin (1899) discovered that the nerve fibers to the neurohypophysis are extensions of the neurons of the hypothalamus. Kopeč found that the substance responsible for metamorphosis in the larva of moths originated in the brain where certain cerebral ganglia served as glands of internal secretion. Kopeč's pioneering studies were largely ignored by vertebrate endocrinologists until the 1950s, when through the studies of B. Scharrer, E. Sharrer, B. Hanström, G.W. Harris, and others it was recognized that vertebrates possess a neurosecretory system (hypothalamo-hypophyseal) analogous to invertebrate systems.

□ **1922:** *Schjelderup-Ebbe, T. Social dominance-subordinance hierarchies.*

This observer found certain types of social hierarchies among birds in which higher-ranking individuals could peck those of lower rank without being pecked in return. Those of the first rank dominated those of the second rank, who dominated those of the third, and so on. Such an organization, once formed, may be permanent.

□ **1922:** *Schmidt, Johann. Life history of the freshwater eel.*

The long, patient work of this oceanographer in solving the mystery of eel migration from the freshwater streams of Europe to their spawning grounds in the Sargasso Sea near Bermuda represents one of the most romantic achievements in natural history.

△ **1923:** *de Hevesy, George. First isotopic tracer method.*

Tracer methodology has proved especially useful in biochemistry and physiology. For instance, it has been possible by the use of these labeled units to determine the fate of the particular molecule in all steps of a metabolic process and the nature of many enzymatic reactions. The exact locations of many elements in the body have been traced by this method.

Nobel Laureate (1943).

△ **1923:** *Warburg, Otto. Manometric methods for studying metabolism of living cells.*

The Warburg apparatus has been useful in measuring gas exchange and other metabolic processes of living tissues. It proved of great value in the study of enzymatic reactions in living systems and was a standard tool in many biochemical laboratories for many years.

Nobel Laureate (1931).

○ **1924:** *Cleveland, L.R. Symbiotic relationships between termites and intestinal flagellates.*

This study was made on one of the most remarkable examples of mutualism known in the animal kingdom. Equally important were the observations this investigator and others made of the symbiosis between the wood-roach (*Cryptocercus*) and its intestinal protozoa.

○ **1924:** *Houssay, Bernardo A. Role of the pituitary gland in regulation of carbohydrate metabolism.*

This investigator showed that, when a dog had been made diabetic by pancreatectomy, the resulting hyperglycemia and glucosuria could be abolished by removing the anterior pituitary gland.

Nobel Laureate (1947).

✕ **1925:** *Dart, Raymond. Discovery of Australopithecus africanus.*

This important fossil, once referred to as the "missing link," bore many human characteristics but had a brain capacity only slightly greater than the higher apes. Most authorities place this hominid on or near the main branch of human ancestry.

△ **1925:** *Mast, S.O. Nature of ameboid movement.*

By studying the reversible sol-gel transformation in the protoplasm of an ameba, Mast not only gave a logical interpretation of ameboid movement but also initiated many fruitful concepts about the contractile nature of cytoplasmic gel systems, such as the furrowing movements (cytokinesis) in cell divisions.

†○ **1925:** *Minot, G.R., M.W.P. Murphy, and G.H. Whipple. Liver treatment of pernicious anemia.*

These investigators discovered that the feeding of raw liver had a pronounced effect in the treatment of pernicious anemia (a serious blood disorder). Much later investigation by numerous workers has led to some understanding of the antipernicious factor, vitamin B_{12}, whose chemical name is cyanocobalamin. This complex vitamin contains, among other components, porphyrin that has a cobalt atom instead of iron or magnesium at its center.

Nobel Laureates (1934).

□ **1925:** *Rowan, William. Photoperiodism hypothesis of bird migration.*

Rowan demonstrated that birds subjected to artificially increased day length in winter increased the size of their gonads and showed a striking tendency to migrate out of season. Other workers, stimulated by Rowan's experiments, showed that naturally increasing day length in spring acts through the brain neurosecretory system to set in motion the migratory disposition in birds.

△ **1926:** *Sumner, James B. Isolation of enzyme urease.*

The isolation of the first enzyme in crystalline form was a key discovery and was followed by others that have helped unravel the complex nature of these important biological substances.

Nobel Laureate (1946).

○ **1927:** *Bozler, E. Analysis of nerve net components.*

Bozler's demonstration that the nerve net of cnidarians was made up of separate cells and contained synaptic junctions resolved the old problem of whether or not the plexus in this group of animals was an actual network.

○ **1927:** *Eggleton, P., G.P. Eggleton, C.H. Fiske, and Y. Subbarow. Role of phosphagen (phosphocreatine) in muscular contraction.*

The demonstration that phosphagen is broken down during muscular contraction and then is resynthesized during recovery gave an entirely new concept of the initial energy necessary for the contraction process. Confirmation of this discovery received a great impetus from the discovery of E. Lungsgaard (1930) that muscles poisoned with monoiodoacetic acid, which inhibits the production of lactic acid from glycogen, would still contract and that the amount of phosphocreatine broken down was proportional to the energy liberated. It is now known that phosphocreatine is a high-energy phosphate storage compound, readily donating its phosphate group to ADP to form ATP.

○ **1927:** *Heymans, Corneille. Role of carotid and aortic reflexes in respiratory control.*

The carotid sinus and aortic areas contain pressoreceptors and chemoreceptors, the former responding to mechanical stimulation, such as blood pressure, and the latter to oxygen lack. When the pressoreceptors are stimulated, respiration is inhibited; when the chemoreceptors are stimulated, the respiratory rate is increased. (A much more potent stimulator of respiration, however, is the effect of carbon dioxide on the respiratory center of the brain.)

Nobel Laureate (1938).

‡ **1927:** *Muller, Hermann J. Artificial induction of mutations.*

By subjecting fruit flies (*Drosophila*) to mild doses of x-rays, Muller found that the rate of mutation could be increased 150 times over the normal rate.

Nobel Laureate (1946).

✕ **1927:** *Stensiö, E.A. Appraisal of the Cephalaspida (ostracoderm) fish fossil.*

The replacement of amphioxus as a prototype of vertebrate ancestry by the ammocoete lamprey larva, currently of great interest, has to a great extent been the result of this careful fossil reconstruction. It is generally believed that living Agnatha (lampreys and hagfishes) are descended from these ancient forms.

✕ **1928:** *Garstang, Walter. Theory of the ascidian ancestry of chordates.*

According to this theory, primitive chordates were sessile, filter-feeding marine organisms very similar to present-day ascidians. The actively swimming prevertebrate was considered a later stage in chordate evolution. The tadpole ascidian larva, with its basic organization of a vertebrate, had evolved within the group by progressive evolution and by neoteny became sexually mature, ceased to metamorphose into a sessile, mature ascidian, and became the true vertebrate.

‡△ **1928:** *Griffith, F. Discovery of the transforming principle (DNA) in bacteria (genetic transduction).*

By injecting living nonencapsulated

bacteria and dead encapsulated bacteria of the *Pneumococcus* strain into mice, it was found that the former acquired the ability to grow a capsule and that this ability was transmitted to succeeding generations. This active agent or transforming principle was isolated from the encapsulated type by other workers later and was found to consist of DNA.

F. Sanfelice (1893) had actually found the same principle when he discovered that nonpathogenic bacilli grown in a culture medium containing the metabolic products of true tetanus bacilli would also produce toxins and would do so for many generations.

△○ **1928:** *Weiland, H., and A. Windaus. Structure of the cholesterol molecule.*

Sterol chemistry has been a focal point in the investigation of such biological products as vitamins, sex hormones, and cortisone. Cholesterol is the precursor of bile acids and steroid hormones in animals.

Nobel Laureates (1927, 1928).

○ **1929:** *Berger, Hans. Demonstration of brain waves.*

The science of electroencephalography, or the electrical recording of brain activity, has revealed much about both the healthy and the diseased brain.

○ **1929:** *Butenandt, A., and E.A. Doisy. Isolation of estrone.*

This discovery was the first isolation of a sex hormone and was arrived at independently by these two investigators. Estrone was found to be the urinary and transformed product of estradiol, the actual hormone. The male hormone testosterone was synthesized by Butenandt and L. Ruzicka in 1931. The second female hormone, progesterone, was isolated from the corpora lutea of sow ovaries in 1934.

Doisy, Nobel Laureate (1943).

† **1929:** *Fleming, Alexander. Discovery of penicillin.*

The chance discovery of this drug from molds and its development by H. Florey a few years later gave us the first of a notable line of antibiotics that have revolutionized medicine.

Nobel Laureate (1945).

○ **1929:** *Heymans, Corneille. Discovery of the role of the carotid sinus and bodies in regulating the respiratory center and arterial blood pressure.*

Heymans found that the carotid sinus contains pressure-sensitive receptors (baroreceptors) that, acting through a nervous reflex to the medulla, help to keep the blood pressure stabilized. He also discovered oxygen-sensitive chemoreceptors in the carotid and aortic bodies. These are the origin of a reflex that responds to a

drop in blood oxygen tension by increasing respiratory rate and blood pressure.

Nobel Laureate (1938).

△ **1929:** *Lohmann, K., C. Fiske, and Y. Subbarow. Discovery of ATP.*

The discovery of ATP (adenosine triphosphate) was the culmination of a long search for the direct source of energy in biochemical reactions of many varieties, such as muscular contraction, vitamin action, and many enzymatic systems.

× **1930:** *Fisher, R.A. Statistical analysis of evolutionary variations.*

With Sewall Wright and J.B.S. Haldane, Fisher analyzed mathematically the interrelationships of the factors of mutation rates, population sizes, selection values, and others in the evolutionary process. Although many of their theories are in the empirical stage, evolutionists in general agree that they have great significance in evolutionary interpretation.

‡ **1931:** *Stern, C., H. Creighton, and B. McClintock. Cytological demonstration of crossing over.*

Proof that crossing over in genes is correlated with exchange of material by homologous chromosomes was independently obtained by Stern in *Drosophila* and by Creighton and McClintock in corn. By using crosses of strains that had homologous chromosomes distinguishable individually, they definitely demonstrated cytologically that genetic crossing over was accompanied by chromosomal exchange.

○□ **1932:** *Bethe, A. Concept of the ectohormone (pheromone).*

An organism secretes these substances to the outside of the body, where they affect the physiology or behavior of another individual of the same species. They have been demonstrated in insects, where they may function in trail making, sex attraction, development control, and the like.

× **1932:** *Danish scientific expedition. Discovery of fossil amphibians (ichthyostegids).*

These fossils were found in the upper Devonian sediments in eastern Greenland and appear to be intermediate between advanced crossopterygians *(Osteolepis)* and early amphibians. They are the oldest known forms that can be considered amphibians. Many of their characters show primitive amphibian conditions.

× **1932:** *Lewis, G. Edward. Discovery of* Ramapithecus *fossil.*

Ramapithecus brevirostris was a small humanlike ape of the Miocene and the earliest known hominid. Since Lewis's initial find in India, other fossil fragments of this genus have been discovered in East Africa, Greece, Turkey, and Hungary.

×‡ **1932:** *Wright, Sewall. Genetic drift as a factor in evolution.*

In small populations the Hardy-Weinberg formula of gene frequency may not apply because of "sampling error." If some genotypes are by chance underrepresented in matings in a small population, gene frequencies in the population may change.

○ **1933:** *Goldblatt, M., and U.S. von Euler. Discovery of prostaglandins.*

These fatty acid derivative compounds have been isolated from many mammalian tissues (such as seminal plasma, pancreas, seminal vesicle, brain, and kidney). They have a variety of hormonelike and pharmacological actions, such as stimulating smooth muscle contractions and relaxation, lowering blood pressure, and inhibiting enzymes and hormones.

× **1933, 1938:** *Haldane, John B.S., and A.I. Oparin. Heterotroph hypothesis of the origin of life.*

This hypothesis is based on the idea that life was generated from nonliving matter under the conditions that existed before the appearance of life and that have not been duplicated since. The hypothesis stresses the idea that living systems at present make it impossible for any incipient life to gain a foothold as primordial life was able to do.

‡ **1933:** *Painter, T.S., E. Heitz, and H. Bauer. Rediscovery of giant salivary chromosomes.*

These interesting chromosomes were first described by Balbiani in 1881, but their true significance was not realized until these investigators rediscovered them. It has been possible in a large measure to establish the chromosome theory of inheritance by comparing the actual cytological chromosome maps of salivary chromosomes with the linkage maps obtained by genetic experimentation.

○ **1933:** *Wald, George. Discovery of vitamin A in the retina.*

The discovery that vitamin A is a part of the visual purple molecule of the rods not only gave a better understanding of an important vitamin but also showed how night blindness can occur when there is a deficiency of this vitamin in the diet.

Nobel Laureate (1967).

○ **1934:** *Dam, Carl P.H., and E.A. Doisy. Identification of vitamin K.*

The isolation and synthesis of this vitamin are important not merely because of the vitamin's practical value in certain forms of hemorrhage but also because of the light they throw on the physiological mechanism of blood clotting.

Nobel Laureates (1943).

△ **1934-1935:** *Danielli, J.F., and H. Davson. Concept of the cell (plasma) membrane.*

Danielli proposed a hypothesis that cell membranes consist of two layers of lipid molecules surrounded on the inner and outer surfaces by a layer of protein molecules. The electron microscope reveals the plasma membrane of a thickness of 7.5 to 10 nm, consisting of two dark (protein) membranes (2.5 to 3 nm thick) separated by a light (lipid) interval membrane of 2.5 to 3 nm thickness. Recent studies confirm the Danielli-Davson model, while demonstrating a greater dynamic role for the peripheral proteins.

○ 1934: *Wigglesworth, V.B. Role of the corpus allatum gland in insect metamorphosis.*

This small gland lies close to the brain of an insect, and it has been shown that during the larval stage this gland secretes a juvenile hormone that causes the larval characters to be retained. Metamorphosis and maturation occur as the gland secretes less and less of the hormone. Removal of the gland causes the larva to undergo precocious metamorphosis; grafting the gland into a mature larva will cause the latter to grow into a giant larval form. The gland was first described by A. Nabert in 1913.

○ 1935: *Hanström, B. Discovery of the X-organ in crustaceans.*

This organ, together with the related sinus gland, constitutes an anatomical complex that has proved of great interest in understanding crustacean endocrinology. The neurosecretory cells in the X-organ (part of the brain) produce a molt-inhibiting hormone that is stored in the sinus gland of the eyestalk, while a molting hormone is produced in the Y-organ. The interrelations of these two hormones control the molting process.

○1935-1936: *Kendall, Edward C., and P.S. Hench. Discovery of cortisone.*

Kendall had first isolated this substance, which he called compound E, from the adrenal glands. Its final stages were prepared by Hench later and involved a long tedious chemical process. A hormone that controls the synthesis and release of cortisone and similar steroids was isolated in 1943 from the pituitary and was called adrenocorticotropic hormone (ACTH).

Nobel Laureates (1950).

△ 1935: *Stanley, Wendell M. Isolation of a virus in crystalline form.*

This achievement of isolating a virus (tobacco mosaic) is noteworthy not only in giving information about these small agencies responsible for many diseases but also in affording much speculation on the differences between the living and the nonliving.

Nobel Laureate (1946).

○ 1936: *Young, J.Z. Demonstration of giant fibers in squid.*

These giant fibers are formed by the fusion of the axons of many neurons whose cell bodies are found in a ganglion near the head. Each fiber is really a tube, up to 1 mm in diameter, consisting of an external sheath filled with liquid axoplasm. Because of their size, they have been a very valuable system in neurophysiology.

△ 1937: *Findlay, G.W.M., and F.O. MacCullum. Discovery of interferon.*

These protein substances, produced by cells in response to viruses and other foreign substances, selectively inhibit virus replication and are one of the body's important defenses against viral infection. They also may play a role in regulation of the immune response.

△ 1937: *Krebs, Hans A. Citric acid (tricarboxylic acid) cycle.*

In a brilliant example of reasoning and deduction, Krebs showed the existence of a cycle of reactions central to aerobic energy production. In the cycle, two carbon fragments from carbohydrate, fatty acids, or amino acids are oxidized to carbon dioxide. The electrons derived from the oxidation reactions in the cycle are passed through a further series of reactions (electron transport system), in which energy is captured in ATP, and finally to oxygen as the final electron acceptor to produce water.

Nobel Laureate (1953).

× 1937: *Sonneborn, T.M. Discovery of mating types in paramecium.*

Sonneborn's discovery that only individuals of complementary physiological classes (mating types) would conjugate opened up a new era of protozoan investigation that promises to shed new light on the problems of species concept and evolution.

△○ 1937: *König, P., and A. Tiselius. Development of electrophoresis.*

Electrophoresis is an extremely valuable method of separating proteins in a solution and, after numerous refinements, is currently in wide use. It depends on the differential migration of proteins on an inert carrier when an electrical field is applied.

□ 1938: *Remane, A. Discovery of the new phylum Gnathostomulida.*

This marine phylum was first described by P. Ax in 1956. The members of the phylum are small wormlike forms (about 0.5 mm long) and show great diversity among the different species. One of their major characteristics is their complicated jaws provided with teeth. They live in sandy substrata and are worldwide in distribution.

○ 1938: *Schoenheimer, R. Use of radioactive isotopes to demonstrate synthesis of bodily constituents.*

By labeling amino acids, fats, carbohydrates, and the like with radioactive isotopes, it was possible to show how these were incorporated into the various constituents of the body. Such experiments demonstrated that parts of the cell were constantly being synthesized and broken down and that the body must be considered a dynamic equilibrium.

□ 1938: *Skinner, B.F. Measurement of motivation in animal behavior.*

Skinner worked out a technique for measuring the rewarding effect of a stimulus, or the effects of learning on voluntary behavior. His experimental animals (rats) were placed in a special box (Skinner's box) containing a lever that the animal could manipulate. When the rat pressed the lever, small pellets of food would or would not be released, according to the experimental conditions.

○△ 1938: *Svedberg, Theodor. Development of ultracentrifuge.*

In biological and medical investigation this instrument has been widely used for the purification of substances, the determination of particle sizes in colloidal systems, the relative densities of materials in living cells, the production of abnormal development, and the study of many problems concerned with electrolytes.

Nobel Laureate (1926).

○ 1939: *Brown, Frank A., Jr., and O. Cunningham. Demonstration of molt-inhibiting hormone in eyestalk of crustaceans.*

Although C. Zeleny (1905) and others had shown that eyestalk removal shortened the intermolt period in crustaceans, Brown and Cunningham were the first to present evidence to explain the effect as being caused by a molt-inhibiting hormone present in the sinus gland.

× 1939: *Discovery of coelacanth fishes.*

The collection of a living specimen of this ancient fish (*Latimeria*), followed later by other specimens, has brought about a complete reappraisal of this "living fossil" with reference to its ancestry of the amphibians and land forms.

✻ 1939: *Hörstadius, S. Analysis of the basic pattern of regulative and mosaic eggs in development.*

The masterful work of this investigator has done much to resolve the differences in the early development of regulative eggs (in which each of the early blastomeres can give rise to a whole embryo) and mosaic eggs (in which isolated blastomeres produce only fragments of an embryo). Regulative eggs were shown to have two kinds of substances, both of which were necessary in proper ratios to produce normal embryos. Each of the early blastomeres has this proper ratio and thus can develop into a complete embryo; in mosaic eggs the regulative power is restricted to a much earlier time scale in development (before cleavage), and thus each isolated blastomere will give rise only to a fragment.

×□ **1939:** *Huxley, Julian. Concept of the cline in evolutionary variation.*

This concept refers to the gradual and continuous variation in character over an extensive area because of adjustments to changing conditions. This idea of character gradients has proved a very fruitful one in the analysis of the mechanism of evolutionary processes, for such a variability helps to explain the initial stages in the transformation of species.

†‡ **1940:** *Landsteiner, Karl, and A.S. Wiener. Discovery of Rh blood factor.*

Not only was a knowledge of the Rh factor of importance in solving a fatal disease of infancy, but it has also yielded a great deal of information about relationships between human races.

Landsteiner, Nobel Laureate (1930).

△‡ **1941:** *Beadle, George W., and E.L. Tatum. Biochemical mutation.*

By subjecting the bread mold *Neurospora* to x-ray irradiation, they found that genes responsible for the synthesis of certain vitamins and amino acids were inactivated (mutated) so that a strain of this mold carrying the mutant genes could no longer grow unless these particular vitamins and amino acids were added to the medium on which the mold was growing. This discovery—that alterations in various genes resulted in loss of a corresponding biosynthetic enzyme—first revealed the precise way in which genes and enzymes are related.

Nobel Laureates (1958).

○ **1941:** *Cori, Carl F., and Gerty T. Cori. Lactic acid metabolic cycle.*

The regeneration of muscle glycogen reserves in mammals involves the passage of lactic acid from the muscles through the blood to the liver, the conversion of lactic acid there to glycogen, the production of blood glucose from the liver glycogen, and the synthesis of muscle glycogen from the blood glucose.

Nobel Laureates (1947).

△○ **1941:** *Martin, A.J.P., and R.L.M. Synge. Development of partition chromatography.*

This is a powerful method for separation of chemically similar substances in mixtures. It depends on differential solubility of a compound in stationary and moving phases of solvents. Variants of the method include column, paper, and thin-layer chromatography.

○ **1941:** *Szent-Györgyi, Albert. Role of ATP in muscular contraction.*

The demonstration showing that muscles get their energy for contraction from ATP (adenosine triphosphate) has done

much to explain many aspects of the puzzling problem of muscle physiology.

Nobel Laureate (1937).

✳ **1942:** *McClean, D., and I.M. Rowlands. Discovery of the enzyme hyaluronidase in mammalian sperm.*

This enzyme dissolves the cement substance of the follicle cells that surround the mammalian egg and facilitates the passage of the sperm to the egg. This discovery not only aided in resolving some of the difficult problems of the fertilization process but also offers a logical explanation of cases of infertility in which too few sperm may not carry enough of the enzyme to afford a passage through the inhibiting follicle cells.

△ **1943:** *Claude, A. Isolation of cell constituents.*

By differential centrifugation, Claude found it possible to separate, in relatively pure form, particulate components, such as mitochondria, microsomes, and nuclei. These investigations led immediately to a more precise knowledge of the chemical nature of these cell constituents and aided the elucidation of the structure and physiology of the mitochondria—one of the great triumphs in the biochemistry of the cell.

Nobel Laureate (1974).

✳ **1943:** *Holtfreter, J. Tissue synthesis from dissociated cells.*

By dissociating the cells of embryonic tissues of amphibians (by dissolving with enzymes or other agents the intercellular cement that holds the cells together) and heaping them in a mass, he found that the cells in time coalesced and formed the type of tissue from which they had come. This is an application to vertebrates of Wilson's discovery with sponge cells. It showed that, by some mechanism, cells could recognize other cells of the same type.

‡ **1943:** *Sonneborn, T.M. Extranuclear inheritance.*

The view that in paramecia cytoplasmic determiners (plasmagenes) that are self-reproducing and capable of mutation can produce genetic variability has thrown additional light on the role of the cytoplasm in hereditary patterns.

△‡ **1944:** *Avery, O.T.C., C.M. MacLeod, and M. McCarty. Agent responsible for bacterial transformation.*

These workers were able to show that the bacterial transformation of nonencapsulated bacteria to encapsulated cells was really attributable to the DNA fraction of debris from disrupted encapsulated cells to which the nonencapsulated cells were exposed. This key demonstration showed for the first time that nucleic acids and not proteins were the basic material of heredity, and initiated the study of molecular genetics. However, the profound significance of Avery's conclusions was only gradually recognized.

△ **1945:** *Cori, Carl F. Hormone influence on enzyme activity.*

The delicate balance that insulin and the diabetogenic hormone of the pituitary exercise over the activity of the enzyme hexokinase in carbohydrate metabolism has opened up a whole new field of the regulative action of hormones on enzymes.

Nobel Laureate (1947).

□ **1945:** *Griffin, D., and R. Galambos. Development of the concept of echolocation.*

Echolocation refers to a type of perception of objects at a distance by which echoes of sound are reflected back from obstacles and detected acoustically. These investigators found that bats generated their own ultrasonic sounds that were reflected back to their own ears so that they were able to avoid obstacles in their flight without the aid of vision. Their work climaxed an interesting series of experiments inaugurated as early as 1793 by Spallanzani, who believed that bats avoided obstacles in the dark by reflection of sound waves to their ears. Others who laid the groundwork for the novel concept were C. Jurine (1794), who proved that ears were the all-important organs in perception; H.S. Maxim (1912), who advanced the idea that the bat made use of low-frequency sounds inaudible to human ears; and H. Hartridge (1920), who proposed the hypothesis that bats emitted sounds of high frequencies and short wavelengths (ultrasonic sounds).

△ **1945:** *Lipmann, Fritz A., and Hans Krebs. Discovery of coenzyme A.*

The discovery of this important coenzyme made possible a better understanding of the breaking down of fatty acid chains and furnished important further knowledge of the reactions in the tricarboxylic acid cycle.

Nobel Laureate (1953).

△ **1945:** *Porter, Keith R. Description of the endoplasmic reticulum.*

The endoplasmic reticulum is a very complex cytoplasmic structure consisting of a lacelike network of irregular anastomosing tubules and vesicular expansions within the cytoplasmic matrix. Associated with the reticulum complex are small, dense granules of ribonucleoprotein and other granules known as microsomes that are fragments of the endoplasmic reticulum. The reticulum complex plays an important role in the synthesis of proteins.

‡ **1946:** *Lederberg, J., and E.L. Tatum. Sexual recombination in bacteria.*

These investigators found that two different strains of bacteria (*Escherichia coli*) could undergo conjugation and exchange genetic material, thereby producing a hereditary strain with characteristics of the two parent strains. W. Hayes (1952) found that recombination still occurred after one parent strain was killed.

Nobel Laureates (1958).

× 1946: *Libby, Willard F. Radiocarbon dating of fossils.*

The radiocarbon age determination is based on the fact that carbon 14 in the dead organism disintegrates at the rate of one half in 5560 years, one half of the remainder in the next 5560 years, and so on. This is based on the assumption that the isotope is mixed equally through all living matter and that the cosmic rays (which form the isotopes) have not varied much in periods of many thousands of years. The limitation of the method is around 40,000 years.

Nobel Laureate (1960).

× 1946: *White, E.I. Discovery of the primitive chordate fossil* Jamoytius.

The discovery of this fossil in the freshwater deposits of Silurian rock in Scotland throws some light on the early ancestry of vertebrates, for this form seems to be intermediate between amphioxus or ammocoete larva (of lampreys) and the oldest known vertebrates, the ostracoderms. Morphologically, *Jamoytius* represents the most primitive vertebrate yet discovered. It could well serve as an ancestor of such forms as amphioxus and the jawless ostracoderms.

○ 1947: *Holtz, P. Discovery of norepinephrine (noradrenaline).*

This hormone (vasoconstriction effects) has since been found in most vertebrates and shares with epinephrine (metabolic effects) the functions of the chromaffin part of the adrenal gland.

× 1947: *Sprigg, R.C. Discovery of Precambrian fossil bed.*

The discovery of a rich deposit of Precambrian fossils in the Ediacara Hills of South Australia has been of particular interest because the scarcity of such fossils in the past has given rise to vague and uncertain explanations about Precambrian life. It was all the more remarkable that the fossils discovered were those of soft-bodied forms, such as jellyfish, soft corals, and segmented worms, including the amazing *Spriggina*, which shows relationship to the trilobites. The fossils are prearthropod but not preannelid.

△ 1947: *Szent-Györgyi, Albert. Concept of the contractile substance actomyosin.*

This protein complex consists of the two components, actin and myosin, and is considered the source of muscular contraction when triggered by ATP. Neither actin nor myosin will contract singly.

Nobel Laureate (1937).

□ 1948: *von Frisch, Karl. Communication mechanisms of honeybees.*

After many years of patient work, von Frisch deciphered the meaning of bee "dances," behavior patterns of individual bees returning to the hive. The dances communicate information to the other bees regarding location of food and water, location and suitability of sites for a new hive, and other information.

Nobel Laureate (1973).

□ 1948: *Hess, Walter R. Localization of instinctive impulse patterns in the brain.*

By inserting electrodes through the skull, fixing them in position, and allowing such holders to heal in place, it was possible to study the brain of an animal in its ordinary activities. When the rat could automatically and at will stimulate itself by pressing a lever, it did so frequently when the electrode was inserted in the hypothalamus region of the brain, indicating a pleasure center. In this way, by placing electrodes at different centers, rats can be made to gratify such drives as thirst, sex, and hunger.

Nobel Laureate (1949).

△ 1948: *Hogeboom, G.H., W.C. Schneider, and G.E. Palade. Separation of mitochondria from the cell.*

This was an important discovery in unraveling the amazing enzymatic activity of the mitochondria in the tricarboxylic acid cycle. The role mitochondria play in the energy transfer of the cell has earned for these rod-shaped bodies the appellation "powerhouse" of the cell.

Palade, Nobel Laureate (1974).

△ 1949: *de Duve, C. Discovery of the lysosome organelle.*

These small particles were first identified chemically, and later (1955) morphologically with the electron microscope. They contain the enzymes for digestion of materials taken into the cell by pinocytosis and phagocytosis and for the digestion of the cell's own cytoplasm. When the cell dies, their enzymes are also released and digest the cell (autolysis).

Nobel Laureate (1974).

† 1949: *Enders, J.F., F.C. Robbins, and T.H. Weller. Cell culture of animal viruses.*

These investigators found that poliomyelitis virus could be grown in ordinary tissue cultures of nonnervous tissue instead of being restricted to host systems of laboratory animals or embryonated chick eggs.

Nobel Laureates (1954).

○ 1949: *von Euler, U.S. Role of norepinephrine as transmitter.*

Von Euler isolated and identified norepinephrine as the neurotransmitter in the sympathetic nervous system (1940). Later

he isolated and characterized norepinephrine storage granules in nerves and described how the substance was taken up, stored, and released by them.

Nobel Laureate (1970).

‡ 1949: *Pauling, Linus. Genic control of protein structure.*

Pauling and his colleagues demonstrated a direct connection between specific chemical differences in protein molecules and alterations in genotypes. Making use of the hemoglobin of patients with sickle cell anemia (which is caused by a homozygous condition of an abnormal gene), Pauling was able by the method of electrophoresis to show a considerable difference in the behavior of this hemoglobin in an electric field compared with that from a heterozygote or from a normal person.

Nobel Laureate (1954).

○ 1949: *Selye, Hans. Concept of the stress syndrome.*

In 1937 Selye began his experiments, which led to what he called the "general adaptation syndrome." This involved the chain reactions of many hormones, such as cortisone and ACTH, in meeting stress conditions faced by an organism. Whenever the stress experience exceeds the limitations of these body defenses, serious degenerative disorders may result.

△ 1950: *Caspersson, T., and J. Brachet. Biosynthesis of proteins.*

Investigations to solve the vital problem of protein synthesis from free amino acids have been under way since Emil Fischer's (1887) outstanding work on protein structure. Many competent research workers, such as Bergmann, Lipmann, and Schoenheimer, have made contributions to an understanding of protein synthesis, but Caspersson and Brachet were the first to point out the significant role of ribonucleic acid (RNA) in the process—and most biochemical investigations of the problem since that time have been directed along this line.

△ 1950: *Chargaff, Erwin. Base composition of DNA.*

The discovery that the amount of purines was equal to the amount of pyrimidines in DNA, the amount of adenine was equal to that of thymine, and the amount of cytosine was equal to that of guanine paved the way for the DNA model of Watson and Crick. The two major functions of DNA are replication and hereditary information storage.

□ 1950: *Lorenz, Konrad. Development of ethology.*

Lorenz is regarded as the founder of ethology, a biological approach to analyzing behavior, emphasizing a comparative method and stressing innate factors in behavior development. His classic studies on the greylag goose first came to the attention of English-speaking scientists during the 1950s, though the work itself commenced in the 1930s.

Nobel Laureate (1973).

□ *1950: von Frisch, Karl. Discovery of polarized light perception by honeybees.*

Honeybees are able to detect, and navigate to, polarized sunlight reaching the earth's surface, using specialized retinular cells in a specific but small area of the compound eyes. Subsequently it has been found that some crustaceans, cephalopod molluscs, and teleost fishes, as well as many other terrestrial arthropods, can orient by polarized light.

✳ *1952: Briggs, Robert, and Thomas J. King. Demonstration of possible differentiated nuclear genotypes.*

The belief that all cells of a particular organism have the same genetic endowment has been questioned as the result of the work of these investigators, who transplanted nuclei of different ages and sources from blastulas and early gastrulas into enucleated zygotes and observed variable and abnormal development.

□ *1952: Kramer, G. Orientation of birds to positional changes of sun.*

Kramer showed that birds (starlings and pigeons) can be trained to find food in accordance with the position of the sun. He found that the general orientation of the birds shifted at a rate (when exposed to a constant artificial sun) that could be predicted on the basis of the birds' correcting for the normal rotation of the earth. Birds were able to orient themselves in a definite direction with references to the sun, whether the light of the sun reached them directly or was reflected by mirrors. They were capable also of finding food at any time of day, indicating an ability to compensate for the sun's motion across the sky.

△ *1952: Palade, G.E. Analysis of the finer structure of the mitochondrion.*

The important role of mitochondria in the enzymatic systems and cellular metabolism has focused much investigation on the structure of these cytoplasmic inclusions. Each mitochondrion is bounded by two membranes; the outer is smooth and the inner is thrown into small folds or cristae that project into a homogeneous matrix in the interior. Some modifications of this pattern are found.

Nobel Laureate (1974).

△ *1952: Zinder, N., and J. Lederberg. Discovery of the transduction principle.*

Transduction is the transfer of DNA from one bacterial cell to another by means of a phage. It occurs when an infective phage picks up from its disintegrated host a small fragment of the host's DNA and carries it to a new host where it becomes a part of the genetic equipment of the new bacterial cell.

Lederberg, Nobel Laureate (1958).

‡△ *1953: Crick, Francis H.C., James D. Watson, and Maurice H.F. Wilkins. Chemical structure of DNA.*

Based on knowledge of the chemical nature of DNA and studies of x-ray diffraction by Wilkins, Crick and Watson formulated the hypothesis that the DNA molecule was made up of two chains twisted around each other in a helical structure with pairs of nitrogenous bases projecting toward each other—adenine opposite thymine and guanine opposite cytosine. Genes are considered to be segments of these molecules, with the sequence of bases coding for the amino acids in a protein. Each of the complementary strands acts as a model or template to form a new strand before cell division. The hypothesis has been widely accepted and is now amply confirmed.

Nobel Laureates (1962).

△ *1953: Palade, G.E. Description of cytoplasmic ribosomes.*

The description of ribonucleic acid–rich granules (usually on the endoplasmic reticulum) represents one of the key links in the unraveling of the mechanism of protein synthesis. The ribosomes (about 250 Å in diameter) serve as the site of protein synthesis; the number of ribosomes (polysomes) involved in the synthesis of a protein depends on the length of messenger RNA and the protein being synthesized.

Nobel Laureate (1974).

✕ *1953: Urey, Harold, and Stanley Miller. Demonstration of the possible primordia of life.*

By exposing a mixture of water vapor, ammonia, methane, and hydrogen gas to electrical discharge (to simulate lightning) for several days, these investigators found that several complex organic substances, such as the amino acids glycine and alanine, were formed when the water vapor was condensed into water. This demonstration offered a very plausible theory to explain how the early beginnings of life substances could have started by the formation of organic substances from inorganic ones.

O† *1953: Sperry, R.W. Independence of brain hemispheric function.*

By severing the bundle of nerve fibers separating the two cortical hemispheres, Sperry developed the "split-brain" technique, which he used to show that the two brain halves govern two sets of activities. He also contributed much to developmental neurobiology.

Nobel Laureate (1981).

△ *1954: Del Castillo, J., and B. Katz. Impulse transmission at nerve junction.*

These researchers demonstrated that the chemical transmitter substance is released from the presynaptic terminal in discrete multimolecular packets, or quanta, each containing several thousand molecules.

Katz, Nobel Laureate (1970).

✳ *1954: Dan, J.C. Acrosome reaction.*

In echinoderms, annelids, and molluscs Dan showed that the acrosome region of the spermatozoon forms a filament and releases an unknown substance at the time of fertilization. Evidence suggests that the filament is associated with the formation of the fertilization cone. Other observers had described similar filaments before Dan made his detailed descriptions. The filament (1 to 75 μm long) may play an important role in the entrance of the sperm into the cytoplasm.

O *1954: Du Vigneaud, V. Synthesis of pituitary hormones.*

This investigator isolated the posterior pituitary hormones oxytocin and vasopressin. Both were found to be polypeptides of amino acids, and oxytocin was the first polypeptide hormone to be produced artificially. Oxytocin contracts the uterus during childbirth and releases the mother's milk; vasopressin raises blood pressure and decreases urine production.

O *1954: Huxley, H.E., A.F. Huxley, and J. Hanson. Theory of muscular contraction.*

By means of electron microscopic studies and x-ray diffraction studies, these investigators showed that the proteins actin and myosin were found as separate filaments that apparently produced contraction by a sliding reaction in the presence of ATP. The concept has been widely accepted.

A.F. Huxley, Nobel Laureate (1963).

△ *1954: Sanger, Frederick. Structure of the insulin molecule.*

Insulin is the important hormone used in the treatment of diabetes. It was the first protein for which a complete amino acid sequence was known. The molecule was found to be made up of 17 different amino acids in 51 amino acid units. Although one of the smallest proteins, its formula contains 777 atoms.

Nobel Laureate (1958).

△ *1955-1957: Kornberg, Arthur, and S. Ochoa. Synthesis of nucleic acids outside of cells (in vitro).*

By mixing the enzyme polymerase, extracted from the bacterium *Escherichia coli*, with a mixture of nucleotides and a tiny amount of DNA, Kornberg was able to produce synthetic DNA. Ochoa obtained the synthesis of RNA in a similar manner by using the enzyme polynucleotide phosphorylase from the bacterium *Azotobacter vinelandii*. This significant work reveals more insight into the mechanism of nucleic acid duplication in the cell.

Nobel Laureates (1959).

× **1955:** *Kettlewell, H.B.D. Natural selection in action: industrial melanism in moths.*

Using field techniques, Kettlewell was able to demonstrate a selective advantage of dark (melanic) mutants in a barklike cryptic moth species in industrial areas of Great Britain, where the tree trunks had been darkened by soot. This demonstration provided an evolutionary explanation for the increasing incidence of melanism in cryptic moths that has been noted throughout the industrialized regions of the world and constitutes a classic example of the effects of a strong selective pressure.

○ **1956:** *von Békésy, Georg. The traveling wave theory of hearing.*

Helmholtz (1868) had proposed the resonance theory of hearing on the basis that each cross fiber of the basilar membrane, which increases in width from the base to the apex of the cochlea, resonates at a different frequency; von Békésy showed that a traveling wave of vibration is set up in the basilar membrane and reaches a maximal vibration in the part of the membrane appropriate for that frequency.

Nobel Laureate (1961).

△ **1956:** *Borsook, H., and P.C. Zamecnik. Site of protein synthesis.*

By injecting radioactive amino acids into an animal, they found that the ribosome of the endoplasmic reticulum is the place where proteins are formed.

‡ **1956:** *Ingram, V.M. Nature of a mutation.*

By tracing the change in one amino acid unit out of more than 300 units that make up the protein hemoglobin, Ingram was able to pinpoint the difference between normal hemoglobin and the mutant form of hemoglobin that causes sickle cell anemia.

△ **1956:** *Sutherland, Earl W., and T.W. Rall. Discovery of cyclic AMP.*

An intracellular mediating agent (cyclic adenosine-3′,5′-monophosphate, or cyclic AMP) is found in all living animal tissues, and changes in cyclic AMP levels (by effects of hormones) cause the hormones to produce different target effects depending on the type of cell in which they are found. Cyclic AMP is formed by a metabolic reaction in which the enzyme adenyl cyclase converts ATP to cyclic AMP.

Sutherland, Nobel Laureate (1971).

‡ **1956:** *Tjio, J.H., and A. Levan. Revision of human chromosome count.*

The time-honored number of chromosomes in humans, 48 (diploid), was found by careful cytological technique to be 46 instead.

‡△ **1957:** *Benzer, S. Concept of the cistron.*

The newer view of the gene has greatly changed the classic concept of the gene as an entity that controlled mutation, hereditary recombination, and function. There are actually several subunits, of which the cistron, the unit of function, is the largest. Many units of recombination may be found in a single cistron. The mutation unit (muton) is variable but usually consists of two to five nucleotides.

△ **1957:** *Calvin, Melvin. Chemical pathways in photosynthesis.*

By using radioactive carbon 14, Calvin and colleagues were able to analyze step by step the incorporation of carbon dioxide and the identity of each intermediate product involved in the formation of carbohydrates and proteins by plants.

Nobel Laureate (1961).

△ **1957:** *Holley, Robert W. The role of transfer RNA in protein synthesis.*

Nucleotides of transfer RNAs differ from each other only in their bases. Holley also devised methods that precisely established the transfer RNAs used in the transfer of certain amino acids to the site of protein synthesis.

Nobel Laureate (1968).

□ **1957:** *Ivanov, A.V. Analysis of phylum Pogonophora (beard worms).*

Specimens of this phylum were collected in 1900 and represent one of the most recent phyla to be discovered and evaluated in the animal kingdom. Collections have been made in the waters of Indonesia, the Okhotsk Sea, the Bering Sea, and the Pacific Ocean. They are found mostly in the abyssal depths. Thought originally to belong to the Deuterostomia division, more recent evidence indicates that they are protostomes. At present 80 species divided into two orders have been described.

△ **1957:** *Perutz, Max F., and J.C. Kendrew. Structure of hemoglobin.*

The mapping of a complex globular protein molecule of 600 amino acids and 10,000 atoms arranged in a three-dimensional pattern represented one of the great triumphs in biochemistry. Myoglobin of muscle, which acts as a storehouse for oxygen and contains only one heme group instead of four (hemoglobin), was found to contain 150 amino acids.

Nobel Laureates (1962).

□ **1957:** *Sauer, E. Celestial navigation by birds.*

By subjecting Old World warblers to various synthetic night skies of star settings in a planetarium, Sauer was able to demonstrate that the birds made use of the stars to guide them in their migrations.

○ **1958:** *Lerner, A.B. Discovery of melatonin in the pineal gland.*

Lerner and associates discovered that the production of melatonin in the pineal gland is increased in darkness and decreased in the light. Activity of the hormone appears important in regulation of gonadal functions affected by photoperiod, and its discovery represented a breakthrough in understanding the function of the pineal gland.

△ **1958:** *Meselson, M., and F.W. Stahl. Confirmation "in vivo" of the duplicating mechanism in DNA.*

This was really confirmation of the self-copying of DNA in accordance with Watson and Crick's scheme of the structure of DNA. These investigators found that, after producing a culture of bacterial cells labeled with heavy nitrogen 15 and then transferring these bacteria to a cultural medium of light nitrogen 14, the resulting bacteria had a DNA density intermediate between heavy and light, as would be expected on the basis of the Watson-Crick hypothesis.

○ **1959:** *Burnet, Frank M. Clonal selection theory of immunity.*

One of the most puzzling aspects of the acquired immune response has been the specificity of the antigen-antibody reaction. Burnet suggested that we have a large variety of antibody-producing cells, each present in such a small number that its product cannot be detected. When exposed to a foreign substance (antigen), a clone of cells that can make antibody to that antigen is "selected" and multiplies rapidly, thus increasing antibody to a detectable level. A corollary to the theory is that antigens present when the organism is embryonic or very young are recognized as "self" and the immune system does not respond. This was confirmed by P. Medawar.

Burnet and Medawar, Nobel Laureates (1960).

‡ **1959:** *Ford, C.E., P.A. Jacobs, and J.H. Tjio. Chromosomal basis of sex determination in humans.*

By discovering that certain genetic defects were associated with an abnormal somatic chromosomal constitution, it was possible to determine that male-determining genes in humans were located on the Y chromosome. Thus, a combination of XXY (47 instead of the normal 46 diploid number) produced sterile males (Klinefelter's syndrome), and those with XO combinations (45 diploid number) gave rise to Turner's disease or immature females.

× **1959:** *Leakey, Mary D. Discovery of Australopithecus (Zinjanthropus) boisei fossil hominid.*

This fossil is a robust form within the small-brained, large-jawed genus *Australopithecus*, first discovered by Dart (1925). Its status is at present controversial: some believe it to be a species distinct from *A. africanus*, while others believe that *A. africanus* and *A. boisei* are females and males within a single, polytypic species.

○ **1959:** *Butenandt, A.F.J. Chemical identification of a pheromone.*

Butenandt and associates chemically analyzed the first pheromone—the sex attractant substance of silk moths *(Bombyx mori)*. Named bombykol, it is a doubly unsaturated fatty alcohol with 16 carbon atoms. The chemical nature of numerous other pheromones has since been determined.

△† **1950s-present:** *Bennacerraf, B., J. Dausset, and G. Snell. Genetics and function of the major histocompatibility complex (MHC).*

This complex of genes codes for cell surface antigens. These antigens are critically important in various interactions between cells, such as rejection of transplanted tissues and control of the immune response. Much work remains to be done before we completely understand the role of the MHC in immunity.

Nobel Laureates (1980).

○ **1959-1960:** *Yalow, Rosalyn, and S.A. Berson. Development of radioimmunoassay.*

The development of this technique made it possible for the first time to measure minute quantities of a hormone directly in a complex mixture of proteins such as serum. A radioactively labeled hormone is mixed with a specific antibody to the hormone, together with a sample of the unknown. The labeled compound competes with the unlabeled in the formation of the antigen-antibody complex, and the amount of unknown is obtained by comparison with a standard curve prepared with known amounts of unlabeled hormone. The technique was originally described for insulin, but it has been rapidly extended to many other hormones and has revolutionized endocrinology.

Yalow, Nobel Laureate (1977).

□ **1960:** *Tinbergen, Niko. Development of the concept of specific searching images in predators.*

Tinbergen's studies of songbird predation in Dutch pinewoods laid the foundation for the science of ethology.

Nobel Laureate (1973).

△ **1960:** *Hurwitz, J., A. Stevens, and S. Weiss. Enzymatic synthesis of messenger RNA.*

The exciting knowledge of the coding system of DNA and its translation to protein synthesis (ribosomes) was further elucidated when it was discovered that an enzyme, RNA polymerase, was responsible for the synthesis of RNA from a template pattern of DNA.

△ **1960:** *Jacob, François, and Jacques Monod. The operon hypothesis.*

The operon hypothesis is a postulated model of how enzyme synthesis is regulated in prokaryotes. The model proposes that refinement in regulation involves an inducible system for allowing structural genes to synthesize needed enzymes and a repressible system that cuts off the synthesis of unneeded enzymes.

Nobel Laureates (1965).

△ **1960:** *Strell, M., and R.B. Woodward. Synthesis of chlorophyll a.*

Strell and Woodward with the aid of many co-workers finally solved this problem, which had been the goal of organic chemists for generations.

Woodward, Nobel Laureate (1965).

△ **1961:** *Hurwitz, J., A. Stevens, and S.B. Weiss. Confirmation of messenger RNA.*

Messenger RNA transcribes directly the genetic message of the nuclear DNA and moves to the cytoplasm, where it becomes associated with a number of ribosomes or submicroscopic particles containing protein and nonspecific structural RNA. Here the messenger RNA molecules serve as templates against which amino acids are arranged in the sequence corresponding to the coded instructions carried by messenger RNA.

‡△ **1961:** *Jacob, François, and Jacques Monod. The role of messenger RNA in the genetic code.*

The transmission of information from the DNA code in the genes to the ribosomes represents an important step in the unraveling of the genetic code, and these investigators proposed certain deductions for confirmation of the hypothesis, which in general has been established by many researchers.

Nobel Laureates (1965).

○ **1961:** *Miller, J.F.A. Function of the thymus gland.*

Long known as a transitory organ that persists during the early growth period of animals, the thymus is now recognized as a vital processing center in the development of certain lymphocytes (T cells). These cells are very important in cell-mediated immunity.

‡△ **1961:** *Nirenberg, Marshall W., and J.H. Matthaei. Deciphering the genetic code.*

By adding a synthetic RNA composed entirely of uracil nucleotides to a mixture of amino acids, these investigators obtained a polypeptide made up solely of a single amino acid, phenylalanine. On the basis of a triplet code, it was concluded that the RNA code word for phenylalanine was UUU and its DNA complement was AAA. This was the beginning of decoding.

Nirenberg, Nobel Laureate (1968).

△ **1961:** *Mitchell, Peter. The chemiosmotic-coupling hypothesis of ATP formation.*

Although it is known that the oxidation of food molecules in the cell results in net synthesis of ATP from ADP and inorganic phosphate, the molecular mechanism to drive the reaction is still unclear. Current evidence supports the chemiosmotic hypothesis, which suggests that the energy derived from electron transport serves to pump hydrogen ions across the inner mitochondrial membrane, actively setting up an electrochemical gradient. The gradient of hydrogen ions is then coupled with an ATPase complex in the inner membrane, providing the free energy to form the high-energy phosphate bond.

○ **1962:** *Copp, Harold. Discovery of calcitonin.*

This peptide hormone is produced by the ultimobranchial glands (lower vertebrates) or their embryological derivatives, the parafollicular cells of the thyroid gland (mammals). It lowers the blood calcium and increases calcium uptake · by bone cells, thus antagonizing the action of parathormone.

△‡ **1962-1972:** *Arber, W., H.O. Smith, and D. Nathans. Discovery, isolation, and characterization of restriction endonucleases.*

Use of these bacterial enzymes has been essential in the recent explosion of knowledge in molecular genetics and recombinant DNA technology. Arber is given credit for predicting the existence of such enzymes, Smith for isolating the first restriction endonuclease and describing its reaction, and Nathans for applying the enzymes in studies of gene regulation and organization.

Nobel Laureates (1978).

× **1964:** *Hamilton, W.D. Concepts of kin selection and inclusive fitness.*

The problem of neuter castes in social insects had destroyed Lamarckian and baffled Darwinian evolutionary explanations. Hamilton, however, demonstrated that the peculiar mode of reproduction in most social insects having neuter castes (haplodiploidy, or males haploid and females diploid) resulted in a situation in which sisters would share more common genes with one another than with their own progeny. Hence, helping to rear "kin" (sisters) could be more adaptive from the point of view of one's genes (inclusive fitness) than rearing one's own young (individual fitness). These ideas have since been extended to social behaviors of many species—vertebrate as well as invertebrate—and provide a fundamental core of the emerging field of sociobiology.

× 1964: *Hoyer, B.H., B.J. McCarthy, and E.T. Bolton. Phylogeny and DNA sequence.*

These investigators presented evidence that certain homologies exist among the polynucleotide sequences in the DNA sequence of such different forms as fishes and humans. Such sequences may represent genes that have been retained with little change throughout vertebrate history. Possible phenotypic expressions may be bilateral symmetry, notochord, hemoglobin, and so on.

△‡ 1966: *Khorana, H.G. Proof of code assignments in the genetic code.*

By using alternating codons (CUC and UCU) in an artificial RNA chain, Khorana was able to synthesize a polypeptide of alternating amino acids (leucine and serine) for which these codons respectively stood.

Nobel Laureate (1968).

△ 1967: *Katz, Bernard, and R. Miledi. Calcium entry at nervous synapses.*

These investigators proposed that the arrival of an action potential at a presynaptic terminal causes calcium influx that facilitates binding of synaptic vesicles with the presynaptic membrane.

△‡ 1967: *Ptashne, M. Isolation of first repressor.*

Repressors are protein substances supposedly formed by regulatory genes and function by preventing a structural gene from making its product when not needed by the cells.

□ 1967: *MacArthur, Robert H., and E.O. Wilson. Theoretical ecology.*

Mathematical models in conjunction with field studies form the basis of theoretical ecology. This is well shown in the *Theory of Island Biogeography* by MacArthur and Wilson. By the methods found in their book and the investigations of many other researchers, it has been possible to determine the equilibrium of species, the number of extinctions, and other factors on islands. This viewpoint has been a revelation in ecological studies.

□ 1968: *Goodall, Jane. Behavior of free-living chimpanzees.*

A long-term, complete study of primate social behavior was done in the field, providing an impetus and stimulus for a large number of similar studies on other primates.

○ 1960s-1970s: *Hubel, D.H., and T.N. Wiesel. Understanding of stereoscopic vision.*

Analysis of processing of images in eyes and brain have opened a new field in vision physiology.

Nobel Laureates (1981).

△† 1960s-1970s: *Bergström, S., B. Samuelsson, and J. Vane. Characterization of prostaglandins.*

Prostaglandins are chemical transmitters of intracellular and intercellular signals. They are involved in a variety of physiological and pathological functions. Bergström is credited with isolating prostaglandins and determining their structures; Samuelsson determined their biosynthesis and metabolism; and Vane found that vascular endothelium produces a prostaglandin (prostacyclin) that inhibits platelet aggregation.

△ 1970: *Temin, H.M., and D. Baltimore. Demonstration of DNA synthesis from an RNA template.*

Many viruses carry RNA rather than DNA as a genetic material, and it was not known how the RNA virus could enter the host cell and induce the host to synthesize more RNA virus particles. Temin and Baltimore independently found an RNA-dependent DNA polymerase in RNA viruses; thus, the RNA virus reproduces by entering a host cell and producing a DNA copy from the RNA template; then the host cell machinery makes new virus particles from the DNA template.

Nobel Laureates (1975).

○△ 1970: *Edelman, Gerald M., and R.R. Porter. The structure of gamma globulin.*

By using myeloma tumors (which contain pure immunoglobulin proteins) the investigators were able to work out after many years a complete analysis of the large gamma globulin molecule, which is made up of 1320 amino acids and 19,996 atoms, with a molecular weight of 150,000.

Nobel Laureates (1972).

△○ 1971: *Cheung, W.Y. Discovery of calmodulin.*

The calcium-binding protein interacts reversibly with intracellular calcium to form a complex that regulates a broad spectrum of cellular activities.

△ 1971: *Berg, P., D. Jackson, and R. Symons. Recombinant DNA.*

A DNA molecule from both a bacterial virus and an animal tumor virus were opened with a restriction endonuclease, then spliced together. This was the first recombinant DNA from two different organisms.

Berg, Nobel Laureate (1980).

† 1971-1973: *Cormack, A.M., and G.N. Hounsfield. Invention of computer-assisted tomography (CAT scanner).*

This x-ray diagnostic technique produces clear images of internal body structures. A basic problem was how to obtain accurate measurements of the x-ray attenuation coefficient for all points in the x-ray section being examined. Cormack and Hounsfield each developed mathematical solutions to the problem.

Nobel Laureates (1979).

△ 1972: *Singer, S.J., and G.L. Nicolson. Fluid-mosaic model of biological membranes.*

The plasma membrane of cells contains a bimolecular leaflet of lipids with the surface interrupted by proteins. Some proteins, called extrinsic proteins, are attached to the lipid surface, whereas others, called intrinsic proteins, penetrate the bilayer and may completely span the membrane. This model remains the most widely accepted model of membrane structure.

× 1972: *Gould, Stephen J., and J. Eldridge. Concept of punctuated equilibrium.*

This hypothesis proposes that species remain virtually unchanged for long periods of time until a sudden spurt of rapid evolution produces a distinct species. Since the hypothesis is an alternative to more orthodox Darwinian gradualism, it has produced lively debate among evolutionists.

○ 1972: *Woodward, R.B., and A. Eschenmoser. The synthesis of vitamin B₁₂.*

Vitamin B_{12} is the last vitamin to be synthesized. This complex molecule is not made up of polymers; new methods of organic chemistry were required before it could be synthesized. It contains the metal ion cobalt.

□ 1973: *The Endangered Species Act.*

This omnibus legislation, created in 1966 and greatly strengthened in 1973, is the first United States domestic law concerned exclusively with wildlife and enacted for purely altruistic motives. Its strength resides in that portion of the act specifically prohibiting federally funded projects from jeopardizing endangered species or their habitats. Some 400 species of plants and animals have been placed on the endangered list.

△† 1975: *Milstein, Cesar, and G. Kohler. Hybridoma technique.*

Hybridomas are cells formed by hybridizing myeloma cells (from immune system tumors) with lymphocytes. Each hybridoma produces a clone of identical daughter cells, all manufacturing identical antibodies. Monoclonal antibodies are of great value in research, are useful diagnostic tools, and have great potential in disease therapy.

△ 1975: *Miller, J., and P. Lu. Alteration of amino acid sequence.*

By inserting known amino acids to replace naturally occurring amino acids in the lac repressor protein, these investigators have been able to determine which amino acids are necessary for the various functions of the lac repressor.

△ 1975: *Sanger, J.W. Chromosome migration on spindle fibers.*

The proteins (actin and myosin) that contract muscles were found to be involved in the migration of chromosomes along the spindle fibers. Actin bundles are present on chromosomal spindle fibers.

△ *1975-1977: Gilbert, W., A. Maxam, and F. Sanger. Methods for determining base sequence in DNA.*

Practical methods for determining the base sequence in DNA have great implications for molecular genetics and DNA technology.

Gilbert and Sanger, Nobel Laureates (1980).

† *1977: Eradication of smallpox.*

The global eradication of variola major, the virulent form of smallpox, was achieved by making preventive immunization available to underdeveloped areas through a World Health Organization campaign.

△ *1981: Complete sequencing of human mitochondrial DNA.*

This landmark research by a group at England's Medical Research Council revealed that the human mitochondrial genome contains 16,569 base pairs. Packed into the genome with remarkable economy are the genes for making two ribosomal RNAs, 22 transfer RNAs, and 13 assorted proteins.

BOOKS AND PUBLICATIONS THAT HAVE GREATLY INFLUENCED DEVELOPMENT OF ZOOLOGY

Aristotle. 336-323 BC. De anima, Historia animalium, De partibus animalium, *and* De generatione animalium. *These biological works of the Greek thinker have exerted an enormous influence on biological thinking for centuries.*

Vesalius, Andreas. 1543. De fabrica corporis humani. *This work is the foundation of modern anatomy and represents a break with the Galen tradition. His representations of some anatomical subjects, such as muscles, have never been surpassed. Moreover, he treated anatomy as a living whole, a viewpoint present-day anatomists are beginning to copy.*

Fabricius of Aquapendente. 1600-1621. De formato foetu *and* De formatione ovi pulli. *This was the first illustrated work on embryology and may be said to be the beginning of the modern study of development.*

Harvey, William. 1628. Essay on the motion of the heart and the blood. *This great work represents one of the first accurate explanations in physical terms of an important physiological process. It initiated an experimental method of observation that gave an impetus to research in all fields of biology.*

Descartes, René. 1637. Discourse on method. *This philosophical essay gave a great stimulus to a mechanistic interpretation of biological phenomena.*

Buffon, Georges. 1749-1804. Histoire naturelle. *This extensive work of many volumes collected together natural history facts in a popular and pleasing style. It had a great influence in stimulating a study of nature. Many eminent biological thinkers, such as Erasmus, Darwin, and Lamarck, were influenced by its generalizations, which here and there suggest an idea of evolution in a crude form.*

Linnaeus, Carolus. 1758. Systema naturae. *This work lays the basis for the classification of animals and plants.*

With few modifications, the taxonomic principles outlined therein have been universally adopted by biologists.

Wolff, Caspar Friedrich. 1759. Theoria generationis. *The theory of epigenesis was here set forth for the first time in opposition to the preformation theory of development so widely held before Wolff's work.*

von Haller, Albrecht. 1760. Elementa physiologiae. *An extensive summary of various aspects of physiology that greatly influenced physiological thinking for many years. Some of the basic concepts laid down therein are still considered valid, especially those on the nervous system.*

Malthus, Thomas R. 1798. Essay on population. *This work stimulated evolutionary thinking among such people as Darwin and Wallace.*

de Lamarck, Jean Baptiste. 1809. Philosophie zoologique. *This publication was of great importance in focusing the attention of biologists on the problem of the role of the environment as a factor in evolution. Lamarck's belief that all species came from other species represented one of the first clear-cut statements on the mutability of species, even though his theory of use and disuse has not been accepted by most biologists.*

Cuvier, Georges. 1817. Le règne animal. *A comprehensive biological work that dealt with classification and a comparative study of animal structures. Its plates are still of value, but the general plan of the work was marred by a disbelief in evolution and a faith in the doctrine of geological catastrophes. The book, however, exerted an enormous influence on contemporary zoological thought.*

von Baer, Karl Ernst. 1828-1837. Entwickelungsgeschichte der Thiere. *In this important work are laid down the fundamental principles of germ layer formation and the similarity of corresponding stages in the development of embryos that have proved to be the foundation studies of modern embryology.*

Audubon, John J. 1828-1838. The birds of America. *The greatest of all ornithological works, it has served as the model for all monographs dealing with a specific group of animals. The plates, the work of a master artist, have seldom been surpassed.*

Lyell, Charles. 1830-1833. Principles of geology. *This great work exerted a profound influence on biological thinking, for it did away with the theory of catastrophism and prepared the way for an evolutionary interpretation of fossils and the forms that arose from them.*

Beaumont, William. 1833. Experiments and observations on the gastric juice and the physiology of digestion. *In this classic work the observations Beaumont made on various functions of the stomach and digestion were accurate and thorough. The work paved the way for the brilliant investigations of Pavlov, Cannon, and Carlson of later generations.*

Müller, Johannes. 1834-1840. Handbook of physiology. *The principles set down in this work by perhaps the greatest of all physiologists have set the pattern for the development of the science of physiology.*

Darwin, Charles. 1839. Journal of researches (Voyage of the Beagle). *This book reveals the training and development of the naturalist and the material that led to the formulation of Darwin's concept of organic evolution.*

Schwann, Theodor. 1839. Mikroskopische Untersuchungen über die Uebereinstimmung in der Struktur und dem Wachstum der Thiere und Pflanzen. *The basic principles concerning the cell doctrine are laid down in this classic work.*

Kölliker, Albrecht. 1852. Mikroskopische

Anatomie. *This was the first textbook in histology and contains contributions of the greatest importance in this field. Many of the histological descriptions Kölliker made have never needed correction. In many of his biological views he was far ahead of his time.*

Maury, Matthew F. 1855. The physical geography of the sea. *This work has often been called the first textbook on oceanography. This pioneer treatise stressed the integration of such knowledge as was then available about tides, winds, currents, depths, circulation, and such matters. Maury's work represents a real starting point in the fascinating study of the oceans and has had a great influence in stimulating investigations in this field.*

Virchow, Rudolf. 1858. Die Cellularpathologie. *In this work Virchow made the first clear distinction between normal and diseased tissues and demonstrated the real nature of pathological cells. The work also represents the death knell of the old humoral pathology, which had held sway for so long.*

Darwin, Charles. 1859. On the origin of species. *One of the most influential books ever published in biology. Although built around the theme that natural selection is the most important factor in evolution, the great influence of the book can be attributed to the extensive array of evolutionary evidence it presented. It also stimulated constructive thinking on a subject that had been vague and confusing before Darwin's time.*

Marsh, George P. 1864. Man and nature: physical geography as modified by human action. *A work that had an early and important influence on the conservation movement in America.*

Mendel, Gregor. 1866. Versuche über Pflanzenhybriden. *Careful, controlled pollination technique and statistical analysis gave a scientific explanation that has influenced all geneticists after the "rediscovery" in 1900 of Mendel's classic paper on the two basic laws of inheritance.*

Owen, Richard. 1866. Anatomy and physiology of the vertebrates. *This work contains an enormous amount of personal observation on the structure and physiology of animals, and some of the basic concepts of structure and function, such as homologue and analogue, are here defined for the first time.*

Brehm, Alfred E. 1869. Tierleben. *The many editions of this work over many years have indicated its importance as a general natural history.*

Bronn, Heinrich G. (ed.). 1873 to present. Klassen und Ordnungen des Tier-Reichs. *This great work is made up of exhaustive treatises on the various groups of animals by numerous authorities. Its growth extends over many years, and it is one of the most valuable works ever published in zoology.*

Balfour, Francis M. 1880. Comparative embryology. *This is a comprehensive summary of embryological work on both vertebrates and invertebrates up to the time it was published. It is often considered the beginning of modern embryology.*

Semper, Karl. 1881. Animal life as affected by the natural conditions of existence. *This work first pointed out the modern ecological point of view and laid the basis for many ecological concepts of existence that have proved important in the further development of this field of study.*

Bütschli, Otto. 1889. Protozoen (Bronn's Klassen und Ordnungen des Tier-Reichs). *This monograph has been of the utmost importance to students of protozoa. No other work on a like scale has ever been produced in this field of study.*

von Hertwig, Richard. 1892. Lehrbuch der Zoologie. *This text has proved to be an invaluable source of material for many generations of zoologists. Its illustrations have been widely used in other textbooks.*

Weismann, August. 1892. Das Keimplasma. *Weismann predicted from purely theoretical considerations the necessity of meiosis or reduction of the chromosomes in the germ cell cycle, a postulate that was quickly confirmed cytologically by others.*

Hertwig, Oskar. 1893. Zelle und Gewebe. *In this work a clear distinction is made between histology as the science of tissues and cytology as the science of cell structure and function. Cytology as a study in its own right dates from this time.*

Korschelt, E., and K. Heider. 1893. Lehrbuch der vergleichende Entwicklungsgeschichte der wirbellosen Thiere, 4 vols. *A treatise that has been a valuable tool for all workers in the difficult field of invertebrate embryology.*

Wilson, Edmund B. 1896. The cell in development and heredity. *This and subsequent editions represented the most outstanding work of its kind in the English language. Its influence in directing the development of cytogenetics cannot be overestimated, and in summarizing the many investigations in cytology, the book has served as one of the most useful tools in the field.*

Pavlov, Ivan. 1897. Le travail des glandes digestives. *This work marks a great landmark in the study of the digestive system, for it describes many of Pavlov's now classic experiments, such as the gastric pouch technique and the rate of gastric secretions.*

De Vries, Hugo. 1901. Die Mutationstheorie. *The belief that evolution is the result of sudden changes or mutations is advanced by one who is commonly credited with the initiation of this line of investigation into the causes of evolution.*

Sherrington, Charles. 1906. The integrative action of the nervous system. *The basic concepts of neurophysiology laid down in this book have been little altered since its publication. Much of the work done in this field has served to confirm the nervous mechanism outlined here.*

Garrod, Archibald. 1909. Inborn errors of metabolism. *This pioneer book showed that certain congenital diseases were caused by defective genes that failed to produce the proper enzymes for normal functioning. It laid the basis for biochemical genetics, which later received a great impetus from the work of Beadle and Tatum.*

Henderson, Lawrence J. 1913. The fitness of the environment. *This book has pointed out in a specific way the reciprocity that exists between living and nonliving nature and how organic matter is fitted to the inorganic environment. It has exerted a considerable influence on the study of ecological aspects of adaptation.*

Shelford, Victor E. 1913. Animal communities in temperate America. *This work was a pioneer in the field of biotic community ecology and has exerted a great influence on ecological study.*

Bayliss, William M. 1915. Principles of general physiology. *If a classic book must meet the requirements of masterly analysis and synthesis of what is known in a particular discipline, then this great work must be called one.*

Wegener, Alfred. 1915. The origin of continents and oceans. *In the first (German) edition of this book, Wegener developed the idea of continental drift, involving the movement of continental masses away from a central common area of origin to their present dispersed positions on the globe. Wegener's interpretation of continental history was out of favor for many decades but was substantiated by geophysical work (plate tectonics) in the 1960s and 1970s. Biogeographers now invoke Wegenerian hypotheses to explain distribution of many groups of plants and animals.*

Matthew, W.D. 1915. Climate and evolution. *Matthew, in contrast to Wegener,* viewed the positions of continents as permanent. He explained distribution of plants and animals by dispersal between continents across land bridges, such as the Bering bridge between Asia and Alaska and the Panamanian bridge between Central and South America. Matthew's ideas dominated biogeographical thinking until the revival of Wegener's hypotheses in the 1960s and 1970s.

Morgan, Thomas H., A.H. Sturtevant, C.B. Bridges, and H.J. Muller. 1915. The mechanism of Mendelian heredity. *This book gave an analysis and synthesis of Mendelian inheritance as formulated from the epoch-making investigations of the authors. This classic work stands as a cornerstone of our modern interpretation of heredity.*

Doflein, F. 1916. Lehrbuch der Protozoenkunde, ed. 6 (revised by E. Reichenow, 1949). *A standard treatise on protozoa. Its many editions have proved helpful to all workers in this field.*

Thompson, D'arcy W. 1917. Growth and form. *In this pioneering work the author attempted to reduce the great diversity of life into common themes and designs.*

Kukenthal, W., and T. Krumbach. 1923. Handbuch der Zoologie. *An extensive treatise on zoology that covers all phyla. The work has been an invaluable tool for all zoologists who are interested in the study of a particular group.*

Fisher, Ronald A. 1930. Genetical basis of natural selection. *This work has exerted an enormous influence on the newer synthesis of evolutionary mechanisms so much in vogue at present.*

Dobzhansky, Theodosius. 1937. Genetics and the origin of species. *The vast change in the explanation of the mechanism of evolution, which emerged about 1930, is well analyzed in this work by a master evolutionist. Other syntheses of this new biological approach to the evolutionary problems have appeared since this work was published, but none of them has surpassed the clarity and fine integration of Dobzhansky's work.*

Spemann, Hans. 1938. Embryonic development and induction. *In this work the*

author summarizes his pioneer investigations that have proved so fruitful in experimental embryology.

Hyman, Libbie H. 1940. The invertebrates: Protozoa through Ctenophora. 1951. Platyhelminthes and Rhynchocoela, The acoelomate Bilateria. 1951. Acanthocephala, Aschelminthes, and Entoprocta, the pseudocoelomate Bilateria. 1955. Echinodermata, the coelomate Bilateria. 1959. Smaller coelomate groups: Chaetognatha, Hemichordata, Pogonophora, Phoronida, Ectoprocta, Brachiopoda, Sipunculida, The coelomate Bilateria. 1967. Mollusca I. *This series of volumes is a monumental work by a single author and is the only such coverage of the invertebrates in the English language. It is a benchmark in completeness, accuracy, and incisive analysis. It is an absolutely essential reference for all teachers and investigators in invertebrate zoology.*

Schrödinger, Erwin. 1945. What is life? *The emphasis placed on the physical explanation of life gave a new point of view of biological phenomena so well expressed in the current molecular biological revolution.*

Grassé, P.P. (ed.). 1948. Traité de zoologie. *This is a series of many treatises by various specialists on both invertebrates and vertebrates. Since it is relatively recent and comprehensive, the work is valuable to all students who desire detailed information on the various groups.*

Allee, W.C., A.E. Emerson, O. Park, T. Park, and K.P. Schmidt. 1949. Principles of animal ecology. *Ecology has become a major field of biological study, and the basic principles laid down in this comprehensive work are a landmark in the field.*

Tinbergen, Niko. 1951. The study of instinct. *The classic statement of the approaches and theoretical interpretations of early ethologists, especially K. Lorenz, is presented. This work brought ethology to the attention of American behavioral scientists, generating both controversy and collaboration.*

Blum, H.F. 1951. Time's arrow and evolution. *In this thoughtful book, Blum*

explores the relation between the second law of thermodynamics ("time's arrow") and organic evolution and recognizes that mutation and natural selection have been restricted to certain channels in accordance with the law, even though these two factors appear to controvert the principle of pointing the direction of events in time.

Simpson, George G. 1953. The major features of evolution. *In a comprehensive synthesis of modern evolutionary theory, the author draws on evidence from paleontology, population genetics, and systematics. This book, along with Simpson's earlier* Tempo and mode in evolution, *have greatly influenced our thinking about the mechanisms of evolution within the framework of natural selection.*

Crick, Francis H.C., and James D. Watson. 1953. Genetic implications of the structure of deoxyribonucleic acid. *The solution of the structure of the DNA molecule has served as the cornerstone for an explanation of genetic replication and control of the cell's attributes and functions.*

Burnet, Frank M. 1959. The clonal selection theory of acquired immunity. *This was an important new theory to explain the specificity of the acquired immune response and has to a great extent replaced the template theory formulated by Haurowitz in 1930.*

Carson, Rachel L. 1962. Silent spring. *Though a polemic addressed to a lay audience, this book was highly valuable in increasing public awareness of the danger to the ecosystem of indiscriminate use of pesticides.*

MacArthur, R.H. 1972. Geographical ecology. *One of the most important theoretical ecology books to have appeared in the 1970s.*

Wilson, Edward O. 1975. Sociobiology: the new synthesis. *The rapidly developing fields of behavioral biology, behavioral ecology, and population genetics are reviewed. Wilson attempts to provide the basis for a new biological science, utilizing concepts developed in these heretofore disparate fields, devoted to analyzing social behaviors at all phylogenetic levels.*

INDEX

Oviparity, 859
Ovis canadensis, aggressive behavior in, 824, *825*
Ovoviviparity, 859
  in fishes, 552-553
Ovulation, 858
Ovum, 854
  mammalian, discovery of, A-3
  penetration of, by a spermatozoon, description of, A-6
  in sexual reproduction, 843, 848
Owen, Richard, A-3, A-4
Owl(s), 631
  great horned, *612*
  life span of, 885
  rod retinas of, 786
  snowy, population cycles of, 628
Oxen, domestication of, 658
Oxidation of acetyl coenzyme A, 109
Oxidation number, 26
Oxidation reactions, 26
Oxidation states, ions and, 25-26
Oxidation water in desert mammals, 649
Oxidation-reduction reaction, 26
  as cell energy source, 105
Oxidative metabolism, appearance of, 66-67
Oxidative phosphorylation, 106-112
  efficiency of, 112-114
Oxygen
  appearance of, 59-60
  arterial, in regulation of respiration, 717
  atmospheric, photosynthesis and, 999
  consumption of, rate of, life span and, 885
  discovery of, A-3
  electron shell of, 25
  extraction of, from water, 711
  generating adenosine triphosphate in presence of, 104-114
  generating adenosine triphosphate without, 114-115
  as requirement for life, 996
  in respired air, 715, 716t,
  transport of, by blood, 717-719
Oxygen content of air, greater, compared to water, 558
Oxygen dissociation curves, 718
Oxyhemoglobin, 718-719
Oxytocin, 859
  actions of, 798t, 800
Oyster, life cycle of, *326*
Oyster borer, 318
Oyster catchers, 631
  stereotyped behavior in, 815

P

Pacemaker of heart, human, development of, 881
Pacinian corpuscles, 780
Paddlefishes, 536
Paedomorphosis in urodeles, 565
Pain, sense of, 779-780
Painted shrimp, 403

Painter, T.S., A-13
Pairing, base, in DNA, 917-918
Palade, G.E., A-16, A-17
Palaeoniscids, 535-536
Paleocortex of vertebrate brain, 772
Paleogenesis, 13
Paleontology, vertebrate, development of, A-3
Pallium in molluscs, 307
Pan troglodytes, 977
Pancreas
  human, development of, 879
  islet cells of
    discovery of, A-5
    insulin from, 807-808
Pancreatectomy, effect of, A-7
Pancreatic enzymes in human digestion, 748-749
Pander, C.H., A-3
Pandion haliaetus, wing of, 620
Pangaea, 1015, *1016*
  formation of, Permian extinction and, 944
Pangolins, 661
Panorpa, 435
Pansy, sea, 244
Panthera
  classification of, 945
  leo, feeding behavior of, *645*
Pantothenic acid, 756
Paper nautilus, 332
Paper wasp, *434*
Papilio krishna, 434
Papio
  anubis, 812, 974
  hamadryas, 974
Papulae
  dermal, of starfish, 711
  of sea stars, 471
Paragonimus
  kellicotti, 265
  westermani, 264-265
Parakeets, 631
  Carolina, extinction of, 1053
Paramecium, 191-197
  aurelia, 193
  bursaria, 193
  caudatum, 192, 193, 194
  contractile vacuole of, 176, 728
  form and function of, 192-194
  mating types in, discovery of, A-14
  multimicronucleatum, 193, 194
  reproduction in, 194-197
  true nature of conjugation in, A-7
Paramylum bodies in *Euglena,* 180
Parapodia on polychaetes, 352, 354, *356,* 357
Parasite(s)
  fluid feeding by, 743
  and host, interaction of, 1035
  intermittent, 1035
  nematode, of humans, 289t, 290-293
  reproduction in, 846
  symbiotic, 1035
Parastichopus californicus, 481, 482, 483

Parasympathetic nervous system, vertebrate, 775-777
Parathyroid glands, 804
Parathyroid hormone (PTH)
  bone growth and, 676
  in mineral metabolism, 804-805
Parazoa, 205; *see also* Sponges
Parchment worms, 357
Parietal cells of stomach, 748
Parkman, Francis, 1043, 1046, 1047
Parrot fish, 533
Parrot snake, *591*
Parrots, 631
  life span of, 885
Parthenogenesis, 844-845
  artificial, discovery of, A-8
  induced, 866
  natural, discovery of, A-2
Particulate matter, feeding on, 741-742
Partition chromatography, development of, A-15
Parturition, 883-884
Passenger pigeon, extinction of, 629, 1046
Passeriformes, 632
Pasteur, Louis, 56-57, A-5, A-6
Pasteur effect, A-6
Patella, 318
Pauling, Linus, A-16
Pauropoda, 365, 407-408
Pauropus, 408
Pavlov, Ivan P., A-10
Pea, Mendel's investigations of, 891-895
Peanut worms, 440
Pearls, production of, 321
Peccaries, 662
Pecten, 321, 326
Pectoral girdle of tetrapods, 679
Pedal disc of hydra, 226
Pedal laceration in sea anemone, 241
Pedicellariae
  of echinoids, 481
  of sea stars, 471
Pedicularia, 310
Peking man, *984, 985*
Pelage
  in adaptation to cold environment, 649, 651
  of mammals, 639
Pelagic forms of life in oceans, 1008
Pelagic zone of marine habitat, 1008
Pelecaniformes, 631
Pelecanus
  occidentalis, 631
  onocrotalus, cooperative feeding behavior of, *623*
Pelecypoda, 306-307, 320, 321-327; *see also* Bivalves
Pelicans, 631
  cooperative feeding behavior of, *623*
Pellicle
  of *Amoeba proteus,* 184
  of ciliates, 191
  of *Euglena,* 180
  of *Paramecium,* 194
Pelomyxa carolinensis, 185

Placenta, human, 876-877
  development of, 876
Placental mammals, reproduction in, 655
Placobdella, 351
Placoderms in vertebrate evolution, 508
Placozoa, 204
Plains Indians, bison culture of, 1043-1044
  destruction of, 1044-1045
Planaria, protonephridium of, 728, 729
Planarians, 257-259
Planetary model of atom, 24
Planets, formation of, 58
Plankton
  feeding on, 741
  nature of, A-3
Planospiral shell in gastropods, *314, 315*
Plantae, 157
Plants
  in food chain, 1026
  net productivity of, 100
Plasma, blood, 692
Plasma membrane of cell, 78, 79, 83-88; *see also* Membrane(s), cell
Plasmalemma in ameboid movement, 679
Plasmids, 912
Plasmodium, 189-191
  faciparum, 189-190
  life history of, A-8
  malariae, 190
  ovale, 190
  vivax, 189, 190
Plastids in eukaryotes, 912
Plate tectonics, theory of, 1015
Platelets in blood coagulation, 702
Plates, comb, of *Pleurobrachia,* 247
Platte River, threat to, 1047
Platyhelminthes, 255-270
  adaptive radiation of, 276
  characteristics of, 255-256
  classification of, 256
  fragmentation in, 843
  phylogeny of, 275-276
Platypus, duck-billed, 659-660
  development of, 875
  reproduction in, 655
Platyrhinii, 663
Plecoptera, 433
Pleiotropic genes, 902
Pleistocene hominids, 985
Pleura in mammals, 715
Pleurobrachia, 247-248
Pleuroploca gigantea, 313
Plexus, nerve, subepidural, in turbellarians, 259
Pliny the Elder, 819-820
Pliohippus in horse evolution, 963, 965
Plovers, 631
  golden, migration of, *621*
Plumatella, 459
  repens, 459
Pneumatophore of Portuguese man-of-war, 233
Pneumostome in gastropods, 316

Poachers, 533
Pocket gophers, 661
Podicipediformes, 631
Podophrya, 198
  feeding method in, *176*
Pogonophora, 442-445
  adaptive radiation of, 445
  analysis of, A-18
  external features of, 443-444
  internal features of, 444-445
  phylogeny of, 445
Pogonophoran worms, giant, in deep-sea vent communities, 1025-1026
Poikilothermy, 647
Poison, skin, of frogs, 568
Polarity in egg, 868
Polarized light perception by honeybees, discovery of, A-17
Polinices lewisii, 315
Polychaeta, 340, 341, 352-357
  clam worms as, 356-357
  form and function of, 352-356
  parchment worms as, 357
Polychaete worms in deep-sea vent communities, 1025
Polycystinea, 170
Polygenic inheritance, 901-902
Polygyny in birds, 625
Polygyra, 320
Polymers, formation of, 63-64
Polymorphism
  in cnidarians, 222-223
  protein, neutral mutations and, 955
Polymorphonuclear leukocytes, phagocytic activity of, 704
Polyodon spatula, 536
Polyorchis penicillatus, 231
Polypeptide chains, structure of, 42-43
Polypeptides, one gene–one polypeptide hypothesis of, 17, 916
Polyphyletic origin of metazoa, 159
Polyphyodont teeth of reptiles, 639
Polyplacophora, 306, 311-312
Polyploidy, 911
  sympathetic speciation and, 961
Polyps
  cnidarian, 222
  sea anemone, 238
Polypterus, 539, 541
  bichir, 536
Polyribosome, 923
Polysaccharides, 37-38
Polysome, 923
Polyspermy, prevention of, 866
Polystoma, 260
Polytene chromosomes, 914
Ponds, 1005-1006
Pongidae, 971
Pongo pygmaeus, 977
Pons of vertebrate brain, 771
Popillia japonica, 431
Population(s), 1035
  allopatric, 1034
  in biosphere, 1022
  genetic changes within, 949-957
  growth of, 1036-1038

Population(s)—cont'd
  growth of—cont'd
    curbing of, 1038-1039
    human, effect of, on food supply, 754
    interactions of, 1035-1036
    mammal, 657-658
    sympatric, 1034
Population biology, 1023
Population genetics, 949
Population growth, logistical theory of, A-4
Porcellio, 399
Porcupines, 661
  spines of, 641
Porifera, 204-216; *see also* Sponges
Porites porites, 242
Pork tapeworm, 266t, 268-269
Porpoises, 661
Porter, Keith R., A-15
Porter, R.R., A-20
Portuguese man-of-war, 233
Posterior pituitary, hormones of, 798t, 800-801
Postsynaptic membrane, 765
Postsynaptic neurons, 765
Posture, upright, evolution of, 978
Potassium
  in nerve action potential, 764-765
  in nerve resting potential, 763-764
Potassium-argon dating of fossils, 944-945
Potential
  action, in nerve impulse, 764-765
  equilibrium, 764
  generator, in touch, 780
  resting
    in nerve impulse, 763-764
    transmembrane, 764
Potentiality, nuclear, constancy of, A-7
Potoroo, *660*
Potto, 663
Pouts, 533
Powder down feathers, 607
Power of flight in insects, 412-414
Prairie, American
  effect of sheep on, 1046
  life on, 1043
Prairie dogs
  communal living of, 656, 657
  social behavior in, 821-822
Praying mantis, legs of, 410, *411*
Preadaptations concept, A-10
Prebiotic synthesis of small organic molecules, 62-63
Precambrian era, life in, evidences for, 943
Precambrian fossil bed, discovery of, A-16
Precambrian life, 67-69
Precocial birds, 626, 627
Predation in population control, 1038
Predators
  confusion of, social behavior in, 822
  control of, extinction and, 1058-1059
  learning discrimination of, 817-818

ORIGIN OF LIFE AND GEOLOGIC TIME TABLE

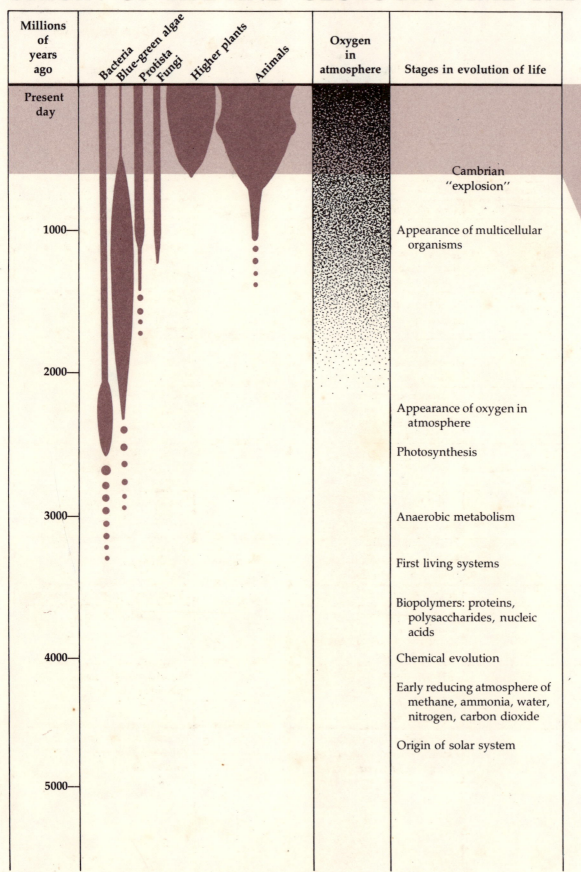